Nursing Diagnosis Handbook

A Guide to Planning Care

Nursing Diagnosis Handbook

A Guide to Planning Care

Betty J. Ackley, MSN, EdS, RN
Gail B. Ladwig, MSN, RN, CHTP, HNC

Sixth edition

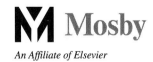

Mosby

An Affiliate of Elsevier

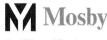

An Affiliate of Elsevier

11830 Westline Industrial Drive
St. Louis, Missouri 63146

NOTICE

Nursing is an ever-changing field. Standard safety precautions must be followed, but as new research and clinical experience broaden our knowledge, changes in treatment and drug therapy may become necessary or appropriate. Readers are advised to check the most current product information provided by the manufacturer of each drug to be administered to verify the recommended dose, the method and duration of administration, and contraindications. It is the responsibility of the licensed prescriber, relying on experience and knowledge of the patient, to determine dosages and the best treatment for each individual patient. Neither the publisher nor the author assumes any liability for any injury and/or damage to persons or property arising from this publication.

Previous editions copyrighted 1993, 1995, 1997, 1999, 2002

Library of Congress Cataloging-in-Publication Data

Nursing diagnosis handbook : a guide to planning care/[edited by] Betty J. Ackley, Gail B. Ladwig.—6th ed.
    p. ; cm.
    Includes bibliographical references and index.
    ISBN 0-323-02551-X
    1. Nursing diagnosis—Handbooks, manuals, etc. 2. Nursing care plans—Handbooks, manuals, etc. I. Ackley, Betty J. II. Ladwig, Gail B.
    [DNLM: 1. Nursing Diagnosis—Handbooks. 2. Patient Care Planning—Handbooks. WY 49 N9745 2004]
RT48.6.A35 2004
6210.73—dc21

Acquisitions Editor: Barbara Nelson Cullen
Senior Developmental Editor: Cindi Anderson
Publishing Services Manager: Deborah L. Vogel
Project Manager: Deon Lee
Design Manager: Mark Bernard

Printed in the United States of America

Last digit is the print number: 9 8 7 6 5 4 3 2

To:

Dale Ackley, the greatest guy in the world, without whose support this book would have never happened, and my daughter, Dr. Goulding, and her husband Cameron. Dale and Dawn have been the joy of my life.

Jerry Ladwig, my wonderful husband, who after 38 years is still supportive and patient—I couldn't have done it without him; my children and their spouses and my grandchildren—Jerry, Kathy Alexandra Elizabeth, and Benjamin; Chrissy, John, Sean, and Ciara; Jenny, Jim, Abby, Katelyn, and Blake; and Amy and Scott—the greatest family anyone could ever hope for.

A special thank you to our nursing students, who teach us every day, and our nursing faculty colleagues—"friends are one of life's most precious gifts." Also, a special thank you to all the contributors who have devoted their time and talent to help "students think like nurses."

Contributors

Betty J. Ackley, MSN, EdS, RN
Professor of Nursing
Consultant in Online Learning
Jackson Community College
Jackson, Michigan

Donna Algase, PhD, RN, FAAN
Professor of Nursing
University of Michigan School of Nursing
Ann Arbor, Michigan

Lisa Burkhart, MPH, PhD, RN
Assistant Professor
Marcella Niehoff School of Nursing
Loyola University Chicago
Chicago, Illinois

Brenda Emick-Herring, RN, MSN, CRRN
Admission Liaison for the Iowa Rehabilitation Network
Staff Development Specialist for Central Iowa Health
  System
Des Moines, Iowa

Arlene Farren
Professor of Nursing
College of Staten Island
City University of New York
Staten Island, New York

Roslyn Fine, MS, CCC, SLP
Preschool Speech Language Pathologist
Goshen Community Schools
Goshen, Indiana
First Step Provider: An Independent Contractor
Private Practitioner
State of Indiana Program

Terri Foster, BSN, CNOR
RN, Unit Educator, Surgery/PACU/CSP/Ortho
  Services
W.A. Foote Memorial Hospital
Jackson, Michigan

Judith R. Gentz, RN, CS, NP
Sole Proprietor
Nurse Practitioner Care
Grass Lake, Michigan

Mikel Gray, PhD, CUNP, CCCN, FAAN
Nurse Practitioner and Professor
Department of Urology and School of Nursing
University of Virginia
Charlottesville, Virginia

T. Heather Herdman, PhD, RN (BSN, MS)
Director of Research and Planning
St. Michaels Hospital and Rice Medical Center
Stevens Point, Wisconsin

Kimberly Hickey, MSN, RN
Clinical Nurse Specialist, Gerontology
University of Michigan Health System
Ann Arbor, Michigan

Teresa Howell, RN, MSN
Assistant Professor of Nursing
Morehead State University
Morehead, Kentucky

Linda Hutson
Assistant Nurse Manager, Staff RN, Sexual Assault
  Nurse Examiner
Emergency Department
Mercy Hospital Anderson, The University Hospital
Cincinnati, Ohio

Ann C. Keeley, RN, MN, CS
Assistant Professor
Georgia Baptist College of Nursing of Mercer
  University
Atlanta, Georgia

Diane Krasner, PhD, RN, CWOCN, CWS, FAAN
Wound Care Consultant and Adjunct Associate
  Professor
Johns Hopkins University
School of Nursing
Baltimore, Maryland

Gail B. Ladwig, MSN, RN, CHTP, HNC
Associate Professor of Nursing
Jackson Community College
Consultant in Guided Imagery
Healing Touch Practitioner
Jackson, Michigan

Marcia LaHaie, MSN, RN, OCN
Hematology/Oncology Nurse Coordinator
Veterans Administration Ann Arbor Health Care
    Center
Ann Arbor, Michigan

Scott Chisholm Lamont, BSN, RN, CCRN, CFRN, ENC(C)
Student, PhD in Nursing Program
Department of Community Health Systems
University of California San Francisco School of
    Nursing
San Francisco, California

Margaret Lunney, PhD, RN, CS
Professor of Nursing
College of Staten Island
City University of New York
Staten Island, New York

Carroll A. Lutz, MA, BSN, RN
Associate Professor Emerita
Consultant in Nutrition
Jackson Community College
Jackson, Michigan

Margo McCaffery, MS, RN, FAAN
Consultant in the Nursing Care of Patients with Pain
Los Angeles, California

Pamela H. Mitchell, PhD, RN, CNRN, FAAN
Elizabeth S. Soule Distinguished Professor of Nursing
    and Health Promotion
Professor of Biobehavioral Nursing and Health Systems
Associate Dean for Research
University of Washington School of Nursing
Seattle, Washington

Leslie H. Nicoll, PhD, MBA, RN
Maine Desk—Professional Editorial Services
Editorial Office for CIN and JHPN
Portland, Maine

Chris Pasero, MS, RN
Pain Management Educator and Consultant
Rocklin, California

P. Ann Solari-Twadell, RN, MPA, PhD
Assistant Professor, Health Promotion, Primary care,
    Health Systems and Dietetics,
Marcella Niehoff School of Nursing,
Loyola University Chicago

Beth Ann Swann PhD, CRNP
Special Projects Coordinator and Adjunct Assistant
    Professor
University of Pennsylvania School of Nursing
Rydal, Pennsylvania

Terry VandenBosch, MS, RN, CS
Research Specialist
Saint Joseph Mercy Health System
Ann Arbor, Michigan

Michele Walters RN, MSN, ARNP
Assistant Professor of Nursing
Morehead State University
Morehead, Kentucky

Linda S. Williams, MSN, RN C, CS
Clinical Nurse Specialist
Jackson Community College
Staff Nurse, Preadmission Testing
W.A. Foote Memorial Hospital
Jackson, Michigan

Consultant in home care—contributor of home care interventions

Kathleen L. Patusky, PhD, APRN-BC
Assistant Professor
Byrdine F. Lewis, School of Nursing
Georgia State University
Atlanta, Georgia

Consultant in culturally competent nursing care

Marina Martinez-Kratz, RN, MS
Associate Professor of Nursing
Jackson Community College
Jackson, Michigan

Consultant in nursing research utilization

Beth Ann Swann PhD, CRNP
Special Projects Coordinator and Adjunct Assistant
    Professor
University of Pennsylvania School of Nursing
Rydal, Pennsylvania

Consultants to previous editions

Elizabeth L. Foster, MS, RN, Consultant in home care—contributor of home care interventions—3ʳᵈ through 5th editions

Ann F. Jacobson, PhD, RN, Consultant in nursing research utilization—3rd edition

Debra Martinez, BSW, Consultant in culturally competent nursing care—5th edition

Brenda J. Wagner, PhD, RN, Consultant in nursing research utilization—3rd edition

Elizabeth H. Winslow, PhD, RN, FAAN, Consultant in nursing research utilization—3rd edition

The authors would also like to thank the following individuals for their contributions to earlier editions:

Jill Barnes, MS, RNCS
Victoria L. Cole-Schonlau, DNSc, MPA, RN
Sandra Cunningham, MS, RN, CCRN, CS
Jane Maria Curtis, MSN, CAN, RN
Gwethalyn B. Edwards, MSN, RN
Pamela M. Emery, BS, RNFA, CNOR, RN
Nancy English, PhD, RN
Mary A. Fuerst-DeWys, BS, RN
J. Keith Hampton, MSN, RN, CS
Mary Henrikson, MN, RNC, ARNP

Kathie D. Hesnan, BSN, RN, CETN
Constance Hollman, MA, EdS
Leslie Kalbach, MN, RN, CETN
Helen Kelley, MSN, RN, CHTP, HNC, NP
Leslie Lysaght RN, MS, CS
Mary Markle, MSN, RNC
Marty J. Martin, MSN, RN
Michelle Masta, RN, BSN
Cathy McClean, RN, BSN
Vicki McClurg, MN, RN
Beverly Pickett, MA, BS, RN, CHTP, HNC
Nancee B. Radtke, MSN, RN
Judith S. Rizzo, MS, RN, CS
Pam B. Schweitzer, MS, RN, CS
Suzanne Skowronski, MSN, RN
Teepa Snow, MS, OTR-L, FAOTA
Martha A. Spies, MSN, RN
Kathy A. Stimac O'Brien, MSN, RN
Linda Straight, MA, RN
Catherine Vincent, MSN, RN
Virginia Wall RN, MN, IBCLC
Peggy A. Wetsch, RN, MSN, CNA
Fran Wistom, MSN, RN, CSW, CPN
Janet Woodruff, BSN, RN
Kathy Wyngarden, MSN, RN

Preface

Nursing Diagnosis Handbook: A Guide to Planning Care is a convenient reference to help the practicing nurse or nursing student make a nursing diagnosis and write a care plan with ease and confidence. This handbook helps nurses correlate nursing diagnoses with known information about clients on the basis of assessment findings, established medical or psychiatric diagnoses, and the current treatment plan.

Making a nursing diagnosis and planning care are complex processes that involve diagnostic reasoning and critical thinking skills. Nursing students and practicing nurses cannot possibly memorize the more than 1200 defining characteristics, related factors, and risk factors for the 169 diagnoses approved by the North American Nursing Diagnosis Association (NANDA). This book correlates suggested nursing diagnoses with what nurses know about clients and offers a care plan for each nursing diagnosis.

Section I, Nursing Diagnosis, the Nursing Process, and Evidence-Based Nursing, explains how the nurse formulates a nursing diagnosis using assessment findings. In Section II, Guide to Nursing Diagnoses, the nurse can look up symptoms and problems and their suggested nursing diagnoses for more than 1200 client symptoms, medical and psychiatric diagnoses, diagnostic procedures, surgical interventions, and clinical states. In Section III, Guide to Planning Care, the nurse can find care plans for all nursing diagnoses suggested in Section II. In this edition, we have included the suggested nursing outcomes from the Nursing Outcomes Classification (NOC) and interventions from the Nursing Interventions Classification (NIC) by the Iowa Intervention Project, as well as a listing of all NOC outcomes labels and NIC intervention labels in Appendixes C and D. We are excited about this work and believe it is a significant addition to the nursing process to further define nursing practice.

New special features of the sixth edition of *Nursing Diagnosis Handbook: A Guide to Planning Care* include the following:

- Twelve new nursing diagnoses recently approved by NANDA
- The changes made by NANDA in existing nursing diagnoses
- Revised NOC outcomes for each nursing diagnosis, including the rating scale
- Revised NIC interventions for each nursing diagnosis
- Even more information about evidenced-based nursing
- Labeling of nursing research and clinical research to identify the source of evidenced-based rationales.
- Even more culturally appropriate interventions added to care plans as relevant
- *evolve* • An associated EVOLVE Course Management System that includes critical thinking case studies; worksheets; and the ability to post a class syllabus and outline and lecture notes, share e-mail, and encourage student participation through chat rooms and discussion boards
- An instructor's manual and PowerPoint lecture slides

The following features of *Nursing Diagnosis Handbook: A Guide to Planning Care* are included from the fifth edition:

- Suggested nursing diagnoses for more than 1200 clinical entities including signs and symptoms, medical diagnoses, surgeries, maternal-child disorders, mental health disorders, and geriatric disorders
- *evolve* • An EVOLVE Courseware System with the Ackley Care Plan Constructor that helps the student or nurse write a nursing care plan, including links to websites for client education
- Rationales for nursing interventions that are based on nursing research and literature

- Nursing references identified for each care plan
- Major clinical practice guidelines of the Agency for Health Care Policy and Research (AHCPR) used in appropriate care plans
- A complete list of NOC outcomes in Appendix C
- A complete list of NIC interventions in Appendix D
- The Taxonomy II organizing framework from NANDA
- Nursing care plans that contain many holistic interventions
- Care plans for **Pain** written by two national experts on pain, Margo McCaffery and Christine Pasero
- Care plans for **Rape-trauma syndrome** written by national expert Linda Hutson
- Care plans for **Spirituality** written by national experts Ann Solari-Twadell and Lisa Burkhart
- Care plans for **Skin integrity** written by national expert Dr. Diane Krasner
- Care plans for **Community** written by national expert Dr. Margaret Lunney
- Care plans for **Incontinence** written by national expert Dr. Mikel Gray
- Care plan for **Decreased Intracranial adaptive capacity** written by national expert Dr. Pamela Mitchell
- Care plan for **Latex Allergy response** written by national expert Dr. Leslie Nicoll
- Care plan for **Wandering** written by national expert Dr. Donna Algase
- A format that facilitates analyzing signs and symptoms by the process already known by nurses, which involves using defining characteristics of nursing diagnoses to make a diagnosis
- Use of NANDA terminology and approved diagnoses
- Inclusion of two additional nursing diagnoses, **Grieving** and **Impaired Comfort**
- An alphabetical format for Sections II and III, which allows rapid access to information
- Nursing care plans for all nursing diagnoses listed in Section II
- Specific geriatric interventions in appropriate plans of care
- Specific client/family teaching interventions in each plan of care
- Information on culturally competent nursing care included where appropriate
- Inclusion of commonly used abbreviations (e.g., AIDS, MI, CHF) and cross-references to the complete term in Section II
- Contributions by leading nurse experts from throughout the United States, who together represent all of the major nursing specialties and have extensive experience with nursing diagnoses and the nursing process

We acknowledge the work of NANDA, which is used extensively throughout this text. In some cases the authors and contributors have modified the NANDA work to increase ease of use. The original NANDA work can be found in *NANDA Nursing Diagnoses: Definitions & Classification 2003-2004.* Several contributors are the original authors of the nursing diagnoses established by NANDA. These contributors include the following:

Dr. Margaret Lunney
Ineffective community Coping
Readiness for enhanced community Coping
Effective Therapeutic regimen management
Ineffective Therapeutic regimen management
Ineffective community Therapeutic regimen management
Ineffective family Therapeutic regimen management

Lisa Burkhart, PhD, RN
Spiritual distress
Readiness for enhanced Spiritual well-being

Dr. Pamela H. Mitchell
Decreased Intracranial adaptive capacity

Brenda Emick-Herring
Impaired bed Mobility
Impaired Transfer ability
Impaired Walking

Vicki E. McClurg, Mary Henrikson, and Virginia R. Wall—1st through 5th editions
Effective Breastfeeding
Ineffective Breastfeeding
Interrupted Breastfeeding

Kathy Wyngarden—1st through 3rd editions
Risk for impaired parent/infant/child Attachment
Impaired wheelchair Mobility

We and the consultants and contributors trust that nurses will find this sixth edition of *Nursing Diagnosis Handbook: A Guide to Planning Care* a valuable tool that simplifies the process of diagnosing clients and planning for their care, thus allowing nurses more time to provide care that speeds each client's recovery.

Acknowledgments

We would like to thank the following people at Mosby: Barbara Nelson Cullen, Executive Editor, who supported us with this sixth edition of the text with intelligence and kindness; Cindi Anderson, who was a continual support and constant source of wise advice and who is frankly wonderful; Amy DeSanto, who helped with the contributors; and a special thank you to Deon Lee for project management of this edition.

We acknowledge with gratitude the nursing students and graduates of Jackson Community College who made us think and shared a very special time with us; the nurses at W.A. Foote Memorial Hospital, Doctors Hospital, Chelsea Hospital, The Jackson County Medical Care Facility, Arbor Manor Care Center, Countryside Care Center, and Lifeways, as well as the professionals in community nursing agencies who have helped us educate students and who have served as role models for excellence in nursing care; and finally, each other, for perseverance, patience, and friendship.

Care has been taken to confirm the accuracy of information presented in this book. However, the authors, editors, and publisher cannot accept any responsibility for consequences resulting from errors or omissions of the information in this book and make no warranty, expressed or implied, with respect to its contents. The reader should use practices suggested in this book in accordance with agency policies and professional standards. Every effort has been made to ensure the accuracy of the information presented in this text.

We hope you find this text useful in your nursing practice.

Betty J. Ackley

Gail B. Ladwig

How to Use Nursing Diagnosis Handbook: A Guide to Planning Care

ASSESS
Assess the client using the format provided by the clinical setting. Collect data including the client's symptoms, clinical state, and known medical or psychiatric diagnoses.

DIAGNOSIS
Turn to Section II, Guide to Nursing Diagnoses, and locate the client's symptoms, clinical state, medical or psychiatric diagnoses, and anticipated or prescribed diagnostic studies or surgical interventions (listed in alphabetical order). Note suggestions for appropriate nursing diagnoses.

Use Section III, Guide to Planning Care, to evaluate each suggested nursing diagnosis and "related to" etiology statement. Section III is a listing of care plans according to NANDA, arranged alphabetically by diagnostic concept, for each nursing diagnosis referred to in Section II. Determine the appropriateness of each nursing diagnosis by comparing the Defining Characteristics and Risk Factors with the client data collected.

DETERMINE OUTCOMES
Use Section III to find appropriate outcomes for the client. Use either the NOC outcomes with the associated rating scales or Client Outcomes as desired.

PLAN INTERVENTIONS
Use Section III to find appropriate interventions for the client. Use either the NIC interventions or Nursing Interventions as found in that section.

GIVE NURSING CARE
The nurse administers nursing care following the plan of care based on the interventions.

EVALUATE NURSING CARE
Evaluate nursing care administered using either the NOC outcomes or Client Outcomes. If the outcomes were not met and the nursing interventions were not effective, it may be appropriate to reassess the client and determine whether the appropriate nursing diagnoses were made.

DOCUMENT
Document all of the previous steps using the format provided in the clinical setting.

Contents

Nursing Diagnosis, the Nursing Process, and Evidence-Based Nursing

Figure I-1

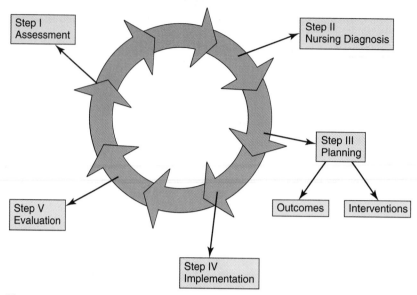

The nursing process.

The nursing process is an organizing framework for professional nursing practice. Components of the process include performing a nursing assessment, making nursing diagnoses, planning, writing outcome/goal statements, determining appropriate nursing interventions, implementing care, and evaluating the nursing care that has been given.

This can be visualized as a circular, continuous process (Figure I-1). A new concept that has been added to this process is basing nursing practice on evidence or research. This new concept is called *evidence-based nursing* (EBN). EBN uses the research of basic nursing interventions and incorporates theory, clinical decision making, knowledge of nursing and the health care milieu, as well as cost-effectiveness to forward nursing practice (Melnyk, 2000).

This book focuses on an essential part of the nursing process: how to make and use a nursing diagnosis.

A nursing diagnosis is a clinical judgment about individual, family, or community responses to actual or potential health problems or life processes. Nursing diagnoses provide the basis for selection of nursing interventions to achieve outcomes for which the nurse is accountable (NANDA, 2003).

The nursing diagnoses that are used throughout this book are taken from North American Nursing Diagnosis Association's (NANDA's) Taxonomy II (NANDA, 2003). The complete nursing diagnosis list by NANDA's domains, classes, and diagnostic concepts is available in Appendix B.

STEP I: ASSESSMENT

Assessment involves performing a thorough holistic nursing assessment of the client. This is the first step needed to make an appropriate nursing diagnosis. This is done using the assessment format adopted by the facility or educational institution in which the practice is situated. Several organizational approaches to assessment are available, including Gordon's Functional Health Patterns and head-to-toe and body systems approaches. Regardless of the approach used, the nurse assesses the client, being alert for symptoms that will help to formulate a nursing diagnosis.

Assessment information is obtained first by taking a medical history. To elicit as many symptoms as possible, the nurse should use open-ended rather than yes/no questions during this part of the assessment. The client should be asked questions such as the following: "Describe what you are feeling." "How long have you been feeling this way?" "When did the symptoms start?" "Describe the symptoms." These types of questions will encourage the client to give more information about his or her situation. Listen carefully for cues and record relevant information that the client shares.

Information is also obtained by performing a physical assessment and noting diagnostic test results. If the client is critically ill or unable to respond verbally, much of the information will be gathered from the physical assessment and diagnostic test results and possibly from the client's significant others. The information from each of these sources is used to formulate a nursing diagnosis.

STEP II: NURSING DIAGNOSIS

A working nursing diagnosis may have two or three parts. The two-part system consists of the nursing diagnosis and the "related to" statement. The three-part system consists of the nursing diagnosis, the "related to" statement, and the defining characteristics.

Some people refer to the three-part diagnostic statement as the PES system:

P (problem)—The nursing diagnosis, the label; a concise term or phrase that represents a pattern of related cues

E (etiology)— "Related to" (r/t) phrase or etiology; related cause or contributor to the problem

S (symptoms)—Defining characteristics phrase; symptoms that the nurse identified in the assessment

Nursing Diagnosis

The first part is the actual nursing diagnosis. When the assessment is completed, common patterns of response to actual or potential health problems are identified. These symptoms may be highlighted, or a short list may be made of the symptoms. Similar symptoms are then put into clusters or groups.

Consider this case study:

A 73-year-old man has been admitted to the unit with a diagnosis of chronic obstructive pulmonary disease (COPD). He states that he has "difficulty breathing when walking short distances." He also states that his "heart feels like it is racing" at the same time. He states that he is "tired all the time," and while talking to you he is continually wringing his hands and looking out the window.

Below is an interpretation of this information:

- "difficulty breathing when walking short distances" = dyspnea
- "heart feels like it is racing" = dysrhythmia
- "tired all the time" = fatigue

In Section II look up *dyspnea* or *dysrhythmia*, and you will find the nursing diagnosis **Activity intolerance** listed with these symptoms.

To validate that the diagnosis **Activity intolerance** is appropriate for the client, turn to Section III, and read the NANDA definition of the nursing diagnosis **Activity intolerance.** When reading the definition, ask *Does this definition describe the symptoms demonstrated by the client?* If the appropriate nursing diagnosis has been selected, the definition should describe the condition that has been observed.

Check to see whether the symptoms that were identified in the assessment are contained in the list of defining characteristics. To help verify the diagnoses made on the basis of client signs and symptoms, you may also look up the client's medical diagnosis in Section II.

This client had a medical diagnosis of COPD. Under the medical diagnosis of COPD, **Activity intolerance** is listed.

The process of identifying significant symptoms, clustering or grouping them into logical patterns, and then choosing an appropriate nursing diagnosis involves diagnostic reasoning (critical thinking) skills that must be learned in the process of becoming a nurse. Our text serves as a tool to help the learner in this process. It is here that you might pose a "clinical question" to incorporate the concept of EBN. *What are some of the ways to help a patient who has intolerance to activity? What does the literature say? What has helped this person in the past? How can the outcomes be measured using standards of practice for a patient with intolerance to activity?*

"Related to" Phrase or Etiology

The second part of the nursing diagnosis is the "related to" (r/t) phrase. This phrase states what may be causing or contributing to the nursing diagnosis, commonly referred to as the etiology. Pathophysiological and psychosocial changes, such as developmental age and cultural and environmental situations, may be causative or contributing factors.

Ideally the etiology, or cause, of the nursing diagnosis is something that can be treated by a nurse. When this is the case, the diagnosis is identified as an independent nursing diagnosis. If medical intervention is also necessary, it might be identified as a collaborative diagnosis. A carefully written, individualized r/t statement enables the nurse to plan nursing interventions that will assist the client in accomplishing goals and return to a state of optimum health.

For each suggested nursing diagnosis, the nurse should refer to the statements listed under the heading "Related Factors (r/t)" in Section III. These r/t factors may or may not be appropriate for the individual client. If they are not appropriate, the nurse should develop and write an r/t statement that is appropriate for the client.

Defining Characteristics Phrase

The defining characteristics phrase is the third part of the three-part diagnostic system. It consists of the signs and symptoms that have been gathered during the assessment phase. Signs and symptoms are labeled as defining characteristics in Section III. The phrase "as evidenced by" (aeb) may be used to connect the etiology (r/t) with the defining characteristics. The use of identifying defining characteristics is similar to the process the physician uses when making a medical diagnosis. For example, the physician who observes the following signs and symptoms—diminished inspiratory and expiratory capacity of the lungs, complaints of dyspnea on exertion, difficulty in inhaling and exhaling deeply, and sometimes, chronic cough—may make the medical diagnosis of COPD. This same process is used to identify the nursing diagnosis of **Activity intolerance.**

Writing a Nursing Diagnosis Statement

P—Choose the label (nursing diagnosis) using the guidelines explained previously. A list of nursing diagnosis labels can be found in Section II.

E—Write an r/t phrase (etiology). These also can be found in Section II.

S—Write the defining characteristics (signs and symptoms). A list of the signs and symptoms associated with each nursing diagnosis can be found in Section III.

Using the information from the above example, the nursing diagnostic statement would be as follows:

P—Activity intolerance

E—Related to imbalance between oxygen supply and demand

S—Verbal reports of fatigue, exertional dyspnea ("difficulty breathing when walking"), and dysrhythmia ("racing heart")

Consider a second case study:

A 45-year-old woman comes to the clinic and asks for medication to help her sleep. She states she is worrying about too much and states, "It takes me about an hour to get to sleep, and it is very hard to fall asleep. I feel like I can't do anything because I am so tired. My husband passed away recently."

- Look up **Sleep** in Section II. Listed under the heading "Sleep Pattern Disorders" in Section II is the following information:

Disturbed Sleep pattern (nursing diagnosis) r/t sensory alterations internal factors (illness, psychological stress), external factors (environmental changes, social cues)

This client states she is worrying too much, which could be considered psychological stress.

- Look up **Disturbed Sleep pattern** in Section III
- Check the definition: Time-limited disruption of sleep (natural periodic suspension of consciousness)
- Does this describe the client in the case study? What are the related factors? What are the symptoms?
- Make the diagnostic statement

P—**Disturbed Sleep pattern**

E—r/t "worrying too much," my husband passed away recently"

S—difficulty falling asleep, I am so tired, I can't do anything

STEP III: PLANNING

This phase consists of writing measurable client outcomes and nursing interventions to accomplish the outcomes. Before this can be done, if the client has more than one diagnosis, the priority of the nursing diagnoses must be determined.

The highest priority nursing diagnoses can be determined by using Maslow's hierarchy of needs. In this hierarchy, priority is generally given to immediate problems that may be life threatening. For example, **Activity intolerance,** a physiological need, may be a higher priority than **Grieving,** a love and belonging need. Refer to Appendix A for assistance in prioritizing nursing diagnoses.

TABLE I-I

NOC Outcome—Sleep

Definition: Extent and pattern of natural periodic suspension of consciousness during which the body is restored.

Sleep	Extremely Compromised 1	Substantially Compromised 2	Moderately Compromised 3	Mildly Compromised 4	Not Compromised 5
Hours of sleep	1	2	3	4	5
Observed hours of sleep	1	2	3	4	5
Sleep pattern	1	2	3	4	5
Sleep quality	1	2	3	4	5
Sleep quantity	1	2	3	4	5
Sleep efficiency (ratio of sleep time/total time trying)	1	2	3	4	5
Uninterrupted sleep	1	2	3	4	5
Sleep routine	1	2	3	4	5
Feelings of rejuvenation after sleep	1	2	3	4	5
Napping appropriate for age	1	2	3	4	5
Wakeful at appropriate times	1	2	3	4	5
EEG IER	1	2	3	4	5
EMG IER	1	2	3	4	5
EOG IER	1	2	3	4	5
Vital signs IER	1	2	3	4	5
Other (specify)	1	2	3	4	5

From Johnson M, Maas M, Moorhead S: *Nursing outcomes classification (NOC)*, ed 2, St Louis, 2000, Mosby.
EEG, Electroencephalogram; *EMG*, electromyogram; *EOG*, electro-oculogram; *IER*, in expected range.

Outcomes

After the appropriate priority of the nursing diagnoses is determined, outcomes are developed. Outcomes are conceptualized as variable client states influenced by nursing intervention. Thus client outcomes represent patient states that vary and that can be measured and compared with a baseline over time (Johnson, Maas, Moorhead, 2000). If at all possible, the nurse involves the client in determining appropriate outcomes.

Development of appropriate outcomes can be done one of two ways: using Nursing Outcomes Classification (NOC) or writing an outcome statement, both of which are included in this book. There are suggested outcome statements for each nursing diagnosis in this text that can be used as written or modified as necessary to meet the needs of the client.

Section III identifies appropriate NOC outcomes for each nursing diagnosis and includes suggested outcomes with indicators. Appendix C includes a listing of additional suggested NOC outcomes.

NOC outcome is defined as follows: An individual, family, or community state; behavior; or perception that is measured along a continuum in response to one or more nursing interventions. Each outcome has a group of indicators that are used to determine patient status in relation to the outcome (Moorhead, 2003). The use of NOC outcomes can be very helpful to the nurse because they contain a five-point Likert-type rating scale that can be used to evaluate progress toward achieving the outcome. In this text the rating scale is listed, along with some of the more common indicators. As an example, the rating scale for the outcome **Sleep** is shown in Table I-1.

Because the NOC outcomes are very specific, they enhance the nursing process by helping the nurse to record change after interventions have been performed. The nurse can choose to have clients rate their own progress using the Likert-type rating scale. This involvement can help increase client motivation to progress toward outcomes.

After client outcomes are selected and discussed with a client, the nurse plans nursing care and establishes a means that will help the client to achieve the selected outcomes. The usual means are nursing interventions.

Interventions

Interventions are like road maps directing the best ways to provide nursing care. The more clearly a nurse writes an intervention, the easier it will be to complete the journey and arrive at the destination of successful client outcomes.

To increase the chance that the chosen interventions will be effective, nurses are now using EBN, which is a set of interventions or guidelines that have been shown to be effective in helping clients. Development of EBN is an ongoing process that should involve all nurses to determine the best methods of doing nursing interventions and providing nursing care. To implement EBN, nurses must work together and follow the strategies outlined in Box I-1.

This text includes EBN interventions whenever possible, along with references to research to validate their usefulness. This is an important part of EBN. It looks at standard protocol and determines whether the protocol is effective based on gathered evidence. This evidence ranges along a continuum from anecdotal experience of provider and consumer, institutional protocols, organizational guidelines, consensus groups, and single-study results to highly structured systematic reviews (Swan, McGinley, and Lang, 2002).

Nurses can find evidence to guide their practice in many places. The Agency for Healthcare Research and Quality (AHRQ, 2003), formerly the Agency for Health Care Policy and Research (AHCPR), began producing clinical practice guidelines in 1989. Clinical practice guidelines are systematically developed statements to help practitioners and clients make decisions about appropriate health care for specific clinical situations. Although AHRQ no longer develops guidelines, it supports the National Guidelines Clearinghouse (NGC). The NGC is a comprehensive database of evidence-based clinical practice guidelines and related documents produced by the AHRQ in partnership with the American Medical Association and the American Association of Health Plans. The NGC mission is to provide physicians, nurses, and other health professionals, health care providers, health plans, integrated delivery systems, purchasers, and others with an accessible mechanism for obtaining objective, detailed information on clinical practice guidelines

---

BOX I-I

Strategies for Implementing Evidence-Based Nursing Practice

1. Pose clinical questions (e.g., What is the best way to provide oral care for clients receiving chemotherapy?).
2. Review and critique literature that is relevant from appropriate studies or systematic reviews in the area of the clinical question. NOTE: Randomized clinical trials are generally the gold standard for producing the best evidence. Systematic reviews can be helpful because they summarize many research studies. Ask a number of questions as part of the review of the research, including the following: How large was the treatment effect? How precise is the estimate of the treatment effect? Will the results help me care for my clients? Is the treatment feasible in our setting? Were all clinically important outcomes considered, including possible harm as well as benefit?
3. Develop practice guidelines using the best evidence currently available.
4. Establish measurable outcomes that can be used to determine the effectiveness of the guidelines.
5. Measure the current outcomes based on existing practice so that there is a "before" measurement to show that evidenced practice made a difference.
6. Implement the practice guidelines.
7. Measure the proposed outcomes after the practice guidelines have been implemented.
8. Evaluate the effectiveness of the practice guidelines and determine where use should be continued or revisions should be made in the guidelines.
9. Pose the next clinical question.

Adapted from Cullum N: Evaluation of studies of treatment or prevention interventions, *Evid Based Nurs* 4:7, 2001; and Melnyk BM et al: Evidenced-based practice: the past, the present, and recommendations for the millennium, *Pediatr Nurs* 26(1):79, 2000.

---

and to further their dissemination, implementation, and use. There are currently 1055 guidelines in the clearinghouse, and new guidelines are added frequently. The guidelines are easily accessed at *www.guideline.gov*. This resource is used by both professionals and consumers to access the guidelines and information for specific health problems.

Evidence-Based Nursing (www.evidencebasednursing.com) is another rich and useful resource. This journal is devoted to helping nurses identify and appraise high-quality, clinically relevant research. The journal selects from the health-related literature both articles reporting studies and reviews that warrant immediate attention by nurses attempting to keep pace with their practice and deliver quality care. The *Annual Review of Nursing Research* is also useful. Many nursing journals now publish practice guidelines based on reviews of nursing research that are helpful to the nurse heading in the direction of EBN.

In an effort to support nursing knowledge worldwide, Sigma Theta Tau International *(www.stti.iupui.edu/library),* through the Virginia Henderson International Library, provides the Registry of Nursing Research (RNR) as a resource to its members. The RNR is an electronic research resource that contains information and abstracts from more than 13,000 studies. As part of an evidence-based practice initiative, the *Online Journal of Knowledge Synthesis for Nursing* has added a new clinical column. This column includes exemplars of EBN practice (Capasso et al, 2002).

A new web-based evidence resource is *www.globalevidence.com.* This website provides a searchable database of online resources, organizations, and institutions related to evidence for practice, research, education, and evaluation, both nationally and internationally. It promotes the advancement of the use of evidence in clinical practice by providing a central information source and communication channel.

Following are helpful websites on evidence-based care:

- Campbell Collaboration—*www.campbellcollaboration.org*. Similar to the Cochrane Collaboration, this international organization aims to produce, disseminate, and continuously update systematic reviews of studies of the effectiveness of social and behavioral interventions.
- Cochrane Collaboration—*www.cochrane.org*. This international collaboration facilitates the creation, maintenance, and dissemination of more than 1000 systematic reviews of the effects of health care interventions in multiple conditions. There are more than 60 interdisciplinary working groups, collaborative review groups comprised of people from around the world who share an interest in developing and maintaining systematic reviews relevant to a particular health area.
- Joanna Briggs Institute—*www.joannabriggs.edu.au*. This site identifies areas in which nurses need summarized evidence on which to base their practice, and it facilitates systematic reviews of international research, undertakes multisite randomized controlled clinical trials in areas in which research is needed, and prepares easy-to-read summaries of best practice in the form of practice information sheets based on the results of systematic reviews.
- University of York: Centre for Evidence-Based Nursing—*www.york.ac.uk/healthsciences/centres/evidence/updindex.htm*. This center works with nurse clinicians, researchers, educators, and managers to identify EBN through research and systematic reviews.

Section III supplies choices of interventions for each nursing diagnosis. The interventions are identified as independent (autonomous actions that are initiated by the nurse in response to a nursing diagnosis) or collaborative (actions that the nurse performs in collaboration with other health care professionals and that may require a physician's order and may be in response to both medical and nursing diagnoses). The nurse may choose the interventions appropriate for the client and individualize them accordingly or determine additional interventions. This text also contains several suggested Nursing Interventions Classification (NIC) activities for each nursing diagnosis to help the reader see how NIC is used along with NOC and nursing diagnoses. The NIC interventions are a comprehensive, standardized classification of treatments that nurses perform. The classification includes both physiological and psychosocial interventions and covers all nursing specialties. A listing of NIC interventions is included in Appendix D. For more information about NIC interventions, refer to the NIC text (McCloskey and Bulechek, 2000).

Putting It All Together—Writing the Care Plan

The final planning phase is writing the actual care plan, including prioritized nursing diagnostic statements, outcomes, and interventions. To ensure continuity of care, the plan must be documented and shared with all health care personnel caring for the client. This text provides rationales, most of which are research based, to validate that the interventions are appropriate and workable. Websites for client and family teaching are available at the EVOLVE website.

A web-based care plan constructor is also available at the EVOLVE website. This site provides a mechanism to electronically create the complete care plan. A sample care plan is included in Figure I-2.

- NOC Outcomes
- Client Outcomes
- NIC Interventions
- Nursing Interventions and Rationales
- Home Care Interventions
- Client/Family Teaching
- Websites for Education
- References

Create the Care Plan

< Main page

Nursing Diagnosis: Activity intolerance

Linda L. Straight

NANDA Definition: Insufficient physiological or psychological energy to endure or complete required or desired daily activities

Defining Characteristics: Verbal report of fatigue or weakness, abnormal heart rate or blood pressure response to activity, exertional discomfort or dyspnea, electrocardiographic changes reflecting dysrhythmias or ischemia

Related Factors: Bed rest or immobility; generalized weakness; sedentary lifestyle; imbalance between oxygen supply and demand

NOC Outcomes (Nursing Outcomes Classification)

Suggested NOC Labels

- ☐ Endurance
- ☐ Energy Conservation
- ☐ Activity Tolerance
- ☐ Self-Care: Activities of Daily Living (ADLs)

Client Outcomes

- ☐ Participates in prescribed physical activity with appropriate increases in heart rate, blood pressure, and breathing rate; maintains monitor patterns (rhythm and ST segment) within normal limits
- ☐ States symptoms of adverse effects of exercise and reports onset of symptoms immediately
- ☐ Maintains normal skin color and skin is warm and dry with activity
- ☐ Verbalizes an understanding of the need to gradually increase activity based on testing, tolerance, and symptoms
- ☐ Expresses an understanding of the need to balance rest and activity
- ☐ Demonstrates increased activity tolerance

NIC Interventions (Nursing Interventions Classification)

Suggested NIC Labels

- ☐ Energy Management
- ☐ Activity Therapy

Nursing Interventions and Rationales

- ☐ Determine cause of activity intolerance (see Related Factors) and determine whether cause is physical, psychological, or motivational. *Determining the cause of a disease can help direct appropriate interventions.*
- ▲ ☐ Assess client daily for appropriateness of activity and bed rest orders. *Inappropriate prolonged bed rest orders may contribute to activity intolerance. A review of 39 studies on bed rest resulting from 15 disorders demonstrated that bed rest for treatment of medical conditions is associated with worse outcomes than early mobilization (Allen, Glasziou, Del Mar, 1999).*

Client/Family Teaching

- ☐ Instruct client on rationale and techniques for avoiding activity intolerance.
- ☐ Teach client to use controlled breathing techniques with activity.
- ☐ Teach client the importance and method of coughing, clearing secretions.
- ☐ Instruct client in the use of relaxation techniques during activity.
- ☐ Help client with energy conservation and work simplification techniques in ADLs.
- ☐ Teach client the importance of proper nutrition.
- ☐ Describe to client the symptoms of activity intolerance, including which symptoms to report to the physician.
- ☐ Explain to client how to use assistive devices or medications before or during activity.
- ☐ Help client set up an activity log to record exercise and exercise tolerance.

Websites for Education: See the EVOLVE website for World Wide Web resources for client education.

References

Create the Care Plan

Figure I-2
Activity intolerance care plan from the Evolve site.

STEP IV: IMPLEMENTATION

The implementation phase of the nursing process is the actual initiation of the nursing care plan. Client outcomes are achieved by the performance of the nursing interventions. During this phase the client is assessed to determine whether the interventions are effective. An important part of this phase is documentation. The facility's tool for documentation should be used to record the results of implementing nursing interventions. Documentation is also necessary for legal reasons because in a legal dispute anything that has not been charted is considered not to have been done.

STEP V: EVALUATION

New Symptoms

Although evaluation is listed as the last phase of the nursing process, it is actually an integral part of each phase and something that is done continually. When evaluation is performed as the last phase, the client's outcomes are evaluated to determine whether they were met. If the outcomes were not met, the nursing process is begun again with assessment to determine the reason the outcomes were not met. Were the outcomes attainable? Was the wrong nursing diagnosis made? Should the interventions be changed? At this point look up any conditions that have been identified and adjust the care plan as needed. When using EBN, determine at this point whether the practice that was followed was effective. Necessary revisions may be made at this time.

Many health care providers are using critical pathways to plan nursing care. The use of nursing diagnoses should be an integral part of any critical pathway to ensure that nursing care needs are being assessed and appropriate nursing interventions are planned and implemented.

The use of nursing diagnoses, NOC outcomes, and NIC interventions ensures that nurses are speaking a common language when providing nursing care. This system also is easily computerized for simplified documentation and analysis of patterns of care. Nursing diagnosis is the essence of nursing, and it is used to ensure that clients receive excellent holistic nursing care.

Just as nurses continually evaluate the interventions and outcomes of care delivered, so too they must continually evaluate the evidence and the quality of the evidence, including both the quality of individual studies and the strength of the body of evidence. Several systems are used to rank the hierarchical levels of evidence by grading/interpreting the strength of individual studies using a numeric or alphabetic rating. The strength of the body of evidence is rated based on quality, quantity, and consistency. *Quality* refers to the aggregate of quality ratings for each research study based on the extent to which bias was minimized. *Quantity* refers to the magnitude of effect and the numbers of studies. For any given topic *consistency* refers to the extent to which similar findings are reported using similar and different study designs (AHRQ, 2002). After rating the quality of the evidence, nurses must ask the following questions: Is the evidence valid? If valid, is this evidence important? If valid and important, can the evidence be applied to a given client using nursing intervention?

The nursing process is continually evolving. In this text our goal is to present state-of-the-art methods and information to assist the nurse and nursing student to provide the best nursing care possible.

REFERENCES

Agency for Healthcare Research and Quality (AHRQ): Evidence based practice outcomes and effectiveness, retrieved from the World Wide Web March 16, 2003, available on-line at: *www.ahcpr.gov/clinic/outcomix.htm.*

Agency for Healthcare Research and Quality: *Systems to rate the strength of scientific evidence. Evidence Report/Technology Assessment No 47.* Washington, DC, 2002, The Agency.

Capasso V et al: Clinical column. Unit-based specialty vascular transitional home care program: an example of evidence-based nursing practice, *Online J Knowl Synth Nurs* 11(3), 2002.

Johnson M, Maas M, Moorhead S: *Nursing outcomes classification (NOC),* ed 2, St Louis, 2000, Mosby.

McCloskey JC, Bulechek GM: *Nursing interventions classification (NIC),* ed 3, St Louis, 2000, Mosby.

Melnyk BM: Evidence-based practice: the past, the present, and recommendations for the millennium, *Pediatr Nurs* 26(1):79, 2000.

Moorhead S: *Measuring outcomes of nursing care using NOC: results & revisions based on 4 years of study,* ACENDIO, 4th European Conference, 2003

North American Nursing Diagnosis Association (NANDA): *Nursing diagnoses: definitions & classification, 2003-2004,* Philadelphia, 2003, The Association.

Guide to Nursing Diagnoses

A

Abdominal Distention

Acute **Pain** r/t retention of air, gastrointestinal secretions

Constipation r/t decreased activity, decreased fluid intake, decreased fiber intake, pathological process

Delayed **Surgical** recovery r/t pain, nausea

Imbalanced **Nutrition**: less than body requirements r/t nausea, vomiting

Nausea r/t irritation to gastrointestinal tract

Abdominal Hysterectomy

See Hysterectomy

Abdominal Pain

Acute **Pain** r/t injury, pathological process

Imbalanced **Nutrition**: less than body requirements r/t unresolved pain

See cause of Abdominal Pain

Abdominal Perineal Resection

Risk for perioperative positioning **Injury** r/t prolonged surgery, lithotomy position

See Abdominal Surgery; Colostomy

Abdominal Surgery

Acute **Pain** r/t surgical procedure

Constipation r/t decreased activity, decreased fluid intake, anesthesia, narcotics

Imbalanced **Nutrition**: less than body requirements r/t high metabolic needs, decreased ability to ingest or digest food

Ineffective **Health** maintenance r/t deficit knowledge regarding self-care after surgery

Risk for ineffective **Tissue** perfusion: peripheral r/t immobility, abdominal surgery resulting in stasis of blood flow

Risk for **Infection** r/t invasive procedure

See Surgery

Abdominal Trauma

Acute **Pain** r/t abdominal trauma

Deficient **Fluid** volume r/t hemorrhage

Disturbed **Body** image r/t scarring, change in body function, need for temporary colostomy

Ineffective **Breathing** pattern r/t abdominal distention, pain

Risk for **Infection** r/t possible perforation of abdominal structures

Abortion, Induced

Acute **Pain** r/t surgical intervention

Chronic **Sorrow** r/t loss of potential child

Compromised family **Coping** r/t unresolved feelings about decision

Ineffective **Health** maintenance r/t deficient knowledge regarding self-care following abortion

Risk for delayed **Development** r/t unplanned or unwanted pregnancy

Risk for imbalanced **Fluid** volume r/t possible hemorrhage

Risk for **Infection** r/t open uterine blood vessels, dilated cervix

Risk for **Post-trauma** syndrome r/t psychological trauma of abortion

Risk for **Spiritual** distress r/t perceived moral implications of decision

Self-esteem disturbance r/t feelings of guilt

Spiritual distress r/t perceived moral implications of decision

Abortion, Spontaneous

Acute **Pain** r/t uterine contractions, surgical intervention

Chronic **Sorrow** r/t loss of potential child

Disabled family **Coping** r/t unresolved feelings about loss

Disturbed **Body** image r/t perceived inability to carry pregnancy, produce child

Fear r/t implications for future pregnancies

Grieving r/t loss of fetus

Ineffective **Coping** r/t personal vulnerability

Ineffective **Health** maintenance r/t deficient knowledge regarding self-care following abortion

Interrupted **Family** processes r/t unmet expectations for pregnancy and childbirth

Risk for deficient **Fluid** volume r/t hemorrhage

Risk for **Infection** r/t septic or incomplete abortion of products of conception, open uterine blood vessels, dilated cervix

Risk for **Post-trauma** syndrome r/t psychological trauma of abortion

Risk for **Spiritual** distress r/t loss of fetus

Self-esteem disturbance r/t feelings of failure, guilt

Abruptio Placentae >36 Weeks

Acute **Pain** r/t irritable uterus, hypertonic uterus

Anxiety r/t unknown outcome, change in birth plans

Death **Anxiety** r/t unknown outcome, hemorrhage/pain

Fear r/t threat to well-being of self and fetus

Impaired **Gas** exchange: placental r/t decreased uteroplacental area

Interrupted **Family** process r/t unmet expectations for pregnancy/childbirth

Ineffective **Health** maintenance r/t deficient knowledge regarding self-care with disorder

Risk for deficient **Fluid** volume r/t hemorrhage

Risk for disproportionate **Growth** r/t uteroplacental insufficiency

Risk for impaired **Tissue** integrity: maternal r/t possible uterine rupture

Risk for ineffective **Tissue** perfusion: fetal r/t uteroplacental insufficiency

Risk for **Infection** r/t partial separation of placenta

Abscess Formation

Impaired **Tissue** integrity r/t altered circulation, nutritional deficit/excess

Ineffective **Health** maintenance r/t deficient knowledge regarding self-care with abscess

Ineffective **Protection** r/t inadequate nutrition, abnormal blood profile, drug therapy, treatment

Abuse, Child

See Child Abuse

Abuse—Spouse, Parent, or Significant Other

Anxiety r/t threat to self-concept, situational crisis of abuse

Caregiver role strain r/t chronic illness, self-care deficits, lack of respite care, extent of caregiving required

Compromised family **Coping** r/t abusive patterns

Defensive **Coping** r/t low self-esteem

Disturbed **Sleep** pattern r/t psychological stress

Impaired verbal **Communication** r/t psychological barriers of fear

Interrupted **Family** process: alcoholism r/t inadequate coping skills

Post-trauma response r/t history of abuse

Powerlessness r/t lifestyle of helplessness

Risk for **Post-trauma** syndrome r/t inadequate social support

Risk for self-directed **Violence** r/t history of abuse

Self-esteem disturbance r/t negative family interactions

Accessory Muscle Use (to Breathe)

Ineffective **Breathing** pattern r/t neuromuscular impairment, pain, musculoskeletal impairment, perception/cognitive impairment, anxiety, decreased energy, fatigue

See Asthma; Bronchitis; COPD; Respiratory Infections, Acute Childhood

Accident Prone

Acute **Confusion** r/t altered level of consciousness

Adult **Failure** to thrive r/t fatigue

Ineffective **Coping** r/t personal vulnerability, situational crises

Risk for **Injury** r/t history of accidents

Achalasia

Impaired **Swallowing** r/t neuromuscular impairment

Ineffective **Coping** r/t chronic disease

Pain r/t stasis of food in esophagus

Risk for **Aspiration** r/t nocturnal regurgitation

Acidosis, Metabolic

Acute **Pain**: headache r/t neuromuscular irritability

Decreased **Cardiac** output r/t dysrhythmias from hyperkalemia

Disturbed **Thought** processes r/t central nervous system depression

Imbalanced **Nutrition**: less than body requirements r/t inability to ingest, absorb nutrients

Impaired **Memory** r/t electrolyte imbalance

Ineffective **Tissue** Perfusion: cardiopulmonary r/t progressive shock

Risk for **Injury** r/t disorientation, weakness, stupor

Acidosis, Respiratory

Activity intolerance r/t imbalance between oxygen supply and demand

Disturbed **Thought** processes r/t central nervous system depression

Impaired **Gas** exchange r/t ventilation perfusion imbalance

Impaired **Memory** r/t hypoxia

Risk for decreased **Cardiac** output r/t dysrhythmias associated with respiratory acidosis

Acne Vulgaris

Disturbed **Body** image r/t biophysical changes associated with skin disorder

Impaired **Skin** integrity r/t hormonal changes (adolescence, menstrual cycle)

A

Ineffective management of **Therapeutic** regimen r/t deficient knowledge (medications, personal care, cause)

Acquired Immunodeficiency Syndrome

See AIDS

Acromegaly

Disturbed **Body** image r/t changes in body function and appearance

Risk for impaired **Mobility** r/t joint pain

Risk for ineffective **Airway** clearance r/t airway obstruction by enlarged tongue

Sexual dysfunction r/t changes in hormonal secretions

Activity Intolerance

Activity intolerance r/t bedrest/immobility, generalized weakness, sedentary lifestyle, imbalance between oxygen supply/demand, pain

Activity Intolerance, Potential to Develop

Risk for **Activity** intolerance r/t deconditioned status, presence of circulatory/respiratory problems, inexperience with activity

Acute Abdomen

Deficient **Fluid** volume r/t fluids trapped in bowel, inability to drink

Pain r/t pathological process

See cause of Acute Abdomen

Acute Alcohol Intoxication

Disturbed **Thought** processes r/t central nervous system depression

Dysfunctional **Family** processes: alcoholism r/t abuse of alcohol

Ineffective **Breathing** pattern r/t depression of the respiratory center

Risk for **Aspiration** r/t depressed reflexes with acute vomiting

Risk for **Infection** r/t impaired immune system from altered nutrition

Acute Back

Acute **Pain** r/t back injury

Anxiety r/t situational crisis, back injury

Constipation r/t decreased activity

Impaired physical **Mobility** r/t pain

Ineffective **Coping** r/t situational crisis, back injury

Ineffective **Health** maintenance r/t deficient knowledge regarding self-care with painful back

Acute Confusion

Acute **Confusion** r/t being >60 years of age, dementia, alcohol abuse, drug abuse, delirium

Acute Respiratory Distress Syndrome

See ARDS

Adams-Stokes Syndrome

See Dysrhythmia

Addiction

See Alcoholism; Drug Abuse

Addison's Disease

Activity intolerance r/t weakness, fatigue

Deficient **Fluid** volume r/t failure of regulatory mechanisms

Disturbed **Body** image r/t increased skin pigmentation

Imbalanced **Nutrition**: less than body requirements r/t chronic illness

Ineffective **Health** maintenance r/t deficient knowledge

Risk for **Injury** r/t weakness

Adenoidectomy

Acute **Pain** r/t surgical incision

Impaired **Comfort** r/t effects of anesthesia, nausea, vomiting

Ineffective **Airway** clearance r/t hesitation/reluctance to cough secondary to pain

Ineffective **Health** maintenance r/t deficient knowledge of postoperative care

Risk for **Aspiration**/suffocation r/t postoperative drainage, impaired swallowing

Risk for deficient **Fluid** volume r/t decreased intake secondary to painful swallowing, effects of anesthesia

Risk for imbalanced **Nutrition**: less than body requirements r/t hesitation/reluctance to swallow

Adhesions, Lysis of

See Abdominal Surgery

Adjustment Disorder

Anxiety r/t inability to cope with psychosocial stressor

Disturbed personal **Identity** r/t psychosocial stressor (specific to individual)

Impaired **Adjustment** r/t assault to self-esteem

Impaired **Social** interaction r/t absence of significant others or peers

Situational low **Self-esteem** r/t change in role function

Adjustment Impairment

Impaired **Adjustment** r/t disability requiring change in lifestyle, inadequate support systems, impaired cognition, sensory overload, assault to self-esteem, altered locus of control, incomplete grieving

Adolescent, Pregnant

Anxiety r/t situational and maturational crisis, pregnancy

Decisional **Conflict**: keeping child vs. giving up child vs. abortion r/t lack of experience with decision-making, interference with decision-making, multiple or divergent sources of information, lack of support system

Deficient **Knowledge** (pregnancy, infant growth and development, parenting)

Delayed **Growth** and development r/t pregnancy

Disturbed **Body** image r/t pregnancy superimposed on developing body

Family **Coping**: disabling r/t highly ambivalent family relationships, chronically unresolved feelings of guilt, anger, despair

Fear r/t labor and delivery

Health-seeking behaviors r/t desire for optimal maternal and fetal outcome

Imbalanced **Nutrition**: less than body requirements r/t lack of knowledge of nutritional needs during pregnancy and as growing adolescent

Impaired **Social** interaction r/t self-concept disturbance

Ineffective **Coping** r/t situational and maturational crisis, personal vulnerability

Ineffective **Denial** r/t fear of consequences of pregnancy becoming known

Ineffective **Health** maintenance r/t deficient knowledge with denial of pregnancy, desire to keep pregnancy secret, fear

Ineffective **Role** performance r/t pregnancy

Interrupted **Family** processes r/t unmet expectations for adolescent, situational crisis

Noncompliance r/t denial of pregnancy

Risk for **Constipation** r/t hormone effect, inadequate fiber in diet, inadequate fluid in diet

Risk for delayed **Development** r/t unplanned or unwanted pregnancy

Risk for impaired parent-infant **Attachment** r/t anxiety associated with the parent role

Risk for impaired **Parenting** r/t adolescent parent, unplanned or unwanted pregnancy, single parent

Risk for urge urinary **Incontinence** r/t pressure on bladder by growing uterus

Situational low **Self-esteem** r/t feelings of shame and guilt about becoming/being pregnant

Social Isolation r/t absence of supportive significant other(s)

Adoption, Giving Child Up for

Chronic **Sorrow** r/t loss of relationship with child

Decisional **Conflict** r/t unclear personal values or beliefs, perceived threat to value system, support system deficit

Disturbed **Sleep** pattern r/t depression or trauma of relinquishment of child

Ineffective **Coping** r/t final decision

Interrupted **Family** processes r/t conflict within family regarding relinquishment of child

Grieving r/t loss of child, loss of role of parent

Readiness for enhanced **Spiritual** well-being r/t harmony with self regarding final decision

Risk for **Post-trauma** syndrome r/t psychological trauma of relinquishment of child

Risk for **Spiritual** distress r/t perceived moral implications of decision

Social isolation r/t making choice that goes against values of significant other(s)

Adrenal Crisis

Deficient **Fluid** volume r/t insufficient ability to reabsorb water

Delayed **Surgical** recovery r/t inability to respond to stress

Ineffective **Protection** r/t inability to tolerate stress

See Addison's Disease; Shock

Advance Directives

Anticipatory **Grieving** r/t possible loss of self, significant other

Death **Anxiety** r/t planning for end-of-life health decisions

Decisional **Conflict** r/t unclear personal values or beliefs, perceived threat to value system, support system deficit

Readiness for enhanced **Spiritual** well-being r/t harmonious interconnectedness with self, others, higher power/God

Affective Disorders

Adult **Failure** to thrive r/t altered mood state

Chronic low **Self-esteem** r/t repeated unmet expectations

Chronic **Sorrow** r/t chronic mental illness

Constipation r/t inactivity, decreased fluid intake

A

Disturbed **Sleep** pattern r/t inactivity

Dysfunctional **Grieving** r/t lack of previous resolution of former grieving response

Fatigue r/t psychological demands

Hopelessness r/t feeling of abandonment, long-term stress

Ineffective **Coping** r/t dysfunctional grieving

Ineffective **Health** maintenance r/t lack of ability to make good judgments regarding ways to obtain help

Risk for **Loneliness** r/t pattern of social isolation, feelings of low self-esteem

Risk for **Suicide** r/t panic state

Self-care deficit: specify r/t depression, cognitive impairment

Sexual dysfunction r/t loss of sexual desire

Social isolation r/t ineffective coping

See specific disorder: Depression; Dysthymic Disorder; Manic Disorder, Bipolar I

Aggressive Behavior

Fear r/t real or imagined threat to own well-being

Risk for other-directed **Violence**: r/t antisocial character, battered woman, catatonic excitement, child abuse, manic excitement, organic brain syndrome, panic states, rage reactions, suicidal behavior, temporal lobe epilepsy, toxic reactions to medication

Risk for self-directed **Violence**: r/t antisocial character, battered woman, catatonic excitement, child abuse, manic excitement, organic brain syndrome, panic states, rage reactions, suicidal behavior, temporal lobe epilepsy, toxic reactions to medication

Aging

Adult **Failure** to thrive r/t depression, apathy, fatigue

Anticipatory **Grieving** r/t multiple losses, impending death

Chronic **Sorrow** r/t multiple losses

Death **Anxiety** r/t fear of unknown, loss of self, impact on significant others

Disturbed **Sensory** perception: visual or auditory r/t aging process

Family **Coping** potential for growth r/t ability to gratify needs, address adaptive tasks

Functional urinary **Incontinence** r/t impaired vision, impaired cognition, neuromuscular limitations, altered environmental factors

Health-seeking behaviors r/t knowledge about medication, nutrition, exercise, coping strategies

Impaired **Dentition** r/t ineffective oral hygiene; barriers to self-care, professional care; nutritional deficits; dietary habits; selected prescription medications; chronic use of tobacco, coffee, tea, red wine; lack of knowledge regarding dental health

Impaired **Memory** r/t fluid and electrolyte imbalance, neurological disturbances, excessive environmental disturbances, anemia, acute or chronic hypoxia, decreased cardiac output

Ineffective management of **Therapeutic** regimen r/t deficient knowledge: medication, nutrition, exercise, coping strategies

Ineffective **Thermoregulation** r/t aging

Readiness for enhanced community **Coping** r/t providing social support and other resources identified as needed for elderly client

Readiness for enhanced **Knowledge** of: specify r/t need to improve health

Readiness for enhanced **Nutrition** r/t need to improve health

Readiness for enhanced **Sleep** r/t need to improve sleep

Readiness for enhanced **Spiritual** well-being r/t one's experience of life's meaning, harmony with self, others, higher power/God, environment

Readiness for enhanced **Urinary** elimination r/t need to improve health

Risk for **Caregiver** role strain r/t inability to handle increasing needs of significant other

Risk for **Injury** r/t disturbed sensory perception

Risk for **Loneliness** r/t inadequate support system, role transition, health alterations, depression, fatigue

Sleep deprivation r/t aging-related sleep stage shifts

Agitation

Acute **Confusion** r/t side effects of medication, alcohol abuse or withdrawal, substance abuse or withdrawal, sensory deprivation, sensory overload

Sleep deprivation r/t sundowner's syndrome

Agoraphobia

Anxiety r/t real or perceived threat to physical integrity

Fear r/t leaving home, going out in public places

Impaired **Social** interaction r/t disturbance in self-concept

Ineffective **Coping** r/t inadequate support systems

Social isolation r/t altered thought process

Agranulocytosis

Delayed **Surgical** recovery r/t abnormal blood profile

Ineffective **Health** maintenance r/t deficient knowledge of protective measures to prevent infection

Ineffective **Protection** r/t abnormal blood profile

AICD (Automatic Implanted Cardioverter Defibrillator)

PREOPERATIVE

Anxiety r/t surgical procedure

Deficient **Knowledge** r/t purpose and function of AICD

POSTOPERATIVE

Ineffective **Health** maintenance r/t deficient knowledge regarding self-care, care of internal cardiac defibrillator

Risk for decreased **Cardiac** output r/t possible dysrhythmia

Risk for **Infection** r/t invasive surgical procedure

AIDS (Acquired Immunodeficiency Syndrome)

Altered **Sexuality** pattern r/t possible transmission of disease

Anticipatory **Grieving**: family/parental r/t potential/impending death of loved one

Anticipatory **Grieving**: individual r/t loss of physiopsychosocial well-being

Disturbed **Body** image r/t chronic contagious illness, cachexia

Caregiver role strain r/t unpredictable illness course, presence of situation stressors

Chronic **Pain** r/t tissue inflammation and destruction

Chronic **Sorrow** r/t living with long-term chronic illness

Death **Anxiety** r/t fear of premature death

Diarrhea r/t inflammatory bowel changes

Disturbed **Energy** field r/t chronic illness

Fatigue r/t disease process, stress, poor nutritional intake

Fear r/t powerlessness, threat to well-being

Hopelessness r/t deteriorating physical condition

Imbalanced **Nutrition**: less than body requirements r/t decreased ability to eat and absorb nutrients secondary to anorexia, nausea, diarrhea

Ineffective **Health** maintenance r/t deficient knowledge regarding transmission of infection, lack of exposure to information, misinterpretation of information

Ineffective **Protection** r/t risk for infection secondary to inadequate immune system

Interrupted **Family** processes r/t distress about diagnosis of human immunodeficiency virus (HIV) infection

Risk for deficient **Fluid** volume r/t diarrhea, vomiting, fever, bleeding

Risk for disturbed **Thought** processes r/t infection in brain

Risk for impaired **Oral** mucous membranes r/t immunological deficit

Risk for impaired **Skin** integrity r/t immunological deficit, diarrhea

Risk for **Infection** r/t inadequate immune system

Risk for **Loneliness** r/t social isolation

Risk for **Spiritual** distress r/t physical illness

Situational low **Self-esteem** r/t crisis of chronic contagious illness

Social isolation r/t self-concept disturbance, therapeutic isolation

Spiritual distress r/t challenged beliefs or moral system

See AIDS in Child; Cancer; Pneumonia

AIDS Dementia

Chronic **Confusion** r/t viral invasion of nervous system

See Dementia

AIDS in Child

Impaired **Parenting** r/t congenital acquisition of infection secondary to intravenous (IV) drug use, multiple sexual partners, history of contaminated blood transfusion

Parental role conflict r/t interruption of family life due to home care regimen, intimidation with invasive or restrictive modalities

Risk for delayed **Development** r/t chronic illness

Risk for disproportionate **Growth** r/t chronic illness

See AIDS; Child with Chronic Condition; Hospitalized Child; Terminally Ill Child

Airway Obstruction/Secretions

Ineffective **Airway** clearance r/t decreased energy; fatigue; tracheobronchial infection, obstruction, secretions; perceptual/cognitive impairment; trauma; decreased force of cough because of aging

Alcohol Withdrawal

Acute **Confusion** r/t effects of alcohol withdrawal

Anxiety r/t situational crisis, withdrawal

Chronic low **Self-esteem** r/t repeated unmet expectations

Disturbed **Sensory** perception: visual, auditory, kinesthetic, tactile, olfactory r/t neurochemical imbalance in brain

Disturbed **Sleep** pattern r/t effect of depressants, alcohol withdrawal, anxiety

Disturbed **Thought** processes r/t potential delirium tremors

Dysfunctional **Family** processes: alcoholism r/t abuse of alcohol

Imbalanced **Nutrition**: less than body requirements r/t poor dietary habits

Ineffective **Coping** r/t personal vulnerability

Ineffective **Health** maintenance r/t deficient knowledge regarding chronic illness or effects of alcohol consumption

Risk for deficient **Fluid** volume r/t excessive diaphoresis, agitation, decreased fluid intake

Risk for other-directed **Violence** r/t substance withdrawal

Risk for self-directed **Violence** r/t substance withdrawal

Alcoholism

Acute **Confusion** r/t alcohol abuse

Anxiety r/t loss of control

Chronic **Confusion** r/t neurological effects of chronic alcohol intake

Compromised/dysfunctional family **Coping** r/t codependency issues

Coping, defensive r/t alcoholism

Denial, ineffective r/t refusal to acknowledge alcoholism

Disturbed **Sleep** pattern r/t irritability, nightmares, tremors

Imbalanced **Nutrition**: less than body requirements r/t anorexia

Impaired adjustment r/t lack of motivation to change behaviors

Impaired **Home** maintenance r/t memory deficits, fatigue

Impaired **Memory** r/t alcohol abuse

Ineffective **Coping** r/t use of alcohol to cope with life events

Ineffective **Protection** r/t malnutrition, sleep deprivation

Interrupted **Family** process: alcoholism r/t alcohol abuse

Powerlessness r/t alcohol addiction

Risk for **Injury** r/t alteration in sensory/perceptual function

Risk for **Loneliness** r/t unacceptable social behavior

Risk for other-directed **Violence** r/t reactions to substances used, impulsive behavior, disorientation, impaired judgment

Risk for self-directed **Violence** r/t reactions to substances used, impulsive behavior, disorientation, impaired judgment

Self-esteem disturbance r/t failure at life events

Social isolation r/t unacceptable social behavior, values

Alcoholism, Altered Family Process

Altered **Family** process, alcoholism r/t abuse of alcohol, genetic predisposition, lack of problem-solving skills, inadequate coping skills, family history of alcoholism, resistance to treatment, biochemical influences, addictive personality

Alkalosis

See Metabolic Alkalosis

Allergies

Ineffective **Health** maintenance r/t deficient knowledge regarding allergies

Latex **Allergy** r/t hypersensitivity to natural rubber latex

Risk for latex **Allergy** r/t repeated exposure to products containing latex

Alopecia

Deficient **Knowledge** r/t self-care needed to promote hair growth

Disturbed **Body** image r/t loss of hair, change in appearance

Altered Mental Status

See Acute Confusion; Chronic Confusion; Impaired Memory

Alzheimer Type Dementia

Adult **Failure** to thrive r/t difficulty in reasoning, judgment, memory, concentration

Disturbed **Thought** processes r/t chronic organic disorder

Caregiver role strain r/t duration and extent of caregiving required

Chronic **Confusion** r/t Alzheimer's disease

Compromised family **Coping** r/t interrupted family processes

Disturbed **Sleep** pattern r/t neurological impairment, daytime naps

Fear r/t loss of self

Hopelessness r/t deteriorating condition

Impaired **Environmental** interpretation syndrome r/t Alzheimer's disease

Impaired **Home** maintenance r/t impaired cognitive function, inadequate support systems

Impaired **Memory** r/t neurological disturbance

Impaired physical **Mobility** r/t severe neurological dysfunction

Ineffective **Health** maintenance r/t deficient knowledge of caregiver regarding appropriate care

Powerlessness r/t deteriorating condition

Risk for **Injury** r/t confusion

Risk for **Loneliness** r/t potential social isolation

Risk for other-directed **Violence** r/t frustration, fear, anger

Risk for **Relocation** stress syndrome r/t impaired psychosocial health, decreased health status

Self-care deficit: specify r/t psychological-physiological impairment

Social isolation r/t fear of disclosure of memory loss

Wandering r/t cognitive impairment, frustration, physiological state

See Dementia

Amenorrhea

Imbalanced **Nutrition**: less than body requirements r/t inadequate food intake

Risk for **Sexual** dysfunction r/t altered body function

See Sexuality, Adolescent

Amnesia

Acute **Confusion** r/t alcohol abuse, delirium, dementia, drug abuse

Altered **Family** process: alcoholism r/t alcohol abuse, inadequate coping skills

Impaired **Memory** r/t excessive environmental disturbance, neurological disturbance

Post-trauma response r/t history of abuse, catastrophic illness, disaster, accident

Amniocentesis

Anxiety r/t threat to self and fetus, unknown future

Decisional **Conflict** r/t choice of treatment pending results of test

Risk for **Infection** r/t invasive procedure

Amnionitis

See Chorioamnionitis

Amniotic Membrane Rupture

See Premature Rupture of Membranes

Amputation

Chronic **Sorrow** r/t grief associated with loss of body part

Disturbed **Body** image r/t negative effects of amputation, response from others

Grieving r/t loss of body part, future lifestyle changes

Impaired physical **Mobility** r/t musculoskeletal impairment, limited movement

Impaired **Skin** integrity r/t poor healing, prosthesis rubbing

Ineffective **Health** maintenance r/t deficient knowledge of care of stump, rehabilitation

Ineffective **Tissue** perfusion: peripheral r/t impaired arterial circulation

Pain r/t surgery, phantom limb sensation

Risk for deficient **Fluid** volume: hemorrhage r/t vulnerable surgical site

Amyotrophic Lateral Sclerosis

Chronic **Sorrow** r/t chronic illness

Death **Anxiety** r/t impending progressive loss of function leading to death

Decisional **Conflict**: ventilator therapy r/t unclear personal values or beliefs, lack of relevant information

Impaired spontaneous **Ventilation** r/t weakness of muscles of respiration

Impaired **Swallowing** r/t weakness of muscles involved in swallowing

Impaired verbal **Communication** r/t weakness of muscles of speech, deficient knowledge of ways to compensate and alternative communication devices

Ineffective **Breathing** pattern r/t compromised muscles of respiration

Risk for **Aspiration** r/t impaired swallowing

Risk for **Spiritual** distress r/t chronic debilitating condition

See Neurological Disorders

Anal Fistula

See Hemorrhoidectomy

Anaphylactic Shock

Impaired spontaneous **Ventilation** r/t acute airway obstruction

Ineffective **Airway** clearance r/t laryngeal edema, bronchospasm

Latex **Allergy** response r/t no immune mechanism response

See Shock

Anasarca

Excess **Fluid** volume r/t excessive fluid intake, cardiac/renal dysfunction, loss of plasma proteins

A

Risk for impaired **Skin** integrity r/t impaired circulation to skin

See Cause of Anasarca

Anemia

Anxiety r/t cause of disease

Delayed **Surgical** recovery r/t decreased oxygen supply to body, increased cardiac workload

Fatigue r/t decreased oxygen supply to the body, increased cardiac workload

Impaired **Memory** r/t anemia

Ineffective **Health** maintenance r/t deficient knowledge regarding nutritional and medical treatment of anemia

Ineffective **Protection** r/t bleeding disorder

Risk for **Injury** r/t alteration in peripheral sensory perception

Anemia in Pregnancy

Anxiety r/t concerns about health of self and fetus

Fatigue r/t decreased oxygen supply to the body, increased cardiac workload

Ineffective **Health** maintenance r/t deficient knowledge regarding nutrition in pregnancy

Risk for delayed **Development** r/t reduction in the oxygen-carrying capacity of blood

Risk for **Infection** r/t reduction in oxygen-carrying capacity of blood

Anemia, Sickle Cell

See Anemia; Sickle Cell Anemia/Crisis

Anencephaly

See Neurotube Defects

Aneurysm, Abdominal Surgery

Risk for deficient **Fluid** volume: hemorrhage r/t potential abnormal blood loss

Risk for ineffective **Tissue** perfusion: peripheral or renal r/t impaired arterial circulation

Risk for **Infection** r/t invasive procedure

See Abdominal Surgery

Aneurysm, Cerebral

See Craniectomy/Craniotomy; Subarachnoid Hemorrhage (if aneurysm has ruptured)

Anger

Anxiety r/t situational crisis

Defensive **Coping** r/t inability to acknowledge responsibility for actions and results of actions

Fear r/t environmental stressor, hospitalization

Grieving r/t significant loss

Impaired **Adjustment** r/t assault to self-esteem, disability requiring change in lifestyle, inadequate support system

Powerlessness r/t health care environment

Risk for other-directed **Violence** r/t history of violence, rage reaction

Risk for **Post-trauma** syndrome r/t inadequate social support

Risk for self-directed **Violence** r/t history of violence, history of abuse, rage reaction

Angina Pectoris

Activity intolerance r/t acute pain, dysrhythmias

Acute **Pain** r/t myocardial ischemia

Altered **Sexuality** pattern r/t disease process, medications, loss of libido

Anxiety r/t situational crisis

Decreased **Cardiac** output r/t myocardial ischemia, medication effect, dysrhythmia

Grieving r/t pain, lifestyle changes

Ineffective **Coping** r/t personal vulnerability to situational crisis of new diagnosis, deteriorating health

Ineffective **Denial** r/t deficient knowledge (delays seeking help when symptoms occur)

Ineffective **Health** maintenance r/t deficient knowledge of care of angina condition

Angiocardiography (Cardiac Catheterization)

See Cardiac Catheterization

Angioplasty, Coronary

Fear r/t possible outcome of interventional procedure

Ineffective **Health** maintenance r/t deficient knowledge regarding care following procedures, measures to limit coronary artery disease

Risk for decreased **Cardiac** output r/t ventricular ischemia, dysrhythmias

Risk for deficient **Fluid** volume r/t possible damage to coronary artery, hematoma formation, hemorrhage

Risk for ineffective **Tissue** perfusion: peripheral/cardiopulmonary r/t vasospasm, hematoma formation

Anomaly, Fetal/Newborn (Parent Dealing with)

Anxiety r/t threat to role functioning, situational crisis

Chronic **Sorrow** r/t loss of ideal child

Decisional **Conflict**: interventions for fetus/newborn r/t lack of relevant information, spiritual distress, threat to value system

Effective **Therapeutic** regimen management r/t verbalized intent to reduce risk factors for progression of illness and sequelae associated with anomaly

Fear r/t real or imagined threat to baby, implications for future pregnancies, powerlessness

Hopelessness r/t long-term stress, deteriorating physical condition of child, lost spiritual belief

Deficient **Knowledge** r/t limited exposure to situation

Disabled family **Coping** r/t chronically unresolved feelings about loss of perfect baby

Ineffective **Coping** r/t personal vulnerability in situational crisis

Impaired **Parenting** r/t interruption of bonding process

Interrupted **Family** processes r/t unmet expectations for perfect baby, lack of adequate support systems

Parental role **Conflict** r/t separation from newborn, intimidation with invasive or restrictive modalities, specialized care center policies

Powerlessness r/t complication threatening fetus/newborn

Risk for dysfunctional **Grieving** r/t loss of perfect child

Risk for disorganized **Infant** behavior r/t congenital disorder

Risk for impaired parent/infant/child **Attachment** r/t ill infant who is unable to effectively initiate parental contact as result of altered behavioral organization

Risk for impaired **Parenting** r/t interruption of bonding process; unrealistic expectations for self, infant, or partner; perceived threat to own emotional survival; severe stress; lack of knowledge

Risk for **Spiritual** distress r/t lack of normal child to raise and carry on family name

Self-esteem disturbance r/t perceived inability to produce a perfect child

Social isolation r/t alterations in child's physical appearance, altered state of wellness

Spiritual distress r/t test of spiritual beliefs

Anorectal Abscess

Acute **Pain** r/t inflammation of perirectal area

Disturbed **Body** image r/t odor and drainage from rectal area

Risk for **Constipation** r/t fear of painful elimination

Anorexia

Deficient **Fluid** volume r/t inability to drink

Delayed **Surgical** recovery r/t inadequate nutritional intake

Imbalanced **Nutrition**: less than body requirements r/t loss of appetite, nausea, vomiting

Anorexia Nervosa

Activity intolerance r/t fatigue, weakness

Altered patterns of **Sexuality** r/t loss of libido from malnutrition

Chronic low **Self-esteem** r/t repeated unmet expectations

Constipation r/t lack of adequate food, fiber, and fluid intake

Defensive **Coping** r/t psychological impairment, eating disorder

Diarrhea r/t laxative abuse

Disabled family **Coping** r/t highly ambivalent family relationships

Disturbed **Body** image r/t misconception of actual body appearance

Disturbed **Thought** processes r/t anorexia

Imbalanced **Nutrition**: less than body requirements r/t inadequate food intake

Ineffective **Denial** r/t fear of consequences of therapy, possible weight gain

Ineffective family **Therapeutic** regimen management r/t family conflict, excessive demands on family associated with complexity of condition and treatment

Interrupted **Family** processes r/t situational crisis

Risk for **Infection** r/t malnutrition resulting in depressed immune system

Risk for **Spiritual** distress r/t low self-esteem

See Maturational Issues, Adolescent

Anosmia (Smell, Loss of Ability to)

Disturbed **Sensory** perception: olfactory r/t altered sensory reception, transmission, integration

Imbalanced **Nutrition**: less than body requirements r/t loss of appetite associated with loss of smell

Antepartum Period

See Pregnancy—Normal; Prenatal Care—Normal

Anterior Repair—Anterior Colporrhaphy

Risk for perioperative positioning **Injury**

Risk for urge urinary **Incontinence** r/t trauma to bladder

Urinary retention r/t edema of urinary structures

See Vaginal Hysterectomy

Anticoagulant Therapy

Anxiety r/t situational crisis

A

Ineffective **Health** maintenance r/t deficient knowledge regarding precautions to take with anticoagulant therapy

Ineffective **Protection** r/t altered clotting function from anticoagulant

Risk for deficient **Fluid** volume: hemorrhage r/t altered clotting mechanism

Antisocial Personality Disorder

Defensive **Coping** r/t excessive use of projection

Disturbed **Thought** processes r/t internal turmoil and conflict (intrusive thinking)

Hopelessness r/t abandonment

Impaired **Social** interaction r/t sociocultural conflict, chemical dependence, inability to form relationships

Ineffective **Coping** r/t frequently violating the norms and rules of society

Ineffective family **Therapeutic** regimen management r/t excessive demands on family

Risk for impaired **Parenting** r/t inability to function as parent or guardian, emotional instability

Risk for **Loneliness** r/t inability to interact appropriately with others

Risk for other-directed **Violence** r/t history of violence

Risk for **Self-mutilation** r/t self-hatred, depersonalization

Spiritual distress r/t separation from religious/cultural ties

Anuria

See Renal Failure

Anxiety

Anxiety r/t threat to or change in role status, unmet needs, interpersonal transmission/contagion, situational/maturational crisis, threat of death, threat to or change in health status, threat to or change in interaction patterns, threat to or change in role function, threat to self-concept, unconscious conflict regarding essential values/goals of life, threat to or change in environment, stress, threat to or change in economic status, substance abuse

Risk for **Powerlessness** r/t anxiety

Risk for situational low **Self-esteem** r/t anxiety

Anxiety Disorder

Anxiety r/t unmet security and safety needs

Death **Anxiety** r/t fears of unknown, powerlessness

Decisional **Conflict** r/t low self-esteem, fear of making a mistake

Defensive **Coping** r/t overwhelming feelings of dread

Disabled family **Coping** r/t ritualistic behavior, actions

Disturbed **Energy** field r/t hopelessness, helplessness, fear

Disturbed **Sleep** pattern r/t psychological impairment, emotional instability

Disturbed **Thought** processes r/t anxiety

Ineffective **Coping** r/t inability to express feelings appropriately

Ineffective **Denial** r/t overwhelming feelings of hopelessness, fear, threat to self

Powerlessness r/t lifestyle of helplessness

Risk for **Spiritual** distress r/t psychological distress

Self-care deficit r/t ritualistic behavior, activities

Sleep deprivation r/t prolonged psychological discomfort

Aortic Aneurysm Repair (Abdominal Surgery)

See Abdominal Surgery; Aneurysm, Abdominal Surgery

Aortic Valvular Stenosis

See Congenital Heart Disease/Cardiac Anomalies

Aphasia

Anxiety r/t situational crisis of aphasia

Impaired verbal **Communication** r/t decrease in circulation to brain

Ineffective **Coping** r/t loss of speech

Ineffective **Health** maintenance r/t deficient knowledge regarding information on aphasia and alternative communication techniques

Aplastic Anemia

Activity intolerance r/t imbalance between oxygen supply and demand

Anxiety r/t deficient knowledge of disease process and treatment

Delayed **Surgical** recovery r/t risk for infection

Impaired **Protection** r/t inadequate immune function

Risk for **Infection** r/t inadequate immune function

Apnea in Infancy

See Premature Infant; SIDS

Apneustic Respirations

Impaired **Breathing** pattern r/t perception/cognitive impairment, neurological impairment

See cause of Apneustic Respirations

Appendectomy

Acute **Pain** r/t surgical incision

A

Deficient **Fluid** volume r/t fluid restriction, hyper-metabolic state, nausea, vomiting

Ineffective **Health** maintenance r/t deficient knowledge regarding self-care following appendectomy

Risk for **Infection** r/t perforation/rupture of appendix, surgical incision, peritonitis

See Hospitalized Child; Surgery

Appendicitis

Acute **Pain** r/t inflammation

Deficient **Fluid** volume r/t anorexia, nausea, vomiting

Delayed **Surgical** recovery r/t risk for infection

Risk for **Infection** r/t possible perforation of appendix

Apprehension

Anxiety r/t threat to self-concept, threat to health status, situational crisis

Death **Anxiety** r/t apprehension over loss of self, consequences to significant others

ARDS (Acute Respiratory Distress Syndrome)

Death **Anxiety** r/t seriousness of physical disease

Delayed **Surgical** recovery r/t complications associated with respiratory difficulty

Impaired **Gas** exchange r/t damage to alveolar-capillary membrane, change in lung compliance

Impaired spontaneous **Ventilation** r/t damage to alveolar capillary membrane

Ineffective **Airway** clearance r/t excessive tracheobronchial secretions

See Child with Chronic Condition; Ventilator Client

Arrhythmia

See Dysrhythmia

Arterial Insufficiency

Delayed **Surgical** recovery r/t ineffective tissue perfusion

Ineffective **Tissue** perfusion: peripheral r/t interruption of arterial flow

Arthritis

Activity intolerance r/t chronic pain, fatigue, weakness

Chronic **Pain** r/t progression of joint deterioration

Chronic **Sorrow** r/t presence of chronic condition

Disturbed **Body** image r/t ineffective coping with joint abnormalities

Impaired physical **Mobility** r/t musculoskeletal impairment

Ineffective **Health** maintenance r/t deficient knowledge regarding care of arthritis

Risk for **Spiritual** distress r/t presence of chronic condition

Self-care deficit: specify r/t pain, musculoskeletal impairment

See Rheumatoid Arthritis, Juvenile

Arthrocentesis

Acute **Pain** r/t invasive procedure

Arthroplasty—Total Hip Replacement

Acute **Pain** r/t tissue trauma associated with surgery

Constipation r/t immobility

Impaired physical **Mobility** r/t decreased muscle strength, surgery

Impaired **Walking** r/t decreased muscle strength, surgery

Risk for **Infection** r/t invasive surgery, foreign object in body, anesthesia, immobility with stasis of respiratory secretions

Risk for **Injury** r/t interruption of arterial blood flow, dislocation of prosthesis

Risk for perioperative positioning **Injury** r/t immobilization, muscle weakness

Risk for **Peripheral** neurovascular dysfunction r/t orthopedic surgery

See Surgery

Arthroscopy

Ineffective **Health** maintenance r/t deficient knowledge regarding procedure, postoperative restrictions

Ascites

Chronic **Pain** r/t altered body function

Imbalanced **Nutrition**: less than body requirements r/t loss of appetite

Ineffective **Breathing** pattern r/t increased abdominal girth

Ineffective **Health** maintenance r/t deficient knowledge of care with condition of ascites

See cause of Ascites; Cancer; Cirrhosis

Asphyxia, Birth

Altered **Tissue** perfusion: cerebral r/t poor placental perfusion or cord compression resulting in lack of oxygen to brain

Anticipatory **Grieving** r/t loss of "perfect" child, concern of loss of future abilities

Fear (parental) r/t concern over safety of infant

Impaired **Gas** exchange r/t poor placental perfusion, lack of initiation of breathing by newborn

Impaired spontaneous **Ventilation** r/t brain injury

A

Ineffective **Breathing** pattern r/t depression of breathing reflex secondary to anoxia

Ineffective **Coping** r/t uncertainty of child outcome

Risk for delayed **Development** r/t lack of oxygen to brain

Risk for disorganized **Infant** behavior r/t lack of oxygen to brain

Risk for disproportionate **Growth** r/t lack of oxygen to brain

Risk for impaired parent/infant **Attachment** r/t ill infant who is unable to initiate parental contact, hospitalization in critical care environment

Risk for **Injury** r/t lack of oxygen to brain

Risk for **Post-trauma** syndrome: parental r/t psychological trauma of sudden potential for loss of newborn

Aspiration, Danger of

Risk for **Aspiration** r/t reduced level of consciousness; depressed cough or gag reflexes; presence of tracheostomy or endotracheal tube; incomplete lower esophageal sphincter; presence of gastrointestinal tubes or tube feedings; medication administration; situations hindering elevation of upper body; increased intragastric pressure; increased gastric residual; decreased gastrointestinal motility; delayed gastric emptying; impaired swallowing; facial, oral, or neck surgery or trauma; wired jaws

Assault Victim

Post-trauma syndrome r/t assault

Rape-trauma syndrome r/t rape

Risk for **Post-trauma** syndrome r/t perception of event, inadequate social support, nonsupportive environment, diminished ego strength, duration of event

Risk for **Spiritual** distress r/t physical, psychological stress

Assaultive Client

Disturbed **Thought** process r/t use of hallucinogenic substance, psychological disorder

Ineffective **Coping** r/t lack of control of impulsive actions

Risk for **Injury** r/t confused thought process, impaired judgment

Risk for other-directed **Violence** r/t paranoid ideation

Asthma

Activity intolerance r/t fatigue, energy shift to meet muscle needs for breathing to overcome airway obstruction

Anxiety r/t inability to breathe effectively, fear of suffocation

Disturbed **Body** image r/t decreased participation in physical activities

Impaired **Home** maintenance r/t deficient knowledge regarding control of environmental triggers

Ineffective **Airway** clearance r/t tracheobronchial narrowing, excessive secretions

Ineffective **Breathing** pattern r/t anxiety

Ineffective **Coping** r/t personal vulnerability to situational crisis

Ineffective **Health** maintenance r/t deficient knowledge regarding physical triggers, medications, treatment of early warning signs

Sleep deprivation r/t ineffective breathing pattern

See Child with Chronic Condition; Hospitalized Child

Ataxia

Anxiety r/t change in health status

Disturbed **Body** image r/t staggering gait

Impaired physical **Mobility** r/t neuromuscular impairment

Risk for **Injury** r/t gait alteration

Atelectasis

Impaired **Gas** exchange r/t decreased alveolar-capillary surface

Ineffective **Breathing** pattern r/t loss of functional lung tissue, depression of respiratory function or hypoventilation because of pain

Athlete's Foot

Impaired **Skin** integrity r/t effects of fungal agent

Ineffective **Health** maintenance r/t deficient knowledge regarding treatment and prevention of athlete's foot

See Itching

Atrial Fibrillation

See Dysrhythmia

Atrial Septal Defect

See Congenital Heart Disease/Cardiac Anomalies

Attention Deficit Disorder

Disabled family **Coping** r/t significant person with chronically unexpressed feelings of guilt, anxiety, hostility, despair, etc.

Impaired **Adjustment** r/t intense emotional state

Risk for delayed **Development** r/t behavior disorders

Risk for impaired **Parenting** r/t lack of knowledge of factors contributing to child's behavior

Risk for **Loneliness** r/t social isolation

Risk for **Spiritual** distress r/t poor relationships

Self-esteem disturbance r/t difficulty in participating in expected activities

Social isolation r/t unacceptable social behavior

Autism

Compromised family **Coping** r/t parental guilt over etiology of disease, inability to accept or adapt to child's condition, inability to help child and other family members seek treatment

Delayed **Growth** and development r/t inability to develop relations with other human beings, inability to identify own body as separate from those of other people, inability to integrate concept of self

Disturbed personal **Identity** r/t inability to distinguish between self and environment, inability to identify own body as separate from those of other people, inability to integrate concept of self

Disturbed **Thought** processes r/t inability to perceive self or others, cognitive dissonance, perceptual dysfunction

Impaired **Social** interaction r/t communication barriers, inability to relate to others

Impaired verbal **Communication** r/t speech and language delays

Risk for delayed **Development** r/t autism

Risk for **Loneliness** r/t health alterations, cognition

Risk for other-directed **Violence** r/t frequent destructive rages toward others secondary to extreme response to changes in routine, fear of harmless things

Risk for self-directed **Violence** r/t frequent destructive rages toward self secondary to extreme response to changes in routine, fear of harmless things

Risk for **Self-mutilation** r/t autistic state

See Child with Chronic Condition; Mental Retardation

Automatic Implanted Cardioverter Defibrillator

See AICD

Autonomic Dysreflexia

Autonomic dysreflexia r/t bladder distention, bowel distention, noxious stimuli

Risk for **Autonomic** dysreflexia r/t bladder distention, bowel distention, noxious stimuli

Autonomic Hyperreflexia

See Autonomic Dysreflexia

B

Back Pain

Acute **Pain** r/t back injury

Anxiety r/t situational crisis, back injury

Chronic **Pain** r/t back injury

Disturbed **Energy** field r/t chronic pain

Impaired physical **Mobility** r/t pain

Ineffective **Coping** r/t situational crisis, back injury

Ineffective **Health** maintenance r/t deficient knowledge regarding prevention of further injury, proper body mechanics

Risk for **Constipation** r/t decreased activity, side effect of pain medication

Risk for **Disuse** syndrome r/t severe pain

Bacteremia

Ineffective **Protection** r/t compromised immune system

See Infection; Infection, Potential for

Barrel Chest

See Aging (if appropriate); COPD

Bathing/Hygiene Problems

Bathing/hygiene **Self-care** deficit r/t intolerance to activity, decreased strength and endurance, pain, discomfort, perceptual or cognitive impairment, neuromuscular impairment, musculoskeletal impairment, depression, severe anxiety

Impaired bed **Mobility** r/t chronic physically limiting condition

Battered Child Syndrome

Acute **Pain** r/t physical injuries

Chronic low **Self-esteem** r/t lack of positive feedback, excessive negative feedback

Chronic **Sorrow** r/t situational crises

Deficient **Diversional** activity r/t diminished/absent environmental or personal stimuli

Delayed **Growth** and development: regression vs. delayed r/t diminished/absent environmental stimuli, inadequate caretaking, inconsistent responsiveness by caretaker

Disturbed **Sleep** pattern r/t hypervigilance, anxiety

Dysfunctional **Family** process: alcoholism r/t inadequate coping skills

Fear r/t threat of punishment for perceived wrongdoing

Imbalanced **Nutrition**: less than body requirements r/t inadequate caretaking

Impaired **Skin** integrity r/t altered nutritional state, physical abuse

Post-trauma syndrome r/t physical abuse, incest, rape, molestation

Risk for delayed **Development** r/t shaken baby, abuse

Risk for disproportionate **Growth** r/t abuse

Risk for **Poisoning** r/t inadequate safeguards, lack of proper safety precautions, accessibility of illicit substances secondary to impaired home maintenance

Risk for **Post-trauma** syndrome r/t physical abuse, incest, rape, molestation

Risk for **Self-mutilation** r/t feelings of rejection, dysfunctional family

Risk for **Suffocation**/aspiration r/t propped bottle, unattended child

Risk for **Trauma** r/t inadequate precautions, cognitive or emotional difficulties

Sleep deprivation r/t prolonged psychological discomfort

Social isolation: family imposed r/t fear of disclosure of family dysfunction and abuse

Battered Person

See Abuse—Spouse, Parent, or Significant Other

Bed Mobility, Impaired

Impaired bed **Mobility** r/t intolerance to activity, decreased strength and endurance, pain or discomfort, perceptual or cognitive impairment, neuromuscular impairment, musculoskeletal impairment, depression, severe anxiety

Bedbugs, Infestation

Impaired **Home** maintenance r/t deficient knowledge regarding prevention of bedbug infestation

Impaired **Skin** integrity r/t bites of bedbugs

See Itching

Bedrest, Prolonged

Deficient **Diversional** activity r/t prolonged bedrest

Disuse syndrome r/t prolonged immobility

Impaired bed **Mobility** r/t neuromuscular impairment

Risk for **Loneliness** r/t prolonged bedrest

Social isolation r/t prolonged bedrest

Bedsores

See Pressure Ulcer

Bedwetting

See Enuresis

Bell's Palsy

Acute **Pain** r/t inflammation of facial nerve

Disturbed **Body** image r/t loss of motor control on one side of face

Imbalanced **Nutrition**: less than body requirements r/t difficulty with chewing

Risk for **Injury** (eye) r/t dysfunction of facial nerve

Benign Prostatic Hypertrophy

See BPH; Prostatic Hypertrophy

Bereavement

Chronic **Sorrow** r/t death of loved one, chronic illness, disability

Disturbed **Sleep** pattern r/t grief

Dysfunctional **Grieving** r/t death of a loved one

Grieving r/t loss of significant person

Risk for **Spiritual** distress r/t death of a loved one

Biliary Atresia

Anxiety r/t surgical intervention, possible liver transplantation

Imbalanced **Nutrition**: less than body requirements r/t decreased absorption of fat and fat-soluble vitamins, poor feeding

Impaired **Comfort** r/t pruritus, nausea

Risk for impaired **Skin** integrity r/t pruritus

Risk for ineffective **Breathing** pattern r/t enlarged liver, development of ascites

Risk for **Injury**: bleeding r/t vitamin K deficiency, altered clotting mechanisms

See Child with Chronic Condition; Cirrhosis (as complication); Hospitalized Child; Terminally Ill Child

Biliary Calculus

See Cholelithiasis

Biliary Obstruction

See Jaundice

Biopsy

Fear r/t outcome of biopsy

Ineffective **Health** maintenance r/t deficient knowledge regarding biopsy site, further needed health care

Bioterrorism

Risk for **Infection** r/t exposure to harmful biological agent

Risk for **Injury** r/t harmful chemical agent exposure

Risk for **Post-Trauma** stress r/t perception of event of bioterrorism

Bipolar Disorder I (Most Recent Episode, Depressed or Manic)

Chronic low **Self-esteem** r/t repeated unmet expectations

Disturbed **Energy** field r/t disharmony of mind, body, spirit

Dysfunctional **Grieving** r/t lack of previous resolution of former grieving response

Fatigue r/t psychological demands

Impaired **Adjustment** r/t low state of optimism

Ineffective **Coping** r/t dysfunctional grieving

Ineffective **Health** maintenance r/t lack of ability to make good judgments regarding ways to obtain help

Risk for **Loneliness** r/t stress, conflict

Risk for **Spiritual** distress r/t mental illness

Self-care deficit: specify r/t depression, cognitive impairment

Social isolation r/t ineffective coping

See Depression; Manic Disorder, Bipolar I

Birth Asphyxia

See Asphyxia, Birth

Birth Control

See Contraceptive Method

Bladder Cancer

Urinary retention r/t clots obstructing urethra

See Cancer; TURP

Bladder Distention

Risk for urge urinary **Incontinence** r/t small bladder capacity

Urge urinary **Incontinence** r/t overdistention of bladder

Urinary retention r/t high urethral pressure caused by weak detrusor, inhibition of reflex arc, blockage, strong sphincter

Bladder Training

Disturbed **Body** image r/t difficulty in maintaining control of urinary elimination

Functional **Incontinence** r/t altered environment; sensory, cognitive, mobility deficit

Ineffective **Health** maintenance r/t deficient knowledge regarding incontinence self-care

Stress urinary **Incontinence** r/t degenerative change in pelvic muscles and structural supports

Urge urinary **Incontinence** r/t decreased bladder capacity, increased urine concentration, overdistention of bladder

Bleeding Tendency

Ineffective **Protection** r/t abnormal blood profile, drug therapies

Risk for delayed **Surgical** recovery r/t bleeding tendency

Blepharoplasty

Disturbed **Body** image r/t effects of surgery

Ineffective **Health** maintenance r/t deficient knowledge regarding postoperative care of surgical area

Blindness

Disturbed **Sensory** perception: visual r/t altered sensory reception, transmission, integration

Impaired **Home** maintenance r/t decreased vision

Ineffective **Role** performance r/t alteration in health status (change in visual acuity)

Interrupted **Family** process r/t shift in health status of family member (change in visual acuity)

Risk for delayed **Development** r/t vision impairment

Risk for **Injury** r/t sensory dysfunction

Self-care deficit r/t inability to see to be able to perform activities of daily living

See Vision Impairment

Blood Disorder

Ineffective **Protection** r/t abnormal blood profile

See cause of Blood Disorder

Blood Pressure Alteration

See Hypertension; Hypotension

Blood Transfusion

Anxiety r/t possibility of harm from transfusion

See Anemia

Body Dysmorphic Disorder

Disturbed **Body** Image r/t over involvement in physical appearance

Body Image Change

Disturbed **Body** image r/t psychosocial, biophysical, cognitive/perceptual, cultural, spiritual, developmental changes; illness; trauma or injury; surgery; illness treatment

Body Temperature, Altered

Risk for imbalanced **Body** temperature r/t extremes of age or weight, exposure to cold or hot environment, dehydration, change in activity, effects of medication, dysfunction of body temperature regulation center

B

Bone Marrow Biopsy

Acute **Pain** r/t bone marrow aspiration

Fear r/t unknown outcome of results of biopsy

Ineffective **Health** maintenance r/t deficient knowledge of expectations following procedure, disease treatment following biopsy

See disease necessitating bone marrow biopsy (e.g., Leukemia)

Borderline Personality Disorder

Anxiety r/t perceived threat to self-concept

Defensive **Coping** r/t difficulty with relationships, inability to accept blame for own behavior

Disturbed **Thought** process r/t poor reality testing

Impaired **Judgment** r/t intense emotional state

Ineffective **Coping** r/t use of maladjusted defense mechanisms (e.g., projection, denial)

Ineffective family **Therapeutic** regimen management r/t manipulative behavior of client

Powerlessness r/t lifestyle of helplessness

Risk for **Caregiver** role strain r/t inability of care receiver to accept criticism, care receiver taking advantage of others to meet own needs or having unreasonable expectations

Risk for self-directed **Violence** r/t feelings of need to punish self, manipulative behavior

Risk for **Self-mutilation** r/t ineffective coping, feelings of self-hatred

Risk for **Spiritual** distress r/t poor relationships associated with behaviors attributed to borderline personality disorder

Social isolation r/t immature interests

Boredom

Deficient **Diversional** activity r/t environmental lack of diversional activity

Social isolation r/t altered state of wellness

Botulism

Deficient **Fluid** volume r/t profuse diarrhea

Ineffective **Health** maintenance r/t deficient knowledge regarding prevention of botulism, care following episode

Bowel Incontinence

Bowel incontinence r/t decreased awareness of need to defecate, loss of sphincter control, fecal impaction

Bowel Obstruction

Constipation r/t decreased motility, intestinal obstruction

Deficient **Fluid** volume r/t inadequate fluid volume intake, fluid loss in bowel

Imbalanced **Nutrition**: less than body requirements r/t nausea, vomiting

Pain r/t pressure from distended abdomen

Bowel Resection

See Abdominal Surgery

Bowel Sounds, Absent or Diminished

Constipation r/t decreased or absent peristalsis

Deficient **Fluid** volume r/t inability to ingest fluids, loss of fluids in bowel

Delayed **Surgical** recovery r/t inability to obtain adequate nutritional status

Bowel Sounds, Hyperactive

Diarrhea r/t increased gastrointestinal motility

Bowel Training

Bowel incontinence r/t loss of control of rectal sphincter

Ineffective **Health** maintenance r/t deficient knowledge regarding treatment of bowel incontinence

BPH (Benign Prostatic Hypertrophy)

Disturbed **Sleep** pattern r/t nocturia

Ineffective **Health** maintenance r/t deficient knowledge regarding self-care with prostatic hypertrophy

Risk for **Infection** r/t urinary residual postvoiding, bacterial invasion of bladder

Risk for urge urinary **Incontinence** r/t detrusor muscle instability with impaired contractility, involuntary sphincter relaxation

Urinary retention r/t obstruction

Bradycardia

Decreased **Cardiac** output r/t slow heart rate supplying inadequate amount of blood for body function

Ineffective **Health** maintenance r/t deficient knowledge of condition, effects of cardiac medications

Ineffective **Tissue** perfusion: cerebral r/t decreased cardiac output secondary to bradycardia

Risk for **Injury** r/t decreased cerebral tissue perfusion

Bradypnea

Ineffective **Breathing** pattern r/t neuromuscular impairment, pain, musculoskeletal impairment, perception/cognitive impairment, anxiety, fatigue/decreased energy, effects of drugs

See cause of Bradypnea

Brain Injury

See Intracranial Pressure, Increased

Brain Surgery

See Craniectomy/Craniotomy

Brain Tumor

Acute **Pain** r/t pressure from tumor

Anticipatory **Grieving** r/t potential loss of physiosocial-psychosocial well-being

Decreased **Intracranial** adaptive capacity r/t presence of brain tumor

Disturbed **Sensory** perception: specify r/t tumor growth compressing brain tissue

Disturbed **Thought** processes r/t altered circulation, destruction of brain tissue

Fear r/t threat to well-being

Risk for **Injury** r/t sensory-perceptual alterations, weakness

See Cancer; Chemotherapy; Child with Chronic Condition; Craniectomy/Craniotomy; Hospitalized Child; Radiation Therapy; Terminally Ill Child

Braxton Hicks Contractions

Activity intolerance r/t increased perception of contractions with increased gestation

Anxiety r/t uncertainty about beginning labor

Disturbed **Sleep** pattern r/t contractions when lying down

Fatigue r/t lack of sleep

Ineffective **Sexuality** patterns r/t fear of contractions

Stress urinary **Incontinence** r/t increased pressure on bladder with contractions

Breast Biopsy

Fear r/t potential for diagnosis of cancer

Ineffective **Health** maintenance r/t deficient knowledge regarding appropriate postoperative care of breasts

Risk for **Spiritual** distress r/t fear of diagnosis of cancer

Breast Cancer

Chronic **Sorrow** r/t diagnosis of cancer, loss of body integrity

Death **Anxiety** r/t diagnosis of cancer

Fear r/t diagnosis of cancer

Ineffective **Coping** r/t treatment, prognosis

Risk for **Spiritual** distress r/t fear of diagnosis of cancer

Sexual dysfunction r/t loss of body part, partner's reaction to loss

See Cancer; Chemotherapy; Mastectomy; Radiation

Breast Lumps

Fear r/t potential for diagnosis of cancer

Ineffective **Health** maintenance r/t deficient knowledge regarding appropriate care of breasts

Breast Pumping

Anxiety r/t interrupted breastfeeding

Decisional **Conflict** r/t infant feeding method

Disturbed **Body** image r/t individual response to breastfeeding process

Ineffective **Health** maintenance r/t deficient knowledge regarding breast milk expression and storage

Risk for impaired **Skin** integrity r/t high suction

Risk for **Infection** r/t contaminated breast pump parts, incomplete emptying of breast

Breastfeeding, Effective

Effective **Breastfeeding** r/t basic breastfeeding knowledge, normal breast structure, normal infant oral structure, infant gestational age >34 weeks, support sources, maternal confidence

Breastfeeding, Ineffective

Impaired **Swallowing** r/t prematurity of infant

Ineffective **Breastfeeding** r/t prematurity, infant anomaly, maternal breast anomaly, previous breast surgery, previous history of breastfeeding failure, infant receiving supplemental feedings with artificial nipple, poor infant sucking reflex, nonsupportive partner/family, deficient knowledge, interruption in breastfeeding, maternal anxiety or ambivalence

Ineffective **Infant** feeding pattern r/t prematurity of infant

See Painful Breasts—Sore Nipples; Painful Breasts—Engorgement

Breastfeeding, Interrupted

Interrupted **Breastfeeding** r/t maternal or infant illness, prematurity, maternal employment, contraindications to breastfeeding (e.g., drugs, true breast milk jaundice), need to abruptly wean infant

Breath Sounds, Decreased or Absent

See Atelectasis; Pneumothorax

Breathing Pattern Alteration

Ineffective **Breathing** pattern r/t neuromuscular impairment, pain, musculoskeletal impairment, perception/cognitive impairment, anxiety, decreased energy/fatigue

Breech Birth

Anxiety: maternal r/t threat to self, infant

Fear: maternal r/t danger to infant, self

Impaired **Gas** exchange: fetal r/t compressed umbilical cord

Ineffective cerebral **Tissue** perfusion r/t compressed umbilical cord

Risk for **Aspiration**: fetal r/t birth of body before head

Risk for delayed **Development** r/t compressed umbilical cord

Risk for impaired **Tissue** integrity: fetal r/t difficult birth

Risk for impaired **Tissue** integrity: maternal r/t difficult birth

Bronchitis

Anxiety r/t potential chronic condition

Health-seeking behavior r/t wish to stop smoking

Ineffective **Airway** clearance r/t excessive thickened mucus secretion

Ineffective **Health** maintenance r/t deficient knowledge regarding care of condition

Bronchopulmonary Dysplasia

Activity intolerance r/t imbalance between oxygen supply and demand

Excess **Fluid** volume r/t sodium and water retention

Imbalanced **Nutrition**: less than body requirements r/t poor feeding, increased caloric needs secondary to increased work of breathing

See Child with Chronic Condition; Hospitalized Child; Respiratory Conditions of the Neonate

Bronchoscopy

Risk for **Aspiration** r/t temporary loss of gag reflex

Risk for **Injury** r/t complication of pneumothorax, laryngeal edema, hemorrhage (if biopsy done)

Bruits, Carotid

Ineffective **Tissue** perfusion: cerebral r/t interruption of carotid blood flow

Risk for **Injury** r/t loss of motor, sensory, visual function

Bryant's Traction

See Traction and Casts

Buck's Traction

See Traction and Casts

Buerger's Disease

See Peripheral Vascular Disease

Bulimia

Chronic low **Self-esteem** r/t lack of positive feedback

Defensive **Coping** r/t eating disorder

Disturbance in **Body** image r/t misperception about actual appearance, body weight

Fear r/t food ingestion, weight gain

Imbalanced **Nutrition**: less than body requirements r/t induced vomiting

Ineffective family **Coping** r/t chronically unresolved feelings of guilt, anger, hostility

Noncompliance r/t negative feelings toward treatment regimen

Powerlessness r/t urge to purge self after eating

See Maturational Issues, Adolescent

Bunion

Ineffective **Health** maintenance r/t deficient knowledge regarding appropriate care of feet

Bunionectomy

Impaired physical **Mobility** r/t sore foot

Impaired **Walking** r/t pain associated with surgery

Ineffective **Health** maintenance r/t deficient knowledge regarding postoperative care of feet

Risk for **Infection** r/t surgical incision, advanced age

Burns

Anticipatory **Grieving** r/t loss of bodily function, loss of future hopes and plans

Anxiety/Fear r/t pain from treatments, possible permanent disfigurement

Deficient **Diversional** activity r/t long-term hospitalization

Delayed **Surgical** recovery r/t ineffective tissue perfusion

Disturbed **Body** image r/t altered physical appearance

Hypothermia r/t impaired skin integrity

Imbalanced **Nutrition**: less than body requirements r/t increased metabolic needs, anorexia, protein and fluid loss

Impaired physical **Mobility** r/t pain, musculoskeletal impairment, contracture formation

Impaired **Skin** integrity r/t injury of skin

Ineffective **Tissue** perfusion: peripheral r/t circumferential burns, impaired arterial/venous circulation

Pain r/t injury, treatments

Post-trauma response r/t life-threatening event

Risk for deficient **Fluid** volume r/t loss from skin surface, fluid shift

Risk for ineffective **Airway** clearance r/t potential tracheobronchial obstruction, edema

Risk for **Infection** r/t loss of intact skin, trauma, invasive sites

Risk for **Peripheral** neurovascular dysfunction r/t eschar formation with circumferential burn

Risk for **Post-trauma** syndrome r/t perception, duration of event that caused burns

See Hospitalized Child; Safety, Childhood

Bursitis

Impaired physical **Mobility** r/t inflammation in joint

Pain r/t inflammation in joint

Bypass Graft

See Coronary Artery Bypass Grafting

Cachexia

Adult **Failure** to thrive r/t imbalanced nutrition: less than body requirements

Imbalanced **Nutrition**: less than body requirements r/t inability to ingest food because of biological factors

Ineffective **Protection** r/t inadequate nutrition

Calcium Alteration

See Hypercalcemia; Hypocalcemia

Cancer

Activity intolerance r/t side effects of treatment, weakness from cancer

Anticipatory **Grieving** r/t potential loss of significant others, high risk for infertility

Chronic **Pain** r/t metastatic cancer

Chronic **Sorrow** r/t chronic illness of cancer

Compromised family **Coping** r/t prolonged disease or disability progression that exhausts supportive ability of significant others

Constipation r/t side effects of medication, altered nutrition, decreased activity

Death **Anxiety** r/t unresolved issues regarding dying

Decisional **Conflict** r/t selection of treatment choices, continuation/discontinuation of treatment, "do not resuscitate" decision

Disturbed **Body** image r/t side effects of treatment, cachexia

Disturbed **Sleep** pattern r/t anxiety, pain

Fear r/t serious threat to well-being

Hopelessness r/t loss of control, terminal illness

Imbalanced **Nutrition**: less than body requirements r/t loss of appetite, difficulty swallowing, side effects of chemotherapy, obstruction by tumor

Impaired physical **Mobility** r/t weakness, neuromusculoskeletal impairment, pain

Impaired **Skin** integrity r/t immunological deficit, immobility

Impaired **Oral** mucous membranes r/t chemotherapy, oral pH changes, decreased/altered oral flora

Ineffective **Coping** r/t personal vulnerability in situational crisis, terminal illness

Ineffective **Denial** r/t dysfunctional grieving process

Ineffective **Health** maintenance r/t deficient knowledge regarding prescribed treatment

Ineffective **Protection** r/t cancer suppressing immune system

Ineffective **Role** performance r/t change in physical capacity, inability to resume prior role

Powerlessness r/t treatment, progression of disease

Readiness for enhanced **Spiritual** well-being r/t desire for harmony with self, others, higher power/God when faced with serious illness

Risk for **Disuse** syndrome r/t severe pain, change in level of consciousness

Risk for impaired **Home** maintenance r/t lack of familiarity with community resources

Risk for **Infection** r/t inadequate immune system

Risk for **Injury** r/t bleeding secondary to bone marrow depression

Risk for **Spiritual** distress r/t physical illness of cancer

Self-care deficit: specify r/t pain, intolerance to activity, decreased strength

Social isolation r/t hospitalization, lifestyle changes

Spiritual distress r/t test of spiritual beliefs

See Chemotherapy; Child with Chronic Condition; Hospitalized Child; Terminally Ill Child

Candidiasis, Oral

Impaired **Oral** mucous membranes r/t overgrowth of infectious agent, depressed immune function

Ineffective **Health** maintenance r/t deficient knowledge regarding care of infected mouth

Capillary Refill Time, Prolonged

Impaired **Gas** exchange r/t ventilation perfusion imbalance

Ineffective **Tissue** perfusion: peripheral r/t interruption of arterial or venous flow

Risk for **Peripheral** neurovascular dysfunction r/t vascular obstruction

See Shock

Cardiac Arrest

Post-Trauma stress response r/t sustaining serious life event

See cause of Cardiac Arrest

Cardiac Catheterization

Anxiety/fear r/t invasive procedure, uncertainty of outcome of procedure

Impaired **Comfort** r/t postprocedure restrictions, invasive procedure

Ineffective **Health** maintenance r/t deficient knowledge regarding procedure, postprocedure care, treatment and prevention of coronary artery disease

Risk for decreased **Cardiac** output r/t ventricular ischemia, dysrhythmia

Risk for ineffective **Tissue** perfusion r/t impaired arterial or venous circulation

Risk for **Injury**: hematoma r/t invasive procedure

Risk for **Peripheral** neurovascular dysfunction r/t vascular obstruction

Cardiac Disorders

Decreased **Cardiac** output r/t cardiac disorder

See specific disorder

Cardiac Disorders in Pregnancy

Activity intolerance r/t cardiac pathophysiology, increased demand secondary to pregnancy, weakness, fatigue

Anxiety r/t unknown outcomes of pregnancy, family well-being

Compromised family **Coping** r/t prolonged hospitalization/maternal incapacitation that exhausts supportive capacity of significant others

Death **Anxiety** r/t potential danger of condition

Fatigue r/t metabolic demands, psychological-emotional demands

Fear r/t potential maternal effects, potential poor fetal/maternal outcome

Ineffective **Coping** r/t personal vulnerability

Ineffective **Health** maintenance r/t deficient knowledge regarding treatment, restrictions with cardiac disorder

Ineffective **Role** performance r/t changes in lifestyle, expectations secondary to disease process with superimposed pregnancy

Interrupted **Family** processes r/t hospitalization, maternal incapacitation, changes in role

Powerlessness r/t illness-related regimen

Risk for delayed **Development** r/t poor maternal oxygenation

Risk for disproportionate **Growth** r/t poor maternal oxygenation

Risk for excess **Fluid** volume r/t compromised regulatory mechanism with increased afterload, preload, circulating blood volume

Risk for imbalanced **Fluid** volume r/t sudden changes in circulation following delivery of placenta

Risk for impaired **Gas** exchange r/t pulmonary edema

Risk for ineffective fetal **Tissue** perfusion r/t poor maternal oxygenation

Risk for **Spiritual** distress r/t fear of diagnosis for self and infant

Situational low **Self-esteem** r/t situational crisis, pregnancy

Social isolation r/t limitations of activity, bedrest/hospitalization, separation from family and friends

Cardiac Dysrhythmia

See Dysrhythmia

Cardiac Output Decrease

Decreased **Cardiac** output r/t cardiac dysfunction

Cardiac Tamponade

Decreased **Cardiac** output r/t fluid in pericardial sac

See Pericarditis

Cardiogenic Shock

Decreased **Cardiac** output r/t decreased myocardial contractility, dysrhythmia

See Shock

Caregiver Role Strain

Caregiver role strain r/t pathophysiological factors, developmental factors, psychosocial factors, situational factors

Risk for **Caregiver** role strain r/t pathophysiological factors, developmental factors, psychosocial factors, situational factors

Carious Teeth

See Cavities in Teeth

Carotid Endarterectomy

Fear r/t surgery in vital area

Ineffective **Health** maintenance r/t deficient knowledge regarding postoperative care

Risk for ineffective **Airway** clearance r/t hematoma compressing trachea

Risk for ineffective **Tissue** perfusion: cerebral r/t hemorrhage, clot formation

Risk for **Injury** r/t possible hematoma formation

Carpal Tunnel Syndrome

Impaired physical **Mobility** r/t neuromuscular impairment

Pain r/t unrelieved pressure on median nerve

Self-care deficit: bathing/hygiene, dressing/grooming, feeding r/t pain

Carpopedal Spasm

See Hypocalcemia

Casts

Deficient **Diversional** activity r/t physical limitations from cast

Ineffective **Health** maintenance r/t deficient knowledge regarding cast care, personal care with cast

Impaired physical **Mobility** r/t limb immobilization

Impaired **Walking** r/t cast(s) on lower extremities, fracture of bones

Risk for impaired **Skin** integrity r/t unrelieved pressure on skin

Risk for **Peripheral** neurovascular dysfunction r/t mechanical compression from cast

Self-care deficit: bathing/hygiene, dressing/grooming, feeding r/t presence of cast(s) on upper extremities

Self-care deficit: toileting r/t presence of cast(s) on lower extremities

Cataract Extraction

Anxiety r/t threat of permanent vision loss, surgical procedure

Disturbed **Sensory** perception: vision r/t edema from surgery

Ineffective **Health** maintenance r/t deficient knowledge regarding postoperative restrictions

Risk for **Injury** r/t increased intraocular pressure, accommodation to new visual field

See Vision Impairment

Cataracts

Disturbed **Sensory** perception: vision r/t altered sensory input

See Vision Impairment

Catatonic Schizophrenia

Imbalanced **Nutrition**: less than body requirements r/t decrease in outside stimulation, loss of perception of hunger, resistance to instructions to eat

Impaired **Memory** r/t cognitive impairment

Impaired physical **Mobility** r/t cognitive impairment, maintenance of rigid posture, inappropriate/bizarre postures

Impaired verbal **Communication** r/t muteness

Social isolation r/t inability to communicate, immobility

See Schizophrenia

Catheterization, Urinary

Ineffective **Health** maintenance r/t deficient knowledge of normal sensation of catheter in place, care of catheter

Risk for **Infection** r/t invasive procedure

Cavities in Teeth

Impaired **Dentition** r/t ineffective oral hygiene, barriers to self-care, economic barriers to professional care, nutritional deficits, dietary habits

Ineffective **Health** maintenance r/t lack of knowledge regarding prevention of dental disease secondary to high-sugar diet, giving infants/toddlers with erupted teeth bottles of milk at bedtime, lack of fluoride treatments, inadequate or improper brushing of teeth

Cellulitis

Impaired **Skin** integrity r/t inflammatory process damaging skin

Ineffective **Tissue** perfusion: peripheral r/t edema

Pain r/t inflammatory changes in tissues from infection

Cellulitis, Periorbital

Disturbed **Sensory** perception: visual r/t decreased visual fields secondary to edema of eyelids

Hyperthermia r/t infectious process

Impaired **Skin** integrity r/t inflammation/infection of skin/tissues

Pain r/t edema and inflammation of skin/tissues

See Hospitalized Child

Central Line Insertion

Ineffective **Health** maintenance r/t deficient knowledge regarding precautions to take when central line in place

Risk for **Infection** r/t invasive procedure

Cerebral Aneurysm

See Craniectomy/Craniotomy; Intracranial Pressure, Increased; Subarachnoid Hemorrhage

C

Cerebral Palsy

Chronic **Sorrow** r/t presence of chronic disability

Deficient **Diversional** activity r/t physical impairments, limitations on ability to participate in recreational activities

Imbalanced **Nutrition**: less than body requirements r/t spasticity, feeding or swallowing difficulties

Impaired physical **Mobility** r/t spasticity, neuromuscular impairment/weakness

Impaired **Social** interaction r/t impaired communication skills, limited physical activity, perceived differences from peers

Impaired verbal **Communication** r/t impaired ability to articulate/speak words secondary to facial muscle involvement

Risk for delayed **Development** r/t chronic illness

Risk for disproportionate **Growth** r/t chronic illness

Risk for **Falls** r/t impaired physical mobility

Risk for impaired **Parenting** r/t caring for child with overwhelming needs resulting from chronic change in health status

Risk for **Injury/Trauma** r/t muscle weakness, inability to control spasticity

Risk for **Spiritual** distress r/t psychic and psychological stress associated with chronic illness

Self-care deficit: specify r/t neuromuscular impairments, sensory deficits

See Child with Chronic Condition

Cerebrovascular Accident

See CVA

Cervicitis

Ineffective **Health** maintenance r/t deficient knowledge regarding care and prevention of condition

Ineffective **Sexuality** pattern r/t abstinence during acute stage

Risk for **Infection** r/t spread of infection, recurrence of infection

Cesarean Delivery

Anxiety r/t unmet expectations for childbirth, unknown outcome of surgery

Disturbed **Body** image r/t surgery, unmet expectations for childbirth

Fear r/t perceived threat to own well-being

Impaired **Comfort**: nausea, vomiting, pruritus r/t side effects of systemic or epidural narcotics

Impaired physical **Mobility** r/t pain

Ineffective **Health** maintenance r/t deficient knowledge regarding postoperative care

Ineffective **Role** performance r/t unmet expectations for childbirth

Interrupted **Family** processes r/t unmet expectations for childbirth

Pain r/t surgical incision, decreased or absent peristalsis secondary to anesthesia, manipulation of abdominal organs during surgery, immobilization, restricted diet

Risk for **Aspiration** r/t positioning for general anesthesia

Risk for deficient **Fluid** volume r/t increased blood loss secondary to surgery

Risk for imbalanced **Fluid** volume r/t loss of blood

Risk for **Infection** r/t surgical incision, stasis of respiratory secretions secondary to general anesthesia

Risk for **Post-trauma** syndrome r/t emergency condition to save life of mother or baby

Risk for **Urinary** retention r/t regional anesthesia

Situational low **Self-esteem** r/t inability to deliver child vaginally

Chemical Dependence

See Alcoholism; Drug Abuse

Chemotherapy

Death **Anxiety** r/t chemotherapy not accomplishing desired results

Delayed **Surgical** recovery r/t compromised immune system

Disturbed **Body** image r/t loss of weight, loss of hair

Fatigue r/t disease process, anemia, drug effects

Imbalanced **Nutrition**: less than body requirements r/t side effects of chemotherapy

Impaired **Oral** mucous membranes r/t effects of chemotherapy

Ineffective **Health** maintenance r/t deficient knowledge regarding action, side effects, way to integrate chemotherapy into lifestyle

Ineffective **Protection** r/t suppressed immune system, decreased platelets

Nausea r/t effects of chemotherapy

Risk for deficient **Fluid** volume r/t vomiting, diarrhea

Risk for ineffective **Tissue** perfusion r/t anemia

Risk for **Infection** r/t immunosuppression

See Cancer

Chest Pain

Fear r/t potential threat of death

Pain r/t myocardial injury, ischemia

Risk for decreased **Cardiac** output r/t ventricular ischemia

See Angina Pectoris; MI

Chest Tubes

Impaired **Gas** exchange r/t decreased functional lung tissue

Ineffective **Breathing** pattern r/t asymmetrical lung expansion secondary to pain

Pain r/t presence of chest tubes, injury

Risk for **Injury** r/t presence of invasive chest tube

Cheyne-Stokes Respiration

Ineffective **Breathing** pattern r/t critical illness

See cause of Cheyne-Stokes Respiration

CHF (Congestive Heart Failure)

Activity intolerance r/t weakness, fatigue

Constipation r/t activity intolerance

Decreased **Cardiac** output r/t impaired cardiac function

Excess **Fluid** volume r/t impaired excretion of sodium and water

Fatigue r/t disease process

Fear r/t threat to one's own well-being

Impaired **Gas** exchange r/t excessive fluid in interstitial space of lungs, alveoli

Ineffective **Health** maintenance r/t deficient knowledge regarding care of disease

Powerlessness r/t illness-related regimen

See Child with Chronic Condition; Congenital Heart Disease/Cardiac Anomalies; Hospitalized Child

Chickenpox

See Communicable Diseases, Childhood

Child Abuse

Anxiety/fear r/t threat of punishment for perceived wrongdoing

Chronic low **Self-esteem** r/t lack of positive feedback, excessive negative feedback

Deficient **Diversional** activity r/t diminished or absent environmental/personal stimuli

Delayed **Growth** and development: regression vs. delayed r/t diminished/absent environmental stimuli, inadequate caretaking, inconsistent responsiveness by caretaker

Disturbed **Sleep** pattern r/t hypervigilance, anxiety

Imbalanced **Nutrition**: less than body requirements r/t inadequate caretaking

Impaired **Parenting** r/t psychological impairment, physical or emotional abuse of parent, substance abuse, unrealistic expectations of child

Impaired **Skin** integrity r/t altered nutritional state, physical abuse

Ineffective community **Therapeutic** regimen management r/t deficits in community regarding prevention of child abuse

Interrupted **Family** process: alcoholism r/t inadequate coping skills

Pain r/t physical injuries

Post-trauma response r/t physical abuse, incest, rape, molestation

Risk for delayed **Development** r/t shaken baby, abuse

Risk for disproportionate **Growth** r/t abuse

Risk for **Poisoning** r/t inadequate safeguards, lack of proper safety precautions, accessibility of illicit substances secondary to impaired home maintenance

Risk for **Suffocation**/aspiration r/t propped bottle, unattended child

Risk for **Trauma** r/t inadequate precautions, cognitive or emotional difficulties

Social isolation: family imposed r/t fear of disclosure of family dysfunction and abuse

Child Neglect

See Child Abuse; Failure to Thrive

Child with Chronic Condition

Activity intolerance r/t fatigue associated with chronic illness

Chronic low **Self-esteem** r/t actual or perceived differences; peer acceptance; decreased ability to participate in physical, school, and social activities

Chronic **Pain** r/t physical, biological, chemical, or psychological factors

Chronic **Sorrow** r/t developmental stages and missed opportunities or milestones that bring comparisons with social or personal norms, unending caregiving as reminder of loss

Compromised family **Coping** r/t prolonged overconcern for child; distortion of reality regarding child's health problem, including extreme denial about its existence or severity

Decisional **Conflict** r/t treatment options, conflicting values

Deficient **Diversional** activity r/t immobility, monotonous environment, frequent/lengthy treatments, reluctance to participate, self-imposed social isolation

C

Deficient **Knowledge**: readiness for enhanced **Health** maintenance r/t knowledge/skill acquisition regarding health practices, acceptance of limitations, promotion of maximal potential of child, self-actualization of rest of family

Delayed **Growth** and development r/t regression or lack of progression toward developmental milestones secondary to frequent or prolonged hospitalization, inadequate or inappropriate stimulation, cerebral insult, chronic illness, effects of physical disability, prescribed dependence

Disabled family **Coping** r/t prolonged disease or disability progression that exhausts supportive capacity of significant people

Disturbed **Sleep** pattern: child or parent r/t time-intensive treatments, exacerbation of condition, 24-hour care needs

Hopelessness: child r/t prolonged activity restriction, long-term stress, lack of involvement in or passively allowing care secondary to parental overprotection

Imbalanced **Nutrition**: less than body requirements r/t anorexia, fatigue secondary to physical exertion

Imbalanced **Nutrition**: more than body requirements r/t effects of steroid medications on appetite

Impaired **Home** maintenance r/t overtaxed family members (e.g., exhausted, anxious)

Impaired **Social** interaction r/t developmental lag/delay, perceived differences

Ineffective **Coping**: child r/t situational or maturational crises

Ineffective **Health** maintenance r/t exhausting family resources (finances, physical energy, support systems)

Ineffective **Sexuality** patterns: parental r/t disrupted relationship with sexual partner

Interrupted **Family** processes r/t intermittent situational crisis of illness, disease, hospitalization

Parental role **Conflict** r/t separation from child as a result of chronic illness, home care of child with special needs, interruptions of family life resulting from home care regimen

Powerlessness: child r/t health care environment, illness-related regimen, lifestyle of learned helplessness

Readiness for enhanced family **Coping** r/t impact of crisis on family values, priorities, goals, or relationships; changes in family choices to optimize wellness

Risk for delayed **Development** r/t chronic illness

Risk for disproportionate **Growth** r/t chronic illness

Risk for impaired **Parenting** r/t impaired/disrupted bonding, caring for child with perceived overwhelming care needs

Risk for **Infection** r/t debilitating physical condition

Risk for **Noncompliance** r/t complex or prolonged home care regimens; expressed intent to not comply secondary to value systems, health beliefs, cultural/religious practices

Social isolation: family r/t actual or perceived social stigmatization, complex care requirements

Childbirth

See Labor—Normal; Postpartum, Normal Care

Chills

Hyperthermia r/t infectious process

Chlamydia Infection

See STD

Choking/Coughing with Feeding

Impaired **Swallowing** r/t neuromuscular impairment

Risk for **Aspiration** r/t depressed cough and gag reflexes

Cholasma

Disturbed **Body** image r/t change in skin color

Cholecystectomy

Imbalanced **Nutrition**: less than body requirements r/t high metabolic needs, decreased ability to digest fatty foods

Ineffective **Health** maintenance r/t deficient knowledge regarding postoperative care

Pain r/t recent surgery

Risk for deficient **Fluid** volume r/t restricted intake, nausea, vomiting

Risk for ineffective **Breathing** pattern r/t proximity of incision to lungs resulting in pain with deep breathing

See Abdominal Surgery

Cholelithiasis

Imbalanced **Nutrition**: less than body requirements r/t anorexia, nausea, vomiting

Ineffective **Health** maintenance r/t deficient knowledge regarding care of disease

Pain r/t obstruction of bile flow, inflammation in gallbladder

Chorioamnionitis

Anticipatory **Grieving** r/t guilt about potential loss of ideal pregnancy and birth

Anxiety r/t threat to self and infant

Hyperthermia r/t infectious process

Risk for delayed **Growth** and development r/t risk of preterm birth

Risk for **Infection** transmission from mother to fetus r/t infection in fetal environment

Situational low **Self-esteem** r/t guilt about threat to infant's health

Chronic Lymphocytic Leukemia

See Leukemia

Chronic Obstructive Pulmonary Disease

See COPD

Chronic Pain

See Pain, Chronic

Chronic Renal Failure

See Renal Failure

Chvostek's Sign

See Hypocalcemia

Circumcision

Ineffective **Health** maintenance r/t deficient knowledge (parental) regarding care of surgical area

Pain r/t surgical intervention

Risk for deficient **Fluid** volume r/t hemorrhage

Risk for **Infection** r/t surgical wound

Cirrhosis

Chronic low **Self-esteem** r/t chronic illness

Chronic **Pain** r/t liver enlargement

Chronic **Sorrow** r/t presence of chronic illness

Diarrhea r/t dietary changes, medications

Disturbed **Thought** processes r/t chronic organic disorder with increased ammonia levels, substance abuse

Fatigue r/t malnutrition

Imbalanced **Nutrition**: less than body requirements r/t loss of appetite, nausea, vomiting

Ineffective **Health** maintenance r/t deficient knowledge regarding correlation between lifestyle habits and disease process

Ineffective management of **Therapeutic** regimen r/t denial of severity of illness

Ineffective **Protection** r/t risk of impaired blood coagulation, bleeding from portal hypertension

Nausea r/t irritation to gastrointestinal system

Risk for deficient **Fluid** volume: hemorrhage r/t abnormal bleeding from esophagus

Risk for impaired **Oral** mucous membranes r/t altered nutrition

Risk for impaired **Skin** integrity r/t altered nutritional state, altered metabolic state

Risk for **Injury** r/t substance intoxication, potential delirium tremors

Cleft Lip/Cleft Palate

Chronic **Sorrow** r/t loss of perfect child, birth of child with congenital defect

Fear: parental r/t special care needs, surgery

Grieving r/t loss of perfect child, birth of child with congenital defect

Imbalanced **Nutrition**: less than body requirements r/t inability to feed with normal techniques

Impaired **Oral** mucous membranes r/t surgical correction

Impaired physical **Mobility** r/t imposed restricted activity, use of elbow restraints

Impaired **Skin** integrity r/t incomplete joining of lip, palate ridges

Impaired verbal **Communication** r/t inadequate palate function, possible hearing loss from infected eustachian tubes

Ineffective **Airway** clearance r/t common feeding and breathing passage, postoperative laryngeal, incisional edema

Ineffective **Breastfeeding** r/t infant anomaly

Ineffective **Health** maintenance r/t lack of parental knowledge regarding feeding techniques, wound care, use of elbow restraints

Ineffective **Infant** feeding pattern r/t cleft lip, cleft palate

Pain r/t surgical correction, elbow restraints

Risk for **Aspiration** r/t common feeding and breathing passage

Risk for deficient **Fluid** volume r/t inability to take liquids in usual manner

Risk for delayed **Development** r/t inadequate nutrition resulting from difficulty feeding

Risk for disproportionate **Growth** r/t inability to feed with normal techniques

Risk for disturbed **Body** image r/t disfigurement, speech impediment

Risk for **Infection** r/t invasive procedure, disruption of eustachian tube development, aspiration

Clotting Disorder

Anxiety/Fear r/t threat to well-being

Ineffective **Health** maintenance r/t deficient knowledge regarding treatment of disorder

Ineffective **Protection** r/t clotting disorder

Risk for deficient **Fluid** volume r/t uncontrolled bleeding

See Anticoagulant Therapy; DIC; Hemophilia

C

Coarctation of Aorta

See Congenital Heart Disease/Cardiac Anomalies

Cocaine Abuse

Disturbed **Thought** processes r/t excessive stimulation of nervous system by cocaine

Ineffective **Breathing** pattern r/t drug effect on respiratory center

Ineffective **Coping** r/t inability to deal with life stresses

See Substance Abuse

Cocaine Baby

See Crack Baby

Codependency

Caregiver role strain r/t codependency

Decisional **Conflict** r/t support system deficit

Denial r/t unmet self-needs

Impaired verbal **Communication** r/t psychological barriers

Ineffective **Coping** r/t inadequate support systems

Powerlessness r/t lifestyle of helplessness

Cognitive Deficit

Disturbed **Thought** processes r/t neurological impairment

Cold, Viral

Impaired **Comfort**: sore throat, aching, nasal discomfort r/t viral infection

Ineffective **Health** maintenance r/t deficient knowledge regarding care of viral condition, prevention of further infections

Colectomy

Constipation r/t decreased activity, decreased fluid intake

Imbalanced **Nutrition**: less than body requirements r/t high metabolic needs, decreased ability to ingest/digest food

Ineffective **Health** maintenance r/t deficient knowledge regarding procedure, postoperative care

Pain r/t recent surgery

Risk for **Infection** r/t invasive procedure

See Abdominal Surgery

Colitis

Deficient **Fluid** volume r/t frequent stools

Diarrhea r/t inflammation in colon

Pain r/t inflammation in colon

See Crohn's Disease; Inflammatory Bowel Syndrome; Ulcerative Colitis

Collagen Disease

See specific disease (e.g., Lupus Erythematosus; Rheumatoid Arthritis, Juvenile)

Colostomy

Disturbed **Body** image r/t presence of stoma, daily care of fecal material

Ineffective **Health** maintenance r/t deficient knowledge regarding care of stoma, integrating colostomy care into lifestyle

Risk for altered **Sexuality** pattern r/t altered body image, self-concept

Risk for **Constipation/Diarrhea** r/t inappropriate diet

Risk for impaired **Skin** integrity r/t irritation from bowel contents

Risk for **Social** isolation r/t anxiety about appearance of stoma and possible leakage

Colporrhaphy, Anterior

See Vaginal Hysterectomy

Coma

Death **Anxiety**: significant others r/t unknown outcome of coma state

Disturbed **Thought** processes r/t neurological changes

Ineffective family **Therapeutic** regimen management r/t complexity of therapeutic regimen

Interrupted **Family** processes r/t illness/disability of family member

Risk for **Aspiration** r/t impaired swallowing, loss of cough/gag reflex

Risk for **Disuse** syndrome r/t altered level of consciousness impairing mobility

Risk for impaired **Oral** mucous membranes r/t dry mouth

Risk for impaired **Skin** integrity r/t immobility

Risk for **Injury** r/t potential seizure activity

Risk for **Spiritual** distress: significant others r/t loss of ability to relate to loved one, unknown outcome of coma

Self-care deficit: specify r/t neuromuscular impairment

Total urinary **Incontinence** r/t neurological dysfunction

See cause of Coma

Comfort, Loss of

Impaired **Comfort** r/t injury agent

Communicable Diseases, Childhood (Measles, Mumps, Rubella, Chickenpox, Scabies, Lice, Impetigo)

Deficient **Diversional** activity r/t imposed isolation from peers, disruption in usual play activities, fatigue, activity intolerance

Impaired **Comfort** r/t hyperthermia secondary to infectious disease process, pruritus secondary to skin rash or subdermal organisms

Ineffective **Health** maintenance r/t nonadherence to appropriate immunization schedules, lack of prevention of transmission of infection

Pain r/t impaired skin integrity, edema

Risk for **Infection**: transmission to others r/t contagious organisms

See Meningitis/Encephalitis; Respiratory Infections, Acute Childhood; Reye's Syndrome

Communication

Readiness for enhanced **Communication** r/t expressed willingness to enhance communication; ability to speak or write a language; ability to form words, phrases, and language; ability to express thoughts and feelings; ability to use and interpret nonverbal cues appropriately; expression of satisfaction with ability to share information and ideas with others

Communication Problems

Impaired verbal **Communication** r/t decrease in circulation to brain, brain tumor, physical barrier (e.g., tracheostomy, intubation), anatomical defect, impaired hearing, cleft palate, psychological barriers (e.g., psychosis, lack of stimuli), cultural difference, developmentally related or age-related factors, side effects of medication, environmental barriers, absence of significant others, altered perceptions, lack of information, stress, alteration of self-esteem or self-concept, physiological conditions, alteration of central nervous system, weakening of musculoskeletal system, emotional conditions

Community Coping

Ineffective community **Coping** r/t natural or manmade disasters; ineffective or nonexistent community systems (e.g., lack of emergency medical, transportation, or disaster planning systems), deficits in community social support services and resources, inadequate resources for problem solving

Readiness for enhanced community **Coping** r/t community sense of power to manage stressors, social supports available, resources available for problem solving

Community Management of Therapeutic Regimen

Ineffective community **Therapeutic** regimen management r/t inadequate community resources

Compartment Syndrome

Fear r/t possible loss of limb, damage to limb

Ineffective **Tissue** perfusion: peripheral r/t increased pressure within compartment

Pain r/t pressure in compromised body part

Compulsion

See Obsessive-Compulsive Disorder

Conduction Disorders (Cardiac)

See Dysrhythmia

Confusion, Acute

Acute **Confusion** r/t >60 years of age, alcohol abuse, delirium, dementia, drug abuse

Adult **Failure** to thrive r/t confusion

Impaired **Memory** r/t fluid and electrolyte imbalance, neurological disturbances, excessive environmental disturbances, anemia, acute or chronic hypoxia, decreased cardiac output

Confusion, Chronic

Adult **Failure** to thrive r/t confusion

Chronic **Confusion** r/t Alzheimer's disease, Korsakoff's psychosis, multiinfarct dementia, cerebrovascular accident, head injury

Disturbed **Thought** processes r/t organic mental disorder, disruption of cerebral arterial blood flow, chemical imbalance, intoxication

Impaired **Memory** r/t fluid and electrolyte imbalance, neurological disturbances, excessive environmental disturbances, anemia, acute or chronic hypoxia, decreased cardiac output

Congenital Heart Disease/Cardiac Anomalies

ACYANOTIC

Patent ductus arteriosus, atrial/ventricular septal defect, pulmonary stenosis, endocardial cushion defect, aortic valvular stenosis, coarctation of aorta

CYANOTIC

Tetralogy of Fallot, tricuspid atresia, transposition of great vessels, truncus arteriosus, total anomalous pulmonary venous return, hypoplastic left lung

Activity intolerance r/t fatigue, generalized weakness, lack of adequate oxygenation

Decreased **Cardiac** output r/t cardiac dysfunction

C

Delayed **Growth** and development r/t inadequate oxygen and nutrients to tissues

Excess **Fluid** volume r/t cardiac defect, side effects of medication

Imbalanced **Nutrition**: less than body requirements r/t fatigue, generalized weakness, inability of infant to suck and feed, increased caloric requirements

Impaired **Gas** exchange r/t cardiac defect, pulmonary congestion

Ineffective **Breathing** pattern r/t pulmonary vascular disease

Interrupted **Family** processes r/t ill child

Risk for deficient **Fluid** volume r/t side effects of diuretics

Risk for delayed **Development** r/t inadequate oxygen and nutrients to tissues

Risk for disproportionate **Growth** r/t inadequate oxygen and nutrients to tissues

Risk for disorganized **Infant** behavior r/t invasive procedures

Risk for ineffective **Thermoregulation** r/t neonatal age

Risk for **Poisoning** r/t potential toxicity of cardiac medications

See Child with Chronic Illness; Hospitalized Child

Congestive Heart Failure

See CHF

Conjunctivitis

Disturbed **Sensory** perception r/t change in visual acuity resulting from inflammation

Pain r/t inflammatory process

Risk for **Injury** r/t change in visual acuity

Consciousness, Altered Level of

Acute **Confusion** r/t alcohol abuse, delirium, dementia, drug abuse

Adult **Failure** to thrive r/t altered level of consciousness

Chronic **Confusion** r/t multiinfarct dementia, Korsakoff's psychosis, head injury, Alzheimer's disease, cerebrovascular accident

Decreased **Intracranial** adaptive capacity r/t brain injury

Disturbed **Thought** processes r/t neurological changes

Impaired **Memory** r/t neurological disturbances

Ineffective **Tissue** perfusion: cerebral r/t increased intracranial pressure, decreased cerebral perfusion

Risk for **Aspiration** r/t impaired swallowing, loss of cough/gag reflex

Risk for **Disuse** syndrome r/t impaired mobility resulting from altered level of consciousness

Risk for impaired **Oral** mucous membranes r/t dry mouth

Risk for impaired **Skin** integrity r/t immobility

Self-care deficit: specify r/t neuromuscular impairment

Total urinary **Incontinence** r/t neurological dysfunction

See cause of Altered Level of Consciousness

Constipation

Constipation r/t decreased fluid intake, decreased intake of foods containing bulk, inactivity, immobility, deficient knowledge of appropriate bowel routine, lack of privacy for defecation

Constipation, Perceived

Perceived **Constipation** r/t cultural or family health beliefs, faulty appraisal, impaired thought processes

Constipation, Risk for

Risk for **Constipation** r/t functional factors impeding defecation, inappropriate diet, psychological factors, physical factors, medications

Continent Ileostomy (Kock Pouch)

Imbalanced **Nutrition**: less than body requirements r/t malabsorption

Ineffective **Coping** r/t stress of disease, exacerbations caused by stress

Ineffective **Health** maintenance r/t deficient knowledge regarding postoperative care

Risk for **Injury** r/t failure of valve, stomal cyanosis, intestinal obstruction

See Abdominal Surgery

Contraceptive Method

Decisional **Conflict**: method of contraception r/t unclear personal values or beliefs, lack of experience or interference with decision-making, lack of relevant information, support system deficit

Health-seeking behavior r/t requesting information about available and appropriate birth control methods

Ineffective **Sexuality** patterns r/t fear of pregnancy

Conversion Disorder

Anxiety r/t unresolved conflict

Disturbed personal **Identity** r/t overwhelming stress

Hopelessness r/t long-term stress

Impaired **Adjustment** r/t multiple stressors

Impaired physical **Mobility** r/t physical conversion symptom

Impaired **Social** interaction r/t altered thought process

Ineffective **Coping** r/t personal vulnerability

Ineffective **Role** performance r/t physical conversion system

Powerlessness r/t lifestyle of helplessness

Risk for **Injury** r/t physical conversion symptom

Self-esteem disturbance r/t unsatisfactory or inadequate interpersonal relationships

Convulsions

Anxiety r/t concern over controlling convulsions

Impaired **Memory** r/t neurological disturbance

Ineffective **Health** maintenance r/t deficient knowledge regarding need for medication and care during seizure activity

Risk for **Aspiration** r/t impaired swallowing

Risk for delayed **Development** r/t seizures

Risk for disturbed **Thought** processes r/t seizure activity

Risk for **Injury** r/t seizure activity

See Seizure Disorders

COPD (Chronic Obstructive Pulmonary Disease)

Activity intolerance r/t imbalance between oxygen supply and demand

Altered **Family** process r/t role changes

Anxiety r/t breathlessness, change in health status

Chronic low **Self-esteem** r/t chronic illness

Chronic **Sorrow** r/t presence of chronic illness

Death **Anxiety** r/t seriousness of medical condition, difficulty being able to "catch breath," feeling of suffocation

Health-seeking behavior r/t wish to stop smoking

Imbalanced **Nutrition**: less than body requirements r/t decreased intake because of dyspnea, unpleasant taste in mouth left by medications

Impaired **Gas** exchange r/t ventilation-perfusion inequality

Impaired **Social** interaction r/t social isolation secondary to oxygen use, activity intolerance

Ineffective **Airway** clearance r/t bronchoconstriction, increased mucus, ineffective cough, infection

Ineffective **Health** maintenance r/t deficient knowledge regarding care of disease

Noncompliance r/t reluctance to accept responsibility for changing detrimental health practices

Powerlessness r/t progressive nature of disease

Risk for **Infection** r/t stasis of respiratory secretions

Self-care deficit: specify r/t fatigue secondary to increased work of breathing

Sleep deprivation r/t breathing difficulties when lying down

Coping

Readiness for enhanced **Coping** r/t defining stressors as manageable; seeking social support; using a broad range of problem-oriented and emotion-oriented strategies; using spiritual resources; acknowledging power; seeking knowledge of new strategies; being aware of possible environmental changes

Coping Problems

Defensive **Coping** r/t superior attitude toward others, difficulty establishing or maintaining relationships, hostile laughter or ridicule of others, difficulty in reality-testing perceptions, lack of follow-through or participation in treatment or therapy

Ineffective **Coping** r/t gender differences in coping strategies, inadequate level of confidence in ability to cope, uncertainty, inadequate social support created by characteristics of relationships, inadequate level of perception of control, inadequate resources available, high degree of threat, disturbance in pattern of tension release, inadequate opportunity to prepare for stressor, inability to conserve adaptive energies, disturbance in appraisal of threat

See Community Coping; Family Problems

Corneal Reflex, Absent

Risk for **Injury** r/t accidental corneal abrasion, drying of cornea

Coronary Artery Bypass Grafting

Decreased **Cardiac** output r/t dysrhythmia, depressed cardiac function, increased systemic vascular resistance

Deficient **Fluid** volume r/t intraoperative fluid loss, use of diuretics in surgery

Fear r/t outcome of surgical procedure

Ineffective **Health** maintenance r/t deficient knowledge regarding postprocedure care, lifestyle adjustment after surgery

Pain r/t traumatic surgery

Risk for perioperative positioning **Injury** r/t hypothermia, extended supine position

C

C

Costovertebral Angle Tenderness

See Kidney Stone; Pyelonephritis

Cough, Effective/Ineffective

Ineffective **Airway** clearance r/t decreased energy, fatigue, normal aging changes

See Bronchitis; COPD; Pulmonary Edema

Crack Abuse

See Cocaine Abuse

Crack Baby

Delayed **Growth** and development r/t effects of maternal use of drugs, neurological impairment, decreased attentiveness to environmental stimuli

Diarrhea r/t effects of withdrawal, increased peristalsis secondary to hyperirritability

Disorganized **Infant** behavior r/t prematurity, pain, lack of attachment

Disturbed **Sensory** perception: specify r/t hypersensitivity to environmental stimuli

Disturbed **Sleep** pattern r/t hyperirritability, hypersensitivity to environmental stimuli

Imbalanced **Nutrition**: less than body requirements r/t feeding problems; uncoordinated/ineffective suck and swallow; effects of diarrhea, vomiting, colic

Impaired **Parenting** r/t impaired/lack of attachment behaviors, inadequate support systems

Ineffective **Airway** clearance r/t pooling of secretions secondary to lack of adequate cough reflex

Ineffective **Infant** feeding r/t prematurity, neurological impairment

Ineffective **Protection** r/t effects of maternal substance abuse

Risk for delayed **Development** r/t substance abuse

Risk for disproportionate **Growth** r/t substance use/abuse

Risk for impaired parent-infant **Attachment** r/t parent's inability to meet infant's needs, substance abuse

Risk for **Infection** (skin, meningeal, respiratory) r/t effects of withdrawal

Crackles in Lungs, Coarse

Ineffective **Airway** clearance r/t excessive secretions in airways, ineffective cough

See cause of Coarse Crackles

Crackles in Lungs, Fine

Ineffective **Breathing** pattern r/t fatigue, surgery, decreased energy

See Bronchitis or Pneumonia (if from pulmonary infection); CHF (if cardiac in origin); Infection

Craniectomy/Craniotomy

Adult **Failure** to thrive r/t altered cerebral tissue perfusion

Decreased **Intracranial** adaptive capacity r/t brain injury, intracranial hypertension

Fear r/t threat to well-being

Impaired **Memory** r/t neurological surgery

Ineffective **Tissue** perfusion: cerebral r/t cerebral edema, decreased cerebral perfusion, increased intracranial pressure

Pain r/t recent surgery, headache

Risk for disturbed **Thought** processes r/t neurophysiological changes

Risk for **Injury** r/t potential confusion

See Coma (if relevant)

Crepitation, Subcutaneous

See Pneumothorax

Creutzfeldt-Jakob Disease (CJD)

Acute **Pain** r/t neck (nuchal) rigidity, inflammation of meninges, headache, kinesthetic

Decreased **Intracranial** adaptive capacity r/t sustained increase in intracranial pressure (10 to 15 mm Hg)

Delayed **Growth** and development r/t brain damage secondary to infectious process, increased intracranial pressure

Disturbed **Sensory** perception: hearing r/t central nervous system infection, ear infection

Disturbed **Sensory** perception: kinesthetic r/t central nervous system infection

Disturbed **Thought** processes r/t inflammation of brain, fever

Excess **Fluid** volume r/t increased intracranial pressure, syndrome of inappropriate secretion of antidiuretic hormone (SIADH)

Impaired **Comfort** r/t central nervous system inflammation

Impaired **Comfort**: photophobia r/t increased sensitivity to external stimuli secondary to central nervous system inflammation

Impaired physical **Mobility** r/t neuromuscular or central nervous system insult

Ineffective **Airway** clearance r/t seizure activity

Ineffective **Tissue** perfusion: cerebral r/t inflamed cerebral tissues and meninges, increased intracranial pressure

Risk for **Aspiration** r/t seizure activity

Risk for **Falls** r/t neuromuscular dysfunction

Risk for **Injury** r/t seizure activity

Crisis

Anticipatory **Grieving** r/t potential significant loss

Anxiety r/t threat to or change in environment, health status, interaction patterns, situation, self-concept, or role-functioning; threat of death of self or significant other

Compromised family **Coping** r/t situational or developmental crisis

Death **Anxiety** r/t feelings of hopelessness associated with crisis

Disturbed **Energy** field r/t disharmony caused by crisis

Fear r/t crisis situation

Ineffective **Coping** r/t situational or maturational crisis

Risk for **Spiritual** distress r/t physical or psychological stress, natural disasters, situational losses, maturational losses

Situational low **Self-esteem** r/t perception of inability to handle crisis

Spiritual distress r/t intense suffering

Crohn's Disease

Anxiety r/t change in health status

Diarrhea r/t inflammatory process

Imbalanced **Nutrition**: less than body requirements r/t diarrhea, altered ability to digest and absorb food

Ineffective **Coping** r/t repeated episodes of diarrhea

Ineffective **Health** maintenance r/t deficient knowledge regarding management of disease

Pain r/t increased peristalsis

Powerlessness r/t chronic disease

Risk for deficient **Fluid** volume r/t abnormal fluid loss with diarrhea

Croup

See Respiratory Infections, Acute Childhood

Cryosurgery for Retinal Detachment

See Retinal Detachment

Cushing's Syndrome

Activity intolerance r/t fatigue, weakness

Disturbed **Body** image r/t change in appearance from disease process

Excess **Fluid** volume r/t failure of regulatory mechanisms

Ineffective **Health** maintenance r/t deficient knowledge regarding needed care

Risk for **Infection** r/t suppression of immune system secondary to increased cortisol

Risk for **Injury** r/t decreased muscle strength, osteoporosis

Sexual dysfunction r/t loss of libido

CVA (Cerebrovascular Accident)

Adult **Failure** to thrive r/t neurophysiological changes

Anxiety r/t situational crisis, change in physical or emotional condition

Caregiver role strain r/t cognitive problems of care receiver, need for significant home care

Chronic **Confusion** r/t neurological changes

Constipation r/t decreased activity

Disturbed **Body** image r/t chronic illness, paralysis

Disturbed **Sensory** perception: visual, tactile, kinesthetic r/t neurological deficit

Disturbed **Thought** processes r/t neurophysiological changes

Grieving r/t loss of health

Impaired **Home** maintenance r/t neurological disease affecting ability to perform activities of daily living (ADLs)

Impaired **Memory** r/t neurological disturbances

Impaired physical **Mobility** r/t loss of balance and coordination

Impaired **Social** interaction r/t limited physical mobility, limited ability to communicate

Impaired **Swallowing** r/t neuromuscular dysfunction

Impaired **Transfer** ability r/t limited physical mobility

Impaired verbal **Communication** r/t pressure damage, decreased circulation to brain in speech center informational sources

Impaired **Walking** r/t loss of balance and coordination

Ineffective **Coping** r/t disability

Ineffective **Health** maintenance r/t deficient knowledge regarding self-care following CVA

Interrupted **Family** process r/t illness, disability of family member

Reflex **Incontinence** r/t loss of feeling to void

Risk for **Aspiration** r/t impaired swallowing, loss of gag reflex

Risk for **Disuse** syndrome r/t paralysis

Risk for impaired **Skin** integrity r/t immobility

Risk for **Injury** r/t disturbed sensory perception

Self-care deficit: specify r/t decreased strength and endurance, paralysis

Total urinary **Incontinence** r/t neurological dysfunction

Unilateral **Neglect** r/t disturbed perception from neurological damage

C

D

Cyanosis, Central with Cyanosis of Oral Mucous Membranes

Impaired **Gas** exchange r/t alveolar-capillary membrane changes

Cyanosis, Peripheral with Cyanosis of Nail Beds

Ineffective **Tissue** perfusion r/t interruption of arterial flow, severe vasoconstriction, cold temperatures

Risk for **Peripheral** neurovascular dysfunction r/t condition causing disruption in circulation

Cystic Fibrosis

Activity intolerance r/t imbalance between oxygen supply and demand

Anxiety r/t dyspnea, oxygen deprivation

Chronic **Sorrow** r/t presence of chronic disease

Disturbed **Body** image r/t changes in physical appearance, treatment of chronic lung disease (clubbing, barrel chest, home oxygen therapy)

Imbalanced **Nutrition**: less than body requirements r/t anorexia; decreased absorption of nutrients, fat; increased work of breathing

Impaired **Gas** exchange r/t ventilation-perfusion imbalance

Impaired **Home** maintenance r/t extensive daily treatment, medications necessary for health, mist/oxygen tents

Ineffective **Airway** clearance r/t increased production of thick mucus

Risk for **Caregiver** role strain r/t illness severity of care receiver, unpredictable course of illness

Risk for deficient **Fluid** volume r/t decreased fluid intake, increased work of breathing

Risk for delayed **Development** r/t chronic illness

Risk for disproportionate **Growth** r/t chronic illness

Risk for **Infection** r/t thick, tenacious mucus; harboring of bacterial organisms; debilitated state

Risk for **Spiritual** distress r/t presence of chronic disease

See Child with Chronic Condition; Hospitalized Child; Terminally Ill Child

Cystitis

Impaired **Urinary** elimination: frequency r/t urinary tract infection

Ineffective **Health** maintenance r/t deficient knowledge regarding methods to treat and prevent urinary tract infections

Pain: dysuria r/t inflammatory process in bladder

Risk for urge urinary **Incontinence** r/t infection in bladder

Cystocele

Ineffective **Health** maintenance r/t deficient knowledge regarding personal care, Kegel exercises to strengthen perineal muscles

Risk for urge urinary **Incontinence** r/t lack of bladder support

Stress urinary **Incontinence** r/t prolapsed bladder

Urge urinary **Incontinence** r/t prolapsed bladder

Cystoscopy

Ineffective **Health** maintenance r/t deficient knowledge regarding postoperative care

Risk for **Infection** r/t invasive procedure

Urinary retention r/t edema in urethra obstructing flow of urine

Deafness

Disturbed **Sensory** perception: auditory r/t alteration in sensory reception, transmission, integration

Impaired verbal **Communication** r/t impaired hearing

Risk for delayed **Development** r/t impaired hearing

Risk for **Injury** r/t alteration in sensory perception

Death

Risk for sudden infant **Death** syndrome r/t modifiable risk factors such as infants placed to sleep in the prone or side-lying position, prenatal and/or postnatal infant smoke exposure, infant overheating/overwrapping, soft underlayment/loose articles in the sleep environment, delayed or nonattendance of prenatal care; potentially modifiable risk factors such as low birth weight, prematurity, young maternal age; nonmodifiable risk factors such as male gender, ethnicity (e.g., African American, Native American race of mother), seasonality of SIDS deaths (higher in winter and fall months); peaking of SIDS mortality between infant ages of 2 and 4 months

Death, Oncoming

Anticipatory **Grieving** r/t loss of significant other

Compromised family **Coping** r/t client's inability to provide support to family

Death **Anxiety** r/t unresolved issues surrounding dying

Fear r/t threat of death

Ineffective **Coping** r/t personal vulnerability

Powerlessness r/t effects of illness, oncoming death

Readiness for enhanced **Spiritual** well-being r/t desire of client and family to be in harmony with each other and higher power/God

Social isolation r/t altered state of wellness

Spiritual distress r/t intense suffering

See Terminally Ill Child

Decisions, Difficulty Making

Decisional **Conflict** r/t support system deficit, perceived threat to value system, multiple or divergent sources of information, lack of relevant information, unclear personal values/beliefs

Decubitus Ulcer

See Pressure Ulcer

Deep Vein Thrombosis

See DVT

Defensive Behavior

Defensive **Coping** r/t nonacceptance of blame, denial of problems or weakness

Ineffective **Denial** r/t inability to face situation realistically

Dehiscence, Abdominal

Delayed **Surgical** recovery r/t altered circulation, malnutrition, opening in incision

Fear r/t threat of death, severe dysfunction

Impaired **Skin** integrity r/t altered circulation, malnutrition, opening in incision

Impaired **Tissue** integrity r/t exposure of abdominal contents to external environment

Pain r/t stretching of abdominal wall

Risk for imbalanced **Fluid** volume r/t altered circulation associated with opening of wound and exposure of abdominal contents

Risk for **Infection** r/t loss of skin integrity

Dehydration

Deficient **Fluid** volume r/t active fluid volume loss

Impaired **Oral** mucous membranes r/t decreased salivation, fluid deficit

Ineffective **Health** maintenance r/t deficient knowledge regarding treatment and prevention of dehydration

See cause of Dehydration

Delirium

Acute **Confusion** r/t effects of medication, response to hospitalization, alcohol abuse, substance abuse, sensory deprivation or overload

Adult **Failure** to thrive r/t delirium

Disturbed **Thought** processes r/t head trauma, altered metabolic state, substance abuse, sleep deprivation, sensory deprivation or overload

Impaired **Memory** r/t delirium

Risk for **Injury** r/t altered level of consciousness

Sleep deprivation r/t nightmares

Delirium Tremens (DT)

See Alcohol Withdrawal

Delivery

See Labor—Normal

Delusions

Acute **Confusion** r/t alcohol abuse, delirium, dementia, drug abuse

Adult **Failure** to thrive r/t delusional state

Anxiety r/t content of intrusive thoughts

Disturbed **Thought** processes r/t mental disorder

Impaired verbal **Communication** r/t psychological impairment, delusional thinking

Ineffective **Coping** r/t distortion and insecurity of life events

Risk for self- or other-directed **Violence** r/t delusional thinking

Dementia

Adult **Failure** to thrive r/t depression, apathy

Altered **Family** process r/t disability of family member

Chronic **Confusion** r/t neurological dysfunction

Chronic **Sorrow** r/t chronic mental illness

Disturbed **Sleep** pattern r/t neurological impairment, naps during the day

Imbalanced **Nutrition**: less than body requirements r/t psychological impairment

Impaired **Environmental** interpretation syndrome r/t dementia

Impaired **Home** maintenance r/t inadequate support system

Impaired physical **Mobility** r/t neuromuscular impairment

Risk for **Caregiver** role strain r/t number of caregiving tasks, duration of caregiving required

Risk for **Falls** r/t diminished mental status

Risk for impaired **Skin** integrity r/t altered nutritional status, immobility

Risk for **Injury** r/t confusion, decreased muscle coordination

D

Self-care deficit: specify r/t psychological or neuro-muscular impairment

Total urinary **Incontinence** r/t neuromuscular impairment

Denial of Health Status

Ineffective **Denial** r/t lack of perception about health status effects of illness

Ineffective management of **Therapeutic** regimen r/t denial of seriousness of health situation

Dental Caries

Impaired **Dentition** r/t ineffective oral hygiene, barriers to self-care, economic barriers to professional care, nutritional deficits, dietary habits

Ineffective **Health** maintenance r/t lack of knowledge regarding prevention of dental disease secondary to high-sugar diet, giving infants or toddlers with erupted teeth bottles of milk at bedtime, lack of fluoride treatments, inadequate or improper brushing of teeth

Dentition Problems

See Dental Caries

Depression (Major Depressive Disorder)

Adult **Failure** to thrive r/t depression

Chronic low **Self-esteem** r/t repeated unmet expectations

Chronic **Sorrow** r/t unresolved grief

Constipation r/t inactivity, decreased fluid intake

Death **Anxiety** r/t feelings of lack of self-worth

Disturbed **Energy** field r/t disharmony

Disturbed **Sleep** pattern r/t inactivity

Dysfunctional **Grieving** r/t lack of previous resolution of former grieving response

Fatigue r/t psychological demands

Hopelessness r/t feeling of abandonment, long-term stress

Impaired **Environmental** interpretation syndrome r/t severe mental functional impairment

Ineffective **Coping** r/t dysfunctional grieving

Ineffective **Health** maintenance r/t lack of ability to make good judgments regarding ways to obtain help

Powerlessness r/t pattern of helplessness

Risk for **Suicide** r/t panic state

Self-care deficit: specify r/t depression, cognitive impairment

Sexual dysfunction r/t loss of sexual desire

Social isolation r/t ineffective coping

Dermatitis

Anxiety r/t situational crisis imposed by illness

Impaired **Comfort**: pruritus r/t inflammation of skin

Impaired **Skin** integrity r/t side effect of medication, allergic reaction

Ineffective **Health** maintenance r/t deficient knowledge regarding methods to decrease inflammation

Despondency

Hopelessness r/t long-term stress

See Depression

Destructive Behavior Toward Others

Impaired **Adjustment** r/t intense emotional state

Ineffective **Coping** r/t situational crises, maturational crises, personal vulnerability

Risk for other-directed **Violence** r/t history of violence, neurological impairment, cognitive impairment, history of childhood abuse, history of witnessing family violence, cruelty to animals, firesetting, history of alcohol/drug abuse, pathological intoxication, psychotic symptomatology, motor vehicle offenses, impulsivity, availability or possession of weapon, body language

Developmental Concerns

Delayed **Growth** and development r/t prescribed dependence, indifference, separation from significant other(s), environmental and stimulation deficiencies, effects of physical disability, inadequate caretaking, inconsistent responsiveness, multiple caretakers

INDIVIDUAL

Risk for delayed **Development** r/t prematurity, seizures, congenital or genetic disorders, positive drug screening test, brain damage (e.g., hemorrhage in postnatal period, shaken baby, abuse, accident), vision impairment, hearing impairment or frequent otitis media, chronic illness, technology dependence, failure to thrive, inadequate nutrition, foster or adopted child, lead poisoning, chemotherapy, radiation therapy, natural disaster, behavior disorders, substance abuse

ENVIRONMENTAL

Risk for delayed **Development** r/t poverty, violence

CAREGIVER

Risk for delayed **Development** r/t abuse, mental illness, mental retardation or severe learning disability

Diabetes in Pregnancy

See Gestational Diabetes

Diabetes Insipidus

Deficient **Fluid** volume r/t inability to conserve fluid

Ineffective **Health** maintenance r/t deficient knowledge regarding care of disease, importance of medications

Diabetes Mellitus

Adult **Failure** to thrive r/t undetected disease process

Disturbed **Sensory** perception r/t ineffective tissue perfusion

Imbalanced **Nutrition**: less than body requirements r/t inability to use glucose (type I [insulin-dependent] diabetes)

Imbalanced **Nutrition**: more than body requirements r/t excessive intake of nutrients (type II diabetes)

Ineffective **Health** maintenance r/t deficient knowledge regarding care of diabetic condition

Ineffective management of **Therapeutic** regimen r/t complexity of therapeutic regimen

Ineffective **Tissue** perfusion: peripheral r/t impaired arterial circulation

Noncompliance r/t restrictive lifestyle; changes in diet, medication, exercise

Powerlessness r/t perceived lack of personal control

Risk for disturbed **Thought** processes r/t hypoglycemia, hyperglycemia

Risk for impaired **Skin** integrity r/t loss of pain perception in extremities

Risk for **Infection** r/t hyperglycemia, impaired healing, circulatory changes

Risk for **Injury**: hypoglycemia or hyperglycemia r/t failure to consume adequate calories, failure to take insulin

Sexual dysfunction r/t neuropathy associated with disease

Diabetes Mellitus, Juvenile (IDDM Type I)

Disturbed **Body** image r/t imposed deviations from biophysical and psychosocial norm, perceived differences from peers

Imbalanced **Nutrition**: less than body requirements r/t inability of body to adequately metabolize and use glucose and nutrients, increased caloric needs of child to promote growth and physical activity participation with peers

Impaired **Adjustment** r/t inability to participate in normal childhood activities

Ineffective **Health** maintenance r/t parental/child deficient knowledge regarding dietary management, medication administration, physical activity, and interaction between the three; daily changes in diet, medications, activity associated with child's growth spurts and needs;

need to instruct other caregivers and teachers regarding signs and symptoms of hypoglycemia or hyperglycemia and treatment

Pain r/t insulin injections, peripheral blood glucose testing

Risk for delayed **Development** r/t chronic illness

Risk for disproportionate **Growth** r/t chronic illness

Risk for **Noncompliance** r/t disturbed body image, impaired adjustment secondary to adolescent maturational crises

See Diabetes Mellitus; Child with Chronic Illness; Hospitalized Child

Diabetic Coma

Deficient **Fluid** volume r/t hyperglycemia resulting in polyuria

Disturbed **Thought** processes r/t hyperglycemia, presence of excessive metabolic acids

Ineffective management of **Therapeutic** regimen r/t lack of understanding of preventive measures, adequate blood sugar control

Risk for **Infection** r/t hyperglycemia, changes in vascular system

See Diabetes Mellitus

Diabetic Ketoacidosis

See Ketoacidosis

Diabetic Retinopathy

Disturbed **Sensory** perception r/t change in sensory reception

Grieving r/t loss of vision

Ineffective **Health** maintenance r/t deficient knowledge regarding preserving vision with treatment if possible, use of low-vision aids

See Vision Impairment

Dialysis

See Hemodialysis; Peritoneal Dialysis

Diaphoresis

Impaired **Comfort** r/t excessive sweating

Diaphragmatic Hernia

See Hiatus Hernia

Diarrhea

Diarrhea r/t infection, change in diet, gastrointestinal disorders, stress, medication effect, impaction

DIC (Disseminated Intravascular Coagulation)

Deficient **Fluid** volume: hemorrhage r/t depletion of clotting factors

Fear r/t threat to well-being

Ineffective **Protection** r/t abnormal clotting mechanism

Risk for ineffective **Tissue** perfusion: peripheral r/t hypovolemia from profuse bleeding, formation of microemboli in vascular system

Digitalis Toxicity

Decreased **Cardiac** output r/t drug toxicity affecting cardiac rhythm, rate

Ineffective management of **Therapeutic** regimen r/t deficient knowledge regarding action, appropriate method of administration of digitalis

Dilation and Curettage (D & C)

Ineffective **Health** maintenance r/t deficient knowledge regarding postoperative self-care

Pain r/t uterine contractions

Risk for deficient **Fluid** volume: hemorrhage r/t excessive blood loss during or after procedure

Risk for ineffective **Sexuality** patterns r/t painful coitus, fear associated with surgery on genital area

Risk for **Infection** r/t surgical procedure

Discharge Planning

Deficient **Knowledge** r/t lack of exposure to information for home care

Impaired **Home** maintenance r/t family member's disease or injury interfering with home maintenance

Ineffective **Health** maintenance r/t lack of material sources

Discomforts of Pregnancy

Acute **Pain**: leg cramps r/t nerve compression, calcium/phosphorus/potassium imbalance

Constipation r/t decreased gastrointestinal tract motility, pressure from enlarged uterus, supplementary iron

Disturbed **Body** image r/t pregnancy-induced body changes

Disturbed **Sleep** pattern r/t psychological stress, fetal movement, muscular cramping, urinary frequency, shortness of breath

Fatigue r/t hormonal, metabolic, body changes

Headache r/t vascular and hormonal changes

Hemorrhoids r/t enlarged uterus, constipation, pelvic venous stasis, decreased gastrointestinal tract motility

Impaired **Comfort** r/t hormonal changes (nausea, ptyalism, leukorrhea, urinary frequency), enlarged uterus (shortness of breath, abdominal distention, pruritus, reduced bladder capacity), increased vascularization (nasal stuffiness, varicosities)

Nausea r/t hormone effect

Risk for **Constipation** r/t decreased intestinal motility, inadequate fiber in diet

Risk for **Injury** r/t faintness and/or syncope secondary to vasomotor lability or postural hypotension, venous stasis in lower extremities

Risk for urge urinary **Incontinence** r/t hormone effect, pressure on bladder from growing uterus

Stress urinary **Incontinence** r/t enlarged uterus, fetal movement

Dissecting Aneurysm

Fear r/t threat to well-being

See Abdominal Surgery; Aneurysm

Disseminated Intravascular Coagulation

See DIC

Dissociative Disorder (Not Otherwise Specified)

Anxiety r/t psychosocial stress

Disturbance in **Self-concept** r/t childhood trauma, childhood abuse

Disturbed personal **Identity** r/t inability to distinguish self caused by multiple personality disorder, depersonalization, disturbance in memory

Disturbed **Sensory** perception: kinesthetic r/t underdeveloped ego

Disturbed **Thought** processes r/t repressed anxiety

Impaired **Memory** r/t altered state of consciousness

Ineffective **Coping** r/t personal vulnerability in crisis of accurate self-perception

Distress

Anxiety r/t situational crises, maturational crises

Death **Anxiety** r/t denial of one's own immortality or impending death

Disturbed **Energy** field r/t disruption in flow of energy as result of pain, depression, fatigue, anxiety, stress

Disuse Syndrome, Potential to Develop

Risk for **Disuse** syndrome r/t paralysis, mechanical immobilization, prescribed immobilization, severe pain, altered level of consciousness

Diversional Activity, Lack of

Deficient **Diversional** activity r/t environmental lack of diversional activity as in frequent hospitalizations, lengthy treatments

Diverticulitis

Constipation r/t dietary deficiency of fiber and roughage

Deficient **Knowledge** r/t diet needed to control disease, medication regimen

Diarrhea r/t increased intestinal motility secondary to inflammation

Imbalanced **Nutrition**: less than body requirements r/t loss of appetite

Pain r/t inflammation of bowel

Risk for deficient **Fluid** volume r/t diarrhea

Dizziness

Decreased **Cardiac** output r/t dysfunctional electrical conduction

Impaired physical **Mobility** r/t dizziness

Ineffective **Tissue** perfusion: cerebral r/t interruption of cerebral arterial blood flow

Risk for **Injury** r/t difficulty maintaining balance

Domestic Violence

Anxiety r/t threat to self-concept, situational crisis of abuse

Caregiver role strain r/t chronic illness, self-care deficits, lack of respite care, extent of caregiving required

Compromised family **Coping** r/t abusive patterns

Defensive **Coping** r/t low self-esteem

Disturbed **Sleep** pattern r/t psychological stress

Impaired verbal **Communication** r/t psychological barriers of fear

Interrupted **Family** process: alcoholism r/t inadequate coping skills

Post-trauma response r/t history of abuse

Powerlessness r/t lifestyle of helplessness

Risk for **Post-trauma** syndrome r/t inadequate social support

Risk for self-directed **Violence** r/t history of abuse

Self-esteem disturbance r/t negative family interactions

Down Syndrome

See Child with Chronic Illness; Mental Retardation

Dress Self (Inability to)

Dressing/grooming **Self-care** deficit r/t intolerance to activity, decreased strength and endurance, pain, discomfort, perceptual or cognitive impairment, neuromuscular impairment, musculoskeletal impairment, depression, severe anxiety

Dribbling of Urine

Stress urinary **Incontinence** r/t degenerative changes in pelvic muscles and structural supports

Drooling

Impaired **Swallowing** r/t neuromuscular impairment, mechanical obstruction

Risk for **Aspiration** r/t impaired swallowing

Drug Abuse

Anxiety r/t threat to self-concept, lack of control of drug use

Disturbed **Sensory** perception: specify r/t substance intoxication

Disturbed **Sleep** pattern r/t effects of medications

Disturbed **Thought** process r/t mind-altering effects of drugs

Imbalanced **Nutrition**: less than body requirements r/t poor eating habits

Impaired **Adjustment** r/t failure to intend to change behavior

Impaired **Social** interaction r/t disturbed thought processes from drug abuse

Ineffective **Coping** r/t situational crisis

Noncompliance r/t denial of illness

Powerlessness r/t feeling unable to change patterns of abuse

Risk for **Injury** r/t hallucinations, drug effects

Risk for **Violence** r/t poor impulse control

Sexual dysfunction r/t actions and side effects of drug abuse

Sleep deprivation r/t prolonged psychological discomfort

Spiritual distress r/t separation from religious, cultural ties

Drug Withdrawal

Acute **Confusion** r/t effects of substance withdrawal

Anxiety r/t physiological withdrawal

Disturbed **Sensory** perception: specify r/t substance intoxication

Disturbed **Sleep** pattern r/t effects of medications

Imbalanced **Nutrition**: less than body requirements r/t poor eating habits

Ineffective **Coping** r/t situational crisis, withdrawal

Noncompliance r/t denial of illness

Risk for **Injury** r/t hallucinations

Risk for **Violence** r/t poor impulse control

See Drug Abuse

DTs (Delirium Tremens)

See Alcohol Withdrawal

D

D

DVT (Deep Vein Thrombosis)

Constipation r/t inactivity, bedrest

Delayed **Surgical** recovery r/t impaired physical mobility

Impaired physical **Mobility** r/t pain in extremity, forced bedrest

Ineffective **Health** maintenance r/t deficient knowledge regarding self-care needs, treatment regimen, outcome

Ineffective **Tissue** perfusion: peripheral r/t interruption of venous blood flow

Pain r/t vascular inflammation, edema

See Anticoagulant Therapy

Dying Client

See Terminally Ill Adult, Terminally Ill Child—Adolescent, Infant/Toddler, Preschool Child, School-Age Child/Preadolescent, Death of Child-Parent

Dysfunctional Eating Pattern

Imbalanced **Nutrition**: less than body requirements r/t psychological factors

Risk for imbalanced **Nutrition**: more than body requirements r/t observed use of food as reward or comfort measure

See Anorexia Nervosa; Bulimia

Dysfunctional Family Unit

See Family Problems

Dysfunctional Grieving

Dysfunctional **Grieving** r/t actual or perceived loss

Dysfunctional Ventilatory Weaning

Dysfunctional **Ventilatory** weaning response r/t physical, psychological, situational factors

Dysmenorrhea

Ineffective **Health** maintenance r/t deficient knowledge regarding prevention and treatment of painful menstruation

Nausea r/t prostaglandin effect

Pain r/t cramping from hormonal effects

Dyspareunia

Sexual dysfunction r/t lack of lubrication during intercourse, alteration in reproductive organ function

Dyspepsia

Anxiety r/t pressures of personal role

Ineffective **Health** maintenance r/t deficient knowledge regarding treatment of disease

Pain r/t gastrointestinal disease, consumption of irritating foods

Dysphagia

Impaired **Swallowing** r/t neuromuscular impairment

Risk for **Aspiration** r/t loss of gag or cough reflex

Dysphasia

Impaired **Social** interaction r/t difficulty in communicating

Impaired verbal **Communication** r/t decrease in circulation to brain

Dyspnea

Activity intolerance r/t imbalance between oxygen supply-demand

Anxiety r/t ineffective breathing pattern

Disturbed **Sleep** pattern r/t difficulty breathing, positioning required for effective breathing

Fear r/t threat to state of well-being, potential death

Impaired **Gas** exchange r/t alveolar-capillary damage

Ineffective **Airway** clearance r/t decreased energy, fatigue

Ineffective **Breathing** pattern r/t decreased lung expansion, neurological impairment affecting respiratory center, extreme anxiety

Sleep deprivation r/t ineffective breathing pattern

Dysrhythmia

Activity intolerance r/t decreased cardiac output

Anxiety/fear r/t threat of death, change in health status

Decreased **Cardiac** output r/t altered electrical conduction

Ineffective **Health** maintenance r/t deficient knowledge regarding self-care with disease

Ineffective **Tissue** perfusion: cerebral r/t interruption of cerebral arterial flow secondary to decreased cardiac output

Dysthymic Disorder

Chronic low **Self-esteem** r/t repeated unmet expectations

Disturbed **Sleep** pattern r/t anxious thoughts

Ineffective **Coping** r/t impaired social interaction

Ineffective **Health** maintenance r/t inability to make good judgments regarding ways to obtain help

Ineffective **Sexuality** pattern r/t loss of sexual desire

Social isolation r/t ineffective coping

See Depression

Dystocia

Anxiety r/t difficult labor, deficient knowledge regarding normal labor pattern

Fatigue r/t prolonged labor

Grieving r/t loss of ideal labor experience

Ineffective **Coping** r/t situational crisis

Pain r/t difficult labor, medical interventions

Powerlessness r/t perceived inability to control outcome of labor

Risk for deficient **Fluid** volume r/t hemorrhage secondary to uterine atony

Risk for delayed **Development** r/t difficult labor and birth

Risk for disproportionate **Growth** r/t difficult labor and birth

Risk for impaired **Tissue** integrity: maternal and fetal r/t difficult labor

Risk for ineffective **Tissue** perfusion: cerebral (fetal) r/t difficult labor and birth

Risk for **Infection** r/t prolonged rupture of membranes

Risk for **Post-trauma** syndrome r/t sudden emergency during delivery of infant

Situational low **Self-esteem** r/t perceived inability to have normal labor and delivery

Dysuria

Impaired **Urinary** elimination r/t urinary tract infection

Risk for urge urinary **Incontinence** r/t detrusor hyperreflexia from cystitis, urethritis

E

Ear Surgery

Disturbed **Sensory** perception: hearing r/t invasive surgery of ears, dressings

Ineffective **Health** maintenance r/t deficient knowledge regarding postoperative restrictions, expectations, care

Pain r/t edema in ears from surgery

Risk for delayed **Development** r/t hearing impairment

Risk for **Injury** r/t dizziness from excessive stimuli to vestibular apparatus

See Hospitalized Child

Earache

Disturbed **Sensory** perception: auditory r/t altered sensory reception, transmission, integration

Pain r/t trauma, edema

Eating Disorder

See Anorexia Nervosa; Bulimia; Obesity

Eclampsia

Fear r/t threat of well-being to self and fetus

Interrupted **Family** processes r/t unmet expectations for pregnancy and childbirth

Risk for **Aspiration** r/t seizure activity

Risk for delayed **Development** r/t uteroplacental insufficiency

Risk for disproportionate **Growth** r/t uteroplacental insufficiency

Risk for excess **Fluid** volume r/t decreased urine output secondary to renal dysfunction

Risk for imbalanced **Fluid** volume r/t retained fluid, decreased renal activity

Risk for ineffective fetal **Tissue** perfusion r/t uteroplacental insufficiency

Risk for **Injury**: maternal r/t seizure activity

ECT (Electroconvulsive Therapy)

Decisional **Conflict** r/t lack of relevant information

Fear r/t real or imagined threat to well-being

Impaired **Memory** r/t effects of treatment

See Depression

Ectopic Pregnancy

Chronic **Sorrow** r/t loss of pregnancy, potential loss of fertility

Death **Anxiety** r/t emergency condition, hemorrhage

Deficient **Fluid** volume r/t loss of blood

Disturbed **Body** image r/t negative feelings about body and reproductive functioning

Fear r/t threat to self, surgery, implications for future pregnancy

Ineffective **Role** performance r/t loss of pregnancy

Pain r/t stretching or rupture of implantation site

Risk for ineffective **Coping** r/t loss of pregnancy

Risk for **Infection** r/t traumatized tissue, blood loss

Risk for interrupted **Family** processes r/t situational crisis

Risk for **Spiritual** distress r/t grief process

Situational low **Self-esteem** r/t loss of pregnancy, inability to carry pregnancy to term

Eczema

Disturbed **Body** image r/t change in appearance from inflamed skin

Impaired **Skin** integrity r/t side effect of medication, allergic reaction

Ineffective **Health** maintenance r/t deficient knowledge regarding how to decrease inflammation and prevent further outbreaks

Pain: pruritus r/t inflammation of skin

ED (Erectile Dysfunction)

See Impotence

Edema

Excess **Fluid** volume r/t excessive fluid intake, cardiac dysfunction, renal dysfunction, loss of plasma proteins

Ineffective **Health** maintenance r/t deficient knowledge regarding treatment of edema

Risk for impaired **Skin** integrity r/t impaired circulation, fragility of skin

See cause of Edema

Elderly

See Aging

Elderly Abuse

See Abuse—Spouse, Parent, or Significant Other

Electroconvulsive Therapy

See ECT

Emaciated Person

Adult **Failure** to thrive r/t imbalanced nutrition: less than body requirements

Imbalanced **Nutrition**: less than body requirements r/t inability to ingest food, digest food, absorb nutrients because of biological, psychological, economic factors

Embolectomy

Fear r/t threat of great bodily harm from embolus

Risk for deficient **Fluid** volume: hemorrhage r/t postoperative complication, surgical area

Risk for **Peripheral** neurovascular dysfunction r/t decreased circulation to extremity

See Surgery—Postoperative Care

Emboli

See Pulmonary Embolism

Emesis

Nausea r/t chemotherapy, irritation of gastrointestinal system, stimulation of neuropharmacological mechanisms

See Vomiting

Emotional Problems

See Coping Problems

Empathy

Health-seeking behaviors r/t desire to attain maximum level of health

Readiness for enhanced community **Coping** r/t social supports, being available for problem solving

Readiness for enhanced family **Coping** r/t basic needs met, desire to move to higher level of health

Readiness for enhanced **Spiritual** well-being r/t desire to establish interconnectedness through spirituality

Emphysema

See COPD

Emptiness

Chronic **Sorrow** r/t unresolved grief

Social isolation r/t inability to engage in satisfying personal relationships

Spiritual distress r/t separation from religious/cultural ties

Encephalitis

See Meningitis/Encephalitis

Endocardial Cushion Defect

See Congenital Heart Disease/Cardiac Anomalies

Endocarditis

Activity intolerance r/t reduced cardiac reserve, prescribed bedrest

Acute **Pain** r/t biological injury, inflammation

Decreased **Cardiac** output r/t inflammation of lining of heart and change in structure of valve leaflets, increased myocardial workload

Ineffective **Health** maintenance r/t deficient knowledge regarding treatment of disease, preventive measures against further incidence of disease

Ineffective **Tissue** perfusion: cardiopulmonary/peripheral r/t high risk for development of emboli

Risk for imbalanced **Nutrition**: less than body requirements r/t fever, hypermetabolic state associated with fever

Endometriosis

Anticipatory **Grieving** r/t possible infertility

Ineffective **Health** maintenance r/t deficient knowledge about disease condition, medications, other treatments

Nausea r/t prostaglandin effect

Pain r/t onset of menses with distention of endometrial tissue

Sexual dysfunction r/t painful coitus

Endometritis

Anxiety r/t prolonged hospitalization, fear of unknown

Hyperthermia r/t infectious process

Ineffective **Health** maintenance r/t deficient knowledge regarding condition, treatment, antibiotic regimen

Pain r/t infectious process in reproductive tract

Enuresis

Ineffective **Health** maintenance r/t unachieved developmental task, neuromuscular immaturity, diseases of urinary system, infections or illnesses such as diabetes mellitus or insipidus, regression in developmental stage secondary to hospitalization or stress, parental deficient knowledge regarding involuntary urination at night after age 6, fluid intake at bedtime, lack of control during sound sleep, male gender

See Toilet Training

Environmental Interpretation Problems

Adult **Failure** to thrive r/t impaired environmental interpretation syndrome

Chronic **Confusion** r/t impaired environmental interpretation syndrome

Disturbed **Thought** processes r/t lack of orientation to person, place, time, circumstances

Impaired **Environmental** interpretation syndrome r/t dementia, Parkinson's disease, Huntington's disease, depression, alcoholism

Impaired **Memory** r/t environmental disturbances

Risk for **Injury** r/t lack of orientation to person, place, time, circumstances

Epididymitis

Anxiety r/t situational crisis, pain, threat to future fertility

Ineffective **Health** maintenance r/t deficient knowledge regarding treatment for pain and infection

Ineffective **Sexuality** patterns r/t edema of epididymis and testes

Pain r/t inflammation in scrotal sac

Epiglottitis

See Respiratory Infections, Acute Childhood

Epilepsy

Anxiety r/t threat to role functioning

Impaired **Memory** r/t seizure activity

Ineffective **Health** maintenance r/t deficient knowledge regarding seizures and seizure control

Ineffective **Therapeutic** regimen management r/t deficient knowledge regarding seizure control

Risk for **Aspiration** r/t impaired swallowing, excessive secretions

Risk for delayed **Development** r/t seizure disorder

Risk for disturbed **Thought** processes r/t excessive, uncontrolled neurological stimuli

Risk for **Injury** r/t environmental factors during seizure

See Seizure Disorders

Episiotomy

Anxiety r/t fear of pain

Disturbed **Body** image r/t fear of resuming sexual relations

Impaired physical **Mobility** r/t pain, swelling, tissue trauma

Impaired **Skin** integrity r/t perineal incision

Pain r/t tissue trauma

Risk for **Infection** r/t tissue trauma

Sexual dysfunction r/t altered body structure, tissue trauma

Epistaxis

Fear r/t large amount of blood loss

Risk for deficient **Fluid** volume r/t excessive fluid loss

Epstein-Barr Virus

See Mononucleosis

Erectile Dysfunction (ED)

See Impotence

Esophageal Varices

Deficient **Fluid** volume: hemorrhage r/t portal hypertension, distended variceal vessels that can easily rupture

Fear r/t threat of death

See Cirrhosis

Esophagitis

Ineffective **Health** maintenance r/t deficient knowledge regarding treatment of disease

Pain r/t inflammation of esophagus

ETOH Withdrawal

See Alcohol Withdrawal

Evisceration

See Dehiscence

Exposure to Hot or Cold Environment

Risk for imbalanced **Body** temperature r/t exposure

E

F

External Fixation

Disturbed **Body** image r/t trauma, change to affected part

Risk for **Infection** r/t pressure of pins on skin surface

See Fracture

Eye Surgery

Anxiety r/t possible loss of vision

Disturbed **Sensory** perception: visual r/t surgical procedure

Ineffective **Health** maintenance r/t deficient knowledge regarding postoperative activity, medications, eye care

Risk for **Injury** r/t impaired vision

Self-care deficit r/t impaired vision

See Hospitalized Child; Vision Impairment

Failure to Thrive, Adult

Adult **Failure** to thrive r/t depression, apathy, fatigue

Failure to Thrive, Nonorganic

Chronic low **Self-esteem**: parental r/t feelings of inadequacy, support system deficiencies, inadequate role model

Delayed **Growth** and development r/t parental deficient knowledge, lack of stimulation, nutritional deficit, long-term hospitalization

Disorganized **Infant** behavior r/t lack of boundaries

Disturbed **Sleep** pattern r/t inconsistency of caretaker, lack of quiet environment

Imbalanced **Nutrition**: less than body requirements r/t inadequate type/amounts of food for infant, inappropriate feeding techniques

Impaired **Parenting** r/t lack of parenting skills, inadequate role modeling

Risk for delayed **Development** r/t failure to thrive

Risk for disproportionate **Growth** r/t failure to thrive

Risk for impaired parent/infant **Attachment** r/t inability of parents to meet infant's needs

Social isolation r/t limited support systems, self-imposed situation

Falls, Risk for

Risk for **Falls** r/t history of falls, physiological factors, cognitive impairment, medication effect, unsafe environment, young child or older adult

Family Problems

Compromised family **Coping** r/t inadequate or incorrect information or understanding by primary person, temporary preoccupation by significant person who is trying to manage emotional conflicts and personal suffering and is unable to perceive or act effectively in regard to client's needs, temporary family disorganization and role changes, other situational or developmental crises the significant person may be facing, little support provided by client for primary person, prolonged disease or disability progression that exhausts supportive capacity of significant people

Disabled family **Coping** r/t significant person with chronically unexpressed feelings such as guilt, anxiety, hostility, despair; dissonant discrepancy of coping styles for dealing with adaptive tasks by significant person and client or among significant people; highly ambivalent family relationships; arbitrary handling of family's resistance to treatment, which tends to solidify defensiveness as it fails to deal adequately with underlying anxiety

Ineffective family **Therapeutic** regimen management r/t complexity of health care system, complexity of therapeutic regimen, decisional conflicts, economic difficulties, excessive demands made on individual or family, family conflict

Interrupted **Family** processes r/t situation transition and/or crises, developmental transition and/or crises

Readiness for enhanced family **Coping** r/t needs sufficiently gratified, adaptive tasks effectively addressed to enable goals of self-actualization to surface

Family Process

Readiness for enhanced **Family Processes** r/t expressed willingness to enhance family dynamics; family functioning that meets physical, social, and psychological needs of family members; activities that support the safety and growth of family members; adequate communication; relationships that are generally positive; interdependence with community; accomplishment of family task; family roles that are flexible and appropriate for developmental stages; evident respect for family members; adaptation of family to change; maintenance of boundaries of family members; energy level of family that supports activities of daily living; evident family resilience; balance between autonomy and cohesiveness

Fatigue

Disturbed **Energy** field r/t disharmony

Fatigue r/t decreased or increased metabolic energy production, overwhelming psychological or emotional demands, increased energy requirements to perform ADLs, excessive social and/or role demands, states of discomfort, altered body chemistry

Fear

Death **Anxiety** r/t fear of death

Fear r/t identifiable physical or psychological threat to person

Febrile Seizures

See Seizure Disorders, Childhood

Fecal Impaction

See Impaction of Stool

Fecal Incontinence

Bowel incontinence r/t neurological impairment, gastrointestinal disorders, anorectal trauma

Feeding Problems—Newborn

Disorganized **Infant** behavior r/t prematurity, immature neurological system

Impaired **Swallowing** r/t prematurity

Ineffective **Breastfeeding** r/t prematurity, infant anomaly, maternal breast anomaly, previous breast surgery, previous history of breastfeeding failure, infant receiving supplemental feedings with artificial nipple, poor infant sucking reflex, nonsupportive partner and family, deficient knowledge, maternal anxiety or ambivalence

Ineffective **Infant** feeding pattern r/t prematurity, neurological impairment or delay, oral hypersensitivity, prolonged NPO

Interrupted **Breastfeeding** r/t maternal or infant illness, prematurity, maternal employment, contraindications to breastfeeding, need to abruptly wean infant

Risk for delayed **Development** r/t inadequate nutrition

Risk for disproportionate **Growth** r/t feeding problems

Risk for imbalanced **Fluid** volume r/t inability to take in adequate amount of fluids

Femoral Popliteal Bypass

Anxiety r/t threat to or change in health status

Pain r/t surgical trauma, edema in surgical area

Risk for deficient **Fluid** volume: hemorrhage r/t abnormal blood loss

Risk for ineffective **Tissue** perfusion: peripheral r/t impaired arterial circulation

Risk for **Infection** r/t invasive procedure

Risk for **Peripheral** neurovascular dysfunction r/t vascular surgery, emboli

Fetal Alcohol Syndrome

See Infant of Substance-Abusing Mother

Fetal Distress/Nonreassuring Fetal Heart Rate Pattern

Fear r/t threat to fetus

Ineffective **Tissue** perfusion: fetal r/t interruption of umbilical cord blood flow

Ineffective **Tissue** perfusion: placental r/t small or old placenta, interference with gas exchange transplacentally

Fever

Hyperthermia r/t infectious process, damage to hypothalamus, exposure to hot environment, medications, anesthesia, inability or decreased ability to perspire

Ineffective **Thermoregulation** r/t fluctuating environmental temperature, trauma, illness

Fibrocystic Breast Disease

See Breast Lumps

Filthy Home Environment

Impaired **Home** maintenance r/t individual or family member disease or injury, insufficient family organization or planning, impaired cognitive or emotional functioning, lack of knowledge, economic factors

Financial Crisis in the Home Environment

Impaired **Home** maintenance r/t insufficient finances

Fistulectomy

See Hemorrhoidectomy (same nursing care)

Flail Chest

Anxiety r/t difficulty breathing

Impaired spontaneous **Ventilation** r/t paradoxical respirations

Ineffective **Breathing** pattern r/t chest trauma

Flashbacks

Post-trauma syndrome r/t catastrophic event

Risk for **Post-trauma** syndrome r/t occupation (e.g., police, fire, rescue, corrections, emergency room staff, mental health), exaggerated sense of responsibility, perception of event, survivor's role in event, displacement from home, inadequate social support, nonsupportive environment, diminished ego strength, duration of event

Flat Affect

Adult **Failure** to thrive r/t apathy

Hopelessness r/t prolonged activity restriction creating isolation, failing or deteriorating physiological condition, long-term stress, abandonment, lost belief in transcendent values or higher power/God

Risk for **Loneliness** r/t social isolation, lack of interest in surroundings

See Dysthymic Disorder

Fluid Balance

Readiness for enhanced **Fluid** balance r/t expressed willingness to enhance fluid balance; stable weight; moist mucous membranes; food and fluid intake adequate for daily needs; straw-colored urine with specific gravity within normal limits; good tissue turgor; no excessive thirst; urine output appropriate for intake; no evidence of edema or dehydration

Fluid Volume Deficit

Deficient **Fluid** volume r/t active fluid loss, failure of regulatory mechanisms

Fluid Volume Excess

Excess **Fluid** volume r/t compromised regulatory mechanism, excess sodium intake

Fluid Volume Imbalance, Risk for

Delayed **Surgical** recovery r/t fluid volume imbalance

Risk for imbalanced **Fluid** volume r/t major invasive surgeries

Foreign Body Aspiration

Impaired **Home** maintenance r/t insufficient family organization or planning, lack of resources or support systems, inability to maintain orderly and clean surroundings

Ineffective **Airway** clearance r/t obstruction of airway

Ineffective **Health** maintenance r/t parental deficient knowledge regarding small toys, pieces of toys, nuts, balloons

Risk for **Suffocation** r/t inhalation of small object

See Safety, Childhood

Formula Feeding

Decisional **Conflict**: maternal r/t multiple or divergent sources of information, values conflict, support system deficit

Grieving: maternal r/t loss of desired breastfeeding experience

Ineffective **Health** maintenance r/t maternal deficient knowledge regarding formula feeding

Risk for **Constipation**: infant r/t iron-fortified formula

Risk for imbalanced **Nutrition**: more than body requirements r/t composition of formula and bottle feeding, overuse of food for reward or comfort measures

Risk for **Infection**: infant r/t lack of passive maternal immunity, supine feeding position

Fracture

Deficient **Diversional** activity r/t immobility

Impaired physical **Mobility** r/t limb immobilization

Impaired **Walking** r/t limb immobility

Ineffective **Health** maintenance r/t deficient knowledge regarding care of fracture

Pain r/t muscle spasm, edema, trauma

Risk for impaired **Skin** integrity r/t immobility, presence of cast

Risk for ineffective **Tissue** perfusion r/t immobility, presence of cast

Risk for **Peripheral** neurovascular dysfunction r/t mechanical compression, treatment of fracture

Fractured Hip

See Hip Fracture

Frequency of Urination

Impaired **Urinary** elimination r/t anatomical obstruction, sensory-motor impairment, urinary tract infection

Risk for urge urinary **Incontinence** r/t effects of medications, caffeine, alcohol

Stress urinary **Incontinence** r/t degenerative change in pelvic muscles and structural support

Urge urinary **Incontinence** r/t decreased bladder capacity, irritation of bladder stretch receptors causing spasm, alcohol, caffeine, increased fluids, increased urine concentration, overdistended bladder

Urinary retention r/t high urethral pressure caused by weak detrusor, inhibition of reflex arc, strong sphincter, blockage

Frostbite

Impaired **Skin** integrity r/t freezing of skin

Pain r/t decreased circulation from prolonged exposure to cold

See Hypothermia

Frothy Sputum

See CHF; Pulmonary Edema; Seizure Disorders

Fusion, Lumbar

Anxiety r/t fear of surgical procedure, possible recurring problems

Impaired physical **Mobility** r/t limitations from surgical procedure, presence of brace

Ineffective **Health** maintenance r/t deficient knowledge regarding postoperative mobility restrictions, body mechanics

Pain r/t discomfort at bone donor site

Risk for **Injury** r/t improper body mechanics

Risk for perioperative positioning **Injury** r/t immobilization

G

Gag Reflex, Depressed or Absent

Impaired **Swallowing** r/t neuromuscular impairment

Risk for **Aspiration** r/t depressed cough/gag reflex

Gallop Rhythm

Decreased **Cardiac** output r/t decreased contractility of heart

Gallstones

See Cholelithiasis

Gangrene

Delayed **Surgical** recovery r/t obstruction of arterial flow

Fear r/t possible loss of extremity

Ineffective **Tissue** perfusion: peripheral r/t obstruction of arterial flow

Gas Exchange, Impaired

Impaired **Gas** exchange r/t ventilation-perfusion imbalance

Gastric Surgery

Risk for **Injury** r/t inadvertent insertion of nasogastric tube through gastric incision line

See Abdominal Surgery

Gastric Ulcer

See Ulcer, Peptic

Gastritis

Imbalanced **Nutrition**: less than body requirements r/t vomiting, inadequate intestinal absorption of nutrients, restricted dietary regimen

Pain r/t inflammation of gastric mucosa

Risk for deficient **Fluid** volume r/t excessive loss from gastrointestinal tract secondary to vomiting, decreased intake

Gastroenteritis

Deficient **Fluid** volume r/t excessive loss from gastrointestinal tract secondary to diarrhea, vomiting

Diarrhea r/t infectious process involving intestinal tract

Imbalanced **Nutrition**: less than body requirements r/t vomiting, inadequate intestinal absorption of nutrients, restricted dietary intake

Ineffective **Health** maintenance r/t deficient knowledge regarding treatment of disease

Nausea r/t irritation to gastrointestinal system

Pain r/t increased peristalsis causing cramping

See Gastroenteritis—Child

Gastroenteritis—Child

Impaired **Skin** integrity: diaper rash r/t acidic excretions on perineal tissues

Ineffective **Health** maintenance r/t lack of parental knowledge regarding fluid and dietary changes

Risk for delayed **Development** r/t inadequate nutrition

See Gastroenteritis; Hospitalized Child

Gastroesophageal Reflux

Anxiety/fear: parental r/t possible need for surgical intervention (Nissen fundoplication, gastrostomy tube)

Deficient **Fluid** volume r/t persistent vomiting

Imbalanced **Nutrition**: less than body requirements r/t poor feeding, vomiting

Ineffective **Airway** clearance r/t reflux of gastric contents into esophagus and tracheal or bronchial tree

Ineffective **Health** maintenance r/t deficient knowledge regarding antireflux regimen (e.g., positioning, oral or enteral feeding techniques, medications), possible home apnea monitoring

Pain r/t irritation of esophagus from gastric acids

Risk for **Aspiration** r/t entry of gastric contents in tracheal or bronchial tree

Risk for impaired **Parenting** r/t disruption in bonding secondary to irritable or inconsolable infant

See Child with Chronic Condition; Hospitalized Child

Gastrointestinal Hemorrhage

See GI Bleed

Gastroschisis/Omphalocele

Anticipatory **Grieving** r/t threatened loss of infant, loss of perfect birth or infant secondary to serious medical condition

Impaired **Gas** exchange r/t effects of anesthesia, subsequent atelectasis

Ineffective **Airway** clearance r/t complications of anesthetic effects

Risk for deficient **Fluid** volume r/t inability to feed secondary to condition, subsequent electrolyte imbalance

Risk for **Infection** r/t disrupted skin integrity with exposure of abdominal contents

G

Risk for **Injury** r/t disrupted skin integrity, ineffective protection

See Hospitalized Child; Premature Infant

Gastrostomy

Risk for impaired **Skin** integrity r/t presence of gastric contents on skin

See Tube Feeding

Genital Herpes

See Herpes Simplex

Genital Warts

See STD

Gestational Diabetes (Diabetes in Pregnancy)

Anxiety r/t threat to self and/or fetus

Impaired fetal **Nutrition**: more than body requirements r/t excessive glucose uptake

Impaired maternal **Nutrition**: less than body requirements r/t decreased insulin production and glucose uptake in cells

Ineffective **Health** maintenance: maternal r/t deficient knowledge regarding care of diabetic condition in pregnancy

Powerlessness r/t lack of control over outcome of pregnancy

Risk for delayed **Development**: fetal r/t endocrine disorder of mother

Risk for disproportionate **Growth**: fetal r/t endocrine disorder of mother

Risk for impaired **Tissue** integrity: fetal r/t macrosomia, congenital defects, birth injury

Risk for impaired **Tissue** integrity: maternal r/t delivery of large infant

See Diabetes Mellitus

GI Bleed (Gastrointestinal Bleeding)

Deficient **Fluid** volume r/t gastrointestinal bleeding

Fatigue r/t loss of circulating blood volume, decreased ability to transport oxygen

Fear r/t threat to well-being, potential death

Imbalanced **Nutrition**: less than body requirements r/t nausea, vomiting

Pain r/t irritated mucosa from acid secretion

Risk for ineffective **Coping** r/t personal vulnerability in crisis, bleeding, hospitalization

Gingivitis

Impaired **Dentition** r/t ineffective oral hygiene, barriers to self-care

Impaired **Oral** mucous membrane r/t ineffective oral hygiene

Glaucoma

Disturbed **Sensory** perception: visual r/t increased intraocular pressure

See Vision Impairment

Glomerulonephritis

Acute **Pain** r/t edema of kidney

Excess **Fluid** volume r/t renal impairment

Imbalanced **Nutrition**: less than body requirements r/t anorexia, restrictive diet

Ineffective **Health** maintenance r/t deficient knowledge regarding care of disease

Gonorrhea

Ineffective **Health** maintenance r/t deficient knowledge regarding treatment and prevention of disease

Pain r/t inflammation of reproductive organs

Risk for **Infection** r/t spread of organism throughout reproductive organs

See STD

Gout

Impaired physical **Mobility** r/t musculoskeletal impairment

Ineffective **Health** maintenance r/t deficient knowledge regarding medications and home care

Pain r/t inflammation of affected joint

Grand Mal Seizure

See Seizure Disorders

Grandiosity

Defensive **Coping** r/t inaccurate perception of self and abilities

Graves' Disease

See Hyperthyroidism

Grieving

Anticipatory **Grieving** r/t anticipated significant loss

Chronic **Sorrow** r/t unresolved grief

Dysfunctional **Grieving** r/t actual or perceived significant loss

Grieving r/t actual significant loss; change in life status, style, or function

Groom Self (Inability to)

Dressing/grooming **Self-care** deficit r/t intolerance to activity, decreased strength and endurance pain, dis-

G

comfort, perceptual or cognitive impairment, neuro-muscular impairment, musculoskeletal impairment, depression, severe anxiety

Growth and Development Lag

Delayed **Growth** and development r/t inadequate caretaking, indifference, inconsistent responsiveness, multiple caretakers, separation from significant others, environmental and stimulation deficiencies, effects of physical disability, prescribed dependence

PRENATAL

Risk for disproportionate **Growth** r/t congenital/genetic disorders, maternal nutrition, multiple gestation, teratogen exposure, substance use/abuse

INDIVIDUAL

Risk for disproportionate **Growth** r/t infection, prematurity, malnutrition, organic and inorganic factors, caregiver and/or individual maladaptive feeding behaviors, anorexia, insatiable appetite, infection, chronic illness, substance abuse

ENVIRONMENTAL

Risk for disproportionate **Growth** r/t deprivation, teratogen, lead poisoning, poverty, violence, natural disasters

See Developmental Concerns

Guillain-Barré Syndrome

Impaired spontaneous **Ventilation** r/t weak respiration muscles

See Neurological Disorders

Guilt

Anticipatory **Grieving** r/t potential loss of significant person, animal, prized material possession

Chronic **Sorrow** r/t unresolved grieving

Dysfunctional **Grieving** r/t actual loss of significant person, animal, prized material possession

Readiness for enhanced **Spiritual** well-being r/t desire to be in harmony with self, others, higher power/God

Risk for **Post-trauma** response r/t exaggerated sense of responsibility for traumatic event

Self-esteem disturbance r/t unmet expectations of self

H

Hair Loss

Disturbed **Body** image r/t psychological reaction to loss of hair

Imbalanced **Nutrition**: less than body requirements r/t inability to ingest food because of biological, psychological, economic factors

Halitosis

Impaired **Dentition** r/t ineffective oral hygiene

Impaired **Oral** mucous membranes r/t ineffective oral hygiene

Hallucinations

Acute **Confusion** r/t alcohol abuse, delirium, dementia, drug abuse

Adult **Failure** to thrive r/t altered mental status

Anxiety r/t threat to self-concept

Disturbed **Thought** processes r/t inability to control bizarre thoughts

Ineffective **Coping** r/t distortion and insecurity of life events

Risk for self- or other-directed **Violence** r/t catatonic excitement, manic excitement, rage/panic reactions, response to violent internal stimuli

Risk for **Self-mutilation** r/t command hallucinations

Head Injury

Acute **Confusion** r/t brain injury

Decreased **Intracranial** adaptive capacity r/t brain injury

Disturbed **Sensory** perception r/t pressure damage to sensory centers in brain

Disturbed **Thought** processes r/t pressure damage to brain

Ineffective **Breathing** pattern r/t pressure damage to breathing center in brain stem

Ineffective **Tissue** perfusion: cerebral r/t effects of increased intracranial pressure

See Neurological Disorders

Headache

Acute **Pain**: headache r/t lack of knowledge of pain control techniques or methods to prevent headaches

Disturbed **Energy** field r/t disharmony

Ineffective management of **Therapeutic** regimen r/t lack of knowledge, identification and elimination of aggravating factors

Health Maintenance Problems

Ineffective **Health** maintenance r/t significant alteration in communication skills, lack of ability to make deliberate and thoughtful judgments, perceptual or cognitive impairment, ineffective coping, dys-

H

functional grieving, unachieved developmental tasks, ineffective family coping, disabling spiritual distress, lack of material resources

Health-Seeking Person

Health-seeking behavior r/t expressed desire for increased control of own personal health

Hearing Impairment

Disturbed **Sensory** perception: auditory r/t altered state of auditory system

Impaired verbal **Communication** r/t inability to hear own voice

Social isolation r/t difficulty with communication

Heart Failure

See CHF

Heart Surgery

See Coronary Artery Bypass Grafting

Heartburn

Ineffective **Health** maintenance r/t deficient knowledge regarding information about factors that cause esophageal reflex

Nausea r/t gastrointestinal irritation

Pain: heartburn r/t gastroesophageal reflux

Risk for imbalanced **Nutrition**: less than body requirements r/t pain after eating

Heat Stroke

Deficient **Fluid** volume r/t profuse diaphoresis

Disturbed **Thought** processes r/t hyperthermia, increased oxygen needs

Hyperthermia r/t vigorous activity, hot environment

Helplessness

Chronic **Sorrow** r/t unresolved grief

Hopelessness r/t prolonged activity restriction creating isolation, failing or deteriorating physiological condition, long-term stress, abandonment, lost belief in transcendent values or higher power/God

Powerlessness r/t lifestyle of helplessness

Hematemesis

See GI Bleed

Hematological Disorder

Ineffective **Protection** r/t abnormal blood profile

See cause of Hematological Disorder

Hematuria

Risk for deficient **Fluid** volume r/t excessive loss of blood through urinary system

Hemianopia

Anxiety r/t change in vision

Disturbed **Sensory** perception r/t altered sensory reception, transmission, integration

Risk for **Injury** r/t disturbed sensory perception

Unilateral **Neglect** r/t effects of disturbed perceptual abilities

Hemiplegia

Anxiety r/t change in health status

Disturbed **Body** image r/t functional loss of one side of body

Impaired physical **Mobility** r/t loss of neurological control of involved extremities

Impaired **Transfer** ability r/t partial paralysis

Impaired **Walking** r/t loss of neurological control of involved extremities

Risk for impaired **Skin** integrity r/t alteration in sensation, immobility

Risk for **Injury** r/t impaired mobility

Risk for unilateral **Neglect** r/t neurological impairment; loss of sensation, vision, movement

Self-care deficit: specify r/t neuromuscular impairment

Unilateral **Neglect** r/t effects of disturbed perceptual abilities

See CVA

Hemodialysis

Excess **Fluid** volume r/t renal disease with minimal urine output

Ineffective **Coping** r/t situational crisis

Ineffective **Health** maintenance r/t deficient knowledge regarding hemodialysis procedure, restrictions, blood access care

Interrupted **Family** processes r/t changes in role responsibilities as a result of therapy regimen

Noncompliance: dietary restrictions r/t denial of chronic illness

Powerlessness r/t treatment regimen

Risk for **Caregiver** role strain r/t complexity of care receiver treatment

Risk for deficient **Fluid** volume r/t excessive removal of fluid during dialysis

Risk for **Infection** r/t exposure to blood products, risk for developing hepatitis B or C

Risk for **Injury**: clotting of blood access r/t abnormal surface for blood flow

See Renal Failure; Renal Failure, Acute/Chronic—Child

Hemodynamic Monitoring

Risk for **Infection** r/t invasive procedure

Risk for **Injury** r/t inadvertent wedging of catheter, dislodgement of catheter, disconnection of catheter with embolism

Hemolytic Uremic Syndrome

Deficient **Fluid** volume r/t vomiting, diarrhea

Impaired **Comfort**: nausea/vomiting r/t effects of uremia

Risk for impaired **Skin** integrity r/t diarrhea

Risk for **Injury** r/t decreased platelet count, seizure activity

See Hospitalized Child; Renal Failure, Acute/Chronic—Child

Hemophilia

Fear r/t high risk for AIDS secondary to contaminated blood products

Impaired physical **Mobility** r/t pain from acute bleeds, imposed activity restrictions

Ineffective **Health** maintenance r/t knowledge and skill acquisition regarding home administration of intravenous clotting factors, protection from injury

Ineffective **Protection** r/t deficient clotting factors

Pain r/t bleeding into body tissues

Risk for **Injury** r/t deficient clotting factors, child's developmental level, age-appropriate play, inappropriate use of toys or sports equipment

See Child with Chronic Condition; Hospitalized Child; Maturational Issues, Adolescent

Hemoptysis

Fear r/t serious threat to well-being

Risk for deficient **Fluid** volume r/t excessive loss of blood

Risk for ineffective **Airway** clearance r/t obstruction of airway with blood and mucus

Hemorrhage

Deficient **Fluid** volume r/t massive blood loss

Fear r/t threat to well-being

See cause of Hemorrhage; Hypovolemic Shock

Hemorrhoidectomy

Anxiety r/t embarrassment, need for privacy

Constipation r/t fear of pain with defecation

Ineffective **Health** maintenance r/t deficient knowledge regarding pain relief, use of stool softeners, dietary changes

Pain r/t surgical procedure

Risk for deficient **Fluid** volume: hemorrhage r/t inadequate clotting

Urinary retention r/t pain, anesthetic effect

Hemorrhoids

Constipation r/t painful defecation, poor bowel habits

Impaired **Comfort**: pruritus r/t inflammation of hemorrhoids

Ineffective **Health** maintenance r/t deficient knowledge regarding care of condition

Hemothorax

Deficient **Fluid** volume r/t blood in pleural space

See Pneumothorax

Hepatitis

Activity intolerance r/t weakness or fatigue secondary to infection

Acute **Pain** r/t edema of liver, bile irritating skin

Deficient **Diversional** activity r/t isolation

Fatigue r/t infectious process, altered body chemistry

Imbalanced **Nutrition**: less than body requirements r/t anorexia, impaired use of proteins and carbohydrates

Ineffective **Health** maintenance r/t deficient knowledge regarding disease process and home management

Risk for deficient **Fluid** volume r/t excessive loss of fluids via vomiting and diarrhea

Social isolation r/t treatment-imposed isolation

Hernia

See Hiatus Hernia; Inguinal Hernia Repair

Herniated Disk

See Low Back Pain

Herniorrhaphy

See Inguinal Hernia Repair

Herpes in Pregnancy

Fear r/t threat to fetus, impending surgery

Impaired **Tissue** integrity r/t active herpes lesion

Impaired **Urinary** elimination r/t pain with urination

Ineffective **Health** maintenance r/t deficient knowledge regarding treatment of disease, protection of fetus

Pain r/t active herpes lesion

Risk for **Infection** transmission r/t transplacental transfer during primary herpes, exposure to active herpes during birth process

H

Situational low **Self-esteem** r/t threat to fetus secondary to disease process

Herpes Simplex I

Impaired **Dentition** r/t impaired oral mucous membranes

Impaired **Oral** mucous membranes r/t inflammatory changes in mouth

Herpes Simplex II

Acute **Pain** r/t active herpes lesion

Impaired **Tissue** integrity r/t active herpes lesion

Impaired **Urinary** elimination r/t pain with urination

Ineffective **Health** maintenance r/t deficient knowledge regarding treatment, prevention of spread of disease

Sexual dysfunction r/t disease process

Situational low **Self-esteem** r/t expressions of shame or guilt

Herpes Zoster

See Shingles

HHNC

See Hyperosmolar Hyperglycemic Nonketotic Coma

Hiatus Hernia

Imbalanced **Nutrition**: less than body requirements r/t pain after eating

Ineffective **Health** maintenance r/t deficient knowledge regarding care of disease

Nausea r/t effects of gastric contents in esophagus

Pain: heartburn r/t gastroesophageal reflux

Hip Fracture

Acute **Confusion** r/t sensory overload, sensory deprivation, medication side effects

Acute **Pain** r/t injury, surgical procedure

Constipation r/t immobility, narcotics, anesthesia

Fear r/t outcome of treatment, future mobility, present helplessness

Impaired physical **Mobility** r/t surgical incision, temporary absence of weight bearing

Impaired **Transfer** ability r/t immobilization of hip

Impaired **Walking** r/t temporary absence of weight bearing

Powerlessness r/t health care environment

Risk for deficient **Fluid** volume: hemorrhage r/t postoperative complication, surgical blood loss

Risk for impaired **Skin** integrity r/t immobility

Risk for **Infection** r/t invasive procedure

Risk for **Injury** r/t dislodged prosthesis, unsteadiness when ambulating

Risk for perioperative positioning **Injury** r/t immobilization, muscle weakness, emaciation

Self-care deficit: specify r/t musculoskeletal impairment

Hip Replacement

See Total Joint Replacement

Hirschsprung's Disease

Acute **Pain** r/t distended colon, incisional postoperative pain

Constipation: bowel obstruction r/t inhibited peristalsis secondary to congenital absence of parasympathetic ganglion cells in distal colon

Grieving r/t loss of perfect child, birth of child with congenital defect even though child expected to be normal within 2 years

Imbalanced **Nutrition**: less than body requirements r/t anorexia, pain from distended colon

Impaired **Skin** integrity r/t stoma, potential skin care problems associated with stoma

Ineffective **Health** maintenance r/t parental deficient knowledge regarding temporary stoma care, dietary management, treatment for constipation or diarrhea

See Hospitalized Child

Hirsutism

Disturbed **Body** image r/t excessive hair

Hitting Behavior

Acute **Confusion** r/t dementia, alcohol abuse, drug abuse, delirium

Impaired **Adjustment** r/t intense emotional state

Ineffective **Coping** r/t situational crises, maturational crises, personal vulnerability

Risk for other-directed **Violence** r/t history of violence, neurological impairment, cognitive impairment, history of childhood abuse, history of witnessing family violence, cruelty to animals, firesetting, history of alcohol/drug abuse, pathological intoxication, psychotic symptomatology, motor vehicle offenses, impulsivity, availability or possession of weapon, body language

HIV (Human Immunodeficiency Virus)

Fear r/t possible death

Ineffective **Protection** r/t depressed immune system

See AIDS

Hodgkin's Disease

See Anemia; Cancer

Home Maintenance Problems

Impaired **Home** maintenance r/t individual or family member disease or injury, insufficient family organization or planning, insufficient finances, unfamiliarity with neighborhood resources, impaired cognitive or emotional functioning, lack of knowledge, lack of role modeling, inadequate support systems

Homelessness

Impaired **Home** maintenance r/t impaired cognitive or emotional functioning, inadequate support system, insufficient finances

Powerlessness r/t interpersonal interactions

Risk for **Trauma** r/t being in high-crime neighborhood

Hopelessness

Chronic **Sorrow** r/t unresolved grief

Hopelessness r/t prolonged activity restriction creating isolation, failing or deteriorating physiological condition, long-term stress, abandonment, lost belief in transcendent values or higher power/God

Powerlessness r/t lifestyle of helplessness

Hospitalized Child

Activity intolerance r/t fatigue associated with acute illness

Anxiety: separation (child) r/t familiar surroundings and separation from family and friends

Compromised family **Coping** r/t possible prolonged hospitalization that exhausts supportive capacity of significant people

Deficient **Diversional** activity r/t immobility, monotonous environment, frequent or lengthy treatments, reluctance to participate, therapeutic isolation, separation from peers

Delayed **Growth** and development r/t regression or lack of progression toward developmental milestones secondary to frequent or prolonged hospitalization, inadequate or inappropriate stimulation, cerebral insult, chronic illness, effects of physical disability, prescribed dependence

Disturbed **Sleep** pattern: child or parent r/t 24-hour care needs of hospitalization

Fear r/t deficient knowledge or maturational level with fear of unknown, mutilation, painful procedures, surgery

Hopelessness: child r/t prolonged activity restriction, uncertain prognosis

Ineffective **Coping**: parent r/t possible guilt regarding hospitalization of child, parental inadequacies

Interrupted **Family** processes r/t situational crisis of illness, disease, hospitalization

Pain r/t treatments, diagnostic or therapeutic procedures

Powerlessness: child r/t health care environment, illness-related regimen

Readiness for enhanced family **Coping** r/t impact of crisis on family values, priorities, goals, relationships in family

Risk for impaired parent/child **Attachment** r/t separation

Risk for delayed **Growth** and development: regression r/t disruption of normal routine, unfamiliar environment or caregivers, developmental vulnerability of young children

Risk for imbalanced **Nutrition**: less than body requirements r/t anorexia, absence of familiar foods, cultural preferences

Risk for **Injury** r/t unfamiliar environment, developmental age, lack of parental knowledge regarding safety (e.g., side rails, IV site/pole)

Hostile Behavior

Risk for self- or other-directed **Violence** r/t antisocial personality disorder

HTN (Hypertension)

Disturbed **Energy** field r/t pain, discomfort

Imbalanced **Nutrition**: more than body requirements r/t lack of knowledge of relationship between diet and disease process

Ineffective **Health** maintenance r/t deficient knowledge regarding treatment and control of disease process

Noncompliance r/t side effects of treatments, lack of understanding regarding importance of controlling hypertension

Human Immunodeficiency Virus

See AIDS; HIV

Hydrocele

Ineffective **Sexuality** pattern r/t recent surgery on area of scrotum

Pain r/t severely enlarged hydrocele

Hydrocephalus

Decisional **Conflict**: cerebral ventricles r/t unclear or conflicting values regarding selection of treatment modality

H

Delayed **Growth** and development r/t sequelae of increased intracranial pressure

Excess **Fluid** volume: cerebral ventricles r/t compromised regulatory mechanism

Imbalanced **Nutrition**: less than body requirements r/t inadequate intake secondary to anorexia, nausea, vomiting, feeding difficulties

Impaired **Skin** (tissue) integrity r/t impaired physical mobility, mechanical irritation

Ineffective **Tissue** perfusion: cerebral r/t interrupted flow, hypervolemia of cerebral ventricles

Interrupted **Family** processes r/t situational crisis

Risk for delayed **Development** r/t sequelae of increased intracranial pressure

Risk for disproportionate **Growth** r/t sequelae of increased intracranial pressure

Risk for **Infection** r/t sequelae of invasive procedure (shunt placement)

See Child with Chronic Condition; Hospitalized Child; Mental Retardation (if appropriate); Premature Infant

Hygiene, Inability to Provide Own

Adult **Failure** to thrive r/t depression, apathy as evidenced by inability to perform self-care

Bathing/hygiene **Self-care** deficit r/t intolerance to activity, decreased strength and endurance, pain, discomfort, perceptual or cognitive impairment, neuromuscular impairment, musculoskeletal impairment, depression, severe anxiety

Hyperactive Syndrome

Compromised family **Coping** r/t unsuccessful strategies to control excessive activity, behaviors, frustration, anger

Decisional **Conflict** r/t multiple or divergent sources of information regarding education, nutrition, medication regimens; willingness to change own food habits; limited resources

Impaired **Social** interaction r/t impulsive and overactive behaviors, concomitant emotional difficulties, distractibility and excitability

Ineffective **Role** performance: parent r/t stressors associated with dealing with hyperactive child, perceived or projected blame for causes of child's behavior, unmet needs for support or care, lack of energy to provide for those needs

Parental role **Conflict**: when siblings present r/t increased attention toward hyperactive child

Risk for delayed **Development** r/t behavior disorders

Risk for impaired **Parenting** r/t disruptive or uncontrollable behaviors of child

Risk for **Violence**: parent or child r/t frustration with disruptive behavior, anger, unsuccessful relationship(s)

Self-esteem disturbance/chronic low **Self-esteem** r/t inability to achieve socially acceptable behaviors; frustration; frequent reprimands, punishment, or scoldings secondary to uncontrolled activity and behaviors; mood fluctuations and restlessness; inability to succeed academically; lack of peer support

Hyperalimentation

See TPN

Hyperbilirubinemia

Anxiety: parent r/t threat to infant, unknown future

Disturbed **Sensory** perception: visual (infant) r/t use of eye patches for protection of eyes during phototherapy

Imbalanced **Nutrition**: less than body requirements (infant) r/t disinterest in feeding because of jaundice-related lethargy

Parental role **Conflict** r/t interruption of family life because of care regimen

Risk for disproportionate **Growth**: infant r/t disinterest in feeding because of jaundice-related lethargy

Risk for **Imbalanced** body temperature: infant r/t phototherapy

Risk for **Injury**: infant r/t kernicterus, phototherapy lights

Hypercalcemia

Decreased **Cardiac** output r/t bradydysrhythmia

Disturbed **Thought** processes r/t elevated calcium levels that cause paranoia, decreased level of consciousness

Imbalanced **Nutrition**: less than body requirements r/t gastrointestinal manifestations of hypercalcemia (nausea, anorexia, ileus)

Impaired physical **Mobility** r/t decreased tone in smooth and striated muscle

Risk for **Trauma** r/t risk for fractures

Hypercapnia

Fear r/t difficulty breathing

Impaired **Gas** exchange r/t ventilation perfusion imbalance

Hyperemesis Gravidarum

Anxiety r/t threat to self and infant, hospitalization

Deficient **Fluid** volume r/t vomiting

Imbalanced **Nutrition**: less than body requirements r/t vomiting

H

Impaired **Home** maintenance r/t chronic nausea, inability to function

Nausea r/t hormonal changes of pregnancy

Powerlessness r/t health care regimen

Social isolation r/t hospitalization

Hyperglycemia

Ineffective management of **Therapeutic** regimen r/t complexity of therapeutic regimen, decisional conflicts, economic difficulties, nonsupportive family, insufficient cues to action, deficient knowledge, mistrust, lack of acknowledgment of seriousness of condition

See Diabetes Mellitus

Hyperkalemia

Risk for **Activity** intolerance r/t muscle weakness

Risk for decreased **Cardiac** output r/t possible dysrhythmia

Risk for excess **Fluid** volume r/t untreated renal failure

Hypernatremia

Risk for deficient **Fluid** volume r/t abnormal water loss, inadequate water intake

Hyperosmolar Hyperglycemic Nonketotic Coma (HHNC)

Deficient **Fluid** volume r/t polyuria, inadequate fluid intake

Disturbed **Thought** processes r/t dehydration, electrolyte imbalance

Risk for **Injury**: seizures r/t hyperosmolar state, electrolyte imbalance

See Diabetes

Hypersensitivity to Slight Criticism

Defensive **Coping** r/t situational crisis, psychological impairment, substance abuse

Hypertension

Imbalanced **Nutrition**: more than body requirements r/t lack of knowledge of relationship between diet and disease process

Ineffective **Health** maintenance r/t deficient knowledge regarding treatment and control of disease process

Noncompliance r/t side effects of treatment

Hyperthermia

Hyperthermia r/t exposure to hot environment, vigorous activity, medications, anesthesia, inappropriate clothing, increased metabolic rate, illness, trauma, dehydration, inability or decreased ability to perspire

Hyperthyroidism

Activity intolerance r/t increased oxygen demands from increased metabolic rate

Anxiety r/t increased stimulation, loss of control

Diarrhea r/t increased gastric motility

Disturbed **Sleep** pattern r/t anxiety, excessive sympathetic discharge

Imbalanced **Nutrition**: less than body requirements r/t increased metabolic rate, increased gastrointestinal activity

Ineffective **Health** maintenance r/t deficient knowledge regarding medications, methods of coping with stress

Risk for **Injury**: eye damage r/t exophthalmos

Hyperventilation

Ineffective **Breathing** pattern r/t anxiety, acid-base imbalance

Hypocalcemia

Activity intolerance r/t neuromuscular irritability

Imbalanced **Nutrition**: less than body requirements r/t effects of vitamin D deficiency, renal failure, malabsorption, laxative use

Ineffective **Breathing** pattern r/t laryngospasm

Hypoglycemia

Disturbed **Thought** processes r/t insufficient blood glucose to brain

Imbalanced **Nutrition**: less than body requirements r/t imbalance of glucose and insulin level

Ineffective **Health** maintenance r/t deficient knowledge regarding disease process, self-care

See Diabetes

Hypokalemia

Activity intolerance r/t muscle weakness

Decreased **Cardiac** output r/t possible dysrhythmia from electrolyte imbalance

Hypomania

Disturbed **Sleep** pattern r/t psychological stimulus

See Manic Disorder

Hyponatremia

Disturbed **Thought** processes r/t electrolyte imbalance

Excess **Fluid** volume r/t excessive intake of hypotonic fluids

Risk for **Injury** r/t seizures, new onset of confusion

H

Hypoplastic Left Lung

See Congenital Heart Disease/Cardiac Anomalies

Hypotension

Decreased **Cardiac** output r/t decreased preload, decreased contractility

Disturbed **Thought** processes r/t decreased oxygen supply to brain

Ineffective **Tissue** perfusion: cardiopulmonary/ peripheral r/t hypovolemia, decreased contractility, decreased afterload

Risk for deficient **Fluid** volume r/t excessive fluid loss

See cause of Hypotension

Hypothermia

Hypothermia r/t exposure to cold environment, illness, trauma, damage to hypothalamus, malnutrition, aging

Hypothyroidism

Activity intolerance r/t muscular stiffness, shortness of breath on exertion

Constipation r/t decreased gastric motility

Disturbed **Thought** processes r/t altered metabolic process

Imbalanced **Nutrition**: more than body requirements r/t decreased metabolic process

Impaired **Gas** exchange r/t possible respiratory depression

Impaired **Skin** integrity r/t edema, dry or scaly skin

Ineffective **Health** maintenance r/t deficient knowledge regarding disease process and self-care

Hypovolemic Shock

See Shock

Hypoxia

Acute **Confusion** r/t decreased oxygen supply to brain

Disturbed **Thought** processes r/t decreased oxygen supply to brain

Fear r/t breathlessness

Impaired **Gas** exchange r/t altered oxygen supply, inability to transport oxygen

Impaired **Memory** r/t hypoxia

Ineffective **Airway** clearance r/t decreased energy and fatigue, increased secretions

Hysterectomy

Acute **Pain** r/t surgical injury

Anticipatory **Grieving** r/t change in body image, loss of reproductive status

Constipation r/t opioids, anesthesia, bowel manipulation during surgery

Ineffective **Coping** r/t situational crisis of surgery

Ineffective **Health** maintenance r/t deficient knowledge regarding precautions and self-care following surgery

Risk for **Constipation** r/t narcotics, anesthesia, bowel manipulation during surgery

Risk for deficient **Fluid** volume r/t abnormal blood loss, hemorrhage

Risk for ineffective **Tissue** perfusion r/t thromboembolism

Risk for urge urinary **Incontinence** r/t edema in area, anesthesia, narcotics, pain

Risk for **Urinary** retention r/t edema in area, anesthesia, opioids, pain

Sexual dysfunction r/t disturbance in self-concept

See Surgery

I

IBS (Irritable Bowel Syndrome)

Chronic **Pain** r/t spasms, increased motility of bowel

Constipation r/t low-residue diet, stress

Diarrhea r/t increased motility of intestines associated with stress

Ineffective **Health** maintenance r/t deficient knowledge regarding self-care with IBS

Ineffective **Therapeutic** regimen management r/t deficient knowledge, powerlessness

Readiness for Enhanced **Therapeutic** regimen management r/t an expressed desire to manage illness and prevention of symptoms

See Inflammatory Bowel Disease

IDDM (Insulin-Dependent Diabetes)

See Diabetes Mellitus

Identity Disturbance

Disturbed personal **Identity** r/t situational crisis, psychological impairment, chronic illness, pain

Readiness for enhanced **Coping** r/t seeking social support

Spiritual distress r/t expression of alienation from others

Idiopathic Thrombocytopenic Purpura

See ITP

Ileal Conduit

Deficient **Knowledge** r/t care of stoma

Disturbed **Body** image r/t presence of stoma

Ineffective **Sexuality** patterns r/t altered body function and structure

Ineffective **Therapeutic** regimen management r/t new skills required to care for appliance and self

Readiness for enhanced **Therapeutic** regimen management r/t expressed desire to care for stoma

Risk for impaired **Skin** integrity r/t difficulty obtaining tight seal of appliance

Risk for natural rubber latex **Allergy** response r/t repeated exposures to latex associated with treatment and management of disease

Social isolation r/t alteration in physical appearance, fear of accidental spill of ostomy contents

Ileostomy

Ineffective **Sexuality** patterns r/t altered body function and structure

Chronic **Sorrow** r/t physical changes associated with presence of stoma

Constipation/Diarrhea r/t dietary changes, change in intestinal motility

Deficient **Knowledge** r/t limited practice of stoma care, dietary modifications

Disturbed **Body** image r/t presence of stoma

Ineffective **Therapeutic** regimen management r/t new skills required to care for appliance and self

Readiness for enhanced **Coping** r/t readiness for enhanced **Therapeutic** regimen management

Risk for impaired **Skin** integrity r/t difficulty obtaining tight seal of appliance, caustic drainage

Social isolation r/t alteration in physical appearance, fear of accidental spill of ostomy contents

Ileus

Acute **Pain** r/t pressure, abdominal distention

Constipation r/t decreased gastric motility

Deficient **Fluid** volume r/t loss of fluids from vomiting, fluids trapped in bowel

Nausea r/t gastrointestinal irritation

Immobility

Adult **Failure** to thrive r/t limited physical mobility

Constipation r/t immobility

Disturbed **Thought** process r/t sensory deprivation from immobility

Impaired physical **Mobility** r/t medically imposed bedrest

Impaired **Transfer** ability r/t limited physical mobility

Impaired **Walking** r/t limited physical mobility

Ineffective **Breathing** pattern r/t inability to deep-breathe in supine position

Ineffective **Tissue** perfusion: peripheral r/t interruption of venous flow

Powerlessness r/t forced immobility from health care environment

Risk for **Disuse** syndrome r/t immobilization

Risk for impaired **Skin** integrity r/t pressure on immobile parts, shearing forces when moving

Immunosuppression

Ineffective **Protection** r/t medications/treatments suppressing immune system function

Risk for **Infection** r/t immunosuppression

Impaction of Stool

Constipation r/t decreased fluid intake, less than adequate amounts of fiber and bulk-forming foods in diet, immobility

Readiness for enhanced **Therapeutic** regimen management r/t to appropriate nutritional choices to prevent constipation

Imperforate Anus

Anxiety r/t ability to care for newborn

Deficient **Knowledge** r/t home care for newborn

Impaired **Skin** integrity r/t pruritus

Risk for impaired **Skin** integrity r/t presence of stool at surgical repair site

Impetigo

Ineffective **Health** maintenance r/t parental deficient knowledge regarding care of impetigo

See Communicable Diseases, Childhood

Impotence

Readiness for enhanced **Knowledge** of treatment information for erectile dysfunction

Self-esteem disturbance r/t physiological crisis, inability to practice usual sexual activity

Sexual dysfunction r/t altered body function

Inactivity

Impaired physical **Mobility** r/t intolerance to activity, decreased strength and endurance, depression, severe anxiety, musculoskeletal impairment, perceptual or cognitive impairment, neuromuscular impairment, pain, discomfort

Risk for **Constipation** r/t insufficient physical activity

Incompetent Cervix

See Premature Dilation of the Cervix

Incontinence of Stool

Bowel incontinence r/t decreased awareness of need to defecate, loss of sphincter control

Deficient **Knowledge** r/t lack of information on normal bowel elimination

Disturbed **Body** image r/t inability to control elimination of stool

Risk for impaired **Skin** integrity r/t presence of stool

Situational low **Self-esteem** r/t inability to control elimination of stool

Toileting **Self-care** deficit r/t toileting needs

Incontinence of Urine

Functional **Incontinence** r/t altered environment; sensory, cognitive, or mobility deficits

Reflex **Incontinence** r/t neurological impairment

Risk for impaired **Skin** integrity r/t presence of urine

Risk for urge urinary **Incontinence** r/t effects of alcohol, caffeine, decreased bladder capacity, irritation of bladder stretch receptors causing spasm, increased urine concentration, overdistention of bladder

Self-care deficit: toileting r/t toileting needs

Situational low **Self-esteem** r/t inability to control passage of urine

Stress urinary **Incontinence** r/t degenerative change in pelvic muscles and structural supports associated with increased age, high intraabdominal pressure (e.g., from obesity, gravid uterus), incompetent bladder outlet, overdistention between voidings, weak pelvic muscles and structural supports

Total urinary **Incontinence** r/t neuropathy preventing transmission of reflex indicating bladder fullness, neurological dysfunction causing triggering of micturition at unpredictable times, independent contraction of detrusor reflex resulting from surgery, trauma or disease affecting spinal cord nerves, anatomical fistula

Urge urinary **Incontinence** r/t decreased bladder capacity (i.e., history of pelvic inflammatory disease, abdominal surgeries, indwelling urinary catheter), irritation of bladder stretch receptors causing spasm (e.g., bladder infection), alcohol, caffeine, increased fluids, increased urine concentration, overdistention of bladder

Indigestion

Imbalanced **Nutrition**: less than body requirements r/t discomfort when eating

Impaired **Comfort** r/t burning, bloating, heaviness, unpleasant sensations experienced when eating

Nausea r/t gastrointestinal irritation

Induction of Labor

Anxiety r/t medical interventions

Decisional **Conflict** r/t perceived threat to idealized birth

Ineffective **Coping** r/t situational crisis of medical intervention in birthing process

Readiness for enhanced **Family** processes r/t family support during induction of labor

Risk for imbalanced **Fluid** volume r/t intravenous fluid therapy

Risk for **Injury**: maternal and fetal r/t hypertonic uterus, potential prematurity of newborn

Self-esteem disturbance r/t inability to carry out normal labor

Infant Apnea

See Premature Infant; Respiratory Conditions of the Neonate; SIDS

Infant Behavior

Disorganized **Infant** behavior r/t pain, oral/motor problems, feeding intolerance, environmental overstimulation, lack of containment/boundaries, prematurity, invasive/painful procedures

Readiness for enhanced organized **Infant** behavior r/t prematurity, pain

Risk for disorganized **Infant** behavior r/t pain, oral/motor problems, environmental overstimulation, lack of containment/boundaries

Infant Feeding Pattern, Ineffective

Disorganized **Infant** behavior r/t prematurity, immature neurological system

Impaired **Swallowing** r/t prematurity

Ineffective **Infant** feeding pattern r/t prematurity, neurological impairment or delay, oral hypersensitivity, prolonged NPO

Risk for imbalanced **Fluid** volume r/t intravenous fluid therapy, inadequate intake or absorption of fluids, regurgitation

Infant of Diabetic Mother

Deficient **Fluid** volume r/t increased urinary excretion and osmotic diuresis

Delayed **Growth** and development r/t prolonged and severe postnatal hypoglycemia

Imbalanced **Nutrition**: less than body requirements r/t hypotonia, lethargy, poor sucking, postnatal metabolic changes from hyperglycemia to hypoglycemia and hyperinsulinism

Risk for decreased **Cardiac** output r/t increased incidence of cardiomegaly

Risk for delayed **Development** r/t prolonged and severe postnatal hypoglycemia

Risk for disproportionate **Growth** r/t prolonged and severe postnatal hypoglycemia

Risk for impaired **Gas** exchange r/t increased incidence of cardiomegaly, prematurity

See Premature Infant; Respiratory Conditions of the Neonate

Infant of Substance-Abusing Mother (Fetal Alcohol Syndrome, Crack Baby, Other Drug Withdrawal Infants)

Delayed **Growth** and development r/t effects of maternal use of drugs, effects of neurological impairment, decreased attentiveness to environmental stimuli or inadequate stimuli

Diarrhea r/t effects of withdrawal, increased peristalsis secondary to hyperirritability

Disturbed **Sensory** perception r/t hypersensitivity to environmental stimuli

Disturbed **Sleep** pattern r/t hyperirritability/ hypersensitivity to environmental stimuli

Imbalanced **Nutrition**: less than body requirements r/t feeding problems; uncoordinated or ineffective suck and swallow; effects of diarrhea, vomiting, or colic associated with maternal substance abuse

Impaired **Parenting** r/t impaired or absent attachment behaviors, inadequate support systems

Ineffective **Airway** clearance r/t pooling of secretions secondary to lack of adequate cough reflex, effects of viral or bacterial lower airway infection secondary to altered protective state

Ineffective **Infant** feeding pattern r/t uncoordinated or ineffective sucking reflex

Ineffective **Protection** r/t effects of maternal substance abuse

Interrupted **Breastfeeding** r/t use of drugs or alcohol by mother

Risk for delayed **Development** r/t substance abuse

Risk for disproportionate **Growth** r/t substance abuse

Risk for **Infection**: skin, meningeal, respiratory r/t effects of withdrawal

See Cerebral Palsy; Failure to Thrive, Nonorganic; Hospitalized Child; Hyperactive Syndrome; SIDS

Infantile Spasms

See Seizure Disorders, Childhood

Infection

Hyperthermia r/t increased metabolic rate

Ineffective **Protection** r/t inadequate nutrition, abnormal blood profiles, drug therapies, treatments

Infection, Potential for

Risk for **Infection** r/t inadequate primary defenses (e.g., broken skin, traumatized tissue, decrease in ciliary action, stasis of body fluids, change in pH secretions, altered peristalsis), inadequate secondary defenses (e.g., decreased hemoglobin, leukopenia suppressed inflammatory response), immunosuppression, inadequate acquired immunity, tissue destruction and increased environmental exposure, chronic disease, invasive procedures, malnutrition, pharmaceutical agents, trauma, rupture of amniotic membranes, insufficient knowledge to avoid exposure to pathogens

Infertility

Chronic **Sorrow** r/t inability to conceive a child

Ineffective **Therapeutic** regimen management r/t deficient knowledge about infertility

Powerlessness r/t infertility

Risk for **Powerlessness** r/t inability to conceive a child

Spiritual distress r/t inability to conceive a child

Inflammatory Bowel Disease (Child and Adult)

Acute **Pain** r/t abdominal cramping and anal irritation

Deficient **Fluid** volume r/t frequent and loose stools

Diarrhea r/t effects of inflammatory changes of the bowel

Imbalanced **Nutrition**: less than body requirements r/t anorexia, decreased absorption of nutrients from gastrointestinal tract

Impaired **Skin** integrity r/t frequent stools, development of anal fissures

Ineffective **Coping** r/t repeated episodes of diarrhea

Social isolation r/t diarrhea

See Child with Chronic Condition; Crohn's Disease; Hospitalized Child; Maturational Issues, Adolescent

Influenza

Acute **Pain** r/t inflammatory changes in joints

Deficient **Fluid** volume r/t inadequate fluid intake

Hyperthermia r/t infectious process

Ineffective **Health** maintenance r/t deficient knowledge regarding self-care

Ineffective **Therapeutic** regimen management r/t lack of knowledge regarding preventive immunizations

Readiness for enhanced **Knowledge** of information to prevent influenza

I

Inguinal Hernia Repair

Acute **Pain** r/t surgical procedure

Impaired physical **Mobility** r/t pain at surgical site and fear of causing hernia to "break open"

Risk for **Infection** r/t surgical procedure

Urinary retention r/t possible edema at surgical site

Injury

Risk for **Falls** r/t orthostatic hypertension, impaired physical mobility, diminished mental status

Risk for **Injury** r/t environmental conditions interacting with client's adaptive and defensive resources

Insomnia

Anxiety r/t actual or perceived loss of sleep

Disturbed **Sleep** pattern r/t sensory alterations, internal factors, external factors

Sleep deprivation r/t sustained inadequate sleep hygiene, prolonged use of pharmacological agents, aging-related sleep stage shifts

Insulin Shock

See Hypoglycemia

Intermittent Claudication

Acute **Pain** r/t decreased circulation to extremities with activity

Deficient **Knowledge** r/t lack of knowledge of cause and treatment of peripheral vascular diseases

Ineffective **Tissue** perfusion: peripheral r/t interruption of arterial flow

Readiness for enhanced **Knowledge** of prevention of pain and impaired circulation

Risk for **Injury** r/t tissue hypoxia

Risk for **Peripheral** neurovascular dysfunction r/t disruption in arterial flow

See Peripheral Vascular Disease

Internal Cardioverter Defibrillator

See AICD

Internal Fixation

Impaired **Walking** r/t repair of fracture

Risk for **Infection** r/t traumatized tissue, broken skin

See Fracture

Interstitial Cystitis

Acute **Pain** r/t inflammatory process

Impaired **Urinary** elimination r/t inflammation of bladder

Risk for **Infection** r/t suppressed inflammatory response

Risk for urge urinary **Incontinence** r/t effects of alcohol, caffeine, decreased bladder capacity, irritation of bladder stretch receptors causing spasm, increased urine concentration, overdistention of bladder

Intervertebral Disk Excision

See Laminectomy

Intestinal Obstruction

See Ileus

Intoxication

Acute **Confusion** r/t alcohol abuse

Anxiety r/t loss of control of actions

Disturbed **Sensory** perception r/t neurochemical imbalance in brain

Disturbed **Thought** processes r/t effect of substance on central nervous system

Impaired **Memory** fluid and electrolyte imbalance

Ineffective **Coping** r/t use of mind-altering substances as a means of coping

Risk for **Falls** r/t diminished mental status

Risk for other-directed **Violence** r/t inability to control thoughts and actions

Intraaortic Balloon Counterpulsation

Anxiety r/t device providing cardiovascular assistance

Compromised family **Coping** r/t seriousness of significant other's medical condition

Decreased **Cardiac** output r/t failing heart needing counterpulsation

Impaired physical **Mobility** r/t restriction of movement because of mechanical device

Risk for **Peripheral** neurovascular dysfunction r/t vascular obstruction of balloon catheter, thrombus formation, emboli, edema

Intracranial Pressure, Increased

Acute **Confusion** r/t increased intracranial pressure

Adult **Failure** to thrive r/t undetected changes from increased intracranial pressure

Decreased **Intracranial** adaptive capacity r/t sustained increase in intracranial pressure (10 to 15 mm Hg)

Disturbed **Sensory** perception r/t pressure damage to sensory centers in brain

Disturbed **Thought** processes r/t pressure damage to brain

Impaired **Memory** r/t neurological disturbance

Ineffective **Breathing** pattern r/t pressure damage to breathing center in brain stem

Ineffective **Tissue** perfusion: cerebral r/t effects of increased intracranial pressure

See cause of Increased Intracranial Pressure

Intrauterine Growth Retardation

Anxiety: maternal r/t threat to fetus

Delayed **Growth** and development r/t insufficient supply of oxygen and nutrients

Imbalanced **Nutrition**: less than body requirements r/t insufficient placenta

Impaired **Gas** exchange r/t insufficient placental perfusion

Ineffective **Coping**: maternal r/t situational crisis, threat to fetus

Risk for delayed **Development** r/t insufficient supply of oxygen and nutrients

Risk for disproportionate **Growth** r/t insufficient supply of oxygen and nutrients

Risk for **Injury** r/t insufficient supply of oxygen and nutrients

Risk for **Powerlessness** r/t unknown outcome of fetus

Situational low **Self-esteem**: maternal r/t guilt about threat to fetus

Spiritual distress r/t unknown outcome of fetus

Intubation—Endotracheal or Nasogastric

Disturbed **Body** image r/t altered appearance with mechanical devices

Imbalanced **Nutrition**: less than body requirements r/t inability to ingest food resulting from presence of tubes

Impaired **Oral** mucous membrane r/t presence of tubes

Impaired verbal **Communication** r/t endotracheal tube

Irregular Pulse

See Dysrhythmia

Irritable Bowel Syndrome

See IBS

Isolation

Adult **Failure** to thrive r/t depression

Risk for **Loneliness** r/t lack of affection, physical isolation, cathectic deprivation, social isolation

Risk for situational low **Self-esteem** r/t decreased power, control over environment

Social isolation r/t factors contributing to absence of satisfying personal relationships, such as delay in accomplishing developmental tasks, immature interests,

alterations in mental status, unacceptable social behavior, unacceptable social values, altered state of wellness, inadequate personal resources, inability to engage in satisfying personal relationships

Itching

Impaired **Comfort** r/t irritation of the skin

Risk for **Infection** r/t potential break in skin

ITP (Idiopathic Thrombocytopenic Purpura)

Deficient **Diversional** activity r/t activity restrictions, safety precautions

Impaired **Home** health maintenance r/t parental lack of ability to follow through with safety precautions secondary to child's developmental stage (active toddler)

Ineffective **Protection** r/t decreased platelet count

Risk for **Injury** r/t decreased platelet count, developmental level, age-appropriate play

See Hospitalized Child

J

Jaundice

Disturbed **Thought** processes r/t toxic blood metabolites

Impaired **Comfort**: pruritus r/t toxic metabolites excreted in the skin

Risk for impaired **Skin** integrity r/t pruritus, itching

See Cirrhosis

Jaw Surgery

Acute **Pain** r/t surgical procedure

Deficient **Knowledge** r/t emergency care for wired jaws (e.g., cutting bands and wires), oral care

Imbalanced **Nutrition**: less than body requirements r/t jaws wired closed

Impaired **Swallowing** r/t edema from surgery

Risk for **Aspiration** r/t wired jaws

Jittery

Anxiety r/t unconscious conflict about essential values and goals, threat to or change in health status

Death **Anxiety** r/t unresolved issues relating to end of life

Risk for **Post-trauma** syndrome r/t occupation, survivor's role in event, inadequate social support

Jock Itch

Ineffective **Therapeutic** regimen management r/t prevention and treatment

See Itching

Joint Replacement

Risk for **Peripheral** neurovascular dysfunction r/t orthopedic surgery

See Total Joint Replacement

JRA (Juvenile Rheumatoid Arthritis)

See Rheumatoid Arthritis, Juvenile

K

Kaposi's Sarcoma

See AIDS

Kawasaki Syndrome (Formerly Mucocutaneous Lymph Node Syndrome)

Acute **Pain** r/t enlarged lymph nodes; erythematous skin rash that progresses to desquamation, peeling, denuding of skin

Anxiety: parental r/t progression of disease, complications of arthritis and cardiac involvement

Hyperthermia r/t inflammatory disease process

Imbalanced **Nutrition**: less than body requirements r/t impaired oral mucous membrane

Impaired **Oral** mucous membrane r/t inflamed mouth and pharynx; swollen lips that become dry, cracked, fissured

Impaired **Skin** integrity r/t inflammatory skin changes

See Hospitalized Child

Kegel Exercise

Health-seeking behavior r/t desire for information to relieve incontinence

Risk for urge urinary **Incontinence** r/t effects of alcohol, caffeine, decreased bladder capacity, irritation of bladder stretch receptors causing spasm, increased urine concentration, overdistention of bladder

Stress urinary **Incontinence** r/t degenerative change in pelvic muscles

Urge urinary **Incontinence** r/t decreased bladder capacity

Ketoacidosis

Deficient **Fluid** volume r/t excess excretion of urine, nausea, vomiting, increased respiration

Imbalanced **Nutrition**: less than body requirements r/t body's inability to use nutrients

Impaired **Memory** r/t fluid and electrolyte imbalance

Ineffective **Therapeutic** regimen management r/t denial of illness, lack of understanding of preventive measures and adequate blood sugar control

Noncompliance: diabetic regimen r/t ineffective coping with chronic disease

Risk for **Powerlessness** r/t illness-related regimen

See Diabetes Mellitus

Kidney Failure

See Renal Failure

Kidney Stone

Acute **Pain** r/t obstruction from renal calculi

Deficient **Knowledge** r/t fluid requirements and dietary restrictions

Impaired **Urinary** elimination: urgency and frequency r/t anatomical obstruction, irritation caused by stone

Risk for deficient **Fluid** volume r/t nausea, vomiting

Risk for **Infection** r/t obstruction of urinary tract with stasis of urine

Knee Replacement

See Total Joint Replacement

Knowledge

Readiness for enhanced **Knowledge** of (specify) r/t the following: expresses an interest in learning, explains knowledge of the topic, displays behaviors congruent with expressed knowledge, describes previous experiences pertaining to the topic

Knowledge, Deficient

Deficient **Knowledge** r/t lack of exposure, lack of recall, information misinterpretation, cognitive limitation, lack of interest in learning, unfamiliarity with information resources

Ineffective **Health** maintenance r/t lack of or significant alteration in communication skills (written, verbal, and/or gestural)

Kock Pouch

See Continent Ileostomy

Korsakoff's Syndrome

Acute **Confusion** r/t alcohol abuse

Impaired **Memory** r/t neurological changes

Risk for imbalanced **Nutrition**: less than body requirements r/t lack of adequate balanced intake

Risk for **Falls** r/t cognitive impairment

Risk for **Injury** r/t sensory dysfunction, lack of coordination when ambulating

L

Labor, Induction of

See Induction of Labor

Labor, Normal

Acute **Pain** r/t uterine contractions, stretching of cervix and birth canal

Anxiety r/t fear of the unknown, situational crisis

Death **Anxiety** r/t threat of maternal mortality

Deficient **Knowledge** r/t lack of preparation for labor

Fatigue r/t childbirth

Health-seeking behaviors r/t healthy outcome of pregnancy, prenatal care, and childbirth education

Impaired **Tissue** integrity r/t passage of infant through birth canal, episiotomy

Risk for deficient **Fluid** volume r/t excessive loss of blood

Risk for **Infection** r/t multiple vaginal examinations, tissue trauma, prolonged rupture of membranes

Risk for **Injury**: fetal r/t hypoxia

Risk for **Post-trauma** syndrome r/t trauma or violence associated with labor pains, birth process, medical/surgical interventions, history of sexual abuse

Risk for **Powerlessness** r/t labor process

Laminectomy

Acute **Pain** r/t localized inflammation and edema

Anxiety r/t change in health status, surgical procedure

Deficient **Knowledge** r/t appropriate postoperative and postdischarge activities

Disturbed **Sensory** perception: tactile r/t possible edema or nerve injury

Impaired physical **Mobility** r/t neuromuscular impairment

Risk for impaired **Tissue** perfusion r/t edema, hemorrhage, or embolism

Risk for perioperative positioning **Injury** r/t prone position

Urinary retention r/t competing sensory impulses, effects of narcotics/anesthesia

See Scoliosis; Surgery

Laparoscopic Laser Cholecystectomy

See Cholecystectomy; Laser Surgery

Laparotomy

See Abdominal Surgery

Laryngectomy

Anticipatory **Grieving** r/t loss of voice, fear of death

Chronic **Sorrow** r/t change in body image

Death **Anxiety** r/t unknown results of surgery

Disturbed **Body** image r/t change in body structure and function

Imbalanced **Nutrition**: less than body requirements r/t absence of oral feeding, difficulty swallowing, increased need for fluids

Impaired **Oral** mucous membrane r/t absence of oral feeding

Impaired **Swallowing** r/t edema, laryngectomy tube

Impaired verbal **Communication** r/t removal of larynx

Ineffective **Airway** clearance r/t surgical removal of glottis, decreased humidification of air

Ineffective **Health** maintenance r/t deficient knowledge regarding self-care with laryngectomy

Interrupted **Family** processes r/t surgery, serious condition of family member, difficulty communicating

Risk for **Infection** r/t invasive procedure, surgery

Risk for **Powerlessness** r/t chronic illness, change in communication

Risk for situational low **Self-esteem** r/t disturbed body image

Laser Surgery

Acute **Pain** r/t heat from laser

Constipation r/t laser intervention in vulval and perianal areas

Deficient **Knowledge** r/t preoperative and postoperative care associated with laser procedure

Risk for **Infection** r/t delayed heating reaction of tissue exposed to laser

Risk for **Injury** r/t accidental exposure to laser beam

Latex Allergy

Latex **Allergy** r/t hypersensitivity to natural latex rubber

Readiness for enhanced **Knowledge** of prevention and treatment of exposure to latex products

Risk for latex **Allergy** response r/t multiple surgical procedures, especially from infancy (e.g., spina bifida); allergies to bananas, avocados, tropical fruits, kiwifruit, chestnuts; professions with daily exposure to latex (e.g., medicine, nursing, dentistry); conditions needing continuous or intermittent catheterization; history of reactions to latex (e.g., balloons, condoms, gloves); allergies to poinsettia plants; history of allergies and asthma

Laxative Abuse

Perceived **Constipation** r/t health belief, faulty appraisal, impaired thought processes

L

Legionnaires' Disease

Risk for **Infection** r/t increased environmental exposure to pathogens (contaminated water in air-conditioning systems and sometime showers)

See Pneumonia

Lens Implant

See Cataract Extraction

Lethargy/Listlessness

Adult **Failure** to thrive r/t apathy

Disturbed **Sleep** pattern r/t internal or external stressors

Fatigue r/t decreased metabolic energy production

Ineffective **Tissue** perfusion: cerebral r/t lack of oxygen supply to brain

See cause of Lethargy/Listlessness

Leukemia

Ineffective **Protection** r/t abnormal blood profile

Risk for deficient **Fluid** volume r/t nausea, vomiting, bleeding, side effects of treatment

Risk for **Infection** r/t ineffective immune system

See Cancer; Chemotherapy

Leukopenia

Risk for **Infection** r/t low white blood cell count

Level of Consciousness, Decreased

See Confusion

Lice

Readiness for enhanced **Therapeutic** regimen management to prevent and treat infestation

See Communicable Diseases, Childhood

Limb Reattachment Procedures

Anticipatory **Grieving** r/t unknown outcome of reattachment procedure

Anxiety r/t unknown outcome of reattachment procedure, use and appearance of limb

Disturbed **Body** image r/t unpredictability of function and appearance of reattached body part

Risk for deficient **Fluid** volume: hemorrhage r/t severed vessels

Risk for perioperative positioning **Injury** r/t immobilization

Risk for **Peripheral** neurovascular dysfunction r/t trauma, orthopedic and neurovascular surgery, compression of nerves and blood vessels

Risk for **Powerlessness** r/t unknown outcome of procedure

Spiritual distress r/t anxiety about condition

See Surgery, Postoperative Care

Liver Biopsy

Anxiety r/t procedure and results

Risk for deficient **Fluid** volume r/t hemorrhage from biopsy site

Risk for **Powerlessness** r/t inability to control outcome of procedure

Liver Disease

See Cirrhosis; Hepatitis

Living Will

Readiness for enhanced **Spiritual** well-being r/t acceptance of and preparation for end of life

See Advanced Directives

Lobectomy

See Thoracotomy

Loneliness

Risk for **Loneliness** r/t lack of affection, physical isolation, cathectic deprivation, social isolation

Risk for situational low **Self-esteem** r/t failure, rejection

Spiritual distress r/t loneliness/social alienation

Loose Stools

Diarrhea r/t increased gastric motility

See cause of Loose Stools

Low Back Pain

Chronic **Pain** r/t degenerative processes, musculotendinous strain, injury, inflammation, congenital deformities

Impaired physical **Mobility** r/t back pain

Ineffective **Health** maintenance r/t deficient knowledge regarding self-care with back pain

Readiness for enhanced **Therapeutic** regimen management r/t expressed desire for information to manage pain

Risk for **Powerlessness** r/t living with chronic pain

Urinary retention r/t possible spinal cord compression

Lumbar Puncture

Acute **Pain**: headache r/t possible loss of cerebrospinal fluid

Anxiety r/t invasive procedure and unknown results

Deficient **Knowledge** r/t information about procedure

Risk for **Infection** r/t invasive procedure

L

Lung Cancer
See Cancer; Thoracotomy

Lupus Erythematosus

Acute **Pain** r/t inflammatory process

Chronic **Sorrow** r/t presence of chronic illness

Disturbed **Body** image r/t change in skin, rash, lesions, ulcers, mottled erythema

Fatigue r/t increased metabolic requirements

Ineffective **Health** maintenance r/t deficient knowledge regarding medication, diet, and activity

Powerlessness r/t unpredictability of course of disease

Risk for impaired **Skin** integrity r/t chronic inflammation, edema, altered circulation

Spiritual distress r/t chronicity of disease, unknown etiology

Lyme Disease

Acute **Pain** r/t inflammation of joints, urticaria, rash

Deficient **Knowledge** r/t lack of information concerning disease, prevention, treatment

Fatigue r/t increased energy requirements

Risk for decreased **Cardiac** output r/t dysrhythmia

Risk for **Powerlessness** r/t possible chronic condition

Lymphedema

Deficient **Knowledge** r/t management of condition

Disturbed **Body** image r/t change in appearance of body part with edema

Excess **Fluid** volume r/t compromised regulatory system; inflammation, obstruction, or removal of lymph glands

Risk for situational low **Self-esteem** r/t disturbed body image

Lymphoma
See Cancer

M

Mad Cow Disease
See Creutzfeldt-Jakob Disease

Magnetic Resonance Imaging
See MRI

Major Depressive Disorder
See Depression

Malabsorption Syndrome

Deficient **Knowledge** r/t lack of information about diet and nutrition

Diarrhea r/t lactose intolerance, gluten sensitivity, resection of small bowel

Imbalanced **Nutrition**: less than body requirements r/t inability of body to absorb nutrients because of biological factors

Risk for deficient **Fluid** volume r/t diarrhea

Maladaptive Behavior
See Crisis; Post-Trauma Syndrome; Risk for Post-Trauma Syndrome; Suicide Attempt

Malaria

Readiness for enhanced **Knowledge** r/t countries requiring malaria prophylaxis, appropriate malaria regimen, use of protective clothing and insecticides

Risk for **Infection** r/t increased environmental exposure (not wearing protective clothing, not using insecticide or repellant on skin and in room in areas where infected mosquitoes are present); inadequate defense mechanisms (inappropriate use of prophylactic regimen)

Malnutrition

Adult **Failure** to thrive r/t undetected malnutrition

Deficient **Knowledge** r/t misinformation about normal nutrition, social isolation, lack of food-preparation facilities

Imbalanced **Nutrition**: less than body requirements r/t inability to ingest food, digest food, or absorb nutrients because of biological, psychological, or economic factors; institutionalization (i.e., lack of menu choices)

Ineffective **Protection** r/t inadequate nutrition

Ineffective **Therapeutic** regimen management r/t economic difficulties

Risk for **Powerlessness** r/t possible inability to provide adequate nutrition

Manic Disorder, Bipolar I

Anxiety r/t change in role function

Deficient **Fluid** volume r/t decreased intake

Disturbed **Sleep** pattern r/t constant anxious thoughts

Disturbed **Thought** processes r/t mania

Imbalanced **Nutrition**: less than body requirements r/t lack of time and motivation to eat, constant movement

Impaired **Home** maintenance r/t altered psychological state, inability to concentrate

M

Ineffective **Coping** r/t situational crisis

Ineffective **Denial** r/t fear of inability to control behavior

Ineffective **Role** performance r/t impaired social interactions

Interrupted **Family** processes r/t family member's illness

Ineffective **Therapeutic** regimen management r/t lack of social supports

Ineffective **Therapeutic** regimen management: families r/t unpredictability of client, excessive demands on family, chronicity of condition

Noncompliance r/t denial of illness

Risk for **Caregiver** role strain r/t unpredictability of condition, mood swings

Risk for **Powerlessness** r/t inability to control changes in mood

Risk for self- or other-directed **Violence** r/t hallucinations, delusions

Risk for **Suicide** r/t bipolar disorder

Sleep deprivation r/t hyperagitated state

Manipulation of Organs, Surgical Incision

Deficient **Knowledge** r/t lack of exposure to information regarding care after surgery and at home

Risk for **Infection** r/t presence of urinary catheter

Urinary retention r/t swelling of urinary meatus

Manipulative Behavior

M

Defensive **Coping** r/t superior attitude toward others

Impaired **Social** interaction r/t self-concept disturbance

Ineffective **Coping** r/t inappropriate use of defense mechanisms

Risk for **Loneliness** r/t inability to interact appropriately with others

Risk for **Self-mutilation** r/t inability to cope with increased psychological or physiological tension in healthy manner

Risk for situational low **Self-esteem** r/t history of learned helplessness

Self-mutilation r/t use of manipulation to obtain nurturing relationship with others

Marasmus

See Failure to Thrive, Nonorganic

Marshall-Marchetti-Krantz Operation

PREOPERATIVE

Stress urinary **Incontinence** r/t weak pelvic muscles and pelvic supports

POSTOPERATIVE

Acute **Pain** r/t manipulation of organs, surgical incision

Deficient **Knowledge** r/t lack of exposure to information regarding care after surgery and at home

Risk for **Infection** r/t presence of urinary catheter

Urinary retention r/t swelling of urinary meatus

Mastectomy

Acute **Pain** r/t surgical procedure

Chronic **Sorrow** r/t disturbed body image, unknown long-term health status

Death **Anxiety** r/t threat of mortality associated with breast cancer

Deficient **Knowledge** r/t self-care activities

Disturbed **Body** image r/t loss of sexually significant body part

Fear r/t change in body image, prognosis

Nausea r/t chemotherapy

Risk for impaired physical **Mobility** r/t nerve or muscle damage, pin

Risk for **Post-trauma** syndrome r/t loss of body part, surgical wounds

Risk for **Powerlessness** r/t fear of unknown outcome of procedure

Sexual dysfunction r/t change in body image, fear of loss of femininity

Spiritual distress r/t change in body image

See Cancer; Surgery

Mastitis

Acute **Pain** r/t infectious disease process, swelling of breast tissue

Anxiety r/t threat to self, concern over safety of milk for infant

Deficient **Knowledge** r/t antibiotic regimen, comfort measures

Ineffective **Breastfeeding** r/t breast pain, conflicting advice from health care providers

Ineffective **Role** performance r/t change in capacity to function in expected role

Maternal Infection

Ineffective **Protection** r/t invasive procedures, traumatized tissue, stress of recent childbirth

See Postpartum Normal Care

Maturational Issues, Adolescent

Deficient **Knowledge**: potential for enhanced health maintenance r/t information misinterpretation, lack of education regarding age-related factors

Impaired **Social** interaction r/t ineffective, unsuccessful, or dysfunctional interaction with peers

Ineffective **Coping** r/t maturational crises

Interrupted **Family** processes r/t developmental crises of adolescence secondary to challenge of parental authority and values, situational crises secondary to change in parental marital status

Readiness for enhanced **Communication** r/t expressing willingness to communicate with parental figures

Risk for **Injury/Trauma** r/t thrill-seeking behaviors

Risk for situational low **Self-esteem** r/t developmental changes

Social isolation r/t perceived alteration in physical appearance, social values not accepted by dominant peer group

See Sexuality, Adolescent; Substance Abuse (if relevant)

Maze III Procedure

See Open Heart Surgery; Dysrhythmia

Measles (Rubeola)

See Communicable Diseases, Childhood

Meconium Aspiration

See Respiratory Conditions of the Neonate

Melanoma

Acute **Pain** r/t surgical incision

Disturbed **Body** image r/t altered pigmentation, surgical incision

Fear r/t threat to well-being

Ineffective **Health** maintenance r/t deficient knowledge regarding self-care and treatment of melanoma

See Cancer

Melena

Fear r/t presence of blood in feces

Risk for deficient **Fluid** volume r/t hemorrhage

See GI Bleed

Memory Deficit

Impaired **Memory** r/t acute or chronic hypoxia, anemia, decreased cardiac output, fluid and electrolyte imbalance, neurological disturbance, excessive environmental disturbances

Meningitis/Encephalitis

Acute **Pain** r/t neck (nuchal) rigidity, inflammation of meninges, headache

Decreased **Intracranial** adaptive capacity r/t sustained increase in intracranial pressure (10 to 15 mm Hg ICP)

Delayed **Growth** and development r/t brain damage secondary to infectious process, increased intracranial pressure

Disturbed **Sensory** perception: hearing r/t central nervous system infection, ear infection

Disturbed **Sensory** perception: kinesthetic r/t central nervous system infection

Disturbed **Sensory** perception: visual r/t photophobia secondary to central nervous system infection

Disturbed **Thought** processes r/t inflammation of brain, fever

Excess **Fluid** volume r/t increased intracranial pressure, syndrome of inappropriate secretion of antidiuretic hormone (SIADH)

Impaired **Comfort** r/t central nervous system inflammation

Impaired **Comfort**: photophobia r/t increased sensitivity to external stimuli secondary to central nervous system inflammation

Impaired **Mobility** r/t neuromuscular or central nervous system insult

Ineffective **Airway** clearance r/t seizure activity

Ineffective **Tissue** perfusion: cerebral r/t inflamed cerebral tissues and meninges, increased intracranial pressure

Risk for **Aspiration** r/t seizure activity

Risk for **Falls** r/t neuromuscular dysfunction

Risk for **Injury** r/t seizure activity

See Hospitalized Child

Meningocele

See Neurotube Defects

Menopause

Health-seeking behavior r/t menopause, therapies associated with change in hormonal levels

Impaired **Memory** r/t change in hormonal levels

Ineffective **Sexuality** patterns r/t altered body structure, lack of physiological lubrication, lack of knowledge of artificial lubrication

Ineffective **Thermoregulation** r/t changes in hormonal levels

Readiness for enhanced **Spiritual** well-being r/t desire for harmony of mind, body, and spirit

Readiness for enhanced **Therapeutic** regimen management r/t verbalized desire to manage menopause

Risk for imbalanced **Nutrition**: more than body requirements r/t change in metabolic rate caused by fluctuating hormone levels

M

Risk for **Powerlessness** r/t changes associated with menopause

Risk for situational low **Self-esteem** r/t developmental changes: menopause

Risk for urge urinary **Incontinence** r/t changes in hormonal levels affecting bladder function

Menorrhagia

Fear r/t loss of large amounts of blood

Risk for deficient **Fluid** volume r/t excessive loss of menstrual blood

Mental Illness

Chronic **Sorrow** r/t presence of mental illness

Compromised family **Coping** r/t lack of available support from client

Defensive **Coping** r/t psychological impairment, substance abuse

Disabled family **Coping** r/t chronically unexpressed feelings of guilt, anxiety, hostility, or despair

Disturbed **Thought** processes r/t head injury, mental disorder, personality disorder, organic mental disorder, substance abuse, severe interpersonal conflict, sleep deprivation, sensory deprivation or overload, impaired cerebral perfusion

Ineffective community **Therapeutic** regimen management r/t inadequate services to care for mentally ill clients, lack of information regarding how to access services

M Ineffective **Coping** r/t situational crisis, coping with mental illness

Ineffective **Denial** r/t refusal to acknowledge abuse problem, fear of the social stigma of disease

Ineffective **Therapeutic** regimen management: families r/t chronicity of condition, unpredictability of client, unknown prognosis

Risk for **Loneliness** r/t social isolation

Risk for **Powerlessness** r/t lifestyle of helplessness

Mental Retardation

Chronic low **Self-esteem** r/t perceived differences

Delayed **Growth** and development r/t cognitive or perceptual impairment, developmental delay

Grieving r/t loss of perfect child, birth of child with congenital defect or subsequent head injury

Impaired **Home** maintenance r/t insufficient support systems

Impaired **Social** interaction r/t developmental lag or delay, perceived differences

Impaired **Swallowing** r/t neuromuscular impairment

Impaired verbal **Communication** r/t developmental delay

Interrupted **Family** processes r/t crisis of diagnosis and situational transition

Parental role **Conflict** r/t home care of child with special needs

Readiness for enhanced family **Coping** r/t adaptation and acceptance of child's condition and needs

Risk for delayed **Development** r/t cognitive or perceptual impairment

Risk for disproportionate **Growth** r/t mental retardation

Risk for **Self-mutilation** r/t separation anxiety, depersonalization

Self-care deficit: bathing/hygiene, dressing/grooming, feeding, toileting r/t perceptual or cognitive impairment

Self-mutilation r/t inability to express tension verbally

Spiritual Distress r/t chronic condition of child with special needs

See Child with Chronic Condition; Safety, Childhood

Metabolic Acidosis

See Ketoacidosis

Metabolic Alkalosis

Deficient **Fluid** volume r/t fluid volume loss, vomiting, gastric suctioning, failure of regulatory mechanisms

MI (Myocardial Infarction)

Acute **Pain** r/t myocardial tissue damage from inadequate blood supply

Anxiety r/t threat of death, possible change in role status

Constipation r/t decreased peristalsis from decreased physical activity, medication effect, change in diet

Death **Anxiety** r/t seriousness of medical condition

Decreased **Cardiac** output r/t ventricular damage, ischemia, dysrhythmias

Fear r/t threat to well-being

Ineffective **Denial** r/t fear, deficient knowledge about heart disease

Ineffective family **Coping** r/t spouse or significant other's fear of partner loss

Ineffective **Health** maintenance r/t deficient knowledge regarding self-care and treatment

Ineffective **Sexuality** patterns r/t fear of chest pain, possibility of heart damage

Interrupted **Family** processes r/t crisis, role change

Readiness for enhanced **Knowledge** of heart problems and rehabilitation and prevention

Risk for **Powerlessness** r/t acute illness

Risk for **Spiritual** distress r/t physical illness: MI

Situational low **Self-esteem** r/t crisis of MI

Midlife Crisis

Ineffective **Coping** r/t inability to deal with changes associated with aging

Powerlessness r/t lack of control over life situation

Readiness for enhanced **Spiritual** well-being r/t desire to find purpose and meaning to life

Spiritual distress r/t questioning belief/value system

Migraine Headache

Acute **Pain**: headache r/t vasodilation of cerebral and extracerebral vessels

Disturbed **Energy** field r/t pain, disruption of normal flow of energy

Ineffective **Health** maintenance r/t deficient knowledge regarding prevention and treatment of headaches

Readiness for enhanced **Therapeutic** regimen management r/t expressed desire to obtain information to prevent and treat pain associated with migraines

Miscarriage

See Pregnancy Loss

Mitral Stenosis

Activity intolerance r/t imbalance between oxygen supply and demand

Anxiety r/t possible worsening of symptoms, activity intolerance, fatigue

Decreased **Cardiac** output r/t incompetent heart valves, abnormal forward or backward blood flow, flow into a dilated chamber, flow through an abnormal passage between chambers

Fatigue r/t reduced cardiac output

Ineffective **Health** maintenance r/t deficient knowledge regarding self-care with disorder

Mitral Valve Prolapse

Acute **Pain** r/t mitral valve regurgitation

Anxiety r/t symptoms of condition: palpitations, chest pain

Fatigue r/t abnormal catecholamine regulation, decreased intravascular volume

Fear r/t lack of knowledge about mitral valve prolapse, feelings of having a heart attack

Ineffective **Health** maintenance r/t deficient knowledge regarding methods to relieve pain and treat

dysrhythmia and shortness of breath, need for prophylactic antibiotics before invasive procedures

Ineffective **Tissue** perfusion: cerebral r/t postural hypotension

Readiness for enhanced **Knowledge** of methods to treat and prevent symptoms associated with condition

Risk for **Infection** r/t invasive procedures

Risk for **Powerlessness** r/t unpredictability of onset of symptoms

Mobility, Impaired Physical

Impaired physical **Mobility** r/t intolerance to activity, decreased strength and endurance, pain, discomfort, perceptual or cognitive impairment, neuromuscular impairment, musculoskeletal impairment, depression, severe anxiety

Risk for **Falls** r/t impaired physical mobility

Modified Radical Mastectomy

Decisional **Conflict** r/t treatment of choice

Readiness for enhanced **Communication** r/t to willingness to discuss options for treatment

See Mastectomy

Mononucleosis

Activity intolerance r/t generalized weakness

Acute **Pain** r/t enlargement of lymph nodes, irritation of oropharyngeal cavity

Fatigue r/t disease state, stress

Hyperthermia r/t infectious process

Impaired **Swallowing** r/t irritation of oropharyngeal cavity

Ineffective **Health** maintenance r/t deficient knowledge concerning transmission and treatment of disease

Risk for **Injury** r/t possible rupture of spleen

Mood Disorders

Caregiver role strain r/t symptoms associated with disorder of care receiver

Impaired **Adjustment** r/t hopelessness, altered locus of control

Readiness for enhanced **Communication** r/t willingness to communicate with others regarding problems associated with mood disorder

Risk for situational low **Self-esteem** r/t unpredictable changes in mood

Social isolation r/t alterations in mental status

See specific disorder: Depression; Dysthymic Disorder; Hypomania; Manic Disorder

M

Moon Face

Disturbed **Body** image r/t change in appearance from disease and medication

Risk for situational low **Self-esteem** r/t change in body image

See Cushing's Syndrome

Moral/Ethical Dilemmas

Decisional **Conflict** r/t questioning personal values and belief which alter decision

Readiness for enhanced **Spiritual** well-being r/t request for interaction with others regarding difficult decisions

Risk for **Powerlessness** r/t lack of knowledge to make a decision

Risk for **Spiritual** distress r/t moral or ethical crisis

Mottling of Peripheral Skin

Ineffective **Tissue** perfusion: peripheral r/t interruption of arterial flow, decreased circulating blood volume

Mouth Lesions

See Mucous Membranes, Impaired Oral

MRI (Magnetic Resonance Imaging)

Anxiety r/t fear of being in closed spaces

Deficient **Knowledge** r/t preparation for examination, contraindications to test, especially presence of any metal in body

Readiness for enhanced **Knowledge** r/t appropriate preparation for exam

Mucocutaneous Lymph Node Syndrome

See Kawasaki Syndrome

Mucous Membranes, Impaired Oral

Impaired **Oral** mucous membrane r/t pathological conditions—oral cavity (radiation to head or neck), dehydration, chemical trauma (e.g., acidic foods, drugs, noxious agents, alcohol), mechanical trauma (e.g., ill-fitting dentures, braces, endotracheal or nasogastric tubes, surgery in oral cavity), NPO for more than 24 hours, ineffective oral hygiene, mouth breathing, malnutrition, infection, lack of or decreased salivation, medication

Multiinfarct Dementia

See Dementia

Multiple Gestation

Anxiety r/t uncertain outcome of pregnancy

Death **Anxiety** r/t maternal complications associated with multiple gestation

Deficient **Knowledge** r/t caring for more than one infant

Disturbed **Sleep** pattern r/t discomforts of multiple gestation or care of infants

Fatigue r/t physiological demands of a multifetal pregnancy and/or care of more than one infant

Imbalanced **Nutrition**: less than body requirements r/t physiological demands of a multifetal pregnancy

Impaired **Home** maintenance r/t fatigue

Impaired physical **Mobility** r/t increased uterine size

Impaired **Transfer** ability r/t enlarged uterus

Readiness for enhanced **Family** processes r/t family adapting to change with more than one infant

Risk for **Constipation** r/t enlarged uterus

Risk for delayed **Development**: fetus r/t multiple gestation

Risk for disproportionate **Growth**: fetus r/t multiple gestation

Risk for ineffective **Breastfeeding** r/t lack of support, physical demands of feeding more than one infant

Stress urinary **Incontinence** r/t increased pelvic pressure

Multiple Personality Disorder (Dissociative Identity Disorder)

Anxiety r/t loss of control of behavior and feelings

Chronic low **Self-esteem** r/t inability to deal with life events, history of abuse

Defensive **Coping** r/t unresolved past traumatic events, severe anxiety

Disturbed **Body** image r/t feelings of powerlessness with personality changes

Disturbed personal **Identity** r/t severe child abuse

Hopelessness r/t long-term stress

Ineffective **Coping** r/t history of abuse

Readiness for enhanced **Communication** r/t willingness to discuss problems associated with condition

Risk for **Self-mutilation** r/t need to act out to relieve stress

See Dissociative Disorder

Multiple Sclerosis (MS)

Chronic **Sorrow** r/t loss of physical ability

Disturbed **Energy** field r/t disruption in energy flow resulting from disharmony between mind and body

Disturbed **Sensory** perception: specify r/t pathology in sensory tracts

Impaired physical **Mobility** r/t neuromuscular impairment

Ineffective **Airway** clearance r/t decreased energy/fatigue

Powerlessness r/t progressive nature of disease

Readiness for enhanced **Spiritual** well-being r/t struggling with chronic debilitating condition

Readiness for enhanced **Therapeutic** regimen management r/t expressing a desire to manage condition

Risk for **Disuse** syndrome r/t physical immobility

Risk for imbalanced **Nutrition**: less than body requirements r/t impaired swallowing, depression

Risk for **Injury** r/t altered mobility, sensory dysfunction

Risk for natural rubber latex **Allergy** response r/t possible repeated exposures to latex associated with intermittent catheterizations

Risk for **Powerlessness** r/t chronic illness

Self-care deficit: specify r/t neuromuscular impairment

Sexual dysfunction r/t biopsychosocial alteration of sexuality

Spiritual distress r/t perceived hopelessness of diagnosis

Urinary retention r/t inhibition of the reflex arc

See Neurological Disorders

Mumps
See Communicable Diseases, Childhood

Murmurs
Decreased **Cardiac** output r/t incompetent heart valves, abnormal forward or backward blood flow, flow into a dilated chamber, flow through an abnormal passage between chambers

Muscular Atrophy/Weakness
Risk for **Disuse** syndrome r/t impaired physical mobility

Risk for **Falls** r/t impaired physical mobility

Muscular Dystrophy (MD)
Activity intolerance r/t fatigue

Constipation r/t immobility

Decreased **Cardiac** output r/t effects of congestive heart failure

Fatigue r/t increased energy requirements to perform activities of daily living

Imbalanced **Nutrition**: less than body requirements r/t impaired swallowing or chewing

Imbalanced **Nutrition**: more than body requirements r/t inactivity

Impaired **Mobility** r/t muscle weakness and development of contractures

Impaired **Transfer** ability r/t muscle weakness

Impaired **Walking** r/t muscle weakness

Ineffective **Airway** clearance r/t muscle weakness and decreased ability to cough

Readiness for enhanced **Self-concept** r/t acceptance of strength and abilities

Risk for **Aspiration** r/t impaired swallowing

Risk for **Disuse** syndrome r/t complications of immobility

Risk for **Falls** r/t muscle weakness

Risk for impaired **Gas** exchange r/t ineffective airway clearance and ineffective breathing pattern secondary to muscle weakness

Risk for impaired **Skin** integrity r/t immobility, braces, or adaptive devices

Risk for ineffective **Breathing** pattern r/t muscle weakness

Risk for **Infection** r/t pooling of pulmonary secretions secondary to immobility and muscle weakness

Risk for **Injury** r/t muscle weakness and unsteady gait

Risk for **Powerlessness** r/t chronic condition

Risk for situational low **Self-esteem** r/t presence of chronic condition

Self-care deficits: feeding, bathing, dressing, toileting r/t muscle weakness and fatigue

See Child with Chronic Condition; Hospitalized Child; Terminally Ill Child

MVA (Motor Vehicle Accident)
See Fracture; Head Injury; Injury; Pneumothorax

Myasthenia Gravis
Fatigue r/t paresthesia, aching muscles

Imbalanced **Nutrition**: less than body requirements r/t difficulty eating and swallowing

Impaired physical **Mobility** r/t defective transmission of nerve impulses at the neuromuscular junction

Impaired **Swallowing** r/t neuromuscular impairment

Ineffective **Airway** clearance r/t decreased ability to cough and swallow

Ineffective **Therapeutic** regimen management r/t lack of knowledge of treatment, uncertainty of outcome

Interrupted **Family** processes r/t crisis of dealing with diagnosis

Readiness for enhanced **Spiritual** well-being r/t heightened coping with serious illness

M

Risk for **Caregiver** role strain r/t severity of illness of client

See Neurological Disorders

Mycoplasma Pneumonia

See Pneumonia

Myelocele

See Neurotube Defects

Myelogram, Contrast

Acute **Pain** r/t irritation of nerve roots

Risk for deficient **Fluid** volume r/t possible dehydration, loss of cerebrospinal fluid

Risk for ineffective **Tissue** perfusion: cerebral r/t hypotension, loss of cerebrospinal fluid

Urinary retention r/t pressure on spinal nerve roots

Myelomeningocele

See Neurotube Defects

Myocardial Infarction

See MI

Myocarditis

Activity intolerance r/t reduced cardiac reserve and prescribed bedrest

Decreased **Cardiac** output r/t impaired contractility of ventricles

Deficient **Knowledge** r/t treatment of disease

Readiness for enhanced **Knowledge** of treatment of disease

See CHF (if appropriate)

Myringotomy

Acute **Pain** r/t surgical procedure

Disturbed **Sensory** perception r/t possible hearing impairment

Fear r/t hospitalization, surgical procedure

Ineffective **Health** maintenance r/t deficient knowledge regarding self-care following surgery

Risk for **Infection** r/t invasive procedure

Myxedema

See Hypothyroidism

N

Narcissistic Personality Disorder

Decisional **Conflict** r/t lack of realistic problem-solving skills

Defensive **Coping** r/t grandiose sense of self

Impaired **Social** interaction r/t self-concept disturbance

Risk for **Loneliness** r/t inability to interact appropriately with others

Risk for **Self-mutilation** r/t inadequate coping

Narcolepsy

Anxiety r/t fear of lack of control over falling asleep

Disturbed **Sleep** pattern r/t uncontrollable desire to sleep

Readiness for enhanced **Sleep** r/t expression of willingness to enhance sleep

Risk for **Trauma** r/t falling asleep during potentially dangerous activity

Narcotic Use

Risk for **Constipation** r/t effects of opioids on peristalsis

See Substance Abuse (if relevant)

Nasogastric Suction

Impaired **Comfort** r/t presence of nasogastric tube

Impaired **Oral** mucous membrane r/t presence of nasogastric tube

Risk for deficient **Fluid** volume r/t loss of gastrointestinal fluids without adequate replacement

Nausea

Nausea r/t gastric irritation secondary to pharmaceuticals (e.g., aspirin, nonsteroidal anti-inflammatory drugs, steroids, antibiotics), alcohol, iron, blood; gastric distention secondary to delayed gastric emptying caused by pharmacological interventions (e.g., narcotics administration, anesthesia agents), pharmaceuticals (e.g., analgesics, antiviral agents for HIV, aspirin, opioids, chemotherapeutic agents), toxins (e.g., radiotherapy); biochemical disorders (e.g., uremia, diabetic ketoacidosis, pregnancy), cardiac pain, cancer of the stomach or intra-abdominal tumors (e.g., pelvic or colorectal cancers), esophageal or pancreatic disease, gastric distention due to delayed gastric emptying, pyloric intestinal obstruction, genitourinary and biliary distension, upper bowel stasis, external compression of the stomach (liver, spleen, or other organ), enlargement that slows the stomach functioning (squashed stomach syndrome), excess food intake, gastric irritation due to pharyngeal and/or peritoneal inflammation, liver or splenetic capsule stretch, local tumors (e.g., acoustic neuroma, primary or secondary brain tumors, bone metastases at base of skull), motion sickness, Meniere's disease or labyrinthitis, physical factors (e.g., increased intracranial pressure, meningitis), toxins (e.g., tumor-produced peptides, abnormal metabolites due to cancer); psychological factors (e.g., pain, fear, anxiety, noxious odors, taste, unpleasant visual stimulation

N (margin tab)

Near-Drowning

Anticipatory/dysfunctional **Grieving** r/t potential death of child, unknown sequelae, guilt about accident

Aspiration r/t aspiration of fluid into the lungs

Fear: parental r/t possible death of child, possible permanent and debilitating sequelae

Hypothermia r/t central nervous system injury, prolonged submersion in cold water

Impaired **Gas** exchange r/t laryngospasm, holding breath, aspiration

Ineffective **Airway** clearance r/t aspiration, impaired gas exchange

Ineffective **Health** maintenance r/t parental deficient knowledge regarding safety measures appropriate for age

Readiness for enhanced **Spiritual** well-being r/t struggle with survival of life-threatening situation

Risk for delayed **Development** and disproportionate growth r/t hypoxemia, cerebral anoxia

Risk for **Infection** r/t aspiration, invasive monitoring

See Child with Chronic Condition; Hospitalized Child; Safety, Childhood; Terminally Ill Child/Death of Child

Neck Vein Distention

Decreased **Cardiac** output r/t decreased contractility of heart and resulting increased preload

Excess **Fluid** volume r/t excess fluid intake, compromised regulatory mechanisms

See CHF

Necrotizing Enterocolitis (NEC)

Deficient **Fluid** volume r/t vomiting, gastrointestinal bleeding

Imbalanced **Nutrition**: less than body requirements r/t decreased ability to absorb nutrients, decreased perfusion to gastrointestinal tract

Ineffective **Breathing** pattern r/t abdominal distention, hypoxia

Ineffective **Tissue** perfusion: gastrointestinal r/t shunting of blood away from mesenteric circulation and toward vital organs secondary to perinatal stress, hypoxia

Risk for **Infection** r/t bacterial invasion of gastrointestinal tract, invasive procedures

See Hospitalized Child; Premature Infant

Negative Feelings About Self

Chronic low **Self-esteem** r/t long-standing negative self-evaluation

Readiness for enhanced **Self-Concept** r/t expressed willingness to enhance self-concept

Self-esteem disturbance r/t inappropriate learned negative feelings about self

Neglect, Unilateral

See Unilateral Neglect of One Side of Body

Neglectful Care of Family Member

Caregiver role strain r/t care demands of family member, lack of social or financial support

Deficient **Knowledge** r/t care needs

Disabled family **Coping** r/t highly ambivalent family relationships, lack of respite care

Ineffective community **Therapeutic** regimen management r/t deficits in community for support of caregivers, detection of client neglect

Interrupted **Family** processes r/t situational transition or crisis

Neoplasm

Fear r/t possible malignancy

See Cancer

Nephrectomy

Acute **Pain** r/t incisional discomfort

Anxiety r/t surgical recovery, prognosis

Constipation r/t lack of return of peristalsis

Impaired **Urinary** elimination r/t loss of kidney

Ineffective **Breathing** pattern r/t location of surgical incision

Risk for deficient **Fluid** volume r/t vascular losses, decreased intake

Risk for **Infection** r/t invasive procedure, lack of deep breathing because of location of surgical incision

Spiritual Distress r/t chronic illness

Nephrostomy, Percutaneous

Acute **Pain** r/t invasive procedure

Impaired **Urinary** elimination r/t nephrostomy tube

Risk for **Infection** r/t invasive procedure

Nephrotic Syndrome

Activity intolerance r/t generalized edema

Disturbed **Body** image r/t edematous appearance and side effects of steroid therapy

Excess **Fluid** volume r/t edema secondary to oncotic fluid shift resulting from serum protein loss and renal retention of salt and water

Imbalanced **Nutrition**: less than body requirements r/t anorexia, protein loss

Imbalanced **Nutrition**: more than body requirements r/t increased appetite secondary to steroid therapy

N

Impaired **Comfort** r/t edema

Risk for impaired **Skin** integrity r/t edema

Risk for **Infection** r/t altered immune mechanisms secondary to disease and effects of steroids

Risk for **Noncompliance** r/t side effects of home steroid therapy

Social Isolation r/t edematous appearance

See Child with Chronic Condition; Hospitalized Child

Nerve Entrapment

See Carpal Tunnel Syndrome

Neuritis

Activity intolerance r/t pain with movement

Acute **Pain** r/t stimulation of affected nerve endings, inflammation of sensory nerves

Ineffective **Health** maintenance r/t deficient knowledge regarding self-care with neuritis

Neurogenic Bladder

Reflex **Incontinence** r/t neurological impairment

Risk for natural rubber latex **Allergy** response r/t repeated exposures to latex associated with possible repeated catheterizations

Urinary retention r/t interruption in the lateral spinal tracts

Neurological Disorders

Acute **Confusion** r/t dementia, alcohol abuse, drug abuse, delirium

Anticipatory **Grieving** r/t loss of usual body functioning

Imbalanced **Nutrition**: less than body requirements r/t impaired swallowing, depression, difficulty feeding self

Impaired **Home** maintenance r/t client's or family member's disease

Impaired **Memory** r/t neurological disturbance

Impaired physical **Mobility** r/t neuromuscular impairment

Impaired **Swallowing** r/t neuromuscular dysfunction

Ineffective **Airway** clearance r/t perceptual or cognitive impairment, decreased energy, fatigue

Ineffective **Coping** r/t disability requiring change in lifestyle

Interrupted **Family** processes r/t situational crisis, illness, or disability of family member

Powerlessness r/t progressive nature of disease

Risk for **Disuse** syndrome r/t physical immobility, neuromuscular dysfunction

Risk for impaired **Skin** integrity r/t altered sensation, altered mental status, paralysis

Risk for **Injury** r/t altered mobility, sensory dysfunction, cognitive impairment

Self-care deficit: specify r/t neuromuscular dysfunction

Sexual dysfunction r/t biopsychosocial alteration of sexuality

Social isolation r/t altered state of wellness

Wandering r/t cognitive impairment

Neurotube Defects (Meningocele, Myelomeningocele, Spina Bifida, Anencephaly)

Chronic low **Self-esteem** r/t perceived differences, decreased ability to participate in physical and social activities at school

Constipation r/t immobility or less than adequate mobility

Delayed **Growth** and development r/t physical impairments, possible cognitive impairment

Disturbed **Sensory** perception: visual r/t altered reception secondary to strabismus

Grieving r/t loss of perfect child, birth of child with congenital defect

Impaired **Mobility** r/t neuromuscular impairment

Impaired **Skin** integrity r/t incontinence

Readiness for enhanced family **Coping** r/t effective adaptive response by family members

Readiness for enhanced **Family** processes r/t family supporting each other

Reflex **Incontinence** r/t neurogenic impairment

Risk for delayed **Development** r/t chronic illness

Risk for disproportionate **Growth** r/t chronic illness

Risk for imbalanced **Nutrition**: more than body requirements r/t diminished, limited, or impaired physical activity

Risk for impaired **Skin** integrity: lower extremities r/t decreased sensory perception

Risk for natural rubber latex **Allergy** response r/t multiple exposures to latex products

Risk for **Powerlessness** r/t debilitating disease

Total urinary **Incontinence** r/t neurogenic impairment

Urge urinary **Incontinence** r/t neurogenic impairment

See Child with Chronic Condition; Premature Infant

Newborn, Normal

Effective **Breastfeeding** r/t normal oral structure and gestational age >34 weeks

Ineffective **Protection** r/t immature immune system

Ineffective **Thermoregulation** r/t immaturity of neuroendocrine system

Readiness for enhanced organized **Infant** behavior r/t appropriate environmental stimuli

Readiness for enhanced **Parenting** r/t providing emotional and physical needs of infant

Risk for **Infection** r/t open umbilical stump

Risk for **Injury** r/t immaturity, need for caretaking

Risk for sudden infant **Death** syndrome r/t lack of knowledge regarding infant sleeping in prone or side-lying position, prenatal or postnatal infant smoke exposure, infant overheating/overwrapping, soft underlayment/loose articles in the sleep environment

Newborn, Postmature

Hypothermia r/t depleted stores of subcutaneous fat

Impaired **Skin** integrity r/t cracked and peeling skin secondary to decreased vernix

Risk for ineffective **Airway** clearance r/t meconium aspiration

Risk for **Injury** r/t hypoglycemia secondary to depleted glycogen stores

Newborn, Small for Gestational Age (SGA)

Imbalanced **Nutrition**: less than body requirements r/t history of placental insufficiency

Ineffective **Thermoregulation** r/t decreased brown fat, subcutaneous fat

Risk for delayed **Development** r/t history of placental insufficiency

Risk for disproportionate **Growth** r/t history of placental insufficiency

Risk for **Injury** r/t hypoglycemia, perinatal asphyxia, meconium aspiration

Risk for sudden infant **Death** syndrome r/t low birth weight

Nicotine Addiction

Ineffective **Health** maintenance r/t lack of ability to make a judgment about smoking cessation

Powerlessness r/t perceived lack of control over ability to give up nicotine

Readiness for enhanced **Therapeutic** regimen management r/t expresses desire to learn measures to stop smoking

NIDDM (Non–Insulin-Dependent Diabetes Mellitus)

Health-seeking behaviors r/t desiring information on exercise and diet to manage diabetes

See Diabetes Mellitus

Nightmares

Disturbed **Energy** field r/t disharmony of body and mind

Post-trauma response r/t disaster, war, epidemic, rape, assault, torture, catastrophic illness or accident

Rape-trauma syndrome: compound reaction/silent reaction r/t forced violent sexual penetration against the victim's will and consent

Nipple Soreness

Acute **Pain** r/t injury to nipples

See Painful Breasts—Sore Nipples

Nocturia

Impaired **Urinary** elimination r/t sensory motor impairment, urinary tract infection

Risk for **Powerlessness** r/t to inability to control nighttime voidings

Total **Urinary** incontinence r/t neuropathy preventing transmission of reflex indicating bladder fullness, neurological dysfunction causing triggering of micturition at unpredictable times, independent contraction of detrusor reflex as result of surgery, trauma or disease affecting spinal cord nerves, anatomical fistula

Urge urinary **Incontinence** r/t decreased bladder capacity, irritation of bladder stretch receptors causing spasm, alcohol, caffeine, increased fluids, increased urine concentration, overdistention of bladder

Nocturnal Paroxysmal Dyspnea

See PND

Noncompliance

Noncompliance r/t client value system, health beliefs, cultural influences, spiritual values, client-provider relationships, deficient knowledge

Non–Insulin-Dependent Diabetes Mellitus (NIDDM)

See Diabetes Mellitus

Nutrition

Readiness for enhanced **Nutrition** r/t the following: expresses willingness to enhance nutrition, eats regularly, consumes adequate food and fluid, expresses knowledge of healthy food and fluid choices, follows an appropriate standard for intake (e.g., the food pyramid or America Diabetic Association guidelines), practices safe preparation and storage for food and fluids, maintains an attitude toward eating and drinking that is congruent with health goals

N

Nutrition, Imbalanced

Imbalanced **Nutrition**: less than body requirements r/t inability to ingest or digest food or absorb nutrients because of biological, psychological, economic factors

Imbalanced **Nutrition**: more than body requirements r/t excessive intake in relation to metabolic need

Risk for imbalanced **Nutrition**: more than body requirements r/t obesity in parents, use of food as reward or comfort measure, dysfunctional eating pattern, eating in response to cues other than hunger

O

Obesity

Chronic low **Self-esteem** r/t ineffective coping, overeating

Disturbed **Body** image r/t eating disorder, excess weight

Imbalanced **Nutrition**: more than body requirements r/t caloric intake exceeding energy expenditure

Readiness for enhanced **Nutrition** r/t expressing willingness to enhance nutrition

Obsessive-Compulsive Disorder

Anxiety r/t threat to self-concept, unmet needs

Decisional **Conflict** r/t inability to make a decision for fear of reprisal

Disabled family **Coping** r/t family process being disrupted by client's ritualistic activities

Disturbed **Thought** processes r/t persistent thoughts, ideas, impulses that seem irrelevant and will not relent

Ineffective **Coping** r/t expression of feelings in an unacceptable way, ritualistic behavior

Powerlessness r/t unrelenting repetitive thoughts to perform irrational activities

Risk for situational low **Self-esteem** r/t inability to control repetitive thoughts and actions

Obstruction, Bowel

See Bowel Obstruction

Older Adult

See Aging

Oligohydramnios

Anxiety: maternal r/t fear of unknown, threat to fetus

Risk for **Injury**: fetal r/t decreased umbilical cord blood flow secondary to compression

Oliguria

Deficient **Fluid** volume r/t active fluid loss, failure of regulatory mechanism

See Cardiac Output Decrease; Renal Failure; Shock

Omphalocele

See Gastroschisis/Omphalocele

Onychomycosis

See Ringworm of Nails

Oophorectomy

Risk for ineffective **Sexuality** patterns r/t altered body function

See Surgery

Open Heart Surgery

Decreased **Cardiac** output r/t altered preload or afterload

Impaired **Gas** exchange r/t cardiac surgery

See Coronary Artery Bypass Grafting; Dysrhythmia

Open Reduction of Fracture with Internal Fixation (Femur)

Anxiety r/t outcome of corrective procedure

Impaired physical **Mobility** r/t postoperative position, abduction of leg, avoidance of acute flexion

Powerlessness r/t loss of control, unanticipated change in lifestyle

Risk for perioperative positioning **Injury** r/t immobilization

Risk for **Peripheral** neurovascular dysfunction r/t mechanical compression, orthopedic surgery, immobilization

See Surgery, Postoperative Care

Opiate Use

Risk for **Constipation** r/t effects of opiates on peristalsis.

See Drug Abuse

Opportunistic Infection

Delayed **Surgical** recovery r/t abnormal blood profiles, impaired healing

Risk for **Infection** r/t abnormal blood profiles

See AIDS

Oral Mucous Membrane, Impaired

Impaired **Oral** mucous membrane r/t pathological conditions—oral cavity (radiation to head or neck), dehydration, chemical trauma (e.g., acidic foods, drugs, noxious agents, alcohol), mechanical trauma (e.g., ill-fitting dentures, braces, endotracheal and nasogastric tubes, surgery in oral cavity), NPO for more than 24 hours, ineffective oral hygiene, mouth breathing, malnutrition, infection, lack of or decreased salivation, medication

Organic Mental Disorders

Adult **Failure** to thrive r/t undetected organic mental disorder

Impaired **Social** interaction r/t disturbed thought processes

Risk for **Injury** r/t disorientation to time, place, person

See Dementia

Orthopedic Traction

Impaired **Social** interaction r/t limited physical mobility

Impaired **Transfer** ability r/t limited physical mobility

Ineffective **Role** performance r/t limited physical mobility

See Traction and Casts

Orthopnea

Decreased **Cardiac** output r/t inability of heart to meet demands of body

Ineffective **Breathing** pattern r/t inability to breathe with head of bed flat

Orthostatic Hypotension

See Dizziness

Osteoarthritis

Activity intolerance r/t pain after exercise or use of joint

Acute **Pain** r/t movement

Impaired **Transfer** ability r/t pain

See Arthritis

Osteomyelitis

Acute **Pain** r/t inflammation in affected extremity

Deficient **Diversional** activity r/t prolonged immobilization, hospitalization

Fear: parental r/t concern regarding possible growth plate damage secondary to infection, concern that infection may become chronic

Hyperthermia r/t infectious process

Impaired physical **Mobility** r/t imposed immobility secondary to infected area

Ineffective **Health** maintenance r/t continued immobility at home, possible extensive casts, continued antibiotics

Risk for **Constipation** r/t immobility

Risk for impaired **Skin** integrity r/t irritation from splint/cast

Risk for spread of **Infection** r/t inadequate primary and secondary defenses

See Hospitalized Child

Osteoporosis

Acute **Pain** r/t fracture, muscle spasms

Deficient **Knowledge** r/t diet, exercise, need to abstain from alcohol and nicotine

Effective **Therapeutic** regimen management: individual r/t appropriate choices for diet and exercise to prevent and manage condition

Imbalanced **Nutrition**: less than body requirements r/t inadequate intake of calcium and vitamin D

Impaired physical **Mobility** r/t pain, skeletal changes

Readiness for enhanced **Therapeutic** regimen management r/t expressing desire to manage the treatment of illness and prevention of complications

Risk for **Injury**: fracture r/t lack of activity, risk of falling resulting from environmental hazards, neuromuscular disorders, diminished senses, cardiovascular responses, responses to drugs

Risk for **Powerlessness** r/t debilitating disease

Ostomy

See Child with Chronic Condition; Colostomy; Ileal Conduit; Ileostomy

Otitis Media

Acute **Pain** r/t inflammation, infectious process

Disturbed **Sensory** perception: auditory r/t incomplete resolution of otitis media, presence of excess drainage in middle ear

Readiness for enhanced **Knowledge** of information relating to treatment and prevent of disease

Risk for delayed **Development** r/t frequent otitis media

Risk for **Infection** r/t eustachian tube obstruction, traumatic eardrum perforation, infectious disease process

Ovarian Carcinoma

Death **Anxiety** r/t unknown outcome, possible poor prognosis

Fear r/t unknown outcome, possible poor prognosis

Ineffective **Health** maintenance r/t deficient knowledge regarding self-care, treatment of condition

See Chemotherapy; Hysterectomy; Radiation Therapy

P

Pacemaker

Acute **Pain** r/t surgical procedure

Anxiety r/t change in health status, presence of pacemaker

Death **Anxiety** r/t worry over possible malfunction of pacemaker

Deficient **Knowledge** r/t self-care program, when to seek medical attention

Readiness for enhanced **Therapeutic** regimen management r/t appropriate health care management of pacemaker

Risk for decreased **Cardiac** output r/t malfunction of pacemaker

Risk for **Infection** r/t invasive procedure, presence of foreign body (catheter and generator)

Risk for **Powerlessness** r/t presence of electronic device to stimulate heart

Paget's Disease

Chronic **Sorrow** r/t chronic condition with altered body image

Deficient **Knowledge** r/t appropriate diet high in protein and calcium, mild exercise

Disturbed **Body** image r/t possible enlarged head, bowed tibias, kyphosis

Risk for **Trauma**: fracture r/t excessive bone destruction

Pain, Acute

Acute **Pain** r/t injury agents (biological, chemical, physical, psychological)

Disturbed **Energy** field r/t unbalanced energy field

Pain, Chronic

Chronic **Pain** r/t chronic physical or psychosocial disability

Disturbed **Energy** field r/t unbalanced energy field

Painful Breasts—Engorgement

Acute **Pain** r/t distention of breast tissue

Impaired **Tissue** integrity r/t excessive fluid in breast tissues

Ineffective **Role** performance r/t change in physical capacity to assume role of breastfeeding mother

Risk for ineffective **Breastfeeding** r/t pain, infant's inability to latch on to engorged breast

Risk for **Infection** r/t milk stasis

Painful Breasts—Sore Nipples

Acute **Pain** r/t cracked nipples

Impaired **Skin** integrity r/t mechanical factors involved in suckling, breastfeeding management

Ineffective **Breastfeeding** r/t pain

Ineffective **Role** performance r/t change in physical capacity to assume role of breastfeeding mother

Risk for **Infection** r/t break in skin

Pallor of Extremities

Ineffective **Tissue** perfusion: peripheral r/t interruption of vascular flow

Pancreatic Cancer

Anticipatory **Grieving** r/t shortened life span

Death **Anxiety** r/t possible poor prognosis of disease process

Deficient **Knowledge** r/t disease-induced diabetes, home management

Fear r/t poor prognosis of the disease

Ineffective family **Coping** r/t poor prognosis

Spiritual distress r/t poor prognosis

See Cancer; Radiation Therapy; Surgery

Pancreatitis

Acute **Pain** r/t irritation and edema of the inflamed pancreas

Chronic **Sorrow** r/t chronic illness

Diarrhea r/t decrease in pancreatic secretions resulting in steatorrhea

Deficient **Fluid** volume r/t vomiting, decreased fluid intake, fever, diaphoresis, fluid shifts

Imbalanced **Nutrition**: less than body requirements r/t inadequate dietary intake, increased nutritional needs secondary to acute illness, increased metabolic needs caused by increased body temperature

Ineffective **Breathing** pattern r/t splinting from severe pain

Ineffective **Denial** r/t ineffective coping, alcohol use

Ineffective **Health** maintenance r/t deficient knowledge concerning diet, alcohol use, medication

Nausea r/t irritation of gastrointestinal system

Panic Disorder

Anxiety r/t situational crisis

Ineffective **Coping** r/t personal vulnerability

Post-trauma syndrome r/t previous catastrophic event

Readiness for enhanced **Coping** r/t seeking problem-oriented and emotion-oriented strategies to manage condition

Risk for **Loneliness** r/t inability to socially interact because of fear of losing control

Risk for **Post-trauma** syndrome r/t perception of the event, diminished ego strength

Risk for **Powerlessness** r/t ineffective coping skills

Social isolation r/t fear of lack of control

P

Paralysis

Acute **Pain** r/t prolonged immobility

Chronic **Sorrow** r/t loss of physical mobility

Constipation r/t effects of spinal cord disruption, inadequate fiber in diet

Disturbed **Body** image r/t biophysical changes, loss of movement, immobility

Impaired **Home** maintenance r/t physical disability

Impaired physical **Mobility** r/t neuromuscular impairment

Impaired **Transfer** ability r/t paralysis

Ineffective **Health** maintenance r/t deficient knowledge regarding self-care with paralysis

Powerlessness r/t illness-related regimen

Reflex **Incontinence** r/t neurological impairment

Risk for **Disuse** syndrome r/t paralysis

Risk for **Falls** r/t to paralysis

Risk for impaired **Skin** integrity r/t altered circulation, altered sensation, immobility

Risk for **Injury** r/t altered mobility, sensory dysfunction

Risk for natural rubber latex **Allergy** response r/t possible repeated urinary catheterizations

Risk for **Post-trauma** syndrome r/t event causing paralysis

Risk for situational low **Self-esteem** r/t change in body image and function

Self-care deficit: specify r/t neuromuscular impairment

Sexual dysfunction r/t loss of sensation, biopsychosocial alteration

See Child with Chronic Condition; Hemiplegia; Hospitalized Child; Neurotube Defects; Spinal Cord Injury

Paralytic Ileus

Acute **Pain** r/t pressure, abdominal distention

Constipation r/t decreased gastric motility

Deficient **Fluid** volume r/t loss of fluids from vomiting, retention of fluid in bowel

Impaired **Oral** mucous membrane r/t presence of nasogastric tube

Nausea r/t gastrointestinal irritation

Paranoid Personality Disorder

Anxiety r/t uncontrollable intrusive, suspicious thoughts

Chronic low **Self-esteem** r/t inability to trust others

Disturbed personal **Identity** r/t difficulty with reality testing

Disturbed **Sensory** perception: specify r/t psychological dysfunction, suspicious thoughts

Disturbed **Thought** processes r/t psychological conflicts

Impaired **Adjustment** r/t intense emotional state

Risk for **Loneliness** r/t social isolation

Risk for other-directed **Violence** r/t being suspicious of others and others' actions

Risk for **Post-trauma** syndrome r/t exaggerated sense of responsibility

Risk for **Suicide** r/t psychiatric illness

Social isolation r/t inappropriate social skills

Paraplegia

See Spinal Cord Injury

Parathyroidectomy

Anxiety r/t surgery

Risk for impaired verbal **Communication** r/t possible laryngeal damage, edema

Risk for ineffective **Airway** clearance r/t edema or hematoma formation, airway obstruction

Risk for **Infection** r/t surgical procedure

See Hypocalcemia

Parent Attachment

Chronic **Sorrow** r/t difficult parent-child relationship

Risk for impaired parent/infant/child **Attachment** r/t inability of parents to meet personal needs; anxiety associated with parental role; substance abuse; premature infant; ill infant/child who is unable to effectively initiate parental contact as a result of altered behavioral organization, separation, physical barriers, or lack of privacy

Risk for **Spiritual** distress r/t altered relationships

Parental Role Conflict

Chronic **Sorrow** r/t difficult parent-child relationship

Parental role **Conflict** r/t separation from child because of chronic illness, intimidation with invasive or restrictive modalities (e.g., isolation, intubation), specialized care center policies, home care of a child with special needs (e.g., apnea monitoring, postural drainage, hyperalimentation), change in marital status, interruptions of family life because of home care regimen (e.g., treatments, caregivers, lack of respite)

Readiness for enhanced **Parenting** r/t willingness to enhance parenting

Risk for **Spiritual** distress r/t altered relationships

P

Parenting

Readiness for enhanced Parenting: r/t the following: expresses willingness to enhance parenting; children or other dependent person(s) express satisfaction with home, environment; emotional and tacit support of children or dependent person(s) evident; bonding or attachment evident; physical and emotional needs of children/dependent person(s) are met; realistic expectations of children/dependent person(s) exhibited

Parenting, Impaired

Chronic **Sorrow** r/t difficult parent-child relationship

Impaired **Parenting** r/t lack of available role model; ineffective role model; physical and psychosocial abuse of nurturing figure; lack of support between and from significant other(s); unmet social, emotional, or maturational needs of parenting figures; interruption in bonding process (e.g., maternal, paternal, other); unrealistic expectations for self, infant, partner; physical illness; presence of stress (e.g., financial, legal, recent crisis, cultural, move); lack of knowledge; limited cognitive functioning; lack of role identity; lack or inappropriate response of child to relationship; multiple pregnancies

Risk for **Spiritual** distress r/t altered relationships

Parenting, Risk for Impaired

Chronic **Sorrow** r/t difficult parent-child relationship

Risk for impaired **Parenting** r/t lack of available role model; ineffective role model; physical and psychosocial abuse of nurturing figure; lack of support between or from significant other(s); unmet social, emotional, or maturational needs of parenting figures; interruption in bonding process (e.g., maternal, paternal, other); unrealistic expectations for self, infant, partner; physical illness; presence of stress (e.g., financial, legal, recent crisis, cultural move); lack of knowledge; limited cognitive functioning; lack of role identity; lack of inappropriate response of child to relationship; multiple pregnancies

Risk for **Spiritual** distress r/t altered relationships

Paresthesia

Disturbed **Sensory** perception: tactile r/t altered sensory reception, transmission, integration

Risk for **Injury** r/t inability to feel temperature changes, pain

Parkinson's Disease

Chronic **Sorrow** r/t loss of physical capacity

Constipation r/t weakness of defecation muscles, lack of exercise, inadequate fluid intake, decreased autonomic nervous system activity

Imbalanced **Nutrition**: less than body requirements r/t tremor, slowness in eating, difficulty in chewing and swallowing

Impaired verbal **Communication** r/t decreased speech volume, slowness of speech, impaired facial muscles

Risk for **Injury** r/t tremors, slow reactions, altered gait

See Neurological Disorders

Paroxysmal Nocturnal Dyspnea

See PND

Patent Ductus Arteriosus (PDA)

See Congenital Heart Disease/Cardiac Anomalies

Patient-Controlled Analgesia

See PCA

Patient Education

Deficient Knowledge r/t lack of exposure to information, information misinterpretation, unfamiliarity with information resources

Effective Therapeutic regimen management r/t verbalized desire to manage illness, prevent complications

Health-seeking behaviors r/t expressed or observed desire to seek a higher level of wellness, control of health practices

Readiness for enhanced **Knowledge** of (specify) r/t interest in learning, knowledge of the topic, behaviors congruent with expressed knowledge, previous experiences pertaining to the topic

Readiness for enhanced **Spiritual** well-being r/t desire to reach harmony with self, others, higher power/God

Readiness for enhanced **Therapeutic** regimen management: r/t the following: expresses a desire to manage the treatment of illness and prevent sequelae, makes choices of daily living that are appropriate for meeting the goals of treatment or prevention, expresses little to no difficulty with regulation/integration of one or more prescribed regimens for treatment of illness or prevention of complications, describes reduction of risk factors for progression of illness and sequelae, shows no unexpected acceleration of illness symptoms

PCA (Patient-Controlled Analgesia)

Deficient **Knowledge** r/t self-care of pain control

Effective **Therapeutic** regimen management r/t ability to manage pain with appropriate use of patient-controlled analgesia

Impaired **Comfort**: pruritus, nausea, vomiting r/t side effects of medication

Readiness for **Knowledge** of appropriate management of PCA

Risk for **Injury** r/t possible complications associated with PCA

Pelvic Inflammatory Disease

See PID

Penile Prosthesis

Health-seeking behavior r/t information regarding use and care of prosthesis

Ineffective **Sexuality** pattern r/t use of penile prosthesis

Risk for **Infection** r/t invasive surgical procedure

Risk for situational low **Self-esteem** r/t Ineffective **Sexuality** patterns

See impotence

Peptic Ulcer

See Ulcer

Percutaneous Transluminal Coronary Angioplasty (PTCA)

See Angioplasty, Coronary Balloon

Pericardial Friction Rub

Acute **Pain** r/t inflammation, effusion

Decreased **Cardiac** output r/t inflammation in pericardial sac, fluid accumulation compressing heart

Delayed **Surgical** recovery r/t complications associated with cardiac problems

Pericarditis

Activity intolerance r/t reduced cardiac reserve, prescribed bedrest

Acute **Pain** r/t biological injury, inflammation

Delayed **Surgical** recovery r/t complications associated with cardiac problems

Deficient **Knowledge** r/t unfamiliarity with information sources

Ineffective **Tissue** perfusion: cardiopulmonary/peripheral r/t risk for development of emboli

Risk for decreased **Cardiac** output r/t inflammation in pericardial sac, fluid accumulation compressing heart function

Risk for imbalanced **Nutrition**: less than body requirements r/t fever, hypermetabolic state associated with fever

Perioperative Positioning

Risk for perioperative positioning **Injury** r/t disorientation; immobilization; muscle weakness; sensory/perceptual disturbances resulting from anesthesia, obesity, emaciation, edema

Peripheral Neurovascular Dysfunction, Risk for

Risk for **Peripheral** neurovascular dysfunction r/t fractures, mechanical compression, orthopedic surgery, trauma, immobilization, burns, vascular obstruction

Peripheral Vascular Disease

Activity intolerance r/t imbalance between peripheral oxygen supply and demand

Chronic **Pain**: intermittent claudication r/t ischemia

Ineffective **Health** maintenance r/t deficient knowledge regarding self-care and treatment of disease

Ineffective **Tissue** perfusion: peripheral r/t interruption of vascular flow

Readiness for enhanced management of **Therapeutic** regimen r/t self-care and treatment of disease

Risk for **Falls** r/t altered mobility

Risk for impaired **Skin** integrity r/t altered circulation or sensation

Risk for **Injury** r/t tissue hypoxia, altered mobility, altered sensation

Risk for **Peripheral** neurovascular dysfunction r/t possible vascular obstruction

Peritoneal Dialysis

Acute **Pain** r/t instillation of dialysate, temperature of dialysate

Chronic **Sorrow** r/t chronic disability

Deficient **Knowledge** r/t treatment procedure, self-care with peritoneal dialysis

Impaired **Home** maintenance r/t complex home treatment of client

Risk for **Fluid** volume excess r/t retention of dialysate

Risk for ineffective **Breathing** pattern r/t pressure from dialysate

Risk for ineffective **Coping** r/t disability requiring change in lifestyle

Risk for **Infection**: peritoneal r/t invasive procedure, presence of catheter, dialysate

Risk for **Powerlessness** r/t chronic condition and care involved

See Child with Chronic Condition; Hospitalized Child; Renal Failure; Renal Failure, Acute/Chronic—Child

Peritonitis

Acute **Pain** r/t inflammation, stimulation of somatic nerves

P

Constipation r/t decreased oral intake, decrease of peristalsis

Deficient **Fluid** volume r/t retention of fluid in bowel with loss of circulating blood volume

Imbalanced **Nutrition**: less than body requirements r/t nausea, vomiting

Ineffective **Breathing** pattern r/t pain, increased abdominal pressure

Nausea r/t gastrointestinal irritation

Persistent Fetal Circulation

See Congenital Heart Disease/Cardiac Anomalies

Personal Identity Problems

Disturbed personal **Identity** r/t situational crisis, psychological impairment, chronic illness, pain

Personality Disorder

Chronic low **Self-esteem** r/t inability to set and achieve goals

Compromised family **Coping** r/t inability of client to provide positive feedback to family, chronicity exhausting family

Decisional **Conflict** r/t low self-esteem, feelings that choices will always be wrong

Disturbed personal **Identity** r/t lack of consistent positive self-image

Impaired **Adjustment** r/t ambivalent behavior toward others, testing of others' loyalty

Impaired **Social** interaction r/t knowledge or skill deficit regarding ways to interact effectively with others, self-concept disturbances

Readiness for enhanced **Self-concept** r/t expressing willingness to enhance self-concept

Risk for **Loneliness** r/t inability to interact appropriately with others

Risk for **Self-mutilation** r/t disturbed interpersonal relationships, borderline personality disorders

Risk for situational low **Self-esteem** r/t history of learned helplessness

Spiritual distress r/t lack of identifiable values, lack of meaning to life

See Antisocial Personality Disorder; Borderline Personality Disorder

Pertussis (Whooping Cough)

See Respiratory Infections, Acute Childhood

Petechiae

See Clotting Disorder

Pharyngitis

See Sore Throat

Pheochromocytoma

Anxiety r/t symptoms from increased catecholamines—headache, palpitations, sweating, nervousness, nausea, vomiting, syncope

Disturbed **Sleep** pattern r/t high levels of catecholamines

Ineffective **Health** maintenance r/t deficient **Knowledge** regarding treatment and self-care

Nausea r/t increased catecholamines

Risk for ineffective **Tissue** perfusion: cardiopulmonary and renal r/t episodes of hypertension

See Surgery

Phobia (Specific)

Anxiety r/t inability to control emotions when dreaded object or situation is encountered

Fear r/t presence or anticipation of specific object or situation

Ineffective **Coping** r/t transfer of fears from self to dreaded object situation

Powerlessness r/t anxiety about encountering unknown or known entity

Readiness for enhanced **Communication** r/t willingness to discuss situation

Risk for **Post-trauma** syndrome r/t exposure to dreaded object or situation

Risk for **Powerlessness** r/t inadequate coping patterns

Risk for situational low **Self-esteem** r/t decreased power/control over fears

See Anxiety; Panic Disorder

Photosensitivity

Ineffective **Health** maintenance r/t deficient knowledge regarding medications inducing photosensitivity

Risk for impaired **Skin** integrity r/t exposure to sun

Physical Abuse

See Abuse

PID (Pelvic Inflammatory Disease)

Acute **Pain** r/t biological injury; inflammation, edema, congestion of pelvic tissues

Ineffective **Health** maintenance r/t deficient knowledge regarding self-care, treatment of disease

Ineffective **Sexuality** patterns r/t medically imposed abstinence from sexual activities until acute infection subsides, change in reproductive potential

Risk for **Infection** r/t insufficient knowledge to avoid exposure to pathogens; proper hygiene, nutrition, other health habits

P

Risk for urge urinary **Incontinence** r/t inflammation, edema, congestion of pelvic tissues

See Maturational Issues, Adolescent

PIH (Pregnancy-Induced Hypertension/ Preeclampsia)

Anxiety r/t fear of the unknown, threat to self and infant, change in role functioning

Death **Anxiety** r/t threat of preeclampsia

Deficient **Diversional** activity r/t bedrest

Deficient **Knowledge** r/t lack of experience with situation

Excess **Fluid** volume r/t decreased renal function

Impaired **Home** maintenance r/t bedrest

Impaired **Parenting** r/t bedrest

Impaired physical **Mobility** r/t medically prescribed limitations

Impaired **Social** interaction r/t imposed bedrest

Ineffective **Role** performance r/t change in physical capacity to assume role of pregnant woman or resume other roles

Interrupted **Family** processes r/t situational crisis

Powerlessness r/t complication threatening pregnancy, medically prescribed limitations

Readiness for enhanced **Knowledge** r/t desire for information on managing condition

Risk for imbalanced **Fluid** volume r/t hypertension, altered renal function

Risk for **Injury**: fetal r/t decreased uteroplacental perfusion, seizures

Risk for **Injury**: maternal r/t vasospasm, high blood pressure

Situational low **Self-esteem** r/t loss of idealized pregnancy

Piloerection

Hypothermia r/t exposure to cold environment

Placenta Previa

Death **Anxiety** r/t threat of mortality associated with bleeding

Deficient **Diversional** activity r/t long-term hospitalization

Disturbed **Body** image r/t negative feelings about body and reproductive ability, feelings of helplessness

Fear r/t threat to self and fetus, unknown future

Impaired **Home** maintenance r/t maternal bed rest, hospitalization

Impaired physical **Mobility** r/t medical protocol, maternal bed rest

Ineffective **Coping** r/t threat to self and fetus

Ineffective **Role** performance r/t maternal bed rest, hospitalization

Ineffective **Tissue** perfusion: placental r/t dilation of cervix, loss of placental implantation site

Interrupted **Family** processes r/t maternal bed rest, hospitalization

Risk for **Constipation** r/t bed rest, pregnancy

Risk for deficient **Fluid** volume r/t maternal blood loss

Risk for imbalanced **Fluid** volume r/t maternal blood loss

Risk for impaired **Parenting** r/t maternal bed rest, hospitalization

Risk for **Injury**: fetal and maternal r/t threat to uteroplacental perfusion, hemorrhage

Risk for **Powerlessness** r/t complications of pregnancy and unknown outcome

Situational low **Self-esteem** r/t situational crisis

Spiritual distress r/t inability to participate in usual religious rituals, situational crisis

Pleural Effusion

Acute **Pain** r/t inflammation, fluid accumulation

Excess **Fluid** volume r/t compromised regulatory mechanisms; heart, liver, or kidney failure

Hyperthermia r/t increased metabolic rate secondary to infection

Ineffective **Breathing** pattern r/t pain

Pleural Friction Rub

Acute **Pain** r/t inflammation, fluid accumulation

Ineffective **Breathing** pattern r/t pain

See cause of Pleural Friction Rub

Pleurisy

Acute **Pain** r/t pressure on pleural nerve endings associated with fluid accumulation or inflammation

Ineffective **Breathing** pattern r/t pain

Risk for impaired **Gas** exchange r/t ventilation perfusion imbalance

Risk for impaired physical **Mobility** r/t activity intolerance, inability to "catch breath"

Risk for ineffective **Airway** clearance r/t increased secretions, ineffective cough because of pain

PMS (Premenstrual Tension Syndrome)

Acute **Pain** r/t hormonal stimulation of gastrointestinal structures

Deficient **Knowledge** r/t methods to deal with and prevent syndrome

P

Excess **Fluid** volume r/t alterations of hormonal levels inducing fluid retention

Fatigue r/t hormonal changes

Readiness for enhanced **Communication** r/t willingness to express thoughts and feelings about PMS

Readiness for enhanced **Therapeutic** regimen management r/t desire for information to manage and prevent symptoms

Risk for **Powerlessness** r/t lack of knowledge and ability to deal with symptoms

PND (Paroxysmal Nocturnal Dyspnea)

Anxiety r/t inability to breathe during sleep

Decreased **Cardiac** output r/t failure of the left ventricle

Disturbed **Sleep** pattern r/t suffocating feeling from fluid in lungs on awakening from sleep

Ineffective **Breathing** pattern r/t increase in carbon dioxide levels, decrease in oxygen levels

Readiness for enhanced **Sleep** r/t expressing willingness to learn measures to enhance sleep

Risk for **Powerlessness** r/t inability to control nocturnal dyspnea

Sleep deprivation r/t inability to breathe during sleep

Pneumonia

Activity intolerance r/t imbalance between oxygen supply and demand

Deficient **Knowledge** r/t risk factors predisposing person to pneumonia, treatment

Hyperthermia r/t dehydration, increased metabolic rate, illness

Imbalanced **Nutrition**: less than body requirements r/t loss of appetite

Impaired **Oral** mucous membrane r/t dry mouth from mouth breathing, decreased fluid intake

Impaired **Gas** exchange r/t decreased functional lung tissue

Ineffective **Airway** clearance r/t inflammation and presence of secretions

Ineffective **Health** maintenance r/t deficient knowledge regarding self-care and treatment of disease

Risk for deficient **Fluid** volume r/t inadequate intake of fluids

See Respiratory Infections, Acute Childhood (for child)

Pneumothorax

Acute **Pain** r/t recent injury, coughing, deep breathing

Fear r/t threat to own well-being, difficulty breathing

Impaired **Gas** exchange r/t ventilation-perfusion imbalance

Risk for **Injury** r/t possible complications associated with closed chest drainage system

Poisoning, Risk for

INTERNAL

Risk for **Poisoning** r/t reduced vision, verbalization of occupational settings without adequate safeguards, lack of safety or drug education, lack of proper precaution, cognitive or emotional difficulties, insufficient finances

EXTERNAL

Risk for **Poisoning** r/t large supplies of drugs in house, medicine stored in unlocked cabinets accessible to children or confused persons, dangerous products placed or stored within the reach of children or confused persons, availability of illicit drugs potentially contaminated by poisonous additives, flaking or peeling paint or plaster in presence of young children, chemical contamination of food and water, unprotected contact with heavy metals or chemicals, paint or lacquer used in poorly ventilated areas or without effective protection, presence of poisonous vegetation, presence of atmospheric pollutants

Polydipsia

Readiness for enhanced **Fluid** balance r/t no excessive thirst when diabetes is controlled

See Diabetes Mellitus

Polyphagia

Readiness for enhanced **Nutrition** r/t knowledge of appropriate diet for diabetes

See Diabetes Mellitus

Polyuria

Readiness for enhanced **Urinary** elimination r/t willingness to learn measures to enhance urinary elimination

See Diabetes Mellitus

Postoperative Care

See Surgery, Postoperative

Postpartum Blues

Anxiety r/t new responsibilities of parenting

Chronic **Sorrow** r/t loss of ideal postpartum experience or ideal parent-infant relationship

Deficient **Knowledge** r/t lifestyle changes

Disturbed **Body** image r/t normal postpartum recovery

Disturbed **Sleep** pattern r/t new responsibilities of parenting

Fatigue r/t childbirth, postpartum state

Impaired **Adjustment** r/t lack of support systems

Impaired **Home** maintenance r/t fatigue, care of newborn

Impaired **Parenting** r/t hormone-induced depression

Impaired **Social** interaction r/t change in role functioning

Ineffective **Coping** r/t hormonal changes, maturational crisis

Ineffective **Role** performance r/t new responsibilities of parenting

Risk for **Post-trauma** syndrome r/t trauma or violence associated with labor and birth process, medical/surgical interventions, history of sexual abuse

Risk for situational low **Self-esteem** r/t decreased power over feelings of sadness

Risk for **Spiritual** distress r/t altered relationships, social isolation

Sexual dysfunction r/t fear of another pregnancy, postpartum pain, lochia flow

Postpartum Hemorrhage

Activity intolerance r/t anemia from loss of blood

Acute **Pain** r/t nursing and medical interventions to control bleeding

Death **Anxiety** r/t threat of mortality associated with bleeding

Decreased **Cardiac** output r/t hypovolemia

Deficient **Fluid** volume r/t uterine atony, loss of blood

Deficient **Knowledge** r/t lack of exposure to situation

Disturbed **Body** image r/t loss of ideal childbirth

Fear r/t threat to self, unknown future

Impaired **Home** maintenance r/t lack of stamina

Ineffective **Tissue** perfusion r/t hypovolemia

Interrupted **Breastfeeding** r/t separation from infant for medical treatment

Risk for imbalanced **Fluid** volume r/t maternal blood loss

Risk for impaired **Parenting** r/t weakened maternal condition

Risk for **Infection** r/t loss of blood, depressed immunity

Risk for **Powerlessness** r/t acute illness

Postpartum, Normal Care

Acute **Pain** r/t episiotomy, lacerations, bruising, breast engorgement, headache, sore nipples, epidural or IV site, hemorrhoids

Anxiety r/t change in role functioning, parenting

Constipation r/t hormonal effects on smooth muscles, fear of straining with defecation, effects of anesthesia

Deficient **Knowledge**: infant care r/t lack of preparation for parenting

Disturbed **Sleep** pattern r/t care of infant

Effective **Breastfeeding** r/t basic breastfeeding knowledge, support of partner and health care provider

Fatigue r/t childbirth, new responsibilities of parenting, body changes

Health-seeking behaviors r/t postpartum recovery and adaptation

Impaired **Skin** integrity r/t episiotomy, lacerations

Impaired **Urinary** elimination r/t effects of anesthesia, tissue trauma

Ineffective **Breastfeeding** r/t lack of knowledge, lack of support, lack of motivation

Ineffective **Role** performance r/t new responsibilities of parenting

Readiness for enhanced family **Coping** r/t adaptation to new family member

Readiness for enhanced **Parenting** r/t expressing willingness to enhance parenting skills

Risk for Impaired **Parenting** r/t lack of role models, deficient knowledge

Risk for **Constipation** r/t hormonal effects on smooth muscles, fear of straining with defecation, effects of anesthesia

Risk for imbalanced **Fluid** volume r/t shift in blood volume, edema

Risk for **Infection** r/t tissue trauma, blood loss

Risk for **Post-trauma** syndrome r/t trauma or violence associated with labor and birth process, medical/surgical interventions, history of sexual abuse

Risk for urge urinary **Incontinence** r/t effects of anesthesia or tissue trauma

Sexual dysfunction r/t fear of pain or pregnancy

Post-Trauma Syndrome

Post-trauma syndrome r/t events outside the range of the usual human experience; physical and psychosocial abuse; tragic occurrence involving multiple deaths; sudden destruction of one's home or community; natural or produced disasters; wars; being held as a prisoner of war or enduring criminal victimization (torture); epidemics; serious accidents; rape; assault; witnessing mutilation, violent death, or other horrors; serious threat or injury to self or loved ones; industrial and motor vehicle accidents; catastrophic illnesses or accidents; military combat

P

Post-Traumatic Stress Disorder

Anxiety r/t exposure to internal or external cues that symbolize or resemble an aspect of the traumatic event

Death **Anxiety** r/t psychological stress associated with traumatic event

Disturbed **Energy** field r/t disharmony of mind, body, spirit

Disturbed **Sensory** perception r/t psychological stress

Disturbed **Sleep** pattern r/t recurring nightmares

Disturbed **Thought** processes r/t sense of reliving the experience (flashbacks)

Ineffective **Breathing** pattern r/t hyperventilation associated with anxiety

Ineffective **Coping** r/t extreme anxiety

Post-trauma syndrome r/t exposure to a traumatic event

Readiness for enhanced **Communication** r/t willingness to express feelings and thoughts

Readiness for enhanced **Spiritual** well-being r/t desire for harmony after stressful event

Risk for **Powerlessness** r/t flashbacks, reliving event

Risk for self- or other-directed **Violence** r/t fear of self or others

Sleep deprivation r/t nightmares associated with traumatic event

Spiritual distress r/t feelings of detachment or estrangement from others

Potassium, Increase/Decrease

See Hyperkalemia/Hypokalemia

Powerlessness

Powerlessness r/t health care environment, illness-related regimen, interpersonal interaction, lifestyle of helplessness

Risk for **Powerlessness** r/t chronic or acute illness, acute injury or progressive debilitating disease process, aging, dying, lack of knowledge of illness or health care style, lifestyle of dependency with inadequate coping patterns, absence of integrality, decreased self-esteem, low or unstable body image

Preeclampsia

See PIH

Pregnancy—Cardiac Disorders

See Cardiac Disorders in Pregnancy

Pregnancy-Induced Hypertension/Preeclampsia

See PIH

Pregnancy Loss

Acute **Pain** r/t surgical intervention

Anxiety r/t threat to role functioning, health status, situational crisis

Chronic **Sorrow** r/t loss of a fetus or child

Compromised family **Coping** r/t lack of support by significant other because of personal suffering

Ineffective **Coping** r/t situational crisis

Ineffective **Role** performance r/t inability to assume parenting role

Ineffective **Sexuality** patterns r/t self-esteem disturbance resulting from pregnancy loss and anxiety about future pregnancies

Readiness for enhanced **Communication** r/t willingness to express feelings and thoughts about loss

Readiness for enhanced **Spiritual** well-being r/t desire for acceptance of loss

Risk for deficient **Fluid** volume r/t blood loss

Risk for dysfunctional **Grieving** r/t loss of pregnancy

Risk for ineffective **Sexuality** patterns r/t self-esteem disturbance, anxiety, grief

Risk for **Infection** r/t retained products of conception

Risk for **Powerlessness** r/t situational crisis

Risk for **Spiritual** distress r/t intense suffering

Spiritual distress r/t intense suffering

Pregnancy—Normal

Deficient **Knowledge** r/t primiparity

Disturbed **Body** image r/t altered body function and appearance

Disturbed **Sleep** pattern r/t sleep deprivation secondary to uncomfortable pregnancy state

Fear r/t labor and delivery

Health-seeking behaviors r/t desire to promote optimal fetal and maternal health

Imbalanced **Nutrition**: less than body requirements r/t growing fetus, nausea

Imbalanced **Nutrition**: more than body requirements r/t deficient knowledge regarding nutritional needs of pregnancy

Ineffective **Coping** r/t personal vulnerability, situational crisis

Interrupted **Family** processes r/t developmental transition of pregnancy

Nausea r/t hormonal changes of pregnancy

Readiness for enhanced family **Coping** r/t satisfying partner relationship, attention to gratification of needs, effective adaptation to developmental tasks of pregnancy

P

Readiness for enhanced **Parenting** r/t expressing willingness to enhance parenting skills

Sexual dysfunction r/t altered body function, self-concept, body image with pregnancy

See Discomforts of Pregnancy

Premature Dilation of the Cervix (Incompetent Cervix)

Anticipatory **Grieving** r/t potential loss of infant

Deficient **Diversional** activity r/t bed rest

Deficient **Knowledge** r/t treatment regimen, prognosis for pregnancy

Fear r/t potential loss of infant

Ineffective **Coping** r/t bed rest, threat to fetus

Ineffective **Role** performance r/t inability to continue usual patterns of responsibility

Impaired physical **Mobility** r/t imposed bed rest to prevent preterm birth

Impaired **Social** interaction r/t bed rest

Powerlessness r/t inability to control outcome of pregnancy

Risk for **Infection** r/t invasive procedures to prevent preterm birth

Risk for **Injury**: fetal r/t preterm birth, use of anesthetics

Risk for **Injury**: maternal r/t surgical procedures to prevent preterm birth (e.g., cerclage)

Risk for **Spiritual** distress r/t physical/psychological stress

Sexual dysfunction r/t fear of harm to fetus

Situational low **Self-esteem** r/t inability to complete normal pregnancy

Premature Infant (Child)

Delayed **Growth** and development: developmental lag r/t prematurity, environmental and stimulation deficiencies, multiple caretakers

Disorganized **Infant** behavior r/t prematurity

Disturbed **Sensory** perception r/t noxious stimuli, noisy environment

Disturbed **Sleep** pattern r/t noisy and noxious intensive care environment

Imbalanced **Nutrition**: less than body requirements r/t delayed or understimulated rooting reflex, easy fatigue during feeding, diminished endurance

Impaired **Gas** exchange r/t effects of cardiopulmonary insufficiency

Impaired **Swallowing** r/t decreased or absent gag reflex, fatigue

Ineffective **Thermoregulation** r/t large body surface/weight ratio, immaturity of thermal regulation, state of prematurity

Readiness for enhanced organized **Infant** behavior r/t prematurity

Risk for delayed **Development** r/t prematurity

Risk for disproportionate **Growth** r/t prematurity

Risk for **Infection** r/t inadequate, immature, or undeveloped acquired immune response

Risk for **Injury** r/t prolonged mechanical ventilation, retrolental fibroplasia (RLF) secondary to 100% oxygen environment

Premature Infant (Parent)

Anticipatory **Grieving** r/t loss of perfect child possibly leading to dysfunctional grieving

Chronic **Sorrow** r/t threat of loss of a child, prolonged hospitalization

Compromised family **Coping** r/t disrupted family roles and disorganization, prolonged condition exhausting supportive capacity of significant persons

Decisional **Conflict** r/t support system deficit, multiple sources of information

Dysfunctional **Grieving** (prolonged) r/t unresolved conflicts

Ineffective **Breastfeeding** r/t disrupted establishment of effective pattern secondary to prematurity or insufficient opportunities

Parental role **Conflict** r/t expressed concerns, expressed inability to care for child's physical, emotional, or developmental needs

Readiness for enhanced **Family** process r/t adaptation to change associated with premature infant

Risk for impaired parent/infant/child **Attachment** r/t separation, physical barriers, lack of privacy

Risk for **Powerlessness** r/t inability to control situation

Risk for **Spiritual** distress r/t challenged belief or value systems regarding moral or ethical implications of treatment plans

Spiritual distress r/t challenged belief or value systems regarding moral or ethical implications of treatment plans

See Child with Chronic Condition; Hospitalized Child

Premature Rupture of Membranes

Anticipatory **Grieving** r/t potential loss of infant

Anxiety r/t threat to infant's health status

Disturbed **Body** image r/t inability to carry pregnancy to term

P

Ineffective **Coping** r/t situational crisis

Risk for **Infection** r/t rupture of membranes

Risk for **Injury**: fetal r/t risk of premature birth

Situational low **Self-esteem** r/t inability to carry pregnancy to term

Premenstrual Tension Syndrome
See PMS

Prenatal Care—Normal

Anxiety r/t unknown future, threat to self secondary to pain of labor

Constipation r/t decreased gastrointestinal motility secondary to hormonal stimulation

Deficient **Knowledge** r/t lack of experience with pregnancy and care

Disturbed **Sleep** pattern r/t discomforts of pregnancy and fetal activity

Fatigue r/t increased energy demands

Health-seeking behaviors r/t consistent prenatal care and education

Imbalanced **Nutrition**: less than body requirements r/t nausea from normal hormonal changes

Impaired **Urinary** elimination r/t frequency caused by increased pelvic pressure and hormonal stimulation

Ineffective **Breathing** pattern r/t increased intrathoracic pressure and decreased energy secondary to enlarged uterus

Interrupted **Family** processes r/t developmental transition

Readiness for enhanced **Knowledge** of appropriate prenatal care

Readiness for enhanced **Nutrition** r/t desire for knowledge of appropriate nutrition during pregnancy

Readiness for enhanced **Parenting** r/t realistic expectations of new role as parent

Readiness for enhanced **Spiritual** well-being r/t oncoming new role as parent

Risk for **Activity** intolerance r/t enlarged abdomen, increased cardiac workload

Risk for **Constipation** r/t decreased gastrointestinal motility secondary to hormonal stimulation

Risk for **Injury**: maternal r/t change in balance and center of gravity secondary to enlarged abdomen

Risk for **Sexual** dysfunction r/t enlarged abdomen, fear of harm to infant

Prenatal Testing

Acute **Pain** r/t invasive procedures

Anxiety r/t unknown outcome, delayed test results

Health-seeking behaviors r/t desire to have information regarding prenatal testing

Risk for **Infection** r/t invasive procedures during amniocentesis or chorionic villi sampling

Risk for **Injury**: fetal r/t invasive procedures

Preoperative Teaching

Health-seeking behaviors r/t preoperative regimens, postoperative precautions, expectations of role of client during preoperative or postoperative time

See Surgery, Preoperative Care

Pressure Ulcer

Acute **Pain** r/t tissue destruction, exposure of nerves

Imbalanced **Nutrition**: less than body requirements r/t limited access to food, inability to absorb nutrients because of biological factors, anorexia

Impaired bed **Mobility** r/t intolerance to activity, pain, cognitive impairment, depression, severe anxiety

Impaired **Skin** integrity: stage I or II pressure ulcer r/t physical immobility, mechanical factors, altered circulation, skin irritants

Impaired **Tissue** integrity: stage III or IV pressure ulcer r/t altered circulation, impaired physical mobility

Risk for **Infection** r/t physical immobility, mechanical factors (shearing forces, pressure, restraint, altered circulation, skin irritants)

Total urinary **Incontinence** r/t neurological dysfunction

Preterm Labor

Anticipatory **Grieving** r/t loss of idealized pregnancy, potential loss of fetus

Anxiety r/t threat to fetus, change in role functioning, change in environment and interaction patterns, use of tocolytic drugs

Deficient **Diversional** activity r/t long-term hospitalization

Disturbed **Sleep** pattern r/t change in usual pattern secondary to contractions, hospitalization, treatment regimen

Impaired **Home** maintenance r/t medical restrictions

Impaired physical **Mobility** r/t medically imposed restrictions

Impaired **Social** interaction r/t prolonged bedrest or hospitalization

Ineffective **Coping** r/t situational crisis, preterm labor

Ineffective **Role** performance r/t inability to carry out normal roles secondary to bedrest or hospitalization, change in expected course of pregnancy

P

Readiness for enhanced **Communication** r/t willingness to discuss thoughts and feelings about situation

Risk for **Injury**: fetal r/t premature birth, immature body systems

Risk for **Injury**: maternal r/t use of tocolytic drugs

Risk for **Powerlessness** r/t lack of control over preterm labor

Sexual dysfunction r/t actual or perceived limitation imposed by preterm labor and/or prescribed treatment, separation from partner because of hospitalization

Situational low **Self-esteem** r/t threatened ability to carry pregnancy to term

Problem-Solving Ability

Defensive **Coping** r/t situational crisis

Impaired **Adjustment** r/t altered locus of control

Ineffective **Coping** r/t situational crisis

Readiness for enhanced **Communication** r/t willingness to share ideas with others

Readiness for enhanced **Spiritual** well-being r/t desire to draw on inner strength and find meaning and purpose to life

Projection

Anxiety r/t threat to self-concept

Chronic low **Self-esteem** r/t failure

Defensive **Coping** r/t inability to acknowledge that own behavior may be a problem, blaming others

Impaired **Social** interaction r/t self-concept disturbance, confrontational communication style

Risk for **Loneliness** r/t blaming others for problems

Risk for **Post-trauma** syndrome r/t diminished ego strength

Prolapsed Umbilical Cord

Fear r/t threat to fetus, impending surgery

Ineffective **Tissue** perfusion: fetal r/t interruption in umbilical blood flow

Risk for **Injury**: fetal r/t cord compression, ineffective tissue perfusion

Risk for **Injury**: maternal r/t emergency surgery

Prolonged Gestation

Anxiety r/t potential change in birthing plans, need for increased medical intervention, unknown outcome for fetus

Defensive **Coping** r/t underlying feeling of inadequacy regarding ability to give birth normally

Imbalanced **Nutrition**: less than body requirements (fetal) r/t aging of placenta

Powerlessness r/t perceived lack of control over outcome of pregnancy

Situational low **Self-esteem** r/t perceived inadequacy of body functioning

Prostatectomy

See TURP

Prostatic Hypertrophy

Disturbed **Sleep** pattern r/t nocturia

Ineffective **Health** maintenance r/t deficient knowledge regarding self-care and prevention of complications

Risk for **Infection** r/t urinary residual after voiding, bacterial invasion of bladder

Risk for urge urinary **Incontinence** r/t small bladder capacity

Urinary retention r/t obstruction

Prostatitis

Ineffective **Health** maintenance r/t deficient knowledge regarding treatment

Ineffective **Protection** r/t depressed immune system

Risk for urge **Incontinence** r/t irritation of bladder

Protection, Altered

Ineffective **Protection** r/t extremes of age, inadequate nutrition, alcohol abuse, abnormal blood profiles (leukopenia, thrombocytopenia, anemia, coagulation), drug therapies (antineoplastic, corticosteroid, immune, anticoagulant, thrombolytic), treatments (surgery, radiation), diseases (e.g., cancer, immune disorders)

Pruritus

Deficient **Knowledge** r/t methods to treat and prevent itching

Impaired **Comfort**: pruritus r/t inflammation in tissues

Risk for impaired **Skin** integrity r/t scratching from pruritus

Psoriasis

Disturbed **Body** image r/t lesions on body

Impaired **Skin** integrity r/t lesions on body

Ineffective **Health** maintenance r/t deficient knowledge regarding treatment modalities

Powerlessness r/t lack of control over condition with frequent exacerbations and remissions

P

Psychosis

Anxiety r/t unconscious conflict with reality

Chronic **Sorrow** r/t chronic mental illness

Disturbed **Sleep** pattern r/t sensory alterations contributing to fear and anxiety

Disturbed **Thought** processes r/t inaccurate interpretations of environment

Fear r/t altered contact with reality

Imbalanced **Nutrition**: less than body requirements r/t lack of awareness of hunger, disinterest toward food

Impaired **Home** maintenance r/t impaired cognitive or emotional functioning, inadequate support systems

Impaired **Social** interaction r/t impaired communication patterns, self-concept disturbance, disturbed thought processes

Impaired verbal **Communication** r/t psychosis, inaccurate perceptions, hallucinations, delusions

Ineffective **Coping** r/t inadequate support systems, unrealistic perceptions, disturbed thought processes, impaired communication

Ineffective **Health** maintenance r/t cognitive impairment, ineffective individual and family coping

Interrupted **Family** processes r/t inability to express feelings, impaired communication

Risk for **Post-trauma** syndrome r/t diminished ego strength

Risk for self- or other-directed **Violence** r/t lack of trust, panic, hallucinations, delusional thinking

Risk for **Suicide** r/t psychiatric illness/disorder

Self-care deficit r/t loss of contact with reality, impairment of perception

Self-esteem disturbance r/t excessive use of defense mechanisms (e.g., projection, denial, rationalization)

Social isolation r/t lack of trust, regression, delusional thinking, repressed fears

See Schizophrenia

PTCA (Percutaneous Transluminal Coronary Angioplasty)

See Angioplasty

Pulmonary Edema

Anxiety r/t fear of suffocation

Impaired **Gas** exchange r/t extravasation of extravascular fluid in lung tissues and alveoli

Ineffective **Breathing** pattern r/t presence of tracheobronchial secretions

Ineffective **Health** maintenance r/t deficient knowledge regarding treatment regimen

Sleep deprivation r/t inability to breathe

See CHF

Pulmonary Embolism

Acute **Pain** r/t biological injury, lack of oxygen to cells

Deficient **Knowledge** r/t activities to prevent embolism, self-care after diagnosis of embolism

Delayed **Surgical** recovery r/t complications associated with respiratory difficulty

Fear r/t severe pain, possible death

Impaired **Gas** exchange r/t altered blood flow to alveoli secondary to lodged embolus

Ineffective **Tissue** perfusion: pulmonary r/t interruption of pulmonary blood flow secondary to lodged embolus

Risk for altered **Cardiac** output r/t right ventricular failure secondary to obstructed pulmonary artery

See Anticoagulant Therapy

Pulmonary Stenosis

See Congenital Heart Disease/Cardiac Anomalies

Pulse Deficit

Decreased **Cardiac** output r/t dysrhythmia

See Dysrhythmia

Pulse Oximetry

Readiness for enhanced **Knowledge** r/t treatment regimen

See Hypoxia

Pulse Pressure, Increased

See Intracranial Pressure, Increased

Pulse Pressure, Narrowed

See Shock

Pulses, Absent or Diminished Peripheral

Ineffective **Tissue** perfusion: peripheral r/t interruption of arterial flow

Risk for **Peripheral** neurovascular dysfunction r/t fractures, mechanical compression, orthopedic surgery trauma, immobilization, burns, vascular obstruction

See Cause of Absent or Diminished Peripheral Pulses

Purpura

See Clotting Disorder

Pyelonephritis

Acute **Pain** r/t inflammation and irritation of urinary tract

Disturbed **Sleep** pattern r/t urinary frequency

Impaired **Comfort** r/t chills and fever

Impaired **Urinary** elimination r/t irritation of urinary tract

Ineffective **Health** maintenance r/t deficient knowledge regarding self-care, treatment of disease, prevention of further urinary tract infections

Risk for urge urinary **Incontinence** r/t irritation of urinary tract

Pyloric Stenosis

Acute **Pain** r/t surgical incision

Deficient **Fluid** volume r/t vomiting, dehydration

Imbalanced **Nutrition**: less than body requirements r/t vomiting secondary to pyloric sphincter obstruction

Ineffective **Health** maintenance r/t parental deficient knowledge regarding home care feeding regimen, wound care

See Hospitalized Child

Q

Quadriplegia

Anticipatory **Grieving** r/t loss of normal lifestyle, severity of disability

Impaired **Transfer** ability r/t quadriplegia

Impaired wheelchair **Mobility** r/t quadriplegia

Ineffective **Breathing** pattern r/t inability to use intercostal muscles

Readiness for enhanced **Spiritual** well being r/t heightened coping associated with disability

Risk for **Autonomic** dysreflexia r/t bladder distention, bowel distention, skin irritation, lack of client and caregiver knowledge

See Spinal Cord Injury

R

Rabies

Acute **Pain** r/t multiple immunization injections

Health-seeking behaviors r/t prophylactic immunization of domestic animals, avoidance of contact with wild animals

Hopelessness r/t poor prognosis

Ineffective **Health** maintenance r/t deficient knowledge regarding care of wound, isolation and observation of infected animal

Radiation Therapy

Activity intolerance r/t fatigue from possible anemia

Deficient **Knowledge** r/t what to expect with radiation therapy

Diarrhea r/t irradiation effects

Disturbed **Body** image r/t change in appearance, hair loss

Imbalanced **Nutrition**: less than body requirements r/t anorexia, nausea, vomiting, irradiation of areas of pharynx and esophagus

Impaired **Oral** mucous membrane r/t irradiation effects

Ineffective **Protection** r/t suppression of bone marrow

Nausea r/t side effects of radiation

Risk for impaired **Skin** integrity r/t irradiation effects

Risk for **Powerlessness** r/t medical treatment and possible side effects

Risk for **Spiritual** distress r/t radiation treatment, prognosis

Radical Neck Dissection

See Laryngectomy

Rage

Risk for other-directed **Violence** r/t panic state, manic excitement, organic brain syndrome

Risk for **Self-mutilation** r/t command hallucinations

Risk for **Suicide** r/t desire to kill oneself

Rape-Trauma Syndrome

Chronic **Sorrow** r/t forced loss of virginity

Rape-trauma syndrome r/t forced, violent sexual penetration against victim's will and consent

Rape-trauma syndrome: compound reaction r/t forced and violent sexual penetration against victim's will and consent, activation of previous health disruptions (e.g., physical illness, psychiatric illness, substance abuse)

Rape-trauma syndrome: silent reaction r/t forced and violent sexual penetration against victim's will and consent, demonstration of repression of incident

Risk for **Post-trauma** syndrome r/t trauma or violence associated with rape

Risk for **Powerlessness** r/t inability to control thoughts about incident

Risk for **Spiritual** distress r/t forced loss of virginity

Rash

Impaired **Comfort**: pruritus r/t inflammation in skin

Impaired **Skin** integrity r/t mechanical trauma

Risk for **Infection** r/t traumatized tissue, broken skin

Risk for latex **Allergy** r/t multiple surgical procedures, allergies to products associated with latex allergy, professions with daily associations with latex, history of reactions to latex

R

Rationalization

Defensive **Coping** r/t situational crisis, inability to accept blame for consequences of own behavior

Ineffective **Denial** r/t fear of consequences, actual or perceived loss

Readiness for enhanced **Communication** r/t expressing desire to share thoughts and feelings

Readiness for enhanced **Spiritual** well-being r/t possibility of seeking harmony with self, others, higher power/God

Risk for **Post-trauma** syndrome r/t survivor's role in event

Rats, Rodents in the Home

Impaired **Home** maintenance r/t lack of knowledge, insufficient finances

Raynaud's Disease

Deficient **Knowledge** r/t lack of information about disease process, possible complications, self-care needs regarding disease process and medication

Ineffective **Tissue** perfusion: peripheral r/t transient reduction of blood flow

RDS (Respiratory Distress Syndrome)

See Respiratory Conditions of the Neonate

Rectal Fullness

Constipation r/t decreased activity level, decreased fluid intake, inadequate fiber in diet, decreased peristalsis, side effects from antidepressant or antipsychotic therapy

Risk for **Constipation** r/t habitual denial/ignoring of urge to defecate

Rectal Pain/Bleeding

Acute **Pain** r/t pressure of defecation

Constipation r/t pain on defecation

Deficient **Knowledge** r/t possible causes of rectal bleeding, pain, treatment modalities

Risk for deficient **Fluid** volume: bleeding r/t untreated rectal bleeding

Rectal Surgery

See Hemorrhoidectomy

Rectocele Repair

Acute **Pain** r/t surgical procedure

Constipation r/t painful defecation

Ineffective **Health** maintenance r/t deficient knowledge of postoperative care of surgical site, dietary measures, exercise to prevent constipation

Risk for **Infection** r/t surgical procedure, possible contamination of site with feces

Risk for urge urinary **Incontinence** r/t edema from surgery

Urinary retention r/t edema from surgery

Reflex Incontinence

Reflex **Incontinence** r/t neurological impairment

Regression

Anxiety r/t threat to or change in health status

Defensive **Coping** r/t denial of obvious problems, weaknesses

Ineffective **Role** performance r/t powerlessness over health status

Powerlessness r/t health care environment

See Hospitalized Child; Separation Anxiety

Regretful

Anxiety r/t situational or maturational crises

Death **Anxiety** r/t feelings of not having accomplished goals in life

Risk for **Spiritual** distress r/t inability to forgive

Rehabilitation

Impaired **Comfort** r/t difficulty in performing rehabilitation tasks

Impaired physical **Mobility** r/t injury, surgery, psychosocial condition warranting rehabilitation

Ineffective **Coping** r/t loss of normal function

Readiness for enhanced **Therapeutic** regimen management r/t expression of desire to manage rehabilitation

Self-care deficit r/t impaired physical mobility

Relaxation Techniques

Anxiety r/t disturbed energy field

Health-seeking behaviors r/t requesting information about ways to relieve stress

Readiness for enhanced **Self-concept** r/t willingness to enhance self-concept

Readiness for enhanced **Spiritual** well-being r/t seeking comfort from higher power

Religious Concern

Readiness for enhanced **Spiritual** well-being r/t desire for increased spirituality

Risk for **Spiritual** distress r/t physical or psychological stress

Spiritual distress r/t separation from religious or cultural ties

Relocation Stress Syndrome

Relocation stress syndrome r/t past, concurrent, recent losses; losses involved with decision to move; feeling of powerlessness; lack of adequate support system; little or no preparation for the impending move; moderate to high degree of environmental change; history and types of previous transfers; impaired psychosocial health status; decreased physical health status; advanced age

Risk for Relocation Stress Syndrome

See Relocation Stress Syndrome

Renal Failure

Activity intolerance r/t effects of anemia, congestive heart failure

Chronic **Sorrow** r/t chronic illness

Death **Anxiety** r/t unknown outcome of disease

Decreased **Cardiac** output r/t effects of congestive heart failure, elevated potassium levels interfering with conduction system

Excess **Fluid** volume r/t decreased urine output, sodium retention, inappropriate fluid intake

Fatigue r/t effects of chronic uremia and anemia

Imbalanced **Nutrition**: less than body requirements r/t anorexia, nausea, vomiting, altered taste sensation, dietary restrictions

Impaired **Comfort**: pruritus r/t effects of uremia

Impaired **Oral** mucous membrane r/t irritation from nitrogenous waste products

Impaired **Urinary** elimination r/t effects of disease, need for dialysis

Ineffective **Coping** r/t depression secondary to chronic disease

Risk for impaired **Oral** mucous membrane r/t dehydration, effects of uremia

Risk for **Infection** r/t altered immune functioning

Risk for **Injury** r/t bone changes, neuropathy, muscle weakness

Risk for **Noncompliance** r/t complex medical therapy

Risk for **Powerlessness** r/t chronic illness

Spiritual distress r/t dealing with chronic illness

Renal Failure, Acute/Chronic—Child

Deficient **Diversional** activity r/t immobility during dialysis

Disturbed **Body** image r/t growth retardation, bone changes, visibility of dialysis access devices (shunt, fistula), edema

See Child with Chronic Illness; Hospitalized Child; Renal Failure

Renal Failure, Nonoliguric

Anxiety r/t change in health status

Risk for deficient **Fluid** volume r/t loss of large volumes of urine

See Renal Failure

Renal Transplantation, Donor

Decisional **Conflict** r/t harvesting of kidney from traumatized donor

Readiness for enhanced **Communication** r/t expressing thoughts and feelings about situation

Readiness for enhanced family **Coping** r/t decision to allow organ donation

Readiness for enhanced **Spirituality** r/t inner peace resulting from allowance of organ donation

Spiritual distress r/t anticipatory grieving from loss of significant person

See Nephrectomy

Renal Transplantation, Recipient

Anxiety r/t possible rejection, procedure

Deficient **Knowledge** r/t specific nutritional needs, possible paralytic ileus, fluid or sodium restrictions

Impaired **Health** maintenance r/t long-term home treatment after transplantation, diet, signs of rejection, use of medications

Impaired **Urinary** elimination r/t possible impaired renal function

Ineffective **Protection** r/t immunosuppression therapy

Readiness for enhanced **Spiritual** well-being r/t acceptance of situation

Risk for **Infection** r/t use of immunosuppressive therapy to control rejection

Risk for **Spiritual** distress r/t obtaining transplanted kidney from someone's traumatic loss

Respiratory Acidosis

See Acidosis, Respiratory

Respiratory Conditions of the Neonate (Respiratory Distress Syndrome [RDS], Meconium Aspiration, Diaphragmatic Hernia)

Fatigue r/t increased energy requirements and metabolic demands

Impaired **Gas** exchange r/t decreased surfactant, immature lung tissue

Ineffective **Airway** clearance r/t sequelae of attempts to breathe in utero resulting in meconium aspiration

Ineffective **Breathing** pattern r/t prolonged ventilator dependence

R

Risk for **Infection** r/t tissue destruction or irritation secondary to aspiration of meconium fluid

See Bronchopulmonary Dysplasia; Hospitalized Child; Premature Infant

Respiratory Distress

See Dyspnea

Respiratory Distress Syndrome (RDS)

See Respiratory Conditions of the Neonate

Respiratory Infections, Acute Childhood (Croup, Epiglottitis, Pertussis, Pneumonia, Respiratory Syncytial Virus)

Activity intolerance r/t generalized weakness, dyspnea, fatigue, poor oxygenation

Anxiety/fear r/t oxygen deprivation, difficulty breathing

Deficient **Fluid** volume r/t insensible losses (fever, diaphoresis), inadequate oral fluid intake

Hyperthermia r/t infectious process

Imbalanced **Nutrition**: less than body requirements r/t anorexia, fatigue, generalized weakness, poor sucking and breathing coordination, dyspnea

Impaired **Gas** exchange r/t insufficient oxygenation secondary to inflammation or edema of epiglottis, larynx, bronchial passages

Ineffective **Airway** clearance r/t excess tracheobronchial secretions

Ineffective **Breathing** pattern r/t inflamed bronchial passages, coughing

Risk for **Aspiration** r/t inability to coordinate breathing, coughing, sucking

Risk for **Infection**: transmission to others r/t virulent infectious organisms

Risk for **Injury** (to pregnant others) r/t exposure to aerosolized medications (e.g., ribavirin, pentamidine), resultant potential fetal toxicity

Risk for **Suffocation** r/t inflammation of larynx, epiglottis

See Hospitalized Child

Respiratory Syncytial Virus

See Respiratory Infections, Acute Childhood

Retching

Imbalanced **Nutrition**: less than body requirements r/t inability to ingest food

Nausea r/t chemotherapy, postsurgical anesthesia, irritation to gastrointestinal system, stimulation of neuropharmacological mechanisms

Retinal Detachment

Anxiety r/t change in vision, threat of loss of vision

Deficient **Knowledge** r/t symptoms, need for early intervention to prevent permanent damage

Disturbed **Sensory** perception: visual r/t changes in vision, sudden flashes of light, floating spots, blurring of vision

Risk for Impaired **Home** maintenance r/t postoperative care, activity limitations, care of affected eye

See Vision Impairment

Reye's Syndrome

Anticipatory **Grieving** r/t uncertain prognosis and sequelae

Compromised family **Coping** r/t acute situational crisis

Deficient **Fluid** volume r/t vomiting, hyperventilation

Disturbed **Sensory** perception r/t cerebral edema

Disturbed **Thought** processes r/t degenerative changes in fatty brain tissue

Excess **Fluid** volume: cerebral r/t cerebral edema

Imbalanced **Nutrition**: less than body requirements r/t effects of liver dysfunction, vomiting

Impaired **Gas** exchange r/t hyperventilation, sequelae of increased intracranial pressure

Impaired **Skin** integrity r/t effects of decorticate or decerebrate posturing, seizure activity

Ineffective **Breathing** pattern r/t neuromuscular impairment

Ineffective **Health** maintenance r/t deficient knowledge regarding use of salicylates during viral illness of child

Risk for **Injury** r/t combative behavior, seizure activity

Situational low **Self-esteem**: family r/t negative perceptions of self, perceived inability to manage family situation, expressions of guilt

See Hospitalized Child

Rh Factor Incompatibility

Anxiety r/t unknown outcome of pregnancy

Deficient **Knowledge** r/t treatment regimen from lack of experience with situation

Health-seeking behaviors r/t prenatal care, compliance with diagnostic and treatment regimen

Powerlessness r/t perceived lack of control over outcome of pregnancy

Risk for fetal **Injury** r/t intrauterine destruction of red blood cells, transfusions

R

Rheumatic Fever

See Endocarditis

Rheumatoid Arthritis, Juvenile (JRA)

Acute **Pain** r/t swollen or inflamed joints, restricted movement, physical therapy

Delayed **Growth** and development r/t effects of physical disability, chronic illness

Fatigue r/t chronic inflammatory disease

Impaired physical **Mobility** r/t pain, restricted joint movement

Risk for impaired **Skin** integrity r/t splints, adaptive devices

Risk for **Injury** r/t impaired physical mobility, splints, adaptive devices, increased bleeding potential secondary to antiinflammatory medications

Risk for situational low **Self-esteem** r/t disturbed body image

Self-care deficits: feeding, bathing/hygiene, dressing/grooming, toileting r/t restricted joint movement, pain

See Child with Chronic Condition; Hospitalized Child

Rib Fracture

Acute **Pain** r/t movement, deep breathing

Ineffective **Breathing** pattern r/t fractured ribs

See Ventilator Client (if relevant)

Ridicule of Others

Defensive **Coping** r/t situational crisis, psychological impairment, substance abuse

Risk for **Post-trauma** syndrome r/t perception of the event

Ringworm of Body

Impaired **Skin** integrity r/t presence of macules associated with fungus

Ineffective **Therapeutic** regimen management r/t deficient knowledge of prevention, treatment

See Itching

Ringworm of Nails

Disturbed **Body** image r/t appearance of nails, removed nails

Ineffective **Therapeutic** regimen management r/t deficient knowledge of prevention, treatment

Ringworm of Scalp

Disturbed **Body** image r/t possible hair loss (alopecia)

Ineffective **Therapeutic** regimen management r/t deficient knowledge of prevention, treatment

See Itching

Roaches, Invasion of Home with

Impaired **Home** maintenance r/t lack of knowledge, insufficient finances

Role Performance, Altered

Ineffective **Role** performance r/t inability to perform role as anticipated

RSV (Respiratory Syncytial Virus)

See Respiratory Infection, Acute Childhood

Rubella

See Communicable Diseases, Childhood

Rubor of Extremities

Ineffective **Tissue** perfusion: peripheral r/t interruption of arterial flow

See Peripheral Vascular Disease

S

Sadness

Dysfunctional **Grieving** r/t actual or perceived loss

Readiness for enhanced **Communication** r/t willingness to share feelings and thoughts

Readiness for enhanced **Spiritual** well-being r/t desire for harmony following actual or perceived loss

Risk for **Powerlessness** r/t actual or perceived loss

Risk for **Spiritual** distress r/t loss of loved one

Spiritual distress r/t intense suffering

Safety, Childhood

Deficient **Knowledge**: potential for enhanced health maintenance r/t parental knowledge and skill acquisition regarding appropriate safety measures

Health-seeking behaviors: enhanced parenting r/t adequate support systems, appropriate requests for help, desire and request for safety information, requests for information or assistance regarding parenting skills

Risk for altered **Health** maintenance r/t parental deficient knowledge regarding appropriate safety needs per developmental stage, childproofing house, infant and child car restraints, water safety, teaching child ways to avoid molestation

Risk for **Aspiration** and/or suffocation r/t pillow or propped bottle placed in infant's crib; sides of playpen/crib being wide enough for child to get head through; child left in car with engine running; enclosed areas; plastic bags or small objects used as toys; toys with small, breakaway parts; refrigerators or freezers with doors accessible as play areas; child left unattended in or near bathtub, pool, spa; low clotheslines; electric ga-

S

rage doors without automatic stop/reopen; pacifier hung around infant's neck; food not cut into small, bite-size, age-appropriate pieces; balloons, hot dogs, nuts, or popcorn given to infant or young child (especially <1 year of age); use of baby powder

Risk for impaired **Parenting** r/t lack of available and effective role model, lack of knowledge, misinformation from other family members (old wives' tales)

Risk for **Injury/Trauma** r/t developmental age, altered home maintenance management (house not childproofed), impaired parenting, hot liquids within child's reach, no infant or child car restraints, no gate at top of stairs, lack of immunization, no fences or pool or spa covers, child left unattended in car with closed windows in hot weather, firearms loaded and within child's reach

Risk for **Poisoning** r/t use of lead-based paint, presence of asbestos or radon gas, drugs not locked in cabinet, household products left in accessible area (bleach, detergent, drain cleaners, household cleaners), alcohol and perfume within reach of child, presence of poisonous plants, atmospheric pollutants

Salmonella
See Gastroenteritis

Salpingectomy
Anticipatory **Grieving** r/t possible loss due to tubal pregnancy

Decisional **Conflict** r/t sterilization procedure

Risk for impaired **Urinary** elimination r/t trauma to ureter during surgery

See Hysterectomy; Surgery

Sarcoidosis
Acute **Pain** r/t possible disease affecting joints

Anxiety r/t change in health status

Impaired **Gas** exchange r/t ventilation-perfusion imbalance

Ineffective **Health** maintenance r/t deficient knowledge regarding home care and medication regimen

Risk for decreased **Cardiac** output r/t dysrhythmias

SARS (Severe Acute Respiratory Syndrome)
Risk for **Infection** r/t increased environmental exposure (travelers in close proximity to infected persons, traveling when a fever is present)

Readiness for Enhanced **Knowledge** of information regarding travel and precautions to avoid exposure to SARS

See Pneumonia

SBE (Self Breast Examination)
Health-seeking behaviors r/t desire to have information about self breast examination

Readiness for enhanced **Knowledge** of self-breast examination

Scabies
See Communicable Diseases, Childhood

Scared
Anxiety r/t threat of death, threat to or change in health status

Death **Anxiety** r/t unresolved issues surrounding end-of-life decisions

Fear r/t hospitalization, real or imagined threat to own well-being

Readiness for enhanced **Communication** r/t willingness to share thoughts and feelings

Schizophrenia
Anxiety r/t unconscious conflict with reality

Chronic **Sorrow** r/t chronic mental illness

Deficient **Diversional** activity r/t social isolation, possible regression

Disturbed **Sleep** pattern r/t sensory alterations contributing to fear and anxiety

Disturbed **Thought** processes r/t inaccurate interpretations of environment

Fear r/t altered contact with reality

Imbalanced **Nutrition**: less than body requirements r/t fear of eating, lack of awareness of hunger, disinterest toward food

Impaired **Home** maintenance r/t impaired cognitive or emotional functioning, insufficient finances, inadequate support systems

Impaired **Social** interaction r/t impaired communication patterns, self-concept disturbance, disturbed thought processes

Impaired verbal **Communication** r/t psychosis, disorientation, inaccurate perception, hallucinations, delusions

Ineffective **Coping** r/t inadequate support systems, unrealistic perceptions, inadequate coping skills, disturbed thought processes, impaired communication

Ineffective **Health** maintenance r/t cognitive impairment, ineffective individual and family coping, lack of material resources

Ineffective **Therapeutic** regimen management: families r/t chronicity and unpredictability of condition

Interrupted **Family** processes r/t inability to express feelings, impaired communication

S

neuromuscular impairment, musculoskeletal impairment, depression, severe anxiety

Self-Care Deficit, Dressing/Grooming

Dressing/grooming **Self-care** deficit r/t intolerance to activity, decreased strength and endurance, pain, discomfort, perceptual or cognitive impairment, neuromuscular impairment, musculoskeletal impairment, depression, severe anxiety

Self-Care Deficit, Feeding

Feeding **Self-care** deficit: r/t intolerance to activity, decreased strength and endurance, pain, discomfort, perceptual or cognitive impairment, neuromuscular impairment, musculoskeletal impairment, depression, severe anxiety

Self-Care Deficit, Toileting

Toileting **Self-care** deficit r/t impaired transfer ability, impaired mobility status, intolerance to activity, decreased strength and endurance, pain, discomfort, perceptual or cognitive impairment, neuromuscular impairment, musculoskeletal impairment, depression, severe anxiety

Self-Concept

Readiness for enhanced **Self-concept** r/t expressed willingness to enhance self-concept; expressed satisfaction with thoughts about self, sense of worthiness, role performance, body image, personal identity; actions congruent with expressed feelings and thoughts; expressed confidence in abilities; acceptance of strengths and limitations

Self-Destructive Behavior

Post-trauma response r/t unresolved feelings from traumatic event

Risk for self-directed **Violence** r/t panic state, history of child abuse, toxic reaction to medication

Risk for **Self-mutilation** r/t feelings of depression, rejection, self-hatred, depersonalization; command hallucinations

Risk for **Suicide** r/t history of self-destructive behavior

Self-Esteem, Chronic Low

Chronic low **Self-esteem** r/t long-standing negative self-evaluation

Self-Esteem, Situational Low

Risk for situational low **Self-esteem** r/t self-esteem disturbance

Self-esteem disturbance r/t inappropriate and learned negative feelings about self

Situational low **Self-esteem** r/t developmental crisis, disturbed body image, functional impairment, loss,

social role changes, lack of recognition/rewards, behavior inconsistent with values, failures/rejections

Self-Mutilation, Risk for

Risk for **Self-mutilation** r/t inability to cope with increased psychological or physiological tension in a healthy manner; feelings of depression, rejection, self-hatred, separation anxiety, guilt, depersonalization; fluctuating emotions; command hallucinations; need for sensory stimuli; parental emotional deprivation; dysfunctional family

Self-mutilation r/t psychotic state (command hallucinations); inability to express tension verbally; childhood sexual abuse; violence between parental figures; family divorce; family alcoholism; family history of self-destructive behaviors; adolescence; peers who self-mutilate; isolation from peers; perfectionism; substance abuse; eating disorders; sexual identity crisis; low or unstable self-esteem; low or unstable body image; labile behavior (mood swings); history of inability to plan solutions or see long-term consequences; use of manipulation to obtain nurturing relationship with others; chaotic/disturbed interpersonal relationships; emotional disturbance; battered child; feels threatened with actual or potential loss of significant relationship (e.g., loss of parent/parental relationship); experiences dissociation or depersonalization; mounting tension that is intolerable; impulsivity; inadequate coping; irresistible urge to cut/damage self; needs quick reduction of stress; childhood illness or surgery; foster, group, or institutional care; incarceration; character disorder; borderline personality disorder; developmental delay or autism; history of self-injurious behavior; feelings of depression, rejection, self-hatred, separation anxiety, guilt, depersonalization; poor parent-adolescent communication; lack of family confidant.

Senile Dementia

See Dementia

Sensory/Perceptual Alterations

Disturbed **Sensory** perceptions: visual, auditory, kinesthetic, gustatory, tactile, olfactory r/t altered, excessive, or insufficient environmental stimuli; altered sensory reception, transmission, and/or integration; endogenous (electrolyte) or exogenous (e.g., drugs) chemical alterations; psychological stress

Separation Anxiety

Ineffective **Coping** r/t maturational and situational crises, vulnerability secondary to developmental age, hospitalization, separation from family and familiar surroundings, multiple caregivers

See Hospitalized Child

S

Risk for **Caregiver** role strain r/t bizarre behavior of client, chronicity of condition

Risk for **Loneliness** r/t inability to interact socially

Risk for **Post-trauma** syndrome r/t diminished ego strength

Risk for **Powerlessness** r/t intrusive, distorted thinking

Risk for self- and other-directed **Violence** r/t lack of trust, panic, hallucinations, delusional thinking

Risk for **Suicide** r/t psychiatric illness

Self-care deficit r/t loss of contact with reality, impairment of perception

Self-esteem disturbance r/t excessive use of defense mechanisms (e.g., projection, denial, rationalization)

Sleep deprivation r/t intrusive thoughts, nightmares

Social isolation r/t lack of trust, regression, delusional thinking, repressed fears

Spiritual distress r/t loneliness/social alienation

Scoliosis

Acute **Pain** r/t musculoskeletal restrictions, surgery, reambulation with cast or spinal rod

Chronic **Sorrow** r/t chronic disability

Disturbed **Body** image r/t use of therapeutic braces, postsurgery scars, restricted physical activity

Impaired **Adjustment** r/t lack of developmental maturity to comprehend long-term consequences of noncompliance with treatment procedures

Impaired **Gas** exchange r/t restricted lung expansion secondary to severe presurgery curvature of spine, immobilization

Impaired physical **Mobility** r/t restricted movement, dyspnea secondary to severe curvature of spine

Impaired **Skin** integrity r/t braces, casts, surgical correction

Ineffective **Breathing** pattern r/t restricted lung expansion secondary to severe curvature of spine

Ineffective **Health** maintenance r/t deficient knowledge regarding treatment modalities, restrictions, home care, postoperative activities

Readiness for enhanced **Therapeutic** regimen management r/t desire for knowledge regarding treatment for condition

Risk for **Infection** r/t surgical incision

Risk for perioperative positioning **Injury** r/t prone position

See Hospitalized Child; Maturational Issues, Adolescent

Sedentary Lifestyle

Activity intolerance r/t sedentary lifestyle

Readiness for enhanced **Coping** r/t seeking knowledge of new strategies to adjust to sedentary lifestyle

Seizure Disorders, Adult

Acute **Confusion** r/t postseizure state

Impaired **Memory** r/t seizure activity

Ineffective **Health** maintenance r/t lack of knowledge regarding anticonvulsive therapy .

Readiness for enhanced **Knowledge** of anticonvulsive therapy

Risk for disturbed **Thought** processes r/t effects of anticonvulsant medications

Risk for **Falls** r/t uncontrolled seizure activity

Risk for ineffective **Airway** clearance r/t accumulation of secretions during seizure

Risk for **Injury** r/t uncontrolled movements during seizure, falls, drowsiness secondary to anticonvulsants

Risk for **Powerlessness** r/t possible seizure

Social isolation r/t unpredictability of seizures, community-imposed stigma

See Epilepsy

Seizure Disorders, Childhood (Epilepsy, Febrile Seizures, Infantile Spasms)

Ineffective **Health** maintenance r/t lack of knowledge regarding anticonvulsive therapy, fever reduction (febrile seizures)

Risk for delayed **Development** and disproportionate growth r/t effects of seizure disorder, parental overprotection

Risk for disturbed **Thought** processes r/t effects of anticonvulsant medications

Risk for **Falls** r/t possible seizure

Risk for ineffective **Airway** clearance r/t accumulation of secretions during seizure

Risk for **Injury** r/t uncontrolled movements during seizure, falls, drowsiness secondary to anticonvulsants

Social isolation r/t unpredictability of seizures, community-imposed stigma

See Epilepsy

Self Breast Examination

See SBE

Self-Care Deficit, Bathing/Hygiene

Bathing/hygiene **Self-care** deficit r/t intolerance to activity, decreased strength and endurance, pain, discomfort, perceptual or cognitive impairment,

S

Sepsis—Child

Delayed **Surgical** recovery r/t presence of infection

Imbalanced **Nutrition**: less than body requirements r/t anorexia, generalized weakness, poor sucking reflex

Impaired **Comfort**: increased sensitivity to environmental stimuli r/t disturbed sensory perceptions: visual, auditory, kinesthetic

Ineffective **Thermoregulation** r/t infectious process, septic shock

Ineffective **Tissue** perfusion: cardiopulmonary, peripheral r/t arterial or venous blood flow exchange problems, septic shock

Risk for impaired **Skin** integrity r/t desquamation secondary to disseminated intravascular coagulation (DIC)

See Hospitalized Child; Premature Infant

Septicemia

Deficient **Fluid** volume r/t vasodilation of peripheral vessels, leaking of capillaries

Imbalanced **Nutrition**: less than body requirements r/t anorexia, generalized weakness

Ineffective **Tissue** perfusion r/t decreased systemic vascular resistance

See Sepsis—Child; Shock; Shock, Septic

Severe acute respiratory syndrome

See SARS; Pneumonia

Sexual Dysfunction

Chronic **Sorrow** r/t loss of ideal sexual experience, altered relationships

Sexual dysfunction r/t biopsychosocial alteration of sexuality, ineffectual or absent role models, physical abuse or harmful relationships, vulnerability, conflicting values, lack of privacy, lack of significant others, altered body structure or function (pregnancy, recent childbirth, drug use, surgery, anomalies, disease process, trauma, radiation), misinformation or lack of knowledge

Sexuality, Adolescent

Decisional **Conflict**: sexual activity r/t undefined personal values or beliefs, multiple or divergent sources of information, lack of relevant information

Deficient **Knowledge**: potential for enhanced health maintenance r/t multiple or divergent sources of information or lack of relevant information regarding sexual transmission of disease, contraception, prevention of toxic shock syndrome

Disturbed **Body** image r/t anxiety secondary to unachieved developmental milestone (puberty) or deficient knowledge regarding reproductive maturation as manifested by amenorrhea or expressed concerns regarding lack of growth of secondary sex characteristics

Risk for **Rape-trauma** syndrome r/t date rape, campus rape, insufficient knowledge regarding self-protection mechanisms

See Maturational Issues, Adolescent

Sexuality Patterns, Ineffective

Ineffective **Sexuality** patterns r/t knowledge or skill deficit regarding alternative responses to health-related transitions, altered body function or structure, illness or medical problems, lack of privacy, lack of significant other, ineffective or absent role models, fear of pregnancy or acquiring a sexually transmitted disease, impaired relationship with a significant other

Sexually Transmitted Disease

See STD

Shakiness

Anxiety r/t situational or maturational crisis, threat of death

Shame

Self-esteem disturbance r/t inability to deal with past traumatic events, blaming of self for events not under one's control

Shingles

Acute **Pain** r/t vesicular eruption along the nerves

Ineffective **Protection** r/t abnormal blood profiles

Risk for **Infection** r/t tissue destruction

Social isolation r/t altered state of wellness, contagiousness of disease

See Itching

Shivering

Hypothermia r/t exposure to cool environment

Shock

Fear r/t serious threat to health status

Ineffective **Tissue** perfusion: cardiopulmonary, peripheral r/t arterial/venous blood flow exchange problems

Risk for **Injury** r/t prolonged shock resulting in multiple organ failure, death

See Shock, Cardiogenic; Shock, Hypovolemic; Shock, Septic

Shock, Cardiogenic

Decreased **Cardiac** output r/t decreased myocardial contractility, dysrhythmia

See Shock

S

Shock, Hypovolemic

Deficient **Fluid** volume r/t abnormal loss of fluid

See Shock

Shock, Septic

Deficient **Fluid** volume r/t abnormal loss of fluid through capillaries, pooling of blood in peripheral circulation

Ineffective **Protection** r/t inadequately functioning immune system

See Sepsis, Child; Septicemia; Shock

Shoulder Repair

Risk for perioperative positioning **Injury** r/t immobility

Self-care deficit: bathing/hygiene, dressing/grooming, feeding r/t immobilization of affected shoulder

See Surgery; Total Joint Replacement

Sickle Cell Anemia/Crisis

Activity intolerance r/t fatigue, effects of chronic anemia

Acute **Pain** r/t viscous blood, tissue hypoxia

Deficient **Fluid** volume r/t decreased intake, increased fluid requirements during sickle cell crisis, decreased ability of kidneys to concentrate urine

Impaired physical **Mobility** r/t pain, fatigue

Risk for ineffective **Tissue** perfusion: renal, cerebral, cardiac, gastrointestinal, peripheral r/t effects of red cell sickling, infarction of tissues

Risk for **Infection** r/t alterations in splenic function

See Child with Chronic Condition; Hospitalized Child

SIDS

Anticipatory **Grieving** r/t potential loss of infant

Anxiety/Fear: parental r/t life-threatening event

Deficient **Knowledge**: potential for enhanced health maintenance r/t knowledge or skill acquisition of CPR and home apnea monitoring

Disturbed **Sleep** pattern: parental/infant r/t home apnea monitoring

Interrupted **Family** processes r/t stress secondary to special care needs of infant with apnea

Risk for **Powerlessness** r/t unanticipated life-threatening event

Risk for sudden infant **Death** syndrome r/t infants placed to sleep in the prone or side-lying position, prenatal and/or postnatal infant smoke exposure, infant overheating/overwrapping, soft underlayment/loose articles in the sleep environment, delayed or nonattendance of prenatal care

See Terminally Ill Child/Death of Child

SIDS (Sudden Infant Death Syndrome), Near Miss (Infant Apnea)

Risk for sudden infant **Death** syndrome r/t modifiable risk factors such as infants placed to sleep in the prone or side-lying position, prenatal and/or postnatal infant smoke exposure, infant overheating/overwrapping, soft underlayment/loose articles in the sleep environment, delayed or nonattendance of prenatal care; potentially modifiable risk factors such as low birth weight, prematurity, young maternal age; nonmodifiable risk factors such as male gender, ethnicity (e.g., African American, Native American race of mother), seasonality of SIDS deaths (higher in winter and fall months); peaking of SIDS mortality between infant ages of 2 and 4 months

See SIDS

Situational Crisis

Ineffective **Coping** r/t situational crisis

Interrupted **Family** processes r/t situational crisis

Readiness for enhanced **Communication** r/t willingness to share feelings and thoughts

Readiness for enhanced **Spiritual** well-being r/t desire for harmony following crisis

Skin Cancer

Impaired **Skin** integrity r/t abnormal cell growth in skin, treatment of skin cancer

Ineffective **Health** maintenance r/t deficient knowledge regarding self-care with skin cancer

Readiness for enhanced **Knowledge** of self-care to prevent and treat skin cancer

Skin Disorders

EXTERNAL

Impaired **Skin** integrity r/t hyperthermia, hypothermia, chemical substances, mechanical factors (shearing forces, pressure, restraint), radiation, physical immobilization, humidity

INTERNAL

Impaired **Skin** integrity r/t medication, altered nutritional state (obesity, emaciation), altered metabolic state, altered circulation, altered sensation, altered pigmentation, skeletal prominence, developmental factors, immunological deficit, alterations in turgor (change in elasticity)

Skin Integrity, Risk for Impaired

Risk for impaired **Skin** integrity r/t internal or external factors that are potentially harmful to skin

Skin Turgor, Change in Elasticity

Deficient **Fluid** volume r/t active fluid loss (NOTE: decreased skin turgor can be a normal finding in the elderly)

Sleep

Readiness for enhanced **Sleep** r/t expressed willingness to enhance sleep, amount of sleep and REM sleep is congruent with developmental needs, expressed feeling of being rested after sleep, following sleep routines that promote sleep habits, occasional or infrequent use of medications to induce sleep

Sleep Apnea

See PND

Sleep Deprivation

Disturbed **Sensory** perception r/t lack of sleep

Fatigue r/t lack of sleep

Sleep deprivation r/t prolonged physical discomfort; prolonged psychological discomfort; sustained inadequate sleep hygiene; prolonged use of pharmacological or dietary antisoporifics; aging-related sleep stage shifts; sustained circadian asynchrony; inadequate daytime activity; sustained environmental stimulation; sustained unfamiliar or uncomfortable sleep environment; non–sleep-inducing parenting practices; sleep apnea; periodic limb movement (e.g., restless leg syndrome, nocturnal myoclonus); sundowner's syndrome; narcolepsy; idiopathic central nervous system hypersomnolence; sleep walking; sleep terror; sleep-related enuresis; nightmares; familial sleep paralysis; sleep-related painful erections; dementia

Sleep Pattern Disorders

Sleep pattern disorders r/t sensory alterations, internal factors (illness, psychological stress), external factors (environmental changes, social cues)

Sleep Pattern, Disturbed—Parent/Child

Disturbed **Sleep** pattern: child r/t anxiety or apprehension secondary to parental deprivation (see Suspected Child Abuse and Neglect), fear, night terrors, enuresis, inconsistent parental responses to child's requests to alter bedtime rules, frequent nighttime awakening, inability to wean from parents' bed, hypervigilance

Disturbed **Sleep** pattern: parent r/t time-intensive home treatments, increased caretaker demands

Slurring of Speech

Impaired verbal **Communication** r/t decrease in circulation to brain, brain tumor, anatomical defect, cleft palate

Situational low **Self-esteem** r/t speech impairment

Small Bowel Resection

See Abdominal Surgery

Smell, Loss of Ability to

See Anosmia

Smoking Behavior

Altered **Health** maintenance r/t denial of effects of smoking, lack of effective support for smoking withdrawal

Readiness for enhanced **Knowledge** of smoking cessation

Social Interaction, Impaired

Social interaction: impaired r/t knowledge or skill deficit regarding ways to enhance mutuality, communication barriers, self-concept disturbance, absence of available significant others or peers, limited physical mobility, therapeutic isolation, sociocultural dissonance, environmental barriers, disturbed thought processes

Social Isolation

Social isolation r/t factors contributing to absence of satisfying personal relationships, such as delay in accomplishing developmental tasks, immature interests, alterations in physical appearance, alterations in mental status, unaccepted social behavior, unaccepted social values, altered state of wellness, inadequate personal resources, inability to engage in satisfying personal relationships, fear

Sociopath

See Antisocial Personality Disorder

Sodium, Decrease/Increase

See Hyponatremia/Hypernatremia

Somatoform Disorder

Anxiety r/t unresolved conflicts channeled into physical complaints or conditions

Chronic **Pain** r/t unexpressed anger, multiple physical disorders, depression

Ineffective **Coping** r/t lack of insight into underlying conflicts

Sore Nipples: Breastfeeding

Ineffective **Breastfeeding** r/t deficient knowledge regarding correct feeding procedure

See Painful Breasts—Sore Nipples

S

Sore Throat
Acute **Pain** r/t inflammation, irritation, dryness

Deficient **Knowledge** r/t treatment, relief of discomfort

Impaired **Oral** mucous membrane r/t inflammation or infection of oral cavity

Impaired **Swallowing** r/t irritation of oropharyngeal cavity

Sorrow
Anticipatory **Grieving** r/t impending loss of significant person or object

Chronic **Sorrow** r/t unresolved grief

Grieving r/t loss of significant person, object, or role

Readiness for enhanced **Communication**

Readiness for enhanced **Spiritual** well-being r/t desire to find purpose and meaning of loss

Spastic Colon
See IBS

Speech Disorders
Anxiety r/t difficulty with communication

Impaired verbal **Communication** r/t anatomical defect, cleft palate, psychological barriers, decrease in circulation to brain

Spina Bifida
Risk for latex **Allergy** response r/t multiple exposures to latex products

See Neurotube Defects

Spinal Cord Injury
Chronic **Sorrow** r/t immobility, change in body function

Constipation r/t immobility, loss of sensation

Deficient **Diversional** activity r/t long-term hospitalization, frequent lengthy treatments

Disturbed **Body** image r/t change in body function

Dysfunctional **Grieving** r/t loss of usual body function

Fear r/t powerlessness over loss of body function

Impaired **Home** maintenance r/t change in health status, insufficient family planning or finances, deficient knowledge, inadequate support systems

Impaired physical **Mobility** r/t neuromuscular impairment

Ineffective **Health** maintenance r/t deficient knowledge regarding self-care with spinal cord injury

Reflex **Incontinence** r/t spinal cord lesion interfering with conduction of cerebral messages

Risk for **Autonomic** dysreflexia r/t bladder or bowel distention, skin irritation, deficient knowledge of patient and caregiver

Risk for **Disuse** syndrome r/t paralysis

Risk for impaired **Skin** integrity r/t immobility, paralysis

Risk for ineffective **Breathing** pattern r/t neuromuscular impairment

Risk for **Infection** r/t chronic disease, stasis of body fluids

Risk for **Loneliness** r/t physical immobility

Risk for **Powerlessness** r/t loss of function

Self-care deficit r/t neuromuscular impairment

Sexual dysfunction r/t altered body function

Urinary retention r/t inhibition of reflex arc

See Child with Chronic Condition; Hospitalized Child; Neurotube Defects

Spiritual Distress
Risk for **Spiritual** distress r/t energy-consuming anxiety, low self-esteem, mental illness, physical illness, blocks to self-love, poor relationships, physical or psychological stress, substance abuse, loss of loved one, natural disasters, situational losses, maturational losses, inability to forgive

Spiritual distress r/t self-alienation, loneliness/social alienation, anxiety, sociocultural deprivation, death and dying of self or others, pain, life change, chronic illness of self or others

Spiritual Well-Being
Readiness for enhanced **Spiritual** well-being r/t desire for harmonious interconnectedness, desire to find purpose and meaning to life

Splenectomy
See Abdominal Surgery

Stapedectomy
Acute **Pain** r/t headache

Disturbed **Sensory** perception: auditory r/t hearing loss caused by edema from surgery

Risk for **Falls** r/t dizziness

Risk for **Infection** r/t invasive procedure

Risk for **Injury**: falls r/t dizziness

Stasis Ulcer
Impaired **Tissue** integrity r/t chronic venous congestion

See Varicose Veins

S

STD (Sexually Transmitted Disease)

Acute **Pain** r/t biological or psychological injury

Ineffective **Health** maintenance r/t deficient knowledge regarding transmission, symptoms, treatment of sexually transmitted disease

Ineffective **Sexuality** patterns r/t illness, altered body function

Fear r/t altered body function, risk for social isolation, fear of incurable illness

Readiness for enhanced **Knowledge** of prevention and treatment of sexually transmitted diseases

Risk for **Infection**/spread of infection r/t lack of knowledge concerning transmission of disease

Social isolation r/t fear of contracting or spreading disease

See Maturational Issues, Adolescent

Stertorous Respirations

Ineffective **Airway** clearance r/t pharyngeal obstruction

Stillbirth

See Pregnancy Loss

Stoma

See Ostomy

Stomatitis

Impaired **Oral** mucous membrane r/t pathological conditions of oral cavity

Stone, Kidney

See Kidney Stone

Stool, Hard/Dry

Constipation r/t inadequate fluid intake, inadequate fiber intake, decreased activity level, decreased gastric motility

Straining with Defecation

Constipation r/t less than adequate fluid intake, less than adequate dietary intake

Risk for decreased **Cardiac** output r/t vagal stimulation with dysrhythmia secondary to Valsalva maneuver

Stress

Anxiety r/t feelings of helplessness, feelings of being threatened

Disturbed **Energy** field r/t low energy level, feelings of hopelessness

Fear r/t powerlessness over feelings

Ineffective **Coping** r/t ineffective use of problem-solving process, feelings of apprehension or helplessness

Readiness for enhanced **Communication** r/t willingness to share thoughts and feelings

Readiness for enhanced **Spiritual** well-being r/t desire for harmony and peace in stressful situation

Risk for **Post-trauma** syndrome r/t perception of event, survivor's role in event

Self-esteem disturbance r/t inability to deal with life events

Stress Urinary Incontinence

Risk for urge urinary **Incontinence** r/t involuntary sphincter relaxation

Stress urinary **Incontinence** r/t degenerative change in pelvic muscles

See Incontinence of Urine

Stridor

Ineffective **Airway** clearance r/t obstruction, tracheobronchial infection, trauma

Stroke

See CVA

Stuttering

Anxiety r/t impaired verbal communication

Impaired verbal **Communication** r/t anxiety, psychological problems

Subarachnoid Hemorrhage

Acute **Pain**: headache r/t irritation of meninges from blood, increased intracranial pressure

Ineffective **Tissue** perfusion: cerebral r/t bleeding from cerebral vessel

See Intracranial Pressure, Increased

Substance Abuse

Anxiety r/t loss of control

Compromised/dysfunctional family **Coping** r/t codependency issues

Defensive **Coping** r/t substance abuse

Disturbed **Sleep** pattern r/t irritability, nightmares, tremors

Dysfunctional **Family** processes: alcohol r/t inadequate coping skills

Imbalanced **Nutrition**: less than body requirements r/t anorexia

Ineffective **Coping** r/t use of substances to cope with life events

Ineffective **Denial** r/t refusal to acknowledge substance abuse problem

Ineffective **Protection** r/t malnutrition, sleep deprivation

S

Powerlessness r/t substance addiction

Readiness for enhanced **Coping** r/t seeking social support and seeking knowledge of new strategies

Readiness for enhanced **Self-concept** r/t accepting strengths and limitations

Risk for impaired parent/infant/child **Attachment** r/t substance abuse

Risk for **Injury** r/t alteration in sensory perception

Risk for self- or other-directed **Violence** r/t reactions to substances used, impulsive behavior, disorientation, impaired judgment

Risk for **Suicide** r/t substance abuse

Self-esteem disturbance r/t failure at life events

Social isolation r/t unacceptable social behavior or values

See Maturational Issues, Adolescent

Substance Abuse, Adolescent

See Alcohol Withdrawal; Maturational Issues, Adolescent; Substance Abuse

Substance Abuse in Pregnancy

Altered **Health** maintenance r/t addiction

Defensive **Coping** r/t denial of situation, differing value system

Deficient **Knowledge** r/t lack of exposure to information regarding effects of substance abuse in pregnancy

Health-seeking behaviors (substance abuse counseling) r/t desire to provide child with substance-free perinatal period

Noncompliance r/t differing value system, cultural influences, addiction

Risk for fetal **Injury** r/t effects of drugs on fetal growth and development

Risk for impaired parent-infant **Attachment** r/t substance abuse, inability of parent to meet infant's/own personal needs

Risk for impaired **Parenting** r/t lack of ability to meet infant's needs

Risk for **Infection** r/t intravenous drug use, lifestyle

Risk for maternal **Injury** r/t drug use

See Substance Abuse

Sucking Reflex

Effective **Breastfeeding** r/t regular and sustained suckling and swallowing at breast

Sudden Infant Death Syndrome

See SIDS

Suffocation, Risk for

INTERNAL

Risk for **Suffocation** r/t reduced olfactory sensation, reduced motor abilities, lack of safety education, lack of safety precautions, cognitive or emotional difficulties, disease or injury process

EXTERNAL

Risk for **Suffocation** r/t pillow or propped bottle placed in infant's crib; vehicle running in closed garage; child playing with plastic bags; child inserting small objects into mouth or nose; accessible discarded or unused refrigerators or freezers with doors; child left unattended in or near bathtub, pool, spa; low clotheslines; pacifier hung around infant's neck; large mouthfuls of food

Suicide Attempt

Hopelessness r/t perceived or actual loss, substance abuse, low self-concept, inadequate support systems

Ineffective **Coping** r/t anger, dysfunctional grieving

Post-trauma response r/t history of traumatic events, abuse, rape, incest, war, torture

Readiness for enhanced **Communication** r/t willingness to share thoughts and feelings

Readiness for enhanced **Spiritual** well-being r/t desire for harmony and inner strength to help redefine purpose for life

Risk for **Post-trauma** syndrome r/t survivor's role in suicide attempt

Risk for **Suicide** r/t history of prior attempt, impulsiveness, gun purchase, medication stockpile, suicide threats, family history of suicide, physical illness, hopelessness, social isolation

Self-esteem disturbance r/t guilt, inability to trust, feelings of worthlessness or rejection

Social isolation r/t inability to engage in satisfying personal relationships

Spiritual distress r/t hopelessness, despair

Support System

Readiness for enhanced family **Coping** r/t ability to adapt to tasks associated with care, support of significant other during health crisis

Readiness for enhanced **Parenting** r/t children or other dependent person(s) expressing satisfaction with home environment

Suppression of Labor

See Preterm Labor; Tocolytic Therapy

S

Surgery, Perioperative Care

Risk for imbalanced Fluid volume r/t surgery

Risk for perioperative positioning Injury r/t predisposing condition, prolonged surgery

Surgery, Postoperative Care

Activity intolerance r/t pain, surgical procedure

Acute Pain r/t inflammation or injury in surgical area

Anxiety r/t change in health status, hospital environment

Deficient Knowledge r/t postoperative expectations, lifestyle changes

Imbalanced Nutrition: less than body requirements r/t anorexia, nausea, vomiting, decreased peristalsis

Nausea r/t manipulation of gastrointestinal tract, postsurgical anesthesia

Risk for Constipation r/t decreased activity, decreased food or fluid intake, anesthesia, pain medication

Risk for deficient Fluid volume r/t hypermetabolic state, fluid loss during surgery, presence of indwelling tubes

Risk for ineffective Breathing pattern r/t pain, location of incision, effects of anesthesia/narcotics

Risk for ineffective Tissue perfusion: peripheral r/t hypovolemia, circulatory stasis, obesity, prolonged immobility, decreased coughing, decreased deep breathing

Risk for Infection r/t invasive procedure, pain, anesthesia, location of incision, weakened cough as a result of aging

Urinary retention r/t anesthesia, pain, fear, unfamiliar surroundings, client's position

Surgery, Preoperative Care

Anxiety r/t threat to or change in health status, situational crisis, fear of the unknown

Deficient Knowledge r/t preoperative procedures, postoperative expectations

Disturbed Sleep pattern r/t anxiety about upcoming surgery

Readiness for enhanced Knowledge of preoperative and postoperative expectations for self-care

Suspected Child Abuse and Neglect (SCAN)—Child

Acute Pain r/t physical injuries

Anxiety/Fear: child r/t threat of punishment for perceived wrongdoing

Chronic low Self-esteem r/t lack of positive feedback, excessive negative feedback

Deficient Diversional activity r/t diminished or absent environmental or personal stimuli

Delayed Growth and development: regression vs. delayed r/t diminished or absent environmental stimuli, inadequate caretaking, inconsistent responsiveness by caretaker

Disturbed Sleep pattern r/t hypervigilance, anxiety

Imbalanced Nutrition: less than body requirements r/t inadequate caretaking

Impaired Skin integrity r/t altered nutritional state, physical abuse

Post-trauma response r/t physical abuse, incest, rape, molestation

Rape-trauma syndrome: compound/silent reaction r/t altered lifestyle secondary to abuse, changes in residence

Readiness for enhanced community Coping r/t obtaining resources to prevent child abuse, neglect

Risk for Poisoning r/t inadequate safeguards, lack of proper safety precautions, accessibility of illicit substances secondary to impaired home maintenance

Risk for Suffocation: secondary to aspiration r/t propped bottle, unattended child

Risk for Trauma r/t inadequate precautions, cognitive or emotional difficulties

Social isolation: family-imposed r/t fear of disclosure of family dysfunction and abuse

See Hospitalized Child; Maturational Issues, Adolescent

Suspected Child Abuse and Neglect (SCAN)—Parent

Chronic low Self-esteem r/t lack of successful parenting experiences

Disabled family Coping r/t dysfunctional family, underdeveloped nurturing parental role, lack of parental support systems or role models

Dysfunctional Family processes: alcoholism r/t inadequate coping skills

Impaired Home maintenance r/t disorganization, parental dysfunction, neglect of safe and nurturing environment

Impaired Parenting r/t unrealistic expectations of child; lack of effective role model; unmet social, emotional, or maturational needs of parents; interruption in bonding process

Ineffective Health maintenance r/t deficient knowledge of parenting skills secondary to unachieved developmental tasks

Powerlessness r/t inability to perform parental role responsibilities

S

Risk for **Violence** toward child r/t inadequate coping mechanisms, unresolved stressors, unachieved maturational level by parent

Suspicion

Impaired **Social** interaction r/t disturbed thought processes, paranoid delusions, hallucinations

Powerlessness r/t repetitive paranoid thinking

Risk for self- or other-directed **Violence** r/t inability to trust

Swallowing Difficulties

Impaired **Swallowing** r/t neuromuscular impairment (e.g., decreased or absent gag reflex, decreased strength or excursion of muscles involved in mastication), perceptual impairment, facial paralysis, mechanical obstruction (e.g., edema, tracheostomy tube, tumor), fatigue, limited awareness, reddened or irritated oropharyngeal cavity, improper feeding or positioning

Syncope

Anxiety r/t fear of falling

Decreased **Cardiac** output r/t dysrhythmia

Impaired physical **Mobility** r/t fear of falling

Ineffective **Tissue** perfusion: cerebral r/t interruption of blood flow

Risk for **Falls** r/t syncope

Risk for **Injury** r/t altered sensory perception, transient loss of consciousness, risk for falls

Social isolation r/t fear of falling

Syphilis
See STD

Systemic Lupus Erythematosus
See Lupus Erythematosus

T

T & A (Tonsillectomy and Adenoidectomy)

Acute **Pain** r/t surgical incision

Deficient **Knowledge**: potential for enhanced health maintenance r/t insufficient knowledge regarding postoperative nutritional and rest requirements, signs and symptoms of complications, positioning

Impaired **Comfort** r/t effects of anesthesia (nausea and vomiting)

Ineffective **Airway** clearance r/t hesitation or reluctance to cough secondary to pain

Risk for **Aspiration**/Suffocation r/t postoperative drainage and impaired swallowing

Risk for deficient **Fluid** volume r/t decreased intake secondary to painful swallowing, effects of anesthesia (nausea, vomiting), hemorrhage

Risk for imbalanced **Nutrition**: less than body requirements r/t hesitation or reluctance to swallow

Tachycardia
See Dysrhythmia

Tachypnea

Ineffective **Breathing** pattern r/t pain, anxiety
See cause of Tachypnea

Taste Abnormality

Adult **Failure** to thrive r/t imbalanced nutrition: less than body requirements associated with taste abnormality

Disturbed **Sensory** perception: gustatory r/t medication side effects; altered sensory reception, transmission, integration; aging changes

TB (Tuberculosis)

Impaired **Gas** exchange r/t disease process

Ineffective **Airway** clearance r/t increased secretions, excessive mucus

Ineffective **Breathing** pattern r/t decreased energy/fatigue

Ineffective **Therapeutic** regimen management r/t deficient knowledge of prevention and treatment regimen

Readiness for enhanced **Therapeutic** regimen management r/t taking medications according to prescribed protocol for prevention and treatment

Risk for **Infection** r/t insufficient knowledge regarding avoidance of exposure to pathogens

TBI (Traumatic Brain Injury)

Acute **Confusion** r/t brain injury

Chronic **Sorrow** r/t change in person's health status and functional ability

Decreased **Intracranial** adaptive capacity r/t brain injury

Disturbed **Sensory** perception: specify r/t pressure damage to sensory centers in brain

Disturbed **Thought** processes r/t pressure damage to brain

Impaired **Memory** r/t neurological disturbances

Ineffective **Tissue** perfusion: cerebral r/t effects of increased intracranial pressure

Ineffective **Breathing** pattern r/t pressure damage to breathing center in brain stem

Interrupted **Family** processes r/t traumatic injury to family member

Risk for **Post-trauma** syndrome r/t perception of event causing traumatic brain injury

TD (Traveler's Diarrhea)

Risk for deficient **Fluid** volume r/t excessive loss of fluids; diarrhea

Risk for **Infection** r/t insufficient knowledge regarding avoidance of exposure to pathogens (water supply, iced drinks, local cheeses, ice cream mile, undercooked meat, fish and shellfish, uncooked vegetables, unclean eating utensils, improper hand washing)

Temperature, Decreased

Hypothermia r/t exposure to cold environment

Temperature, Increased

Hyperthermia r/t dehydration, illness, trauma

Temperature Regulation, Impaired

Ineffective **Thermoregulation** r/t trauma, illness

Tension

Anxiety r/t threat to or change in health status, situational crisis

Disturbed **Energy** field r/t change in health status, discouragement, pain

Readiness for enhanced **Communication** r/t willingness to share feelings and thoughts

Terminally Ill Adult

Anticipatory **Grieving** r/t loss of self or significant other

Compromised family **Coping** r/t inability to discuss impending death

Death **Anxiety** r/t unresolved issues relating to death and dying

Decisional **Conflict** r/t planning for advance directives

Disturbed **Energy** field r/t impending disharmony of mind, body, spirit

Readiness for enhanced **Spiritual** well-being r/t desire to achieve harmony of mind, body, spirit

Risk for **Spiritual** distress r/t impending death

Spiritual distress r/t suffering before death

Terminally Ill Child—Adolescent

Disturbed **Body** image r/t effects of terminal disease, already critical feelings of group identity and self-image

Impaired **Social** interaction/social isolation r/t forced separation from peers

Ineffective **Coping** r/t inability to establish personal and peer identity secondary to threat of being different or not being, inability to achieve maturational tasks

See Child with Chronic Condition; Hospitalized Child

Terminally Ill Child—Infant/Toddler

Ineffective **Coping** r/t separation from parents and familiar environment secondary to inability to grasp external meaning of death

Terminally Ill Child—Preschool Child

Fear r/t perceived punishment, bodily harm, feelings of guilt secondary to magical thinking (i.e., believing that thoughts cause events)

Terminally Ill Child—School-Age Child/Preadolescent

Fear r/t perceived punishment, body mutilation, feelings of guilt

Terminally Ill Child/Death of Child—Parent

Anticipatory **Grieving** r/t possible, expected, or imminent death of child

Compromised family **Coping** r/t inability or unwillingness to discuss impending death and feelings with child or to support child through terminal stages of illness

Decisional **Conflict** r/t continuation or discontinuation of treatment, do not resuscitate decision, ethical issues regarding organ donation

Disturbed **Sleep** pattern r/t grieving process

Grieving r/t death of child

Hopelessness r/t overwhelming stresses secondary to terminal illness

Impaired **Parenting** r/t risk for overprotection of surviving siblings

Impaired **Social** interaction r/t dysfunctional grieving

Ineffective **Denial** r/t dysfunctional grieving

Interrupted **Family** processes r/t situational crisis

Powerlessness r/t inability to alter course of events

Readiness for enhanced family **Coping** r/t impact of crisis on family values, priorities, goals, or relationships; expressed interest or desire to attach meaning to child's life and death

Risk for dysfunctional **Grieving** r/t prolonged, unresolved, obstructed progression through stages of grief and mourning

Social isolation: imposed by others r/t feelings of inadequacy in providing support to grieving parents

Social isolation: self-imposed r/t unresolved grief, perceived inadequate parenting skills

T

Spiritual distress r/t sudden and unexpected death, prolonged suffering before death, questioning the death of youth, questioning the meaning of one's own existence

Tetralogy of Fallot

See Congenital Heart Disease/Cardiac Anomalies

Therapeutic Regimen, Effective Management

Effective **Therapeutic** regimen management r/t adequate ability to manage needed health care

Therapeutic Regimen, Ineffective Management

Ineffective **Therapeutic** regimen management r/t complexity of health care system; complexity of therapeutic regimen; decisional conflicts; economic difficulties; excessive demands made on individual or family; family conflict; family patterns of health care; inadequate number and types of cues to action; deficient knowledge; mistrust of regimen or health care personnel; perceived seriousness, susceptibility, barriers, or benefits; powerlessness; social support deficits

Therapeutic Regimen, Ineffective Management: Community

Ineffective community **Therapeutic** regimen management r/t illness symptoms above the norm expected for the number and type of population, unexpected acceleration of illness(es), number of health care resources insufficient for the incidence or prevalence of illness(es), deficits in advocates for aggregates, deficits in people and programs to be accountable for illness care of aggregates, deficits in community activities for secondary and tertiary prevention, unavailable health care resources for illness care

Therapeutic Regimen, Ineffective Management: Family

Ineffective family **Therapeutic** regimen management r/t complexity of health care system, complexity of therapeutic regimen, decisional conflicts, economic difficulties, excessive demands on individual or family, family conflict

Therapeutic Regimen Management, Readiness for Enhanced

Readiness for enhanced **Therapeutic** regimen management r/t the following: expresses desire to manage the treatment of illness and prevention of sequelae, makes choices of daily living that are appropriate for meeting the goals of treatment or prevention, expresses little to no difficulty with regulation/integration of one or more prescribed regimens for treatment of illness or prevention of complications, describes reduction of risk factors for progression of illness and sequelae, shows no unexpected acceleration of illness symptoms

Therapeutic Touch

Disturbed **Energy** field r/t low energy levels, disturbance in energy fields, pain, depression, fatigue

Thermoregulation, Ineffective

Ineffective **Thermoregulation** r/t trauma, illness, immaturity, aging, fluctuating environmental temperature

Thoracotomy

Activity intolerance r/t pain, imbalance between oxygen supply and demand, presence of chest tubes

Acute **Pain** r/t surgical procedure, coughing, deep breathing

Deficient **Knowledge** r/t self-care, effective breathing exercises, pain relief

Ineffective **Airway** clearance r/t drowsiness, pain with breathing and coughing

Ineffective **Breathing** pattern r/t decreased energy, fatigue, pain

Risk for **Infection** r/t invasive procedure

Risk for **Injury** r/t disruption of closed-chest drainage system

Risk for perioperative positioning **Injury** r/t lateral positioning, immobility

Thought Disorders

Disturbed **Thought** processes r/t disruption in cognitive thinking, processing

See Schizophrenia

Thought Processes, Disturbed

Disturbed **Thought** processes r/t head injury, mental disorder, personality disorder, organic mental disorder, substance abuse, severe interpersonal conflict, sleep deprivation, sensory deprivation or overload, impaired cerebral perfusion

Thrombocytopenic Purpura

See ITP

Thrombophlebitis

Acute **Pain** r/t vascular inflammation, edema

Constipation r/t inactivity, bedrest

Deficient **Diversional** activity r/t bedrest

Deficient **Knowledge** r/t pathophysiology of condition, self-care needs, treatment regimen and outcome

Delayed **Surgical** recovery r/t complication associated with inactivity

Impaired physical **Mobility** r/t pain in extremity, forced bedrest

T

Ineffective **Tissue** perfusion: peripheral r/t interruption of venous blood flow

Risk for **Injury** r/t possible embolus

See Anticoagulant Therapy

Thyroidectomy

Risk for altered verbal **Communication** r/t edema, pain, vocal cord of laryngeal nerve damage

Risk for ineffective **Airway** clearance r/t edema or hematoma formation, airway obstruction

Risk for **Injury** r/t possible parathyroid damage or removal

See Surgery

TIA (Transient Ischemic Attack)

Acute **Confusion** r/t hypoxia

Health-seeking behaviors r/t obtaining knowledge regarding treatment, prevention of inadequate oxygenation

Ineffective **Tissue** perfusion: cerebral r/t lack of adequate oxygen supply to brain

Risk for decreased **Cardiac** output r/t dysrhythmia contributing to inadequate oxygen supply to brain

Risk for **Falls** r/t hypoxia

Risk for **Injury** r/t possible syncope

See Syncope

Tinea Capitis

See Ringworm of Scalp

Tinea Corporis

See Ringworm of Body

Tinea Cruris

See Jock Itch

Tinea Pedis

See Athlete's Foot

Tinea Unguium (Onychomycosis)

See Ringworm of Nails

Tinnitus

Disturbed **Sensory** perception: auditory r/t altered sensory reception, transmission, integration

Ineffective **Health** maintenance r/t deficient knowledge regarding self-care with tinnitus

Tissue Damage—Corneal, Integumentary, or Subcutaneous

Impaired **Tissue** integrity r/t altered circulation, nutritional deficit or excess, fluid deficit or excess, deficient knowledge, impaired physical mobility, chemical irritants (including body excretions, secretions, medica-

tions), thermal irritants (temperature extremes), mechanical irritants (pressure, shear, friction), radiation irritants (including therapeutic radiation)

Tissue Perfusion, Decreased

Ineffective **Tissue** perfusion r/t arterial or venous interruption of flow, exchange problems, hypovolemia, hypervolemia

Tocolytic Therapy

Ineffective **Health** maintenance r/t deficient knowledge regarding management of preterm labor, treatment regimen

Risk for **Fluid** volume excess r/t effects of tocolytic drugs

See Preterm Labor

Toilet Training

Health-seeking behaviors: bladder/bowel training r/t achievement of developmental milestone secondary to enhanced parenting skills

Toileting Problems

Impaired **Transfer** ability r/t neuromuscular deficits

Self-care deficit: toileting r/t impaired transfer ability, impaired mobility status, intolerance of activity, neuromuscular impairment, cognitive impairment

Tonsillectomy and Adenoidectomy

See T & A

Toothache

Impaired **Dentition** r/t ineffective oral hygiene, barriers to self-care, economic barriers to professional care, nutritional deficits, lack of knowledge regarding dental health

Total Anomalous Pulmonary Venous Return

See Congenital Heart Disease/Cardiac Anomalies

Total Joint Replacement— Total Hip/Total Knee

Acute **Pain** r/t possible edema, physical injury, surgery

Deficient **Knowledge** r/t self-care, treatment regimen, outcomes

Disturbed **Body** image r/t large scar, presence of prosthesis

Impaired physical **Mobility** r/t musculoskeletal impairment, surgery, prosthesis

Risk for **Infection** r/t invasive procedure, anesthesia, immobility

Risk for **Injury**: neurovascular r/t altered peripheral tissue perfusion, altered mobility, prosthesis

T

Total Parenteral Nutrition

See TPN

Total Urinary Incontinence

Total urinary **Incontinence** r/t neuropathy, neurological dysfunction, compromised contraction of detrusor reflex, anatomical incontinence (fistula)

Toxemia

See PIH

TPN (Total Parenteral Nutrition)

Imbalanced **Nutrition**: less than body requirements r/t inability to ingest or digest food or absorb nutrients as a result of biological or psychological factors

Risk for **Fluid** volume excess r/t rapid administration of TPN

Risk for **Infection** r/t concentrated glucose solution, invasive administration of fluids

Tracheoesophageal Fistula

Imbalanced **Nutrition**: less than body requirements r/t difficulties in swallowing

Ineffective **Airway** clearance r/t aspiration of feeding secondary to inability to swallow

Risk for **Aspiration** r/t common passage of air and food

See Respiratory Conditions of the Neonate; Hospitalized Child

Tracheostomy

Acute **Pain** r/t edema, surgical procedure

Anxiety r/t impaired verbal communication, ineffective airway clearance

Deficient **Knowledge** r/t self-care, home maintenance management

Disturbed **Body** image r/t abnormal opening in neck

Impaired verbal **Communication** r/t presence of mechanical airway

Risk for **Aspiration** r/t presence of tracheostomy

Risk for ineffective **Airway** clearance r/t increased secretions, mucus plugs

Risk for **Infection** r/t invasive procedure, pooling of secretions

Traction and Casts

Acute **Pain** r/t immobility, injury, or disease

Constipation r/t immobility

Deficient **Diversional** activity r/t immobility

Impaired physical **Mobility** r/t imposed restrictions on activity secondary to bone or joint disease injury

Impaired **Transfer** ability r/t presence of traction, casts

Risk for **Disuse** syndrome r/t mechanical immobilization

Risk for impaired **Skin** integrity r/t contact of traction or cast with skin

Risk for **Peripheral** neurovascular dysfunction r/t mechanical compression

Self-care deficit: feeding, dressing/grooming, bathing/hygiene, toileting r/t degree of impaired physical mobility, body area affected by traction or cast

Transfer Ability

Impaired **Transfer** ability r/t intolerance of activity, decreased strength and endurance, pain or discomfort, perceptual or cognitive impairment, neuromuscular impairment, musculoskeletal impairment, depression, severe anxiety

Transient Ischemic Attack

See TIA

Transposition of Great Vessels

See Congenital Heart Disease/Cardiac Anomalies

Transurethral Resection of the Prostate

See TURP

Trauma in Pregnancy

Acute **Pain** r/t trauma

Anxiety r/t threat to self or fetus, unknown outcome

Deficient **Knowledge** r/t lack of exposure to situation

Impaired **Skin** integrity r/t trauma

Risk for deficient **Fluid** volume r/t blood loss

Risk for fetal **Injury** r/t premature separation of placenta

Risk for **Infection** r/t traumatized tissue

Trauma, Risk for

INTERNAL

Risk for **Trauma** r/t weakness, poor vision, balancing difficulties, reduced temperature and/or tactile sensation, reduced large or small muscle coordination, reduced hand-eye coordination, lack of safety education, lack of safety precautions, insufficient finances to purchase safety equipment or effect repairs, cognitive or emotional difficulties, history of previous trauma

EXTERNAL

Risk for **Trauma** r/t slippery floors or walkways, unanchored rugs, bathtub without hand grip or anti-slip equipment, use of unsteady ladders or chairs, entering unlighted rooms, unsturdy or absent stair rails, unanchored electrical wires, litter or liquid spills on floors or stairways, high beds, children playing at top of

T

ungated stairs, obstructed passageways, unsafe window protection in home with young children, inappropriate call-for-aid mechanisms for client on bedrest, pot handles facing toward front of stove, bathing in very hot water, unsupervised bathing of young children, potentially ignitable gas leaks, delayed lighting of gas burner or oven, experimenting with chemicals or gasoline, unscreened fires or heaters, wearing plastic apron or flowing clothes around open flame, children playing with dangerous objects (e.g., matches, candles, cigarettes), inadequately stored combustible items or corrosives, highly flammable children's toys or clothing, overloaded fuse box, contact with rapidly moving objects (e.g., machinery, industrial belts, pulleys), sliding on coarse bed linen or struggling within bed restraints, faulty electrical plugs, frayed wires, defective appliances, contact with acids or alkalis, playing with fireworks or gunpowder, contact with intense cold, overexposure to sun or radiotherapy, misuse of sun lamps, use of cracked dishware or glasses, knives stored uncovered, guns or ammunition stored unlocked, large icicles hanging from the roof, exposure to dangerous machinery, children playing with sharp-edged toys, high-crime neighborhoods and vulnerable clients, driving a mechanically unsafe vehicle, driving after consuming alcoholic beverages or drugs, driving at excessive speeds, driving without necessary visual aids, children riding in the front seat of a vehicle, smoking in bed or near oxygen, overloaded electrical outlets, grease waste collected on stoves, use of thin or worn potholders, misuse of necessary headgear for motorized cyclists, young children carried on adult bicycles, unsafe road or road-crossing conditions, playing or working near vehicle pathways, nonuse or misuse of seat restraints

Traumatic Brain Injury (TBI)

See TBI; Intracranial Pressure, Increased

Traumatic Event

Post-trauma syndrome r/t previously experienced trauma

Traveler's Diarrhea

See TD

Trembling of Hands

Anxiety/Fear r/t threat to or change in health status, threat of death, situational crisis

Tricuspid Atresia

See Congenital Heart Disease/Cardiac Anomalies

Trigeminal Neuralgia

Acute **Pain** r/t irritation of trigeminal nerve

Imbalanced **Nutrition**: less than body requirements r/t pain when chewing

Ineffective **Therapeutic** regimen management r/t deficient knowledge regarding prevention of stimuli that trigger pain

Risk for **Injury** (eye) r/t possible decreased corneal sensation

Truncus Arteriosus

See Congenital Heart Disease/Cardiac Anomalies

TSE (Testicular Self-Examination)

Health-seeking behavior r/t procedure for doing testicular self-examinations

Tube Feeding

Risk for **Aspiration** r/t improperly administered feeding, improper placement of tube, improper positioning of client during and after feeding, excessive residual feeding or lack of digestion, altered gag reflex

Risk for deficient **Fluid** volume r/t inadequate water administration with concentrated feeding

Risk for Imbalanced **Nutrition**: less than body requirements r/t intolerance to tube feeding, inadequate calorie replacement to meet metabolic needs

Tuberculosis

See TB

TURP (Transurethral Resection of the Prostate)

Acute **Pain** r/t incision, irritation from catheter, bladder spasms, kidney infection

Deficient **Knowledge** r/t postoperative self-care, home maintenance management

Risk for deficient **Fluid** volume r/t fluid loss, possible bleeding

Risk for **Infection** r/t invasive procedure, route for bacteria entry

Risk for urge urinary **Incontinence** r/t edema from surgical procedure

Risk for **Urinary** retention r/t obstruction of urethra or catheter with clots

U

Ulcer, Peptic or Duodenal

Acute **Pain** r/t irritated mucosa from acid secretion

Fatigue r/t loss of blood, chronic illness

Ineffective **Health** maintenance r/t lack of knowledge regarding health practices to prevent ulcer formation

Nausea r/t gastrointestinal irritation

See GI Bleed

U

Ulcerative Colitis

See Inflammatory Bowel Disease

Ulcers, Stasis

See Stasis Ulcers

Unilateral Neglect of One Side of Body

Unilateral **Neglect** r/t effects of disturbed perceptual abilities (e.g., hemianopsia), one-sided blindness, neurological illness or trauma

Unsanitary Living Conditions

Impaired **Home** maintenance r/t impaired cognitive or emotional functioning, lack of knowledge, insufficient finances

Urgency to Urinate

Risk for urge urinary **Incontinence** r/t effects of alcohol, caffeine, decreased bladder capacity, irritation of bladder stretch receptors causing spasm, increased urine concentration, overdistention of bladder

Urge urinary **Incontinence** r/t decreased bladder capacity, irritation of bladder stretch receptors causing spasm, alcohol, caffeine, increased fluids, increased urine concentration, overdistention of bladder

Urinary Diversion

See Ileal Conduit

Urinary Elimination, Altered

Impaired **Urinary** elimination r/t anatomical obstruction, sensory motor impairment, urinary tract infection

Urinary Incontinence

See Incontinence of Urine

Urinary Readiness

Readiness for enhanced **Urinary** elimination

Urinary Retention

Urinary retention r/t high urethral pressure caused by weak detrusor, inhibition of reflex arc, strong sphincter, blockage

Urinary Tract Infection

See UTI

Urolithiasis

See Kidney Stone

Uterine Atony in Labor

See Dystocia

Uterine Atony in Postpartum

See Postpartum Hemorrhage

Uterine Bleeding

See Hemorrhage; Postpartum Hemorrhage; Shock

UTI (Urinary Tract Infection)

Acute **Pain**: dysuria r/t inflammatory process in bladder

Impaired **Urinary** elimination: frequency r/t urinary tract infection

Ineffective **Health** maintenance r/t deficient knowledge regarding methods to treat and prevent UTIs

Risk for urge urinary **Incontinence** r/t hyperreflexia from cystitis

Vaginal Hysterectomy

Risk for **Infection** r/t surgical site

Risk for **Perioperative** positioning injury r/t lithotomy position

Risk for urge urinary **Incontinence** r/t edema, congestion of pelvic tissues

Urinary retention r/t edema at surgical site

See Hysterectomy

Vaginitis

Acute **Pain**: pruritus r/t inflamed tissues, edema

Ineffective **Health** maintenance r/t deficient knowledge regarding self-care with vaginitis

Ineffective **Sexuality** patterns r/t abstinence during acute stage, pain

Risk for **Infection** r/t spread of infection, risk of reinfection

Vagotomy

See Abdominal Surgery

Value System Conflict

Readiness for enhanced **Spiritual** well-being r/t desire for harmony with self, others, higher power/God

Spiritual distress r/t challenged value system

Varicose Veins

Chronic **Pain** r/t impaired circulation

Ineffective **Health** maintenance r/t deficient knowledge regarding health care practices, prevention, treatment regimen

Ineffective **Tissue** perfusion: peripheral r/t venous stasis

Risk for impaired **Skin** integrity r/t altered peripheral tissue perfusion

V

Vascular Dementia (Formerly Called Multiinfarct Dementia)

See Dementia

Vascular Obstruction—Peripheral

Acute **Pain** r/t vascular obstruction

Anxiety r/t lack of circulation to body part

Ineffective **Tissue** perfusion: peripheral r/t interruption of circulatory flow

Risk for **Peripheral** neurovascular dysfunction r/t vascular obstruction

Venereal Disease

See STD

Ventilation, Inability to Sustain Spontaneous

Impaired spontaneous **Ventilation** r/t metabolic factors, respiratory muscle fatigue

Ventilator Client

Dysfunctional **Ventilatory** weaning response r/t psychological, situational, physiological factors

Fear r/t inability to breathe on own, difficulty communicating

Impaired **Gas** exchange r/t ventilation-perfusion imbalance

Impaired spontaneous **Ventilation** r/t metabolic factors, respiratory muscle fatigue

Impaired verbal **Communication** r/t presence of endotracheal tube, decreased mentation

Ineffective **Airway** clearance r/t increased secretions, decreased cough and gag reflex

Ineffective **Breathing** pattern r/t decreased energy and fatigue secondary to possible altered nutrition: less than body requirements

Powerlessness r/t health treatment regimen

Risk for **Infection** r/t presence of endotracheal tube, pooled secretions

Risk for latex **Allergy** r/t repeated exposure to latex products

Social isolation r/t impaired mobility, ventilator dependence

See Child with Chronic Condition; Hospitalized Child; Respiratory Conditions of the Neonate

Ventilatory, Dysfunctional Weaning Response (DVWR)

Dysfunctional **Ventilatory** weaning response r/t perceived inefficacy about the ability to wean, powerlessness, decreased motivation, adverse environment, inadequate social support, inadequate nutrition, sleep pattern disturbance, uncontrolled pain, ineffective airway clearance

Vertigo

Disturbed **Sensory** perception: kinesthetic r/t altered sensory reception, transmission, integration; medications

Ineffective **Tissue** perfusion: cerebral r/t decreased blood supply to brain

Risk for **Falls** r/t vertigo

Risk for **Injury** r/t disturbed sensory perception

Violent Behavior

Risk for other-directed **Violence** r/t body language, history of violence against others, history of violent antisocial behavior, history of violence, indirect (e.g., tearing off clothes, ripping objects off walls), neurological impairment, cognitive impairment, history of childhood abuse, history of witnessing family violence, cruelty to animals, firesetting, prenatal/perinatal complications and abnormalities, history of drug/alcohol abuse, pathological intoxication, psychotic symptomatology, motor vehicle offenses, suicidal behavior, impulsivity, availability/possession of weapon(s)

Risk for self-directed **Violence** r/t suicidal ideation, suicidal plan, history of multiple suicide attempts, behavioral clues of suicide, verbal clues of suicide, emotional status, mental health, physical health, unemployment, age 15 to 19 years, age >45 years, marital status, occupation, conflictual interpersonal relationships, family background, sexual orientation, personal resources, social resources, engaging in autoerotic sexual acts

Vision Impairment

Disturbed **Sensory** perception r/t altered sensory reception associated with impaired vision

Fear r/t loss of sight

Risk for **Injury** r/t disturbed sensory perception

Self-care deficit: specify r/t perceptual impairment

Social isolation r/t altered state of wellness, inability to see

See Blindness

Vomiting

Nausea r/t chemotherapy, postsurgical anesthesia, irritation to the gastrointestinal system, stimulation of neuropharmacological mechanisms

Risk for deficient **Fluid** volume r/t decreased intake, loss of fluids with vomiting

Risk for imbalanced **Nutrition**: less than body requirements r/t inability to ingest food

V

W

Walking Impairment

Impaired **Walking** r/t intolerance to activity, decreased strength and endurance, pain or discomfort, perceptual or cognitive impairment, neuromuscular impairment, musculoskeletal impairment, depression, severe anxiety, lower extremity amputation

Wandering

Wandering r/t cognitive impairment, specifically memory and recall deficits, disorientation, poor visuoconstructive (or visuospatial) ability, language (primarily expressive) defects; cortical atrophy; premorbid behavior (e.g., outgoing, sociable personality; premorbid dementia); separation from familiar people and places; sedation; emotional state, especially frustration, anxiety, boredom, or depression (agitation); overstimulating/understimulating social or physical environment; physiological state or need (e.g., hunger/thirst, pain, urination, constipation); time of day

Weakness

Fatigue r/t decreased or increased metabolic energy production

Risk for **Falls** r/t weakness

Weight Gain

Imbalanced **Nutrition**: more than body requirements r/t excessive intake in relation to metabolic need

Weight Loss

Imbalanced **Nutrition**: less than body requirements r/t inability to ingest food because of biological, psychological, economic factors

Wellness-Seeking Behavior

Health-seeking behavior r/t expressed desire for increased control of health practice

Wheelchair Use Problems

Impaired wheelchair **Mobility** r/t intolerance to activity, decreased strength and endurance, pain or discomfort, perceptual or cognitive impairment, neuromuscular impairment, musculoskeletal impairment, depression, severe anxiety, amputation

Wheezing

Ineffective **Airway** clearance r/t tracheobronchial obstructions, secretions

Withdrawal from Alcohol

See Alcohol Withdrawal

Withdrawal from Drugs

See Drug Withdrawal

Wound Débridement

Acute **Pain** r/t débridement of wound

Impaired **Tissue** integrity r/t débridement, open wound

Risk for **Infection** r/t open wound, presence of bacteria

Wound Dehiscence, Evisceration

Fear r/t client fear of body parts falling out, surgical procedure not going as planned

Imbalanced **Nutrition**: less than body requirements r/t inability to digest nutrients, need for increased protein for healing

Risk for deficient **Fluid** volume r/t inability to ingest nutrients, obstruction, fluid loss

Risk for delayed **Surgical** recovery r/t separation of wound, exposure of abdominal contents

Risk for **Injury** r/t exposed abdominal contents

Wound Infection

Disturbed **Body** image r/t dysfunctional open wound

Hyperthermia r/t increased metabolic rate, illness, infection

Imbalanced **Nutrition**: less than body requirements r/t biological factors, infection, hyperthermia

Impaired **Tissue** integrity r/t wound, presence of infection

Risk for deficient **Fluid** volume r/t increased metabolic rate

Risk for delayed **Surgical** recovery r/t presence of infection

Risk for **Infection**: spread of r/t imbalanced nutrition: less than body requirements

W

Guide to Planning Care

Activity intolerance

Betty J. Ackley and Linda Straight

NANDA   Definition

Insufficient physiological or psychological energy to endure or complete required or desired daily activities

Defining Characteristics

Verbal report of fatigue or weakness; abnormal heart rate or blood pressure response to activity; exertional discomfort or dyspnea; electrocardiographic changes reflecting dysrhythmias or ischemia

Related Factors (r/t)

Bed rest or immobility; generalized weakness; sedentary lifestyle; imbalance between oxygen supply and demand

NOC   Outcomes (Nursing Outcomes Classification)

Suggested NOC Outcomes

Activity Tolerance; Endurance; Energy Conservation; Self-Care: Instrumental Activities of Daily Living (IADLs)

> **Example NOC Outcome with Indicators**
>
> **Endurance** as evidenced by the following indicators: Performance of usual routine/Activity/Rested appearance/Blood oxygen level within normal limits/Expresses feelings about loss/Verbalizes acceptance of loss/Describes meaning of the loss or death/Reports decreased preoccupation with loss/Expresses positive expectations about the future (Rate each indicator of **Endurance:** 1 = extremely compromised, 2 = substantially compromised, 3 = moderately compromised, 4 = mildly compromised, 5 = not compromised [see Section I].)

Client Outcomes

Client Will (Specify Time Frame):

- Participate in prescribed physical activity with appropriate increases in heart rate, blood pressure, and breathing rate; maintains monitor patterns (rhythm and ST segment) within normal limits
- State symptoms of adverse effects of exercise and reports onset of symptoms immediately
- Maintain normal skin color and skin is warm and dry with activity
- Verbalize an understanding of the need to gradually increase activity based on testing, tolerance, and symptoms
- Express an understanding of the need to balance rest and activity
- Demonstrate increased activity tolerance

NIC   Interventions (Nursing Interventions Classification)

Suggested NIC Interventions

Activity Therapy; Energy Management

- = Independent; ▲ = Collaborative

Example NIC Activities—Energy Management

Monitor cardiorespiratory response to activity; Monitor location and nature of discomfort or pain during movement/activity

Nursing Interventions and Rationales

- Determine cause of activity intolerance (see Related Factors) and determine whether cause is physical, psychological, or motivational. *Determining the cause of a disease can help direct appropriate interventions.*
- Assess the client daily for appropriateness of activity and bed rest orders. *Inappropriate prolonged bed rest orders may contribute to activity intolerance.* **Clinical Research:** *A review of 39 studies on bed rest resulting from 15 disorders demonstrated that bed rest for treatment of medical conditions is associated with worse outcomes than early mobilization (Allen et al, 1999).*
- If the client is able to walk and has chronic obstructive pulmonary disease (COPD), consider the use of an accelerometer to assess walking ability. **Nursing Research:** *Use of the accelerometer was very predictive of maximum distance walked during a 6-minute walk test (Belza et al, 2001).*
- If the client is able to walk and has heart failure, consider use of the 6-minute walk test to determine physical ability. **Clinical Research:** *The 6-minute walk test was shown to be highly reproducible in determining ability to ambulate in a client in heart failure (Demers et al, 2001).*
- If mainly on bed rest, minimize cardiovascular deconditioning by positioning a client as close to the upright position as possible several times daily. *The hazards of bed rest in the elderly are multiple, serious, quick to develop, and slow to reverse. Deconditioning of the cardiovascular system occurs within days and involves fluid shifts, fluid loss, decreased cardiac output, decreased peak oxygen uptake, and increased resting heart rate (Resnick, 1998).*
- When appropriate, gradually increase activity, allowing the client to assist with positioning, transferring, and self-care as possible. Progress from sitting in bed to dangling, to standing, to ambulation. *Always have the client dangle at the bedside before trying standing to evaluate for postural hypotension. Watch the client closely for dizziness during increased activity (Fried and Fried, 2001). Increasing activity helps to maintain muscle strength, tone, and endurance.*
- Ensure that the client changes position slowly. Consider using a chair-bed (stretcher-chair) for a client who cannot get out of bed. Monitor for symptoms of activity intolerance. *Bed rest in the supine position results in loss of plasma volume, which contributes to postural hypotension and syncope (Creditor, 1994; Fried and Fried, 2001).*
- When getting up a client, observe for symptoms of intolerance such as nausea, pallor, dizziness, visual dimming, and impaired consciousness, as well as changes in vital signs. *Heart rate and blood pressure responses to orthostasis vary widely. Vital sign changes by themselves should not define orthostatic intolerance (Winslow et al, 1995).*
- ▲ If a client experiences syncope with activity, refer for evaluation by a physician. *Syncope has many causes, including benign vasovagal, but can also be due to serious cardiac disease, resulting in death (Hauer, 2003).*
- Perform range-of-motion exercises if the client is unable to tolerate activity or is mostly immobile. *Inactivity rapidly contributes to muscle shortening and changes in periar-*

- **•** = **Independent; ▲** = **Collaborative**

ticular and cartilaginous joint structure. These factors contribute to contracture and limitation of motion (Creditor, 1994; Fried and Fried, 2001).

▲ Refer the client to physical therapy to help increase activity levels and strength.

• Monitor and record the client's ability to tolerate activity: note pulse rate, blood pressure, monitor pattern, dyspnea, use of accessory muscles, and skin color before and after activity. If the following signs and symptoms of cardiac decompensation develop, activity should be stopped immediately (Wenger, 2001):

  ■ Onset of chest discomfort
  ■ Dyspnea
  ■ Palpitations
  ■ Excessive fatigue
  ■ Lightheadedness, confusion, ataxia, pallor, cyanosis, dyspnea, nausea, or any peripheral circulatory insufficiency
  ■ Dysrhythmia (symptomatic supraventricular tachycardia, ventricular tachycardia, exercise-induced intraventricular conduction defect, second- or third-degree atrioventricular block, frequent premature ventricular contractions)
  ■ Exercise hypotension (drop in systolic blood pressure of >10 mm Hg from baseline blood pressure despite an increase in workload)
  ■ Excessive rise in blood pressure (systolic >180 mm Hg or diastolic >110 mm Hg). note: These are upper limits; activity may be stopped before reaching these values
  ■ Inappropriate bradycardia (drop in heart rate >10 beats/min or <50 beats/min)
  ■ Increased heart rate above 100 beats/min

▲ Instruct the client to stop the activity immediately and report to the physician if the client is experiencing the following symptoms: new or worsened intensity or increased frequency of discomfort; tightness or pressure in chest, back, neck, jaw, shoulders, and/or arms; palpitations; dizziness; weakness; unusual and extreme fatigue; excessive air hunger. *These are common symptoms of angina and are caused by a temporary insufficiency of coronary blood supply. Symptoms typically last for minutes as opposed to momentary twinges. If symptoms last longer than 5 to 10 minutes, the client should be evaluated by a physician. The client should be evaluated before resuming activity.*

• Allow for periods of rest before and after planned exertion periods such as meals, baths, treatments, and physical activity. *Rest periods decrease oxygen consumption (Prizant-Weston and Castiglia, 1992).*

• Observe and document skin integrity several times a day. *Activity intolerance may lead to pressure ulcers. Mechanical pressure, moisture, friction, and shearing forces all predispose to their development (Resnick, 1998).*

• Assess urinary incontinence related to functional ability. Assess independent ability to get to the toilet and to remove and adjust clothing. *The loss of functional ability that accompanies disease often leads to continence problems. The cause may not be the person's bladder instability but his or her ability to get to the toilet quickly.*

• Assess for constipation. If present, refer to care plan for **Constipation.** *Impaired mobility is associated with increased risk of bowel dysfunction, including constipation. Constipation increases the risk of urinary tract infection and urge incontinence (Nazarko, 1997).*

▲ Consider dietitian referral to assess nutritional needs related to activity intolerance. *Severe malnutrition can lead to activity intolerance. Dietitians can recommend dietary changes that can improve the client's health status.*

▲ Refer the cardiac client to cardiac rehabilitation for assistance in developing safe exercise guidelines based on testing and medications. Cardiac rehabilitation exercise

  • = Independent; ▲ = Collaborative

training improves objective measures of exercise tolerance in both men and women, including elderly clients with coronary heart disease and heart failure. This functional improvement occurs without significant cardiovascular complications or other adverse outcomes (Wenger, 2001). **Clinical Research:** *Exercise-based cardiac rehabilitation is effective in reducing the number of cardiac deaths (Joliffe et al, 2002).*

▲ Ensure that the chronic pulmonary client has oxygen saturation testing with exercise. Use supplemental oxygen to keep oxygen saturation 90% or above or as prescribed with activity. *Supplemental oxygen increases circulatory oxygen levels and improves activity tolerance (Casaburi and Petty, 1993).*

• Monitor a COPD client's response to activity by observing for symptoms of respiratory intolerance such as increased dyspnea, loss of ability to control breathing rhythmically, use of accessory muscles, and skin tone changes such as pallor and cyanosis.

• Instruct and assist a COPD client in using conscious controlled breathing techniques such as pursing their lips and diaphragmatic breathing. *Training a client with COPD to slow his or her respiratory rate with a prolonged exhalation (with or without pursed lips) helps control dyspnea and results in improved ventilation, increased tidal volume, decreased respiratory rate, and a reduced alveolar-arterial oxygen difference. This breathing pattern not only helps relieve dyspnea but also can improve the ability to exercise and carry out ADLs (Casaburi and Petty, 1993).*

• Provide emotional support and encouragement to the client to gradually increase activity. *Fear of breathlessness, pain, or falling may decrease willingness to increase activity.*

▲ Refer the COPD client to a pulmonary rehabilitation program. **Clinical Research:** *Pulmonary rehabilitation has been shown to relieve dyspnea and fatigue and enhance the client's sense of control over his or her disease. Rehabilitation is an important component of the management of COPD (Lacasse et al, 2002).*

▲ Observe for pain before activity. If possible, treat pain before activity, and ensure that the client is not heavily sedated. *Pain restricts the client from achieving a maximal activity level and is often exacerbated by movement.*

• Obtain any necessary assistive devices or equipment needed before ambulating the client (e.g., walkers, canes, crutches, portable oxygen). *Assistive devices can increase mobility by helping the client overcome limitations.*

• Use a walking belt when ambulating a client who is unsteady. *With a walking belt the client can walk independently, but the nurse can provide support if the client's knees buckle.*

• Work with the client to set mutual goals that increase activity levels.

▲ If the client is scheduled for a surgical intervention that will result in bed rest in intensive care, consider referring to physical therapy for a prehabilitation program including warm-up, aerobic conditioning, strength building, and flexibility enhancement. *Increasing a client's functional capacity before hospitalization can be a helpful means of modifying the predictable deconditioning that happens with ICU admission (Topp et al, 2002).*

Geriatric

• Slow the pace of care. Allow the client extra time to carry out activities.

• Encourage families to help/allow an elderly client to be independent in whatever activities possible. *Sometimes families believe they are assisting by allowing clients to be sedentary. Encouraging activity not only enhances good functioning of the body's systems but also promotes a sense of worth by providing an opportunity for productivity (Eliopoulous, 1997).*

▲ If the client has heart disease causing activity intolerance, refer for cardiac rehabilita-

• = Independent; ▲ = Collaborative

tion. **Clinical Research:** *Elderly clients with coronary artery disease in exercise regimens after hospitalization have exercise trainability comparable to that of younger clients participating in similar experiences (Williams et al, 1985; Shepard, 1990).*

▲ Refer the client to physical therapy for resistance exercise training as able, including abdominal crunch, leg press, leg extension, leg curl, calf press, and more. **Clinical Research:** *A study demonstrated that 6 months of resistance exercise for the elderly greatly increased their aerobic capacity, possibly from increased skeletal muscle strength (Vincent et al, 2002).*

• When mobilizing the elderly client, watch for orthostatic hypotension accompanied by dizziness and fainting. *Orthostatic hypotension is common in the elderly as a result of cardiovascular changes, chronic diseases, and medication effects (Mobily and Kelley, 1991).*

• Once the client is able to walk independently and needs an exercise program, suggest the client enter an exercise program with a friend. **Nursing Research:** *Findings from a study of exercise behavior found that friends have the strongest influence to keep on an exercise program, more than family members or experts (Resnick et al, 2002).*

Home care

▲ Begin discharge planning as soon as possible with case manager or social worker to assess need for home support systems and the need for community or home health services.

▲ Assess the home environment for factors that precipitate or contribute to decreased activity tolerance: stairs; lack of assistive bed or bathroom devices; distance to bathroom; presence of allergens such as dust, smoke, and those associated with pets; temperature; energy-intensive activity patterns; and furniture placement. Refer to occupational therapy if needed to assist the client in restructuring the home and activities of daily living patterns. *During hospitalization, clients and families often estimate energy requirements at home inaccurately because the hospital's availability of staff support distorts the level of care that will be needed.*

▲ Refer to physical therapy for strength training, possible weight training. *Physical therapists can initiate a program of exercise for the client, with family assistance, to regain strength, increase endurance, and improve balance. Use of hand weights or stretch bands can be used to increase muscle strength. If the client is homebound, physical therapist can also initiate cardiac rehabilitation.*

▲ Support strength training program prescribed by physical therapist. *A client may resist exercise in light of low energy level; reminders and positive feedback by other care providers will help the client maintain prescribed exercises.*

• Normalize the client's activity intolerance; encourage progress with positive feedback. The client's experience should be validated as within expected norms. Recognition of progress enhances motivation. **Nursing Research:** *In a qualitative study, fatigued women reported that they felt distressed when health care providers invalidated their experiences of fatigue (Patusky, 2002).*

• Teach the client/family the importance of and methods for setting priorities for activities, especially those having a high energy demand (e.g., home/family events). Instruct in realistic expectations. The client and/or family may assume a more rapid rate of energy recovery than actually occurs. Assistance may be needed to ensure accuracy of expectations for the client. **Nursing Research:** *Unrealistic expectations provoke guilt feelings in the client, leading to efforts that can exceed the client's energy capacity (Patusky, 2002).*

• = Independent; ▲ = Collaborative

- Provide the client/family with resources such as senior centers, exercise classes, educational and recreational programs, and volunteer opportunities that can aid in promoting socialization and appropriate activity. *Social isolation can be an outcome of and contribute to activity intolerance.*
- Discuss the importance of sexual activity as part of daily living. Instruct the client in adaptive techniques to conserve energy during sexual interactions. *Families may make unsafe choices for sexual activity or place added stress on themselves trying to cope with this issue without proper support or teaching.*
- Instruct the client and family in the importance of maintaining proper nutrition, rest, and behavioral pacing for energy conservation and rehabilitation. Instruct in use of dietary supplements as indicated. *Illness may suppress appetite, leading to inadequate nutrition. Pacing activities to energy capacity and need for rest are important to ensure the client does not overdo his or her capability.*
- ▲ Refer to medical social services as necessary to assist the family in adjusting to major changes in patterns of living.
- ▲ Assess the need for long-term supports for optimal activity tolerance of priority activities (e.g., assistive devices, oxygen, medication, catheters, massage), especially for a hospice client. Evaluate intermittently. *Assessments ensure the safety and appropriate use of these supports.*
- ▲ Refer to home health aide services to support the client and family through changing levels of activity tolerance. Introduce aide support early. Instruct the aide to promote independence in activity as tolerated. *Home health aides provide initial assistance with ADLs that may involve experience with safe body mechanics. Changes in the amount of support necessary as the client progresses are important because providing unnecessary assistance with transfers and bathing activities may promote dependence and a loss of mobility (Mobily and Kelley, 1991).*
- Be aware of increased risk of bone fracture even after muscle strength is normalized, especially in osteoporosis-prone individuals such as estrogen-deficient women and the elderly. *Reduction in weight-bearing muscle activity during bed rest invariably produces significant changes in calcium balance and, in weeks, changes in bone mass (Bloomfield, 1997).*
- Allow terminally ill clients and their families to guide care. *Control by the client or family respects their autonomy and promotes effective coping.*
- Provide increased attention to comfort and dignity of the terminally ill client in care planning. *Interventions should be provided as much for psychological effect as for physiological support. For example, oxygen may be more valuable as a support to the client's psychological comfort than as a booster of oxygen saturation.*
- ▲ Institute case management of frail elderly to support continued independent living. *Difficulties with activity intolerance can lead to increasing needs for assistance in using the health care system effectively. Case management combines nursing activities of the client and family assessment, planning and coordination of care among all health care providers, delivery of direct nursing care, and monitoring of care and outcomes. These activities are able to address continuity of care, mutual goal setting, behavior management, and prevention of worsening health problems (Guttman, 1999).*
- ▲ In the presence of psychiatric illness, refer for psychiatric home health care services for client reassurance and implementation of a therapeutic regimen. *Psychiatric home care nurses can address issues relating to the client's depression with activity intolerance. Behavioral interventions in the home can assist the client to participate more effectively in treatment plan (Patusky et al, 1996).*

- **= Independent; ▲ = Collaborative**

Client/Family Teaching

- Instruct the client on rationale and techniques for avoiding activity intolerance.
- Teach the client to use controlled breathing techniques with activity.
- Teach the client the importance and method of coughing, clearing secretions.
- Instruct the client in the use of relaxation techniques during activity.
- Help client with energy conservation and work simplification techniques in ADLs.
- Teach the client the importance of proper nutrition.
- Describe to the client the symptoms of activity intolerance, including which symptoms to report to the physician.
- Explain to the client how to use assistive devices or medications before or during activity.
- Help client set up an activity log to record exercise and exercise tolerance.

evolve WEBSITES FOR EDUCATION

See the EVOLVE website for World Wide Web resources for client education.

REFERENCES

Allen C, Glasziou P, Del Mar C: Bed rest: a potentially harmful treatment needing more careful evaluation, *Lancet* 354(9186):1229, 1999.

Belza B et al: Correlates of physical activity in chronic obstructive pulmonary disease, *Nurs Res* 50(4):195, 2001.

Bloomfield SA: Changes in musculoskeletal structure and function with prolonged bed rest, *Med Sci Sports Exerc* 29(2):197, 1997.

Casaburi R, Petty T: *Principles and practice of pulmonary rehabilitation,* Philadelphia, 1993, WB Saunders.

Creditor M: Hazards of hospitalization of the elderly, *Ann Intern Med* 118(3):219, 1994.

Demers C et al: Reliability, validity, and responsiveness of the six-minute walk test in patients with heart failure, *Am Heart J* 142(4):698, 2001.

Eliopoulous C: *Gerontological nursing,* ed 4, Philadelphia, 1997, Lippincott.

Fried KM, Fried GW: Immobility. In Derstine JB, Hargrove SD, editors: *Comprehensive rehabilitation nursing,* Philadelphia, 2001, WB Saunders.

Guttman R: Case management of the frail elderly in the community, *Clin Nurs Spec* 13(4):174, 1999.

Hauer KE: Discovering the cause of syncope, *Postgrad Med* 113(1):31, 2003.

Joliffe JA et al: Exercise-based rehabilitation for coronary heart disease, *Cochrane Library* CD001800, 2002.

Lacasse Y et al: Pulmonary rehabilitation for chronic obstructive pulmonary disease, *Cochrane Library* CD003793, 2002.

Mobily PR, Kelley LS: Iatrogenesis in the elderly: factors of immobility, *J Gerontol Nurs* 17(9):5, 1991.

Nazarko L: The whole story: continence in people with dementia, *Nurs Times* 93(4):63, 1997.

Patusky KL: Relatedness theory as a framework for the treatment of fatigued women, *Arch Psychiatr Nurs* 5:224, 2002.

Patusky KL, Rodning C, Martinez-Kratz M: Clinical lessons in psychiatric home care: a case study approach, *J Home Health Case Manage* 9:18, 1996.

Prizant-Weston M, Castiglia K: Hemodynamic regulation. In Bulechek GM, McCloskey JC, editors: *Nursing interventions: essential nursing treatments,* Philadelphia, 1992, WB Saunders.

Resnick B, Orwig D, Magaziner J. The effect of social support on exercise behavior in older adults, *Clin Nurs Res* 11(1):52, 2002.

Resnick N: Geriatric medicine. In Tierney L Jr, McPhee S, Papadakis M, editors: *Current medical diagnosis and treatment,* ed 37, Stamford, Conn, 1998, Appleton and Lange.

Shepard RJ. The scientific basis of exercise prescribing for the very old, *J Am Geriatr Soc* 38:62, 1990.

Topp R et al: The effect of bed rest and potential of prehabilitation on patients in the intensive care unit, *AACN Clin Issues* 13(2):263, 2002.

Vincent KR et al: Improved cardiorespiratory endurance following 6 months of resistance exercise in elderly men and women, *Arch Intern Med* 162:673, 2002.

• = Independent; ▲ = Collaborative

Wenger NK: Rehabilitation of the patient with coronary heart disease. In Fuster V et al, editors: *Hurst's the heart,* ed 10, New York, 2001, McGraw-Hill.

Williams MA et al: Early exercise training in patients older than age 65 years compared with that in younger patients after acute myocardial infarction or coronary artery bypass grafting, *Am J Cardiol* 55:263, 1985.

Winslow EH, Lane LD, Woods RJ: Dangling: a review of relevant physiology, research, and practice, *Heart Lung* 24(4):263, 1995.

Risk for Activity intolerance

Betty J. Ackley and Linda Straight

NANDA Definition

At risk for experiencing insufficient physiological or psychological energy to endure or complete required or desired daily activities

Risk Factors

History of intolerance to activity; deconditioned status; presence of circulatory or respiratory problems; inexperience with activity

Related Factors (r/t)

See Risk Factors

NOC Outcomes (Nursing Outcomes Classification)

Suggested NOC Outcomes

Activity Tolerance; Endurance; Energy Conservation

Example NOC Outcome with Indicators

Endurance as evidenced by the following indicators: Performance of usual routine/Activity/Rested appearance/Blood oxygen level within normal limits/Expresses feelings about loss/Verbalizes acceptance of loss/Describes meaning of the loss or death/Reports decreased preoccupation with loss/Expresses positive expectations about the future (Rate each indicator of **Endurance:** 1 = extremely compromised, 2 = substantially compromised, 3 = moderately compromised, 4 = mildly compromised, 5 = not compromised [see Section I].)

NIC Interventions (Nursing Interventions Classification)

Suggested NIC Interventions

Energy Management; Exercise Promotion: Strength Training; Activity Therapy

Example NIC Activities—Energy Management

Monitor cardiorespiratory response to activity; Monitor location and nature of discomfort or pain during movement/activity

Client Outcomes, Nursing Interventions and Rationales, and Client/Family Teaching

See care plan for **Activity intolerance.**

• = Independent; ▲ = Collaborative

evolve WEBSITES FOR EDUCATION

See the EVOLVE website for World Wide Web resources for client education.

Impaired Adjustment

Ann Keeley

NANDA Definition

Inability to modify lifestyle/behavior in a manner consistent with a change in health status

Defining Characteristics

Denial of health status change; failure to achieve optimal sense of control; failure to take actions that would prevent further health problems; demonstration of nonacceptance of health status change, occurs within a recent time period of notification of alteration in health status requiring a change in client behavior

Related Factors (r/t)

Expressed negativity; intense emotional state; negative attitude toward health behavior; failure to intend to change behavior; multiple stressors; absence of social support for change in beliefs and practices; disability or health status change requiring change in lifestyle; lack of motivation to change behaviors, family system pressure to remain status quo

NOC Outcomes (Nursing Outcomes Classification)

Suggested NOC Outcomes

Acceptance: Health Status; Coping; Grief Resolution; Health-Seeking Behavior; Participation in Health Care Decisions; Psychosocial Adjustment: Life Change; Treatment Behavior: Illness or Injury

> #### Example NOC Outcome with Indicators
>
> **Acceptance: Health Status** as evidenced by the following indicators: Peacefulness/Relinquishment of previous concept of health/Expressed reactions to health status/Recognition of reality of health situation/Coping with health status (Rate each indicator of **Acceptance: Health Status:** 1 = none, 2 = limited, 3 = moderate, 4 = substantial, 5 = extensive [see Section I].)

Client Outcomes

Client Will (Specify Time Frame):

- State acceptance of change in health status
- Request assistance in altering behaviors to adapt to change
- State personal goals for dealing with change in health status and means to prevent further health problems

- = Independent; ▲ = Collaborative

- State experience of a period of grief that is proportional to the actual or perceived effect of the loss
- Report and/or demonstrate behavior changes mutually agreed upon with nurse as evidence of positive adaptation

NIC   Interventions (Nursing Interventions Classification)

Suggested NIC Intervention
Coping Enhancement

> **Example NIC Activities—Coping Enhancement**
>
> Assist the client with developing an objective appraisal of the event; Explore with the client previous methods of dealing with life problems

Nursing Interventions and Rationales

- Assess the client's perception about the illness/event. Ask the client to state feelings related to the change in health status. **Nursing Research:** *Negative responses to a need for change in behavior related to an alteration in health status can be understood only following a thorough assessment of the client's appraisal framework (Dudley-Brown, 2002).*
- Assess the client and family for the presence of additional stressors (e.g., financial difficulty, health of other family members, occupational changes). *Additional stressors have been found to hinder the client's and/or family's adjustment (Dibartolo, 2002).*
- Assess the client's feelings about whether change in health status is personally being dealt with effectively. **Nursing Research:** *Psychological distress can negatively affect positive adaptation (Dudley-Brown, 2002).*
- Assess for negative affect and internalization of problems. **Nursing Research:** *Exploring the meaning of health status change and the adjustments required for a successful adaptation within the client's life experience fosters positive growth (Norris and Spelic, 2002; Richer and Ezer, 2002).*
- Assess the socioeconomic status of all clients. *Clients of low socioeconomic status have been found to have more difficulty with adjustment in social functioning, mental health, pain, fatigue, and physical fitness than do clients of high socioeconomic status (Sykes et al, 1999).*
- Allow the client adequate time to express feelings about the change in health status. **Nursing Research:** *Nurses need to provide an opportunity for clients to address all aspects of the impact of a health status change on their lives (Richer and Ezer, 2002)*
- Help the client work through the stages of grief. Denial is usually the initial response. Acknowledge that grief takes time, and give the client permission to grieve; accept crying. *The process of grieving is integral to adaptation to a disruption of health status (Norris and Spelic, 2002).* **Nursing Research:** *Cognitive dysfunction is a manifestation of grieving a change in health status (Wassem et al, 2001).*
- Recognize that denial may be adaptive at certain stages of a threatening encounter. *Denial is the initial phase of the grieving response and would be expected when a client is told of a significant change in health status (Norris and Spelic, 2002).*
- Discuss resources (e.g., the client's support system) that have worked previously when

• = **Independent;** ▲ = **Collaborative**

dealing with changes in lifestyle or health status. *As a client adjusts to a change in health status, he or she will call on previous behaviors that proved successful in a crisis situation (Norris and Spelic, 2002).* **Nursing Research:** *Integration of a client's repertoire of coping strategies into an intervention program to facilitate adaptation to a change in health status will facilitate positive coping (Wassem et al, 2001).*

▲ Refer to community resources. Provide general and contact information for ease of use. Available resources should be integrated in to any intervention aimed at facilitating a positive adjustment to a change in health status (Norris and Spelic, 2002). **Nursing Research:** *Social support is necessary to coordinate all possible resources that may assist the client and/or family in their adjustment to a change in health status (Wassem et al, 2001)*

• Use open-ended questions to allow the client free expression (e.g., "Tell me about your last hospitalization" or "How does this time compare?"). **Nursing Research:** *Active listening aimed at clarifying family concerns regarding the change in health status will facilitate nursing interventions that promote positive coping behaviors (Weiss and Chan, 2002).*

• Discuss the client's current goals. If appropriate, have the client list goals so that they can be referred to and steps can be taken to accomplish them. **Nursing Research:** *Clarification of the client/family goals and expectations will allow the nurse to clarify what is possible and to identify measures that can facilitate achievement of the goals (Northouse et al, 2002).*

• List the client activities that may require assistance and those that can be performed independently. **Nursing Research:** *Clarification of behaviors conducive to a positive adjustment to a change in health status and the resources available to the client facilitates positive coping behaviors toward adaptation (Northouse et al, 2002).*

• Allow the client choices in daily care, particularly choices that result from the change in health status. **Nursing Research:** *A client will demonstrate a more positive adaptation if the resources and interventions offered by the nurse are adapted to the client's perceived circumstances and needs (LeClere et al, 2002).*

• Allow the client time to adjust to new situations. Introduce new material gradually to prevent overload. Ask for frequent feedback. *The stress of changes in health care can be overwhelming. New material takes longer to learn and absorb; thus, clarification of information and frequent repetition may be necessary.*

• Give the client positive feedback for accomplishments, no matter how small. **Nursing Research:** *The nurse's provision of a climate of acceptance and encouragement facilitates a positive adaptation (Riche and Ezer, 2002).*

• Manipulate the environment to decrease stress; allow the client to display personal items that have meaning. **Nursing Research:** *Appraisal uncertainty is a risk factor for a negative adaptation to health change (Dudley-Brown, 2002).*

• Maintain consistency and continuity in daily schedule. When possible, provide the same caregiver. **Nursing Research:** *The predictability of interaction with the same nurses as a part of treatment facilitates trust, confidence, and positive adaptation (Riche and Ezer, 2002).*

▲ Foster communication between the client/family and medical staff. **Nursing Research:** *Perceived ability to access a variety of resources promotes self-efficacy and positive adaptation to health status changes (Czuchta and McCay, 2001).*

• Promote use of positive spiritual influences. *Spiritual coping strategies may facilitate a positive adaptation to a change in health status (Baldacchino and Draper, 2001).*

• = Independent; ▲ = Collaborative

Geriatric

▲ Assess for signs of depression resulting from illness-associated changes and make appropriate referral. **Nursing Research:** *Signs and symptoms of depression when evident would assist the nurse in the individualization of interventions to a particular client (Reynaud and Meeker, 2002).*

• Monitor the client for agitation. *The elderly often use agitation to express an inability to accept change.*

• Increase and mobilize support available to the elderly client. Encourage interaction with family and friends. **Nursing Research:** *Relationships are pivotal in supporting coping of older adults (Cutcliff and Grant, 2001). Maintain continuity of care by keeping the number of caregivers to a minimum.*

Multicultural

• Assess for the influence of cultural beliefs, norms, and values on the client's ability to modify health behavior. **Nursing Research:** *What the client considers normal and abnormal health behavior may be based on cultural perceptions (Cochran, 1998; Doswell and Erlen, 1998; Leininger and McFarland, 2002).*

• Encourage spirituality as a source of support for coping. **Nursing Research:** *Many African Americans and Latinos identify spirituality, religiousness, prayer, and church-based approaches as coping resources (Samuel-Hodge et al, 2000).*

• Discuss with the client those aspects of their health behavior/lifestyle that will remain unchanged by their health status.

• Negotiate with the client regarding the aspects of health behavior which will need to be modified. **Nursing Research:** *Give and take with the client will lead to culturally congruent care (Leininger and McFarland, 2002).*

• Assess the role of fatalism on the client's ability to modify health behavior. *Fatalistic perspectives, which involve the belief that you cannot control your own fate, may influence health behaviors in some African American and Latino populations (Phillips et al, 1999).*

• Identify which family members the client can rely on for support. **Nursing Research:** *A variety of different cultures rely on family members to cope with stress (Aziz and Rowland, 2002; Donnelly, 2002; Gleeson-Kreig et al, 2002; White et al, 2002).*

• Validate the client's feelings regarding the impact of health status on current lifestyle. *Validation lets the client know that the nurse has heard and understands what was said, thus promoting the nurse-client relationship (Stuart and Laraia, 2001).*

Home care

• Include a spiritual assessment in overall assessment of client and family resources. **Nursing Research:** *Many African Americans and Latinos identify spirituality, religiousness, prayer, and church-based approaches as coping resources (Samuel-Hodge et al, 2000).*

▲ Refer to medical social services to facilitate the listed interventions and support client care goals. *Support for transition to the home setting can facilitate acceptance of the changes required to maintain the client in the home setting.*

• Assess affective climate within family and family support system. *Positive family affective climate and family support have been found to enhance social adjustment (Langfitt et al, 1999).*

▲ Observe for signs of caregiver stress on an ongoing basis. Refer to necessary support

• = **Independent;** ▲ = **Collaborative**

services. **Nursing Research:** *Support groups provide an essential resource to clients and their families when adapting to health status change (Fung and Chien, 2002).*

▲ Refer the client to counselor or therapist for follow-up care. Initiate community referrals as needed (e.g., grief counseling, self-help groups). **Nursing Research:** *Families need assistance in coping with health changes. The nurse is often perceived as the individual who can help them obtain necessary social support (Northouse et al, 2002; Tak and McCubbin, 2002). Support groups can provide families with a close setting that allows for minor problems and fears to be resolved readily (Herranz and Gavilan, 1999).*

Client/Family Teaching

- Teach the client to maintain a positive outlook by listing current strengths. *Successful adaptation requires a coordination of efforts to fit the nursing interventions to the client's perception of the threat, personal values and beliefs and recognition of personal strengths (Norris and Spelic, 2002).*
- Teach a client and his or her family relaxation techniques (controlled breathing, guided imagery) and help them practice. **Nursing Research:** *Relaxation training has been demonstrated to improve self-efficacy in Alzheimer family caregivers (Fisher and Laschinger, 2001).*
- Allow the client to proceed at own pace in learning; provide time for return demonstrations (e.g., self-injection of insulin). *Use clear and distinct language free of medical jargon and meaningless values.*
- Involve significant others in planning and teaching. **Nursing Research:** *Client's ability to cognitively absorb new information will vary according to his or her perceived threat, prior coping successes, and support (Northouse et al, 2002).*
- If long-term deficits are expected, inform the family as soon as possible. **Nursing Research:** *An honest assessment shared by the nurse of a particular situation is important to the family's sense of what is expected of them in adapting to a health care change (Weiss and Chen, 2002).*
- Teach families intervention techniques for family members such as setting limits, communicating acceptable behavior, and having time-outs. *Psychological, social, and behavioral interventions are effective in mediating aggressive behavior (Harper-Jaques and Reimer, 2002).*
- Educate and prepare families regarding the appearance of the client and the environment before initial exposure. *Appearance and unfamiliar environment may be a source of distress leading to maladjustment (Doering et al, 1999).*

evolve WEBSITES FOR EDUCATION

See the EVOLVE website for World Wide Web resources for client education.

REFERENCES

Baldacchino D, Draper P: Spiritual coping strategies: a review of the nursing research literature, *J Adv Nurs* 34(6):833, 2001.
Cochran M: Tears have no color, *Am J Nurs* 98(6):53, 1998.
Czuchta DM, McCay E: Help-seeking for parents of individuals experiencing a first episode of schizophrenia, *Arch Psychiatr Nurs* 15(4):159, 2001.
Doering LV, Dracup K, Moser D: Comparison of psychosocial adjustment of mothers and fathers of high-risk infants in the neonatal intensive care unit, *J Perinatol* 19(2):132, 1999.

• = Independent; ▲ = Collaborative

Doswell W, Erlen J: Multicultural issues and ethical concerns in the delivery of revising care interventions, *Nurs Clin North Am* 33(2):353, 1998.

Dudley-Brown S: Prevention of psychological distress in persons with inflammatory bowel disease, *Issues Ment Health Nurs* 23:403, 2002.

Giger JN, Davidhizar RE: *Transcultural nursing*, ed 3, St Louis, 1999, Mosby.

Harper-Jaques S, Reimer M: Management of aggression. In Boyd MA, editor: *Psychiatric nursing in contemporary practice*, ed 2, Philadelphia, 2002, Lippincott.

Herranz J, Gavilan J: Psychosocial adjustment after laryngeal cancer surgery, *Ann Otol Rhinol Laryngol* 108(10): 990, 1999.

Langfitt JT et al: Family interactions as targets for intervention to improve social adjustment after epilepsy surgery, *Epilepsia* 40(6):735, 1999.

LeClerc CM et al: Falling short of the mark, *Clin Nurs Res* 11(3):242, 2002.

Leininger MM, McFarland MR: *Transcultural nursing: concepts, theories, research and practices*, ed 3, New York, 2002, McGraw-Hill.

Mazur E et al: Cognitive moderators of children's adjustment to stressful divorce events: the role of negative cognitive errors and positive illusions, *Child Dev* 70(1):231, 1999.

Northouse L et al: A family-based program of care for women with recurrent breast cancer and their family members, *Oncol Nurs Forum* 29(10):1411, 2002.

Phillips JM, Cohen MZ, Moses G: Breast cancer screening and African American women: fear, fatalism, and silence, *Oncol Nurs Forum* 26(3):561, 1999.

Reynaud SN, Meeker BJ: Coping styles of older adults with ostomies, *J Gerontol Nurs* 30, 2002.

Richer MC, Ezer H: Living in it, living with it, and moving on: dimensions of meaning during chemotherapy, *Oncol Nurs Forum* 29(1):113, 2002.

Stuart GW, Laraia MT: Therapeutic nurse-client relationship. In Stuart GW, Laraia MT, editors: *Principles and practice of psychiatric nursing*, St Louis, 2001, Mosby.

Sykes DH et al: Socioeconomic status, social environment, depression and postdischarge adjustment of the cardiac client, *J Psychosom Res* 46(1):83, 1999.

Ineffective Airway clearance

Betty J. Ackley

NANDA Definition

Inability to clear secretions or obstructions from the respiratory tract to maintain a clear airway

Defining Characteristics

Dyspnea; diminished breath sounds; orthopnea; adventitious breath sounds (crackles, wheezes); cough, ineffective or absent; sputum production; cyanosis; difficulty vocalizing; wide-eyed; changes in respiratory rate and rhythm; restlessness

Related Factors (r/t)

Environmental

Smoking; smoke inhalation; second-hand smoke; obstructed airway; airway spasm; retained secretions; excessive mucus; presence of artificial airway; foreign body in airway; secretions in bronchi; exudate in alveoli

Physiological

Neuromuscular dysfunction; hyperplasia of bronchial walls; COPD; infection; asthma; allergic airways

• = Independent; ▲ = Collaborative

NOC   Outcomes (Nursing Outcomes Classification)

Suggested NOC Outcomes

Aspiration Prevention; Respiratory Status: Airway Patency, Gas Exchange, Ventilation

---

Example NOC Outcome with Indicators

Respiratory Status: Ventilation as evidenced by the following indicators: Respiratory rate/Moves sputum out of airway/Adventitious breath sounds not present/SOB not present/Auscultated breath sounds IER/ Auscultated vocalization IER/Chest x-ray findings IER (Rate each indicator of **Respiratory Status: Ventilation:** 1 = extremely compromised, 2 = substantially compromised, 3 = moderately compromised, 4 = mildly compromised, 5 = not compromised [see Section I].)

IER, In expected range; *SOB,* shortness of breath.

Client Outcomes

Client Will (Specify Time Frame):

- Demonstrate effective coughing and clear breath sounds; is free of cyanosis and dyspnea
- Maintain a patent airway at all times
- Relate methods to enhance secretion removal
- Relate the significance of changes in sputum to include color, character, amount, and odor
- Identify and avoid specific factors that inhibit effective airway clearance

NIC   Interventions (Nursing Interventions Classification)

Suggested NIC Interventions

Airway Management; Airway Suctioning; Cough Enhancement

Example NIC Activities—Airway Management

Instruct how to cough effectively; Auscultate breath sounds, noting areas of decreased or absent ventilation and presence of adventitious sounds

---

Nursing Interventions and Rationales

- Auscultate breath sounds q 1 to 4 h(rs). Breath sounds are normally clear or scattered fine crackles at bases, which clear with deep breathing. *The presence of coarse crackles during late inspiration indicates fluid in the airway; wheezing indicates an airway obstruction.*
- Monitor respiratory patterns, including rate, depth, and effort. A normal respiratory rate for an adult without dyspnea is 12 to 16. *With secretions in the airway, the respiratory rate will increase.*
- Monitor blood gas values and pulse oxygen saturation levels as available. *An oxygen saturation of less than 90% (normal: 95% to 100%) or a partial pressure of oxygen of less than 80 (normal: 80 to 100) indicates significant oxygenation problems (Grap, 2002; Berry and Pinard, 2002).*

• = Independent; ▲ = Collaborative

- Position the client to optimize respiration (e.g., head of bed elevated 45 degrees and repositioned at least every 2 hours). *An upright position allows for maximal lung expansion; lying flat causes abdominal organs to shift toward the chest, which crowds the lungs and makes it more difficult to breathe.* **Clinical Research:** *Studies have shown that in a mechanically ventilated client, there is a decreased incidence of pneumonia if the client is positioned at a 45-degree semirecumbent position as opposed to a supine position (Collard et al, 2003; Drakulovic et al, 1999; Torres et al, 1992).*

- If the client has unilateral lung disease, alternate a semi-Fowler's position with a lateral position (with a 10- to 15-degree elevation and "good lung down") for 60 to 90 minutes. This method is contraindicated for a client with a pulmonary abscess or hemorrhage or with interstitial emphysema. *Gravity and hydrostatic pressure allow the dependent lung to become better ventilated and perfused, which increases oxygenation (Smith-Sims, 2001; Yeaw, 1992).*

- Help the client to deep breathe and perform controlled coughing. Have the client inhale deeply, hold breath for several seconds, and cough two or three times with mouth open while tightening the upper abdominal muscles. *This technique can help increase sputum clearance and decrease cough spasms (Celli, 1998; Donahue, 2002). Controlled coughing uses the diaphragmatic muscles, making the cough more forceful and effective.*

- If the client has COPD, cystic fibrosis, or bronchiectasis, consider helping the client use the forced expiratory technique, the "huff cough." The client does a series of coughs while saying the word "huff." *This technique prevents the glottis from closing during the cough and is effective in clearing secretions in the central airways (Goodman and Jones, 2002; Hess, 2001).*

- Encourage the client to use incentive spirometer. *The incentive spirometer is an effective tool that can help prevent atelectasis and retention of bronchial secretions (Peruzzi and Smith, 1995; Smith-Sims, 2001).*

- Assist with clearing secretions from pharynx by offering tissues and gentle suction of the oral pharynx if necessary. Do not do nasotracheal suctioning. It is preferable for the client to cough up secretions. *In the debilitated client, gentle suctioning of the posterior pharynx may stimulate coughing and help remove secretions; nasotracheal suctioning is dangerous because the nurse is unable to hyperoxygenate before, during, and after to maintain adequate oxygenation (Peruzzi and Smith, 1995).*

- Observe sputum, noting color, odor, and volume. *Normal sputum is clear or gray and minimal; abnormal sputum is green, yellow, or bloody; malodorous; and often copious.*

- When suctioning an endotracheal tube or tracheostomy tube for a client on a ventilator, do the following:
  - Explain the process of suctioning before and ensure the client is not in pain or overly anxious. *Suctioning can be a frightening experience, an explanation along with adequate pain relief or needed sedation can reduce stress, anxiety, and pain (Day, Farnell, and Wilson-Barnett, 2002).*
  - Hyperoxygenate before and between endotracheal suction sessions. **Nursing Research:** *Studies have demonstrated that hyperoxygenation helps prevent oxygen desaturation in a suctioned client (Adlkofer and Powaser, 1978; Harshbarger et al, 1992).*
  - Use a closed, in-line suction system. **Clinical Research:** *The closed, in-line suction system is associated with a decrease in nosocomial pneumonia (Deppe et al, 1990; Johnson et al, 1994).*

- = **Independent;** ▲ = **Collaborative**

- ▪ Avoid saline instillation during suctioning. **Nursing Research:** *Repeated studies have demonstrated that saline instillation before suctioning has an adverse effect on oxygen saturation (Ackerman, 1993; Ackerman and Mick, 1998; Kinloch and Rock, 1999).* **Clinical Research:** *A study demonstrated that instillation of a small amount of saline into the endotracheal tube increased greatly the number of colonies of bacteria dislodged from the tube to enter the lower airways, which can result in pneumonia (Hagler and Traver, 1994).*
  - ▪ Document results of coughing and suctioning, particularly client tolerance and secretion characteristics such as color, odor, and volume.
- • Provide oral care every 4 hours. *Oral care freshens the mouth after respiratory secretions have been expectorated. Research is promising on the use of chlorhexidine oral rinses after oral care to reduce bacteria, and possibly reduce the incidence of nosocomial pneumonia (Kollef, 1999).*
- • Encourage activity and ambulation as tolerated. If unable to ambulate the client, turn the client from side to side at least every 2 hours. *Body movement helps mobilize secretions and can be a powerful means to maintain lung health (Fink, 2002). The supine position and immobility have been shown to predispose a postoperative client to pneumonia (Brooks-Brunn, 1995). See interventions for **Impaired Gas exchange** for further information on positioning a respiratory client.*
- • Encourage increased fluid intake of up to 2500 ml/day within cardiac or renal reserve. *Fluids help minimize mucosal drying and maximize ciliary action to move secretions (Carroll, 1994; Smith-Sims, 2001). Some clients cannot tolerate increased fluids because of underlying disease.*
- ▲ Administer oxygen as ordered. *Oxygen has been shown to correct hypoxemia, which can be caused by retained respiratory secretions.*
- ▲ Administer medications such as bronchodilators or inhaled steroids as ordered. *Watch for side effects such as tachycardia or anxiety with bronchodilators, or inflamed pharynx with inhaled steroids. Bronchodilators decrease airway resistance secondary to bronchoconstriction.*
- ▲ Provide postural drainage, percussion, and vibration only as ordered. Chest physical therapy should be used only when prescribed because it can cause harm if the client has underlying conditions such as cardiac disease or increased intracranial pressure (Peruzzi and Smith, 1995). *Postural draining provides improved secretion clearance only in clients with cystic fibrosis of excessive sputum production (Fink, 2002).* **Clinical Research:** *In most clinical trials, bronchial hygiene physical therapy produced no significant effects on pulmonary function, other than clearing sputum in COPD and bronchiectasis (Jones and Rowe, 2002).*
- ▲ Refer for physical therapy or respiratory therapy for further treatment.

Geriatric

- • Encourage ambulation as tolerated without causing exhaustion. *Immobility is often harmful to the elderly because it decreases ventilation and increases stasis of secretions, leading to atelectasis or pneumonia (Hoyt, 1992; Tempkin et al, 1997).*
- • Actively encourage the elderly to deep breathe and cough. *Cough reflexes are blunted and coughing is decreased in the elderly (Sparrow and Weiss, 1988).*
- • Ensure adequate hydration within cardiac and renal reserves. *The elderly are prone to dehydration, and therefore more viscous secretions, because they frequently use diuretics or laxatives and forget to drink adequate amounts of water (Hoyt, 1992).*

- • = **Independent;** ▲ = **Collaborative**

Home care

- Some of the above interventions may be adapted for home care use.
- ▲ Begin discharge planning as soon as possible with case manager or social worker to assess need for home support systems, assistive devices, and community or home health services.
- Assess home environment for factors that exacerbate airway clearance problems (e.g., presence of allergens, lack of adequate humidity in air, poor air flow, stressful family relationships).
- Assess affective climate within family and family support system. *Problems with respiratory function and resulting anxiety can provoke anger and frustration in the client. Feelings may be displaced onto caregiver and require intervention to ensure continued caregiver support. Refer to care plan for* **Caregiver role strain.**
- Provide the client with emotional support in dealing with symptoms of respiratory distress.
- Provide family with support for care of a client with chronic or terminal illness. *Breathing difficulty can provoke extreme anxiety, which can interfere with the client's ability or willingness to adhere to the treatment plan. Refer to care plan for* **Anxiety.** Witnessing breathing difficulties and facing concerns of dealing with chronic or terminal illness can create fear in caregiver. Fear inhibits effective coping.
- Instruct the client to avoid exposure to persons with upper respiratory infections.
- ▲ Provide/teach percussion and postural drainage per physician orders. Teach adaptive breathing techniques. *Adaptive breathing, percussion, and postural drainage loosen secretions and allow more effective oxygenation.*
- Determine client adherence to medical regimen. Instruct the client and family in importance of reporting effectiveness of current medications to physician. *Inappropriate use of medications (too much or too little) can influence amount of respiratory secretions.*
- Teach the client when and how to use inhalant or nebulizer treatments at home.
- Teach the client/family importance of maintaining regimen and having prn drugs easily accessible at all times. *Success in avoiding emergency or institutional care may rest solely on medication compliance or availability.*
- Teach the client/family the importance of and methods for setting priorities for activities, especially those having a high energy demand (e.g., home/family events). Instruct in realistic expectations. **Nursing Research:** *Client and/or family may assume a higher degree of energy than is actually present. Assistance may be needed to ensure accuracy of expectations for the client. Unrealistic expectations provoke guilt feelings in the client, leading to efforts that can exceed the client's energy capacity (Patusky, 2002).*
- Instruct the client and family in the importance of maintaining proper nutrition, adequate fluids, rest, and behavioral pacing for energy conservation and rehabilitation. Instruct in use of dietary supplements as indicated. *Illness may suppress appetite, leading to inadequate nutrition. Pacing activities to energy capacity and rest are important to ensure the client does not overdo his or her capability. Low fluid intake can increase the thickness of respiratory secretions.*
- Identify an emergency plan, including criteria for use. *Ineffective airway clearance can be life threatening.*
- ▲ Refer for home health aide services for assist with ADLs. Clients with decreased oxygenation and copious respiratory secretions are often unable to maintain energy for ADLs.

• = **Independent;** ▲ = **Collaborative**

▲ Assess family for role changes and coping skills. Refer to medical social services as necessary. *Clients with decreased oxygenation are unable to maintain role activities and therefore experience frustration and anger, which may pose a threat to family integrity. Family counseling to adapt to role changes may be needed.*

▲ Institute case management of frail elderly to support continued independent living. *Respiratory difficulties represent and can lead to increasing needs for assistance in using the health care system effectively. Case management combines nursing activities of the client and family assessment, planning and coordination of care among all health care providers, delivery of direct nursing care, and monitoring of care and outcomes. These activities are able to address continuity of care, mutual goal setting, behavior management, and prevention of worsening health problems (Guttman, 1999).*

Client/Family Teaching

▲ Teach importance of not smoking. Be aggressive in approach, ask to set a date for smoking cessation, and recommend nicotine replacement therapy (nicotine patch or gum). Refer to smoking cessation programs, and encourage clients who relapse to keep trying to quit. *All health care clinicians should be aggressive in helping smokers quit (AHCPR Guidelines, 1996).*

▲ Teach the client how to use a flutter clearance device if ordered, which vibrates to loosen mucus and gives positive pressure to keep airways open. **Clinical Research:** *This device has been shown to effectively decrease mucous viscosity and elasticity (App et al, 1998), increase amount of sputum expectorated (Bellone et al, 2000), and increase peak expiratory flow rate (Burioka et al, 1998). Daily use of the flutter device was shown to be as effective as the active cycle of breathing technique and was a preferred technique by clients (Thompson et al, 2002).*

▲ Teach the client how to use peak expiratory flow rate (PEFR) meter if ordered and when to seek medical attention if PEFR reading drops. Also teach how to use metered dose inhalers and self-administer inhaled corticosteroids following precautions to decrease side effects (Owen, 1999).

• Teach the client how to deep breathe and cough effectively. Teach how to use the ELTGOL method—an airway clearance method that uses lateral posture and different lung volumes to control expiratory flow of air to avoid airway compression. **Clinical Research:** *Controlled coughing uses the diaphragmatic muscles, making the cough more forceful and effective. The ELTGOL method was shown to be more effective in secretion removal in chronic bronchitis than postural drainage (Bellone et al, 2000).*

• Teach the client/family to identify and avoid specific factors that exacerbate ineffective airway clearance, including known allergens and especially smoking (if relevant) or exposure to second-hand smoke.

• Educate the client and family about the significance of changes in sputum characteristics, including color, character, amount, and odor. *With this knowledge, the client and family can identify early the signs of infection and seek treatment before acute illness occurs.*

• Teach the client/family need to take antibiotics until the prescription has run out. *Taking the entire course of antibiotics helps to eradicate bacterial infection, which decreases lingering, chronic infection.*

• = **Independent;** ▲ = **Collaborative**

WEBSITES FOR EDUCATION

See the EVOLVE website for World Wide Web resources for client education.

REFERENCES

Ackerman MH: The effect of saline lavage prior to suctioning, *Am J Crit Care* 2(4):326, 1993.

Ackerman MH, Mick DJ: Instillation of normal saline before suctioning in patients with pulmonary infections: a prospective randomized controlled trial, *Am J Crit Care* 7(4):261, 1998.

Adlkofer R, Powaser M: The effect of endotracheal suctioning on arterial blood gases in patients after cardiac surgery, *Heart Lung* 7(6):1011, 1978.

Agency for Health Care Policy and Research: *Smoking cessation, clinical practice guideline,* Washington, DC, 1996, U.S. Government Printing Office.

App EM et al: Sputum rheology changes in cystic fibrosis lung disease following two different types of physiotherapy: flutter vs autogenic drainage, *Chest* 114(1):171, 1998.

Bellone A et al: Chest physical therapy in patients with acute exacerbation of chronic bronchitis: effectiveness of three modes, *Arch Phys Med Rehabil* 81(5):558, 2000.

Berry BE, Pinard AE: Assessing tissue oxygenation, *Crit Care Nurs* 22(3):22, 2002.

Brooks-Brunn JA: Postoperative atelectasis and pneumonia: risk factors, *Am J Crit Care* 4(5):340, 1995.

Burioka N et al: Clinical efficacy of the FLUTTER device for airway mucus clearance in patients with diffuse panbronchiolitis, *Respirology* 3(3):183, 1998.

Carroll P: Safe suctioning prn, *RN* 57(5):32, 1994.

Carroll P: Spotting the difference in respiratory care, *RN* 96(6):26, 1998.

Celli BR: Pulmonary rehabilitation for COPD, *Postgrad Med* 103(4):159, 1998.

Collard HR, Saint S, Matthay MA: Prevention of ventilator-associated pneumonia: an evidenced-based systemic review, *Ann Intern Med* 138(6):494, 2003.

Day T, Farnell S, Wilson-Barnett J: Suctioning: a review of current research recommendations, *Intensive Crit Care Nurs* 18(2):79, 2002.

Deppe SA et al: Incidence of colonization, nosocomial pneumonia, and mortality in critically ill patients using a Trach Care closed-suction system: prospective, randomized study, *Crit Care Med* 18:1389, 1990.

Drakulovic MB et al: Supine body position as a risk factor for nosocomial pneumonia in mechanically ventilated patients: a randomised trial, *Lancet* 354(9193):1851, 1999.

Fink JB: Positioning versus postural drainage, *Respir Care* 47(7):769, 2002.

Goodman LT, Jones M: Bronchial hygiene therapy, *Am J Nurs* 102(1):37, 2002.

Grap MJ: Protocols for practice: applying research at the bedside: pulse oximetry, *Crit Care Nurs* 22(3):69, 2002.

Guttman R: Case management of the frail elderly in the community, *Clin Nurs Spec* 13(4):174, 1999.

Hagler DA, Traver GA: Endotracheal saline and suction catheters: sources of lower airway contamination, *Am J Crit Care* 3(6):444, 1994.

Hess DR: The evidence for secretion clearance techniques. *Respir Care* 46(11):1276, 2001.

Hoyt MM: Impaired gas exchange in the elderly, *Geriatr Nurs* 13:262, 1992.

Johnson KL et al: Closed versus open endotracheal suctioning: costs and physiologic consequences, *Crit Care Med* 22(4):658, 1994.

Jones AP, Rowe BH: Bronchopulmonary hygiene physical therapy for chronic obstructive pulmonary disease and bronchiectasis, *Cochrane Library,* CD000045, 2002.

Kinloch D, Rock L: Instillation of normal saline during endotracheal suctioning; effects on mixed venous oxygen saturation. *Am J Crit Care* 8(4):231, 1999.

Kollef MH: Epidemiology and risk factors for nosocomial pneumonia, *Clin Chest Med* 20(3):653, 1999.

Mathews PJ, Mathews LM: Reducing the risks of ventilator-associated infections, *Dimens Crit Care Nurs* 19(1): 17, 2000.

Owen CL: New directions in asthma management, *Am J Nurs* 99(3):27, 1999.

Patusky KL: Relatedness theory as a framework for the treatment of fatigued women, *Arch Psychiatr Nurs* 5:224, 2002.

Peruzzi WT, Smith B: Bronchial hygiene therapy, *Crit Care Clin* 11(1):79, 1995.

Raymond SJ: Normal saline instillation before suctioning: helpful or harmful? A review of the literature, *Am J Crit Care* 4(4):267, 1995.

Smith-Sims K: Hospital-acquired pneumonia, *Am J Nurs* 101(1):24AA, 2001.

• = **Independent;** ▲ = **Collaborative**

Sparrow D, Weiss S: Pulmonary system. In Rose JW, Besdine RS, editors: *Geriatric medicine,* Boston, 1988, Little, Brown.

Tempkin T, Tempkin A, Goodman H: Geriatric rehabilitation, *Nurse Pract Forum* 8(2):59, 1997.

Thompson CS, Harrison S, Ashley J: Randomised crossover study of the flutter device and the active cycle of breathing technique in noncystic fibrosis bronchiectasis, *Thorax* 57:446, 2002.

Torres A et al: Pulmonary aspiration of gastric contents in patients receiving mechanical ventilation: the effect of body position, *Ann Intern Med* 116:540, 1992.

Winslow EH: Open-and-closed debate on hyperoxygenation: working smart, *Am J Nurs* 93:16, 1993a.

Winslow EH: Save the saline, *Am J Nurs* 93:16, 1993b.

Yeaw P: Good lung down, *Am J Nurs* 92:27, 1992.

Latex Allergy response

Leslie H. Nicoll and Gail B. Ladwig

NANDA   Definition

An immunological reaction to natural rubber latex (NRL)

Defining Characteristics

Type I reactions: Immediate hypersensitivity response, which is IgE mediated. Symptoms include contact urticaria progressing to systemic urticaria, angioedema, rhinitis, conjunctivitis, bronchospasm, and anaphylaxis (Toraason et al, 2000).

May also include: Orofacial characteristics: edema of sclera or eyelids, erythema and/or itching of the eyes, tearing of the eyes, nasal congestion, itching and/or erythema, rhinorrhea, facial erythema, facial itching; gastrointestinal characteristics: abdominal pain, nausea; generalized characteristics: flushing, general discomfort, generalized edema, increasing complaint of total body warmth, restlessness.

Type IV reactions: Allergic contact dermatitis (delayed hypersensitivity, also sometimes called chemical sensitivity dermatitis):eczema; irritation; may progress to oozing skin blisters; rash usually begins 24 to 48 hours after contact.

Irritant contact dermatitis: Dry, itchy, irritated areas on the skin; chapped or cracked skin; blisters. Irritant dermatitis is not a true allergy.

Related Factors (r/t)

No immune mechanism response

NOC   Outcomes (Nursing Outcomes Classification)

Suggested NOC Outcomes

Allergic Response: Localized, Systemic; Immune Hypersensitivity Response; Symptom Severity; Tissue Integrity: Skin and Mucous Membranes

> ### Example NOC Outcome with Indicators
>
> **Immune Hypersensitivity Response** as evidenced by the following indicators: Respiratory, cardiac, gastrointestinal, renal and neurological function status IER/Free of allergic reactions (Rate each indicator of **Immune Hypersensitivity Response:** 1 = not controlled, 2 = slightly controlled, 3 = moderately controlled, 4 = well controlled, 5 = very well controlled [see Section I].)

IER, In expected range.

- = Independent; ▲ = Collaborative

Client Outcomes

Client Will (Specify Time Frame):
- Identify presence of NRL allergy
- List history of risk factors
- Identify type of reaction
- State reasons not to use or to have anyone use latex products
- Experience a latex-free environment for all health care procedures
- Avoid areas where there is powder from NRL gloves
- State the importance of wearing a Medic-Alert bracelet and wear one
- State the importance of carrying an emergency kit with a supply of nonlatex gloves, antihistamines, and an autoinjectable epinephrine syringe (Epi-pen), and carry one

NIC   Interventions (Nursing Interventions Classification)

Suggested NIC Interventions
Allergy Management; Latex Precautions

Example NIC Activities—Latex Precautions

Question client or appropriate other about history of systemic reaction or sensitization to NRL (e.g., facial or scleral edema, tearing eyes, urticaria, rhinitis, and wheezing); Place an allergy band on client

---

Nursing Interventions and Rationales

- Identify clients at risk: those persons who are most likely to exhibit a sensitivity to NRL that may result in varying degrees of reactivity. Consider the following client groups:
  - Persons with neural tube defects including spina bifida, myelomeningocele/ meningocele. **Clinical Research:** *Patients with spina bifida represent the highest-risk group for developing NRL hypersensitivity. Recognized risk factors for these clients are repeated surgeries and an atopic disposition (Buck et al, 2000).*
  - Children who have experienced three or more surgeries, particularly as a neonate. **Clinical Research:** *A significant correlation between the total number of surgeries, particularly during the first year of life, and degree of sensitization has been established (Degenhardt et al, 2001).*
  - Atopic individuals (persons with a tendency to have multiple allergic conditions) including allergies to food products. Particular allergies to fruits and vegetables including bananas, avocado, celery, fig, chestnut, papaya, potato, tomato, melon, and passion fruit are significant. **Clinical Research:** *Children with atopic dermatitis are a high-risk group for NRL sensitization and latex-associated foods (Tucke et al, 1999).* **Clinical Research:** *Class I chitinases, related to plant defense, are the panallergens in these foods and are associated with latex-fruit syndrome (Perkin, 2000; Salcedo et al, 2001; Sanchez-Monge et al, 2000).* **Clinical Research:** *Atopic persons with increasing years of occupational exposure have an increased risk of developing NRL allergy (Galobardes et al, 2001).*
  - Persons who possess a known or suspected NRL allergy by having exhibited an allergic or anaphylactic reaction, positive skin testing, or positive IgE antibodies against latex. **Clinical Research:** *Persons who are sensitized or have demonstrated an*

• = Independent; ▲ = Collaborative

NRL allergy are at risk, even when a latex-free environment is adopted (Mazon et al, 2000).

▪ Persons who have had an ongoing occupational exposure to NRL, including health care workers, rubber industry workers, bakers, laboratory personnel, food handlers, hairdressers, janitors, policemen, and firefighters. **Clinical Research:** *The predominant pattern of allergen reactivity in health care workers and others with occupational exposure is different from that among children with spina bifida; it has been suggested that occupational exposure is from NRL glove proteins inhaled through powders as opposed to particle bound latex proteins in urinary catheters (Sutherland et al, 2002).* **Clinical Research:** *Ongoing exposure by health care workers has been shown to be associated with an increased risk of IgE sensitization to NRL (Galobardes et al, 2001; Weissman and Lewis, 2002).* **Clinical Research:** *Allergic reactions to NRL have increased during the past 10 years, especially in health care workers who have high exposure to latex allergens both by direct skin contact and by inhalation of latex particles from powdered gloves (Nielsen et al, 2000).*

• Take a thorough history of the client at risk. **Nursing Research:** *A complete and thorough history remains as the most reliable screening test to predict the likelihood of an anaphylactic reaction (American Association of Nurse Anesthetists, 1998).* **Clinical Research:** *Skin prick tests and serum IgE are of limited value in epidemiological studies of NRL allergy; questionnaires about local symptoms are more relevant (Galobardes et al, 2001).* **Clinical Research:** *It is possible to make a diagnosis of type I NRL allergy by taking an accurate history, including questions on atopic status, food allergy, and possible reactions to latex devices (Toraason et al, 2000).*

• Question the client about associated symptoms of itching, swelling, and redness after contact with rubber products such as rubber gloves, balloons, and barrier contraceptives, or swelling of the tongue and lips after dental examinations. **Clinical Research:** *Dermatitis, itching, erythema, contact urticaria, asthma and/or rhinitis were significantly related to skin prick tests that were positive for latex (Larese Filon et al, 2001; Ylitalo et al, 2000).*

• Consider a skin prick test with NRL extracts to identify IgE-mediated immunity. **Clinical Research:** *Although a standardized, commercial skin test reagent for NRL is not yet available, many allergy centers have prepared latex extracts for clinical testing (Joint Task Force on Practice Parameters, 1998).*

• All latex-sensitive clients are treated as if they have NRL allergy. **Clinical Research:** *Even if a person has not experienced an NRL reaction, if it can be documented that he or she has been sensitized, then he or she should be treated as if he or she has an NRL allergy. NRL allergy in the workplace can result in potentially serious health problems for workers, who are often unaware of the risk of latex exposure (National Institute for Occupational Safety and Health, 1998).*

▲ Patients with spina bifida and others with a positive history of NRL sensitivity or NRL allergy should have all medical/surgical/dental procedures performed in a latex-controlled environment. **Clinical Research:** *A latex-controlled environment is defined as one in which no latex gloves are used in the room or surgical suite and no latex accessories (catheters, adhesives, tourniquet, and anesthesia equipment) come in contact with the client (Joint Task Force on Practice Parameters, 1998).*

▲ The most effective approach to preventing NRL anaphylaxis is complete latex avoidance. Medications may reduce certain symptoms. **Clinical Research:** *Safe and read-*

• = **Independent;** ▲ = **Collaborative**

ily available immunotherapy for NRL allergy is currently lacking (Brehler and Kutting, 2001; Sutherland et al, 2002).

▲ Materials and items that contain NRL must be identified, and latex-free alternatives must be found. **Clinical Research:** *A wide variety of products contain NRL: medical supplies, personal protective equipment, and numerous household objects (National Institute for Occupational Safety and Health, 1998).*

▲ In health care settings, general use of latex gloves having negligible allergen content, powder-free latex gloves, and nonlatex gloves and medical articles should be considered in an effort to minimize exposure to latex allergen. **Clinical Research:** *The risk of NRL allergy appears to be largely linked to occupational exposure and NRL-associated occupational asthma is due almost solely to powdered glove use. Airborne NRL is dependent on the use of powdered NRL gloves; conversion to non-NRL or nonpowdered NRL substitutes results in predictable rapid disappearance of detectable levels of aeroallergen (Charous et al, 2002).*

• See Box III-1 for examples of products that may contain NRL. **Clinical Research:** *Anaphylaxis from NRL allergy is a medical emergency and must be treated as such. Latex is a potent allergen and a type I anaphylactic reaction may be immediate in sensitized individuals. Acute treatment must be carried out in a latex-free environment (Holzman, 1997).*

Home care

• Assess the home environment for presence of NRL products (e.g., balloons, condoms, gloves, and products of related allergies, such as bananas, avocados, and poinsettia plants). **Clinical Research:** *Latex avoidance measures in the home setting is the key to prevention (Mazon et al, 2000).*

• At onset of care, assess client history and current status of NRL allergy response. *A complete and thorough history remains as the most reliable screening test to predict the likelihood of an anaphylactic reaction (American Association of Nurse Anesthetists, 1998).*

▲ Seek medical care as necessary.

• Do not use NRL products in caregiving.

• Assist the client in identifying and obtaining alternatives to NRL products. **Nursing Research:** *Preventing exposure to latex is the key to managing and preventing this allergy. Providing a safe environment for clients with NRL allergy is the responsibility of all health care professionals (American Association of Nurse Anesthetists, 1998).* **Clinical Research:** *Avoidance management should be individualized, taking into consideration factors such as age, activity, occupation, hobbies, residential conditions, and the client's level of personal anxiety (Joint Task Force on Practice Parameters, 1998).*

Client/Family Teaching

• Provide written information about NRL allergy and sensitivity. **Clinical Research:** *Patient education is the most important preventive strategy. Patients should be carefully instructed about "hidden" latex, cross reactions, particularly foods, and unforeseen risks during medical procedures (Joint Task Force on Practice Parameters, 1998).*

▲ Instruct the client to inform health care professionals if he or she has an NRL allergy, particularly if they are scheduled for surgery. **Clinical Research:** *To prevent problems associated with exposure to products containing latex, it is essential that clients with NRL allergy are identified (Dakin and Yentis, 1998).*

• Teach the client what products contain NRL and to avoid direct contact with all latex

• = Independent; ▲ = Collaborative

BOX III-1   PRODUCTS THAT MAY CONTAIN LATEX

Emergency Equipment
Blood pressure cuffs
Stethoscopes
Disposable gloves
Oral and nasal airways
Endotracheal tubes
Tourniquets
IV solutions and tubing systems
Bulb syringes
Medication syringes
Electrode pads
Ambu (bag-valve) masks
Instrument pads

Personal Protective Equipment
Gloves
Surgical masks
Goggles
Respirators
Rubber aprons

Hospital Supplies
Anesthesia masks
Urinary catheters and drainage systems
Wound drains
Injection ports
Rubber tops of multidose vials
Dental dams
Mattresses on stretchers
Adhesive tape (porous), Band-Aids
    and other similar bandage products
Elastic bandages and wraps
Stomach and intestinal tubes
Chest tubes and drainage systems
Protective sheets
Enema tubing kits
Fluid-circulating thermal blankets
Hemodialysis equipment
Surgical drapes
Patient controlled analgesia syringes

Objects Outside the Home
Grocery store checkout belts
Restaurants that use latex gloves for food
    preparation
Auto races that emit tire and rubber
    particles
ATM machine buttons—often made of
    rubber

Household Objects
Automobile tires
Motorcycle and bicycle handgrips
Carpeting
Swimming goggles
Racquet handles
Shoe soles
Expandable fabric (waistbands) in
    underwear, bathing suits, socks
Dishwashing gloves
Hot water bottles
Condoms and diaphragms
Balloons
Pacifiers
Baby bottle nipples
Rubber bands, mouse and keyboard cords,
    desktop and chair pads, rubber stamps
Erasers
Remote controllers with rubber grips
    or keys
Pens with comfort grip or any rubber
    coating
Rubber tub toys
Rubber sink stoppers, sink mats, grip
    utensils
Adhesives such as glue, paste, art supplies,
    glue pens
Camera, telescope, or binocular eye pieces

Data from American Association of Nurse Anesthetists: *AANA latex protocol,* Park Ridge, Ill, 1998, The Association, pp 1-9; National Institute for Occupational Safety and Health: *Preventing allergic reactions to natural rubber latex in the workplace,* Cincinnati, July 1998, The Institute; The Cleveland Clinic Health Information Center: *Latex allergy,* available on-line at www.clevelandclinic.org/health/health-info/docs/1900/1955.asp, accessed Dec 27, 2002.

• = Independent; ▲ = Collaborative

products and foods that trigger allergic reactions. **Clinical Research:** *Once NRL allergy has developed, the client is at risk for anaphylaxis and needs to be informed as to what products contain latex (Tarlo, 1998).*

- Teach the client to avoid areas where powdered latex gloves are used, as well as where latex balloons are inflated or deflated. **Nursing Research:** *Powder from gloves acts as a carrier for latex protein (American Association of Nurse Anesthetists, 1998).*
- Instruct the client with NRL allergy to wear a medical identification bracelet and/or carry a medical identification card. **Clinical Research:** *Identification of the client with NRL allergy is critical for preventing problems and for early intervention with appropriate treatment if an exposure occurs (Joint Task Force on Practice Parameters, 1998; Kelly and Walsh-Kelly, 1998).*
- Instruct the client to carry an emergency kit with a supply of nonlatex gloves, antihistamines, and an autoinjectable epinephrine syringe (Epi-Pen). **Clinical Research:** *An autoinjectable epinephrine syringe should be prescribed to sensitized clients who are at risk for an anaphylactic episode with accidental latex exposure (Joint Task Force on Practice Parameters, 1998; National Institute for Occupational Safety and Health, 1998; Tarlo, 1998).*

evolve WEBSITES FOR EDUCATION

See the EVOLVE website for World Wide Web resources for client education.

REFERENCES

American Association of Nurse Anesthetists: *AANA latex protocol,* Park Ridge, Ill, 1998, The Association.

Baumann NH: Latex allergy. An orthopaedic case presentation and considerations in patient care, *Orthop Nurs* 18(3):15, 1999.

Brehler R, Kutting B: Natural rubber latex allergy: a problem of interdisciplinary concern in medicine, *Arch Intern Med* 161(8):1057, 2001.

Buck D et al: Ventricular shunts and the prevalence of sensitization and clinically relevant allergy to latex in patients with spina bifida, *Pediatr Allergy Immunol* 11(2):111, 2000.

Charous BL et al: Natural rubber latex allergy after 12 years: recommendations and perspectives, *J Allergy Clin Immunol* 109(1):31, 2002.

Dakin MJ, Yentis SM: Latex allergy: a strategy for management, *Anaesthesia* 53(8):774, 1998.

Degenhardt P et al: Latex allergy in pediatric surgery is dependent on repeated operations in the first year of life, *J Pediatr Surg* 36(10):1535, 2001.

Galobardes B et al: Influence of occupational exposure to latex on the prevalence of sensitization and allergy to latex in a Swiss hospital, *Dermatology* 203 (3):226, 2001.

Holzman RS: Clinical management of latex-allergic children, *Anesth Analg* 85(3):529, 1997.

Joint Task Force on Practice Parameters; American Academy of Allergy, Asthma and Immunology; American College of Allergy, Asthma and Immunology; and the Joint Council of Allergy, Asthma and Immunology: The diagnosis and management of anaphylaxis, *J Allergy Clin Immunol* 101(6 Pt 2):S465, 1998.

Kelly KJ, Walsh-Kelly CM: Latex allergy: a patient and health care system emergency, *Ann Emerg Med* 32(6): 723, 1998.

Larese Filon F et al: Latex symptoms and sensitisation in health care workers, *Int Arch Occup Environ Health* 74(3):219, 2001.

Mazon A et al: Latex sensitization in children with spina bifida: follow-up comparative study after two years, *Ann Allergy Asthma Immunol* 84(2):207, 2000.

National Institute for Occupational Safety and Health: *Preventing allergic reactions to natural rubber latex in the workplace,* Cincinnati, 1998, The Institute.

Nielsen PS et al: Assessment of IgE allergen specificity among latex-allergic health care workers: review of IgE-binding components of various latex extracts, *Ann Allergy Asthma Immunol* 85(6 Pt 1):489, 2000.

Perkin JE: The latex and food allergy connection, *J Am Diet Assoc* 100(11):1381, 2000.

- = **Independent;** ▲ = **Collaborative**

Salcedo G, Diaz-Perales A, Sanchez-Monge R: The role of plant panallergens in sensitization to natural rubber latex, *Curr Opin Allergy Clin Immunol* 1(2):177, 2001.

Sanchez-Monge R et al: Class I chitinases, the panallergens responsible for the latex-fruit syndrome, are induced by ethylene treatment and inactivated by heating, *J Allergy Clin Immunol* 106(1 Pt 1):190, 2000.

Sutherland MF et al: Latex allergy: towards immunotherapy for health care workers, *Clin Exp Allergy* 32(5): 667, 2002.

Tarlo SM: Latex allergy: a problem for both health care professionals and patients, *Ostomy Wound Manage* 44(8):80, 1998.

Toraason M et al: Latex allergy in the workplace, *Toxicol Sci* 58(1):5, 2000.

Tucke J et al: Latex type I sensitization and allergy in children with atopic dermatitis. Evaluation of cross-reactivity to some foods, *Pediatr Allergy Immunol* 10(3):160, 1999.

Weissman DN, Lewis DM: Allergic and latex-specific sensitization: route, frequency, and amount of exposure that are required to initiate IgE production, *J Allergy Clin Immunol* 110(2 suppl):S57, 2002.

Ylitalo L et al: Natural rubber latex allergy in children: a follow-up study, *Clin Exp Allergy* 30(11):1611, 2000.

Risk for latex Allergy response

Leslie H. Nicoll and Gail B. Ladwig

NANDA Definition

At risk for allergic response to natural rubber latex (NRL) products

Risk Factors

Children with three or more surgeries, especially as a neonate; neural tube defects (e.g., spina bifida); allergies to bananas, avocados, tropical fruits, kiwis, chestnuts, apples, carrots, celery, potatoes, tomatoes; professions with daily exposure to latex (e.g., health care workers, rubber industry workers, food handlers, hairdressers, janitors, police, firefighters); conditions needing continuous or intermittent catheterization; history of re-actions to latex (e.g., balloons, condoms, gloves); atopic individuals (persons with a tendency to have multiple allergic conditions).

NOC Outcomes (Nursing Outcomes Classification)

Suggested NOC Outcomes

Allergic Response: Systemic; Immune Hypersensitivity Response; Knowledge: Health Behavior; Risk Control; Risk Detection; Tissue Integrity: Skin and Mucous Membranes

Example NOC Outcome with Indicators

Immune Hypersensitivity Response as evidenced by the following indicators: Respiratory, cardiac, gastrointestinal, renal and neurological function status IER/Free of allergic reactions (Rate each indicator of **Immune Hypersensitivity Response:** 1 = not controlled, 2 = slightly controlled, 3 = moderately controlled, 4 = well controlled, 5 = very well controlled [see Section I].)

IER, In expected range.

• = Independent; ▲ = Collaborative

Client Outcomes

Client Will (Specify Time Frame):
- State risk factors for NRL allergy
- Request latex-free environment
- Demonstrate knowledge of plan to treat NRL allergic reaction

NIC Interventions (Nursing Interventions Classification)

Suggested NIC Interventions
Allergy Management; Latex Precautions

Example NIC Activities—Latex Precautions

Question client or appropriate other about history of systemic reaction to NRL (e.g., facial or scleral edema, tearing eyes, urticaria, rhinitis, and wheezing); Place an allergy band on client

---

Nursing Interventions and Rationales

- Clients at high risk need to be identified, such as those with frequent bladder catheterizations, occupational exposure to latex, past history of atopy (hay fever, asthma, dermatitis, or food allergy to fruits such as bananas, avocados, papaya, chestnut, or kiwi); those with a history of anaphylaxis of uncertain etiology, especially if associated with surgery; health care workers; and females exposed to barrier contraceptives and routine examinations during gynecological and obstetric procedures. **Clinical Research:** *Health care professionals, hospital patients, and rubber industry workers have noted a marked increase in allergic reactions to NRL in the past 10 years (Nielsen et al, 2000).* **Clinical Research:** *Recent studies have shown that allergy to NRL is significantly associated with hypersensitivity to certain foods, including avocados, chestnuts, papayas, kiwis, potatoes, tomatoes, and bananas (Perkin, 2000; Salcedo et al, 2001; Sanchez-Monge et al, 2000).* **Nursing Research:** *A latex-directed history is the primary method of identifying latex sensitivity, although both skin and serum testing are available and are increasingly accurate (American Association of Nurse Anesthetists, 1998; Galobardes et al, 2001; Toraason et al, 2000).*
- Clients with spina bifida are a high-risk group for NRL allergy and should remain latex free from the first day of life. **Clinical Research:** *Clients with spina bifida represent the highest risk group for developing NRL hypersensitivity. Recognized risk factors for these clients are repeated surgeries and an atopic disposition (Buck et al, 2000).*
- Children who are on home ventilation should be assessed for NRL allergy. **Clinical Research:** *This study showed a high incidence of NRL allergy in children on home ventilation. All children on home ventilation should be screened for NRL allergy to prevent untoward reactions from exposure to latex (Nakamura et al, 2000).*
- Assess for NRL allergy in clients who are exposed to "hidden" latex. **Clinical Research:** *Case studies have reported on serious complications in clients exposed to latex through hair glue (Cogen and Beezhold, 2002) and microdermabrasion (Farris and Rietschel, 2002).*
- See care plan for **Latex Allergy response**.

Home care
▲ Ensure that the client has a medical plan if a response develops. Prompt treatment decreases potential severity of response.

• = Independent; ▲ = Collaborative

- See care plan for **Latex Allergy response**. Note client history and environmental assessment.

Client/Family Teaching

▲ A client who has had symptoms of NRL allergy or who suspects he or she is allergic to latex should tell his or her employer and contact his or her institution's occupational health services. **Clinical Research:** *Occupational health services can arrange testing by an allergist. If an allergy is present, measures to protect the client's well-being in the workplace should be instituted (National Institute for Occupational Safety and Health, 1998).*

- Provide written information about latex allergy and sensitivity. **Clinical Research:** *Patient education is the most important preventive strategy. Patients should be carefully instructed about "hidden" latex; cross reactions, particularly foods; and unforeseen risks during medical procedures (Joint Task Force on Practice Parameters, 1998).*

- Health care workers should avoid the use of latex gloves and seek alternatives such as gloves made from nitrile. **Clinical Research:** *The risk of NRL allergy appears to be largely linked to occupational exposure and NRL-associated occupational asthma is due almost solely to powdered glove use. Airborne NRL is dependent on the use of powdered NRL gloves; conversion to non-NRL or nonpowdered NRL substitutes results in predictable rapid disappearance of detectable levels of aeroallergen (Charous et al, 2002).* **Clinical Research:** *Preliminary reports of primary preventive strategies suggest that avoidance of high-protein, powdered gloves in health care facilities can be cost-effective and is associated with a decline in sensitized workers (Tarlo et al, 2001).* **Nursing Research:** *Nitrile examination gloves offer better protection than latex types when handling lipid-soluble substances and chemicals (Russell-Fell 2000).*

REFERENCES

American Association of Nurse Anesthetists: *AANA latex protocol,* Park Ridge, Ill, 1998, The Association.

Buck D et al: Ventricular shunts and the prevalence of sensitization and clinically relevant allergy to latex in patients with spina bifida, *Pediatr Allergy Immunol* 11(2):111, 2000.

Charous BL et al: Natural rubber latex allergy after 12 years: recommendations and perspectives, *J Allergy Clin Immunol* 109(1):31, 2002.

Cogen FC, Beezhold DH: Hair glue anaphylaxis: a hidden latex allergy, *Ann Allergy Asthma Immunol* 88(1):61, 2002.

Farris PK, Rietschel RL: An unusual acute urticarial response following microdermabrasion, *Dermatol Surg* 28(7):606, 2002.

Galobardes B et al: Influence of occupational exposure to latex on the prevalence of sensitization and allergy to latex in a Swiss hospital, *Dermatology* 203(3):226, 2001.

Joint Task Force on Practice Parameters; American Academy of Allergy, Asthma and Immunology; American College of Allergy, Asthma and Immunology; and the Joint Council of Allergy, Asthma and Immunology: The diagnosis and management of anaphylaxis, *J Allergy Clin Immunol* 101(6 Pt 2):S465, 1998.

Nakamura CT et al: Latex allergy in children on home mechanical ventilation, *Chest* 118(4):1000, 2000.

National Institute for Occupational Safety and Health: *Preventing allergic reactions to natural rubber latex in the workplace,* Cincinnati, 1998, The Institute.

Nielsen PS et al: Assessment of IgE allergen specificity among latex-allergic health care workers: review of IgE-binding components of various latex extracts, *Ann Allergy Asthma Immunol* 85(6 Pt 1):489, 2000.

Perkin JE: The latex and food allergy connection, *J Am Diet Assoc* 100(11):1381, 2000.

Russell-Fell R: Avoiding problems: evidence-based selection of medical gloves, *Br J Nurs* 9(3):144, 2000.

Salcedo G, Diaz-Perales A, Sanchez-Monge R: The role of plant panallergens in sensitization to natural rubber latex, *Curr Opin Allergy Clin Immunol* 1(2):177, 2001.

• = Independent; ▲ = Collaborative

Sanchez-Monge R et al: Class I chitinases, the panallergens responsible for the latex-fruit syndrome, are induced by ethylene treatment and inactivated by heating, *J Allergy Clin Immunol* 106(1 Pt 1):190, 2000.

Tarlo SM et al: Outcomes of a natural rubber latex control program in an Ontario teaching hospital, *J Allergy Clin Immunol* 108(4):628, 2001.

Toraason M et al: Latex allergy in the workplace, *Toxicol Sci* 58(1):5, 2000.

Anxiety

Pam B. Schweitzer, Teresa Howell, and Gail B. Ladwig

NANDA Definition

A vague, uneasy feeling of discomfort or dread accompanied by an autonomic response, with the source often nonspecific or unknown to the individual; a feeling of apprehension caused by anticipation of danger. Anxiety is an alerting signal that warns of impending danger and enables the individual to take measures to deal with threat.

Defining Characteristics

Behavioral
Diminished productivity; scanning and vigilance; poor eye contact; restlessness; glancing about; extraneous movement (e.g., foot shuffling, hand/arm movements); expressed concerns resulting from change in life events; insomnia; fidgeting

Affective
Regretful; irritability; anguish; scared; jittery; overexcited; painful and persistent increased helplessness; rattled; uncertainty; increased wariness; focus on self; feelings of inadequacy; fearful; distressed; apprehension; anxious

Physiological
Voice quivering

Objective
Trembling/hand tremors; insomnia

Subjective
Shakiness; worried; regretful

Physiological-sympathetic
Increased pulse; increased blood pressure; increased tension; cardiovascular excitation; heart pounding; superficial vasoconstriction; respiratory difficulties; increased respiration; increased perspiration; facial flushing; facial tension; pupil dilation; anorexia; dry mouth; weakness; increased reflexes; twitching

Physiological-parasympathetic
Decreased pulse; decreased blood pressure; abdominal pain; nausea; diarrhea; urinary urgency; urinary hesitancy; urinary frequency; tingling in extremities; fatigue; faintness; sleep disturbance

• = Independent; ▲ = Collaborative

Cognitive

Blocking of thoughts; confusion; preoccupation; forgetfulness; rumination; impaired attention; decreased perceptual field; fear of nonspecific consequences; tendency to blame others; difficulty concentrating; diminished ability to problem solve; diminished learning ability; awareness of physiological symptoms

Related Factors (r/t)

Unconscious conflict regarding essential values or life goals; threat to self-concept; threat of death; threat to or change in health status, environment, interaction patterns; situational or maturational crises; interpersonal transmission of contagion; unmet needs

NOC   Outcomes (Nursing Outcomes Classification)

Suggested NOC Outcomes

Aggression Self-Control; Anxiety Level; Anxiety Self-Control; Coping; Impulse Self-Control

---

Example NOC Outcome with Indicators

Anxiety Self-Control as evidenced by the following indicators: Eliminates precursors of anxiety/Reports absence of physical manifestations of anxiety/Controls anxiety response (Rate each indicator of **Anxiety Self-Control:** 1 = never demonstrated, 2 = rarely demonstrated, 3 = sometimes demonstrated, 4 = often demonstrated, 5 = consistently demonstrated [see Section I].)

Client Outcomes

Client Will (Specify Time Frame):

- Identify and verbalize symptoms of anxiety
- Identify, verbalize, and demonstrate techniques to control anxiety
- Verbalize absence of or decrease in subjective distress
- Have vital signs that reflect baseline or decreased sympathetic stimulation
- Have posture, facial expressions, gestures, and activity levels that reflect decreased distress
- Demonstrate improved concentration and accuracy of thoughts
- Identify and verbalize anxiety precipitants, conflicts, and threats
- Demonstrate return of basic problem-solving skills
- Demonstrate increased external focus
- Demonstrate some ability to reassure self

NIC   Interventions (Nursing Interventions Classification)

Suggested NIC Intervention

Anxiety Reduction

Example NIC Activities—Anxiety Reduction

Use a calm, reassuring approach; Explain all procedures, including sensations likely to be experienced

---

• = Independent; ▲ = Collaborative

Nursing Interventions and Rationales

- Assess the client's level of anxiety and physical reactions to anxiety (e.g., tachycardia, tachypnea, nonverbal expressions of anxiety). Use the Sheehan Patient-Rated Anxiety Scale (SPRAS). Validate observations by asking the client, "Are you feeling anxious now?" Consider the use of a "faces scale" to assess anxiety in critically ill clients. **Clinical Research:** *The collection of symptoms, the stages of presentation, and the duration of symptoms help the clinician identify residents who are suffering from persistent anxiety (Neel, 1996).* **Nursing Research:** *SPRAS was more effective in detecting asthmatics likely to be suffering from coexisting anxiety disorders (Davis et al, 2002).* **Nursing Research:** *The Faces Anxiety Scale has minimal subject burden and elicits self-report from intensive care patients more often than do other simple scales (McKinley, 2003)*
- Use presence, touch (with permission), verbalization, and demeanor to remind clients that they are not alone and to encourage expression or clarification of needs, concerns, unknowns, and questions. *Being supportive and approachable encourages communication (Olson and Sneed, 1995).*
- Accept the client's defenses; do not confront, argue, or debate. *If defenses are not threatened, the client may feel safe enough to look at behavior (Rose et al, 1994).*
- Allow and reinforce the client's personal reaction to or expression of pain, discomfort, or threats to well-being (e.g., talking, crying, walking, other physical or nonverbal expressions). *Talking or otherwise expressing feelings sometimes reduces anxiety (Johnson, 1972).*
- Help the client identify precipitants of anxiety that may indicate interventions. *Gaining insight enables the client to reevaluate the threat or identify new ways to deal with it (Damrosch, 1991).*
- If the situational response is rational, use empathy to encourage the client to interpret the anxiety symptoms as normal. **Nursing Research:** *The way a nurse interacts with a client influences his/her quality of life. Enhancing self-esteem and providing information and psychological support promotes the client's well-being and his or her quality of life (Di Giulio, 2001).*
- If irrational thoughts or fears are present, offer the client accurate information and encourage him or her to talk about the meaning of the events contributing to the anxiety. **Nursing Research:** *During the diagnosis and management of cancer, highlighting the importance of the meaning of events to an individual is an important factor in helping clients to identify what makes them anxious. Acknowledgment of this meaning may help to reduce anxiety (Stark and House, 2000).*
- Encourage the client to use positive self-talk such as, "Anxiety won't kill me," "I can do this one step at a time," "Right now I need to breathe and stretch," "I don't have to be perfect." *Cognitive therapies focus on changing behaviors and feelings by changing thoughts. Replacing negative self-statements with positive self-statements helps to decrease anxiety (Fishel, 1998).*
- Avoid excessive reassurance; this may reinforce undue worry. **Nursing Research:** *Reassurance is not helpful for the anxious individual (Garvin et al, 1992).*
- Intervene when possible to remove sources of anxiety. *Anxiety is a normal response to actual or perceived danger; if the threat is removed, the response will stop.* **Nursing Research:** *One study on children's posthospital adjustment suggests that mothers who know what behavior changes to expect in their children experienced less anxiety and participated more in their children's care during hospitalization (Melnyk and Feinstein, 2001).*
- Explain all activities, procedures, and issues that involve the client; use nonmedical

• = **Independent;** ▲ = **Collaborative**

terms and calm, slow speech. Do this in advance of procedures when possible, and validate the client's understanding. *With preadmission client education, clients experience less anxiety and emotional distress and have increased coping skills because they know what to expect (Review, 2000).* **Nursing Research:** *Uncertainty and lack of predictability contribute to anxiety (Garvin et al, 1992).*

- Explore coping skills previously used by client to relieve anxiety; reinforce these skills and explore other outlets. *Methods of coping with anxiety that have been successful in the past are likely to be helpful again. Listening to clients and helping them to sort through their fears and expectations encourages them to take charge of their lives (Fishel, 1998).*

- Provide backrubs for the client to decrease anxiety. **Nursing Research:** *Anxiety was measured prior to back massage, immediately following, and 10 minutes later on four consecutive evenings. There was a statistically significant difference in the mean anxiety (STAI) score between the back massage group and the no-intervention group (Fraser and Kerr, 1993).* **Nursing Research:** *Massage significantly decreased anxiety or perception of tension (Richards et al, 2000).*

- Provide massage before procedures to decrease anxiety. **Clinical Research:** *Parents performed massage on their hospitalized preschoolers and school-age children before venous puncture. The results obtained indicate that massage had a significant effect on nonverbal reactions, especially those related to muscular relaxation (Garcia et al, 1997).*

- Use therapeutic touch and healing touch techniques. *Various techniques that involve intention to heal, laying on of hands, clearing the energy field surrounding the body, and transfer of healing energy from the environment through the healer to the subject can reduce anxiety (Fishel, 1998).* **Nursing Research:** *Anxiety was significantly reduced in a therapeutic touch placebo condition. Healing touch may be one of the most useful nursing interventions available to reduce anxiety (Gagne and Toye, 1998).*

- Provide clients with a means to listen to music of their choice. Provide a quiet place and encourage clients to listen for 20 minutes. **Nursing Research:** *Immediately and 1 hour after listening to music for 20 minutes in a quiet environment, reductions in heart rate, respiratory rate, and myocardial oxygen demand were significantly greater in the experimental group of clients with myocardial infarction (MI) than in the control group (White, 1999).* **Nursing Research:** *Music therapy has the potential to reduce physiological signs of anxiety (heart rate and blood pressure) and the need for sedation among individuals undergoing colonoscopy (Smolen et al, 2002).*

- For the client experiencing preoperative anxiety, provide music of their choice for listening. **Nursing Research:** *Patients who listened to their choice of music before surgery in addition to receiving preoperative instruction had significantly lower heart rates than the clients in the control group who received only preoperative instruction (Augustin and Hains, 1996).*

- Animal-assisted therapy (AAT) can be incorporated into the care of perioperative clients. **Nursing Research:** *A study of perioperative clients has shown that interaction with animals reduces blood pressure and cholesterol, decreases anxiety, and improves a person's sense of well-being (Miller and Ingram, 2000).*

- Rule out withdrawal from alcohol, sedatives, or smoking as the cause of anxiety. **Clinical Research:** *One third of respondents in this study with an alcohol use disorder (abuse or dependence) were three times more likely to have an anxiety disorder (Burns and Teeson, 2002).*

▲ Identify and limit, discontinue, or be aware of the use of any stimulants such as caf-

- = Independent; ▲ = Collaborative

feine, nicotine, theophylline, terbutaline sulfate, amphetamines, and cocaine. *Many substances cause or potentially cause anxiety symptoms.*

Geriatric
▲ Monitor the client for depression. Use appropriate interventions and referrals. *Anxiety often accompanies or masks depression in elderly adults. Patients who have depression and anxiety, are socially isolated or severely ill should be asked whether they've been thinking about ending their life or wanting to die (Bartels, 2002).*
- Provide a protective and safe environment. Use consistent caregivers and maintain the accustomed environmental structure. *Elderly clients tend to have more perceptual impairments and adapt to changes with more difficulty than younger clients, especially during illness (Halm and Alpen, 1993).*
- Observe for adverse changes if antianxiety drugs are taken. *Age renders clients more sensitive to both the clinical and toxic effects of many agents.*
- Provide a quiet environment with diversion. *Excessive noise increases anxiety; involvement in a quiet activity can be soothing to the elderly.*

Multicultural
- Assess for the presence of culture-bound anxiety states. **Nursing Research:** *The context in which anxiety is experienced, its meaning, and responses to it are culturally mediated. The following culture-bound syndromes are related to anxiety: Susto—Latin America; Nervios—Latin America; Dhat—Asia; Koro—Southeast Asia; Kayak angst—Eskimo; Taijin kyousho—Japan; Nervous breakdown or bad nerves—African Americans (Charron, 1998; Kavanagh, 1999).*
- Assess for the influence of cultural beliefs, norms, and values on the client's perspective of a stressful situation. **Nursing Research:** *What the client considers stressful may be based on cultural perceptions (Cochran, 1998; Doswell and Erlen, 1998; Leininger and McFarland, 2002).*
- Identify how anxiety is manifested in the culturally diverse client. **Nursing Research:** *Anxiety is manifested differently from culture to culture through cognitive to somatic symptoms (Charron, 1998).*
- Acknowledge that value conflicts from acculturation stresses may contribute to increased anxiety. **Nursing Research:** *Challenges to traditional beliefs and values are anxiety provoking (Charron, 1998).*
- Acknowledge that socioeconomic factors may contribute to increased stress and anxiety. **Nursing Research:** *Job and marital instability, female-headed households, unstable finances, and housing issues create additional sources of stress (Lewis and Bernstein, 1996).*
- For the diverse client experiencing preoperative anxiety, provide music of their choice. **Nursing Research:** *Music intervention was found to have cross-cultural validity in the reduction of preoperative anxiety in Chinese male clients (Yung et al, 2002).*

Home care
- Above interventions may be adapted for home care use.
- Approach the client's anxiety in nonjudgmental fashion. *The inability of others to perceive the source of the client's anxiety does not make it any less distressing for the client.*
- Assist family to be supportive of the client in the face of anxiety symptoms. **Nursing Research:** *Social support, self-esteem, and optimism were all positively related to posi-*

• = Independent; ▲ = Collaborative

tive health practices, and social support was positively related to self-esteem and optimism (McNicholas, 2002).

- Adapt treatment needs to specific anxiety type. *Changes in usual approach may be needed to achieve same objective; for example, limiting physician visits and accompanying the client may be necessary if the client is agoraphobic.*
- Assess for presence of depression. *Depression and anxiety co-occur frequently.*
- ▲ Consider referral for the prescription of antianxiety or antidepressant medications for clients who have panic disorder (PD) or other anxiety-related psychiatric disorders. **Nursing Research:** *PD may be treated with drugs, psychosocial intervention, or both. In a recent study, the combination of imipramine and cognitive-behavioral therapy appeared to offer limited advantage in the short term but more substantial advantage by the end of maintenance (Barlow et al, 2000). In a study of older adults, anxiety was associated with increased disability and decreased well-being; although the use of health services was increased, appropriate care was often not received (de Beurs et al, 1999).*
- ▲ Assist the client/family to institute medication regimen appropriately. Instruct in side effects, importance of taking medications as ordered, and effects to report immediately to nurse or physician. *Antianxiety and antidepressant medications have side effects that may prompt the client to discontinue use, sometimes with additional uncomfortable effects. Some medications may be used to overdose. Antidepressant medications can take up to several weeks for full effect, and the client may discontinue use prematurely if there is little effect or if the medication is effective and the client considers it no longer necessary.*
- ▲ Assess for suicidal ideation. Implement emergency plan as indicated. *Suicidal ideation may occur in response to co-occurring depression or a sense of hopelessness over severe anxiety symptoms or once antidepressant medications have been started. Refer to care plan for* **Risk of Suicide**.
- ▲ Encourage use of appropriate community resources: family, friends, neighbors, self-help and support groups, volunteer agencies, churches, clubs and centers for recreation, and other persons with similar interests. *One of the most reassuring elements of care includes access to the family (Fishel, 1998). Vicarious experience provided through dyadic support is effective in helping clients undergoing cardiac surgery to cope with surgical anxiety and in improving self-efficacy expectations and self-reported activity after surgery (Parent and Fortin, 2000).*
- ▲ Refer for psychiatric home health care services for client reassurance and implementation of a therapeutic regimen. *Psychiatric home care nurses can address issues relating to the client's anxiety, including agoraphobia, with or without coexisting depression. Behavioral interventions in the home can assist the client to participate more effectively in the treatment plan (Patusky et al, 1996).*

Client/Family Teaching

- Teach the client/family the symptoms of anxiety. *If the client/family can identify anxious responses, they can intervene earlier than otherwise (Reider, 1994). Information is empowering and reduces anxiety (Fishel, 1998).*
- Because intensive care unit (ICU) stays are increasingly shorter, provide written teaching information that is readily available to clients when they are transferred out. *Time constraints have become a barrier to effective teaching. A pamphlet (available in Spanish and English) has been developed to ease the move for clients, families, and critical care and medical nurses from a medical ICU (MICU) to a general floor. Reading this pamphlet has helped to reduce symptoms of anxiety (Maillet et al, 1993).*

- • = Independent; ▲ = Collaborative

- Help client to define anxiety levels (from "easily tolerated" to "intolerable") and select appropriate interventions. *Mild anxiety enhances learning and adaptation, but moderate to severe anxiety may impede or immobilize progress (Peplau, 1963).*
- Teach the client techniques to self-manage anxiety. *Mental health interventions during hospitalization should emphasize teaching clients to manage their own anxiety, instead of directly intervening to reduce current levels of anxiety (Rose et al, 1994).*
- Teach the client to identify and use distraction or diversion tactics when possible. *Early interruption of the anxious response prevents escalation.*
- Teach the client to allow anxious thoughts and feelings to be present until they dissipate. *Allowing and even devoting time and energy to a thought, purposefully and repetitively, reduces associated anxiety (Beck and Emery, 1985).*
- Teach progressive muscle relaxation techniques. **Nursing Research:** *A significant reduction in anxiety level was obtained by using progressive muscle relaxation interventions (Weber, 1996).*
- Teach relaxation breathing for occasional use: client should breathe in through nose, fill slowly from abdomen upward while thinking "re," and then breathe out through mouth, from chest downward, and think "lax." *Anxiety management training effectively treats both specific and generalized anxiety (Fishel, 1998).*
- Teach the client to visualize or fantasize about the absence of anxiety or pain, successful experience of the situation, resolution of conflict, or outcome of procedure. **Nursing Research:** *Use of guided imagery has been useful for reducing anxiety (Weber, 1996).*
- Teach relationship between a healthy physical and emotional lifestyle and a realistic mental attitude. Health and well-being are influenced by how well-defined and well-met needs are in areas of safety, diet, exercise, sleep, work, pleasure, and social belonging. Exercise is an excellent means of decreasing anxiety (Fishel, 1998). **Clinical Research:** *Aerobic exercise training has antidepressant and anxiolytic effects and protects against harmful consequences of stress (Salmon, 2001).*
- ▲ Teach use of appropriate community resources in emergency situations (e.g., suicidal thoughts), such as hotlines, emergency departments, law enforcement, and judicial systems. *The method of suicide prevention found to be most effective is a systematic, direct-screening procedure that has a high potential for institutionalization (Shaffer and Craft, 1999).*
- ▲ Provide family members with information to help them to distinguish between a panic attack and serious physical illness symptoms. Instruct family members to consult a health care professional if they have questions. *Education on managing anxiety disorders must include family members because they are the ones usually called on to take the client for emergency care. Family members can be expert informants because of their familiarity with the client's history and symptoms (Fishel, 1998).*

evolve WEBSITES FOR EDUCATION

See the EVOLVE website for World Wide Web resources for client education.

• = **Independent;** ▲ = **Collaborative**

REFERENCES

American Psychiatric Association: *Diagnostic and statistical manual of mental disorders*, ed 4-TR, Washington DC, 2000, The Association.

Augustin P, Hains AA: Effect of music on ambulatory surgery patients' preoperative anxiety, *AORN J* 63(4): 750, 1996.

Barlow DH et al: Cognitive-behavioral therapy, imipramine, or their combination for panic disorder: a randomized controlled trial, *JAMA* 283(19):2529, 2000.

Bartels SJ: Patients with depression and anxiety might be contemplating suicide, *Geriatrics* 57:8, 2002.

Beck AT, Emery G: *Anxiety disorders and phobias: a cognitive perspective,* New York, 1985, Basic Books.

Burns L, Teeson M: Alcohol use disorders comorbid with anxiety, depression and drug use disorders: findings from the Australian National Survey of Mental Health and Well Being, *Drug Alcohol Depend* 68(3):299, 2002.

Charron HS: Anxiety disorders. In Varcarolis EM, editor: *Foundations of psychiatric mental health nursing,* ed 3, Philadelphia, 1998, WB Saunders.

Cochran M: Tears have no color, *Am J Nurs* 98(6):53, 1998

Damrosch S: General strategies for motivating people to change their behavior, *Nurs Clin North Am* 26:833, 1991.

Davis TMA, Rocc CJM, MacDonald GF: Screening and assessing adult asthmatics for anxiety disorders, *Clin Nurs Res* 11(2):173, 2002.

De Beurs E et al: Consequences of anxiety in older persons: its effect on disability, well-being and use of health services, *Psychol Med* 29:583, 1999.

Di Giuli P: Cancer care: the unique contribution of nursing, *Int Nurs Perspect* 1(1):39, 2001

Doswell W, Erlen J: Multicultural issues and ethical concerns in the delivery of revising care interventions, *Nurs Clin North Am* 33(2):353, 1998.

Fishel A: Nursing management of anxiety and panic, *Nurs Clin North Am* 33(1):135, 1998.

Fraser J, Kerr JR: Psychophysiological effects of back massage on elderly institutionalized patients, *J Adv Nurs* 18(2):238, 1993.

Gagne D, Toye FC: Nursing management of anxiety and panic, *Nurs Clin North Am* 33(1):135, 1998.

Garcia RM, Horta AL, Farias F: The effect of massage before venipuncture on the reaction of pre-school and school children, *Rev Esc Enferm USP* 31(1):119, 1997.

Garvin BJ, Huston GP, Baker CF: Information used by nurses to prepare patients for a stressful event, *Appl Nurs Res* 5:158, 1992.

Halm MA, Alpen MA: The impact of technology on patients and families, *Nurs Clin North Am* 28:443, 1993.

Johnson J: Effects of structuring patients' expectations on their reactions to threatening events, *Nurs Res* 21(6):499, 1972.

Kavanagh KH: The role of cultural diversity in mental health nursing. In Fontaine KL, Fletcher JS, editors: *Mental health nursing,* ed 4, Menlo Park, Calif, 1999, Addison Wesley.

Leininger MM, McFarland MR: *Transcultural nursing: concepts, theories, research and practices,* ed 3, New York, 2002, McGraw-Hill.

Lewis JA, Bernstein J: *Women's health: a relational perspective across the life cycle,* Sudbury, Mass, 1996, Jones and Bartlett.

Maillet RJ, Pata I, Grossman S: A strategy for decreasing anxiety of ICU transfer patients and their families, *Nurs Connect* 6(4):5, 1993.

McKinley S: Development and testing of a Faces Scale for the assessment of anxiety in critically ill patients, *J Adv Nurs* 41(1):73, 2003.

McNicholas SL: Social support and positive health practices, *West J Nurs Res* 24(7):772, 2002.

Melnyk BM, Feinstein NF: Mediating functions of maternal anxiety and participation in care on young children's posthospital adjustment, *Res Nurs Health* 24:18, 2000.

Miller J, Ingram L: Perioperative nursing and animal-assisted therapy, *AORN J* 72(3):477, 2000.

Neel AB Jr: Comorbid disorders: anxiety and depression in the nursing home resident, *J Am Soc Consult Pharm* 11(suppl), 1996. Available on-line at http://www.ascp.com/public/pubs/cc/supp4.shtml, retrieved March 12, 2003.

Olson M, Sneed N: Anxiety and therapeutic touch, *Issues Ment Health Nurs* 16:97, 1995.

Parent N, Fortin F: A randomized, controlled trial of vicarious experience through peer support for male first-time cardiac surgery patients: impact on anxiety, self-efficacy expectation, and self-reported activity, *Heart Lung* 29(6):389, 2000.

• = **Independent;** ▲ = **Collaborative**

Patusky KL, Rodning C, Martinez-Kratz M: Clinical lessons in psychiatric home care: a case study approach, *J Home Health Case Manage* 9:18, 1996.

Peplau H: A working definition of anxiety. In Burd S, Marshall M, editors: *Some clinical approaches to psychiatric nursing,* New York, 1963, Macmillan.

Reider JA: Anxiety during critical illness of a family member, *Dimens Crit Care Nurs* 13:272, 1994.

Review: A practical guide to improving patient outcomes, *Orthop Nurs* 19(suppl):22, 2000.

Richards KC, Gibson R, Overton-McCoy AL: Effects of massage in acute and critical care, *AACN Clin Issues* 11(1):77, 2000.

Rose SK, Conn VS, Rodeman BJ: Anxiety and self-care following myocardial infarction, *Issues Ment Health Nurs* 15(4):433, 1994.

Salmon P: Effects of physical exercise on anxiety, depression, and sensitivity to stress: a unifying theory, *Clin Psychol Rev* 21(1):33, 2001.

Shaffer D, Craft L: Methods of adolescent suicide prevention, *J Clin Psychiatry* 60(suppl 2):70, 1999; discussion 60(suppl 2):75, 113, 1999.

Smolen D, Topp R, Singer L: The effect of self-selected music during colonoscopy on anxiety, heart rate, and blood pressure, *Appl Nurs Res* 15(3):126, 2002.

Stark DP, House A: Anxiety in cancer patients, *Br J Cancer* 83(10):1261, 2000.

Weber S: The effects of relaxation exercises on anxiety levels in psychiatric inpatients, *J Holist Nurs* 14(3):196, 1996.

White J: Effects of relaxing music on cardiac autonomic balance and anxiety after acute myocardial infarction, *Am J Crit Care* 8(4):220, 1999.

Yung PMB et al: A controlled trial of music and pre-operative anxiety in Chinese men undergoing transurethral resection of the prostate, *J Adv Nurs* 39(4):352, 2002.

Death Anxiety

Teresa Howell and Gail B. Ladwig

NANDA   Definition

The apprehensions, worry, or fear related to death or dying

Defining Characteristics

Worrying about impact of one's own death on significant others; powerless over issues related to dying; fear of loss of physical and/or mental abilities when dying; anticipated pain related to dying; deep sadness; fear of process of dying; concerns of overworking caregiver as terminal illness incapacitates self; concern about meeting one's creator or feeling doubtful about existence of God or higher being; total loss of control over any aspect of one's own death; negative death images or unpleasant thoughts about any event related to death or dying; fear of delayed demise; fear of premature death because it prevents accomplishment of important life goals; worrying about being the cause of others' grief and suffering; fear of leaving family alone after death; fear of developing a terminal illness; denial of one's own mortality or impending death

Related Factors (r/t)

To be developed—see Defining Characteristics

NOC   Outcomes (Nursing Outcomes Classification)

Suggested NOC Outcomes

Dignified Life Closure; Fear Self-Control; Health Beliefs: Perceived Threat

• = Independent; ▲ = Collaborative

Client Outcomes

Client Will (Specify Time Frame):
- State concerns about impact of death on others
- Express feelings associated with dying
- Seek help in dealing with feelings
- Discuss concerns about God or higher being
- Discuss realistic goals
- Use prayer or other religious practice for comfort

NIC   Interventions (Nursing Interventions Classification)

Suggested NIC Interventions
Dying Care; Grief Work Facilitation; Spiritual Support

Nursing Interventions and Rationales
- Assess the psychosocial maturity of the individual. Erikson's scale of task accomplishment may be used. **Clinical Research:** *A study using the framework of Erikson indicates that the higher the ego integrity, the lower is the death anxiety (Fishman, 1992). As psychosocial maturity and age increase, death anxiety decreases. Findings have shown that psychosocial maturity is a better predictor of death anxiety than is age (Rasmussen and Brems, 1996).*
- Assist clients to identify with their culture and its values. *The process of identification with one's culture is identified as a coping mechanism that may protect the individual from increased death anxiety (Tomer and Eliason, 1996).*
- Assess clients for pain and provide pain relief measures. **Nursing Research:** *Barriers to optimal care of the dying, according to family members contacted by phone interview, include level of pain and management of pain (Tolle et al, 2000).*
- Assess client for fears related to death. **Nursing Research:** *Saunders (1995) indicated that clients with terminal illnesses commonly fear suffering from pain, suffocation, or abandonment before death. Acknowledging and responding to these fears is the core of end-of-life palliative care (Tarzian, 2000).*
- Assist clients with life planning: consider and redefine main life goals, focus on areas of strength and/or goals that will provide satisfaction, adopt realistic goals and recognize those that are impossible to achieve. *Life planning processes affect self-esteem and self-concept. By changing unrealistic goals, the individual may be able to reduce the amount*

• = **Independent;** ▲ = **Collaborative**

of future-related regret that the prospect of a not-too-distant death may produce (Tomer and Eliason, 1996).

- Assist clients with life review and reminiscence. *Life reviewing can foster the integration of past conflicts. It can improve ego integrity and life satisfaction, lower depression, and reduce stress (Tomer and Eliason, 1996).*
- Provide music of a client's choosing. *Music therapy is a nonpharmacological nursing intervention that may be used to promote relaxation (Chlan, 2000).*
- Provide social support for families receiving CPR training to save the life of a family member at risk for sudden death. **Clinical Research:** *Findings support tailoring family CPR training so that instruction does not result in negative psychological states in clients. The findings also illustrate the efficacy of a simple intervention that combines CPR training with social support (Dracup et al, 1997).*
- Encourage clients to pray. **Nursing Research:** *Participants in one study stated their belief that God listened to their prayers and answered them when they were seeking comfort. It was this reassurance that gave them the strength to face uncertainty and possible death (Hawley and Irurita, 1998).*

Geriatric

- Carefully assess older adults for issues regarding death anxiety. **Clinical Research:** *Lower ego integrity, more physical problems, and more psychological problems are predictive of higher levels of death anxiety in the elderly (Fortner and Neimeyer, 1999). Elders differ in their readiness for death. Some still have goals that they want to reach. These goals may not always be realistic (Burgess, 1997).*
- Provide back massage for clients who have anxiety regarding issues such as death. **Nursing Research:** *Back massage used on elderly residents in a long-term care facility reduced anxiety levels (Fraser and Kerr, 1993).* **Nursing Research:** *Massage significantly decreased anxiety or perception of tension (Richards et al, 2000).*
- Refer to care plan for **Anticipatory Grieving**.

Multicultural

- Refer to care plans for **Anxiety** and **Anticipatory Grieving.**

Home care

- Above interventions may be adapted for home care.
- Identify times and places when anxiety is greatest. Provide for psychological support at those times, using such strategies as personal contact, telephone contact, diversionary activities, or therapeutic self. *Anxiety may be related to earlier events associated with home setting or daily patterns that created pain and now serve as triggers.*
- Support religious beliefs; encourage client to participate in services and activities of choice. *Belief in a supreme being/higher power provides a feeling of ever-present help.*
- ▲ Refer to medical social services or mental health services, including support groups as appropriate (e.g., anticipatory grieving groups from hospice, visiting volunteers of hospice). *Referral to specialty groups may be a key part of the nursing plan.*
- Encourage the client to verbalize feelings to family/caregivers, counselors, and self. Expression of feelings relieves fear burden and allows examination and validation of feelings.
- Assist the client in making contact with death-related planning organizations, if appropriate, such as the Cremation Society and funeral homes. *Planning and direct action*

- = Independent; ▲ = Collaborative

(contracting for afterdeath care) often relieve anxiety and provide the client with a measure of control.

- With client, create a memento book reflecting life achievements. Leave in the home for regular review by client. If family will be the recipient, a memento book serves as both an opportunity for life review and a means of proactively leaving something behind for survivors. *It gives client a sense of focus, decreasing feelings of powerlessness over death. Refer to care plan for* **Powerlessness.**
- With client/caregivers, establish realistic life goals for anticipated lifespan of self or others. Create manageable, tangible steps that client can refer to and use to measure activity. Memento books and written life goals are tangible milestones related to life and death. *They provide comfort, reassurance, hope, and direction for the client and more definition for client/caregiver expectations.*
- ▲ Refer for psychiatric home health care services for client reassurance and implementation of a therapeutic regimen. Psychiatric home care nurses can address issues relating to client's death anxiety, including family relationships. *Behavioral interventions in the home can assist client to participate more effectively in the treatment plan (Patusky et al, 1996).*

Client/Family Teaching

- Promote more effective communication to family members engaged in the caregiving role. Encourage them to talk to their loved one about areas of concern. *One study investigated both the content and avoidance of communication between 84 spousal and filial caregivers and care receivers. The study findings indicate that both caregivers and care receivers avoid discussing issues of concern. Nurses working with families are well placed to promote more effective communication (Edwards and Forster, 1999).* **Nursing Research:** *A study by Tarzian (2000) indicates that increasing the knowledge of and access to palliative care decreases suffering before death.*
- Allow family members to be physically close to their dying loved one, giving them permission, instruction, and opportunities to touch. Keep family members informed. **Nursing Research:** *Tertiary care centers are criticized for not providing a peaceful death experience. A qualitative study was undertaken to ascertain suggestions of family members (N = 29) (Pierce, 1999). The suggestions mentioned came out of this study.* **Nursing Research:** *One study relayed the importance of preparing clients and family members for what to expect during the dying process, including the possibility of the client developing air hunger (Tarzian, 2000).*
- To increase clients' knowledge about end-of-life issues, teach them and their family members about options for care, such as advance directives. **Clinical Research:** *A survey of 1000 clients suggests that greater public knowledge about end-of-life care is needed, and advance care planning must be preceded by education about options (Silveira et al, 2000).*

evolve WEBSITES FOR EDUCATION

See the EVOLVE website for World Wide Web resources for client education.

• = **Independent;** ▲ = **Collaborative**

REFERENCES

Burgess AW: *Psychiatric nursing: promoting mental health,* Stamford, Conn, 1997, Appleton and Lange.

Chlan LL: Music therapy as a nursing intervention for patients supported by mechanical ventilation, *AACN Clin Issues* 11(1):128, 2000.

Dracup K et al: The psychological consequences of cardiopulmonary resuscitation training for family members of patients at risk for sudden death, *Am J Public Health* 87(9):1434, 1997.

Edwards H, Forster E: Avoidance of issues in family care giving, *Contemp Nurse* 8(2):5, 1999.

Fishman S: Relationships among an older adult's life review, ego integrity, and death anxiety, *Int Psychogeriatr* 4(suppl 2):267, 1992.

Fortner BV, Neimeyer RA: Death anxiety in older adults: a quantitative review, *Death Stud* 23(5):387, 1999.

Fraser J, Kerr JR: Psychophysiological effects of back massage on elderly institutionalized patients, *J Adv Nurs* 18(2):238, 1993.

Hawley G, Irurita V: Seeking comfort through prayer, *Int J Nurs Pract* 4(1):9, 1998.

Patusky KL, Rodning C, Martinez-Kratz M: Clinical lessons in psychiatric home care: a case study approach, *J Home Health Case Manage* 9:18, 1996.

Pierce SF: Improving end-of-life care: gathering suggestions from family members, *Nurs Forum* 34(2):5, 1999.

Rasmussen CA, Brems C: The relationship of death anxiety with age and psychosocial maturity, *J Psychol* 130(2):141, 1996.

Richards KC, Gibson R, Overton-McCoy AL: Effects of massage in acute and critical care, *AACN Clin Issues* 11(1):77, 2000.

Silveira MJ et al: Patients' knowledge of options at the end of life: ignorance in the face of death, *JAMA* 284(19):2483, 2000.

Tarzian AJ: Caring for dying patients who have air hunger, *J Nurs Scholarship* 32(2):137, 2000.

Tolle SW et al: Family reports of barriers to optimal care of the dying, *Nurs Res* 49(6):310, 2000.

Tomer A, Eliason G: Toward a comprehensive model of death anxiety, *Death Stud* 20:343, 1996.

Risk for Aspiration

Betty J. Ackley

NANDA Definition

At risk for entry of gastrointestinal secretions, oropharyngeal secretions, solids, or fluids into the tracheobronchial passages

Risk Factors

Increased intragastric pressure; tube feedings; situations hindering elevation of upper body; reduced level of consciousness; presence of tracheostomy or endotracheal tube; medication administration; wired jaws; increased gastric residual; incomplete lower esophageal sphincter; impaired swallowing; gastrointestinal tubes; facial, oral, or neck surgery or trauma; depressed cough and gag reflexes; decreased gastrointestinal motility; delayed gastric emptying

NOC Outcomes (Nursing Outcomes Classification)

Suggested NOC Outcomes

Aspiration Prevention; Respiratory Status: Ventilation; Swallowing Status

• = Independent; ▲ = Collaborative

Example NOC Outcome with Indicators

Respiratory Status: Ventilation as evidenced by the following indicators: Respiratory rate IER/Moves sputum out of airway/Adventitious breath sounds not present/SOB not present/Auscultated breath sounds IER/Auscultated vocalization IER/Chest x-ray findings IER (Rate each indicator of **Respiratory Status: Ventilation:** 1 = extremely compromised, 2 = substantially compromised, 3 = moderately compromised, 4 = mildly compromised, 5 = not compromised [see Section I].)

IER, In expected range.

Client Outcomes

Client Will (Specify Time Frame):
- Swallow and digest oral, nasogastric, or gastric feeding without aspiration
- Maintain patent airway and clear lung sounds

NIC   Interventions (Nursing Interventions Classification)

Suggested NIC Intervention
Aspiration Precautions

Example NIC Activities—Aspiration Precautions

Monitor level of consciousness, cough reflex, gag reflex, and swallowing ability; Check nasogastric or gastrostomy residual before feeding

Nursing Interventions and Rationales

- Monitor respiratory rate, depth, and effort. Note any signs of aspiration such as dyspnea, cough, cyanosis, wheezing, or fever. *Signs of aspiration should be detected as soon as possible to prevent further aspiration and to initiate treatment that can be lifesaving. Because of laryngeal pooling and residue in clients with dysphagia, silent aspiration (i.e., not manifested by choking or coughing) may occur.*
- Auscultate lung sounds frequently and before and after feedings; note any new onset of crackles or wheezing.
- Take vital signs frequently, noting onset of a temperature.
- Before initiating oral feeding, check client's gag reflex and ability to swallow by feeling the laryngeal prominence as the client attempts to swallow. *It is important to check client's ability to swallow before feeding. A client can aspirate even with an intact gag reflex (Baker, 1993).*
- When feeding client, watch for signs of impaired swallowing or aspiration, including coughing, choking, spitting food, or excessive drooling. If client is having problems swallowing, see Nursing Interventions for **Impaired Swallowing**.
- Have suction machine available when feeding high-risk clients. If aspiration does occur, suction immediately. *A client with aspiration needs immediate suctioning and will need further lifesaving interventions such as intubation (Fater, 1995).*
- Keep head of bed elevated when feeding and for at least an hour afterward. *Maintaining a sitting position after meals may help decrease aspiration pneumonia in the elderly (Sasaki et al, 1997).*

- **• = Independent; ▲ = Collaborative**

▲ Note presence of any nausea, vomiting, or diarrhea. Treat nausea promptly with antiemetics.

• Listen to bowel sounds frequently, noting if they are decreased, absent, or hyperactive. *Decreased or absent bowel sounds can indicate an ileus with possible vomiting and aspiration; increased high-pitched bowel sounds can indicate mechanical bowel obstruction with possible vomiting and aspiration.*

• Note new onset of abdominal distention or increased rigidity of abdomen. *Abdominal distention or rigidity can be associated with paralytic or mechanical obstruction and an increased likelihood of vomiting and aspiration.*

▲ If client has a tracheostomy, ask for referral to speech pathologist for swallowing studies before attempting to feed. After evaluation, decision should be made to have cuff either inflated or deflated when client eats. **Nursing and Clinical Research:** *The presence of a tracheostomy tube increases the incidence of aspiration (Elpern et al, 1993). One study demonstrated that clients who had aspiration following a tracheostomy had aspiration before the tracheostomy, and if the client did not aspirate before the tracheostomy, they also did not aspirate after the tracheostomy procedure was done (Leder and Ross, 2000) For some clients, inflating the cuff may help decrease aspiration; for others, the inflated cuff will interfere with swallowing. This decision should be made following swallowing studies for the safety of the client's airway (Murray and Brzozowski, 1998).*

• Feed client only during formal rest periods from restraints.

• If client shows symptoms of nausea and vomiting, position on side.

• If client needs to be fed, feed slowly and allow adequate time for chewing and swallowing. Position upright during and after feedings.

Enteral feedings

▲ Check to make sure initial nasogastric feeding tube placement was confirmed by x-ray, especially if a small-bore feeding tube is used. If unable to use x-ray for verification, check the pH of the aspirate. If pH reading is 4 or less, the tube is probably in the stomach. Also check bilirubin level of aspirate if possible. *X-ray verification of placement remains the gold standard for determining safe placement of feeding tubes (Metheny et al, 1998).* **Nursing Research:** *Small-bore feeding tubes have been inadvertently placed in the respiratory tract, and clients did not demonstrate any signs of respiratory distress (Metheny et al, 1990a). Use of pH and bilirubin measurement has been found to be predictive of correct placement of feeding tubes, both gastric and intestinal. Bilirubin testing is done using urinary bilirubin test strip and a developed visual bilirubin scale (Metheny et al, 2000).*

• Keep nasogastric tube securely taped. Use pink tape to secure the tube. **Nursing Research:** *Use of pink tape as opposed to clear tape or butterfly tape increases the length of time a tube stays taped (Burns et al, 1995).*

• Determine placement of feeding tube before each feeding or every 4 hours if client is on continuous feeding. Check pH of aspirate and note characteristic appearance of aspirate; do not rely on air insufflation method. **Nursing Research:** *The auscultatory air insufflation method is often not reliable for differentiating between gastric or respiratory placement (Metheny et al, 1990b). Testing the pH generally predicts feeding tube position in the gastrointestinal tract, especially if combined with identification of appearance of aspirate (Metheny et al, 1993, 1998).*

• Check for gastric residual every 4 hours during continuous feedings or before feedings; if residual is greater than 100 ml for gastrostomy feedings or greater than 200 ml for

• = **Independent;** ▲ = **Collaborative**

nasogastric tube feedings (McClave et al, 1992), hold feedings following institutional protocol. *Increased intragastric pressure from retained feeding can result in regurgitation and aspiration, but holding feeding unnecessarily can also result in an inadequate caloric intake (Edwards, Metheny, 2000).* **Nursing Research:** *A study of the effectiveness of either returning gastric residual volumes to the client, or discarding it resulted in inconclusive findings with complications when either action was taken, more research is needed in the area (Booker et al, 2000).*

- Test for the presence of glucose in tracheobronchial secretions or the presence of pepsin to detect aspiration of enteral feedings. Recognize that the glucose test may not be accurate if there is blood in the aspirate or if a low glucose feeding is being used (St John, 2000). **Nursing Research:** *Tracheobronchial secretions that test positive for glucose can indicate aspiration of enteral feedings (Metheny et al, 1998). The detection of pepsin in tracheal secretions is considered an indicator of aspiration of gastric contents, a flat position is strongly associated with the presence of pepsin in secretions (Metheny et al, 2002).*

- Do not use blue dye to tint enteral feedings. *The presence of blue and green skin and urine and serum discoloration has been associated with the death of two clients; the use of blue dye in feedings should be stopped (Maloney et al, 2002). This technique is not reliable and use of a multiple-use bottle may result in contamination of feedings and spread bacteria (Fellows et al, 2000).*

- During enteral feedings, position client with head of bed elevated 30 to 40 degrees; maintain for 30 to 45 minutes after feeding. **Nursing and Clinical Research:** *A study of mechanically ventilated clients receiving tube feedings demonstrated there was an increase of the presence of pepsin (from gastric contents) in pulmonary secretions if the client was in a flat position versus being positioned with head elevated (Metheny et al, 2000). A study of mechanically ventilated clients receiving enteral feedings demonstrated a decreased incidence of nosocomial pneumonia if the client was positioned at a 45-degree semirecumbent position as opposed to a supine position (Drakulovic et al, 1999).*

- Use a closed versus an open enteral delivery system if possible. **Clinical Research:** *A study demonstrated that the closed delivery system did not result in contamination of the feeding, use of the open bags resulted in several tube feeding formulas becoming contaminated (Vanek, 2000).*

- Stop continual feeding temporarily when turning or moving client. *When turning or moving a client, it is difficult to keep the head elevated to prevent regurgitation and possible aspiration.*

Geriatric

- Carefully check elderly client's gag reflex and ability to swallow before feeding. *Laryngeal nerve endings are reduced in the elderly, which diminishes the gag reflex (Close and Woodson, 1989).*

- Watch for signs of aspiration pneumonia in the elderly with cerebrovascular accidents, even if there are no apparent signs of difficulty swallowing or of aspiration. *Bedside evaluation for swallowing and aspiration can be inaccurate; silent aspiration can occur in this population (Smithard et al, 1998).*

- ▲ Use central nervous system depressants cautiously; elderly clients may have an increased incidence of aspiration with altered levels of consciousness. *Elderly clients have altered metabolism, distribution, and excretion of drugs. Some medications can interfere with the swallowing reflex.*

- Keep the elderly, mostly bedridden client sitting upright for 2 hours following meals.

- **● = Independent; ▲ = Collaborative**

Clinical Research: *A study demonstrated that the number of clients developing a fever was significantly reduced when kept sitting upright after eating (Matsui et al, 2002).*

Home care

- Above interventions may be adapted for home care use.
- For clients at high risk for aspiration, obtain complete information from the discharging institution regarding institutional management. *Continuity of care can prevent unnecessary stress for the client and family and can facilitate successful management in the home setting.*
- Assess the client and family for willingness and cognitive ability to learn and cope with swallowing, feeding, and related disorders. *Food and feeding habits may be strongly tied to family cultural values. Acknowledgment and/or adjustment to cultural values can facilitate compliance and successful family coping.*
- Assess caregiver understanding and reinforce teaching regarding positioning and assessment of the client for possible aspiration. *Caregiver is in the position to prevent and respond to aspiration difficulties.*
- Provide the client with emotional support in dealing with fears of aspiration. *Fear of choking can provoke extreme anxiety, which can interfere with the client's ability or willingness to adhere to the treatment plan. Refer to care plan for* **Anxiety.**
- Establish emergency and contingency plans for care of client. *Clinical safety of client between visits is a primary goal of home care nursing (Stanhope and Lancaster, 1996).*
- ▲ Have a speech and occupational therapist assess client's swallowing ability and other physiological factors and recommend strategies for working with client in the home (e.g., pureeing foods served to client; providing adaptive equipment for independence in eating). *Successful strategies allow the client to remain part of the family.*
- Obtain suction equipment for the home as necessary.
- Teach caregivers safe, effective use of suctioning devices. Inform client and family that only individuals instructed in suctioning should perform the procedure.
- ▲ Institute case management of frail elderly to support continued independent living. Swallowing difficulties represent and can lead to increasing needs for assistance in using the health care system effectively. Case management combines nursing activities of client and family assessment, planning and coordination of care among all health care providers, delivery of direct nursing care, and monitoring of care and outcomes. *These activities are able to address continuity of care, mutual goal setting, behavior management, and prevention of worsening health problems (Guttman, 1999).*

Client/Family Teaching

- Teach the client and family signs of aspiration and precautions to prevent aspiration.
- Teach the client and family how to safely administer tube feeding.

ⓔⓥⓞⓛⓥⓔ WEBSITES FOR EDUCATION

See the EVOLVE website for World Wide Web resources for client education.

• = Independent; ▲ = Collaborative

REFERENCES

Ackerman MI: Ask the experts, *Crit Care Nurse* 13:103, 1993.

Baker DM: Assessment and management of impairments in swallowing, *Nurs Clin North Am* 28:793, 1993.

Booker KJ, Niedringhaus L, Eden B: Comparison of 2 methods of managing gastric residual volumes from feeding tubes, *Am J Crit Care* 9(5):318, 2000.

Burns SM et al: Comparison of nasogastric tube securing methods and tube types in medical intensive care patients, *Am J Crit Care* 4:198, 1995.

Close LG, Woodson GE: Common upper airway disorders in the elderly and their management, *Geriatrics* 44:67, 1989.

Drakulovic MB et al: Supine body position as a risk factor for nosocomial pneumonia in mechanically ventilated patients: a randomised trial, *Lancet* 354(9193):1851, 1999.

Edwards SJ, Metheny NA: Measurement of gastric residual volume: state of the science, *MedSurg Nurs* 9(3):125, 2000.

Elpern EH, Jacobs ER, Bone RC: Incidence of aspiration in tracheally intubated adults, *Heart Lung* 16:527, 1993.

Fater KH: Determining nasoenteral feeding tube placement, *MedSurg Nurs* 4:27, 1995.

Fellows LS et al: Evidence-based practice for enteral feedings: aspiration prevention strategies, bedside detection, and practice change, *MedSurg Nurs* 9(1):27, 2000.

Guttman R: Case management of the frail elderly in the community, *Clin Nurs Spec* 13(4):174, 1999.

Leder SB, Ross DA: Investigation of the causal relationship between tracheostomy and aspiration in the acute care setting, *Laryngoscope* 100(4):641, 2000.

Maloney JP et al: Food dye use in enteral feedings: a review and a call for a moratorium, *Nutr Clin Pract* 17(3):169, 2002.

Matsui T et al: Sitting position to prevent aspiration in bed-bound patients, *Gerontology* 48:194, 2002.

McClave SA et al: Use of residual volume as a marker for enteral feeding intolerance: prospective blinded comparison with physical examination and radiographic findings, *JPEN J Parenter Enteral Nutr* 16(2):99, 1992.

Metheny NA, Smith L, Stewart BJ: Development of a reliable and valid bedside test for bilirubin and its utility for improving prediction of feeding tube location, *Nurs Res* 49(6):302, 2000.

Metheny NA, St John RE, Clouse RE: Measurement of glucose in tracheobronchial secretions to detect aspiration of enteral feedings, *Heart Lung* 27(5):285, 1998.

Metheny N et al: Detection of inadvertent respiratory placement of small-bore feeding tubes: a report of 10 cases, *Heart Lung* 19(6):631, 1990a.

Metheny N et al: Effectiveness of the auscultatory method in predicting feeding tube location, *Nurs Res* 39(5):262, 1990b.

Metheny N et al: Effectiveness of pH measurements in predicting feeding tube placement: an update, *Nurs Res* 42(6):324, 1993.

Metheny N et al: Visual characteristics of aspirates from feeding tubes as a method for predicting tube location, *Nurs Res* 43(5):282, 1994.

Metheny NA et al: pH, color and feeding tubes, *RN* 1(1):25, 1998.

Metheny NA et al: Pepsin as a marker for pulmonary aspiration, *Am J Crit Care* 11(2):150, 2002.

Murray KA, Brzozowski LA: Swallowing in patients with tracheotomies, *AACN Clin Issues* 9(3):416, 1998.

Rakel BA et al: Nasogastric and nasointestinal feeding tube placement: an integrative review of research, *AACN Clin Issues Crit Care Nurs* 5(2):194, 1994.

Sasaki H et al: New strategies for aspiration pneumonia, *Intern Med* 36(12):851, 1997.

Smithard et al: Can bedside assessment reliably exclude aspiration following acute stroke? *Age Ageing* 27(2):99, 1998.

St John RE: Ask the experts, *Crit Care Nurse* 20(4):100, 2000.

Stanhope M, Lancaster J, editors: *Community health nursing: promoting health of aggregates, families, and individuals*, ed 4, St Louis, Mosby, 1996.

Vanek VW: Closed versus open enteral delivery systems: a quality improvement study, *Nutr Clin Pract* 15(5):234, 2000.

• = **Independent**; ▲ = **Collaborative**

Risk for impaired parent/infant/child Attachment

T. Heather Herdman, Kathy Wyngarden, Mary A. Fuerst-DeWys, and Gail B. Ladwig

NANDA | Definition

Disruption of the interactive process between parent/significant other and infant/child that fosters the development of a protective and nurturing reciprocal relationship

Risk Factors

Physical barriers; anxiety associated with the parent role; substance abuse; premature infant, ill infant/child who is unable to effectively initiate parental contact as a result of altered behavioral organization; lack of privacy; inability of parents to meet personal needs; separation

NOC | Outcomes (Nursing Outcomes Classification)

Suggested NOC Outcomes

Caregiver Adaptation to Patient Institutionalization; Child Development: 2 Months, 4 Months, 6 Months, 12 Months, 2 Years, 3 Years, 4 Years, Preschool; Coping; Parent-Infant Attachment; Family Physical Environment; Parenting Performance; Parenting: Psychosocial Safety; Safe Home Environment

---

Example NOC Outcome with Indicators

Demonstrates appropriate **Child Development: 2 Months** as evidenced by the following indicators: Coos and vocalizes/Shows interest in visual stimuli/Shows interest in auditory stimuli/Smiles/Shows pleasure in interactions, especially with parent(s) (Rate each indicator with regard to delay from expected range: 1 = extreme delay, 2 = substantial delay, 3 = moderate delay, 4 = mild delay, 5 = no delay [see Section I].)

Client Outcomes

Client Will Demonstrate (Specify Time Frame):

- Infant/child development appropriate for age
- Parent(s) able to participate in caregiving for infant/child
- Parent(s) visit nursery/hospital unit
- Parent(s) respond to infant/child cues
- Parent(s) eliminate controllable environmental hazards
- Parent(s) use community and other resources as appropriate

NIC | Interventions (Nursing Interventions Classification)

Suggested NIC Interventions

Anticipatory Guidance; Attachment Process; Attachment Promotion; Coping Enhancement; Developmental Care; Developmental Enhancement: Child; Environmental Management: Attachment Process; Family Integrity Promotion; Parent Education: Infant; Parenting Promotion; Role Enhancement

• = Independent; ▲ = Collaborative

> ### Example NIC Activities—Anticipatory Guidance
>
> Instruct parent(s) about normal infant/child development and behavior, as appropriate; Provide information on realistic expectations related to the infant/child's behavior; Use case examples and/or model appropriate parenting behaviors to enhance the parent(s)' problem-solving skills, as appropriate

Nursing Interventions and Rationales

Family

- Establish a trusting relationship with the parents. *If trust is established with family members, they are more likely to openly share the real difficulties of integrating therapeutic regimens with family processes (Clemen-Stone et al, 1998).*
- Assist parents in recognizing behaviors used by infant/child to communicate avoidance/stress and approach/engagement. *Understanding infant behaviors gives meaning to these behaviors and provides parents with a guideline for choosing their own behaviors (Boris et al, 1999; Oehler et al, 1993). Providing nursing interventions that focus on supporting positive appraisal and promoting knowledge of infant crying promotes later adaptive functioning of parents (Elliott et al, 1996).*
- Support parents' ability to alleviate infant's/child's distress. *When parents respond quickly to alleviate stress, the child is more likely to calm down than to be spoiled. In this way parents are building a foundation for security and trust. Assist parents in recognizing how their own interactions affect their infant/child (Hedlund, 1986).*
- If necessary, allow parents to verbalize their fears of "ghosts in the nursery" that may influence attachment to their infant/child. Ghosts in the nursery are parents' early memories of painful experiences (e.g., unanswered cries, feeling abandoned, being abused) and are real and powerful. *"Hearing a mother's cries" is necessary to help her "hear her child's cries," an important aspect of therapeutic healing (Frailberg et al, 1975).*
- Listen to the parents' stories to understand their struggle to attach. Acknowledge the parents' point of view and stories as worthy of respect; important truths can be learned, such as what they think and how they feel about themselves and their infant (Trout, 1987). **Nursing Research:** *One study indicated that health care providers may recommend storytelling as the central mechanism of interactions in support groups that help participants to cope with daily anxieties of living (Dickerson et al, 2000).*
- Assist parents with recognizing how their infant/child learns through the senses (e.g., visual, auditory, tactile/kinesthetic) and with strategies that can be used, such as timing, intensity, imitation, repetition, to initiate interactions. Encourage parents of premature infants to interact with infants through the systems that are more mature (tactile and vestibular) while decreasing stimulation of the least mature systems (auditory and visual) (White-Traut, 1996). *By recognizing infant likes and dislikes based on their behavioral responses to stimuli, parents can generate their own strategies regarding which stimuli are most effective (McCollum and Stayton, 1985).*
- Guide parents in adapting to infant/child cues and changing needs. Give anticipatory guidance to parents about what infant/child behaviors are possible in given situations. *Model calming interventions to provide parents with tools for positive interactions with their infant/child (Karl, 1999). Premature infants respond more positively to less intense maternal stimulation (Lozoff et al, 1977).*
- Nurture parents so that they in turn can nurture their infant/child. Establish a nurturing environment in which parents can interact with their infant/child (Goulet et al,

• = **Independent;** ▲ = **Collaborative**

1998). Offer a safe, nonjudgmental environment in which parents can express their feelings. *If parents are unable to focus on infant, nurse should focus on parents' feelings (Zabielski, 1994). Acknowledge and support the strengths of the infant/child, parent, and family (Goodfriend, 1993).*

- Provide child development guidance and peer support. The unrealistic expectations of parents regarding infant/child abilities can negatively influence the parent-child relationship. *Offer another parent as peer support (Lindsay et al, 1993).*
- Attend to both the parents and infant/child in an effort to strengthen the early developing attachment relationship. *Identifying the infant's/child's strengths and limitations can provide parents with more information regarding how they can encourage optimal growth and development (Denehy, 1992).*
- Encourage parents of hospitalized infants to "personalize" their infant by bringing in baby clothes, pictures of themselves, toys, and tapes of their voices. *These actions help parents claim the infant as their own.*
- Encourage skin-to-skin experience for parents and infants as appropriate. The mothers studied perceived skin-to-skin contact with their very immature infants as a positive and helpful intervention. *Skin-to-skin contact took place regularly and for increasing periods (Bauer et al, 1999). Skin-to-skin care has been found to increase a favorable perception of the infant by the caregiver, and result in parents who feel more competent in caring for their infant (Tessier et al, 1998). Parents who participate in bonding and skin-to-skin activities are less likely to reject their infant (Hamelin and Ramachandran, 1993).*
- Encourage parents and caregivers to massage their infants and children. **Clinical Research:** *One study demonstrated that massage therapy on infants and children with various medical conditions resulted in lower anxiety and stress hormones and improved clinical course. Having grandparent volunteers and parents provide the therapy enhances their own wellness and provides a cost-effective treatment for the infants/children (Field, 1995).*
- Assist parents in developing new caregiving practice competencies and/or revising and extending old ones. One model to consider for use with parents is guided participation, a process in which an experienced person helps another with less experience to become competent in practices that are personally and socially meaningful for everyday life (Pridham et al, 1998). *Caregiving competencies foster a child's development. A caregiving practice is a patterned and customary act of giving care that involves activities addressed to a child's physical, physiological, psychological needs and includes functions concerned with health needs. Five domains of caregiving activities have been identified: (1) being with the infant, (2) knowing the infant as a person, (3) giving care to the infant, (4) communicating and engaging with others about needs (infant and parental), and (5) problem solving/decision-making/learning (Pridham et al, 1998).*
- Plan ways for parents to interact with/assist with caregiving for their infant/child. **Nursing Research:** *One nursing research study indicates that the ability to see an infant in the delivery room prior to transporting the infant to an intensive care unit may decrease parental stress, which can be a significant barrier to attachment (Shields-Poe and Pinelli, 1997). Research has shown that the most stressful aspect of parental role alteration is the feeling of helplessness in not being able to protect or help the infant/child during hospitalization/institutionalization. Finding ways to help parents feel important as parents and allowing touching/holding as soon as possible are important interventions in strengthening the attachment process (Miles et al, 1991).*

- **= Independent; ▲ = Collaborative**

Infant

- Provide lyrical, soothing music in the nursery as appropriate (be aware that this may not be an appropriate intervention for premature infants). **Clinical Research:** *The results from one study suggest that soothing music may be a feasible intervention to help newborns demonstrate fewer high-arousal states and less state lability (Kaminski and Hall, 1996). Premature infants may find auditory and visual stimulation stressful (White-Traut, 1996).*
- Protect and enhance infant's interactive capacities through organization of the environment. *Minimizing meaningless, unpatterned stimuli (noise, light, procedures, etc.) enhances depth and duration of sleep, which allows infants to retain more energy for use during interaction with parents. Well-regulated sleep and wake states contribute to a more satisfying parent-child interaction (Goldson, 1992).*
- Provide therapeutic touch for children with anxiety. **Nursing Research:** *In one study the therapeutic touch (TT) intervention resulted in lower overall mean anxiety scores, whereas the mimic TT did not. These findings provide preliminary support for the use of TT in reducing the anxiety level of children with HIV infection (Ireland, 1998).*

Multicultural

- Discuss cultural norms with families to provide care that is appropriate for enhancing attachment with the infant/child. **Nursing Research:** *Misinterpretation of parenting behaviors can occur when the nurse and parent are from different cultures. It is inappropriate to pressure parents to relate to the infant/child in a way that is culturally unacceptable/abnormal for the family (Coffman, 1992; Guarnaccia, 1998). This limits family choice and sets up a tense environment rather than a trusting, supportive one.*
- Encourage a reciprocal attachment process. **Nursing Research:** *Parents who develop a sensitivity to their infant's/child's communication patterns and behavioral cues will respond appropriately to the infant's/child's desire for increased interaction; the infant may then attempt to obtain the parent's attention. This encourages a process of mutual feedback that enhances the attachment process (Goulet et al, 1998).*
- Promote the attachment process by providing a treatment environment that is culturally based and women centered. **Nursing Research:** *Pregnant and post-partum Asian/Pacific Islander women in substance abuse treatment identified provisions for the newborn, infant health care, parent education, and infant mother bonding as conducive to their treatment (Morelli et al, 2001).*

Home care

- Above interventions may be adapted for home care use.
- Assess quality of interaction between parent and infant/child. *Attachment provides the infant with a source of comfort when anxious and is a precursor to social interaction. Social interaction, beginning with parents, is important to child development.*
- Use interaction coaching: teach mother about infant's behavioral cues and how to match infant's preferences; have mother position infant in direct line of sight; demonstrate responsive behaviors that can be modulated (e.g., facial, expression, voice, touch); encourage practice by trial and error; reinforce sensitive responsiveness as it occurs; give positive reinforcement for success. **Nursing Research:** *Mothers with post-partum depressive symptoms who received interaction coaching demonstrated significantly greater maternal-infant responsiveness (Censullo, 1994; Horowitz et al, 2001).*

- = Independent; ▲ = Collaborative

WEBSITES FOR EDUCATION

See the EVOLVE website for World Wide Web resources for client education.

REFERENCES

Bauer K, Uhrig C, Versmold H: How do mothers experience skin contact with their very immature (gestational age 27-30 weeks), only days old premature infants? *Geburtshilfe Neonatol* 203(6), 1999 (in German).

Bialoskurski M, Cox C, Hayes J: The nature of attachment in a neonatal intensive care unit, *J Perinat Neonat Nurs* 13(1):66, 1999.

Boris N, Aoki Y, Zeanah C: The development of infant-parent attachment: considerations for assessment, *Infants Young Children* 11(4):1, 1999.

Censullo M: Strategy for promoting greater responsiveness in adolescent parent/child relationships: report of a pilot study, *J Pediatr Nurs* 9:326, 1994.

Clemen-Stone S, McGuire SL, Eigsti DG: *Comprehensive community health nursing: family aggregate and community practice,* ed 5, St Louis, Mosby, 1998.

Coffman S: Parent and infant attachment: review of nursing research: 1981-1990, *Pediatr Nurs* 18(4):421, 1992.

Denehy J: Interventions related to parent-infant attachment, *Nurs Clin North Am* 27(2):425, 1992.

Elliott M, Drummond J, Barnard K: Subjective appraisal of infant crying, *Clin Nurs Res* 5(2):37, 1996.

Field T: Massage therapy for infants and children, *J Dev Behav Pediatr* 16(2):105, 1995.

Frailberg S, Adelson E, Shapiro V: Ghosts in the nursery: a psychoanalytic approach to the problems of impaired infant-mother relationships, *J Am Acad Child Psychiatry* 14:387, 1975.

Goldson E: The neonatal intensive care unit: premature infants and parents, *Infants Young Children* 4(3):31, 1992.

Goodfriend MS: Treatment of attachment disorders of infancy in a neonatal intensive care unit, *Pediatrics* 91: 139, 1993.

Goulet C et al: A concept analysis of parent-infant attachment, *J Adv Nurs* 28(5):1071, 1998.

Guarnaccia P: Multicultural experiences of family caregiving: a study of African American, European American, and Hispanic American families, *New Direct Ment Health Serv* 77:45, 1998.

Hamelin K, Ramachandran C: Kangaroo care, *Can Nurse* 89:15, 1993.

Hedlund R: Fostering positive social interactions between parents and infants, *Teaching Exceptional Children* p 43, 1986.

Ireland M: Therapeutic touch with HIV-infected children: a pilot study, *J Assoc Nurses AIDS Care* 9(4):68, 1998.

Kaminski J, Hall W: The effect of soothing music on neonatal behavioral states in the hospital newborn nursery, *Neonat Netw* 15(1):45, 1996.

Karl D: The interactive newborn bath: using infant neurobehavior to connect parents and newborns, *MCN Am J Matern Child Nurs* 24(6):280, 1999.

Lindsay JK et al: Creative caring in the NJCO parent to parent support, *Neonat Netw* 12:37, 1993.

Lozoff B et al: The mother-newborn relationship: limits of adaptability, *J Pediatr* 91:1, 1977.

McCollum J, Stayton V: Infant/parent interaction: studies and intervention guidelines based on the SIAI model, *J Dev Early Childhood* 9:123, 1985.

Mercer R, Ferketich S: Predictors of parental attachment during early parenthood, *J Adv Nurs* 15(3):268, 1990.

Miles S, Funk S, Kasper M: The neonatal intensive care unit environment: sources of stress for parents, *AACN Clin Issues* 2(2):346, 1991.

Morelli PT, Fong R, Oliveria J: Culturally competent substance abuse treatment for Asian/Pacific Islander women, *J Hum Behav Soc Environ* 3(3/4):263, 2001.

Oehler J, Hannan T, Catlett A: Maternal views of preterm infants' responsiveness to social interaction, *Neonat Netw* 12:67, 1993.

Pridham K et al: Guided participation and development of caregiving competencies for families of low birth-weight babies, *J Adv Nurs* 28(5):948, 1998.

Schuengel C, Bakermans-Kranenbur M, van Ijzendoorn M: Frightening maternal behavior linking unresolved loss and disorganized infant attachment, *J Consult Clin Psychol* 67(1):54, 1999.

Shields-Poe D, Pinelli J: Variables associated with parental stress in neonatal intensive care units, *Neonat Netw* 16(1):29, 1997.

• **= Independent;** ▲ **= Collaborative**

Tessier R et al: Kangaroo mother care and the bonding hypothesis, *Pediatrics* 102(2):e17, 1998.

Trout M: *Working papers on process in infant mental health assessment and intervention,* Champaign, Ill, 1987, The Infant-Parent Institute.

van Ijzendoorn M et al: The relative effects of maternal and child problems on the quality of attachment: a meta-analysis of attachment in clinical samples, *Child Dev* 63(4):850, 1992.

White-Traut R: Environmental factors and alternative therapies in nursing, *Voice* 4(9):1, 1996.

Zabielski M: Recognition of maternal identity in preterm and fullterm mothers, *Matern Child Nurs J* 22:2, 1994.

Autonomic dysreflexia

Betty J. Ackley

NANDA Definition

Life-threatening, uninhibited sympathetic response of the nervous system to a noxious stimulus after a spinal cord injury at T7 or above

Defining Characteristics

Pallor (below the injury); paroxysmal hypertension (sudden, periodic elevated blood pressure where systolic pressure is >140 mm Hg and diastolic is >90 mm Hg); red splotches on skin (above the injury); bradycardia or tachycardia (pulse rate of <60 or >100 beats/min); diaphoresis above the injury; headache (diffuse pain in different parts of the head, not confined to any nerve distribution area); blurred vision; chest pain; chilling; conjunctival congestion; Horner's syndrome (contraction of pupil on one side, partial ptosis of the eyelid, recession of eyeball into the head, occasional loss of sweating over the affected side of the face); metallic taste in mouth; nasal congestion; paresthesia; pilomotor reflex (gooseflesh formation when skin is cooled)

Related Factors (r/t)

Bladder distention; bowel distention; skin irritation; lack of client and caregiver knowledge

NOC Outcomes (Nursing Outcomes Classification)

Suggested NOC Outcomes

Neurological Status; Neurological Status: Autonomic; Vital Signs

> **Example NOC Outcome with Indicators**
>
> **Neurological Status: Autonomic** as evidenced by the following indicators: Systolic blood pressure WNL/Diastolic blood pressure WNL/Heart rate WNL/Perspiration pattern/Goose bumps when appropriate/Pupil size/Peripheral tissue perfusion (Rate each indicator of **Neurological Status: Autonomic:** 1 = extremely compromised, 2 = substantially compromised, 3 = moderately compromised, 4 = mildly compromised, 5 = not compromised [see Section I].)

WNL, Within normal limits.

• = Independent; ▲ = Collaborative

Client Outcomes/Goals

Client Will (Specify Time Frame):

- Maintain normal vital signs
- Remain free of dysreflexia symptoms
- Explain symptoms, prevention, and treatment of dysreflexia

NIC Interventions (Nursing Interventions Classification)

Suggested NIC Intervention

Dysreflexia Management

Example NIC Activities—Dysreflexia Management

Identify and minimize stimuli that may precipitate dysreflexia; Monitor for signs and symptoms of autonomic dysreflexia

Nursing Interventions and Rationales

- Monitor the client for symptoms of dysreflexia. See Defining Characteristics
- ▲ Observe with physician the cause of dysreflexia (e.g., distended bladder, impaction, pressure ulcer, urinary calculi, bladder infection, acute condition in the abdomen, penile pressure, ingrown toenail, or other source of noxious stimuli). *Noxious stimuli cause an uncontrolled sympathetic nervous system response (Autonomic Dysreflexia, 2002; Kavchak-Keyes, 2000).*
- Use the following interventions to prevent dysreflexia:
  - Ensure that drainage from Foley catheter is good and that bladder is not distended.
  - Ensure a regular pattern of defecation to prevent fecal impaction. *Bladder distention and bowel impaction are the most common causes of dysreflexia (Autonomic Dysreflexia, 2002; Karlsson, 1999).*
  - Frequently change position of client to relieve pressure and prevent the formation of pressure ulcers.
  - If ordered, apply an anesthetic agent to any wound below level of injury before performing wound care.
  - If symptoms of dysreflexia are present, place client in high Fowler's position, remove all support hoses or binders, and immediately determine the identity of the noxious stimuli causing the response. If blood pressure cannot be decreased within 1 minute, notify the physician STAT (Autonomic Dysreflexia, 2002; Karlsson, 1999).
  These steps promote venous pooling, decrease venous return, and decrease blood pressure. A large number of different stimuli can cause dysreflexia (Adsit and Bishop, 1995). The client should be rapidly evaluated by both the physician and nurse to find the possible cause (Kavchak-Keyes, 2000).
- To determine the stimulus for dysreflexia:
  - First, assess bladder function. Check for distention, and if present catheterize using an anesthetic jelly as a lubricant. Do not use Valsalva maneuver or Crede's method to empty the bladder. Ensure existing catheter patency (Travers, 1999).
  - Second, assess bowel function. Numb the bowel area with a topical anesthetic as ordered, and once agent is effective (5 minutes), check for impaction (Travers, 1999).

- **• = Independent; ▲ = Collaborative**

- Third, assess the skin looking for any points of pressure (Travers, 1999). *The stimulus for dysreflexia is most commonly bladder distention, then bowel impaction, then pressure on the skin (Travers, 1999).*
▲ Initiate antihypertensive therapy as soon as ordered. *A severely elevated blood pressure needs to be decreased for client safety (Autonomic Dysreflexia, 2002; Kavchak-Keyes, 2000).*
▲ Be careful not to increase noxious sensory stimuli. If numbing agent is ordered, use it on anus and 1 inch of rectum before attempting to remove a fecal impaction. Also spray pressure ulcer with it. If necessary to replace an obstructed catheter, use an anesthetic jelly as ordered. *Increased noxious sensory stimuli can exacerbate the abnormal response and worsen the client's prognosis (Autonomic Dysreflexia, 2002; Travers, 1999).* **Clinical Research:** *In one study the use of topical lidocaine did not limit the development of autonomic dysreflexia during anorectal procedures in spinal cord injury clients (Cosman et al, 2002).*
- Monitor vital signs every 3 to 5 minutes during acute event; continue to monitor vital signs after event is resolved. *It is possible for the client to develop rebound hypotension after the acute event because of the use of antihypertensive medications, or symptoms of dysreflexia may reoccur (Travers, 1999).*
- Watch for complications of dysreflexia, including signs of cerebral hemorrhage, seizures, MI, or intraocular hemorrhage. *Extremely high blood pressure can cause rupture of cerebral vessels, myocardial damage, and bleeding within the eye (Wirtz et al, 1996).*
- Accurately and completely record any incidences of dysreflexia; especially note the precipitating stimuli. *It is imperative to determine both the causes of the condition and whether the condition is persistent, requiring the client to take medications routinely to prevent repeat incidences (Kavchak-Keyes, 2000).*
▲ Because episodes can reoccur, notify all health care team members of the possibility of a dysreflexia episode. *All health care personnel working with the client should be aware of the condition because symptoms could begin while the client is away from the nursing unit (Travers, 1999).*

Home care
- Above interventions may be adapted for home care use.
- Instruct the client with any known proclivity toward dysreflexia to wear a Medic-Alert bracelet and carry a Medic-Alert wallet card when not in a safe environment (i.e., not with someone who knows client has the condition and can respond appropriately). *Autonomic dysreflexia is life-threatening response (Kavchak-Keyes, 2000).*
▲ Establish an emergency plan: obtain physician orders for medications to be used in situations in which first aid does not work (e.g., nifedipine, nitroglycerin ointment) (Wirtz et al, 1996). *Medication administered immediately can reverse early stage dysreflexia. Dysreflexia that is not recognized and treated can result in death (Tepper, 1997).*
- If orders have not been obtained or client does not have medications, use emergency medical services.
- If episode of dysreflexia is resolved, monitor blood pressure every 30 to 60 minutes for next 4 to 5 hours or admit to institution for observation. *After an episode of autonomic dysreflexia, it is not uncommon for a second episode or rebound to occur (Hammond et al, 1989).*
▲ Institute case management of frail elderly to support continued independent living. Nervous system difficulties represent and can lead to increasing needs for assistance in using the health care system effectively. Case management combines nursing activi-

• = Independent; ▲ = Collaborative

ties of client and family assessment, planning and coordination of care among all health care providers, delivery of direct nursing care, and monitoring of care and outcomes. *These activities are able to address continuity of care, mutual goal setting, behavior management, and prevention of worsening health problems (Guttman, 1999).*

Client/Family Teaching

- Teach recognition of the earliest symptoms of dysreflexia, the actions that should be taken when they occur, and the need to summon help immediately. Give client a written card that contains this information. *The client must know the symptoms and treatment well enough to instruct people in his or her environment how to relieve the symptoms (Kavchak-Keyes, 2000).*
- Teach steps to prevent dysreflexia episodes: care of bladder, bowel, and skin and prevention of other forms of noxious stimuli (i.e., not wearing clothing that is too tight). *Dysreflexia can occur anytime after discharge (Spoltore and O'Brien, 1995). Prevention of dysreflexia is the most effective treatment (Nolan, 1994).*

evolve WEBSITES FOR EDUCATION

See the EVOLVE website for World Wide Web resources for client education.

REFERENCES

Adsit PA, Bishop C: Autonomic dysreflexia: let it be a surprise, *Orthop Nurs* 14(3):17, 1995.
Autonomic dysreflexia—fact file. *Prof Nurse* 17(9):519, 2002.
Bergman SB, Yarkony RM, Stiens SA: Spinal cord injury rehabilitation: medical complications, *Arch Phys Med Rehabil* 78(3 suppl):S53, 1997.
Cosman BC, Vu TT, Plowman BK: Topical lidocaine does not limit autonomic dysreflexia during anorectal procedures in spinal cord injury: a prospective, double-blind study. *Int J Colorectal Dis,* 17(2):104, 2002.
Curt A et al: Assessment of autonomic dysreflexia in patients with spinal cord injury, *J Neurol Neurosurg Psychiatry* 62(5):473, 1997.
Guttman R: Case management of the frail elderly in the community, *Clin Nurs Spec* 13(4):174, 1999.
Hammond M et al, editors: *Yes you can: a guide to self-care for persons with spinal cord injury,* 1989, Paralyzed Veterans of America.
Karlsson AK: Autonomic dysreflexia, *Spinal Cord* 37(6):383, 1999.
Kavchak-Keyes MA: Autonomic hyperreflexia, *Rehabil Nurs* 25(1):31, 2000.
Nolan S: Current trends in the management of acute spinal cord injury, *Crit Care Nurse* 17(1):64, 1994.
Spoltore TA, O'Brien AM: Rehabilitation of the spinal cord injured patient, *Orthop Nurs* 14(3):7, 1995.
Tepper K: Management of autonomic dysreflexia in a home care setting, *Clin Excell Nurse Pract* 1(3):163, 1997.
Travers PL: Autonomic dysreflexia: a clinical rehabilitation problem, *Rehabil Nurs* 24(1):19, 1999.
Wirtz KM, LaFavor KM, Ang R: Managing chronic spinal cord injury: issues in critical care, *Crit Care Nurse* 16(4):24, 1996.

Risk for Autonomic dysreflexia

Betty J. Ackley

NANDA Definition

At risk for life-threatening, uninhibited response of the sympathetic nervous system; post–spinal shock; in an individual with spinal cord injury or lesion at T6 or above (has been demonstrated in clients with injuries at T7 or T8)

- **• = Independent; ▲ = Collaborative**

Defining Characteristics (Risk Factors)

- An injury/lesion at T6 or above and at least one of the following noxious stimuli:
- Neurological stimuli: Painful/irritating stimuli below the level of injury
- Urological stimuli: Bladder distention; detrusor sphincter dyssynergia; bladder spasms; instrumentation or surgery; epididymitis; urethritis; urinary tract infection; calculi; cystitis; catheterization
- Gastrointestinal stimuli: Bowel distention; fecal impaction; digital stimulation; suppositories; hemorrhoids; difficult passage of feces; constipation; enemas; gastrointestinal system pathology; gastric ulcers; esophageal reflux; gallstones
- Reproductive stimuli: Menstruation; sexual intercourse; pregnancy; labor and delivery; ovarian cyst; ejaculation
- Regulatory stimuli: Temperature fluctuations; extreme environmental temperatures
- Musculoskeletal-integumentary stimuli: Cutaneous stimulations (e.g., pressure ulcer, ingrown toenail, dressings, burns, rash); heterotrophic bone; pressure over bony prominences or genitalia; spasm; fractures; range-of-motion exercises; wounds; sunburns
- Situational stimuli: Positioning; drug reactions (e.g., decongestants, sympathomimetics, vasoconstrictors, narcotic withdrawal); constrictive clothing (e.g., straps, stockings, shoes); surgical procedures
- Cardiac/pulmonary problems: Pulmonary emboli; deep vein thrombosis

NOC   Outcomes (Nursing Outcomes Classification)

Suggested NOC Outcomes
Neurological Status; Neurological Status: Autonomic; Vital Signs

---

Example NOC Outcome with Indicators

Neurological Status: Autonomic as evidenced by the following indicators: Systolic blood pressure WNL/Diastolic blood pressure WNL/Heart rate WNL/Perspiration pattern/Goose bumps when appropriate/Pupil size/Peripheral tissue perfusion (Rate each indicator with regard to **Neurological Status: Autonomic:** 1 = extremely compromised, 2 = substantially compromised, 3 = moderately compromised, 4 = mildly compromised, 5 = not compromised [see Section I].)

WNL, Within normal limits.

NIC   Interventions (Nursing Interventions Classification)

Suggested NIC Intervention
Dysreflexia Management

Example NIC Activities—Dysreflexia Management

Identify and minimize stimuli that may precipitate dysreflexia; Monitor for signs and symptoms of autonomic dysreflexia

---

• = Independent; ▲ = Collaborative

Client Outcomes, Nursing Interventions and Rationales, Websites for Education

Refer to care plan for **Autonomic dysreflexia.**

Disturbed Body image

Teresa Howell and Gail B. Ladwig

NANDA Definition

Confusion in mental picture of one's physical self

Defining Characteristics

Nonverbal response to actual or perceived change in structure and/or function; verbalization of feelings that reflect an altered view of one's body in appearance, structure, or function; verbalization of perceptions that reflect an altered view of one's body in appearance, structure, or function; behaviors of avoidance, monitoring, or acknowledgment of one's body

Objective

Missing body part; actual change in structure or function; avoidance of looking at or touching body part; intentional or unintentional hiding or overexposure of body part; trauma to nonfunctioning part; change in social involvement; change in ability to estimate spatial relationship of body to environment

Subjective

Change in lifestyle; fear of rejection or reaction by others; focus on past strength, function, or appearance; negative feelings about body; feelings of helplessness, hopelessness, or powerlessness; preoccupation with change or loss; emphasis on remaining strengths and heightened achievement; extension of body boundary to incorporate environmental objects; personalization of part or loss by name; depersonalization of part or loss by impersonal pronouns; refusal to verify actual change

Related Factors (r/t)

Psychosocial, biophysical, cognitive/perceptual, cultural, spiritual, or developmental changes; illness; trauma or injury; surgery; illness treatment

NOC   Outcomes (Nursing Outcomes Classification)

Suggested NOC Outcomes

Body Image; Child Development: 2 Years, 3 Years, 4 Years, Preschool, Middle Childhood, Adolescence; Distorted Thought Self-Control; Grief Resolution; Psychosocial Adjustment: Life Change; Self-Esteem

• = Independent; ▲ = Collaborative

NOC Outcome with Indicators

Body Image as evidenced by the following indicators: Congruence between body reality, body ideal, and body presentation/Satisfaction with body appearance/Adjustment to changes in physical appearance (Rate each indicator of **Body Image:** 1 = never positive, 2 = rarely positive, 3 = sometimes positive, 4 = often positive, 5 = consistently positive [see Section I].)

Client Outcomes

Client Will (Specify Time Frame):
- State or demonstrate acceptance of change or loss and an ability to adjust to lifestyle change
- Call body part or loss by appropriate name
- Look at and touch changed or missing body part
- Care for changed or nonfunctioning part without inflicting trauma
- Return to previous social involvement
- Correctly estimate relationship of body to environment

NIC   Interventions (Nursing Interventions Classification)

Suggested NIC Intervention
Body Image Enhancement

Example NIC Activities—Body Image Enhancement

Determine client's body image expectations based on developmental stage; Assist the client to identify activities that will enhance appearance

---

Nursing Interventions and Rationales

- Use a tool such as the Body Image Instrument (BII) to identify clients who have concerns about changes in body image. The five BII subscales—General Appearance, Body Competence, Others' Reaction to Appearance, Value of Appearance, and Body Parts—exhibited moderate to high internal reliability and concurrent validity (Kopel et al, 1998). **Nursing Research:** *Using a body image scale can help nurses to identify possible body image disturbances and to plan individual nursing interventions (Souto and Garcia, 2002).*
- ▲ Assess for body dysmorphic disorder (BDD) and make appropriate referrals. The severity of BDD varies. Some youth experience manageable distress about their appearance and are able to function well, although not up to their potential. Psychiatric treatment is often effective in decreasing BDD symptoms and the suffering they cause (Phillips, 2003). **Evidence-Based Research:** *In delusional and nondelusional clients with body dysmorphic disorder, fluoxetine hydrochloride was more effective than placebo (Rao, 2002).*
- Observe client's usual coping mechanisms during times of extreme stress and reinforce their use in the current crisis. **Nursing Research:** *In this study of clients on hemodialysis, more psychosocial stressors were associated with greater use of problem-solving, social sup-*

• = Independent; ▲ = Collaborative

port, and avoidance coping; avoidance coping was found to explain much of the relationship between psychosocial stressors and depression (Welch and Austin, 2001).

- Acknowledge denial, anger, or depression as normal feelings when adjusting to changes in body and lifestyle. **Clinical Research:** *The influence of emotion-focused coping (venting emotions and mental disengagement) on distress following disfiguring injury was associated with less body image disturbance (Fauerbach et al, 2002).*

- Identify clients at risk for body image disturbance (e.g., body builders, cancer survivors). **Clinical Research:** *Male body builders are at risk for body image disturbance and the associated psychological characteristics that have been commonly reported among eating disorder clients. These psychological characteristics also appear to predict steroid use in this group of males. Steroid users reported an elevated drive to put on muscle mass in the form of bulk (Blouin and Goldfield, 1995).*

- Clients should not be rushed into sharing their feelings. *Feelings associated with complicated and emotionally powerful issues involving an altered body image take time to work through and express (Johnson, 1994).*

- Do not ask clients to explore feelings unless they have indicated a need to do so. **Nursing Research:** *Patients reported keeping their feelings to themselves as a frequently used coping strategy (Zacharia et al, 1994).*

- Explore strengths and resources with client. Discuss possible changes in weight and hair loss; select a wig before hair loss occurs. **Nursing Research:** *Nurses play an important role in assisting the client to cope with alopecia and help clients move through a potentially devastating experience to a renewed sense of well-being (Bachelor, 2001).*

- Encourage the client to purchase clothes that are attractive and that deemphasize their disability. *Individuals with osteoporosis are not usually disabled but may perceive themselves as unattractive and experience social isolation as a result of ill-fitting clothes that accentuate the physical changes (Sedlak and Doheny, 2000).*

- Allow client and others gradual exposure to the body change. Begin by having the client touch the affected area; then use a mirror to look at it. Go to a hospital shop with a nurse or support person and discuss feelings associated with the reaction of others to the body change. *Part of the rehabilitation process is graded exposure—the client moves from a protected to an unprotected environment with the support of the nurse (MacGinley, 1993).*

- Encourage the client to discuss interpersonal and social conflicts that may arise. *Changes in physical appearance and function associated with disease processes (and sometimes treatment) need to be integrated into the interaction that occurs between clients and lay caregivers (Price, 2000).*

- Encourage the client to make own decisions, participate in plan of care, and accept both inadequacies and strengths. **Nursing Research:** *It has been found that support given to women with breast cancer has a positive effect on their reactions to the illness and may even prolong their survival (Lindrop and Cannon, 2001).* **Clinical Research:** *The results of this study of clients with severe psoriasis indicate that the criterion for the management of psoriasis should be the clients' own perception of the consequences of the disease (Wahl et al, 2002).* **Nursing Research:** *Data from one study suggest that satisfaction with body image is disturbed by surgery for breast cancer despite active participation in decisions regarding selection of treatment. These outcomes suggest that women need assistance in adjusting to alterations in body image from nurses (Newell, 1999).*

▲ Help client accept help from others; provide a list of appropriate community resources (e.g., Reach to Recovery, Ostomy Association). *Motivation, sharing of experiences, ca-*

- • = **Independent;** ▲ = **Collaborative**

maraderie with and support from peers, and knowledge of not being alone have been identified as advantages of group learning (Payne, 1993).

- Help client describe self-ideal, identify self-criticisms, and be accepting of self. *The perception of self-image involves knowing the self and what is important and valued. Disability causes individuals to live as changed human beings regardless of whether they are willing to do so (Pohl and Winland-Brown, 1992).*

- Encourage the client to write a narrative description of their changes. **Clinical Research:** *One's experience of coping or adjustment to a disability is represented as narratives about himself or herself. Each person with traumatic brain injury (TBI) reconstructed certain self-narratives when coping with their changed self-images and daily lives (Nochi, 2000).*

- Avoid looks of distaste when caring for clients who have had disfiguring surgery or injuries. Provide privacy; care should be completed without unnecessary exposure. *Nurses must be aware of their nonverbal behavior; clients often become acutely aware of nurses' feelings as a result of the nurses' facial expressions, tone of voice, touch, or other behaviors (MacGinley, 1993).*

- Encourage the client to continue same personal care routine that was followed before the change in body image. It is preferable that this care be completed in the bathroom and not in bed. **Nursing Research:** *This routine gives the client privacy and also prevents the client from settling into an "invalid" role. Research has shown that women who resume familiar routines and habits heal better and suffer less depression than those who settle into the role of client (Johnson, 1994).*

Geriatric

- Focus on remaining abilities. Have client make a list of strengths. **Clinical Research:** *Results from unstructured interviews with women aged 61 to 92 years regarding their perceptions and feelings about their aging bodies suggest that women exhibit the internalization of ageist beauty norms, even as they assert that health is more important to them than physical attractiveness and comment on the "naturalness" of the aging process (Hurd, 2000).*

Multicultural

- Assess for the influence of cultural beliefs, norms, and values on the client's body image. **Nursing Research:** *The client's body image may be based on cultural perceptions, as well as influences from the larger social context (Cochran, 1998; Doswell and Erlen, 1998; Leininger and McFarland, 2002).*

- Validate the client's feelings with regard to the impact of health status on disturbances in body image. **Nursing Research:** *Validation is a therapeutic communication technique that lets the client know that the nurse has heard and understands what was said and promotes the nurse-client relationship (Heineken, 1998).*

- Acknowledge that body image disturbances can affect all individuals regardless of culture, race, or ethnicity. **Nursing Research:** *Body image disturbances are pervasive across western cultures and appear to increase in other cultures with acculturation to western ideals (Thomas and Ricciardelli, 2000).*

- Assess for the presence of conflicting cultural demands. **Nursing Research:** *Poor peer socialization and family rigidity were found to be related to the preoccupation with body size and slimness in a young female Mexican American population (Kuba and Harrisi, 2001).*

- • = Independent; ▲ = Collaborative

Home care

- Above interventions may be adapted for home care use.
- Assess client's stage of grieving or acceptance of body change on return to home setting. Include the future role of sexuality in the psychological assessment of acceptance as appropriate. *Body change or loss of a body part raises multiple issues relating to self-concept as well as continuing functional ability and dealing with responses of others.*
- Assess family/caregiver level of acceptance of client's body changes. *Negative feedback from family/caregiver can influence client's reactions and ability to adjust to body changes negatively.*
- Recognize that older women may continue their younger preoccupation with weight and recurrent dieting, despite being at normal weight. Assess source of low weight or weight loss with this in mind. **Clinical Research:** *Reports suggest that elderly women continue to be preoccupied with being thin. Increased awareness of eating habits and weight preoccupation in elderly women has been recommended (Fallaz et al, 1999).*
- Be accepting of body changes in all interactions with client and family/caregivers. *Acceptance promotes trust and assures client that others can be accepting of him or her.*
- Help client to see new or changing roles in family. Point out ways in which the community can help support client and family strengths.
- ▲ Refer to medical social services to address level of acceptance and possible financial impact of changes. *Social worker visits can support the client or caregivers with dedicated time and can work with the nurse to be supportive and adapt interventions to promote acceptance. The nurse or social worker can introduce or reinforce use of community resources.*
- Teach all aspects of care. Involve client and caregivers in self-care as soon as possible. Do this in stages if client still has difficulty looking at or touching changed body part. *The quicker the involvement in self-care, the greater are the chances for permanent acceptance and positive self-esteem.*
- ▲ Teach family and client complications of medical condition and when to contact physician.
- ▲ Refer to occupational therapy if necessary to evaluate home setting for safety and adaptive equipment and to assist client with return to normal activities. *The quicker the reinvolvement in daily living activities and self-care, the greater are the chances for permanent acceptance and positive self-esteem.*
- ▲ If appropriate, provide home health aide support to help the client and family through ADL transition.
- ▲ Refer to physical therapy if necessary to build range-of-joint motion, flexibility and strength, prevent contractures, assist with transfer/ambulation safety, or obtain use of a prosthetic device in the home setting.
- Assess for and promote good nutrition and sleep patterns. Adapt nutrition to specific physiological situations (e.g., client with ostomy). *Good nutrition and sleep patterns promote faster healing and better coping.*
- ▲ Assist family with obtaining needed supplies. *Cost of ostomy supplies and adaptive equipment can be an added stressor for the client. Community resources can assist.*
- ▲ Refer for psychiatric home health care services for client reassurance and implementation of a therapeutic regimen. Psychiatric home care nurses can address issues relating to client's distorted body image. *Behavioral interventions in the home can assist client to participate more effectively in treatment plan (Patusky et al, 1996).*

- = **Independent;** ▲ = **Collaborative**

Client/Family Teaching

- Teach appropriate care of surgical site (e.g., mastectomy site, amputation site, ostomy site). *Patient teaching by ET nurses may alleviate problems associated with altered body image in relation to the presence of an ostomy (Tomaselli et al, 1991).*
- Inform client of available community support groups; offer to make initial phone call. *Motivation, sharing of experiences, camaraderie with and support from peers, and knowledge of not being alone have been identified as advantages of group learning (Payne, 1993).*
- ▲ Refer the client to counseling for help adjusting to body change. *Counseling is important for a client who is trying to create a new body ideal or work through a grief process (Price, 1990).*
- Provide printed material and didactic information for significant others. *Some significant others prefer to receive didactic material rather than vent their feelings as a way of showing support (Northouse and Peters-Golden, 1993).*
- Encourage significant others to offer support. *Social support from significant others enhances both emotional and physical health (Badger, 1990).*
- Direct social support as follows: instruct regarding practical care (bandaging), encourage appraisal support (listening), encourage self-esteem support (favorable comparisons between client's and others' appearance), and encourage sense of belonging (assist with socializing). The preceding are four categories of support recognized in the body-image care model. *Clients with an active social support network are likely to make better progress than those without support (Price, 1990).*
- ▲ Refer an interdisciplinary team to clients with ostomies who are having difficulty with personal acceptance, personal and social body-image disruption, sexual concerns, reduced self-care skills, and the management of surgical complications. **Clinical Research:** *Many clinical studies have found clients with ostomies to be a group facing multiple adjustment demands. One of these demands is coping with a significant change in body image. At the Medical College of Wisconsin, a team approach has been initiated; the ET nurse, the psychologist, and the surgeon deal with body image concerns together. The multidisciplinary approach has been demonstrated to be successful in facilitating adaptation to an altered body image (Walsh et al, 1995).*

evolve WEBSITES FOR EDUCATION

See the EVOLVE website for World Wide Web resources for client education.

REFERENCES

Bachelor D: Hair and cancer chemotherapy: consequences and nursing care—a literature study, *Eur J Cancer Care* 10(3):147, 2001.

Badger V: Men with cardiovascular disease and their spouses: coping, health and marital adjustment, *Arch Psychiatr Nurs* 4:319, 1990.

Blouin AG, Goldfield GS: Body image and steroid use in male bodybuilders, *Int J Eat Disord* 18(2):159, 1995.

Cochran M: Tears have no color, *Am J Nurs* 98(6):53, 1998.

Doswell W, Erlen J: Multicultural issues and ethical concerns in the delivery of revising care interventions, *Nurs Clin North Am* 33(2):353, 1998.

Fallaz AF et al: Weight loss preoccupation in aging women: a review, *J Nutr Health Aging* 3:177, 1999.

Fauerbach JA et al: Coping with body image changes following a disfiguring burn injury, *Health Psychology* 21(2):115, 2002.

- = Independent; ▲ = Collaborative

Heineken J: Patient silence is not necessarily client satisfaction: communication in home care nursing, *Home Health Care Nurse* 16(2):115, 1998.

Hurd LC: Older women's body image and embodied experience: an exploration, *J Women Aging* 12(3-4):77, 2000.

Johnson J: Caring for the woman who's had a mastectomy, *Am J Nurs* 94:25, 1994.

Kopel SJ et al: Brief report: assessment of body image in survivors of childhood cancer, *J Pediatr Psychol* 23(2): 141, 1998.

Kuba SA, Harris DJ: Eating disturbances in women of color: an exploratory study of contextual factors in the development of disordered eating in Mexican American women, *Health Care Women Int* 22(3):281, 2001.

Leininger MM, McFarland MR: *Transcultural nursing: concepts, theories, research and practices,* ed 3, New York, 2002, McGraw-Hill.

Lindrop, Cannon S: Evaluating the self-assessed support needs of women with breast cancer, *J Adv Nurs* 34(6): 760, 2001.

MacGinley K: Nursing care of the patient with altered body image, *Br J Nurs* 2:1098, 1993.

Newell RJ: Altered body image: a fear-avoidance model of psycho-social difficulties following disfigurement, *J Adv Nurs* 30(5):1230, 1999.

Nochi M: Reconstructing self-narratives in coping with traumatic brain injury, *Soc Sci Med* 51(12):1795, 2000.

Northouse L, Peters-Golden H: Cancer and the family: strategies to assist spouses, *Semin Oncol Nurs* 9:74, 1993.

Patusky KL, Rodning C, Martinez-Kratz M: Clinical lessons in psychiatric home care: a case study approach, *J Home Health Case Manage* 9:18, 1996.

Payne J: The contribution of group learning to the rehabilitation of spinal cord injured adults, *Rehabil Nurs* 18: 375, 1993.

Phillips K: Child and Adolescent Action Center, Nami E-News, 2003. Available on-line at http://www.nami.org/youth/dysmorphic.html, retrieved March 12, 2003.

Pohl C, Winland-Brown J: The meaning of disability in a caring environment, *J Nurs Adm* 22:29, 1992.

Price B: A model for body-image care, *J Adv Nurs* 15:585, 1990.

Price B: Altered body image: managing social encounters, *Int J Palliat Nurs* 6(4):179, 2000.

Rao S: Fluoxetine was safe and effective for body dysmorphic disorder, *Evidence-Based Ment Health* 5(4):119, 2002.

Sedlak CA, Doheny MO: Fashion tips for women with osteoporosis, *Orthop Nurs* 19(5):31, 2000.

Souto CMR, Garcia TR: Construction and validation of a Body Image Rating Scale: a preliminary study *Int J Nurs Terminol Class* 13(4):117, 2002.

Thomas K, Ricciardelli I: Gender traits and self-concept as indicators of problem eating and body dissatisfaction among children, *Sex Roles* 43(7/8):441, 2000.

Tomaselli N, Jenks J, Morin K: Body image in patients with stomas: a critical review of the literature, *J ET Nurs* 18:95, 1991.

Wahl AK, Gjengedal E, Hanestad BR: The bodily suffering of living with severe psoriasis: in-depth interviews with 22 hospitalized patients with psoriasis, *Q Health Res* 12(2):250, 2002.

Walsh BA et al: Multidisciplinary management of altered body image in the patient with an ostomy, *J Wound Ostomy Continence Nurs* 22(5):227, 1995.

Welch JL, Austin JK: Stressors, coping and depression in haemodialysis patients, *J Adv Nurs* 33(2):200, 2001.

Zacharias DR, Gilig CA, Foxall MJ: Quality of life and coping in patients with gynecologic cancer and their spouses, *Oncol Nurs Forum* 21:1699, 1994.

Risk for imbalanced Body temperature

Betty J. Ackley

NANDA Definition

At risk for failure to maintain body temperature within a normal range

• = Independent; ▲ = Collaborative

Risk Factors

Altered metabolic rate; extremes of age or weight; exposure to cool/cold or hot/warm environments; dehydration; inactivity or vigorous activity; medications that cause vasoconstriction or vasodilatation; sedation; clothing inappropriate for environmental temperature; illness or trauma that affects body temperature regulation

Related Factors (r/t)

See Risk Factors

NOC   Outcomes (Nursing Outcomes Classification)

Suggested NOC Outcomes

Thermoregulation; Thermoregulation: Newborn

Example NOC Outcome with Indicators

Thermoregulation as evidenced by the following indicators: Body temperature WNL/Skin temperature IER/Skin color changes not present/Hydration adequate/Reported thermal comfort (Rate each indicator of **Thermoregulation:** 1 = extremely compromised, 2 = substantially compromised, 3 = moderately compromised, 4 = mildly compromised, 5 = not compromised [see Section I].)

IER, In expected range; *WNL*, within normal limits.

Client Outcomes

Client Will (Specify Time Frame):

- Maintain temperature within normal range of 97° to 99° F in the adult
- Explain measures needed to maintain normal temperature
- Identify symptoms of hypothermia or hyperthermia

NIC   Interventions (Nursing Interventions Classification)

Suggested NIC Interventions

Temperature Regulation; Temperature Regulation: Intraoperative; Vital Signs Monitoring

---

Example NIC Activities—Temperature Regulation

Institute a continuous core temperature monitoring device as appropriate; Promote adequate fluid and nutritional intake

---

Nursing Interventions and Rationales

- Monitor temperature q 1 to 4 h(rs) or use continuous temperature monitoring as appropriate. Normal adult temperature is usually identified at 98.6° F (37° C), but in actuality the normal temperature fluctuates throughout the day. In the early morning it may be as low as 96.4° F (35.8° C) and in the late afternoon or evening as high as 99.1° F (37.3° C) (Bates, 1998). *Disease, injury, or pharmacological agents may impair regulation of body temperature (Dennison, 1995; Holtzclaw, 1993).*

• = Independent; ▲ = Collaborative

- If client is awake, take the temperature orally in the adult, instead of by use of a tympanic thermometer or an axillary temperature. **Nursing Research:** *Oral temperatures provide a more accurate temperature than tympanic thermometers (Fisk and Arcona, 2001; Giuliano et al, 2000; Lee et al, 1999). Axillary temperatures are often inaccurate (Fulbrook, 1997). The oral temperature is usually accurate even in the intubated client (Fallis, 2002).*
- Take vital signs q 1 to 4 h(rs), noting changes associated with hypothermia: first, increased blood pressure, pulse, and respirations; then, decreased values as hypothermia progresses (Edwards, 1999).
- Monitor the client for signs of hypothermia (e.g., shivering, cool skin, piloerection, pallor, slow capillary refill, cyanotic nailbeds, decreased mentation, dysrhythmias) (Edwards, 1999).
- Note changes in vital signs associated with hyperthermia: rapid, bounding pulse; increased respiratory rate; and decreased blood pressure with orthostatic hypotension present (Worfolk, 2000). *Consistent monitoring promotes prevention and early intervention in clients with altered cardiopulmonary status associated with hypothermia or hyperthermia.*
- Monitor the client for signs of hyperthermia (e.g., headache, nausea and vomiting, weakness, absence of sweating, delirium, and coma) (Worfolk, 2000). *Monitoring for defining characteristics of hypothermia and hyperthermia allows for prevention and/or early intervention.*
- Maintain a consistent room temperature (72° F). *A consistent temperature limits environmental effects on thermoregulation.*
- Promote adequate nutrition and hydration. *These measures help maintain a normal body temperature.*
- Adjust clothing to facilitate passive warming or cooling as appropriate. *This will help maintain a normal body temperature.*
- See Nursing Interventions and Rationales for **Hypothermia** or **Hyperthermia** as appropriate.

Geriatric
- Do not allow geriatric clients to become chilled. Keep covered when giving a bath or doing a procedure. Offer socks to wear when in bed and a head covering if desired. *Older adults have a decreased ability to adapt to temperature extremes and need protection from extreme environmental temperatures. Older adults have a higher threshold of central temperature for sweating, diminished or absent sweating, impaired warmth or cold perception, impaired shiver response, diminished thermogenesis, abnormal peripheral blood flow response to warmth or cold, and compromised cardiovascular reserve (Ballester and Harchelroad, 1999; Florez-Duquet and McDonald, 1998).*
- Assess medication profile for potential risk of drug-related altered body temperature. *Anesthetics, barbiturates, salicylates, nonsteroidal anti-inflammatory drugs (NSAIDs), diuretics, antihistamines, anticholinergics, beta-blockers, and thyroid hormones have been linked to altered body temperatures (Carroll, 2002; Haskell et al, 1997).*
- Ensure that elderly clients receive sufficient fluids during hot days and stay out of the sun. *The elderly may have trouble walking independently to obtain fluids, have decreased thirst sensation, and have chronic illnesses that predispose to heat stroke (Carroll, 2002).*

- = **Independent;** ▲ = **Collaborative**

Pediatric

- Recognize that pediatric clients have a decreased ability to adapt to temperature extremes. Take the following actions to maintain body temperature in the infant/child:
  - Keep the head covered.
  - Use blankets to keep the client warm.
  - Keep client covered during procedures, transport, and diagnostic testing.
  - Maintain a consistent room temperature of 72° F.

  These measures can help prevent hypothermia, which is highly possible, especially in the pediatric trauma client (Bernardo and Henker, 1999). The combination of a relatively large body surface area, small body-fluid volume, less well-developed temperature control mechanisms, and a small amount of protective body fat limits the pediatric client's ability to maintain normal temperatures (Roncoli and Medoff-Cooper, 1992; Noerr, 1997).
- Recognize that the infant and small child are vulnerable to develop heat stroke in hot weather and ensure they receive sufficient fluids and are protected from hot environments. *Infants and young children are at risk for heat stroke for many reasons including a decreased thermoregulatory ability in the young body and the inability to obtain their own fluids (Carroll, 2002).*

Home care

- Above interventions may be adapted for home care use.

Prevention of Hypothermia in Cold Weather

- Avoid prolonged exposure outside. Wear a hat and gloves. Wool or fleece clothing can help to maintain body heat.
- Keep room temperature at 68° to 72° F.
- Ensure adequate source of heat; refer to social services if client is low income and heat could be turned off.
- Help elderly client determine a warm environment they can go to for safety in cold weather if his or her home environment is no longer warm.

Prevention of Hyperthermia in Hot Weather

- Encourage the client to wear lightweight loose-fitting cotton clothing. Help the elderly remove their usual sweaters.
- Ensure that client drinks adequate amounts of fluids (2000 ml/day), avoiding caffeine and alcohol. *Adequate fluids are needed during hot weather to replace fluids lost from sweating. Fluids containing caffeine and alcohol can serve as diuretics and decrease fluid volume in the body.*
- Help client obtain a fan to increase evaporation, or an air conditioner as needed, using social services if needed. *Air moving across the skin enhances evaporative cooling if the temperature is below the high 90s° F (Carroll, 2002).*
- Take the temperature of the elderly in hot weather. *The elderly may not be able to tell that they are hot because of decreased sensation (Worfolk, 2000).*
- Help elderly client determine a cool environment they can go to for safety in hot weather.

Client/Family Teaching

- Teach the client and family the signs of hypothermia and hyperthermia and the appropriate actions they should take if either condition develops. *Adequate teaching improves compliance and reduces anxiety.*

• = Independent; ▲ = Collaborative

- Teach the client and family proper method for taking temperature. *Optimal placement of the appropriate device is essential for accurate monitoring.*
- Teach to avoid alcohol and medications that depress cerebral function. *When the client is sedated or under the influence of alcohol, mentation is depressed, resulting in decreased activities to maintain an adequate body temperature. In addition, traumatic injuries are associated with alcohol and illicit drug use (Ruffolo, 2002).*

evolve WEBSITES FOR EDUCATION

See the EVOLVE website for World Wide Web resources for client education.

REFERENCES

Ballester JM, Harchelroad FP: Hypothermia: an easy-to-miss, dangerous disorder in winter weather, *Geriatrics* 54(2):51, 1999.

Bates B, Bickley LS, Hoekelman RA: *A guide to physical examination and history taking,* ed 7, Philadelphia, 1998, Lippincott.

Bernardo LM, Henker R: Thermoregulation in pediatric trauma: an overview, *Int J Trauma Nurs* 5(3):101, 1999.

Carroll P: The heat is one: protecting your patients from Nature's silent killer, *Home Health Care Nurse* 20(6): 376, 2002.

Dennison D: Thermal regulation of patients during the perioperative period, *AORN J* 61:827, 1995.

Edwards SL: Hypothermia, *Prof Nurse* 14(4):253, 1999.

Fisk J, Arcona S: Comparing tympanic membrane and pulmonary artery catheter temperatures, *DDCN* 20(2), 2001.

Florez-Duquet M, McDonald RB: Cold-induced thermoregulation and biological aging, *Physiol Rev* 78(2):339, 1998.

Fulbrook P: Core body temperature measurement: a comparison of axilla, tympanic membrane and pulmonary artery blood temperature, *Intensive Crit Care Nurs* 13(5), 1997.

Giuliano KK et al: Temperature measurement in critically ill adults: a comparison of tympanic and oral methods, *Am J Crit Care* 9(4), 2000.

Haskell RM et al: Hypothermia, *AACN Clin Issues* 8(3):368, 1997.

Holtzclaw BJ: Monitoring body temperature, *AACN Clin Issues Crit Care Nurs* 4:44, 1993.

Lee VK, McKenzie NE, Cathcart M: Ear and oral temperatures under usual practice conditions, *Res Nurs Pract* 1(1), 1999.

Noerr B: Keeping the newborn warm: understanding thermoregulation, *Mother Baby J* 2(5):6, 1997.

Roncoli M, Medoff-Cooper B: Thermoregulation in low-birth-weight infants, *NAACOG Clin Issues* 3:25, 1992.

Ruffolo D: Hypothermia in trauma: the cold hard facts, *RN* 65(2), 2002.

Worfolk JB: Heat waves: their impact on the health of elders, *Geriatr Nurs* 21(2):70, 2000.

Bowel incontinence

Mikel Gray

NANDA Definition

Change in normal bowel elimination habits characterized by involuntary passage of stool.

Defining Characteristics

Constant dribbling of soft stool, fecal odor; inability to delay defecation; rectal urgency; self-report of inability to feel rectal fullness or presence of stool in bowel; fecal staining of underclothing; recognition of rectal fullness but reported inability to expel formed

- = **Independent;** ▲ = **Collaborative**

stool; inattention to urge to defecate; inability to recognize urge to defecate; red perineal skin

Related Factors (r/t)

Change in stool consistency (diarrhea, constipation, fecal impaction); abnormal motility (metabolic disorders, inflammatory bowel disease, infectious disease, drug induced motility disorders, food intolerance); defects in rectal vault function (low rectal compliance from ischemia, fibrosis, radiation, infectious proctitis, Hirschprung's disease, local or infiltrating neoplasm, severe rectocele); sphincter dysfunction (obstetric or traumatic induced incompetence, fistula or abscess, prolapse, third-degree hemorrhoids, pseudodyssynergia of the pelvic muscles); neurological disorders impacting gastrointestinal motility, rectal vault function and sphincter function (cerebrovascular accident, spinal injury, traumatic brain injury, central nervous system tumor, advanced stage dementia, encephalopathy, profound mental retardation, multiple sclerosis, myelodysplasia and related neural tube defects, gastroparesis of diabetes mellitus, heavy metal poisoning, chronic alcoholism, infectious or autoimmune neurological disorders, myasthenia gravis)

NOC Outcomes (Nursing Outcomes Classification)

Suggested NOC Outcomes

Bowel Continence; Bowel Elimination

> ### Example NOC Outcomes with Indicators
>
> **Bowel Continence** as evidenced by the following indicators: Predictable evacuation of stool/ Maintains control of passage of stool/ Regular evacuation of stool at least every 3 days (Rate each indicator of **Bowel Continence:** 1 = never demonstrated, 2 = rarely demonstrated, 3 = sometimes demonstrated, 4 = often demonstrated, 5 = consistently demonstrated [see Section I].)

Client Outcomes

Client Will (Specify Time Frame):

- Have regular, complete evacuation of fecal contents from the rectal vault (pattern may vary from every day to every 3 to 5 days) (Roig et al, 1993)
- Have regulation of stool consistency (soft, formed stools)
- Reduce or eliminate frequency of incontinent episodes
- Demonstrate intact skin in the perianal/ perineal area
- Demonstrate the ability to isolate, contract and relax pelvic muscles (when incontinence related to sphincter incompetence, pseudodyssynergia)
- Increase pelvic muscle strength (when incontinence related to sphincter incompetence)

NIC Interventions (Nursing Interventions Classification)

Suggested NIC Interventions

Bowel Incontinence Care; Bowel Incontinence Care: Encopresis; Bowel Training

• = Independent; ▲ = Collaborative

Determine physical or psychological cause of fecal incontinence; Instruct client family to record fecal output, as appropriate

Nursing Interventions and Rationales

- In a reasonably private setting, directly question any client at risk about the presence of fecal incontinence. If the client reports altered bowel elimination patterns, problems with bowel control or "uncontrollable diarrhea," complete a focused nursing history including previous and present bowel elimination routines, dietary history, frequency and volume of uncontrolled stool loss, aggravating and alleviating factors. *Unless questioned directly, clients are unlikely to report the presence of fecal incontinence (Schultz et al, 1997). The nursing history determines the patterns of stool elimination, to characterize involuntary stool loss, and the likely etiology of the incontinence (Norton and Chelvanaygam, 2000).*
- Complete a focused physical assessment including inspection of perineal skin, pelvic muscle strength assessment, digital examination of the rectum for presence of impaction and anal sphincter strength, and evaluation of functional status (mobility, dexterity, visual acuity). *A focused physical examination assists in determining the severity of fecal leakage, and its likely etiology. A functional assessment provides information concerning the impact of functional status on stool elimination patterns and incontinence (Gray and Burns, 1996).*
- Complete an assessment of cognitive function. *Dementia, acute confusion, and mental retardation are risk factors for fecal incontinence (O'Donnell et al, 1992; Norton and Chelvanaygam, 2000).*
- Document patterns of stool elimination and incontinent episodes via a bowel record including frequency of bowel movements, stool consistency, frequency and severity of incontinent episodes, precipitating factors, dietary and fluid intake. *This document, used to confirm the verbal history, assists in determining the likely etiology of stool incontinence and serves as a baseline to evaluate treatment efficacy (Norton and Chelvanaygam, 2000).*
- Assess stool consistency and its influence on risk for stool loss. *Several classification systems for stool have been promulgated (Bliss et al, 2001). They assist the nurse and client to differentiate between normal soft, formed stool, hardened stools associated with constipation, and liquid stools associated with diarrhea.* **Nursing Research:** *A study of stool consistency found good reliability when evaluated by professional nurses, student nurses, and clients. Word-only descriptors yielded equivocal consistency when assessed by subjects as did tools that combined words with illustrations of various stool consistencies (Bliss et al, 2001).*
- Identify conditions contributing to or causing fecal incontinence. *Fecal incontinence is frequently multifactorial. Accurate assessment of the probable etiology of fecal incontinence is necessary to select a treatment plan likely to control or eliminate the condition (Norton and Chelvanaygam, 2000).*
- Improve access to toileting:
  - Identify usual toileting patterns among persons in the acute care or long-term care facility and plan opportunities for toileting accordingly.

- = **Independent; ▲ = Collaborative**

- Provide assistance with toileting for clients with limited access or impaired functional status (mobility, dexterity, access).
- Institute a prompted toileting program for persons with impaired cognitive status (retardation, dementia).
- Provide adequate privacy for toileting.
- Respond promptly to requests for assistance with toileting.

Acute or transient fecal incontinence frequently occurs in the acute care or long-term care facility because of inadequate access to toileting facilities, insufficient assistance with toileting, or inadequate privacy when attempting to toilet (Bliss et al, 2000; Gray and Burns, 1996).

- Counsel clients with fecal incontinence associated with liquid stools (diarrhea) about methods to normalize stool consistency via dietary fiber or fiber supplements. *A liquid stool is associated with an increased likelihood of fecal incontinence (Bliss et al, 2000).* **Nursing Research:** *Daily supplementation of dietary fiber using a product containing psyllium, improved stool consistency and reduced frequency of incontinent stools (Bliss et al, 2001).*
- For the client with intermittent episodes of fecal incontinence related to acute changes in stool consistency, begin a bowel re-education program consisting of:
  - Cleansing the bowel of impacted stool if indicated
  - Normalizing stool consistency by adequate intake of fluids (30 ml/kg of body weight/day) and dietary or supplemental fiber
  - Establishing a regular routine of fecal elimination based on established patterns of bowel elimination (patterns established prior to onset of incontinence)

Bowel reeducation is designed to re-establish normal defecation patterns and to normalize stool consistency in order to reduce or eliminate the risk of recurring fecal incontinence associated with changes in stool consistency (Doughty, 1996).

- Begin a prompted defecation program for the adult with dementia, mental retardation, or related learning disabilities. *Prompted urine and fecal elimination programs have been shown to reduce or eliminate incontinence in the long-term care facility and in community settings (Doughty, 1996; Smith et al, 1994).*
- Begin a scheduled, stimulation defecation program for persons with neurological conditions causing fecal incontinence including the following steps:
  - Cleanse the bowel of impacted fecal material before beginning the program
  - Implement strategies to normalize stool consistency including adequate intake of fluid and fiber and avoidance of foods associated with diarrhea
  - Determine a regular schedule for bowel elimination (typically every day or every other day) based on prior patterns of bowel elimination whenever feasible
  - Provide a stimulus prior to assisting the client to a position on the toilet; digital stimulation, a stimulating suppository, "mini-enema" or pulsed evacuation enema may be used for stimulation.

The scheduled, stimulated program relies on consistency of stool, and a mechanical or chemical stimulus to produce a bolus contraction of the rectum with evacuation of fecal material (Doughty, 1996; Dunn and Galka; 1994; King et al, 1994, Munchiando and Kendall, 1993).

- Begin a pelvic floor re-education or muscle exercise program for the person with sphincter incompetence or pseudodyssynergia of the pelvic muscles, or refer persons with fecal incontinence related to sphincter dysfunction to a nurse specialist or other therapist with clinical expertise in these techniques of care. *Although the evidence*

• = Independent; ▲ = Collaborative

remains quite weak, existing research suggests that pelvic muscle rehabilitation may improve fecal control in selected clients with fecal incontinence, particularly when it is associated with anal sphincter damage or dysfunction (Norton et al, 2003).

▲ Begin a pelvic muscle biofeedback program among clients with urgency to defecate and fecal incontinence related to recurrent diarrhea. *Pelvic muscle re-education, including biofeedback, can reduce uncontrolled loss of stool among persons who experience urgency and diarrhea as provocative factors for fecal incontinence (Chiarioni et al, 1993).*

• Cleanse the perineal and perianal skin following each episode of fecal incontinence. When incontinence is frequent, use an incontinence-cleansing product specifically designed for this purpose. *Frequent cleaning with soap and water may compromise perianal skin integrity and enhance the irritation produced by fecal leakage (Gray et al, 2002).*

• Apply mineral oil or a petroleum-based ointment to the perianal skin when frequent episodes of fecal incontinence occur. *These products form a moisture and chemical barrier to the perianal skin that may prevent or reduce the severity of compromised skin integrity with severe fecal incontinence (Fiers and Thayer, 2000).*

• Assist the client to select and apply a containment device for occasional episodes of fecal incontinence. *A fecal containment device will prevent soiling of clothing and reduce odors in the client with uncontrolled stool loss (Brazelli et al, 2000).*

• Teach the caregiver of the client with frequent episodes of fecal incontinence and limited mobility to regularly monitor the sacrum and perineal area for pressure ulcerations. *Limited mobility, particularly when combined with fecal incontinence, increases the risk of pressure ulceration. Routine cleansing, pressure reduction techniques, and management of fecal and urinary incontinence reduce this risk (Johanson et al, 1997; Schnelle et al, 1997).*

▲ Teach the client with more frequent stool loss to apply an anal continence plug in consultation with the physician. *The anal continence plug is a device that can reduce or eliminate persistent liquid or solid stool incontinence in selected clients.*

• Apply a fecal pouch to the client with frequent stool loss, particularly when fecal incontinence produces altered perianal skin integrity. *Fecal pouches contain stool loss, reduce odor and protect the perianal skin for chemical irritation related to contact with stool (Fiers and Thayer, 2000; Waldrop and Doughty, 2000).*

▲ Consult the physician concerning the use of a rectal tube for the client with severe fecal incontinence. *A large French-sized indwelling catheter or nasopharyngeal airway device (nasal trumpet) has been used for fecal containment when incontinence is severe and perianal skin integrity is significantly compromised (Grogan and Kramer, 2002; Waldrop and Doughty, 2000).*

Geriatric

• Evaluate all elderly clients for established or acute fecal incontinence when the elderly client enters the acute or long-term care facility and intervene as indicated. *The rate of fecal incontinence in the acute care facility is as high as 3% and as high as 50% of residents in long-term care facilities (Egan et al, 1983).*

• Evaluate cognitive status in the elderly person with a NEECHAM confusion scale (Neelan et al, 1992) for acute cognitive changes, a Folstein Mini-Mental Status Examination (Folstein et al, 1975), or other tool as indicated. *Acute or established dementias increase the risk of fecal incontinence among elderly persons.*

• = **Independent;** ▲ = **Collaborative**

Home care

- Above interventions may be adapted for home care use.
- Assess and teach a bowel management program to support continence. Address timing, diet, fluids, and actions taken independently to deal with bowel incontinence. *Identifying factors that change level of incontinence may guide interventions. If client has been taking over-the-counter medications or home remedies, it is important to consider their influence.*
- Instruct caregiver to provide clothing that is nonrestrictive, can be manipulated easily for toileting, and can be changed with ease. *Avoidance of complicated maneuvers increases the chance of success in toileting programs and decreases the client's risk for embarrassing incontinent episodes.*
- Assist the family in arranging care in a way that allows the client to participate in family or favorite activities without embarrassment. *Careful planning can both help client retain dignity and maintain integrity of family patterns.*
- ▲ If the client is limited to bed (or bed and chair), provide a commode or bedpan that can be easily accessed. If necessary, refer the client to physical therapy services to learn side transfers and to build strength for transfers.
- ▲ If the client is frequently incontinent, refer for home health aide services to assist with hygiene and skin care.

Client/ Family Teaching

- Teach the client and family to perform a bowel reeducation program, scheduled, stimulated program, or other strategies to manage fecal incontinence.
- Teach the client and family about common dietary sources for fiber, as well as supplemental fiber or bulking agents as indicated.
- ▲ Refer the family to support services to assist with in-home management of fecal incontinence as indicated.
- Teach nursing colleagues and nonprofessional care providers the importance of providing toileting opportunities and adequate privacy for the client in an acute or long-term care facility.

NOTE: Refer to nursing diagnoses **Diarrhea** and **Constipation** for detailed management of these related conditions.

REFERENCES

Bliss D et al: Reliability of a stool consistency classification system, *J Wound Ostomy Cont Nurs* 28(6):305, 2001.

Bliss DZ et al: Fecal incontinence in hospitalized patients who are acutely ill, *Nurs Res* 49(2):101, 2000.

Bliss DZ et al: Supplementation with dietary fiber improves fecal incontinence, *Nurs Res* 50(4):203, 2001.

Brazzelli M, Shirran E, Vale L: Absorbent products for containing urinary and/or fecal incontinence in adults, *J Wound Ostomy Cont Nurs* 29(1):45, 2002.

Chiarinoni G et al: Liquid stool incontinence with severe urgency: anorectal function and effective biofeedback treatment, *Gut* 34:1576, 1993.

Doughty DB: A physiologic approach to bowel training, *J Wound Ostomy Cont Nurs* 23:46, 1996.

Dunn KL, Galka ML: A comparison of the effectiveness of Therevac SB and bisacodyl suppositories in SCI patients' bowel programs, *Rehabil Nurs* 19:334, 1994.

Egan M, Plymad K, Thomas T: Incontinence in patients in two district general hospitals, *Nurs Times* 79:22, 1983.

Fiers S, Thayer D: Management of intractable incontinence. In: Doughty DB, editor: *Urinary and fecal incontinence: nursing management,* ed 2, St Louis, 2000, Mosby.

Folstein MF, Folstein EF, McHugh P: Mini Mental State: a practical method of grading the cognitive status of the patient for the clinician, *J Psychiatric Rev* 12:189, 1975.

• = **Independent;** ▲ = **Collaborative**

Gray M, Ratliff C, Donovan A: Perineal skin care for the incontinent patient, *Adv Skin Wound Care* 15:170, 2002.

Gray ML, Burns SM: Continence management, *Crit Care Nurs Clin North Am* 8:29, 1996.

Grogan TA, Kramer DJ: The rectal trumpet: use of a nasopharyngeal airway to contain fecal incontinence in critically ill patients, *J Wound Ostomy Cont Nurs* 29(4):193, 2002.

Johanson JF, Irizarry F, Doughty A: Risk factors for fecal incontinence in a nursing home population, *J Clin Gastroenterol* 24:156, 1997.

King JC, Currie DM, Wright E: Bowel training in spina bifida: importance of education, patient compliance, age, and anal reflexes, *Arch Phys Med Rehabil* 75:243, 1994.

Munchiando JF, Kendall K: Comparison of the effectiveness of two bowel programs for CVA patients, *Rehabil Nurs* 18:168, 1993.

Neelan VJ et al: Use of the NEECHAM confusion scale to assess acute confusional states of hospitalized older patients. In: Funk SG et al, editors: *Key aspects of elder care: managing falls, incontinence and cognitive impairment*, New York, 1992, Springer.

Norton C, Chelvanayagam S: A nursing assessment tool for adult with fecal incontinence, *J Wound Ostomy Cont Nurs* 27:279, 2000.

Norton C, Hosker G, Brazzelli M: Biofeedback and/or sphincter exercises for the treatment of fecal incontinence in adults, *Cochrane Incontinence Group Cochrane Database of Systematic Rev* 1, 2003.

O'Donnell BF et al: Incontinence and troublesome behaviors predict institutionalization in dementia, *J Geriatr Psychiatry Neurol* 5:45, 1992.

Roig Vila JV et al: The defecation habits in a normal working population, *Rev Esp Enfermed Dig* 84:224, 1993.

Schnelle JF et al: Skin disorders and moisture in incontinent nursing home residents: intervention implications, *J Am Geriatr Soc* 45:1182, 1997.

Schultz A, Dickey G, Skoner M: Self-report of incontinence in acute care, *Urol Nurs* 17:23, 1997.

Smith LJ et al: A behavioral approach to retraining bowel function after long-standing constipation and fecal impaction in people with learning disabilities, *Dev Med Child Neurol* 36:41, 1994.

Waldrop J, Doughty DB: Pathophysiology of bowel dysfunction and fecal incontinence. In: Doughty DB, editor: *Urinary and fecal incontinence: nursing management*, ed 2, St Louis, 2000, Mosby.

Effective Breastfeeding

Arlene Farren

NANDA Definition

Mother-infant dyad/family exhibits adequate proficiency and satisfaction with the breastfeeding process

Defining Characteristics

Effective mother/infant communication patterns; regular and sustained suckling/swallowing at the breast; appropriate infant weight pattern for age; infant content after feeding; mother able to position infant at breast to promote a successful latch-on response; signs and/or symptoms of oxytocin release; adequate infant elimination patterns for age; eagerness of infant to nurse; maternal verbalization of satisfaction with the breastfeeding process

Related Factors (r/t)

Basic breastfeeding knowledge/normal breast structure/normal infant oral structure/infant gestational age >34 weeks/support sources (e.g., encouraging partner, history of positive breastfeeding experiences among relatives and friends, access to support groups such as La Leche League)/maternal confidence

• = Independent; ▲ = Collaborative

NOC   Outcomes (Nursing Outcomes Classification)

Suggested NOC Outcomes
Breastfeeding Establishment: Infant, Maternal; Breastfeeding Maintenance

> **Example NOC Outcome with Indicators**
>
> **Breastfeeding Establishment: Infant** as evidenced by the following indicators: Proper alignment and latch-on/Proper areolar grasp/Proper areolar compression/Correct suck and tongue placement/Swallowing a minimum of 5 to 10 minutes per breast/minimum, eight feedings per day/Six or more urinations per day/Age-appropriate weight gain (Rate each indicator of **Breastfeeding Establishment: Infant:** 1 = not adequate, 2 = slightly adequate, 3 = moderately adequate, 4 = substantially adequate, 5 = Totally adequate [see Section I].)

Client Outcomes

Client Will (Specify Time Frame):
- Maintain effective breastfeeding
- Maintain normal growth patterns (infant)
- Verbalize satisfaction with breastfeeding process (mother)

NIC   Interventions (Nursing Interventions Classification)

Suggested NIC Interventions
Breastfeeding Assistance, Lactation Counseling

> **Example NIC Activities—Breastfeeding Assistance**
>
> Discuss with parents an estimate of effort and length of time they would like to put toward breastfeeding; Provide early mother/infant contact opportunity to breastfeed within 2 hours after birth

Nursing Interventions and Rationales

- Encourage rooming-in and breastfeeding on demand. *Rooming-in and breastfeeding on demand are positively associated with breastfeeding success (US Department of Health and Human Services, 2000; Janken et al, 1999; Renfrew et al, 2001).* **Nursing Research:** *Demand feedings have been associated with the continuation of breastfeeding 4 to 6 weeks postpartum in comparison to restricted feeding intervals (Renfrew et al, 2001).*
- Monitor the breastfeeding process. *The nurse's presence and involvement allows for early detection of areas in need of clarification and fosters breastfeeding success in primiparous and multiparas women (Association of Women's Health Obstetric and Neonatal Nurses, 2000; Gill, 2001; Hong et al, 2003; Patistea and Siamantha, 1999).* **Nursing Research:** *Nurses provide assistance with technique and informational needs while observing mothers. Breastfeeding mothers expect nurses to observe and provide feedback during breastfeeding (Gill, 2001).*
- Identify opportunities to enhance knowledge and experience regarding breastfeeding. Support and teaching must be individualized to the client's level of understanding.

• = Independent; ▲ = Collaborative

Exposure to a variety of sources of information is an important predictor of breastfeeding duration (Dennis, 2002; deOlivera et al, 2001; Lauver et al, 2002; Susin et al, 1999; Tiedje et al, 2002). **Nursing Research:** *Primiparous, postpartum women participating in the experimental group of a clinical trial involving video, printed material, and open discussion were more knowledgeable and more likely to be exclusively breastfeeding at 3 and 6 months than those in the control groups (Susin et al, 1999).*

- Give encouragement/positive feedback related to breastfeeding mother-infant interactions. *These activities foster maternal satisfaction with care and promote maternal confidence which can predict breastfeeding outcomes (Blyth et al, 2002; Gill, 2001).* **Nursing Research:** *High breastfeeding self-efficacy (maternal confidence) was associated with breastfeeding initiation, continuing to breastfeed at 4 months, and exclusive breastfeeding (Blyth et al, 2002).*

- Monitor for signs and symptoms of nipple pain and/or trauma. *These factors have been identified as impacting the continuation of breastfeeding in the first weeks of motherhood. Early detection and treatment of problems are important for successful breastfeeding (Association of Women's Health Obstetric and Neonatal Nurses, 2000; Smith and Tully, 2001; Riordan et al, 2001).* **Nursing Research:** *Women with breast/nipple comfort continued to breastfeed longer in comparison to women with less breast/nipple comfort (Riordan et al, 2001).*

- Discuss prevention and treatment of common breastfeeding problems. Permits the nurse to identify the need for information and clarification. *Common problems that can lead to early termination of breastfeeding are mainly preventable or can be overcome with assistance and support (Association of Women's Health Obstetric and Neonatal Nurses, 2000; Tiedje et al, 2002).* **Nursing Research:** *Evidence-based practice guidelines support the need to evaluate breastfeeding women's knowledge regarding the prevention and management of common problems (e.g., sore nipples, breast engorgement) associated with breastfeeding (Association of Women's Health Obstetric and Neonatal Nurses, 2000).*

- Monitor infant responses to breastfeeding. *Ongoing evaluation of the adequacy of infant intake such as weight, number of excretions (urine and stool) per 24 hours, and assessment of the presence of jaundice is important to support ongoing effective breastfeeding and for early detection of problems (Association of Women's Health Obstetric and Neonatal Nurses, 2000; International Lactation Consultant Association, 1999).* **Nursing Research:** *Evidence-based practice guidelines include monitoring infant responses as described above (Association of Women's Health Obstetric and Neonatal Nurses, 2000; International Lactation Consultant Association, 1999).*

- Identify current support person network and opportunities for continued breastfeeding support. *Support from family, professionals, and peer support have been found to improve outcomes such as postpartal complications (psychosocial), duration of breastfeeding and satisfaction with breastfeeding (Adams et al, 2001; Association of Women's Health Obstetric and Neonatal Nurses, 2000; Dennis et al, 2002; McKeever et al, 2002; Pugh et al, 2001).* **Nursing Research:** *In a randomized controlled trial, mothers receiving support through a peer support program were continuing to breastfeed longer and reported greater satisfaction with their breastfeeding experience than their counterparts receiving conventional care (Dennis et al, 2002).*

- Avoid supplemental bottle feedings and do not provide samples of formula on discharge. *Supplemental/formula/bottle feedings can interfere with the infant's desire to breastfeed, increases the risk of allergies, and conveys the subtle message that the mother's breast milk is not adequate. These practices are associated with poor breastfeeding success (Dennis,*

• = **Independent;** ▲ = **Collaborative**

2002; DiGirolamo et al, 2001; Donnelly et al, 2000). **Nursing Research:** *Supplemental feedings were identified as one of two strong risk factors for early breastfeeding termination (DiGirolamo et al, 2001).*

▲ Provide follow-up contact; as available provide home visits and/or peer counseling. *Outreach of this type is associated with better outcomes including breastfeeding duration (Adams et al, 2001; Association of Women's Health Obstetric and Neonatal Nurses, 2000; McKeever et al, 2002; Pugh et al, 2002).* **Nursing Research:** *Breastfeeding women receiving nurse and peer counselor support had longer duration of breastfeeding and infants had fewer sick visits and reported use of fewer medications than those receiving usual care (Pugh et al, 2002).*

Multicultural

- Assess for the influence of cultural beliefs, norms, and values on current breastfeeding practices. **Nursing Research:** *The client's knowledge of breastfeeding may be based on cultural perceptions, as well as influences from the larger social context (Cochran, 1998; Doswell and Erlen, 1998; Leininger and McFarland, 2002).*
- Assess for when the mother wishes to begin breastfeeding. **Nursing Research:** *Usual hospital practice is to begin breastfeeding immediately, but some cultures do not regard colostrum as appropriate for newborns and may prefer to wait until milk is present at about 3 days of age (Galanti, 1997; Pillitteri, 1999).*
- Validate the client's concerns about the amount of milk taken. **Nursing Research:** *Some cultures may add semisolid food within the first month of life as a result of concerns that the infant is not getting enough to eat and the perception that "big is healthy" (Bentley et al, 1999; Higgins, 2000).*

Client/Family Teaching

- Include the father and other family members in education about breastfeeding. *Allaying the misconceptions and the social embarrassment associated with breastfeeding can encourage fathers to be more supportive (DDHS, 2000; Shepherd et al, 2000; Susin et al, 1999).* **Nursing Research:** *Paternal knowledge was associated with frequency and duration of breastfeeding (Susin et al, 1999).*
- Teach the client the importance of maternal nutrition. Generally, no special diet is required but drinking to satisfy thirst and a healthy diet using foods from a variety of sources is recommended (International Lactation Consultant Association, 1999). **Nursing Research:** *Health-enhancing behaviors such as consuming five or more fruits and vegetables daily has been associated with breastfeeding (Pesa and Shelton, 1999).*
- Reinforce the infant's subtle hunger cues (e.g., quiet-alert state, rooting, sucking, hand-to-mouth activity) and encourage the client to nurse whenever signs are apparent. *Parents need to know infant characteristics and the early feeding readiness cues of infants so that they can respond appropriately (Association of Women's Health Obstetric and Neonatal Nurses, 2000; International Lactation Consultant Association, 1999; Milligan et al, 2000).* **Nursing Research:** *Evidence-based practice guidelines support the teaching/reinforcement of these skills as important to effective breastfeeding (Association of Women's Health Obstetric and Neonatal Nurses, 2000; International Lactation Consultant Association, 1999).*
- Review guidelines for frequency (every 2 to 3 hours, or at least eight feedings per 24 hours) and duration (until suckling and swallowing slow down and satiety is reached) of feeding times. *In the first few days, frequent and regular stimulation of the breasts is im-*

• = Independent; ▲ = Collaborative

portant to establish an adequate milk supply (Association of Women's Health Obstetric and Neonatal Nurses, 2000; International Lactation Consultant Association, 1999; Janken et al, 1999). **Nursing Research:** *In a research utilization project, early initiation, frequency of feeding, unlimited suckling time, and avoidance of supplementation were associated with reduced need for bilirubin tests (Janken et al, 1999).*

- Provide anticipatory guidance about common infant behaviors. *Being able to anticipate and manage behaviors and problems promote parental confidence (Association of Women's Health Obstetric and Neonatal Nurses, 2000; Milligan et al, 2000).* **Nursing Research:** *Lack of knowledge about infant growth spurts, temperament, sleep/wake cycles, and introduction of other foods can create parental anxiety and lead to premature termination of breastfeeding (Milligan et al, 2000).*

- Provide information about additional breastfeeding resources. *Breastfeeding books, materials, websites, and breastfeeding support groups, which provide current and accurate information, can enhance maternal success and satisfaction with the breastfeeding process (Association of Women's Health Obstetric and Neonatal Nurses, 2000; International Lactation Consultant Association, 1999; Zimmerman, 1999).* **Nursing Research:** *Continuation of breastfeeding (2 weeks) rates were increased for those participating in an intervention including written materials, gifts, and support groups (Zimmerman, 1999).*

evolve WEBSITES FOR EDUCATION

See the EVOLVE website for World Wide Web resources for client education.

REFERENCES

Adams C et al: Breastfeeding trends at a community breastfeeding center: an evaluative survey, *J Gynecol Neonat Nurs* 30:392, 2001.

Association of Women's Health Obstetric and Neonatal Nurses: *Evidence-based clinical practice guideline: breastfeeding support: prenatal care through the first year (practice guideline),* Washington, DC, 2000, The Association.

Bentley M et al: Infant feeding practices of low-income, African American, adolescent mothers: an ecological, multigenerational perspective, *Soc Sci Med* 49(8):10850, 1999.

Blyth R et al: Effect of maternal confidence on breastfeeding duration: An application of breastfeeding self-efficacy theory, *Birth* 29:278, 2002.

Cochran M: Tears have no color, *Am J Nurs* 98(6):53, 1998.

de Oliveira MIC, Comacho LAB, Tedstone AE: Extending breastfeeding duration through primary care: a systematic review of prenatal and postnatal interventions, *J Hum Lact* 17(4):326, 2001.

Dennis CL: Breastfeeding initiation and duration: a 1990-2000 literature review, *J Gynecol Neonat Nurs* 31:12, 2002a.

Dennis CL: Breastfeeding peer support: maternal and volunteer perceptions from a randomized controlled trial, *Birth* 29:169, 2002b.

Dennis CL et al: The effect of peer support on breast-feeding duration among primiparous women: a randomized controlled trial, *CMAJ* 166:21, 2002.

DiGirolamo AM, Grummer-Strawn LM, Fein S: Maternity care practices: implications for breastfeeding, *Birth* 28:94, 2001.

Donnelly A et al: The influence of discharge packs on breastfeeding. In J. Neilson et al, editors: *Pregnancy and childbirth module of the Cochrane Database of Systematic Reviews.* Available in the Cochrane Library [database on disk and CD ROM]. The Cochrane Collaboration, Issue 1. Oxford, UK: Updata Software (updated quarterly), 2001.

Doswell W, Erlen J: Multicultural issues and ethical concerns in the delivery of revising care interventions, *Nurs Clin North Am* 33(2):353, 1998.

- = Independent; ▲ = Collaborative

Galanti G: *Caring for patients from different cultures: case studies from American hospitals,* ed 2, Philadelphia, 1997, University of Pennsylvania Press.

Gill SL: The little things: perceptions of breastfeeding support, *J Gynecol Neonat Nurs* 30:401, 2001.

Higgins B: Puerto Rican cultural beliefs: influence on infant feeding practices in western New York, *J Transcultural Nurs* 11(1), 2000.

Hong TM, Callister LC, Schwartz R: First-time mothers' views of breastfeeding support from nurses, *MCN Am J Matern Child Nurs* 28:10:2003.

International Lactation Consultant Association: *Evidence-based guidelines for breastfeeding management during the first fourteen days,* Raleigh, NC, 1999, The Association.

Janken JK, Blythe G, Campbell PT, Carter RH: Changing nursing practice through research utilization: Consistent support for breastfeeding mothers, *Appl Nurs Res* 12:22, 1999.

Lauver DR et al: Patient-centered interventions, *Res Nurs Health* 25:246, 2002.

Leininger MM, McFarland MR: *Transcultural nursing: concepts, theories, research and practices,* ed 3, New York, 2002, McGraw-Hill.

McKeever P et al: Home versus hospital breastfeeding support for newborns: a randomized controlled trial, *Birth* 29:258, 2002.

Milligan RA et al: Breastfeeding duration among low income women, *J Midwif Womens Health* 45:246, 2000.

Pesa JA, Shelton MM: Health-enhancing behaviors correlated with breastfeeding among a national sample of mothers, *Public Health Nurs* 16:120, 1999.

Pillitteri A: Nutritional needs of the newborn. In Pillitteri A, editor: *Maternal and child health nursing: care of the childbearing and childrearing family,* Philadelphia, 1999, Lippincott.

Pugh LC et al: Breastfeeding duration, costs, and benefits of a support program for low-income breastfeeding women, *Birth* 29:95, 2002.

Renfrew M et al: Feeding schedules in hospitals for newborn infants. In J Neilson et al, editors: *Pregnancy and childbirth module of the Cochrane Database of Systematic Reviews.* Available in The Cochrane Library [database on disk and CD ROM]. The Cochrane Collaboration, Issue 1. Oxford, UK: Updata Software (updated quarterly), 2001.

Riordan J et al: Predicting breastfeeding duration using the LATCH breastfeeding assessment tool, *J Hum Lact* 17:20, 2001.

Shepherd CK, Power KG, Carter H: Examining the correspondence of breastfeeding and bottle-feeding couples' infant feeding attitudes, *J Adv Nurs* 31:651, 2000.

Smith JW, Tully MR: Midwifery management of breastfeeding: using the evidence, *J Midwif Womens Health* 46:423, 2001.

Susin LR et al: Does parental breastfeeding knowledge increase breastfeeding rates? *Birth* 26:149, 1999.

Tiedja LB et al: An ecological approach to breastfeeding, *MCN Am J Matern Child Nurs* 27:154, 2002.

US Department of Health and Human Services: *HHS Blueprint for Action on Breastfeeding,* Washington, DC, 2000, US Department of Health and Human Services, Office on Women's Health.

Zimmerman DR: You can make a difference: increasing breastfeeding rates in an inner-city clinic, *J Hum Lact* 15:217, 1999.

Ineffective Breastfeeding

Arlene Farren

NANDA Definition

Dissatisfaction or difficulty a mother, infant, or child experiences with the breastfeeding process

Defining Characteristics

Unsatisfactory breastfeeding process; nonsustained suckling at the breast; resisting latching on; unresponsive to comfort measures; persistence of sore nipples beyond first week of breastfeeding; observable signs of inadequate infant intake; insufficient emptying of each breast per feeding; infant inability to latch on to maternal breast correctly; infant arching and crying at the breast; infant exhibiting fussiness and crying within the first

• = Independent; ▲ = Collaborative

hour after breastfeeding; actual or perceived inadequate milk supply; no observable signs of oxytocin release; insufficient opportunity for suckling at the breast

Related Factors (r/t)

Non-supportive partner/family; previous breast surgery; infant receiving supplemental feedings with artificial nipple; prematurity; previous history of breastfeeding failure; poor infant sucking reflex; maternal breast anomaly; maternal anxiety or ambivalence; interruption in breastfeeding; infant anomaly; knowledge deficit

NOC   Outcomes (Nursing Outcomes Classification)

Suggested NOC Outcomes

Breastfeeding Establishment: Infant, Maternal; Breastfeeding Maintenance; Breastfeeding Weaning; Knowledge: Breastfeeding

---

Example NOC Outcome with Indicators

Breastfeeding Establishment: Infant as evidenced by the following indicators: Proper alignment and latch-on/Proper areolar grasp/Proper areolar compression/Correct suck and tongue placement/Swallowing a minimum of 5 to 10 minutes per breast/Minimum eight feedings per day/Six or more urinations per day/Age-appropriate weight gain (Rate each indicator of **Breastfeeding Establishment: Infant**: 1 = not adequate, 2 = slightly adequate, 3 = moderately adequate, 4 = substantially adequate, 5 = totally adequate [see Section I].)

Client Outcomes

Client Will (Specify Time Frame):
- Achieve effective breastfeeding (dyad)
- Verbalize/demonstrate techniques to manage breastfeeding problems (mother)
- Manifest signs of adequate intake at the breast (infant)
- Manifest positive self-esteem in relation to the infant feeding process (mother)
- Explain alternative method of infant feeding if unable to continue exclusive breastfeeding (mother)

NIC   Interventions (Nursing Interventions Classification)

Suggested NIC Interventions

Breastfeeding Assistance; Lactation Counseling

Example NIC Activities—Breastfeeding Assistance

Discuss with parents an estimate of effort and length of time they would like to put toward breastfeeding; Provide early mother/infant contact opportunity to breastfeed within 2 hours after birth

---

Nursing Interventions and Rationales

- Identify women with risk factors for lower breastfeeding initiation and continuation rates (age <20 years, low socioeconomic status) as well as factors contributing to ineffective breastfeeding as early as possible in the perinatal experience. *Early identifica-*

• = Independent; ▲ = Collaborative

tion of potential problems make individualized, targeted interventions that are culturally sensitive possible (Association of Women's Health Obstetric and Neonatal Nurses, 2000a; Mozingo et al, 2000; Schwartz et al, 2002). **Nursing Research:** *A prospective cohort study of more than 900 revealed younger and less educated women, those with nipple/breast pain, mastitis, and bottle use were among those more likely to discontinue breastfeeding early. The researchers concluded that these women need additional assistance and counseling (Schwartz et al, 2002).*

- Use valid and reliable tools to measure breastfeeding performance and to predict early discontinuance of breastfeeding whenever possible/feasible. *Using instruments to measure clinically relevant constructs in a consistent manner permits identification of women/infants at risk and provides for systematic clinical outcome measurement (Dennis and Faux, 1999; Dick et al, 2002; Hall et al, 2002; Kirchhoff and Rakel, 1999).* **Nursing Research:** *Researchers estimated internal consistency reliability and predictive validity of the Breastfeeding Attrition Prediction Tool (BAPT) in a sample of postpartal women and concluded that the BAPT (modified version) showed promise for clinical use (Dick et al, 2002).*

- Encourage rooming-in and feeding on demand. *These approaches have been positively associated with breastfeeding success (US Department of Health and Human Services, 2000; Janken et al, 1999; Renfrew et al, 2001).* **Nursing Research:** *Rooming-in and breastfeeding on demand were associated with full breastfeeding at 4 months (Centuori et al, 1999).*

- Evaluate the breast and nipple structures and provide appropriate measures as needed. *Normal nipple and breast structure and early detection and treatment of abnormalities with continuing support are important for successful breastfeeding. Nipple trauma is associated with latch-on problems and increased risk for mastitis (Association of Women's Health Obstetric and Neonatal Nurses, 2000b; Foxman et al, 2002; International Lactation Consultant Association, 1999; Smith and Tully, 2001).* **Nursing Research:** *Sore/cracked nipples were found to be strongly associated with mastitis (Foxman et al, 2002). Breast/nipple comfort has been linked to continuation of breastfeeding (Riordan et al, 2001).*

- Observe a full breastfeeding session (every 8 hours in the early postpartum and once per visit on follow-up). *The nurse's presence and involvement allows for identification of those areas of the breastfeeding process for which assistance and support are needed and promotes maternal confidence (Association of Women's Health Obstetric and Neonatal Nurses, 2000a; Gill, 2001; Hong et al, 2003; Raisler, 2000).* **Nursing Research:** *Women identified nurses' activities such as assessment, teaching, and assistance as being sources of emotional, informational, and tangible support (Hong et al, 2003).*

- Provide evidence-based teaching and breastfeeding assistance appropriate to the client's individualized needs (see Client/Family Teaching). *Accurate, consistent information and providing practical assistance with breastfeeding techniques that are based on evidence and in response to individualized client needs are associated with successful breastfeeding, longer duration breastfeeding, promotion of maternal confidence, and client satisfaction (Association of Women's Health Obstetric and Neonatal Nurses, 2000b; Gill, 2001; Hailes and Wellard, 2000; Janken et al, 1999; Lauver et al, 2002; Mozingo et al, 2000; Raisler, 2000).* **Nursing Research:** *In a qualitative study, mothers described factors contributing to early termination of breastfeeding (e.g., incomplete and inconsistent information about breastfeeding). Mothers experiencing confusion, frustration, and dissatisfaction discontinued breastfeeding (Hailes and Wellard, 2000; Mozingo et al, 2000).*

- Promote comfort and relaxation to reduce pain and anxiety. *Discomfort and increased*

- = Independent; ▲ = Collaborative

tension are factors associated with reduced let-down reflex and premature discontinuance of breastfeeding. Anxiety and fear are associated with decreased milk production (Association of Women's Health Obstetric and Neonatal Nurses, 2000a; Mezzacappa and Katkin, 2002; Tait, 2000). **Nursing Research:** *Evidence-based practice guidelines include employing comfort measures for breastfeeding mothers such as providing analgesia approximately 30 minutes before feeding (Association of Women's Health Obstetric and Neonatal Nurses, 2000a).*

- Provide time for clients to express their expectations and concerns and give emotional support. *Discussing concerns and differences between expectations and experiences provide an opportunity for mothers to ventilate and may contribute to positive coping strategies and increase breastfeeding duration (Boettcher et al, 1999; Porteous et al, 2000; Vari et al, 2000).* **Nursing Research:** *In an intervention study examining a social support intervention, women receiving the intervention (professionally mediated peer support) were more satisfied, were exclusively breastfeeding, and breastfeeding duration was longer than those receiving the usual care (Vari et al, 2000).*

- Avoid supplemental feedings. *Supplementation with formula feedings has been associated with higher risk of discontinuance of breastfeeding (DiGirolamo et al, 2001; Hall et al, 2002).* **Nursing Research:** *Supplementing breast milk with formula was one of 8 factors that significantly predicted breastfeeding cessation within 7 to 10 days of age in a large sample of mothers who intended to breastfeed their infants (Hall et al, 2002).*

- Monitor infant behavioral cues and responses to breastfeeding. *Infant behaviors contribute to oxytocin release and let down, contribute to effective feeding, indicate effective breastfeeding, manifest satiety, and indicate adequacy of the feeding while contributing to positive maternal-infant attachment (Association of Women's Health Obstetric and Neonatal Nurses, 2000a, 2000b; Matthiesen et al, 2001; Pridham et al, 1999; White et al, 2002).* **Nursing Research:** *In a small sample, researchers analyzed videotaped behaviors from birth to 2 hours and measured maternal oxytocin levels. The findings suggest that infants use their hands and mouths to stimulate maternal oxytocin release thereby influencing milk ejection (Matthiesen et al, 2001).*

- Collect data and monitor signs of adequate infant intake/nutrition. *Signs such as number of feedings in 24 hours, weight loss/gain pattern, elimination patterns indicate that the infant is getting sufficient infant nutrition for normal patterns of growth and development and permit early identification and treatment of problems (Association of Women's Health Obstetric and Neonatal Nurses, 2000a; International Lactation Consultant Association, 1999; Locklin and Jansson, 1999).* **Nursing Research:** *Evidence-based practice guidelines include assessment and monitoring of the above noted signs of adequate infant intake (Association of Women's Health Obstetric and Neonatal Nurses, 2000a; International Lactation Consultant Association, 1999).*

- Provide necessary equipment/instruction/assistance for milk expression as needed. *While infant suckling is optimal, expressing human milk is done to stimulate the breasts, when the infant is unable to suckle, or when mother and baby are separated (such as mother returning to work). Expression of human milk is done either by hand or pump (Association of Women's Health Obstetric and Neonatal Nurses, 2000a; Biancuuzzo, 1999; Jones et al, 2001; Phillips and Merewood, 2003).* **Nursing Research:** *In a randomized control trial, researchers found that a combination of breast massage and simultaneous (both breasts at the same time) pumping increased the volume of milk produced and also increased maternal satisfaction (Jones et al, 2001).*

- Provide anticipatory guidance in relation to home management of breastfeeding.

- **= Independent; ▲ = Collaborative**

Mothers who are prepared for the needs of home management and possible problems (such as fatigue) can institute self-care measures, will feel more confident, and be less likely to discontinue breastfeeding (Blyth et al, 2002; Ertem et al, 2001; International Lactation Consultant Association, 1999; Pugh et al, 1999; Schwartz et al 2002). **Nursing Research:** *Maternal confidence (breastfeeding self-efficacy) is a significant predictor of breastfeeding duration. The researchers identified implications for practice such as the use of self-efficacy enhancing strategies (Blyth et al, 2002).*

- Assist the client to identify and utilize support network. *Support from family, significant others, professionals, and peer support has been found to improve outcomes such as postpartal complications (psychosocial), duration of breastfeeding, and satisfaction with breastfeeding (Adams et al, 2001; Association of Women's Health Obstetric and Neonatal Nurses, 2000a; Dennis et al, 2002; McKeever et al, 2002).* **Nursing Research:** *In a randomized controlled trial, mothers receiving support through a peer support program were continuing to breastfeed longer and reported greater satisfaction with their breastfeeding experience than their counterparts receiving conventional care (Dennis et al, 2002).*

- Do not provide samples of formula on discharge. *Supplemental/formula/bottle feeding are associated with poor breastfeeding success and can interfere with the infant's desire to breastfeed and increase the risk of allergies, and these practices convey subtle messages that the mother's breast milk is not adequate (Dennis, 2002; DiGirolamo et al, 2001; Donnelly et al, 2000).* **Nursing Research:** *Supplemental feeding was identified as one of two strong risk factors for early breastfeeding termination (DiGirolamo et al, 2001).*

- Initiate breastfeeding follow-up after hospital discharge. *Follow-up provides the opportunity for review of information, feedback about proper technique, and identification of and assistance with problems, and promotes maternal confidence and satisfaction (Escobar et al, 2001; Hogan, 2001; Johnson et al, 1999; Pugh et al, 2002).* **Nursing Research:** *Breastfeeding women receiving nurse and peer counselor support had longer duration of breastfeeding and infants had fewer sick visits and reported use of fewer medications than those receiving usual care (Pugh et al, 2002).*

- ▲ Provide referrals and resources. *Lactation consultants, nurse and peer support programs, community organizations, and written and electronic sources of information contribute to successful breastfeeding and have been supported through outcomes such as knowledge, maternal confidence, duration of breastfeeding, and client satisfaction (Ahluwalia et al, 2000; Association of Women's Health Obstetric and Neonatal Nurses, 2000a; Tarkka et al, 1999; Sikorsk and Renfrew, 1999).* **Nursing Research:** *Evidenced-based guidelines and systematic reviews support the use of professionals with special skills in breastfeeding and other support programs to promote continued breastfeeding (Association of Women's Health Obstetric and Neonatal Nurses, 2000a; Sikorsk, and Renfrew, 1999).*

- If unsuccessful in achieving effective breastfeeding, help client accept and learn an alternate method of infant feeding. *Once the decision has been made to provide an alternate method of infant feeding, the mother needs support and education (Mozingo et al, 2000).* **Nursing Research:** *In a qualitative study of women's experiences with short-term breastfeeding, researchers uncovered women's concerns about breastfeeding failure and their feelings of relief versus guilt and shame for which women may need assistance and support (Mozingo et al, 2000).*

Multicultural

- Assess for the influence of cultural beliefs, norms, and values on breastfeeding attitudes. **Nursing Research:** *The client's knowledge of breastfeeding may be based on cultural*

- **= Independent; ▲ = Collaborative**

perceptions, as well as influences from the larger social context (Cochran, 1998; Doswell and Erlen, 1998; Leininger and McFarland, 2002).

- Assess whether the client's concerns about the amount of milk taken during breastfeeding is contributing to dissatisfaction with the breastfeeding process. **Nursing Research:** *Some cultures may add semisolid food within the first month of life as a result of concerns that the infant is not getting enough to eat and the perception that "big is healthy" (Bentley et al, 1999; Higgins, 2000).*
- Assess the influence of family support on the decision to continue or discontinue breastfeeding. **Nursing Research:** *Women are the keepers and transmitters of culture in families. Female family members can play a dominant role in how infants are fed (Cesario, 2001; Guranaccia, 1998; Pillitteri, 1999).*
- Validate the client's feelings regarding the difficulty or dissatisfaction with breastfeeding. **Nursing Research:** *Validation is a therapeutic communication technique that lets the client know that the nurse has heard and understands what was said and promotes the nurse-client relationship (Heineken, 1998).*

Home care

- Above interventions may be adapted for home care use.
- ▲ Investigate availability/refer to public health department or hospital home follow-up breastfeeding program. Some hospitals and public health departments have follow-up breastfeeding programs, particularly for high-risk mothers (e.g., older mothers, past history substance use, risk of physical abuse). Instructions initiated during hospitalization are continued.
- Monitor for specific difficulties contributing to bonding difficulties between mother and infant. *Refer to care plan for* **Risk for impaired parent/infant/child Attachment.**

Client/Family Teaching

- Review maternal and infant benefits of breastfeeding. *Information about benefits of breastfeeding can assist women/families to make informed decisions about breastfeeding (Association of Women's Health Obstetric and Neonatal Nurses, 2000a,b; Dennis and Faux, 1999; Duckett et al, 1998; Janken et al, 1999; US Department of Health and Human Services, 2000).* **Nursing Research:** *In a large sample, full breastfeeding was associated with the lowest infant illness rates (Raisler et al, 1999).*
- Instruct the client on maternal breastfeeding behaviors/techniques (preparation for, positioning, initiation of/promoting latch-on, burping, completion of session, and frequency of feeding). Difficulties in these practices contribute to ineffective breastfeeding. *Teaching behaviors/techniques of importance to breastfeeding will provide the woman with the necessary information and skills to initiate and continue breastfeeding and instill maternal confidence (Association of Women's Health Obstetric and Neonatal Nurses, 2000a,b; Ertem et al, 2001; Johnson et al, 1999; Susin et al, 1999; US Department of Health and Human Services, 2000).* **Nursing Research:** *A teaching intervention (video, discussion, and written material) was tested in a sample of postpartal mothers and fathers of healthy newborns and researchers found that there was an increase in knowledge and duration of breastfeeding in the group receiving the intervention (Susin et al, 1999).*
- Teach the client self-care measures for the breastfeeding woman (e.g., Breast care, Management of breast/nipple discomfort, Nutrition/fluid, rest/activity). *Nipple trauma, pain, mastitis, and fatigue are some of the problems a breastfeeding woman may experience. Developing knowledge and skill facilitates prevention and self-care management*

• = Independent; ▲ = Collaborative

of these potential problems, fosters maternal confidence, and improves breastfeeding duration (Association of Women's Health Obstetric and Neonatal Nurses, 2000a; Foxman et al, 2002; Ruchala, 2000; Smith and Tully, 2001; Tait, 2000). **Nursing Research:** *In a sample of low-risk early postpartum women, the researcher found mothers perceived that receiving teaching regarding their own care (in contrast to newborn care) was the priority (Ruchala, 2000).*

- Provide information regarding infant cues and behaviors related to breastfeeding and appropriate maternal responses (e.g., cues that infant is ready to feed, behaviors during feeding that contribute to effective breastfeeding, measures of infant feeding adequacy). *Mothers who correctly interpret the infant's behaviors/responses and are able to provide comfort measures are more likely to continue to breastfeed, experience maternal confidence and satisfying maternal-infant interaction (Association of Women's Health Obstetric and Neonatal Nurses, 2000a,b; Bryan, 2000; Dennis and Faux, 1999; Schwartz et al, 2002; Smith and Tully, 2001; White et al, 2002).* **Nursing Research:** *In a research utilization project, researchers asserted that nurses are vital to helping parents understand infant states, cues, and behaviors and by providing that information postnatally, will foster a mutually satisfying interaction between parent and infant (White et al, 2002).*

- Provide education to father/family/significant others as needed. *Informed support people have a desire to learn, may be needed to assist mothers with breastfeeding management issues (for example, fatigue), and may have an impact on breastfeeding duration (Association of Women's Health Obstetric and Neonatal Nurses, 2000a; Moore, 2000; Pollock et al, 2002; Susin et al, 1999; Tarkka et al, 1999).* **Nursing Research:** *In a descriptive study, men present at perinatal settings indicated a preference for their babies to be breastfed and wanted to be included in decisions concerning breastfeeding (Pollock et al, 2002).*

evolve WEBSITES FOR EDUCATION

See the EVOLVE website for World Wide Web resources for client education.

REFERENCES

Adams C et al: Breastfeeding trends at a community breastfeeding center: an evaluative survey, *J Gynecol Neonat Nurs* 30:392, 2001.

Ahluwalia IB et al: Georgia's breastfeeding promotion program for low-income women, *Pediatrics* 105:e85, 2000.

Association of Women's Health Obstetric and Neonatal Nurses: *Evidence-based clinical practice guideline: breastfeeding support: prenatal care through the first year (practice guideline),* Washington, DC, 2000a, The Association.

Association of Women's Health Obstetric and Neonatal Nurses: *Evidence-based clinical practice guideline: breastfeeding support: prenatal care through the first year (monograph),* Washington, DC, 2000b, The Association.

Bentley M et al: Infant feeding practices of low-income, African American, adolescent mothers: an ecological, multigenerational perspective, *Soc Sci Med* 49(8):10850, 1999.

Biancuzzo M: Selecting pumps for breastfeeding mothers, *J Gynecol Neonat Nurs* 28:417, 1999.

Blyth R et al: Effect of maternal confidence on breastfeeding duration: an application of breastfeeding self-efficacy theory, *Birth* 29:278, 2002.

Boettcher JP et al: Interaction of factors related to lactation duration, *J Perinat Educ* 8 (2):11, 1999.

Centuori S et al: Nipple care, sore nipples, and breastfeeding: a randomized trial, *J Hum Lact* 15:125, 1999.

Cesario S: Care of the Native American woman: strategies for practice, education, and research, *J Gynecol Neonat Nurs* 30(1):13, 2001.

Cochran M: Tears have no color, *Am J Nurs* 98(6):53, 1998.

- = **Independent;** ▲ = **Collaborative**

Dennis C, Faux S: Development and psychometric testing of the Breastfeeding Self-Efficacy Scale, *Res Nurs Health* 22:399, 1999.

Dennis CL et al: The effect of peer support on breast-feeding duration among primiparous women: A randomized controlled trial, *CMAJ* 166(1):21, 2002.

Dick MJ et al: Predicting early breastfeeding attrition, *J Hum Lact* 18:21, 2002.

DiGirolamo AM, Grummer-Strawn LM, Fein S: Maternity care practices: implications for breastfeeding, *Birth* 28:94, 2001.

Donnelly A et al: The influence of discharge packs on breastfeeding. In J. Neilson C et al, editors: *Pregnancy and childbirth module of the Cochrane Database of Systematic Reviews.* Available in the Cochrane Library [database on disk and CD ROM]. The Cochrane Collaboration, Issue 1. Oxford, UK: Updata Software (updated quarterly), 2001.

Doswell W, Erlen J: Multicultural issues and ethical concerns in the delivery of revising care interventions, *Nurs Clin North Am* 33(2):353, 1998.

Duckett L et al: A theory of planned behavior-based structural model for breast-feeding, *Nurs Res* 47:325, 1998.

Ertem IO, Votto N, Leventhal JM: The timing and predictors of the early termination of breastfeeding, *Pediatrics* 107:543, 2001.

Escobar GJ et al: A randomized comparison of home visits and hospital-based group follow-up visits after early postpartum discharge, *Pediatrics* 108:719, 2001.

Foxman B et al: Lactation mastitis: Occurrence and medical management among 946 breastfeeding women in the United States, *Am J Epidemiol* 155:103, 2002.

Gill SL: The little things: perceptions of breastfeeding support, *J Gynecol Neonat Nurs* 30:401, 2001.

Guarnaccia P: Multicultural experiences of family caregiving: a study of African American, European American, and Hispanic American families, *New Direct Ment Health Serv* 77:45, 1998.

Hailes JE, Wellard SJ: Support for breastfeeding in the first postpartum month: perceptions of breastfeeding women, *Breastfeed Rev* 8 (3):5, 2000.

Hall RT et al: A breast-feeding assessment score to evaluate the risk for cessation of breast-feeding by 7 to 10 days of age, *J Pediatr* 141:659, 2002.

Heineken J: Patient silence is not necessarily client satisfaction: communication in home care nursing, *Home Health Care Nurse* 16(2):115, 1998.

Higgins B: Puerto Rican cultural beliefs: influence on infant feeding practices in western New York, *J Transcultural Nurs* 11(1), 2000.

Hogan SE: Overcoming barriers to breastfeeding: suggested breastfeeding promotion programs for communities in eastern Nova Scotia, *Can J Public Health* 92:105, 2001.

Hong TM, Callister LC, Schwartz R: First-time mothers' views of breastfeeding support from nurses. *MCN Am J Matern Child Nurs* 28:10, 2003.

International Lactation Consultant Association: *Evidence-based guidelines for breastfeeding management during the first fourteen days,* Raleigh, NC, 1999, The Association.

Janken JK et al: Changing nursing practice through research utilization: consistent support for breastfeeding mothers, *Appl Nurs Res* 12:22, 1999.

Johnson TS, Brennan RA, Flynn-Tymkow CD: A home visit program for breastfeeding education and support, *J Gynecol Neonat Nurs* 28:480, 1999.

Jones E, Dimmock PW, Spencer SA: A randomized controlled trial to compare methods of milk expression after preterm delivery, *Arch Dis Child* 85:F91, 2001.

Kirchhoff KT, Rakel BA: Outcomes evaluation. In Mateo MA, Kirchhoff KT, editors: *Using and conducting nursing research in the clinical setting,* 2nd ed.. Philadelphia, 1999, WB Saunders.

Lauver DR et al: Patient-centered interventions, *Res Nurs Health* 25:246.

Leininger MM, McFarland MR: *Transcultural nursing: concepts, theories, research and practices,* ed 3, New York, 2002, McGraw-Hill.

Locklin MP, Jansson MJ: Home visits: strategies to protect the breastfeeding newborn at risk, *J Gynecol Neonat Nurs* 28:33, 1999.

Matthiesen AS et al: Postpartum maternal oxytocin release by newborns: effects of infant hand massage and sucking, *Birth* 28:13, 2001.

McKeever P et al: Home versus hospital breastfeeding support for newborns: a randomized controlled trial, *Birth* 29:258, 2002.

Meier PP et al: Nipple shields for preterm infants: effect on milk transfer and duration of breastfeeding, *J Hum Lact* 16(2):106, quiz 129, 2000.

Mezzacappa ES, Katkin ES: Breast-feeding is associated with reduced perceived stress and negative mood in mothers, *Health Psychol* 21:187, 2002.

• = **Independent**; ▲ = **Collaborative**

Moore ML: Perinatal nursing research: a 25-year review—1976-2000, *MCN Am J Matern Child Nurs* 25:305, 2000.

Mozingo JN et al: "It wasn't working": women's experiences with short-term breastfeeding, *MCN Am J Matern Child Nurs* 25:120, 2000.

Philipp BL, Merewood A: Encouraging patients to use a breast pump. *Cont OB/GYN* 48:88, 2003.

Pillitteri A: Nutritional needs of the newborn. In Pillitteri A, editor: *Maternal and child health nursing: care of the childbearing and childrearing family,* Philadelphia, 1999, Lippincott.

Pollock CA, Bustamante-Forest R, Giarratano G: Men of diverse cultures: knowledge and attitudes about breastfeeding, *J Gynecol Neonat Nurs* 31:673, 2002.

Porteous R, Kaufman K, Rush J: The effect of individualized professional support on duration of breastfeeding: a randomized controlled trial, *J Hum Lact* 16:303, 2000.

Pridham K, Lin CY, Brown R: Mothers' evaluation of their caregiving for premature and full-term infants through the first year: contributing factors, *Res Nurs Health* 24:157, 2001.

Pugh LC et al: Clinical approaches in the assessment of childbearing fatigue, *J Gynecol Neonat Nurs* 28:74, 1999.

Pugh LC et al: Breastfeeding duration, costs, and benefits of a support program for low-income breastfeeding women, *Birth* 29:95, 2002.

Raisler J: Against the odds: breastfeeding experiences of low income mothers, *J Midwif Women's Health* 45:253, 2000.

Raisler J, Alexander C, O'Campo P: Breast-feeding and infant illness: a dose-response relationship?, *Am J Pub Health* 89:25, 1999.

Riordan J et al: Predicting breastfeeding duration using the LATCH breastfeeding assessment tool, *J Hum Lact* 17:20, 2001.

Ruchala PL: Teaching new mothers: priorities of nurses and postpartum women, *J Gynecol Neonat Nurs* 29:265, 2000.

Schwartz K et al: Factors associated with weaning in the first 3 months postpartum, *J Fam Pract* 51:439, 2002.

Sikorsk J, Renfrew MJ: Support for breastfeeding mothers, *Birth* 26:131, 1999.

Smith JW, Tully MR: Midwifery management of breastfeeding: using the evidence, *J Midwif Women's Health* 46:423, 2001.

Susin LR et al: Does parental breastfeeding knowledge increase breastfeeding rates? *Birth* 26:149, 1999.

Tait P: Nipple pain in breastfeeding women: causes, treatment, and prevention strategies, *J Midwif Women's Health* 45:212, 2000.

Tarkka MT, Paunonen M, Laippala P: Factors related to successful breastfeeding by first-time mothers when the child is 3 months old, *J Adv Nurs* 29(1):113, 1999.

US Department of health and Human Services: *HHS blueprint for action on breastfeeding,* Washington, DC, 2000, US Department of Health and Human Services, Office on Women's Health.

Vari PM, Camburn J, Henly SJ: Professionally mediated peer support and early breastfeeding success, *J Perinat Educ* 9:22, 2000.

White C, Simon M, Bryan A: Using evidence to educate birthing center nursing staff: about infant states, cues, and behaviors, *MCN Am J Matern Child Nurs* 27:294, 2002.

Interrupted Breastfeeding

Arlene Farren

NANDA Definition

Break in the continuity of the breastfeeding process as a result of inability or inadvisability to putting the infant to the breast for feeding

Defining Characteristics

Infant does not receive nourishment at the breast for some or all feedings; maternal desire to maintain lactation and provide (or eventually provide) her breast milk for her infant's nutritional needs; separation of mother and infant; lack of knowledge regarding expression and storage of breast milk

- • = Independent; ▲ = Collaborative

Related Factors (r/t)

Maternal or infant illness; prematurity; maternal employment; contraindications to breastfeeding (e.g., drugs, true breast milk jaundice); need to abruptly wean infant (with intent to resume at later date)

NOC   Outcomes (Nursing Outcomes Classification)

Suggested NOC Outcomes

Breastfeeding Establishment: Infant, Maternal; Breastfeeding Maintenance; Knowledge: Breastfeeding; Parent-Infant Attachment

> **Example NOC Outcome with Indicators**
>
> **Breastfeeding Establishment: Infant** as evidenced by the following indicators: Proper alignment and latch on/Proper areolar grasp/Proper areolar compression/Correct suck and tongue placement/Swallowing a minimum of 5 to 10 minutes per breast/Minimum eight feedings per day/Six or more urinations per day/Age appropriate weight gain (Rate each indicator of **Breastfeeding Establishment: Infant:** 1 = not adequate, 2 = slightly adequate, 3 = moderately adequate, 4 = substantially adequate, 5 = totally adequate [see Section I].)

Client Outcomes

Client Will (Specify Time Frame):

Infant

- Receive mother's breast milk if not contraindicated by maternal conditions (e.g., certain drugs, infections) or infant conditions (e.g., true breast milk jaundice)

Maternal

- Maintain lactation
- Achieve effective breastfeeding or satisfaction with the breastfeeding experience
- Demonstrate effective methods of breast milk collection and storage

NIC   Interventions (Nursing Interventions Classification)

Suggested NIC Interventions

Bottle Feeding; Breastfeeding Assistance; Emotional Support; Kangaroo Care; Lactation Counseling

> **Example NIC Activities—Lactation Counseling**
>
> Instruct parents on how to differentiate between perceived and actual insufficient milk supply; Encourage employers to provide opportunities for and private facilities for lactating mothers to pump and store breast milk during work times

Nursing Interventions and Rationales

- Discuss mother's desire/intention to begin or resume breastfeeding (breastfeeding). *Mothers' commitment/attitude about breastfeeding are associated with breastfeeding success (Kloeblen-Tarver et al, 2002; Mozingo et al, 2000; Pinelli et al, 2001).* **Nursing Re-**

- • = Independent; ▲ = Collaborative

search: *Researchers examining the efficacy of an intervention to improve duration of breast-feeding in very low-birth-weight infants suggested that high motivation to breast feed may have accounted for the lack of demonstrated differences in breastfeeding duration of parents who did and did not receive the intervention (Pinelli et al, 2001).*

- Provide anticipatory guidance to the mother/family regarding potential duration of the interruption when possible/feasible. *When conditions (e.g., certain maternal drugs/substances; setting/maternal or infant illness) require a temporary interruption of breastfeeding, having an approximate duration of the interruption will assist the mother/family to plan and will provide reassurance of the temporary nature of the interruption (Auerbach, 1999; Davis et al, 2000; International Lactation Consultant Association, 1999; Ito, 2000; Nystrom and Axelsson, 2002; Ward et al, 2001; US Department of Health and Human Services, 2000).* **Nursing Research:** *Mothers who experienced separation from their infants due to the infant needing to go to the NICU shared that they desired someone to speak with them and provide explanations about what was happening with their baby (Nystrom and Axelsson, 2002).*

- Reassure mother/family that early measures to sustain lactation and promote parent-infant attachment can make it possible to resume breastfeeding when the condition/situation requiring interruption is resolved. *Early breast stimulation assists in establishing lactation, and efforts to maintain lactation during interrupted breastfeeding can assist in the resumption of breastfeeding (Association of Women's Health Obstetric and Neonatal Nurses, 2000a; Hill et al, 1999, 2001; Jones et al, 2001; Jones and Spencer, 2001).* **Nursing Research:** *Researchers found that delays in suckling and milk expression may cause maternal prolactin levels to decrease suggesting the chance for difficulty in resuming lactation unless early measures are taken (Jones et al, 2001).*

- Reassure the mother/family that the infant will benefit from any amount of breast milk provided. *The benefits of breast milk include protection (immunity, reduced risk of allergies, etc.). Breast milk is the preferable nutrition source (Association of Women's Health Obstetric and Neonatal Nurses, 2000a,b; International Lactation Consultant Association, 1999; Raisler et al, 1999; Shanler et al, 1999; US Department of Health and Human Services, 2000).* **Nursing Research:** *In a large sample focused on high-risk groups, breastfeeding's protective effects against diarrhea, cough, and ear infection were found with doses other than full breastfeeding (Raisler et al, 1999).*

- Provide time for mother/family to express their expectations and concerns and give emotional support. Emotional responses regarding events leading to the interruption that may arise include feelings of grief/loss, guilt, anxiety, and failure. *Discussing concerns and differences between expectations and experiences provide an opportunity for the client to ventilate and may contribute to positive coping strategies (Boettcher et al, 1999; Mozingo et al, 2000; Nystrom and Axelsson, 2002; Porteous et al, 2000, Vari et al, 2000).* **Nursing Research:** *In a qualitative study, mothers who were separated from their newborns revealed emotional strain and anxiety regardless of the presence of serious illness (Nystrom and Axelsson, 2002).*

▲ Collaborate with the mother/family/health care providers/employers (as needed) to develop a plan for expression of breast milk/infant feeding/and kangaroo care/skin-to-skin contact (KC). *Clients' participation will assure the success of the plan, promote maternal confidence and self-esteem, and/or facilitate maternal role performance (Charpak et al, 2001; Griffin et al, 2000; Hill et al, 1999; Libbus and Bullock, 2002; Matthiesen et al, 2001; Pugh et al, 1999).* **Nursing Research:** *In a small study of mothers of preterm infants, mothers who pumped more frequently and participated in KC had adequate milk*

• = **Independent;** ▲ = **Collaborative**

weights more frequently than those who pumped less and participated less in KC (Hill et al, 1999).

- Monitor for signs indicating infants' ability to and interest in breastfeeding. *The infant must be able to demonstrate the ability to breastfeed and demonstrate responsiveness for the mother to begin/ resume breastfeeding. The interplay between mother and baby is an important factor in maternal confidence and breastfeeding success (Mennella, 2001; Pridham et al, 2001; Thomas, 2000).* **Nursing Research:** *Researchers found that an infant's contentedness and soothability (aspects of responsiveness) contribute to mothers' evaluation of self in relation to confidence and competence (Pridham et al, 2001).*

- Provide evidence-based teaching and practical assistance with milk expression, storage, temporary feeding techniques, and breastfeeding techniques appropriate to the client's individualized needs (see Client/Family Teaching). *Accurate, consistent information and providing practical assistance based on evidence and in response to individualized needs are associated with maternal confidence, client satisfaction, and successful breastfeeding (Association of Women's Health Obstetric and Neonatal Nurses, 2000b; Hattori and Hattori, 1999; Jones et al, 2001; Lauver et al, 2002; Meier et al, 2000; Nyqvist, 2002; Philipp and Merewood, 2003; Pugh et al, 1999).* **Nursing Research:** *In a prospective study of a small number of mothers delivering preterm twins, the researcher elicited mothers' need for special support and nurses practical assistance, encouragement, and emotional support (Nyqvist, 2002).*

- Observe mother performing psychomotor skill (expression, storage, alternative feeding, KC, and/or breastfeeding) and assist as needed. *The nurse's presence and involvement allow for identification of those areas for which assistance, clarification, and/or support are needed and promotes maternal confidence (Association of Women's Health Obstetric and Neonatal Nurses, 2000a; Gill, 2001; Hong, Callister, and Schwartz, 2003; US Department of Health and Human Services, 2000).* **Nursing Research:** *Evidence-based guidelines include observation and practical assistance with psychomotor skills for all women/families (Association of Women's Health Obstetric and Neonatal Nurses, 2000a; US Department of Health and Human Services, 2000).*

- ▲ Provide and/or assist with arrangements for necessary equipment. *Pumping and other equipment recommendations should be based on each mother's/infant's situation and needs (Biancuzzo, 1999a; Dowling, 1999; Hill et al, 1999; Meier et al, 2000).* **Nursing Research:** *The researcher found that for some infants orthodontic nipple use for bottle-feeding resulted in physiological stability and effective feeding behaviors when preterm infants could not be breastfed (Dowling, 1999).*

- ▲ Use supplementation only as medically indicated. *If human milk can be provided and fed to the infant, it is preferable (Association of Women's Health Obstetric and Neonatal Nurses, 2000a; Fenton et al, 2000; International Lactation Consultant Association, 1999; Schanler et al, 1999).* **Nursing Research:** *Researchers found that mothers of very-low-birth-weight infants who used commercial breast milk enhancing powder products with expressed breast milk were able to achieve lactation durations closer to their stated goals (Fenton et al, 2000).*

- Provide anticipatory guidance for common problems associated with interrupted breastfeeding (e.g., incomplete emptying of milk glands, diminishing milk supply, infant difficulty with resuming breastfeeding, or infant refusal of alternative feeding method). *Mothers who are know what to expect will feel more confident and be more likely to cope with any difficulties that may arise (Blyth et al, 2002; Libbus and Bullock, 2002; Pugh et al, 1999; Thoyre, 2000).* **Nursing Research:** *Researchers found that the most com-*

• = Independent; ▲ = Collaborative

mon reason for discontinuation of breastfeeding was insufficient milk supply (Blyth et al, 2002).

▲ Initiate follow-up and make appropriate referrals. *Follow-up provides the opportunity for review of information, feedback about techniques, identification of and assistance with problems, and promotes maternal confidence and satisfaction (Association of Women's Health Obstetric and Neonatal Nurses, 2000a; Locklin and Jansson, 1999; Pugh et al, 2002).* **Nursing Research:** *Breastfeeding women receiving nurse and peer counselor support had longer duration of breastfeeding and infants had fewer sick visits and reported use of fewer medications than those receiving usual care (Pugh et al, 2002).*

• Assist the client to accept and learn an alternative method of infant feeding if effective breastfeeding is not achieved. *If it is clear that breastfeeding cannot be achieved following the interruption and an alternative feeding method must be instituted, the mother needs support and education (Mozingo et al, 2000).* **Nursing Research:** *In a qualitative study of women's experiences with short-term breastfeeding, researchers uncovered women's concerns about breastfeeding failure and their feelings of relief versus guilt and shame for which women may need assistance and support (Mozingo et al, 2000).*

Multicultural

• Assess for the influence of cultural beliefs, norms, and values on current decision to stop breastfeeding. **Nursing Research:** *The client's decision to halt breastfeeding may be based on cultural perceptions, as well as influences from the larger social context (Cochran, 1998; Doswell and Erlen, 1998; Leininger and McFarland, 2002).*

• Assess the influence of family support on the decision to continue or discontinue breastfeeding. **Nursing Research:** *Women are the keepers and transmitters of culture in families. Female family members can play a dominant role in how infants are fed (Cesario, 2001; Guarnaccia, 1998; Pillitteri, 1999).*

• Assess whether the client's concerns about the amount of milk taken during breastfeeding is contributing to decision to stop breastfeeding. **Nursing Research:** *Some cultures may add semisolid food within the first month of life as a result of concerns that the infant is not getting enough to eat and the perception that "big is healthy" (Bentley et al, 1999; Higgins, 2000).*

• Validate the client's feelings with regard to the difficulty of or her dissatisfaction with breastfeeding. **Nursing Research:** *Validation is a therapeutic communication technique that lets the client know that the nurse has heard and understands what was said and promotes the nurse-client relationship (Heineken, 1998).*

Client/Family Teaching

• Teach mother effective methods to express breast milk. *There are a variety of methods of expression and these involve psychomotor skills requiring instruction; breast stimulation is essential to continuing lactation (Association of Women's Health Obstetric and Neonatal Nurses, 2000a; Biancuzzo, 1999a; Fewtrell et al, 2001; International Lactation Consultant Association, 1999; Jones et al, 2001; Matthiesen et al, 2001; Phillip and Merewood, 2003).* **Nursing Research:** *In a sample of women who delivered preterm infants, researchers testing the use of electric and manual pumps found that those using the electric pump had shorter expression times but produced no more milk than those using the manual pump (Fewtrell et al, 2001).*

• Teach mother/parents about kangaroo care. *Indirect stimulation of lactation through close contact with the infant can occur and KC has been associated with positive neonatal out-*

• = Independent; ▲ = Collaborative

comes (Charpak et al, 2001; Daley and Kennedy, 2000; Mellien, 2001). **Nursing Research:** *In a small study of very-low-weight preterm infants, the infants maintained a stable temperature in their mothers' arms with no indication of increased metabolic activity (Mellien, 2001).*

- Instruct mother on safe breast milk handling techniques. *Storage and handling practices can optimize the nutritional value and provide protection against contaminants (Association of Women's Health Obstetric and Neonatal Nurses, 2000a; Biancuzzo, 1999b; International Lactation Consultant Association, 1999; Phillipp and Merewood, 2003; Tully, 2000).* **Nursing Research:** *Evidence-based guidelines address the importance of expression, storage, and provision of stored human milk in cases of mother-infant separation particularly as it relates to women returning to work (Association of Women's Health Obstetric and Neonatal Nurses, 2000a,b; International Lactation Consultant Association, 1999).*

- Provide education to father/family/significant others as needed. *Informed support people have a desire to learn, may be needed to assist mothers who are separated from their infants, and may have an impact on breastfeeding duration (Association of Women's Health Obstetric and Neonatal Nurses, 2000a; Guttman and Zimmerman, 2000; Hill, 2000; Moore, 2000; Pollock et al, 2002; Susin et al, 1999).* **Nursing Research:** *Paternal knowledge was associated with frequency and duration of breastfeeding (Susin et al, 1999).*

evolve WEBSITES FOR EDUCATION

See the EVOLVE website for World Wide Web resources for client education.

REFERENCES

Association of Women's Health Obstetric and Neonatal Nurses: *Evidence-based clinical practice guideline: breastfeeding support: prenatal care through the first year (practice guideline)*, Washington, DC, 2000a, The Association.

Association of Women's Health Obstetric and Neonatal Nurses: *Evidence-based clinical practice guideline: breastfeeding support: prenatal care through the first year (monograph)*, Washington, DC, 2000b, The Association.

Auerbach KG: Breastfeeding and maternal medication use, *J Gynecol Neonat Nurs* 28:554, 1999.

Bentley M et al: Infant feeding practices of low-income, African American, adolescent mothers: an ecological, multigenerational perspective, *Soc Sci Med* 49(8):10850, 1999.

Biancuzzo M: Selecting pumps for breastfeeding mothers, *J Gynecol Neonat Nurs* 28:417, 1999a.

Biancuzzo M: *Breastfeeding the newborn: clinical strategies for nurses*, St Louis, 1999b, Mosby.

Blyth R et al: Effect of maternal confidence on breastfeeding duration: an application of breastfeeding self-efficacy theory, *Birth* 29:278, 2002.

Boettcher JP et al: Interaction of factors related to lactation duration, *J Perinat Educ* 8 (2):11, 1999.

Cesario S: Care of the Native American woman: strategies for practice, education, and research, *J Gynecol Neonat Nurs* 30(1):13, 2001.

Charpak N et al: A randomized, controlled trial of kangaroo mother care: results of follow-up at 1 year of corrected age, *Pediatrics* 108:10729, 2001.

Cochran M: Tears have no color, *Am J Nurs* 98(6):53, 1998.

Daley HK, Kennedy CM: Meta analysis: effects of interventions on premature infants feeding, *J Perinat Neonat Nurs* 14:62, 2000.

Davis LJ, Okuboye S, Ferguson SL: Healthy people 2010: examining a decade of maternal and infant health, *Association of Women's Health Obstetric and Neonatal Nurses Lifelines* 4(3):26, 2000.

Doswell W, Erlen J: Multicultural issues and ethical concerns in the delivery of revising care interventions, *Nurs Clin North Am* 33(2):353, 1998.

Dowling DA: Physiological responses of preterm infants to breast-feeding and bottle-feeding with the orthodontic nipple, *Nurs Res* 48:78, 1999.

● = **Independent;** ▲ = **Collaborative**

Fenton TR, Tough SC, Belik J: Breast milk supplementation for preterm infants: parental preferences and postdischarge lactation duration, *Am J Perinatol* 17:329, 2000.

Fewtrell MS et al: Randomized trial comparing the efficacy of a novel manual breast pump with a standard electric breast pump in mothers who delivered preterm infants, *Pediatrics* 107:12917, 2001.

Gill SL: The little things: perceptions of breastfeeding support, *J Gynecol Neonat Nurs* 30:401, 2001.

Griffin TL et al: Mothers' performing creamatocrit measures in the NICU: accuracy, reactions, and cost, *J Gynecol Neonat Nurs* 29:249, 2000.

Guarnaccia P: Multicultural experiences of family caregiving: a study of African American, European American, and Hispanic American families, *New Direct Ment Health Serv* 77:45, 1998.

Guttman N, Zimmerman DR: Low-income mothers' views on breastfeeding, *Soc Sci Med* 50:14573, 2000.

Hattori R, Hattori H: Breastfeeding twins: guidelines for success, *Birth* 26:37, 1999.

Heineken J: Patient silence is not necessarily client satisfaction: communication in home care nursing, *Home Health Care Nurse* 16(2):115, 1998.

Higgins B: Puerto Rican cultural beliefs: influence on infant feeding practices in western New York, *J Transcult Nurs* 11(1), 2000.

Hill PD: Update on breastfeeding: Healthy People 2010 objectives, *MCN Am J Matern Child Nurs* 25:248, 2000.

Hill PD, Aldag JC, Chatterton RT: Effects of pumping style on milk production in mothers of nonnursing preterm infants, *J Hum Lact* 15:209, 1999a.

Hill PD, Aldag JC, Chatterton RT: Breastfeeding experience and milk weight in lactating mothers pumping for preterm infants, *Birth* 26:233, 1999b.

Hong TM, Callister LC, Schwartz R: First-time mothers' views of breastfeeding support from nurses, *MCN Am J Matern Child Nurs* 28:10, 2003.

International Lactation Consultant Association: *Evidence-based guidelines for breastfeeding management during the first fourteen days,* Raleigh, NC, 1999, The Association.

Ito S: Drug therapy: drug therapy for breast-feeding women, *N Engl J Med* 343:118, 2000.

Jones E, Dimmock PW, Spencer SA: A randomized controlled trial to compare methods of milk expression after preterm delivery, *Am Dis Child* 85, F91-F95, 2001.

Jones E, Spencer SA: Promoting successful breastfeeding for mothers of preterm infants, *Prof Care Mother Child* 10:145, 2001.

Kloeblen-Tarver AS, Thompson NJ, Miner KR: Intent to breast-feed: the impact of attitudes, norms, parity, and experience, *Am J Health Behav* 26:182, 2002.

Lauver DR et al: Patient-centered interventions, *Res Nurs Health* 25:246, 2002.

Leininger MM, McFarland MR: *Transcultural nursing: concepts, theories, research and practices,* ed 3, New York, 2002, McGraw-Hill.

Libbus MK, Bullock LFC: Breastfeeding and employment: an assessment of employers' attitudes, *J Hum Lact* 18:247, 2002.

Locklin MP, Jansson MJ: Home visits: strategies to protect the breastfeeding newborn at risk, *J Gynecol Neonat Nurs* 28:33, 1999.

Matthiesen AS et al: Postpartum maternal oxytocin release by newborns: effects of infant hand massage and sucking, *Birth* 28:13, 2001.

Meier PP et al: Nipple shields for preterm infants: effect on milk transfer and duration of breastfeeding, *J Hum Lact* 16:106, 2000.

Mellien AC: Incubators versus mothers' arms: body temperature conservation in very-low-birth-weight premature infants, *J Gynecol Neonat Nurs* 30:157, 2001.

Mennella JA: Regulation of milk intake after exposure to alcohol in mothers' milk, *Alcoholism* 25:590, 2001.

Meyer K, Anderson GC: Using kangaroo care in a clinical setting with full-term infants having breastfeeding difficulties, *MCN Am J Matern Child Nurs* 24:190, 1999.

Mozingo JN et al: "It wasn't working": women's experiences with short-term breastfeeding, *MCN Am J Matern Child Nurs* 25:120, 2000.

Nyqvist KH: Breast-feeding in preterm twins: development of feeding behavior and milk intake during hospital stay and related caregiving practices, *J Pediatr Nurs* 17:246, 2002.

Nystrom K, Axelsson K: Mothers' experience of being separated from their newborns, *J Gynecol Neonat Nurs* 31, 275, 2002.

Philipp BL, Merewood A: Encouraging patients to use a breast pump, *Cont OB/GYN* 48:88, 2003.

Pillitteri A: Nutritional needs of the newborn. In Pillitteri A, editor: *Maternal and child health nursing: care of the childbearing and childrearing family,* Philadelphia, 1999, Lippincott.

• = **Independent**; ▲ = **Collaborative**

Pinelli J, Atkinson SA, Saigal S: Randomized trial of breastfeeding support in very low-birth-weight infants, *Arch Pediatr Adolesc Med* 155:548, 2001.

Pollock CA, Bustamante-Forest R, Giarratano G: Men of diverse cultures: knowledge and attitudes about breastfeeding, *J Gynecol Neonat Nurs* 31:673, 2002.

Porteous R, Kaufman K, Rush J: The effect of individualized professional support on duration of breastfeeding: a randomized controlled trial, *J Hum Lact* 16:303, 2000.

Pridham K, Lin CY, Brown R: Mothers' evaluation of their caregiving for premature and full-term infants through the first year: contributing factors, *Res Nurs Health* 24:157, 2001.

Pugh LC et al: Clinical approaches in the assessment of childbearing fatigue, *J Gynecol Neonat Nurs* 28:74, 1999.

Pugh LC et al: Breastfeeding duration, costs, and benefits of a support program for low-income breastfeeding women, *Birth* 29:95, 2002.

Raisler J, Alexander C, O'Campo P: Breast-feeding and infant illness: a dose-response relationship? *Am J Public Health* 89:25, 1999.

Schanler RJ, Shulman RJ, Chantal D: Feeding strategies for premature infants: beneficial outcomes of feeding fortified human milk versus preterm formula (part 1), *Pediatrics* 103:11507, 1999.

Susin LR et al: Does parental breastfeeding knowledge increase breastfeeding rates? *Birth* 26:149, 1999.

Thomas KA: Differential effects of breast- and formula-feeding on preterm infants sleep-wake patterns, *J Gynecol Neonat Nurs* 29:145, 2000.

Thoyre SM: Mothers' ideas about their role in feeding their high-risk infants, *J Gynecol Neonat Nurs* 29:613, 2000.

Tully MR: Recommendations for handling of mothers' own milk, *J Hum Lact* 16:149, 2000.

US Department of Health and Human Services: *HHS blueprint for action on breastfeeding,* Washington, DC, 2000, US Department of Health and Human Services, Office on Women's Health.

Vari PM, Camburn J, Henly SJ: Professionally mediated peer support and early breastfeeding success, *J Perinat Educ* 9:22, 2000.

Ward RM et al: The transfer of drugs and other chemicals into human milk, *Pediatrics* 108:776, 2001.

Ineffective Breathing pattern

Betty J. Ackley

NANDA Definition

Inspiration and/or expiration that does not provide adequate ventilation

Defining Characteristics

Decreased inspiratory/expiratory pressure; decreased minute ventilation; use of accessory muscles to breathe; nasal flaring; dyspnea; altered chest excursion; shortness of breath; assumption of a three-point position; pursed-lip breathing; prolonged expiration phases; increased anteroposterior diameter; respiratory rate (adults <11 or >24; infants <25 or >60; ages 1 to 4 <20 or >30; ages 5 to 14 <14 or >25); depth of breathing (adults ventilation 500 ml at rest; infants 6 to 8 ml/kg); timing ratio; decreased vital capacity

Related Factors (r/t)

Hyperventilation; hypoventilation syndrome; bony deformity; pain; chest wall deformity; anxiety; decreased energy/fatigue; neuromuscular dysfunction; musculoskeletal impairment; perception/cognitive impairment; obesity; spinal cord injury; body position; neurological immaturity; respiratory muscle fatigue

• = Independent; ▲ = Collaborative

Outcomes (Nursing Outcomes Classification)

Suggested NOC Outcomes

Respiratory Status: Airway Patency, Ventilation; Vital Signs

Example NOC Outcome with Indicators

Respiratory Status: Ventilation as evidenced by the following indicators: Respiratory rate IER/Respiratory rhythm IER/Depth of inspiration/Chest expansion symmetrical/Ease of breathing/Accessory muscle use not present/Chest retraction not present/Auscultated breath sounds IER/Tidal volume IER/Vital capacity IER (Rate each indicator of **Respiratory Status: Ventilation:** 1 = extremely compromised, 2 = substantially compromised, 3 = moderately compromised, 4 = mildly compromised, 5 = not compromised [see Section I].)

IER, In expected range.

Client Outcomes

Client Will (Specify Time Frame):
- Demonstrate a breathing pattern that supports blood gas results within the client's normal parameters
- Report ability to breathe comfortably
- Demonstrate ability to perform pursed-lip breathing and controlled breathing and use relaxation techniques effectively
- Identify and avoid specific factors that exacerbate episodes of ineffective breathing patterns

NIC   Interventions (Nursing Interventions Classification)

Suggested NIC Interventions

Airway Management; Respiratory Monitoring

Example NIC Activities—Airway Management

Encourage slow, deep breathing; turning; and coughing; Monitor respiratory and oxygenation status as appropriate

---

Nursing Interventions and Rationales

- Monitor respiratory rate, depth, and ease of respiration. Normal respiratory rate is 12 to 16 breaths/min in the adult. *When the respiratory rate exceeds 24 breaths/min, there is often significant respiratory or cardiovascular disease. See Defining Characteristics for guidelines for children.*
- Note pattern of respiration. If client is dyspneic, note what seems to cause the dyspnea, the way in which the client deals with the condition, and how the dyspnea resolves or gets worse. *A normal respiratory pattern is regular in a healthy adult. To assess dyspnea, it is important to consider all of its dimensions, including antecedents, mediators, reactions, and outcomes (McCord and Cronin-Stubbs, 1992; Meek, 1999).*
- Attempt to determine if client's dyspnea is physiological or psychogenic in cause. *There are two distinct categories of antecedents to dyspnea: physiological and psychogenic.*

• = Independent; ▲ = Collaborative

Psychogenic dyspnea includes dyspnea caused by anxiety, fear, or anger (McCord and Cronin-Stubbs, 1992). Psychogenic dyspnea is commonly known as hyperventilation.

Psychogenic Dyspnea—Hyperventilation

- Assess cause of hyperventilation by asking client about current emotions and psychological state. *Hyperventilation can be caused by factors including anxiety, fear, pain, and anger (McCord and Cronin-Stubbs, 1992).*
- Ask the client to breathe with you to slow down respiratory rate. Maintain eye contact and give reassurance. *By making the client aware of respirations and giving support, the client may gain control of the breathing rate.*
- Consider having client use a paper bag to breathe into and rebreathe expired air or help to do diaphragmatic breathing. *Rebreathing air with increased levels of carbon dioxide helps raise the carbon dioxide level in the body and combats the respiratory alkalosis that follows hyperventilation (Forrest and Ricketts, 1995).*
- ▲ If pain is the cause of hyperventilation, provide medication routinely as ordered to prevent severe pain. Use distraction techniques to help client deal with pain. See interventions for **Acute Pain.** *An increased respiratory rate is one sign of pain. Providing pain relief will cause the respiratory rate to return to normal.*
- ▲ If client has chronic problems with hyperventilation, numbness and tingling in extremities, dizziness, and other signs of panic attacks, refer for counseling. *Cognitive behavioral therapy for hyperventilation and panic attacks has been shown to be beneficial (Forrest and Ricketts, 1995).*

Physiological Dyspnea

- ▲ Ensure that client in acute dyspneic state has received medications, oxygen, and any other treatment needed. *Pharmacological treatment of dyspnea exists but may not suffice to relieve dyspnea (Bruera et al, 2000; Janssens, 2000).*
- Determine severity of dyspnea using a rating scale such as the modified Borg scale, rating dyspnea 0 (best) to 10 (worst) in severity. An alternative scale is the Visual Analogue Scale (VAS) with dyspnea rated as 0 (best) to 100 (worst). **Nursing and Clinical Research:** *In a study in an emergency room, the modified Borg scale correlated well with clinical measurements of respiratory function and was found helpful by both clients and nurses (Kendrick et al, 2000). Another study comparing the Borg and the VAS scales found that they measured symptoms reproducibly during steady-state exercise and can detect the effect of a drug intervention (Grant et al, 1999).*
- Note abdominal breathing, use of accessory muscles, nasal flaring, retractions, irritability, confusion, or lethargy. *These symptoms signal increasing respiratory difficulty and increasing hypoxia.*
- Observe color of tongue, oral mucosa, and skin. *Cyanosis of the tongue and oral mucosa is central cyanosis and generally represents a medical emergency. Peripheral cyanosis of nail beds or lips may or may not be serious (Carpenter, 1993).*
- Auscultate breath sounds, noting decreased or absent sounds, crackles, or wheezes. *These abnormal lung sounds can indicate a respiratory pathology associated with an altered breathing pattern.*
- ▲ Monitor client's oxygen saturation and blood gases. *An oxygen saturation of less than 90% (normal: 95% to 100%) or a partial pressure of oxygen of less than 80 (normal: 80 to 100) indicates significant oxygenation problems (Berry and Pinard, 2002; Grap, 2002).*
- ▲ Monitor for presence of pain and provide pain medication for comfort as needed. *Pain*

• = Independent; ▲ = Collaborative

causes the client to hypoventilate and take shallow breaths that predispose the client to atelectasis.

- Using touch on the shoulder, coach the client to slow respiratory rate, demonstrating slower respirations; making eye contact with the client; and communicating in a calm, supportive fashion. *The nurse's presence, reassurance, and help in controlling the client's breathing can be very beneficial in decreasing anxiety (Truesdell, 2000).* **Nursing Research:** *Anxiety can exacerbate dyspnea, causing the client to enter into a dyspneic panic state (Gift et al, 1992).*

- Demonstrate and encourage the client to use pursed-lip breathing. *Pursed-lip breathing results in increased use of intercostal muscles, decreased respiratory rate, increased tidal volume, and improved oxygen saturation levels (Collins et al, 2001). Pursed-lip breathing can result in increased exercise performance, and it empowers the client to self-manage dyspneic incidences (Truesdell, 2000).*

- Position the client in an upright or semi-Fowler's position. *An upright position facilitates lung expansion. See nursing interventions for* **Impaired Gas exchange** *for further information on positioning.*

▲ Administer oxygen as ordered. *Oxygen therapy helps decrease dyspnea through reduction in the central drive mediated via peripheral chemoreceptors in the carotid body (Meek, 1999).*

- Increase client's activity to walking three times per day as tolerated. Assist the client to use oxygen during activity as needed. *See nursing interventions for* **Activity intolerance.** Supervised exercise has been shown to decrease dyspnea and increase tolerance to activity (Meek, 1999). **Nursing Research:** *A group of COPD clients who participated in a systematic movement program used less emotion-focused coping than did nonexercisers (Gift and Austin, 1992).*

- Schedule rest periods before and after activity. *Respiratory clients with dyspnea are easily exhausted and need additional rest.*

▲ Evaluate the client's nutritional status. Refer to a dietitian if needed. Use nutritional supplements to increase nutritional level if need indicated. *Improved nutrition may help increase inspiratory muscle function and decrease dyspnea (Meek, 1999).*

- Provide small, frequent feedings. Small feedings are given to avoid compromising ventilatory effort and to conserve energy. *Clients with dyspnea often do not eat sufficient amounts of food because their priority is breathing.*

- Offer a fan to move the air in the environment. *The movement of cool air on the face may help relieve dyspnea in pulmonary clients (Meek, 1999).*

- Encourage the client to take deep breaths at prescribed intervals and do controlled coughing. Help the client with chronic respiratory disease to evaluate dyspnea experience to determine if similar to previous incidences of dyspnea and to recognize that he or she made it through those incidences. Encourage the client to be self-reliant if possible, use problem solving skills, and maximize use of social support. *The focus of attention on sensations of breathlessness has an impact on judgment used to determine the intensity of the sensation (Meek, 2000).* **Nursing Research:** *One study demonstrated that the most frequently used coping styles for clients with COPD were being optimistic and self-reliant, using problem-solving skills, and receiving social support (Baker and Scholz, 2002).*

- See **Ineffective Airway clearance** if client has a problem with increased respiratory secretions.

▲ Refer COPD client for pulmonary rehabilitation. **Clinical Research:** *Pulmonary rehabilitation has been shown to relieve dyspnea and fatigue, and enhance clients' sense of con-*

- = Independent; ▲ = Collaborative

trol over their disease. *Rehabilitation is an important component of the management of COPD (Lacasse et al, 2002).*

Geriatric

- Encourage ambulation as tolerated. *Immobility is often harmful to the elderly because it decreases ventilation and increases stasis of secretions (Foyt, 1992; Tempkin et al, 1997).*
- Encourage elderly clients to sit upright or stand and to avoid lying down for prolonged periods during the day. *Thoracic aging results in decreased lung expansion; an erect position fosters maximal lung expansion.*

Home care

- Above interventions may be adapted for home care use.
- Assist the client and family with identifying other factors that precipitate or exacerbate episodes of ineffective breathing patterns (i.e., stress, allergens, stairs, activities that have high energy requirements). *Awareness of precipitating factors helps clients avoid them and decreases risk of ineffective breathing episodes.*
- Assess client knowledge of and compliance with medication regimen. *Client/family may need repetition of instructions received at hospital discharge, and may require reiteration as fear of a recent crisis decreases. Fear interferes with the ability to assimilate new information.*
- Teach the client and family the importance of maintaining regimen and having prn drugs easily accessible at all times. *Appropriate and timely use of medications can decrease the risk of exacerbating ineffective breathing.*
- Provide the client with emotional support in dealing with symptoms of respiratory difficulty. Provide family with support for care of a client with chronic or terminal illness. *Breathing difficulty can provoke extreme anxiety, which can interfere with the client's ability or willingness to adhere to the treatment plan. Refer to care plan for* **Anxiety.** *Witnessing breathing difficulties and facing concerns of dealing with chronic or terminal illness can create fear in caregiver. Fear inhibits effective coping.*
- ▲ Identify an emergency plan including when to call the physician or 911. *Having a ready emergency plan reassures the client and promotes client safety.*
- ▲ Refer the client to an outpatient pulmonary rehabilitation program or a home-based training program for COPD. **Clinical Research:** *Outpatient rehabilitation programs can achieve worthwhile benefits including decreased perception of dyspnea, increased walking distance, and less fatigue (Glell et al, 2000; Lacasse et al, 2002). A simple home-based program of exercise training can help COPD clients achieve improvement in exercise tolerance, dyspnea, and quality of life (Hernandez et al, 2000).*
- ▲ Refer to occupational therapy for evaluation and teaching of energy conservation techniques.
- ▲ Refer to home health aide services as needed to support energy conservation. *Energy conservation decreases the risk of exacerbating ineffective breathing.*
- ▲ Institute case management of frail elderly to support continued independent living. Respiratory difficulties represent and can lead to increasing needs for assistance in using the health care system effectively. Case management combines nursing activities of client and family assessment, planning and coordination of care among all health care providers, delivery of direct nursing care, and monitoring of care and outcomes. *These activities are able to address continuity of care, mutual goal setting, behavior management, and prevention of worsening health problems (Guttman, 1999).*

- • = **Independent;** ▲ = **Collaborative**

Client/Family Teaching

- Teach pursed-lip and controlled breathing techniques. *Pursed-lip breathing results in increased use of intercostal muscles, decreased respiratory rate, increased tidal volume, and improved oxygen saturation levels (Collins et al, 2001).*
- Using a prerecorded tape, teach client progressive muscle relaxation techniques. **Nursing Research:** *Relaxation therapy can help reduce dyspnea and anxiety (Gift et al, 1992).*
- Teach about dosage, actions, and side effects of medications. *Inhaled steroids and bronchodilators can have undesirable side effects, especially when taken in inappropriate doses.*
- Teach the client to identify and avoid specific factors that exacerbate ineffective breathing patterns, such as exposure to other sources of air pollution (especially smoking).

evolve WEBSITES FOR EDUCATION

See the EVOLVE website for World Wide Web resources for client education.

REFERENCES

Baker CF, Scholz JA: Coping with symptoms of dyspnea in chronic obstructive pulmonary disease, *Rehabil Nurs* 27(2):67, 2002.

Breslin EH: The pattern of respiratory muscle recruitment during pursed-lip breathing, *Chest* 101(1):75, 1992.

Bruera E et al: The frequency and correlates of dyspnea in patients with advanced cancer, *J Pain Symptom Manage* 19(5):357, 2000.

Carpenter KD: A comprehensive review of cyanosis, *Crit Care Nurse* 13:66, 1993.

Collins EG et al: Breathing pattern retraining and exercise in person with chronic obstructive pulmonary disease. *AACN Clin Issues* 12(2):202, 2001.

Forrest J, Ricketts T: A cognitive approach to panic disorder, *Nurs Times* 91(45):27, 1995.

Foyt MM: Impaired gas exchange in the elderly, *Geriatr Nurs* 13:262, 1992.

Gift A, Austin D. The effects of a program of systematic movement on COPD patients, *Rehabil Nurs* 17:6, 1992.

Gift A, Moore T, Soeken K: Relaxation to reduce dyspnea and anxiety in COPD patients, *Nurs Res* 41(4):242, 1992.

Glell R et al: Long-term effects of outpatient rehabilitation of COPD: a randomized trial, *Chest* 117(4), 2000.

Grant S et al: A comparison of the reproducibility and the sensitivity to change of visual analogue scales, Borg scales, and Likert scales in normal subjects during submaximal exercise, *Chest* 116(5), 1999.

Guttman R: Case management of the frail elderly in the community, *Clin Nurs Spec* 13(4):174, 1999.

Hernandez MTE et al: Results of a home-based training program for patients with COPD, *Chest* 188(1), 2000.

Janssens JP, Muralt BD, Titelion V: Management of dyspnea in severe chronic obstructive pulmonary disease, *J Pain Symptom Manage* 19(5):378, 2000.

Kendrick KR, Baxi SC, Smith RM: Usefulness of the modified 1-10 Borg scale in assessing the degree of dyspnea in patients with COPD and asthma, *J Emerg Nurs* 26(3):216, 2000.

Lacasse Y et al: Pulmonary rehabilitation for chronic obstructive pulmonary disease, *Cochrane Database Syst Rev* CD003793(3), 2002.

McCord M, Cronin-Stubbs D: Operationalizing dyspnea: focus on measurement, *Heart Lung* 21(2):167, 1992.

Meek PM: Influence of attention and judgment on perception of breathlessness in healthy individuals and patients with chronic obstructive pulmonary disease, *Nurs Res* 49(1):11, 2000.

Meek PM et al: Dyspnea: mechanisms, assessment, and management: a consensus statement, *Am J Respir Crit Care Med* 159:321, 1999.

Tempkin T, Tempkin A, Goodman H: Geriatric rehabilitation, *Nurse Pract Forum* 8(2):59, 1997.

Truesdell S: Helping patients with COPD manage episodes of acute shortness of breath, *MedSurg Nurs* 9(4):178, 2000.

• = **Independent;** ▲ = **Collaborative**

Decreased Cardiac output

Betty J. Ackley and Linda L. Straight

NANDA Definition

Inadequate blood pumped by the heart to meet metabolic demands of the body

Defining Characteristics

Altered heart rate/rhythm: Dysrhythmias (tachycardia, bradycardia); palpitations; electrocardiographic changes

Altered preload: Jugular vein distention; fatigue; edema; murmurs; increased/decreased central venous pressure (CVP); increased/decreased pulmonary artery wedge pressure (PAWP); weight gain

Altered afterload: Cold/clammy skin; shortness of breath/dyspnea; oliguria; prolonged capillary refill; decreased peripheral pulses; variations in blood pressure readings; increased/decreased systemic vascular resistance (SVR); increased/decreased pulmonary vascular resistance (PVR); skin color changes

Altered contractility: Crackles; cough; orthopnea/paroxysmal nocturnal dyspnea; cardiac output less than 4 L/min; cardiac index less than 2.5 L/min; decreased ejection fraction; stroke volume index (SVI); left ventricular stroke work index (LVSWI); S3 or S4 sounds

Behavioral/emotional: Anxiety; restlessness

Related Factors (r/t)

Altered heart rate/rhythm; altered stroke volume: altered preload, altered afterload, altered contractility

NOC   Outcomes (Nursing Outcomes Classification)

Suggested NOC Outcomes

Cardiac Pump Effectiveness; Circulation Status; Tissue Perfusion: Abdominal Organs, Peripheral; Vital Signs

---

Example NOC Outcome with Indicators

Cardiac Pump Effectiveness as evidenced by the following indicators: blood pressure IER/Heart rate IER/Cardiac index IER/Ejection fraction IER/Activity tolerance IER/Peripheral pulses strong/NVD not present/ Dysrhythmias not present/Abnormal heart sounds not present/Angina not present/Peripheral edema not present/ Pulmonary edema not present (Rate each indicator of **Cardiac Pump Effectiveness:** 1 = extremely compromised, 2 = substantially compromised, 3 = moderately compromised, 4 = mildly compromised, 5 = not compromised [see Section I].)

IER, In expected range; *NVD,* neck vein distention.

• = Independent; ▲ = Collaborative

Client Outcomes

Client Will (Specify Time Frame):

- Demonstrate adequate cardiac output as evidenced by blood pressure and pulse rate and rhythm within normal parameters for client; strong peripheral pulses; and an ability to tolerate activity without symptoms of dyspnea, syncope, or chest pain
- Remain free of side effects from the medications used to achieve adequate cardiac output
- Explain actions and precautions to take for cardiac disease

NIC ₀ Interventions (Nursing Interventions Classification)

Suggested NIC Interventions

Cardiac Care; Cardiac Care: Acute

Example NIC Activities—Cardiac Care

Evaluate chest pain (e.g., intensity, location, radiation, duration, and precipitating and alleviating factors); Document cardiac dysrhythmias

---

Nursing Interventions and Rationales

- Monitor for symptoms of heart failure and decreased cardiac output; listen to heart sounds, lung sounds, note symptoms including paroxysmal nocturnal dyspnea, neck vein distention, crackles in lung bases, S3 gallop, increased venous pressure greater than 16 cm H_2O, and positive hepatojugular reflex. *These are major criteria for diagnosis of heart failure—the Framingham Criteria (Braunwald et al, 2001).*
- Observe for symptoms of cardiogenic shock including impaired mentation, hypotension with blood pressure lower than 90 mm Hg, decreased peripheral pulses, cold clammy skin, signs of pulmonary congestion and decreased organ function. If present, notify physician immediately. *Cardiogenic shock is a state of circulatory failure from loss from cardiac function associated with inadequate organ perfusion with a high mortality rate (Clark and Kruse, 2003).* **Nursing Research:** *In a study the defining characteristics of decreased cardiac output were best indicated by decreased peripheral pulses and decreased peripheral perfusion (Oliva and Cruz, 2003).*
- If shock is present, monitor hemodynamic parameters for an increase in pulmonary wedge pressure, an increase in systemic vascular resistance, or a decrease in cardiac output and index. *Hemodynamic parameters give a good indication of cardiac function (Sole et al, 2001).*
- Titrate inotropic and vasoactive medications within defined parameters to maintain contractility, preload, and afterload per physician's order. *By following parameters, the nurse ensures maintenance of a delicate balance of medications that stimulate the heart to increase contractility, while maintaining adequate perfusion of the body.*
- Observe for chest pain or discomfort; note location, radiation, severity, quality, duration, associated manifestations such as nausea, indigestion, and diaphoresis, also note precipitating and relieving factors. *Chest pain/discomfort is generally indicative of an inadequate blood supply to the heart, which can compromise cardiac output. Clients with heart failure can continue to have chest pain with angina or can reinfarct.*
- If chest pain is present, have client lie down, monitor cardiac rhythm, give oxygen, check vital signs, run a strip, medicate for pain, and notify the physician. *Prompt assess-*

• = Independent; ▲ = Collaborative

ment of the client with acute coronary symptoms is critical because the incidence of ventricular fibrillation is 15 times greater during the first hour after symptoms of an acute myocardial infection (Newberry, 2003).

- Monitor intake and output. If client is acutely ill, measure hourly urine output and note decreases in output. *Decreased cardiac output results in decreased perfusion of the kidneys, with a resulting decrease in urine output.*

- Note results of electrocardiography and chest radiography. *An electrocardiogram can reveal previous MI, or evidence of left ventricular hypertrophy, indicating aortic stenosis or chronic systemic hypertension. Radiography may provide information on pulmonary edema, pleural effusions, or enlarged cardiac silhouette found in dilated cardiomyopathy or large pericardial effusion (Fuster et al, 2001).*

- Note results of diagnostic imaging studies such as echocardiogram, radionuclide imaging, or dobutamine stress echocardiography. *The echocardiogram is the most important imaging tool for evaluating clients with symptoms of heart failure because overall systolic function and chamber size can be evaluated quickly. In addition, global versus regional left ventricular function, valvular abnormalities, and diastolic function can be defined, assisting in differential diagnosis (Fuster et al, 2001). An ejection fraction in a healthy heart is approximately 50%. Most clients experiencing heart failure have an ejection fraction of less than 40% (Janowski, 1996).*

- Watch laboratory data closely, especially arterial blood gases, electrolytes including potassium, and B-type natriuretic peptide (BNP assay). *Client may be receiving cardiac glycosides and the potential for toxicity is greater with hypokalemia; hypokalemia is common in heart clients because of diuretic use (Lessig and Lessig, 1998).* **Clinical Research:** *Rapid measurement of BNP is useful in establishing or eliminating the diagnosis of heart failure in the client with dyspnea (Maisel et al, 2002).*

- Monitor lab work such as complete blood count, sodium level, and serum creatinine. *Routine blood work can provide insight into the etiology of heart failure and extent of decompensation. A low serum sodium level often is observed with advanced heart failure and can be a poor prognostic sign (Fuster et al, 2001). Serum creatinine levels will elevate in clients with severe heart failure because of decreased perfusion to the kidneys.*

▲ Administer oxygen as needed per physician's order. *Supplemental oxygen increases oxygen availability to the myocardium.*

- Place client in semi-Fowler's position or position of comfort. *Elevating the head of the bed may decrease the work of breathing, and also decrease venous return and preload.*

- Check blood pressure, pulse, and condition before administering cardiac medications such as angiotensin-converting enzyme (ACE) inhibitors, digoxin, and beta-blockers such as carvedilol. Notify physician if heart rate or blood pressure is low before holding medications. *It is important that the nurse evaluate how well the client is tolerating current medications before administering cardiac medications; do not hold medications without physician input. The physician may decide to have medications administered even though the blood pressure or pulse rate has lowered.*

- During acute events, ensure client remains on short-term bed rest or maintains activity level that does not compromise cardiac output. *In severe heart failure, restriction of activity reduces the workload of the heart (Braunwald et al, 2001).*

- Gradually increase activity when client's condition is stabilized by encouraging slower paced activities or shorter periods of activity with frequent rest periods following exercise prescription; observe for symptoms of intolerance. Take blood pressure and

● = **Independent;** ▲ = **Collaborative**

pulse before and after activity and note changes. *Activity of the cardiac client should be closely monitored. See **Activity intolerance.***

- Serve small sodium-restricted, low-cholesterol meals. Sodium-restricted diets help decrease fluid volume excess. Low-cholesterol diets help decrease atherosclerosis, which causes coronary artery disease. Clients with cardiac disease tolerate smaller meals better because they require less cardiac output to digest. *Serve only small amounts of coffee or caffeine-containing beverages if requested (no more than four cups per 24 hours) if no resulting dysrhythmia. note: it is common practice to still restrict caffeine in the cardiac client.* **Nursing and Clinical Research:** *Moderate amounts of caffeine when ingested by the person used to caffeine, does not cause an increase in dysrhythmias (Myers and Harris, 1990; Schneider, 1987).*

- Monitor bowel function. Provide stool softeners as ordered. Caution client not to strain when defecating. *Decreased activity can cause constipation. Straining when defecating that results in the Valsalva maneuver can lead to dysrhythmia, decreased cardiac function, and sometimes death.*

- Have clients use a commode or urinal for toileting and avoid use of a bedpan. *Getting out of bed to use a commode or urinal does not stress the heart any more than staying in bed to toilet. In addition, getting the client out of bed minimizes complications of immobility and is often preferred by the client (Winslow, 1992).*

- Provide a restful environment by minimizing controllable stressors and unnecessary disturbances. Schedule rest periods after meals and activities. *Rest periods decrease oxygen consumption (Prizant-Weston and Castiglia, 1992).*

- Weigh client at same time daily (after voiding). *An accurate daily weight is a good indicator of fluid balance. Increased weight and severity of symptoms can signal decreased cardiac function with retention of fluids.*

- Assess for presence of anxiety. Consider using music to decrease anxiety and improve cardiac function. See Nursing Interventions and Rationales for **Anxiety** to facilitate reduction of anxiety in clients and family. **Nursing Research:** *Music has been shown to reduce heart rate, blood pressure, anxiety, and cardiac complications (Guzzetta, 1994).*

- ▲ Watch for signs of depression: flat affect, poor sleeping, loss of appetite, listlessness. Refer for treatment if present. *Depression is very common in heart failure clients and can result in increased mortality (Thomas et al, 2003).*

- ▲ Closely monitor fluid intake, including intravenous lines. Maintain fluid restriction if ordered. *In clients with decreased cardiac output, poorly functioning ventricles may not tolerate increased fluid volumes.*

- ▲ Refer to heart failure program or cardiac rehabilitation program for education, evaluation, and guided support to increase activity and rebuild life. **Clinical Research:** *Exercise can help many clients with heart failure. Whereas rest was commonly recommended a few years ago, it has become clear that inactivity can worsen the skeletal muscle myopathy in these clients. A carefully monitored exercise program can improve both functional capacity (Bellardinelli et al, 1999) and left ventricular function (Giannuzzi et al, 1997). Exercise-based cardiac rehabilitation is effective in reducing the number of cardiac deaths (Joliffe et al, 2002).*

Geriatric

- Observe for atypical pain; the elderly often have jaw pain instead of chest pain or may have silent MIs with symptoms of dyspnea or fatigue. *The elderly have altered pain*

• = Independent; ▲ = Collaborative

pathways and often do not experience the usual chest pain of cardiac patients (Carnevali and Patrick, 1993).

▲ If client has heart disease causing activity intolerance, refer for cardiac rehabilitation. **Clinical Research:** *Elderly clients with coronary artery disease in exercise regimens after hospitalization have exercise trainability comparable to that of younger clients participating in similar experiences (Shepard, 1990; Williams et al, 1985).*

▲ Observe for syncope, dizziness, palpitations, or feelings of weakness associated with an irregular heart rhythm. *Dysrhythmias are common in the elderly (Carnevali and Patrick, 1993).*

▲ Observe for side effects from cardiac medications. *The elderly have difficulty with metabolism and excretion of medications due to decreased function of the liver and kidneys; therefore toxic side effects are more common.*

Home care

• Some of the above interventions may be adapted for home care use.

▲ Begin discharge planning as soon as possible with case manager or social worker to assess home support systems and the need for community or home health services. Support services may be needed to assist with home care, meal preparations, housekeeping, personal care, transportation to doctor visits, or emotional support. *Clients often need help upon discharge. The existing social support network needs to be assessed and assistance provided as needed to meet client needs and to keep the support persons from being overwhelmed (Campbell, 1998).* **Nursing Research:** *Being discharged to home without adequate support may result in readmission of elderly clients (Jaarsma, 1996).*

• Consider development of a clinical pathway to address focused interventions with congestive heart failure (CHF), coronary artery bypass graft (CABG). *National Practice Guidelines for Cardiac Home Care are available to direct intervention for the client post-CABG who is recovering at home (Frantz and Walters, 2001a).* **Nursing Research:** *Study of the outcome of a CHF clinical pathway revealed a 45% reduction in rehospitalization (Hoskins et al, 2001).*

▲ Assess or refer to case manager or social worker to evaluate client ability to pay for prescriptions. *The cost of drugs may be a factor in filling prescriptions and adhering to a treatment plan (Campbell, 1998).*

• Continue to monitor client for exacerbation of heart failure when discharged home. *Transition to home can create increased stress and physiological instability related to diagnosis.*

• Monitor women for differential symptoms of MI and institute emergency treatment measures as indicated. **Nursing Research:** *Continuing research is exploring differences in MI symptoms between men and women. A qualitative study of 40 women following MI noted prodromal symptoms (0 to 11 per woman) a few weeks to 2 years prior. Most frequent were unusual fatigue, discomfort in the shoulder blade area, and chest sensations. Most frequent acute symptoms were chest sensations, shortness of breath, feeling hot and flushed, and unusual fatigue. Severe pain during the acute phase was experienced by only 11 women (McSweeney and Crane, 2000).*

• Assess client for understanding of and compliance with medical regimen, including medications, activity level, and diet. Client/family may need repetition of instructions received at hospital discharge, and may require reiteration as fear of a recent crisis decreases. *Fear interferes with the ability to assimilate new information.*

▲ Assess and monitor for signs of depression (particularly in adults age 65 years or older)

• = **Independent;** ▲ = **Collaborative**

or social isolation. Refer for mental health treatment as indicated. **Nursing and Clinical Research:** *Depression has been noted as prevalent after acute MI in clients over age 65. Depressed older adults post–MI had greater comorbidity than those who were nondepressed and almost 4 times the risk of dying within 4 months of hospital discharge. Inability to follow recommendations to reduce cardiac risk may have been the cause (Romanelli et al, 2002). Mood disturbance, social isolation, low socioeconomic status, and nonwhite ethnicity predicted lower functional status of clients with left ventricular dysfunction after 1 year (Clarke et al, 2000). Depression has been shown to be an independent risk factor for heart failure in elderly women but not in elderly men (Williams et al, 2002).*

- Instruct family and client about the disease process, complications of disease process, information on medications, need for weighing daily, and when it is appropriate to call doctor. *Early recognition of symptoms facilitates early problem solving and prompt treatment (Janowski, 1996).* **Nursing Research:** *Clients with heart failure need intensive education about these topics to help prevent readmission to the hospital (Moser, 2000). Home instruction (covering physical sensations and their management) regarding CABG recovery was found to be an effective intervention to prepare clients for home recovery. Women experienced positive effects on physical functioning; men experienced positive effects on psychological distress, vigor, and fatigue (Moore and Dolansky, 2001). Decreased cardiac output can be life threatening.*

- Help family adapt daily living patterns to establish life changes that will maintain improved cardiac functioning in the client. *Transition to the home setting can cause risk factors such as inappropriate diet to reemerge.*

- Support client self-efficacy to increase physical activity by creating a supportive environment, offering encouragement, providing anticipatory guidance, and supplying a realistic assessment of the client's abilities. *Increasing self-efficacy takes time, but can lead to increased physical activity, decreased symptomatology, and improved quality of life for the client (Borsody et al, 1999).*

- ▲ Explore barriers to medical regimen adherence. Review medications and treatment regularly for needed modifications. Take complaints of side effects seriously and serve as client advocate to address changes as indicated. *The presence of uncomfortable side effects frequently motivates clients to deviate from the medication regimen. A discussion of treatment regimen with coronary heart disease noted that physicians do not always adhere to guideline recommendations; adherence to guidelines and long-term strategies would prompt use of the most effective agents with the lowest incidence of side effects (Erhardt, 1999).*

- ▲ Refer to physical therapy for cardiac rehabilitation, strengthening exercises if client is not involved in outpatient cardiac rehabilitation. Refer to agency cardiac care program if available. *Cardiac rehabilitation safely increases aerobic capacity, muscular strength, and endurance in older clients (Ades, 1999). Specialized cardiac care programs have addressed the needs to CABG clients discharged from the hospital early (Frantz and Walters, 2001b).*

- ▲ Refer to medical social services as necessary for counseling about the impact of severe or chronic cardiac disease. *Social workers can assist the client and family with acceptance of life changes.*

- ▲ Institute case management of frail elderly to support continued independent living. *Difficulties with cardiac output represent and can lead to increasing needs for assistance in using the health care system effectively. Case management combines nursing activities of client and family assessment, planning and coordination of care among all health care providers, delivery of direct nursing care, and monitoring of care and outcomes. These activities*

- **• = Independent; ▲ = Collaborative**

are able to address continuity of care, mutual goal setting, behavior management, and prevention of worsening health problems (Guttman, 1999).

▲ As client condition warrants, refer to hospice. *The multidisciplinary hospice team can reduce hospital readmission, increase functional capacity, and improve quality of life in end-stage heart failure (Coviello et al, 2002).*

▲ Provide specific written materials and self-care plan for client/caregivers to use for reference. Consult dietitian or assist client in understanding the need for a sodium-restricted diet. Provide alternatives for salt such as spices, herbs, lemon juice, or vinegar. *Although the initial elimination of salt from the diet is very difficult for a person used to its taste, the taste of salt can be unlearned. The above can enhance the taste appeal of food while the preference for salt is changing (Peckenpaugh and Poleman, 1999).*

▲ Identify emergency plan, including use of CPR. Encourage family members to become certified in cardiopulmonary resuscitation. **Nursing Research:** *CPR training significantly increased perceived control in spouses of recovering cardiac clients (Moser and Dracup, 2000).*

Client/Family Teaching

- Teach symptoms of heart failure and appropriate actions to take if client becomes symptomatic.
- Teach importance of smoking cessation and avoidance of alcohol intake. *Clients who continue to smoke increase their chance of dying by at least 50%, and alcohol depresses heart contractility (Janowski, 1996).* **Clinical Research:** *Smoking cessation advice and counsel given by nurses can be effective, and should be available to clients to help stop smoking (Rice and Stead, 2000).*
- Teach stress reduction (e.g., imagery, controlled breathing, muscle relaxation techniques).
- Explain necessary restrictions, including consumption of a sodium-restricted diet, guidelines on fluid intake, and the avoidance of Valsalva's maneuver. Teach the importance of pacing activities, work simplification techniques, and the need to rest between activities to prevent becoming overly fatigued. *Sodium retention leading to fluid overload is a common cause of hospital readmission (Bennett et al, 2000).*
- ▲ Assist the client in understanding the need for and how to incorporate lifestyle changes. Refer to cardiac rehabilitation for assistance with coping and adjustment. *Psychoeducational programs including information on stress management and health education have been shown to reduce long-term mortality and recurrence of myocardial infarction in heart patients (Benson, 2000).*
- ▲ Teach the client actions, side effects, and importance of consistently taking cardiovascular medications. *Medications can prolong the lives of heart failure clients but often are not taken, resulting in hospital readmissions (Agency for Health Care Policy and Research, 1994).* **Nursing Research:** *A research study demonstrated that heart failure clients were not knowledgeable of the medications, but also the need for weight monitoring and recognizing the definition for heart failure (Artinian et al, 2002).*
- Provide client/family with advance directive information to consider. Allow client to give advance directions about medical care or designate who should make medical decisions if he or she should lose decision-making capacity (Alspach, 1998).
- Instruct the client on importance of getting a pneumonia shot (usually one per lifetime) and yearly flu shots as prescribed by physician. *Clients with decreased cardiac out-*

• = **Independent;** ▲ = **Collaborative**

put are considered higher risk for complications or death if they do not get immunization injections.

- Instruct client/family on the need to weigh daily and keep a weight log. Ask if client has a scale at home; if not, assist in getting one. Instruct on establishing baseline weight on own scale when gets home. *Daily weighing is an essential aspect of self-management. A scale is necessary (Campbell, 1998). Scales vary; the client needs to establish a baseline weight on his or her home scale.*
- Provide specific written materials and self-care plan for client/caregivers to use for reference.
▲ Consult dietitian or assist client in understanding the need for a sodium-restricted diet. Provide alternatives for salt such as spices, herbs, lemon juice, or vinegar. *Although the initial elimination of salt from the diet is very difficult for a person use to its taste, the taste of salt can be unlearned. The above can enhance the taste appeal of food while the preference for salt is changing (Peckenpaugh and Poleman, 1999).*
- Instruct family regarding cardiopulmonary resuscitation.

evolve WEBSITES FOR EDUCATION

See the EVOLVE website for World Wide Web resources for client education.

REFERENCES

Ades PA: Cardiac rehabilitation in older coronary patients, *J Am Geriatr Soc* 47:98, 1999.

Agency for Health Care Policy and Research (AHCPR): *Guidelines for patients with heart failure,* AHCPR Publication No 942, Rockville, Md, 1994, US Department of Health and Human Services.

Ahrens SG: Managing heart failure: a blueprint for success, *Nursing* 25:26, 1995.

Alspach JG, editor: *Core curriculum for critical care nursing,* ed 5, Philadelphia, 1998, WB Saunders.

Artinian NT et al: What do patients know about their heart failure? *Appl Nurs Res* 15(4):200, 2002.

Bellardinelli R et al: A randomized, controlled trial of long-term moderate exercise training in chronic heart failure: effects on functional capacity, quality of life, and clinical outcome, *Circulation* 99(9):11732, 1999.

Bennett SJ et al: Self-care strategies for symptom management in patients with chronic heart failure, *Nurs Res* 49(3):139, 2000.

Benson G: Review: psychoeducational programmes reduce long term mortality and recurrence of myocardial infarction in cardiac patients, *Evidence-Based Nurs* 3(3):80, 2000.

Borsody JM et al: Using self-efficacy to increase physical activity in patients with heart failure, *Home Healthc Nurse* 17:113, 1999.

Braunwald E, Fauci AS, Kasper DL. *Harrison's principles of internal medicine,* ed 15, New York, 2001, McGraw-Hill.

Campbell R et al: Discharge planning and home follow-up of the elderly patient with heart failure, *Geriatr Nurs* 33(3):497, 1998.

Carnevali DL, Patrick M: *Nursing management for the elderly,* ed 3, Philadelphia, 1993, Lippincott.

Clark VL, Kruse JA: Cardiogenic shock. In Kruse JA, Fink MP, Carlson RW, editors: *Saunders manual of critical care,* Philadelphia, 2003, WB Saunders.

Clarke SP et al: Psychosocial factors as predictors of functional status at 1 year in patients with left ventricular dysfunction, *Res Nurs Health* 23:290, 2000.

Coviello JS, Hricz L, Masulli PS: Client challenge. Accomplishing quality of life in end-stage heart failure: a hospice multidisciplinary approach, *Home Healthc Nurs* 20:195, 2002.

Erhardt ER: The essence of effective treatment and compliance is simplicity, *Am J Hypertens* 12(10 Pt 2):105SS, 1999.

Frantz AK, Walters JI: Recovery from coronary artery bypass grafting at home: is your practice current? *Home Healthc Nurs* 19:417, 2001a.

Frantz AK, Walters JI: Cardiac home care programs impact patients after coronary artery bypass grafting, *Home Healthc Nurs* 19:495, 2001b.

- **= Independent;** ▲ **= Collaborative**

Fuster V et al: *Hurst's the heart*, ed 10, New York, 2001, McGraw-Hill.

Giannuzzi P et al: Attenuation of unfavorable modeling by exercise training in postinfarction patients with left ventricular dysfunction: results of the Exercise in Left Ventricular Dysfunction (ELVD) Trial, *Circulation* 96(6):17907, 1997.

Guttman R: Case management of the frail elderly in the community, *Clin Nurs Spec* 13(4):174, 1999.

Guzzetta CE: Soothing the ischemic heart, *Am J Nurs* 94:24, 1994.

Hoskins LM et al: A clinical pathway for congestive heart failure—clinical pathways versus a usual plan of care: what's the difference? Part 2, *Home Healthc Nurs* 19:207, 2001.

Jaarsma T et al: Readmission of older heart failure patients, *Prog Cardiovasc Nurs* 11(1):15, 1996.

Janowski MJ: Managing heart failure, *RN* 59:34, 1996.

Joliffe JA et al: Exercise-based rehabilitation for coronary heart disease, *Cochrane Library* (CD001800), 2002.

Lessig ML, Lessig PM: The cardiovascular system. In Alspach JG, editor: *Core curriculum for critical care nursing*, ed 5, Philadelphia, 1998, WB Saunders.

Maisel AS et al: Rapid measurement of B-type natriuretic peptide in the emergency diagnosis of heart failure. *N Engl J Med* 347(3), 161, 2002.

Massie B, Amidon TM: Heart. In Tierney L, McPhee S, Papadakis M, editors: *Current medical diagnosis and treatment*, ed 37, Stamford, Conn, 1998, Appleton and Lange.

McSweeney JC, Crane PB: Challenging the rules: women's prodromal and acute symptoms of myocardial infarction, *Res Nurs Health* 23:135, 2000.

Moore SM, Dolansky MA: Randomized trial of a home recovery intervention following coronary artery bypass surgery, *Res Nurs Health* 24:93, 2001.

Moser DK: Heart failure management: optimal health care delivery programs, *Annu Rev Nurs* Res 18:91, 2000.

Moser DK, Dracup K: Impact of cardiopulmonary resuscitation training on perceived control in spouses of recovering cardiac patients, *Res Nurs Health* 23:270, 2000.

Murphy T, Bennett EJ: Low-tech, high-touch perfusion assessment, *Am J Nurs* 92:36, 1992.

Myers MG, Harris L: High dose caffeine and ventricular arrhythmias *Can J Cardiol* 6(3):95, 1990.

Newberry L: *Sheehy's emergency nursing*, ed 5, St Louis, 2003, Mosby.

Oliva PC, Cruz DD. Decreased cardiac output: validation with postoperative heart surgery patients. *Dimens Crit Care Nurs* 22(1):39, 2003.

Peckenpaugh NJ, Poleman C: *Nutrition essentials and diet therapy*, ed 8, Philadelphia, 1999, WB Saunders.

Prizant-Weston M, Castiglia K: Hemodynamic regulation. In Bulechek GM, McCloskey JC, editors: *Nursing interventions: essential nursing treatments*, Philadelphia, 1992, WB Saunders.

Rice VH, Stead LF: Nursing interventions for smoking cessation (Cochrane Review), *Cochrane Library* (2): CD001188, 2000.

Rolfson DB et al: Incidence and risk factors for delirium and other adverse outcomes in older adults after coronary artery bypass graft surgery, *Can J Cardiol* 15:771, 1999.

Romanelli J et al: The significance of depression in older patients after myocardial infarction, *J Am Geriatr Soc* 50:817, 2002.

Schneider JR: Effects of caffeine ingestion on heart rate, blood pressure, myocardial oxygen consumption, and cardiac rhythm in acute myocardial infarction patients, *Heart Lung* 16:167, 1987.

Sole ML, Lamborn ML, Hartshorn JC. *Introduction to critical care nursing*, ed 3, Philadelphia, 2001, WB Saunders.

Thomas SA et al: Depression in patients with heart failure, *AACN Clin Issues* 14(1):3, 2003.

Williams SA et al: Depression and risk of heart failure among the elderly: a prospective community-based study, *Psychosom Med* 64:6, 2002.

Winslow EH: Panning bedpans, *Am J Nurs* 92:16G, 1992.

Caregiver role strain

Betty J. Ackley

NANDA Definition

Difficulty in performing family caregiver role

• = **Independent;** ▲ = **Collaborative**

Defining Characteristics

Caregiving activities
Apprehension about possible institutionalization of care receiver; apprehension about the future regarding care receiver's health and caregiver's ability to provide care; difficulty performing/completing required tasks; apprehension about care receiver's care if caregiver becomes ill or dies; preoccupation with care routine

Caregiver health status—physical
Gastrointestinal upset; weight change; rash; hypertension; cardiovascular disease; diabetes; fatigue; headaches

Caregiver health status—emotional
Impaired individual coping; feeling of depression; disturbed sleep; anger; stress; somatization; increased nervousness; increased emotional lability; impatience; lack of time to meet personal needs; frustration

Caregiver health status—socioeconomic
Withdrawal from social life; changes in leisure activities; low work productivity; refusal of career advancement

Caregiver–care receiver relationship
Grief and/or uncertainty regarding changed relationship with care receiver; difficulty watching care receiver go through the illness

Family processes
Family conflict; concerns about family members

Related Factors (r/t)

Care receiver health status
Illness severity; illness chronicity; increasing care needs/dependency; unpredictability of illness course; instability of care receiver's health; problem behaviors; psychological or cognitive problems; addiction or codependency

Caregiving activities
Amount of activities; complexity of activities; 24-hour care responsibilities; ongoing changes in activities; discharge of family members to home with significant care needs; years of caregiving; unpredictability of care situation

Caregiver health status
Physical problems; psychological or cognitive problems; addiction or codependency; marginal coping patterns; unrealistic expectations of self; inability to fulfill one's own or others' expectations

Socioeconomic factors
Isolation from others; competing role commitments; alienation from family, friends, and coworkers; insufficient recreational resources

• = Independent; ▲ = Collaborative

Caregiver–care receiver relationship

History of poor relationship; presence of abuse or violence; unrealistic expectations of caregiver by care receiver; mental status of elder that inhibits conversation

Family processes

History of marginal family coping; history of family dysfunction

Resources

Inadequate physical environment for providing care; inadequate equipment for providing care; inadequate transportation; inadequate community resources; insufficient finances; lack of support; lack of developmental readiness of caregiver for caregiving role; inexperience with caregiving; insufficient time; lack of knowledge of or difficulty with accessing community resources; lack of caregiver privacy, emotional strength, physical energy, assistance, and support

NOC   Outcomes (Nursing Outcomes Classification)

Suggested NOC Outcomes

Caregiver Emotional Health; Caregiver Lifestyle Disruption; Caregiver Performance: Direct Care, Indirect Care; Caregiver Physical Health; Caregiver Stressors; Caregiver Well-Being; Role Performance

> **Example NOC Outcome with Indicators**
>
> **Caregiver Emotional Health** with plans for a positive future as evidenced by the following indicators: Satisfaction with life/Sense of control/Self-esteem/Free of anger/Free of guilt/Free of depression/Perceived social connectedness/Perceived spiritual well-being (Rate each indicator of **Caregiver Emotional Health:** 1 = extremely compromised, 2 = substantially compromised, 3 = moderately compromised, 4 = mildly compromised, 5 = not compromised [see Section I].)

Client Outcomes

- Caregiver will maintain physical and psychological health.
- Caregiver will identify resources available to help in giving care.
- Care receiver will obtain appropriate care.

NIC   Interventions (Nursing Interventions Classification)

Suggested NIC Intervention

Caregiver Support

> **Example NIC Activities—Caregiver Support**
>
> Determine caregiver's acceptance of role; Accept expressions of negative emotion

Nursing Interventions and Rationales

- Use an evaluation tool to determine caregiver coping and strain. Various instruments have been developed, including the Burden Interview, the Caregiver Strain Index, the Caregiver Burden Inventory, and the Subjective and Objective Burden Scale

- • = Independent; ▲ = Collaborative

(Montgomery, Gonyea, and Hooyman, 1985). **Nursing and Clinical Research:** *Research has validated the effectiveness of a number of evaluation tools for caregiver stress, including the Burden Interview (Zarit et al, 1980), the Caregiver Strain Index (Robinson, 1983), the Caregiver Burden Inventory (Novak and Guest, 1989), and the Subjective and Objective Burden Scale (Montgomery, Gonyea, and Hooyman, 1985).*

- Watch for signs of depression in the caregiver, especially if the marital relationship is poor. Intervene to help the caregiver cope. If signs are present, refer to the care plan for **Hopelessness.** *Caregiving may weaken the immune system and predispose the caregiver to illness in some situations. The incidence of depression in family caregivers is estimated to be 40% to 50% (Stevens, Walsh, and Baldwin, 1993; Knop, Bergman-Evans, and McCabe, 1998).* **Nursing Research:** *Intervening early to help the caregiver can result in improved care for the stroke client and, it is hoped, improved health for the caregiver (Teel, Duncan, and Lai, 2001). Psychiatric nurses can play an important role in the assessment and treatment of caregiver depression (Buckwalter, 1999).*
- Monitor the quality of care by the caregiver for adequacy and need for improvement.
- Observe for signs of addiction or codependency in the caregiver or care receiver.
- ▲ Arrange for a home health nurse to provide nursing care and case management following discharge. *Home health nurses can decrease the burden of caregiving and depression in elderly caregivers (Mignor, 2000).*
- Arrange for intervals of respite care for the caregiver; encourage use if available. *Respite care is beneficial to caregivers, if they can be convinced to use it (Sayles-Cross and DeLorme, 1995; Hayes, 1999).*
- Help the caregiver to identify supports and be assertive in using them. *Caregivers sometimes feel abandoned (Given et al, 1990) and need assistance to activate their support systems (Kleffel, 1998).*
- Encourage the caregiver to grieve over loss of the care receiver's function. Give the caregiver permission to share angry feelings in a safe environment. Refer to nursing interventions for **Grieving.** *Caregivers grieve the loss of function of their loved one, especially when dementia is involved (Liken and Collins, 1993; Narayan et al, 2001).*
- Identify with the caregiver the factors that can and cannot be controlled.
- Help the caregiver find personal time to meet his or her own needs and learn stress management techniques. *Self-care is important for the caregiver. Practicing personal wellness measures can increase stamina, energy, and self-esteem and enhance the quality of care given (Ruppert, 1996).*
- Support the female caregiver in setting boundaries, determining the legitimate caregiving role, trusting her own judgment, and attending to her own voice—being true to herself as well as to the care receiver. **Nursing Research:** *Women in caregiving roles can develop "fraying connections" and lose sense of self when own needs are not met (Wuest, 1998).*
- Encourage the caregiver to use humor to cope when appropriate, including cartoons, stories, and jokes. **Nursing Research:** *Humor is a healthy distancing technique, helping the caregiver to feel liberated from oppressive stimuli. It can help relieve pain, loss, grief, or unpleasantness (Buffum and Brod, 1998).*
- Encourage the caregiver to talk about feelings, concerns, and fears. Acknowledge the frustration associated with caregiver responsibilities. *Professionals need to listen to caregiving spouses and note expressions of positive and negative responses to caregiving (Narayan et al, 2001).*
- Observe for any evidence of caregiver or care receiver violence; if evidence is present,

- • = Independent; ▲ = Collaborative

speak with the caregiver and care receiver separately. *Caregiver violence is possible, especially if the care receiver was violent to the caregiver in the past (Brandle and Raymond, 1997).*

▲ Involve the family in discharge planning; utilize a multidisciplinary team to provide medical and social serves for discharge instruction and planning. **Nursing Research:** *Caregivers who reported involvement in discharge planning reported better acceptance of the caregiving role and better health (Bull, Hansen, and Gross, 2000). Use of an interdisciplinary team to provide discharge planning was seen by elders as a "proper discharge" (Bull and Roberts, 2001).*

• Give the caregiver permission to arrange custodial care in an extended care facility if necessary; support both caregiver and care receiver during this difficult transition. Help the caregiver deal with predictable elements of pretending that the move is temporary, dawning realization that the move is permanent, putting on a brave face to handle the stress, and seeking solace in support from others. *Placing a loved one in an extended care facility can relieve the burden of care but does not relieve the stress resulting from financial concerns, guilt, loss of control, or lack of support (Stevens, Walsh, and Baldwin, 1993).* **Nursing Research:** *The process of separation experienced by a caregiver after placing a spouse in an extended care facility includes four elements: pretending, dawning, putting on a brave front, and seeking solace (Sandberg, Lundh, and Nolan, 2001).*

Geriatric

• Monitor the caregiver for psychological distress and signs of depression, especially if caring for a mentally impaired elder or if there was an unsatisfactory marital relationship before caregiving. **Nursing Research:** *Those caring for mentally impaired elders for an extended time with minimal social support are at high risk for psychological distress or depression (Baille, Norbeck, and Barnes, 1988). A difficult marriage before caregiving predisposes the caregiver to depression (Knop, Bergman-Evans, and McCabe, 1998).*

• Assess the health of the caregiver at intervals, especially if he or she has chronic illness in addition to caregiving role. *The elderly can be overly self-sufficient, especially if they live in rural areas, and elderly caregivers can develop poor health as a result (Silveira and Winstead-Fry, 1997).* **Clinical Research:** *If caregiving is associated with self-reported physical or emotional strain, the older caregiver has an increased risk of mortality (Schulz and Beach, 1999).*

• Recognize that it is hard for the elderly to accept any change in caregivers or in the environment. *Help the caregiver identify ways to equitably distribute workload among family or significant others.*

Multicultural

• Assess for the influence of cultural beliefs, norms, values, and expectations on the family's experience of caregiving. **Nursing Research:** *How the family views caregiving may be based on cultural perceptions (Leininger and McFarland, 2002; Cochran, 1998; Doswell and Erlen, 1998; Guarnaccia, 1998).*

• Assess for conflicts between the caregiver's cultural obligations to provide care and competing factors like employment. **Nursing Research:** *Conflicts between cultural expectations and competing factors can increase caregiver stress (Jones, 1996).*

• Negotiate with the client regarding the aspects of caregiving that can be modified

• = **Independent;** ▲ = **Collaborative**

while still honoring cultural beliefs. **Nursing Research:** *Give and take with the client will lead to culturally congruent care (Leininger and McFarland, 2002).*

▲ Refer the family to social services or other supportive services to assist with the impact of caregiving. **Nursing Research:** *African American caregivers of dementia clients evidence less desire than others to institutionalize their family members and are more likely to report unmet service needs (Hinrichsen and Ramirez, 1992). African American and white families of dementia clients report restricted social activity (Haley et al, 1995).*

▲ Assist the family/caregiver in identifying barriers that would prevent the use of social services or other supportive services that could help reduce the impact of caregiving. **Nursing Research:** *Expectations of discrimination, lack of knowledge about services, expectations embedded in familism, lack of sense of prevention, lack of health insurance, preference for traditional remedies, and neglect or abuse were barriers identified by researchers studying the low utilization of skilled home care nursing services among elderly Hispanic individuals (Crist, 2002). Language may present another barrier to the access of supportive services (McGrath, Vun, and McLeod, 2001).*

• Encourage the family to use support groups or other service programs. **Nursing Research:** *Studies indicate that minority families of clients with dementia use few support programs even though these programs could have a positive impact on caregiver well-being (Cox, 1999).*

• Encourage caregiver use of spirituality or religion as a source of support for the caregiver. **Nursing Research:** *Studies indicate that African American caregivers cited religion and spirituality as their greatest source of support (Poindexter and Linsk, 1998).*

• Validate the family's feelings regarding the impact of caregiving on family and personal lifestyle. **Nursing Research:** *Validation is a therapeutic communication technique that lets the individual know that the nurse has heard and understood what was said (Heineken, 1998).*

Home care

• Identify client and caregiver factors that necessitated the use of formal home care services and that may affect provision of care or need to be addressed before the client can be safely discharged. **Nursing Research:** *A study noted predictors of caregivers' use of home care services. On the part of the care recipient, limitations in the ability to perform the activities of daily living (ADLs) predicted referral to home care, while diagnosis and presence of physical impairment did not. Elders living alone or with fewer household members were more likely to use home care. On the part of the caregiver, factors included lack of mobility outside of the home, need to rearrange work schedules, and need for provision of bowel or bladder care (Houde, 1998). Problem solving should address each of these elements as possible prior to discharge from home care.*

• Assess the client and caregiver at every visit for quality of relationship, quality of care provided, functional disability of care recipient, and signs of caregiver stress. Document all observations objectively. **Nursing Research:** *The changing level of support from institutional care to home care and the length of time that care is needed may contribute to cumulative caregiver burden (Silveira and Winstead-Fry, 1997). Greater caregiver burden and decreased quality of life have been associated with more serious illness and a higher degree of functional disability on the part of the client, and with greater differences in reciprocity between the past and present relationship with the client. However, caregiver overload did not itself lead to deterioration in the quality of care the client received (Clark, 1997).*

• Assess family caregiving skill. *The identification of caregiver difficulty with any of a core*

• = **Independent;** ▲ = **Collaborative**

set of processes highlights areas for intervention. **Nursing Research:** *The ability to engage effectively and smoothly in nine processes has been identified as constituting family caregiving skill: monitoring client behavior, interpreting changes accurately, making decisions, taking action, making adjustment to care, accessing resources, providing hands-on care, working together with the ill person, and negotiating the health care system (Schumacher et al, 2000).*

- Assess perceived level of power experienced by the caregiver in daily activities. **Nursing Research:** *Decreased perceived power level can lead to caregiver overload, possibly because of a burden of financial management the caregiver must assume when ill prepared (Clark, 1997).*

- Assess preexisting strengths and weaknesses the caregiver brings to the situation, as well as current responses, depression, and fatigue levels. **Nursing Research:** *Low individual and family hardiness was found to foster depression and fatigue in caregivers; coping strategies did not mediate the relationship (Clark, 2002). The type of empathy shown by caregivers can influence outcomes. Caregivers with high cognitive empathy (i.e., ability to understand another's feelings while maintaining emotional distance) viewed caregiving as less stressful, were less depressed, and reported higher life satisfaction than those with low cognitive empathy. Emotional empathy (i.e., vicarious emotional response to the perceived feelings of others) was associated with lower life satisfaction, presumably because caregivers were unable to detach themselves from the clients' feelings (Lee, Brennan, and Daly, 2001).*

- Identify strengths of the caregiver and efforts to gain control of unpredictable situations.

- Help the caregiver to stay connected with the client who may be behaving differently than usual, to make life as routine as possible, to help the client set goals and sustain hope, and to allow the client space to experience progress. *Identifying and acknowledging positive caregiver responses to the client's illness will help the caregiver to maintain a positive relationship with the client.* **Nursing Research:** *Family members of persons with severe mental illness have found it helpful to work at staying connected to the person with mental illness, finding a role that they can feel comfortable with, and helping the relative move forward (Rose, 1998).*

- Recognize that caregiver disabilities may not prevent them from providing care; assess each situation individually. *Caregivers with mental illness need not be considered incapable of the caregiving role.* **Nursing Research:** *Adult children with mental illness have been shown to provide their mothers help with a range of daily living tasks, thus decreasing maternal subjective burden (Greenberg, 1995).*

- Form a trusting and supportive relationship with the caregiver. Allow the caregiver to verbalize frustrations. *Providing attention to the caregiver can decrease caregiver stress and reduce the risk of caregiver violence.*

- Assist the caregiver in identifying sources of concern and areas of stress in dealing with the client's illness. **Nursing Research:** *A study identified the need for support of heart transplantation clients' spouses (Bohachick et al, 2001). Prior to transplantation, spouses experienced high levels of distress because of an inability to participate in social activities, as their time was spent in caregiving and maintaining the home. Anxiety, depression, worry, vocational disruption, and sexual adjustment difficulties occurred. Improvements in all of these areas were found by 1 year after transplantation, in part due to relief of fears that the client might die before a donor could be found. After transplantation, spouses were more relaxed and able to resume social activities.*

- Instruct the caregiver in the care needs of the client, disease processes, medications, and what to expect; use a variety of instructional techniques (e.g., explanations, demonstrations, visual aids) until the caregiver is able to express a degree of comfort with

• = Independent; ▲ = Collaborative

care delivery. *Knowledge and confidence are separate concepts. Self-assurance in caregiving will improve performance of the role in client maintenance that caregivers assume (Clark, 1997).*

- Assist the caregiver and client in arranging care so that it is compatible with other household patterns. **Nursing Research:** *Caregivers of elders have been identified as using home environmental modification strategies for specific purposes: organizing the home, supplementing the elder's function, structuring the elder's day, protecting the elder, working around limitations or deficits in the home environment, enriching the home environment, and transitioning to a new home setting (Messecar et al, 2002).*

- Explore the state of the relationship between the client and the caregiver before the onset of chronic illness or dementia; identify the strengths and weaknesses of each party. Formulate a plan to assist the couple in dealing with likely worsening of dementia. *Chronic illness, especially dementia, can represent a gradual and devastating loss of the marital relationship as it existed formerly. An understanding of the prior relationship is needed before the couple can be helped to anticipate continuing care needs or deterioration (Zarit, 2001). In a study of cancer clients and spousal caregivers, past relationships characterized by mutual concern and responsiveness (communal) led to caregiver depression, as loss of intimacy and affection predicted restriction of caregiver's routine activity. When past relationships were less communal, activity restriction was predicted by the severity of client symptoms and led to resentment of the care recipient and the caregiving role (Williamson, Shaffer, and Schultz, 1998).*

- Explore with the spouse the process of understanding the client's behavior that the spouse has been undergoing; assist with reframing that understanding to be as realistic and positive as possible. Consider use of the Progressively Lowered Stress Threshold psychoeducational nursing intervention to help the spouse understand and handle the behavior changes associated with Alzheimer's disease. **Nursing Research:** *In a qualitative study, wives of clients with Alzheimer's disease described a process of recognizing changes; drawing inferences about their observations; rewriting identities for themselves and their husbands as they took on the husbands' roles and responsibilities; and constructing a new daily life. Reframing interventions can help caregivers to consider positive aspects of caring along with grief and frustration (Perry, 2002). Nurses can help caregivers normalize events, making these events more manageable and less threatening (Ayres, 2000a, 2000b). The Progressively Lowered Stress Threshold psychoeducational nursing intervention has been shown to have a positive effect in decreasing the frequency of disruptive behavior and improving the response of the caregiver to the behaviors of the Alzheimer's client (Gerdner, Buckwalter, and Reed, 2002).*

- ▲ Refer the client to home health aide services for assistance with ADLs and light housekeeping. Allow the caregiver to gain confidence in the respite provider. *Home health aide services can provide physical relief and respite for the caregiver (Boland and Sims, 1996).*

- ▲ Identify appropriate individual and group interventions for the caregiver; assess for appropriateness of referrals given the caregiver's needs and mobility. **Nursing Research:** *Individual interventions (family-focused individual therapy, cognitive behavioral therapy, cognitive stimulation training, professional and peer counseling, stress management and problem solving) and group interventions (professional versus self-help support groups, stress management, respite care, multimedia training groups, caregiver training in behavior management and social skills) have been identified as effective in reducing caregiver stress (Yin, Zhou, and Bashford, 2002).*

- ▲ Refer to a caregivers support group if available or recommend an online support

• = Independent; ▲ = Collaborative

group—see suggested websites listed on the EVOLVE website. **Nursing Research:** *Sharing concerns with others can mitigate loneliness. Increased caregiver loneliness has been associated with depression, relational deprivation, and poorer quality of the current caregiver-client relationship (Beeson et al, 2000). Because members read and send messages 24 hours a day every day of the week, online support groups offer the advantage of immediate communication with others offering support. When nurses assist with online support groups, the groups can help caregivers learn, give them a sense of community, and encourage a sense of empowerment (White and Dorman, 2000).*

- Assess the caregiver for overinvolvement with the client and client's illness. Encourage the caregiver to address an enmeshed relationship with the client prompted by concerns over the client's illness and altered quality of life by discussing the issue, seeking respite, and attending support groups. Assist with identification of the spouse's needs and verbalization of the caregiving experience. **Nursing Research:** *In one study of women caring for husbands with chronic obstructive pulmonary disease, women had difficulty separating themselves from their husbands (Bergs, 2002).*

▲ Refer to case managers as necessary for community resource assistance, financial planning, and supportive counseling for both client and caregiver. **Nursing Research:** *Individualized counseling in problem solving by nurses was shown to be effective in reducing the number of admissions to nursing homes (Roberts et al, 1999).*

▲ Refer for homemaker or psychiatric home health care services for respite, client reassurance, and implementation of a therapeutic regimen. *Taking responsibility for a person needing extensive care results in high caregiver stress. Respite decreases caregiver stress. The presence of caring individuals is reassuring to both the client and caregivers, especially during periods of client anxiety or agitation. Counseling may be necessary to address unresolved family relationship issues that threaten to impede the delivery of care.*

▲ As indicated by deterioration of the client's condition, assist the caregiver in examining options for institutional placement. **Nursing Research:** *Caregiver overload leads to decreased physical health and increased anxiety over time. The caregiver may require instruction in the client's need for formal supports as condition deteriorates (Winslow, 1997). Caregiver burden has been shown to decrease following institutional placement (Winslow et al, 1999).*

- Assess the caregiver's emotional response to placement of the client and provide support, cognitive interventions, and problem solving as needed. *A variety of difficulties may impede the caregiver's acceptance of the need for the client's placement, including financial concerns, inability to accept the client's level of need for increased supervision, guilt, or unresolved relationship issues. It is important to identify the relevant concerns and options, as well as to address psychological issues.* **Nursing Research:** *Placement of a family member involves a struggle to make a decision, find reassurance, and remain connected to the client (Butcher et al, 2001).*

NOTE: Families of terminally ill clients are especially vulnerable to caregiver role strain because the timing of the impending death is unpredictable, and caregiver effort and resources are disproportionately spent early in the caregiving process.

Client/Family Teaching

- Teach the caregiver methods for managing behavioral symptoms if the care receiver has dementia. Refer to the care plan for **Chronic Confusion.** *Caregivers can be taught to understand and manage problem behavior (Mastrian, Ritter, Diemling, 1996).*
- Teach the caregiver how to provide the physical care needed.
▲ Refer to counseling or support groups to assist in adjusting to the caregiver role.

- **= Independent; ▲ = Collaborative**

evolve WEBSITES FOR EDUCATION

See the EVOLVE website for World Wide Web resources for client education.

REFERENCES

Ayres L: Narratives of family caregiving: four story types, *Res Nurs Health* 23:359, 2000a.

Ayres L: Narratives of family caregiving: the process of making meaning, *Res Nurs Health* 23:424, 2000b.

Baille V, Norbeck JS, Barnes LE: Stress, social support, and psychological distress of family caregivers of the elderly, *Nurs Res* 37(4):217, 1988.

Beeson R et al: Loneliness and depression in caregivers of persons with Alzheimer's disease or related disorders, *Issues Ment Health Nurs* 21:779, 2000.

Bergs D: "The hidden client"—women caring for husbands with COPD: their experience of quality of life, *J Clin Nurs* 11:613, 2002.

Bohachick P et al: Psychosocial impact of heart transplantation on spouses, *Clin Nurs Res* 10:6, 2001.

Boland D, Sims S: Family caregiving at home as a solitary journey, *Image J Nurs Sch* 28:55, 1996.

Brandle B, Raymond J: Unrecognized elder abuse victims: older abused women, *J Case Manage* 6(2):62, 1997.

Buckwalter KC et al: A nursing intervention to decrease depression in family caregivers of person with dementia, *Arch Psychiatr Nurs* 13(2):80, 1999.

Buffum MD, Brod M: Humor and well-being in spouse caregivers of patients with Alzheimer's disease, *Appl Nurs Res* 11(1):12, 1998.

Bull MJ, Hansen HE, Gross CR: Differences in family caregiver outcomes by their level of involvement in discharge planning, *Appl Nurs Res* 13(2):76, 2000.

Bull MJ, Roberts J: Components of a proper hospital discharge for elders, *J Adv Nurs* 35(4):571, 2001.

Butcher HK et al: Thematic analysis of the experience of making a decision to place a family member with Alzheimer's disease in a special care unit, *Res Nurs Health* 24:470, 2001.

Clark MC: A causal functional explanation of maintaining a dependent elder in the community, *Res Nurs Health* 20:515, 1997.

Clark PC: Effects of individual and family hardiness on caregiver depression and fatigue, *Res Nurs Health* 25:37, 2002.

Cochran, M: Tears have no color, *Am J Nurs* 98(6):53, 1998.

Cox C: Race and caregiving: patterns of service use by African-American and white caregivers of persons with Alzheimer's, *J Gerontol Soc Work* 32(2):5, 1999.

Crist JD: Mexican American elders' use of skilled home care nursing services, *Public Health Nurs* 19(5):366, 2002.

Doswell W, Erlen J: Multicultural issues and ethical concerns in the delivery of nursing care interventions, *Nurs Clin North Am* 33(2):353, 1998.

Gerdner LA, Buckwalter KC, Reed D: Impact of a psychoeducational intervention on caregiver response to behavior problems, *Nurs Res* 51(6):363, 2002.

Given B et al: Responses of elder spouse caregivers, *Res Nurs Health* 13:77, 1990.

Greenberg JS: The other side of caring: adult children with mental illness as supports to their mothers in late life, *Soc Work* 40:414, 1995.

Guarnaccia P: Multicultural experiences of family caregiving: a study of African American, European American, and Hispanic American families, *New Dir Ment Health Serv* 77:45, 1998.

Haley WE et al: Psychological, social, and health impact of caregiving: a comparison of black and white dementia family caregivers and noncaregivers, *Psychol Aging* 10(4):540, 1995.

Hayes JM: Respite for caregivers: a community-based model in a rural setting, *J Gerontol Nurs* 25(1):22, 1999

Heineken J: Patient silence is not necessarily client satisfaction: communication in home care nursing, *Home Healthc Nurse* 16(2):115, 1998.

Hinrichsen GA, Ramirez M: Black and white dementia caregivers: a comparison of their adaptation, *Gerontologist* 32(3):375, 1992.

Houde SC: Predictors of elders' and family caregivers' use of formal home services, *Res Nurs Health* 21:533, 1998.

Jones PS: Asian American women caring for elderly parents, *J Fam Nurs* 2(1):56, 1996.

Kleffel D: Lives on hold: evaluation of a caregivers' support program, *Home Healthc Nurse* 16(7):465, 1998.

• = **Independent;** ▲ = **Collaborative**

Knop DS, Bergman-Evans B, McCabe BW: In sickness and in health: an exploration of the perceived quality of the marital relationship, coping, and depression in caregivers of spouses with Alzheimer's disease, *J Psychosoc Nurs Ment Health Serv* 36(1):16, 1998.

Lee HS, Brennan PF, Daly BJ: Relationship of empathy to appraisal, depression, life satisfaction, and physical health in informal caregivers of older adults, *Res Nurs Health* 24:44, 2001.

Leininger MM, McFarland MR: *Transcultural nursing: concepts, theories, research and practices,* ed 3, New York, 2002, McGraw-Hill.

Liken MA, Collins CE: Grieving: facilitating the process for dementia caregivers, *J Psychosoc Nurs Ment Health Serv* 31(1):21, 1993.

Mastrian KG, Ritter C, Diemling GT: Predictors of caregiver health strain, *Home Healthc Nurse* 14(3):209, 1996.

McGrath P, Vun M, McLeod L: Needs and experiences on non-English speaking hospice patients and families in an English speaking country, *Am J Hosp Palliat Care* 18(5):305, 2001.

Messecar DC et al: Home environmental modification strategies used by caregivers of elders, *Res Nurs Health* 25:357, 2002.

Mignor D: Effectiveness of use of home health nurses to decrease burden and depression of elderly caregivers, *J Psychosoc Nurs* 38(7):34, 2000.

Montgomery RJV, Gonyea JG, Hooyman NR: Caregiving and the experience of subjective and objective burden, *Fam Relat* 34:19, 1985.

Narayan S et al: Subjective responses to caregiving for a spouse with dementia, *J Gerontol Nurs* 27(3):19, 2001.

Novak M, Guest C. Application of a multidimensional caregiver burden inventory, *Gerontologist* 29(6):798, 1989.

Perry J: Wives giving care to husbands with Alzheimer's disease: a process of interpretive caring, *Res Nurs Health* 25:307, 2002.

Poindexter CC, Linsk NL: Sources of support in a sample of HIV-affected older minority caregivers, *Fam Soc J Contemp Hum Serv* Sept/Oct:491, 1998.

Roberts J et al: Problem-solving counseling for caregivers of the cognitively impaired: effective for whom? *Nurs Res* 48(3):162, 1999.

Robinson BC: Validation of a caregiver strain index, *J Gerontol* 38(3):344, 1983.

Rose LE: Gaining control: family members relate to persons with severe mental illness, *Res Nurs Health* 21(4):363, 1998.

Ruppert RA: Caring for the lay caregiver, *Am J Nurs* 96(3):40, 1996.

Sandberg J, Lundh U, Nolan MR: Placing a spouse in a care home: the importance of keeping, *J Clin Nurs* 10(3):406, 2001.

Sayles-Cross S, DeLorme J: Worried, worn out, and angry: providing relief for caregivers, *ABNF J* 6:74, 1995.

Schulz R, Beach SR: Caregiving as a risk factor for mortality: the Caregiver Health Effects Study. *JAMA* 282(23):2215, 1999.

Schumacher KL et al: Family caregiving skill: development of the concept, *Res Nurs Health* 23:191, 2000.

Silveira JM, Winstead-Fry P: The needs of patients with cancer and their caregivers in rural areas, *Oncol Nurs Forum* 24(1):71, 1997.

Stevens GL, Walsh RA, Baldwin BA: Family caregivers of institutionalized and noninstitutionalized elderly individuals, *Nurs Clin North Am* 28(2):349, 1993.

Teel CS, Duncan P, Lai SM: Caregiving experiences after stroke, *Nurs Res* 50(1):53, 2001.

White MH, Dorman SM: Online support for caregivers: analysis of an internet Alzheimer mailgroup, *Comput Nurs* 18(4):168, 2000.

Williamson GM, Shaffer DR, Schulz R: Activity restriction and prior relationship history as contributors to mental health outcomes among middle-aged and older spousal caregivers, *Health Psychol* 17:152, 1998.

Winslow BW: Effects of formal supports on stress outcomes in family caregivers of Alzheimer's patients, *Res Nurs Health* 20:527, 1997.

Winslow BW et al: Patterns of burden in wives who care for husbands with dementia, *Nurs Clin North Am* 34:275, 1999.

Wuest J: Setting boundaries: a strategy for precarious ordering of women's caring demands, *Res Nurs Health* 21(1):39, 1998.

Yin T, Zhou Q, Bashford C: Burden on family members. Caring for frail elderly: a meta-analysis of interventions, *Nurs Res* 51:199, 2002.

Zarit J: A tribute to adaptability: mental illness and dementia in intimate late-life relationships, *Generations* 25(2):70, 2001.

Zarit SH et al: Relatives of the impaired elderly: correlates of feelings of burden, *Gerontologist* 20(6):649, 1980.

• = Independent; ▲ = Collaborative

Risk for Caregiver role strain

Betty J. Ackley

NANDA Definition

Caregiver vulnerability for felt difficulty in performing family caregiver role

Risk Factors

Lack of developmental readiness on part of caregiver for caregiving role (e.g., young adult needing to provide care for middle-aged person); inadequate physical environment for providing care (e.g., housing, transportation, community services, equipment); unpredictable illness course or instability in care receiver's health; psychological or cognitive problems in care receiver; presence of situational stressors that normally affect families (e.g., significant loss, disaster, or crisis; economic vulnerability; major life events); presence of abuse or violence; premature birth or congenital defect; past history of poor relationship between caregiver and care receiver; marginal family adaptation or dysfunction before caregiving situation; marginal coping patterns on part of caregiver; lack of respite and recreation for caregiver; inexperience with caregiving; female gender of caregiver; addiction or codependency; demonstration of deviant or bizarre behavior by care receiver; competing role commitments of caregiver; caregiver health impairment; illness severity of care receiver; spousal status of caregiver; high complexity/amount of caregiving tasks; developmental delay or retardation of care receiver or caregiver; discharge of family member with significant home care needs; long duration of caregiving; family/caregiver isolation

NOC Outcomes (Nursing Outcomes Classification)

Suggested NOC Outcomes

Caregiver Emotional Health; Caregiver Lifestyle Disruption; Caregiver Performance: Direct Care, Indirect Care; Caregiver Physical Health; Caregiver Stressors; Caregiver Well-Being; Role Performance

Example NOC Outcome with Indicators

Caregiver Emotional Health with plans for a positive future as evidenced by the following indicators: Satisfaction with life/Sense of control/Self-esteem/Free of anger/Free of guilt/Free of depression/Perceived social connectedness/Perceived spiritual well-being (Rate each indicator of **Caregiver Emotional Health:** 1 = extremely compromised, 2 = substantially compromised, 3 = moderately compromised, 4 = mildly compromised, 5 = not compromised [see Section I].)

Client Outcomes

Client/Caretaker Will (Specify Time Frame):
- Maintain physical and psychological health
- Identify resources available to help in giving care
- Obtain appropriate care

• = Independent; ▲ = Collaborative

| NIC | Interventions (Nursing Interventions Classification) |

Suggested NIC Interventions

Caregiver Support; Family Support; Home Maintenance Assistance; Normalization Promotion; Respite Care; Support Group

> **Example NIC Activities—Caregiver Support**
>
> Determine caregiver's acceptance of role; Accept expressions of negative emotion

Nursing Interventions and Rationales and Client/Family Teaching

- See the care plan for **Caregiver role strain.**

evolve WEBSITES FOR EDUCATION

See the EVOLVE website for World Wide Web resources for client education.

Impaired Comfort

Scott C. Lamont

| NANDA | Definition |

State in which an individual experiences an uncomfortable sensation in response to a noxious stimulus (Carpenito, 2000). Unpleasant sensation of being physically ill at ease that may be localized or generalized but is not described in terms of tissue damage (Lamont, 2002).

Defining Characteristics

Verbalization of discomfort (specific examples include aches, pruritus); observed behaviors indicative of discomfort; shifting and/or restlessness; tenseness; shivering and covering up or removing of covers; avoidance; malaise; aching; stiffness; distention; hunger and thirst; reduced mobility; itching; reddened, irritated skin (pruritus)

Related Factors (r/t)

Reaction to chemical irritants (including allergies); dry skin; illness and/or immobility; unmet physical needs (food, fluid, bathing, etc.); fever; disease processes; pregnancy; immobility; musculoskeletal disorders; inflammation; intestinal gas, colic; medication side effects; contagious diseases (chickenpox, etc.)

| NOC | Outcomes (Nursing Outcomes Classification) |

Suggested NOC Outcomes

Comfort Level; Symptom Control

• = Independent; ▲ = Collaborative

Example NOC Outcome with Indicators

Comfort Level as evidenced by the following indicators: Reported physical well-being/Reported satisfaction with symptom control (Rate each indicator of **Comfort Level:** 1 = none, 2 = limited, 3 = moderate, 4 = substantial, 5 = extensive [see Section I].)

Client Outcomes

Client Will (Specify Time Frame):

- State he or she is comfortable
- State that his or her uncomfortable sensations (aches, itching, etc.) are relieved
- Explain methods to decrease own discomfort
- Display improved physical mobility
- Appear less restless and more at ease

NIC   Interventions (Nursing Interventions Classification)

Suggested NIC Interventions

Acupressure; Bathing; Distraction; Exercise Promotion; Exercise Promotion: Stretching; Heat/Cold Application; Medication Administration; Music Therapy; Positioning; Progressive Muscle Relaxation; Pruritus Management; Simple Guided Imagery; Simple Massage; Simple Relaxation Therapy; Skin Care: Topical Treatments

---

Example NIC Activities—Pruritus Management

Apply medicated creams and lotions as appropriate; Instruct client to limit bathing to once or twice a week as appropriate

---

Nursing Interventions and Rationales

- Assess client needs holistically. Physical discomfort often coexists with and is exacerbated by emotional and spiritual discomfort; therefore addressing nonphysical needs can improve the client's perception of physical comfort. The nurse's therapeutic approach and demeanor can have a profound impact on perception of comfort. **Nursing Research:** *One small quantitative study found that female breast cancer clients undergoing radiation therapy rated their overall comfort as being greater than the sum of the hypothesized components of comfort, which lent support to the theory of the holistic nature of comfort (Kolcaba and Steiner, 2000). A grounded theory study of clients' perceptions of nurses' comfort work found that, although physical care provided was important, empathy and interpersonal skills were the dominant issue for clients (Walker, 2002).*
- ▲ Consult with the physician for medication to reduce discomforting symptoms such as aching. *Medications can reduce many discomforting sensations.*
- Provide distraction techniques such as music, television, or games. *These activities help to temporarily distract the client from discomforting sensations.* **Nursing Research:** *Music therapy was found to reduce reported discomfort and anxiety compared to a control condition of no music in a study of individuals undergoing flexible sigmoidoscopy (Chlan et al, 2000).*
- Encourage early mobilization to decrease physical discomforts associated with bed rest. **Nursing Research:** *A study of the comfort and complications associated with a 6-hour*

• = Independent; ▲ = Collaborative

Assist patient when performing ADLS

bed rest versus a 4-hour bed rest after cardiac catheterization found no significant differences and concluded that shorter periods may be acceptable (Wang et al, 2001). A quality improvement study to improve the comfort of clients after cardiac catheterization found no increase in complications after reducing the bed rest period from 6 hours to 2 hours (Vlasic and Almond, 1999).

- Provide simple massage. *Massage may be helpful by reducing discomfort and anxiety, and promoting relaxation and sleep.* **Nursing Research:** *A review of 22 articles on the effects of massage in acute care settings noted that the majority of studies found a significant decrease in anxiety or perception of tension. Some studies found decreased discomfort, but the outcomes related to sleep were unclear. More research on these effects is needed (Richards, Gibson, and Overton-McCoy, 2000). A quasi-experimental study of subjects in a rehabilitation facility found that subjects provided with 3 days of massage had improved physiological measures and reported a positive response to the massage (Holland and Pokorny, 2001).*

- Provide gentle, soothing touch, which may be well suited for clients who cannot tolerate more stimulating interventions such as simple massage. **Nursing Research:** *A study of 1- to 3-week-old neonates in a level III NICU found that clients receiving gentle human touch showed evidence of being soothed compared to a control group but that the intervention must be carefully monitored in this client group because episodes of physiological instability were experienced by some subjects (Harrison et al, 2000).*

- Position the client to maximize comfort. **Nursing Research:** *A qualitative study reported that some clients found positioning by nurses, such as leg elevation following injury, to be helpful (Hawley, 2000).*

- Inform the client of options for control of discomfort such as self-hypnosis and guided imagery, and provide these interventions if appropriate. **Nursing Research:** *A study found that female breast cancer clients treated with guided imagery while undergoing radiation therapy had significant improvements in comfort (using one of two scales) compared with the control group (Kolcaba and Steiner, 2000).*

- Individualize the timing and type of bathing for each client; bathing may be distressing or comforting. **Nursing Research:** *Clients in labor may find discomfort and anxiety reduced if allowed to bathe for approximately 60 minutes early in labor (Benfield et al, 2001). This study and a second study found no maternal or neonatal ill effects associated with early labor bathing (Benfield et al, 2001; Ohlsson et al, 2001). Conversely, an experiment comparing a modified type of bed bathing using a no-rinse cleanser with standard tub bathing for elderly clients with dementia found that agitated behaviors were significantly lower for the bed-bathing group and that the effect was greater for men than for women. These clients may therefore experience less discomfort if not subjected to tub baths (Dunn, Thiru-Chelvam, and Beck, 2002).*

- Limit potentially uncomfortable interventions. Implement only when clearly needed and include the impetus for or timing of discontinuation in the plan of care. **Nursing Research:** *A descriptive study of clients who had urinary catheters placed found that for 15 of 51 observed individuals there was no plan of care associated with their urinary catheterization, and for only 8 was there a plan for the discontinuation of catheter use (Brennan and Evans, 2001).*

- Tailor uncomfortable interventions to individual client needs or responses to therapy. Be aware of current research on alternatives to uncomfortable therapies that may benefit specific client groups or subgroups. **Nursing Research:** *A descriptive study of two specific groups of individuals experiencing leg ulcers found that reduced compression bandaging resulted in little or no discomfort without compromising wound healing (Arthur and*

• = **Independent;** ▲ = **Collaborative**

Lewis, 2000). An experimental study of pressure bandaging to reduce bleeding after coronary angiography found that, although the incidence of femoral bleeding was higher and the time of its onset was earlier in the nonbandage group, the overall incidence was low, the extent of bruising was the same for both groups, and the incidence of severe physical discomfort was higher in the bandage group. Based on these findings, the authors did not recommend the routine application of pressure bandaging after angiography (Botti et al, 1998).

Geriatric

- Comforting touch is helpful for elders because they respond to touch more than to verbal comforting. **Nursing Research:** *A study of outcomes of comfort touch with elderly institutionalized women found that perceptions of self-esteem, well-being, health status, and other measures improved significantly in the experimental group (Butts, 2001).*
- Frail elderly clients should be protected from cold discomfort. *Frail elders are at risk for cold discomfort and hypothermia even in warm environments and may not be able to meet their own needs by means such as adding a layer of clothing (Worfolk, 1997).*

Multicultural

- Assess for the influence of cultural beliefs, norms, and values on the client's perceptions of skin and/or hair status and practices. **Nursing Research:** *What the client considers normal and abnormal skin and hair condition may be based on cultural perceptions (Leininger and McFarland, 2002; Cochran, 1998; Doswell and Erlen, 1998).*
- Identify and clarify cultural language used to describe skin and hair. **Nursing Research:** *Clients may interchange words meaning discomfort and pain, may refer to minor discomforts as pain, or may not discuss nonpainful discomforts at all (Lamont, 2002). Specific words and nonverbal expression are related to health beliefs, practices, and values (Leininger and McFarland, 2002).*
- Assess skin for ashy appearance. **Nursing Research:** *Black skin and the skin of other people of color will appear ashy as a result of the flaking off of the top layer of the epidermis (Smith and Burns, 1999; Jackson, 1998).*
- Encourage the use of lanolin-based lotions for African American clients with dry skin. **Nursing Research:** *Vaseline may clog the pores and cause cellulitis or other skin problems (Jackson, 1998).*
- Offer hair oil and lanolin-based lotion for dry scalp and skin. **Nursing Research:** *Black skin seems to produce less oil than lighter colored skin; therefore African Americans may use more lubricants as a normal part of skin hygiene (Smith, Burns, 1999).*
- Use soap sparingly if the skin is dry. **Nursing Research:** *Black skin tends to be dry, and soap will exacerbate this condition (Jackson, 1998).*

Home care

- Assist the client and family in identifying and providing comfort measures that are effective and safe for the condition and situation.
- Encourage mobilization as frequently as is appropriate for the client.
- Keep the temperature of the home moderate to warm for frail clients.

Client/Family Teaching

- Teach techniques to use when the client is uncomfortable, including relaxation techniques, guided imagery, hypnosis, and music therapy. *Interventions such as progres-*

• = **Independent;** ▲ = **Collaborative**

sive muscle relaxation training, guided imagery, hypnosis, and music therapy can effectively decrease the perception of uncomfortable sensations.
- Instruct the client and family on prescribed medications and therapies that improve comfort.
- ▲ Teach the client to follow up with the physician or other practitioner if discomfort persists.

Pruritus
- Perform a complete assessment to determine the cause of pruritus (e.g., dry skin, contact with irritating substance, medication side effect, insect bite, infection, healing burns, underlying systemic disease). *The cause of pruritus helps direct treatment (Bueller and Bernhard, 1998). Pruritus may be caused by serious illnesses such as renal failure, liver failure, malignancy, or diabetes (Eaglestein, McKay, and Pariser, 1994; Bueller and Bernhard, 1998), as well as by dry skin and various skin conditions. Treatment should be individualized (Bueller and Bernhard, 1998).*
- Assess for sleep disturbances. **Nursing Research:** *One study found that a majority of clients reported difficulty falling asleep and that itching was more frequent at night (Yosipovitch et al, 2002).*
- Implement soaks with cool or cold washcloths or offer cool baths if appropriate. **Nursing Research:** *Some clients report that bathing with cool or cold water can depress the itching sensation (Yosipovitch et al, 2002). Bathing with salts may improve skin barrier protection and have an emollient effect. Baking soda, colloidal oatmeal (with and without oil), and bath oils may also be comforting.* **Nursing Research:** *A study with an experimental irritant design demonstrated reduced transepidermal water loss and improved skin water capacitance with the use of sea water and water containing NaCl and KCl (Yoshizawa et al, 2001). A study comparing postburn itching in individuals showering with either a 5% colloidal oatmeal and liquid paraffin combination or a plain liquid paraffin bath oil found the colloidal oatmeal and oil combination significantly more effective (Matheson, Clayton, and Muller, 2001).*
- Keep the client's fingernails short; have the client wear mitts if necessary. *Scratching with fingernails can excoriate the area and increase skin damage and risk of cellulitis.*
- Leave pruritic area open to the air if possible. *Covering the area with a nonventilated dressing can increase itching sensation and warmth in the area.*
- Use nonallergenic mild soap and use it sparingly. *Many soaps can be irritating to the skin and increase the itching sensation (Bueller and Bernhard, 1998).*
- Keep skin well lubricated. After bathing, while the skin is still moist, apply nonallergenic moisturizers such as Medilan that are alcohol free and available in cream or ointment form. Apply moisturizers daily. *These agents lubricate the skin surface and make the skin feel smoother and less dry (Hardy, 1996). Medilan is a hypoallergenic lanolin that has soothing and hydrating properties. It can be helpful for the treatment of eczema and other dry skin conditions (Stone, 2000). Creams and ointments are more effective than lotions because they contain more oil and less water (Bueller, Bernhard, 1998). Apply emollients within 3 to 5 minutes of exiting bath to trap absorbed water; pat rather than rub dry after application (Koblenzer, 1999).* **Nursing Research:** *Daily application of moisturizers can have the persistent clinical effect of relieving dry skin (Tabata et al, 2000).*
- Provide simple massage for select client groups, such as those recovering from burns. **Nursing Research:** *Two studies of the effects of massage on burn wounds demonstrated*

• = **Independent;** ▲ = **Collaborative**

reduced pruritus; one involved the remodeling phase of wound healing (Field et al, 2000) and the other involved hypertrophic scars (Patino et al, 1999).

- Behavior modification may reduce self-injury due to scratching and improve quality of life. *Incorporating a behavioral model for care using a habit reversal technique into nursing care plans for clients with atopic eczema has been advocated (Buchanan, 2001).*

▲ Advocate for altering or substituting medications if pruritus is potentially a side effect of the current regimen.

▲ Consult with the physician for appropriate medications to relieve itching. Be aware of current research regarding medications best suited to relieving the pruritus associated with different causes. *Many medications are potentially useful for pruritic conditions (Buchanan, 2001; Bueller and Bernhard, 1998). Medications such as topical steroids or antihistamines can be helpful (Buchanan, 2001; Koblenzer, 1999).* **Nursing Research:** *A study of burn wound itch found that an oral cetirizine/cimetidine combination was superior to a diphenhydramine/placebo combination, even after controlling for the effect of topical medications (Baker et al, 2001). A review of trials involving the use of antihistamines to control pruritus in atopic dermatitis found evidence of efficacy to be insufficient, but the sedative effects of some medications may be useful at bedtime (Klein, 1999).*

Geriatric

- Limit the number of complete baths to no more than one every other day. Consider the use of no-rinse skin cleansers as a bathing alternative for select clients. *Excessive bathing, especially in hot water, depletes aging skin of moisture and increases dryness. Use a tepid water temperature (e.g., 90° to 105° F or 32° C) for bathing and limit immersion to less than 20 minutes (Bueller and Bernhard, 1998).* **Nursing Research:** *One study showed no clinical difference in outcome between use of a regular skin detergent for bathing and use of a no-rinse cleanser in a long-term care setting, but the no-rinse cleanser is more than double the cost. Selected clients with pruritus may benefit from the no-rinse preparations, but further research is required (Dawson et al, 2001).*
- Use a superfatted soap such as Dove, Tone, Basis, or Caress. *Superfatted soaps help retain moisture in dry skin of elderly clients (Hardy, 1996). Dove is reported to be the mildest soap available (Bueller and Bernhard, 1998).*
- Increase fluid intake within cardiac or renal limits to a minimum of 1500 ml/day. *Dry skin is caused by loss of fluid through the skin; increasing fluid intake rehydrates the skin. Adequate hydration helps decrease itching (Koblenzer, 1999).*
- Use a humidifier or place a container of water on a heat source to increase humidity in the environment, especially during winter. *Increasing moisture in the air helps to keep moisture in the skin (Hardy, 1996; Bueller and Bernhard, 1998). During times of cold weather and low humidity, dermatitis of the hands is common (Uter, Gefeller, and Schwanitz, 1998).*

Home care

- Assist the client and family in identifying and avoiding irritants that exacerbate pruritus (e.g., wool, cleansers, allergens). *Avoidance of irritants decreases discomfort of pruritus (Koblenzer, 1999).*
- Teach the family to use mild, nonscented, and non–bleach-containing laundry products. *Chemical irritants increase the discomfort of pruritus.*
- Keep the temperature of the home moderate to cool. Use a humidifier. *Overheated home environments increase sweating, which adds salts to the skin and increases irritation.*

- **= Independent; ▲ = Collaborative**

Raising the moisture in the air helps to keep moisture in the skin (Hardy, 1996). **Nursing Research:** *Cool ambient temperature has been reported to reduce pruritus in some clients (Yosipovitch et al, 2002).*

- Support the use of the client's preferred body lotion, as long as it has not been found to exacerbate pruritus. Have the client apply lotion after bathing before blotting skin dry. *Clients are more likely to continue past practices. Applying lotion while the skin is still wet increases the moisturizing action of the lotion.*

Client/Family Teaching

- Teach techniques to use when the client is uncomfortable, including relaxation techniques, guided imagery, hypnosis, and music therapy. *Interventions such as progressive muscle relaxation, guided imagery, hypnosis, and music therapy can effectively decrease the itching sensation.*
- Teach the client with pruritus and the family to substitute rubbing, massage, pressure, or vibration for scratching when itching is severe and irrepressible. *Scratching may be self-injurious and may not relieve the pruritus (Buchanan, 2001).*
- Teach the client and the family correct application or administration of prescribed medications or therapies. *Some clients may benefit from education regarding the link between stress and pruritus caused by certain conditions (Koblenzer, 1999).*
- ▲ Instruct the client to see the primary care practitioner if itching persists and no cause is found. *Itching can be a symptom of other conditions (Eaglestein, McKay, and Pariser, 1994; Koblenzer, 1999).*

⟨evolve⟩ WEBSITES FOR EDUCATION

See the EVOLVE website for World Wide Web resources for client education.

REFERENCES

Arthur J, Lewis P: When is reduced-compression bandaging safe and effective? *J Wound Care* 9(10):469, 2000.

Baker RA et al: Burn wound itch control using H1 and H2 antagonists, *J Burn Care Rehabil* 22(4):263, 2002.

Benfield RD et al: Hydrotherapy in labor, *Res Nurs Health* 24(1):57, 2001.

Botti M et al: The effect of pressure bandaging on complications and comfort in patients undergoing coronary angiography: a multicenter randomized trial, *Heart Lung* 27(6):360, 1998.

Brennan ML, Evans A: Why catheterize? Audit findings on the use of urinary catheters, *Br J Nurs* 10(9):580, 2001.

Buchanan PI: Behavior modification: a nursing approach for young children with atopic eczema, *Dermatol Nurs* 13(1):15, 2001.

Bueller HA, Bernhard JD: Review of pruritus therapy, *Dermatol Nurs* 10(2):101, 1998.

Butts JB: Outcomes of comfort touch in institutionalized elderly female residents, *Geriatr Nurs* 22(4):180, 2001.

Carpenito JL: *Nursing diagnosis: application to clinical practice*, ed 8, Philadelphia, 2000, Lippincott.

Chlan L et al: Effects of a single music therapy intervention on anxiety, discomfort, satisfaction, and compliance with screening guidelines in outpatients undergoing flexible sigmoidoscopy, *Gastroenterol Nurs* 23(4):148, 2000.

Cochran M: Tears have no color, *Am J Nurs* 98(6):53, 1998.

Dawson M et al: An evaluation of two bathing products in a chronic care setting, *Geriatr Nurs* 22(2):91, 2001.

Doswell W, Erlen J: Multicultural issues and ethical concerns in the delivery of nursing care interventions, *Nurs Clin North Am* 33(2):353, 1998.

Dunn JC, Thiru-Chelvam B, Beck CH: Bathing. Pleasure or pain? *J Gerontol Nurs* 28(11):6, 2002.

Eaglestein WH, McKay M, Pariser DM: The problems that plague aging skin, *Patient Care* 28:89, 1994.

- = Independent; ▲ = Collaborative

Field T et al: Postburn itching, pain, and psychological symptoms are reduced with massage therapy, *J Burn Care Rehabil* 21(3):189, 2000.

Hardy MA: What can you do about your patient's dry skin? *J Gerontol Nurs* 5:11, 1996.

Harrison LL et al: Physiologic and behavioral effects of gentle human touch on preterm infants, *Res Nurs Health* 23(6):435, 2000.

Hawley MP: Nurse comforting strategies: perceptions of emergency department patients, *Clin Nurs Res* 9(4): 441, 2000.

Holland B, Pokorny ME: Slow stroke back massage: its effect on patients in a rehabilitation setting, *Rehabil Nurs* 26(5):182, 2001.

Jackson F: The ABC's of black hair and skin care, *ABNF J* 9(5):100, 1998.

Klein PA: An evidence-based review of the efficacy of antihistamines in relieving pruritus in atopic dermatitis, *Arch Dermatol* 135(12):1522, 1999.

Koblenzer CS: Itching and the atopic skin, *J Allergy Clin Immunol* 104(3):S109, 1999.

Kolcaba K, Steiner R: Empirical evidence for the nature of holistic comfort, *J Holist Nurs* 18(1):46, 2000.

Lamont SC: "Discomfort" as a potential nursing diagnosis: a concept analysis and review of the literature, Paper presented at the NNN'02 Conference, April 10–13, 2002, Chicago, Ill.

Leininger MM, McFarland MR: *Transcultural nursing: concepts, theories, research and practices,* ed 3, New York, 2002, McGraw-Hill.

Matheson JD, Clayton J, Muller MJ: The reduction of itch during burn wound healing, *J Burn Care Rehabil* 22(1):76, 2001.

Ohlsson G et al: Warm tub bathing during labor: maternal and neonatal effects, *Acta Obstet Gynecol Scand* 80(4):311, 2001.

Patino O et al: Massage in hypertrophic scars, *J Burn Care Rehabil* 20(3):268, 1999.

Richards KC, Gibson R, Overton-McCoy AL: Effects of massage in acute and critical care, *AACN Clin Issues* 11(1):77, 2000.

Smith W, Burns C: Managing the hair and skin of African-American pediatric clients, *J Pediatr Health Care* 13: 72, 1999.

Stone L: Product focus: Medilan—a hypoallergenic lanolin for emollient therapy, *Br J Nurs* 9(1)54, 2000.

Tabata N et al: Biophysical assessment of persistent effects of moisturizers after their daily applications: evaluation of corneotherapy, *Dermatology* 200(4):308, 2000.

Uter W, Gefeller O, Schwanitz HJ: An epidemiological study of the influence of season on the occurrence of irritant skin changes of the hands, *Br J Dermatol* 138(2):266, 1998.

Vlasic W, Almond D: Research-based practice: reducing bedrest following cardiac catheterization, *Can J Cardiovasc Nurs* 10(1-2):19, 1999.

Walker AC: Safety and comfort work of nurses glimpsed through patient narratives, *Int J Nurs Pract* 8: 42, 2002.

Wang S et al: Comparison of comfort and local complications after cardiac catheterization, *Clin Nurs Res* 10(1):29, 2001.

Worfolk JB: Keep frail elders warm! *Geriatr Nurs* 18(1):7, 1997.

Yoshizawa, Y et al: Sea water or its components alter experimental irritant dermatitis in man, *Skin Res Technol* 7(1):36, 2001.

Yosipovitch G et al: Itch characteristics in Chinese patients with atopic dermatitis using a new questionnaire for the assessment of pruritus, *Int J Dermatol* 41(4):212, 2002.

Readiness for enhanced Communication

Gail B. Ladwig

NANDA Definition

Pattern of exchanging information and ideas with others that is sufficient for meeting one's needs and life's goals and can be strengthened

Defining Characteristics

Expresses willingness to enhance communication; able to speak or write a language; forms words, phrases, and language; expresses thoughts and feelings; uses and interprets

• = Independent; ▲ = Collaborative

nonverbal cues appropriately; expresses satisfaction with ability to share information and ideas with others

Related Factors (r/t)

To be developed

| NOC | Outcomes (Nursing Outcomes Classification) |

Suggested NOC Outcomes

Communication; Communication: Expressive, Receptive

> **Example NOC Outcome with Indicators**
>
> **Communication** as evidenced by the following indicators: Use of spoken language/Use of written language/Acknowledgment of messages received/Exchange of messages with others (Rate each indicator of **Communication:** 1 = extremely compromised, 2 = substantially compromised, 3 = moderately compromised, 4 = mildly compromised, 5 = not compromised [see Section I].)

Client Outcomes

Client Will (Specify Time Frame):

- Express willingness to enhance communication
- Demonstrate ability to speak or write a language
- Form words, phrases, and language
- Express thoughts and feelings
- Use and interpret nonverbal cues appropriately
- Express satisfaction with ability to share information and ideas with others

| NIC | Interventions (Nursing Interventions Classification) |

Suggested NIC Interventions

Active Listening; Communication Enhancement: Hearing Deficit, Speech Deficit

> **Example NIC Activities—Communication Enhancement: Hearing Deficit**
>
> Listen attentively; Validate understanding of messages by asking client to repeat what was said

Nursing Interventions and Rationales

- Establish a good nurse-client relationship: provide appropriate education for the client, demonstrate caring by being present to the client. **Clinical Research:** *A good nurse-client relationship is essential to meet the clinical, psychological, and social needs of the client to optimize treatment in clients with renal disease. In this context, the importance of effective client education to increase client compliance played a vital role (Jenkins et al, 2002).* **Nursing Research:** *Studies have demonstrated the importance of presence and caring communication (Sundin, Jansson, and Norberg, 2002).*
- Carefully assess the client's readiness to communicate. **Nursing Research:** *Best practice with regard to communication in palliative care was achieved by using a sensitive assessment of how each client chooses to cope with his or her situation rather than a uniform approach to care (Dean, 2002).*

• = Independent; ▲ = Collaborative

- Assess the client's literacy level. **Clinical Research:** *Health literacy is increasingly recognized as a critical factor affecting communication across the continuum of cancer care. According to the National Adult Literacy Survey, considered the most accurate portrait of literacy in our society, about one in five American adults may lack the necessary literacy skills to function adequately in our society (Davis et al, 2002).*
- Listen attentively and provide a comfortable environment for communicating; use these practical guidelines to assist in communication:
  - Slow down and listen to the client's story.
  - Use "living room" language.
  - Use pictures and stories to illustrate important points.
  - Repeat instructions; limit the amount of information given.
  - Have the client "teach back" to confirm understanding.
  - Avoid asking, "Do you understand?"
  - Be respectful, caring, and sensitive.

  Clinical Research: *Practical communication aids can help bridge the cancer communication gap (Davis et al, 2002).* **Nursing Research:** *A descriptive qualitative study of the nurse-client relationship identified helping influences that included consistency, pacing, listening, positive initial impressions, and attention to comfort and control (Forchuk et al, 2000). Listening was identified as positive communication in the nurse-client relationship (Gilbert, 1998).*
- ▲ Provide communication with specialty nurses who have knowledge about the client's situation. **Nursing Research:** *Evidence suggests that clients supported by a nurse specialist are well informed and have a high degree of satisfaction (Greenhill, Betts, and Pickard, 2002).*
- ▲ Refer couples in maladjusted relationships to psychosocial intervention and social support to strengthen communication; consider nurse specialists. **Clinical Research:** *One study examined the relationship between coping and distress in couples faced with prostate cancer. Findings suggest that the relationship between coping and distress depends on the quality of dyadic functioning. Being part of a strong dyad may serve as a buffering factor; this implies the need for psychosocial intervention for couples in maladjusted relationships (Banthia et al, 2003).* **Nursing Research:** *Social support intervention may be most useful when delivered by clinical nurse specialists who have additional education, training in communication, and teaching and consulting skills (Daugherty et al, 2002).*

Geriatric

- ▲ Assess for hearing and vision impairments and make appropriate referrals for hearing aids. **Clinical Research:** *One study recommended that clinicians assess each client's vision and conversational performance along with hearing thresholds before considering directions for rehabilitation. During face-to-face interaction, many people with adequate vision can compensate for a high-frequency hearing loss through lip reading, which precludes the need for hearing aids; many people with poor vision cannot compensate for a high-frequency hearing loss through lip reading and may require hearing aids (Erber, 2002).*
- Use touch if culturally acceptable when communicating with older clients and their families. *Touch can be useful for improving comfort and communication among terminally ill older adults and their loved ones (Bush, 2001).* **Nursing Research:** *Provision of comfort touch to 45 institutionalized elderly women significantly improved perceptions of self-esteem, well-being and social processes, health status, life satisfaction and self-actualization, faith or belief, and self-responsibility (Butts, 2001).*

- = **Independent;** ▲ = **Collaborative**

- Caregivers may sing when delivering care and instructions. **Nursing Research:** *During caregiver singing, the client communicated with an increased understanding of the situation, both verbally and behaviorally (Gtell, Brown, and Ekman, 2002).*

Multicultural

- Nurses should become more sensitive to the meaning of a culture's nonverbal communication modes, such as eye contact, facial expression, touching, body language, and distancing practices, in cross-cultural encounters.
- Nurses should realize that their good intentions and their usual nonverbal communication style may sometimes be interpreted as offensive and insulting by a specific cultural group. *To give a client a positive signal during a therapy session, a nurse may display the American sign of thumbs up. In Iran, however, thumbs extended upward are considered a vulgar gesture (Campinha-Bacote, 1998).*
- Assess for the influence of cultural beliefs, norms, and values on the client's communication process. **Nursing Research:** *What the client considers normal and abnormal communication may be based on cultural perceptions (Leininger and McFarland, 2002; Johnson, 1999; Cochran, 1998; Doswell and Erlen, 1998). An affirmative answer does not necessarily mean "yes"; a client may be showing respect to the caregiver or avoiding the embarrassment of saying "no" (Galanti, 1997).*
- Assess personal space needs, acceptable communication styles, acceptable body language, interpretation of eye contact, perception of touch, and use of paraverbal modes when communicating with the client. **Nursing Research:** *Nurses need to consider multiple factors when interpreting verbal and nonverbal messages (Purnell, 2000). Native Americans may consider avoiding direct eye contact to be a sign of respect and asking questions to be rude and intrusive (Seiderman et al, 1996).*
- Take extreme care when using touch. **Nursing Research:** *Touch is largely culturally defined (Leininger and McFarland, 2002). Touch is believed by some cultures to be a source of illness. Touching a baby's head requires parental permission in some Southeast Asian cultures. Many Latinos believe that excessive admiration of a child without touching will result in physical illness of the child (mal de ojo—"evil eye"). In some Islamic and Latino cultures, physical touch between a nurse and client is acceptable only if the individuals are of the same sex (Kelley, 1998). Some Asian cultures believe that touching the head is a sign of disrespect (Galanti, 1997).*
- Modify the communication approach in keeping with the client's particular culture. **Nursing Research:** *Modification of communication will convey respect to the client (Purnell, 2000).*
- ▲ Use an interpreter if the client speaks a different language. **Nursing Research:** *An experienced interpreter will allow for accurate translation (Maltby, 1999).*
- ▲ Use therapeutic communication techniques that emphasize acceptance, offer the self, validate the client's concerns, and convey respect. **Nursing Research:** *Validation is a therapeutic communication technique that lets the client know that the nurse has heard and understood what was said, and it promotes the nurse-client relationship (Heineken, 1998). Studies show that, even when language is not a barrier, some ethnic clients may be reluctant to discuss their beliefs and practices because of fear of criticism or ridicule (Evans and Cunningham, 1996).*
- ▲ Use reminiscence therapy as a language intervention. **Nursing Research:** *Reminiscence therapy is well suited as a language intervention for older adults from culturally and linguistically diverse backgrounds (Harris, 1997).*

- • = **Independent;** ▲ = **Collaborative**

Home care
- The interventions described previously may be used in home care.
- Refer to the care plan **Impaired verbal Communication.**

REFERENCES

Banthia R et al: The effects of dyadic strength and coping styles on psychological distress in couples faced with prostate cancer, *J Behav Med* 26(1):31, 2003.

Bush E: The use of human touch to improve the well-being of older adults: a holistic nursing intervention, *J Holist Nurs* 19(3):256, 2001.

Butts JB: Outcomes of comfort touch in institutionalized elderly female residents, *Geriatr Nurs* 22(4):180, 2001.

Campinha-Bacote J: *A model of practice to address cultural competence in rehabilitation nursing,* continuing education, Association of Rehabilitation Nurses, 1998, available online at http://www.rehabnurse.org/ce/010201/010201_a.htm, accessed Feb 12, 2003.

Cochran M: Tears have no color, *Am J Nurs* 98(6):53, 1998.

Daugherty J et al: Can we talk? Developing a social support nursing intervention for couples, *Clin Nurse Spec* 16:211, 2002.

Davis TC et al: Health literacy and cancer communication, *CA Cancer J Clin* 52(3):130, 2002.

Dean A: Talking to dying clients of their hopes and needs, *Nurs Times* 98(43):34, 2002.

Doswell W, Erlen J: Multicultural issues and ethical concerns in the delivery of nursing care interventions, *Nurs Clin North Am* 33(2):353, 1998.

Erber NP: Hearing, vision, communication, and older people, *Semin Hearing* 23(1):35, 2002.

Evans CA, Cunningham BA: Caring for the ethnic elder, *Geriatr Nurs* 17(3):105, 1996.

Forchuk C et al: The developing nurse-client relationship: nurses' perspectives. *J Am Psychiatr Nurses Assoc* 6(1):3, 2000.

Galanti G: *Caring for patients from different cultures: case studies from American hospitals,* ed 2, Philadelphia, 1997, University of Pennsylvania Press.

Gilbert DA: Relational message themes in nurses' listening behavior during brief client-nurse interactions, *Sch Inq Nurs Pract* 12(1):5, 1998.

Greenhill L, Betts T, Pickard N: The epilepsy nurse specialist—expendable handmaiden or essential colleague? *Seizure* 11(suppl A):615, 2002.

Gtell E, Brown S, Ekman S: Caregiver singing and background music in dementia car, *West J Nurs Res* 24(2):195, 2002.

Harris JL: Clinical focus: Reminiscence: a culturally and developmentally appropriate language intervention for older adults, *Am J Speech Lang Pathol* 6(3):19, 1997.

Heineken J: Patient silence is not necessarily client satisfaction: Communication in home care nursing, *Home Healthc Nurse* 16(2):115, 1998.

Jenkins K et al: Improving the nurse-patient relationship: a multi-faceted approach, *EDTNA ERCA J* 28(3):145, 2002.

Johnson M: Focus. Communication in healthcare: a review of some key issues, *NT Res* 4(1):18, 1999.

Kelley J: Cultural and ethnic considerations. In Frisch NC, Frisch LE, editors: *Psychiatric mental health nursing,* Albany, NY, 1998, Delmar.

Leininger MM, McFarland MR: *Transcultural nursing: concepts, theories, research and practices,* ed 3, New York, 2002, McGraw-Hill.

Maltby HJ: Interpreters: a double-edged sword in nursing practice, *J Transcult Nurs* 10(3):248, 1999.

Purnell L: A description of the Purnell model for cultural competence, *J Transcult Nurs* 11(1):40, 2000.

Seiderman RY et al: Assessing American Indian families, *MCN Am J Matern Child Nurs* 21(6):274, 1996.

Sundin K, Jansson L, Norberg A: Understanding between care providers and patients with stroke and aphasia: a phenomenological hermeneutic inquiry, *Nurs Inq* 9(2):9, 2002.

• = Independent; ▲ = Collaborative

Impaired verbal Communication

Gail B. Ladwig

NANDA Definition

Decreased, delayed, or absent ability to receive, process, transmit, and use a system of symbols

Defining Characteristics

Willful refusal to speak; disorientation in the three spheres of time, space, and person; inability to speak dominant language; failure or inability to speak; speaking or verbalization with difficulty; inappropriate verbalizations; difficulty forming words or sentences (e.g., aphonia, dyslalia, dysarthria); difficulty expressing thoughts verbally (e.g., aphasia, dysphasia, apraxia, dyslexia); stuttering; slurring; dyspnea; absence of eye contact or difficulty in selectively attending; difficulty in comprehending and maintaining usual communication pattern; partial or total visual deficit; inability to use or difficulty in using facial or body expressions

Related Factors (r/t)

Decrease in circulation to brain; brain tumor; physical barrier (e.g., tracheostomy, intubation); anatomical defect; cleft palate; alteration of neuromuscular visual system, auditory system, phonatory apparatus; psychological barriers (e.g., psychosis, lack of stimuli); cultural difference; differences related to developmental age; side effects of medication; environmental barriers; absence of significant others; altered perceptions; lack of information; stress; alteration of self-esteem or self-concept; physiological conditions; alteration of central nervous system; weakening of musculoskeletal system; emotional conditions

NOC Outcomes (Nursing Outcomes Classification)

Suggested NOC Outcomes

Communication; Communication: Expressive, Receptive

> **Example NOC Outcome with Indicators**
>
> **Communication** as evidenced by the following indicators: Use of spoken language/Use of written language/Acknowledgment of messages received/Exchange of messages with others (Rate each indicator of **Communication:** 1 = extremely compromised, 2 = substantially compromised, 3 = moderately compromised, 4 = mildly compromised, 5 = not compromised [see Section I].)

Client Outcomes

Client Will (Specify Time Frame):
- Use effective communication techniques
- Use alternative methods of communication effectively
- Demonstrate congruency of verbal and nonverbal behavior
- Demonstrate understanding even if not able to speak
- Express desire for social interactions

• = Independent; ▲ = Collaborative

NIC   Interventions (Nursing Interventions Classification)

Suggested NIC Interventions

Active Listening; Communication Enhancement: Hearing Deficit, Speech Deficit

> **Example NIC Activities—Communication Enhancement: Hearing Deficit**
>
> Listen attentively; Validate understanding of messages by asking client to repeat what was said

Nursing Interventions and Rationales

▲ When the client is having difficulty communicating, assess and refer for consultation for hearing problems. Hearing loss might be suspected when a person does not always hear sounds such as a ringing telephone or doorbell, turns his or her ear toward the source of sound, frequently asks the speaker to repeat, turns the volume on the television or radio up too loud, or shows obvious signs of confusion or misunderstanding of speech. *People with hearing disorders do not hear sounds clearly. Such disorders may range from hearing speech sounds faintly or in a distorted way to profound deafness (American Speech-Language-Hearing Association, 2001).*

• Involve a familiar person when attempting to communicate with a person who has difficulty with communication. Ask about deviations in behaviors. *The involvement of a familiar person may be reassuring and assist in interpretation of communications, whether behavior is typical or new. Sometimes deviations from normal behavior indicate a change in health status or a need (Hahn, 1999).*

▲ Determine the language spoken; obtain a language dictionary or interpreter if possible and accepted by the client. **Nursing Research:** *The lack of fluency in the English language of many clients and the lack of bilingual or multilingual nurses are major sources of miscommunication, even with the use of interpreters and translated health information. Many immigrant women find the use of interpreters unacceptable, and nurses are concerned with legal issues (Maltby, 1999).*

• Listen carefully. Validate verbal and nonverbal expressions. **Nursing Research:** *In a study of caring behavior involving 200 nurse practitioners, listening was identified as one of the top ten caring behaviors (Brunton and Beaman, 2000). Listening carefully to clients gives nurses valuable tools for intervening in the lives of their clients (Walden-McBride and McBride, 2000).*

• Spend time communicating with the client. **Nursing Research:** *In a qualitative study, psychological well-being was found to be enhanced by humanistic and personal interaction with the nurse (Richardson, 2002).*

• Use simple communication, speak in a well-modulated voice, smile, and show concern for the client. Such techniques have been described by clients as demonstrating caring (Clark, 1993). **Clinical Research:** *Verbal and nonverbal techniques can be used to soften the delivery of grave news and convey information more clearly. Know when it may be better not to say anything but just to listen (Travaline, 2002).*

• Involve clients with mental retardation in communication when possible by asking open-ended questions to elicit answers. *Sometimes people with mental retardation answer "yes" to both yes and no questions. If you ask many yes and no questions, validate the answers by asking pertinent open-ended questions (Hahn, 1999).*

• = Independent; ▲ = Collaborative

- Recognize behavioral cues for pain (e.g., hair pulling, face slapping, facial grimacing). *Accurately reading cues may help to identify pain (Hahn, 1999).*
- Observe behavioral communication cues in infants. **Nursing Research:** *In one study, greater pain was strongly associated with tears, stiff posture, guarding, and fisting in infants up to 12 months of age (Fuller et al, 1996).*
- Maintain eye contact at the client's level. **Nursing Research:** *Good communication involves many familiar concepts, including good eye contact (Summers, 2002).*
- When working with the hearing impaired, remove masks and reduce background noise whenever possible. **Clinical Research:** *One study of hearing-impaired children receiving dental care indicated that removing masks while talking, reducing background noise, and learning to use simple signs may improve communication with these children (Champion and Holt, 2000).*
- Assess whether a person is averse to touch (tactile defensiveness), which is common among children or adults with pervasive developmental delays or autism. *The use of touch may not be effective if someone experiences tactile defensiveness (Hahn, 1999).*
- Use touch as appropriate. **Clinical Research:** *Physicians in a qualitative study who showed interest in their clients as persons and who used touch to communicate caring were perceived as supportive communicators (Harris and Templeton, 2001).* **Nursing Research:** *Physical touch in caring has physical, emotional, social, and spiritual significance and needs to be treated in a holistic way. It is possible to enrich the meanings and methods of physical touch in nursing so that its application may produce positive impacts on clients' well-being and comfort (Chang, 2001).*
- Use presence. Spend time with the client, allow time for responses, and make the call light readily available. **Nursing Research:** *Providing nursing presence, interacting one on one, connecting with the client's experience, going beyond the scientific data, and knowing what will work and when to act all support the nurse-client relationship and affirm the client's self. As a result, the client grows in awareness of his or her own being (Doona, Chase, and Haggerty, 1999).*
- Explain all health care procedures. *The nurse cannot assume that a person will not understand, even if that person is nonverbal. A person's receptive language skills may be better than his or her expressive language skills (Hahn, 1999).*
- Obtain communication equipment such as electronic devices, letter boards, picture boards, and magic slates. **Nursing Research:** *A study demonstrated that communication technology enables humanness (Dickerson et al, 2002).*
- Establish an alternative method of communication such as writing or pointing to letters, word phrases, picture cards, or simple drawings of basic needs. **Clinical Research:** *Alternative methods of communication are necessary when the client is unable to use verbal communication. A booklet of drawings (visual language) representing the most common needs was used with a group of 34 clients affected by severe dysarthria or motor aphasia causing severe language disorders. Most of these clients used this booklet to express their basic needs (Marquez-Rebollo and Tornel-Costa, 1997).*
- Provide pencil and paper for letter writing to facilitate expression of feelings. *Letter writing has been used with clients who have had amputations to help them successfully express feelings (Hatipoglu and Temiz, 1995).*
- ▲ Consultation with a speech therapist may be helpful. Supplement the work of the speech therapist with appropriate exercises. **Evidence-Based Research:** *Consultation and collaboration with a specialist may be necessary to provide the best approach to improving communication. The main conclusion of one review is that speech and language ther-*

• = Independent; ▲ = Collaborative

apy for people with aphasia after a stroke has not been shown to be either clearly effective or clearly ineffective in a randomized controlled trial (Greener, Enderby, and Whurr, 2000).

- Give praise for progress noted. Ignore mistakes and watch for frustration or fatigue. *Positive reinforcement raises confidence, which can increase communication (Boss, 1991).*
- Encourage the family to bring in familiar pictures or calendars.
- Establish an understanding of the client's symbolic speech (especially with schizophrenic clients). Ask the client to clarify particular statements. *Clarification is a necessary communication skill. Psychoeducation covers the practical problems of living with schizophrenia. Families learn when to ignore problem behaviors and when to intervene (Huddleston, 1992).*
- If a comprehension deficit is present, keep the environment quiet when communicating and get the client's attention before attempting to communicate (e.g., touch the client's shoulder, call the client's name). *When the client is confused, a distracting environment interferes with communication. It is necessary to get the client's full attention before any communication can take place (Boss, 1991).*
- Use "affection therapy" when the client cannot express thoughts or ideas. Provide frequent and regular reminders that the client is wanted and cared about (e.g., physical signs of affection such as a hug or a friendly comment before and after every interaction regardless of the client's performance). *When clients are unable to communicate their thoughts and feelings adequately, they may whistle, swear, and make other noises incessantly. "Affection therapy" works when behavior modification techniques do not (Armstrong, 1991).*
- Do not raise your voice or shout at the client. *A loud voice can be frightening and decrease communication.*

Geriatric

- Initiate communication with the client with dementia. **Nursing Research:** *In a qualitative study participants were more often responders than initiators in social interactions (Fitzgerald, 2001).*
- Carefully assess the client for hearing difficulty using an audiometer. **Clinical Research:** *The prevalence of hearing impairment in hospitalized elderly clients was found to be very high during screening with an audiometer (Lim and Yap, 2000).* **Clinical Research:** *One study demonstrated that decreases in speech understanding in noise and declines in central auditory processing are common in the growing population of older women (Garstecki and Erler, 2001).*
- Encourage the client to wear prescribed eyeglasses and hearing aids. *Auditory and visual disorders are prevalent among older people. About 40% of adults aged 65 and older have a hearing loss sufficient to interfere with daily conversation (Erber, 1994). About 20% in the same age range experience low vision and reduced visual fields, which can prevent clear perception of a communication partner at a conversational distance (Erber, 1994).*
- When communicating with a client, face toward his or her unaffected side or better ear. *Correct positioning increases the client's awareness of the interaction and enhances the client's ability to interact.*
- Provide sufficient light and remove distractions such as glare and background noise. *Background noise further impairs the elderly client's hearing.*
- Use low voice tones and recognize that perception of the sounds *f, s, th, ch, sh, b, t, p, k,* and *d* is impaired with age-related hearing loss. *Presbycusis decreases the ability to hear high-pitched sounds and the consonant sounds listed earlier. Perception of consonants is important to understanding language.*

- = Independent; ▲ = Collaborative

- Allow time for thought comprehension when communicating with the client. *Older clients do not like to be rushed. They fare much better in a calm, consistent environment that functions at a moderately slow pace (Bailey and Bailey, 1993).*
- Schedule time to listen to the client's life story. **Nursing Research:** *This is a means of finding out what is important to the client. The practice of nursing comes alive by listening to individual stories. Each person's story is created out of personal life experiences (Running, 1996).*
- Use touch as culturally appropriate. **Nursing Research:** *A number of studies suggest that the appropriate use of touch by nurses can be useful for improving comfort and communication in terminally ill older adults and their loved ones (Bush, 2001).*

Multicultural

- Assess for the influence of cultural beliefs, norms, and values on the client's communication process. **Nursing Research:** *What the client considers normal and abnormal communication may be based on cultural perceptions (Leininger and McFarland, 2002; Johnson, 1999; Cochran, 1998; Doswell and Erlen, 1998). An affirmative answer does not necessarily mean "yes"; a client may be showing respect to the caregiver or avoiding the embarrassment of saying "no" (Galanti, 1997).*
- Assess personal space needs, acceptable communication styles, acceptable body language, interpretation of eye contact, perception of touch, and use of paraverbal modes when communicating with the client. **Nursing Research:** *Nurses need to consider multiple factors when interpreting verbal and nonverbal messages (Purnell, 2000). Native Americans may consider avoiding direct eye contact to be a sign of respect and asking questions to be rude and intrusive (Seiderman et al, 1996).*
- Take extreme care when using touch. **Nursing Research:** *Touch is largely culturally defined (Leninger and McFarland, 2002). Touch is believed by some cultures to be a source of illness. Touching a baby's head requires parental permission in some Southeast Asian cultures. Many Latinos believe that excessive admiration of a child without touching will result in physical illness of the child (mal de ojo—"evil eye"). In some Islamic and Latino cultures, physical touch between a nurse and client is acceptable only if the individuals are of the same sex (Kelley, 1998). Some Asian cultures believe that touching the head is a sign of disrespect (Galanti, 1997).*
- Modify the communication approach in keeping with the client's particular culture. **Nursing Research:** *Modification of communication will convey respect to the client (Purnell, 2000).*
- ▲ Use an interpreter if the client speaks a different language. **Nursing Research:** *An experienced interpreter will allow for accurate translation (Maltby, 1999).*
- Use therapeutic communication techniques that emphasize acceptance, offer the self, validate the client's concerns, and convey respect. **Nursing Research:** *Validation is a therapeutic communication technique that lets the client know that the nurse has heard and understood what was said, and it promotes the nurse-client relationship (Heineken, 1998). Studies show that, even when language is not a barrier, some ethnic clients may be reluctant to discuss their beliefs and practices because of fear of criticism or ridicule (Evans and Cunningham, 1996).*
- Use reminiscence therapy as a language intervention. **Nursing Research:** *Reminiscence therapy is well suited as a language intervention for older adults from culturally and linguistically diverse backgrounds (Harris, 1997).*

- = Independent; ▲ = Collaborative

Home care

- The interventions described previously may be adapted for home care use.
- ▲ Begin discharge planning as soon as possible with the case manager or social worker to assess the need for home support systems, assistive devices, and community or home health services.
- ▲ Continue with speech therapy services per the physician's order. Support the speech therapy plan of care. *With appropriate support, clients can continue to make significant progress toward resuming normal or improved communication function.*
- ▲ Assess the cause of communication difficulty and the psychological response to communication difficulty. Refer for mental health assessment as indicated. **Clinical Research:** *Seemingly willful refusal to speak may indicate a psychiatric disorder or a medication reaction (e.g., severe dystonia). Major depression has been diagnosed in an average of 20% of poststroke clients (Tateno, Kimura, and Robinson, 2002). Impaired communication as a result of stroke may increase depressed mood.*
- ▲ Use an understanding of the client's specific physiological changes to implement actions that will assist client communication, provide support, and decrease stress. *Inability to express oneself and be understood by others is frustrating and stressful. Acknowledging the experience for the client can be helpful. The specific pathophysiological cause can indicate appropriate expectations of the client; for example, an expressive aphasic condition will interfere with coherent speech but does not mean that the client does not understand what is said to him or her. It is inappropriate to assume that the client has lost global communication functions.*
- ▲ Assess the family for possible role changes resulting from communication impairment of a family member. *An impairment that prevents a family member from fulfilling the usual role can change the family constellation.*
- ▲ When possible, encourage the family to include the client in family activities using enhanced communication techniques with sensitivity. *Involving the client in family activities promotes earlier return to normal life patterns, but doing so in an awkward or embarrassing way can diminish interest.*
- ▲ Refer to medical social services as necessary for help in obtaining funds for communication devices and counseling for dealing with the long-term impact of the communication changes in the family.
- ▲ Institute case management of the frail elderly to support continued independent living. *Difficulties with communication can lead to increasing needs for assistance in using the health care system effectively. Case management combines the nursing activities of client and family assessment, planning and coordination of care among all health care providers, delivery of direct nursing care, and monitoring of care and outcomes. These activities can address continuity of care, mutual goal setting, behavior management, and prevention of worsening health problems (Guttman, 1999).*
- ▲ Refer for psychiatric home health care services for client reassurance and implementation of a therapeutic regimen. *Psychiatric home care nurses can address issues relating to the client's ability to adjust to communication difficulties. Behavioral interventions in the home can assist the client in participating more effectively in the treatment plan (Patusky, Rodning, and Martinez-Kratz, 1996).*

Client/Family Teaching

- Teach the client and family techniques to increase communication. *Alternative methods of communication are necessary when the client is unable to use verbal communication.*

- **•** = **Independent;** ▲ = **Collaborative**

- Teach basic signs to indicate needs, such as "eat," "drink," "toilet," "more," "finished." *Sometimes clients with mental retardation are taught basic signs for communication (Hahn, 1999).*
- Encourage significant others to use touch, such as holding the client's hand or stroking the arm. *Involving relatives in this aspect of care provides continuity with the client's real life and fulfills relatives' need to demonstrate care (MacGinley, 1993).*
- Teach the client how to use communication devices.
- ▲ Refer the client to a speech-language pathologist or audiologist. *A thorough evaluation by a speech-language pathologist or audiologist is needed to determine a person's communication strengths and weaknesses. After this evaluation, the speech-language pathologist or audiologist will be able to provide a plan for meeting individual needs (American Speech-Language-Hearing Association, 2001).*
- ▲ Refer to a specialist for possible surgical intervention when clients have surgical defects caused by cancer of the maxillary sinus and alveolar ridge. **Clinical Research:** *Obturators have been developed for surgical defects caused by cancer of the maxillary sinus and alveolar ridge. In a study of 32 consecutively treated maxillectomy clients with the obturator inserted, mean speech intelligibility was 94%, speaking rate was 164 words per minute, and nasality was rated as 1.6. Clients' mean self-perceived communication effectiveness was 75% of what it was before the diagnosis of cancer (Sullivan et al, 2002).*

evolve WEBSITES FOR EDUCATION

See the EVOLVE website for World Wide Web resources for client education.

REFERENCES

American Speech-Language-Hearing Association: *Stroke,* available online at http://www.asha.org/speech/disabilities/Stroke.cfm, accessed May 29, 2001.

Armstrong C: Emotional changes following brain injury: psychological and neurological components of depression, denial and anxiety, *J Rehabil* 57:15, 1991.

Bailey DS, Bailey DR: *Therapeutic approaches to the care of the mentally ill,* ed 3, Philadelphia, 1993, FA Davis.

Boss BJ: Managing communication disorders in stroke, *Nurs Clin North Am* 26:985, 1991.

Brunton B, Beaman M: Nurse practitioners' perceptions of their caring behaviors, *J Am Acad Nurse Pract* 11:451, 2000.

Bush E: The use of human touch to improve the well-being of older adults: a holistic nursing intervention, *J Holist Nurs* 19(3):256, 2001.

Champion J, Holt R: Dental care for children and young people who have a hearing impairment, *Br Dent J* 189(3):155, 2000.

Chang SO: The conceptual structure of physical touch in caring, *J Adv Nurs* 33(6):820, 2001.

Clark S: Challenges in critical care nursing: helping patients and families cope, *Crit Care Nurs* S2:2, 1993.

Cochran M: Tears have no color, *Am J Nurs* 98(6):53, 1998.

Dickerson SS et al: The meaning of communication: experiences with augmentative communication devices, *Rehabil Nurs* 27(6):215, 2002.

Doona M, Chase S, Haggerty L: Nursing presence, as real as a Milky Way Bar, *J Holist Nurs* 17(1):54, 1999.

Doswell W, Erlen J: Multicultural issues and ethical concerns in the delivery of nursing care interventions, *Nurs Clin North Am* 33(2):353, 1998.

Erber N: Conversation as therapy for older adults in residential care: the case for intervention, *Eur J Disord Commun* 29:269, 1994.

Evans CA, Cunningham BA: Caring for the ethnic elder, *Geriatr Nurs* 17(3):105, 1996.

Fitzgerald DC: Descriptive study of the social interactions of older adults diagnosed with dementia, doctoral dissertation, Washington, DC, 2001, The Catholic University of America.

Fuller B et al: Relationship of cues to assessed infant pain level, *Clin Nurs Res* 5(1):43, 1996.

- = **Independent;** ▲ = **Collaborative**

Galanti G: *Caring for patients from different cultures: case studies from American hospitals,* ed 2, Philadelphia, 1997, University of Pennsylvania Press.

Garstecki D, Erler SF: Personal and social conditions potentially influencing women's hearing loss management, *Am J Audiol* 10(2):78, 2001.

Greener J, Enderby P, Whurr R: Speech and language therapy for aphasia following stroke, *Cochrane Library,* CD000425, 2000.

Guttman R: Case management of the frail elderly in the community, *Clin Nurs Spec* 13(4):174, 1999.

Hahn J: Cueing in to patient language, *Reflections* 25(1):8, 1999.

Harris JL: Clinical focus: Reminiscence: a culturally and developmentally appropriate language intervention for older adults, *Am J Speech Lang Pathol* 6(3):19, 1997.

Harris SR, Templeton E: Who's listening? Experiences of women with breast cancer in communicating with physicians, *Breast J* 7(6):444, 2001.

Hatipoglu S, Temiz Z: Nurse's notes from Turkey. Amputee's diary, *Image J Nurs Sch* 27:248, 1995.

Heineken J: Patient silence is not necessarily client satisfaction: communication in home care nursing, *Home Healthc Nurse* 16(2):115, 1998.

Huddleston J: Family and group psychoeducational approaches in the management of schizophrenia, *Clin Nurs Spec* 6:118, 1992.

Johnson M: Focus. Communication in healthcare: a review of some key issues, *NT Res* 4(1):18, 1999.

Kelley J: Cultural and ethnic considerations. In Frisch NC, Frisch LE, editors: *Psychiatric mental health nursing,* Albany, NY, 1998, Delmar.

Leininger MM, McFarland MR: *Transcultural nursing: concepts, theories, research and practices,* ed 3, New York, 2002, McGraw-Hill.

Lim JK, Yap KB: Screening for hearing impairment in hospitalised elderly, *Ann Acad Med Singapore* 29(2):237, 2000.

MacGinley K: Nursing care of the patient with altered body image, *Br J Nurs* 2:1098, 1993.

Maltby HJ: Interpreters: a double-edged sword in nursing practice, *J Transcult Nurs* 10(3):248, 1999.

Marquez-Rebollo MC, Tornel-Costa MC: Design of a non-verbal method of communication using cartoons, *Rev Neurol* 25(148):2045, 1997.

Patusky KL, Rodning C, Martinez-Kratz M: Clinical lessons in psychiatric home care: a case study approach, *J Home Health Case Manag* 9:18, 1996.

Purnell L: A description of the Purnell model for cultural competence, *J Transcult Nurs* 11(1):40, 2000.

Richardson J: Health promotion in palliative care: the patients' perception of therapeutic interaction with the palliative nurse in the primary care setting, *J Adv Nurs* 40(4):432, 2002.

Running AF: "The measure of my days" critiqued by the oldest old, *Image J Nurs Sch* 28:71, 1996.

Seiderman RY et al: Assessing American Indian families, *MCN Am J Matern Child Nurs* 21(6):274, 1996.

Sullivan M et al: Impact of palatal prosthodontic intervention on communication performance of patients' maxillectomy defects: a multilevel outcome study, *Head Neck* 24(6):530, 2002.

Summers LC: Mutual timing: an essential component of provider/patient communication, *J Am Acad Nurse Pract* 14(1):19, 2002.

Tateno A, Kimura M, Robinson RG: Phenomenological characteristics of poststroke depression. Early- versus late-onset, *Am J Geriatr Psychiatry* 10:575, 2002.

Travaline JM: Communication in the ICU: an essential component of patient care: strategies for communicating with patients and their families, *J Crit Illness* 17(11):451, 2002.

Walden-McBride DL, McBride JL: Listening for the patient's story: the psychosocial story of a patient with end-stage heart disease, *J Psychosoc Nurs Ment Health Serv* 38(11):26, 2000.

Decisional Conflict (specify)

Gail B. Ladwig

NANDA Definition

Uncertainty about course of action to be taken when choice among competing actions involves risk, loss, or challenge to personal life values

• = **Independent;** ▲ = **Collaborative**

Defining Characteristics

Verbalization of uncertainty about choices; verbalization of undesired consequences of alternative actions being considered; vacillation between alternative choices; delayed decision making; verbalization of feelings of distress while attempting to make a decision; self-focusing; physical signs of distress or tension (e.g., increased heart rate, increased muscle tension, restlessness); questioning of personal values and beliefs while attempting to make a decision

Related Factors (r/t)

Support system deficit; perceived threat to value system; lack of experience or interference with decision making; multiple or divergent sources of information; lack of relevant information; unclear personal values/beliefs

NOC   Outcomes (Nursing Outcomes Classification)

Suggested NOC Outcomes
Decision Making; Information Processing; Participation in Health Care Decisions

> **Example NOC Outcome with Indicators**
>
> **Decision Making** as evidenced by the following indicators: Identifies relevant information/Identifies alternatives/Identifies potential consequences of each alternative/Identifies resources necessary to support each alternative (Rate each indicator of **Decision Making:** 1 = severely compromised, 2 = substantially compromised, 3 = moderately compromised, 4 = mildly compromised, 5 = not compromised [see Section I].)

Client Outcomes

Client Will (Specify Time Frame):
- State the advantages and disadvantages of choices
- Share fears and concerns regarding choices and responses of others
- Make an informed choice

NIC   Interventions (Nursing Interventions Classification)

Suggested NIC Intervention
Decision-Making Support

> **Example NIC Activities—Decision-Making Support**
>
> Inform client of alternative views or solutions; Facilitate client's articulation of goals for care

Nursing Interventions and Rationales

- Observe for factors causing or contributing to conflict (e.g., value conflicts, fear of outcome, poor problem-solving skills). *Baseline data are important in directing interventions; no single set of values is appropriate for all individuals. Values clarification emphasizes the client's capacity for intelligent, self-directed behavior (Dossey et al, 1988).*
- Work with and allow the client to make decisions in a way that is comfortable for the client, such as deferring (allowing others to decide), delaying (choosing an alternative that meets basic requirements), or deliberating (looking at all alternatives).

- **= Independent; ▲ = Collaborative**

Nursing Research: *Individual clients confronting health care choices have unique decision-making styles (Pierce, 1993).* **Clinical Research:** *Involving clients in health care decisions makes a potentially significant and enduring difference to health care outcomes (Elwyn et al, 2000).*

- Give the client time and permission to express feelings associated with decision making. *Decisions become more difficult when feelings are repressed. Once the client relieves some of the stress by talking through problems and releasing pent-up emotions, the decision process often becomes easier (Burnard, 1992).*
- Explore the client's perception of the future with regard to different decisions. *Perceiving the future helps the client focus on what is important. Accurate time orientation (the ability to view the future on the basis of present and past experience) indicates that the client will have better coping skills (Haber et al, 1992).*
- Demonstrate reassurance with unconditional respect for and acceptance of the client's values, spiritual beliefs, and cultural norms. **Nursing Research:** *Good communication with and reassurance of the client are nursing skills that promote trust and orientation and reduce anxiety (Harvey, 1996).*
- Encourage the client to list the advantages and disadvantages of each alternative. *Listing alternatives helps clients learn how to problem solve. Clients might not believe they have alternatives and may need assistance exploring options (Chez, 1994).*
- ▲ Initiate health teaching and referrals when needed. *Advanced practice nurses as case managers can make a positive contribution toward individualizing care for the elderly (Mick and Ackerman, 2002).*
- ▲ Facilitate communication between the client and family members regarding the final decision; offer support to the person actually making the decision. **Nursing Research:** *Studies suggest that clients' decisions are rarely the same as those of their friends and family members; therefore, when possible, clients are best suited to determine their own life support treatment (Beland and Froman, 1995).* **Clinical Research:** *Formulation of an advance proxy plan is important to ensure that the client's previous wishes or best interests are considered when decisions about treatment strategies are made (Volicer, 2001).*
- ▲ Provide detailed information on benefits and risks using functional terms and probabilities tailored to clinical risk, plus steps for considering the issues and means for making a decision, including values clarification and decision aides, when clients are faced with difficult treatment choices. **Clinical Research:** *Tailored decision aids prepare women for decision making better than do general pamphlets (O'Connor et al, 1998).* **Clinical Research:** *Decision aids improve knowledge, reduce decisional conflict, and stimulate clients to be more active in decision making without increasing their anxiety (O'Connor et al, 1999).*

Geriatric

- Work with the clients in setting goals for the plans of care. **Clinical Research:** *Goal-centered advance medical planning can be initiated in nursing homes by asking residents or their surrogates to prioritize their goals of care. These prioritizations can form the foundation for specific patterns of care (Gillick, Berkman, and Cullen, 1999).*
- Review with the client and family the importance of discussing and recording end-of-life decisions. *These decisions are of extreme importance to an aging client. Discussing these issues gives the client both a sense of control and the opportunity to prepare for the inevitable (Dossey et al, 1988).*
- If end-of-life discussions are being avoided, describe the possible consequences. **Nurs-**

• = **Independent;** ▲ = **Collaborative**

ing Research: *Participants in one study thought that a "do not resuscitate" decision should be discussed with clients and also with relatives if appropriate. However, there was ambivalence about whether individuals would like to be involved personally in such a decision because of the anxiety this would produce (Phillips and Woodward, 1999).*

▲ Discuss the purpose of a living will and advance directives. **Nursing Research:** *Elderly clients and their significant others need to know how to legally make end-of-life decisions. (NOTE: Laws differ in each state.) Research has demonstrated that the presence of an advance directive can be very helpful in decreasing family stress when end-of-life decisions need to be made (Tilden et al, 2001).*

• Discuss choices or changes to be made (e.g., moving in with children, into a nursing home, or into an adult foster care home). **Nursing Research:** *Exploring options gives the client and family a sense of control. For a change to be effective, it must be accepted and owned by the client (Fleury, 1991). Caregivers need to provide support when the client and family are facing difficult decisions (Hurley and Volicer, 2002).*

• Teach family members how to be supportive of the final decision or how to refrain from being destructive if they are unable to be supportive. *It is important to support the decisions that the client makes.*

Multicultural

• Assess for the influence of cultural beliefs, norms, and values on the client's decision-making conflict. **Nursing Research:** *Cultural influences may interfere with the client's decision-making process (Leininger and McFarland 2002; Cochran, 1998; Doswell and Erlen, 1998; Wright, Cohen, and Caroselli, 1997). Individuals of Chinese and Korean descent, as well as individuals of the Muslim religion, may accept the health provider's decision regarding medical needs rather than assert their own wishes (Valle, 2001; Moazam, 2000).*

• Identify who will be involved in the decision-making process. **Nursing Research:** *In a group of frail elderly clients, ethnic variations were found with regard to the family member identified as the decision maker (Hornug et al, 1998). Contrary to expectations, Latinas will often make decisions related to prenatal care and services (Browner, Preloran, and Cox, 1999). Korean American clients and other Asian clients may consider some decisions to be a family affair (D'Avanzo et al, 2001; Blackhall et al, 1999). Elders may play a key role in decision making in some Asian populations (Davis, 2001). Some Native American societies are matriarchal in structure, and the matriarch's approval and support may be required for compliance with a treatment plan (Cesario, 2001).*

• Use cross-cultural decision aids whenever possible. **Nursing Research:** *Consumer-based cross-cultural decision aids inform clients of potential risks and benefits so that they can make value- and evidence-integrated decisions (Lawrence et al, 2000). In one study, Latinas' assessment of risk and uncertainty with procedures was associated with decisions to refuse certain procedures (Browner, Preloran and Cox, 1999).*

• Validate the client's feelings regarding the decisional conflict. **Nursing Research:** *Validation is a therapeutic communication technique that lets the client know that the nurse has heard and understood what was said, and it promotes the nurse-client relationship (Heineken, 1998).*

Home care

NOTE: Before addressing decisional conflict, nurses should be aware of their existing biases and preconceptions, and avoid superimposing them on the client's decision-making pro-

• **= Independent; ▲ = Collaborative**

cess. For example, clients making end-of-life decisions must process multiple issues regarding their choices; nurses' discomfort with end-of-life issues could interfere with clients' ability to reflect on choices.

- The interventions described previously may be adapted for home care use.
- ▲ Before providing any home care, assess the client plan for advance directives (living will and power of attorney). If a plan exists, place a copy in the client file. If no plan exists, offer information on advance directives according to agency policy. Refer for assistance in completing advance directives as necessary. Do not witness a living will. *This is a legal requirement of the Consolidated Omnibus Budget Reconciliation Act (COBRA).*
- Determine the relevance of the decisional conflict to the plan of care.
- Assess the client and family for consensus (or lack thereof) regarding the issue in conflict. When the conflict involves end-of-life decisions, work to shift the client's and family's expectations from curative to palliative. **Nursing Research:** *A study of the means by which providers worked with clients and families at the end of life revealed that the focus was on changing expectations from unrealistic (curative) to realistic (palliative). Helping the client and family accurately understand the client's condition involved the following: laying the groundwork (teaching, planting the seeds), shifting the picture (working together, arranging family meetings, creating new expectations, changing the scope of choice, changing the value of treatment options, changing indicators), and accepting the new picture (involving others, redirecting hope, repeating and reiterating information) (Norton and Bowers, 2001).*
- ▲ If a decision is relevant to the plan of care, the primary nurse or medical social services may evaluate the need for a family conference and call such a conference. If a consensus cannot be reached, continue efforts to resolve the conflict. Clients, unless medically incompetent (by legal guidelines) or under authorized power of attorney, may make their own decisions. *Guided family conferences allow all persons affected by the decision to be heard and the value system of the client to be validated. The nurse or social worker serves as the facilitator and client advocate.*
- Assist the client and family in initiating problem solving and in identifying options, pros and cons, and consequences of choices. *Situations involving illness may create tunnel vision or a sense of being overwhelmed. Assistance is needed to help the client and family perceive that options do exist and to help them evaluate these options.* Refer to the care plan for **Anxiety** as indicated.
- ▲ If the decision is not relevant to the plan of care, refer to community support services appropriate to the type of decision and client need.

Client/Family Teaching

- ▲ Instruct the client and family members to provide advance directives in the following areas:
  - Person to contact in an emergency
  - Preference (if any) to die at home or in the hospital
  - Desire to sign a living will
  - Desire to donate an organ
  - Funeral arrangements (i.e., burial, cremation)

  Clinical Research: *A large discrepancy exists between the wishes of dying patients and their actual end-of-life care. However, retrospective clinical experience suggests that early advance care planning can markedly reduce this discrepancy (Schwartz et al, 2002).*

- • = Independent; ▲ = Collaborative

▲ Inform the family of treatment options; encourage and defend self-determination. **Nursing Research:** *The Patient Self-Determination Act, effective since December 1991, has changed the importance of introducing life support options to clients (Beland and Froman, 1995).*

• Identify reasons for family decisions regarding care. Explore ways in which family decisions can be respected. **Nursing Research:** *A high proportion of elders and their caregivers report substantial unmet transitional care needs, with the need for information and increased access to services consistently among the top priorities. Differences in expectations between and among clients, families, and health care providers, and the need for increased client and family involvement in decision making, are common themes in discharge planning studies (Naylor, 2002).*

• Recognize and allow the client to discuss the selection of complementary therapies available, such as spiritual support, relaxation, imagery, exercise, lifestyle changes, diet (e.g., macrobiotic, vegetarian), and nutritional supplementation. **Nursing Research:** *A study of cancer clients found that the clients unanimously believed that complementary therapies helped to improve their quality of life by helping them to cope more effectively with stress, decreasing the discomforts of treatment and illness, and giving them a sense of control (Sparber et al, 2000).* **Clinical Research:** *One study demonstrated that the use of complementary/alternative medicine for cancer care is widespread. There is clearly an expressed need for complementary/alternative medical treatments by clients and a willingness to pay for them (Lewith, Broomfield, and Prescott, 2002).*

• Include families in client care conferences. As a client's condition changes, it may be necessary to rethink the goal of treatment. The goal may change from restoration and cure to stabilization of functioning or preparation for comfortable and dignified death. *Families who are consistently apprised of changes in a client's condition and assist in exploring what these changes mean are more likely than others to trust the recommendation of the care team to withdraw or withhold further aggressive treatment (Taylor, 1995).*

evolve WEBSITES FOR EDUCATION

See the EVOLVE website for World Wide Web resources for client education.

REFERENCES

Beland K, Froman R: Preliminary validation of a measure of life support preferences, *Image J Nurs Sch* 27:307, 1995.

Blackhall LJ et al: Ethnicity and attitudes towards life sustaining technology, *Soc Sci Med* 48(12):1779, 1999.

Browner CH, Preloran HM, Cox SJ: Ethnicity, bioethics, and prenatal diagnosis: the amniocentesis decisions of Mexican-origin women and their partners, *Am J Public Health* 89(11):1658, 1999.

Burnard PL: *Counseling: a guide to practice in nursing,* Oxford, England, 1992, Butterworth–Heinemann.

Cesario S: Care of the Native American woman: strategies for practice, education, and research, *J Obstet Gynecol Neonatal Nurs* 30(1):13, 2001.

Chez N: Helping the victim of domestic violence, *Am J Nurs* 94:33, 1994.

Cochran M: Tears have no color, *Am J Nurs* 98(6):53, 1998.

D'Avanzo CE et al: Developing culturally informed strategies for substance-related interventions. In Naegle MA, D'Avanzo CE, editors: *Addictions and substance abuse: strategies for advanced practice nursing,* St Louis, 2001, Mosby.

Davis R: The convergence of health and family in the Vietnamese culture, *J Fam Nurs* 6(2):136, 2001.

Dossey B et al: *Holistic nursing: a handbook for practice,* Gaithersburg, Md, 1988, Aspen Publishers.

• = **Independent;** ▲ = **Collaborative**

Doswell W, Erlen J: Multicultural issues and ethical concerns in the delivery of nursing care interventions, *Nurs Clin North Am* 33(2):353, 1998.

Elwyn G et al: Shared decision making and the concept of equipoise: the competences of involving patients in healthcare choices, *Br J Gen Pract* 50(460):892, 2000.

Fleury J: Empowering potential: a theory of wellness motivation, *Nurs Res* 40:268, 1991.

Gillick M, Berkman S, Cullen L: A patient-centered approach to advance medical planning in the nursing home, *J Am Geriatr Soc* 47(2):227, 1999.

Haber J et al: *Comprehensive psychiatric nursing*, ed 4, St Louis, 1992, Mosby.

Harvey M: Managing agitation in critically ill patients, *Am J Crit Care* 5:7, 1996.

Heineken J: Patient silence is not necessarily client satisfaction: communication in home care nursing, *Home Healthc Nurse* 16(2):115, 1998.

Hornug CA et al: Ethnicity and decision makers in a group of frail elderly, *J Am Geriatr Soc* 46(3):280, 1998.

Hurley AC, Voicer L: Alzheimer disease: "It's okay, Mama, if you want to go, it's okay," *JAMA* 288(18):2324, 2002.

Lawrence VA et al: A cross-cultural consumer based decision aid for screening mammography, *Prev Med* 30(3):200, 2000.

Leininger MM, McFarland MR: *Transcultural nursing: concepts, theories, research and practices*, ed 3, New York, 2002, McGraw-Hill.

Lewith GT, Broomfield J, Prescott P: Complementary cancer care in Southampton: a survey of staff and patients, *Complement Ther Med* 10(2):100, 2002.

Mick DJ, Ackerman MH: New perspectives on advanced practice nursing case management for aging patients, *Crit Care Nurs Clin North Am* 14(3):281, 2002.

Moazam F: Families, patients, and physicians in medical decision making, *Hastings Cent Rep* 30(6):28, 2000.

Naylor MD: Transitional care of older adults, *Annu Rev Nurs Res* 20:127, 2002.

Norton SA, Bowers BJ: Working toward consensus: providers' strategies to shift patients from curative to palliative treatment choices, *Res Nurs Health* 24:258, 2001.

O'Connor A et al: Randomized trial of a portable, self-administered decision aid for postmenopausal women considering long-term preventive hormone therapy, *Med Decis Making* 18(3):295, 1998.

O'Connor AM et al: Decision aids for patients facing health treatment or screening decisions: systematic review, *BMJ* 319(7212):731, 1999.

Phillips K, Woodward V: The decision to resuscitate: older people's views, *J Clin Nurs* 8(6):753, 1999.

Pierce P: Deciding on breast cancer treatment: a description of decision behavior, *Nurs Res* 42:1, 1993.

Schwartz CE et al: Early intervention in planning end-of-life care with ambulatory geriatric patients: results of a pilot trial, *Arch Intern Med* 162(14):1611, 2002.

Sparber A et al: Use of complementary medicine by adult patients participating in cancer clinical trials, *Oncol Nurs Forum* 27(4):623, 2000.

Taylor C: Medical futility and nursing, *Image J Nurs Sch* 27:301, 1995.

Tilden VP et al: Family decision making to withdraw life-sustaining treatments from hospitalized patients, *Nurs Res* 50(2):105, 2001.

Valle R: Cultural assessment in bioethical advocacy: toward cultural competency and bioethical practice, *Bioethics Forum* 17(1):15, 2001.

Voicer L: Management of severe Alzheimer's disease and end-of-life issues, *Clin Geriatr Med* 17(2):377, 2001.

Wright F, Cohen S, Caroselli C: Diverse decisions: how culture affects ethical decision-making, *Crit Care Nurs Clin North Am* 9(1):63, 1997.

Parental role Conflict

T. Heather Herdman, Peggy A. Wetsch, and Mary Markle

NANDA Definition

Parent's experience of role confusion and conflict in response to crisis

Defining Characteristics

Expresses concerns about changes in parental role, family functioning, family communication, family health; expresses concerns/feelings of inadequacy with regard to provid-

• = Independent; ▲ = Collaborative

ing for child's physical and emotional needs during hospitalization or at home; shows reluctance to participate in usual caregiving activities, even with encouragement and support; demonstrates disruption in care and caregiving routines; expresses concern about perceived loss of control regarding decisions relating to child; verbalizes or demonstrates feelings of guilt, anger, fear, anxiety, and frustration concerning effect of child's illness on family processes

Related Factors (r/t)

Change in marital status; home care of child with special needs (e.g., apnea monitoring, postural drainage, hyperalimentation); interruptions of family life as a result of home care regimens (e.g., treatments, caregivers, lack of respite, specialized care center policies); separation from child as a result of chronic illness; intimidation by invasive or restrictive modalities (e.g., isolation, intubation)

NOC   Outcomes (Nursing Outcomes Classification)

Suggested NOC Outcomes

Acceptance: Health Status; Caregiver Adaptation to Patient Institutionalization; Caregiver Home Care Readiness; Caregiver Lifestyle Disruption; Coping; Grief Resolution; Hope; Parent-Infant Attachment; Parenting Performance; Psychosocial Adjustment: Life Change; Role Performance

---

Example NOC Outcome with Indicators

Caregiver Adaptation to Patient Institutionalization as evidenced by the following indicators: Participation in care as desired/Trust in nonfamily caregivers/Caregiver's resolution of guilt/Caregiver's comfort with role transition (Rate each indicator of **Caregiver Adaptation to Patient Institutionalization:** 1 = no adaptation, 2 = limited adaptation, 3 = moderate adaptation, 4 = substantial adaptation, 5 = extensive adaptation [see Section I].)

Client Outcomes

Client Will (Specify Time Frame):

- Express feelings and perceptions regarding impacts of illness, disability, and/or hospitalization on parental role
- Participate in hospital and home care as much as able to given the availability of resources and support systems
- Exhibit assertiveness and responsibility in active family decision making regarding care of the child
- Describe and select available resources to support parental management of the child's and family's needs

NIC   Interventions (Nursing Interventions Classification)

Suggested NIC Interventions

Abuse Protection Support: Child; Caregiver Support; Counseling; Crisis Intervention; Decision-Making Support; Environmental Management: Attachment Process; Family Process Maintenance; Family Therapy; Role Enhancement

• = Independent; ▲ = Collaborative

> **Example NIC Activities—Role Enhancement**
>
> Teach new behaviors needed by parent to fulfill a role; Serve as role model for learning new behaviors

Nursing Interventions and Rationales

- Assess parents' previous coping behaviors. *Having previous success with coping gives parents a feeling of competence. Identification of ineffective or absent coping behaviors allows development of interventions.* **Nursing Research:** *Research indicates that parents who cope successfully are better able to promote the adjustment and recovery of the child (Ladebauche, 1992).*

- Explore parent/family sources of stress, usual methods of coping, and perceptions of illness/condition. Capitalize on the strengths identified. Involve both parents in the assessment. *Identification of parents' perceptions of the magnitude of circumstances, perceived degree of adequacy, and usual coping methods can support strategies that promote active constructive coping or help the nurse to develop approaches to build or strengthen coping ability. Maintaining an optimistic outlook is important for parents who are caring for a chronically ill child at home (Ray and Ritchie, 1993; Bond, Phillips, and Rollins, 1994; Heaman, 1995; Melnyk, 1995).*

- Consider the use of family theory as a framework to help guide interventions (e.g., family stress theory, role theory, social exchange theory). *Theory helps to identify the focus, means, and goals of nursing practice. It enhances communication and increases autonomy and accountability for care (Gillis et al, 1989; Meleis, 1991).*

- Sustain parental involvement in shared decision making with regard to care by using the following steps:
  - Incorporate parents' information concerning the child's typical routines, behaviors, fears, likes, and dislikes.
  - Provide clear and direct firsthand information concerning the child's condition and progress.
  - Normalize the home/hospital environment as much as possible.
  - Collaborate in care by providing choices when possible.

  Involving parents in a child's caregiving and in decision making helps increase parental feelings of control and decrease feelings of stress. Noting parents' questions and nonverbal cues to determine need for improved communication is important (Sims et al, 1992; Shellabarger and Thompson, 1993; Bond, Phillips, and Rollins, 1994).

- Seek and support parental participation in care. *As parents of disabled children gain knowledge and become more involved in caregiving activities, their caregiver identity comes forth. Parents eventually emerge as the central persons in their children's lives. Parental participation has been demonstrated to have a positive effect on a child's reactions to procedures, resulting in improved cooperation and decreases in upset behaviors and the child's level of disturbed activity (Moynihan, Nalcerio, and Kiley, 1995; Perkins, 1993; Jones, Maestri, and McCoy, 1994).*

- Provide support for each parent's primary coping strategies. *Mothers tend to focus more on strategies related to social support, whereas fathers are inclined to analyze situations (Heaman, 1995). Mothers may require additional support in their role in caring for chronically ill children. Mothers exhibit greater efforts than fathers in coping patterns, including strategies to acquire social support outside the family, increase self-worth, and decrease psychological tensions (Brazil and Krueger, 2002).*

- **● = Independent; ▲ = Collaborative**

- Evaluate the family's perceived strength of its social support system. Encourage the family to use social support to increase its resiliency and to moderate stress. *Perceived social support is a factor influencing resiliency and ability to cope with stress (Tak and McCubbin, 2002).*
- Offer respite care to assist parents in maintaining sufficient energy and personal resources to continue caregiving responsibilities. *Medically fragile or technology-dependent children and children with chronic health problems and resultant disabilities receive most of their care at home from family members, frequently at severe economic and psychological costs (Coffman and Folden, 1992; Folden and Coffman, 1993).*
- Determine the older-than-average mother's support systems and self-expectations for motherhood. Pay particular attention to the relationships with spouse or partner, family, and friends. *Social support has a positive influence on early parenting for primiparas older than 35 years of age. Older primiparas with high self-expectations, low satisfaction with parenting, or inadequate social support systems may be at risk (Ferris and Reece, 1994).*
- Be available to discuss concerns and be a good listener. *The parent is more likely to verbalize concerns when the nurse is not hurried. Open communication is essential for the identification of potential coping problems (Ladebauche, 1992).*
- Encourage the parent to meet his or her own needs for rest, nutrition, and hygiene. Provide facilities so that the parent may stay with the sick child (e.g., cot, reclining chair). *A parent is unable to meet the child's needs when his or her basic self-needs are unmet.*
- Demonstrate safe places where the parent may touch or stroke the child. Encourage the parent to talk or sing to the child. Adjust equipment so that the parent is able to hold the child, and provide a comfortable chair, preferably a rocking chair. Provide opportunities and offer praise for successful caregiving. *Involvement in the child's care will give parents a sense of control in the hospital environment.*
- ▲ Refer parents to available telephone counseling services. *Telephone counseling services can provide confidential advice to families who might otherwise have no access to help for dealing with a child's problems (Jones, Maestri, and McCoy, 1994).*

Multicultural

- Acknowledge racial/ethnic differences at the onset of care. **Nursing Research:** *Acknowledgment of race/ethnicity issues will enhance communication, establish rapport, and promote treatment outcomes (D'Avanzo et al, 2001; Ludwick and Siva, 2000).*
- Assess for the influence of cultural beliefs, norms, and values on the client's perceptions of the parental role. **Nursing Research:** *What the client considers a normal or abnormal parental role may be based on cultural perceptions (Leininger and McFarland, 2002; Cochran, 1998; Doswell and Erlen, 1998). Some Mexican American families may engage in an intergenerational family ritual called* La Cuarentena, *which lasts for 40 days after birth and involves prescriptions for maternal food, clothing, and paternal role (Niska, Snyder, and Lia-Hoagberg, 1998).*
- Acknowledge that value conflicts arising from acculturation stresses may contribute to increased anxiety and significant conflict with the parental role. **Nursing Research:** *Challenges to traditional beliefs and values are anxiety provoking (Charron, 1998). Less acculturated parents may experience conflict with their more acculturated children as the children demand greater independence and freedom (True, 1995).*
- Promote the female parenting role by providing a treatment environment that is culturally based and woman centered. **Nursing Research:** *Pregnant and postpartum Asian and Pacific Islander women in substance abuse treatment identified provisions for the*

- = **Independent;** ▲ = **Collaborative**

newborn, infant health care, parent education, and infant-mother bonding as conducive to their treatment (Morelli, Fong, and Oliveria, 2001).

- Validate the client's feelings with regard to parental role confusion and conflict. **Nursing Research:** *Validation is a therapeutic communication technique that lets the client know that the nurse has heard and understood what was said, and it promotes the nurse-client relationship (Heineken, 1998).*

Home care

- The interventions described previously may be adapted for home care use.
- Assess family adjustment prenatally and postpartum; assist new parents to renegotiate behavior around issues such as amount of time spent together, sexual relationship, resolution of disagreements, and provision of sufficient time for leisure/recreational activities. Encourage the father to take an active role in infant care. **Nursing Research:** *Declining satisfaction in family function indicates a need for supportive nursing intervention. Most decline has been shown to occur during the first 4 months postpartum, with little change thereafter. Less decline was evident when fathers were involved in infant care and household tasks. Prenatal satisfaction with family functioning influenced mothers' sense of competence at 4 and 8 months postpartum (Knauth, 2000).*
- Assess interference with family functioning. Refer for family counseling as indicated. *Parental role conflict can influence all areas of family life, creating additional stress and family dysfunction. Family therapy or counseling provides an opportunity to address stressors and improve family functioning.*

Client/Family Teaching

- Furnish clear explanations about condition, disease or disability, associated treatments, and prognosis. Describe circumstances involving emotional and physical reactions of the child and types of family member reactions that might be anticipated in response to the condition or crisis. Provide ample time for skill practice. *Providing information to families decreases confusion and anxiety, increases understanding, and allows a feeling of competence and control. Providing information about the disease and treatment process helps build parents' feelings of confidence (Baker, 1994).*
- For parents of children with chronic disabilities, tailor educational opportunities based on the experiential phase of the parents (protection, survival, or development of the parent as a central person) as parents develop an identity as the central caregivers for their child. *As parents of physically and/or cognitively disabled children gain knowledge and become more involved in caregiving activities, their caregiver identity emerges (Perkins, 1993).*
- Involve parents in formal and/or informal social support situations, including parent-to-parent groups, community agencies, and counseling resources. *Parents of children with special health care needs are uniquely equipped to help each other learn day-to-day coping skills. Use of available social supports in the community can help parents to achieve successful outcomes (Coffman and Folden, 1992; Hartman, Radin, and McConnell, 1992).*

evolve WEBSITES FOR EDUCATION

See the EVOLVE website for World Wide Web resources for client education.

- • = Independent; ▲ = Collaborative

REFERENCES

Baker NA: Avoid collisions with challenging families, *MCN Am J Matern Child Nurs* 19:97, 1994.

Bond N, Phillips P, Rollins JA: Family centered care at home for families with children who are technology dependent, *Pediatr Nurs* 20:123, 1994.

Brazil K, Krueger P: Patterns of family adaptation to childhood asthma, *J Pediatr Nurs* 17(3):167, 2002.

Charron HS: Anxiety disorders. In Varcarolis EM, editor: *Foundations of psychiatric mental health nursing,* ed 3, Philadelphia, 1998, WB Saunders.

Cochran, M: Tears have no color, *Am J Nurs* 98(6):53, 1998.

Coffman S, Folden SL: Respite care for medically fragile children, *J Home Health Care Pract* 5:16, 1992.

D'Avanzo CE et al: Developing culturally informed strategies for substance-related interventions. In Naegle MA, D'Avanzo CE, editors: *Addictions and substance abuse: strategies for advanced practice nursing,* St Louis, 2001, Mosby.

Doswell W, Erlen J: Multicultural issues and ethical concerns in the delivery of nursing care interventions, *Nurs Clin North Am* 33(2):353, 1998.

Ferris A, Reece C: Nutritional consequences of chronic maternal conditions during pregnancy and lactation: lupus and diabetes, *J Clin Nutr* 59:4658, 1994.

Folden SL, Coffman S: Respite care for families of children with disabilities, *J Pediatr Health Care* 7:103, 1993.

Gillis C et al: *Toward a science of family nursing,* Menlo Park, Calif, 1989, Addison-Wesley.

Hartman AF, Radin MB, McConnell B: Parent-to-parent support: a critical component of health care services for families, *Issues Compr Pediatr Nurs* 15(1):55, 1992.

Heaman DJ: Perceived stressors and coping strategies of parents who have children with developmental disabilities: a comparison of mothers with fathers, *J Pediatr Nurs* 10:311, 1995.

Heineken J: Patient silence is not necessarily client satisfaction: communication in home care nursing, *Home Healthc Nurse* 16(2):115, 1998.

Jones LC, Maestri BO, McCoy K: Why parents use the warm line, *MCN Am J Matern Child Nurs* 18:258, 1994.

Knauth DG: Predictors of parental sense of competence for the couple during the transition to parenthood, *Res Nurs Health* 23:496, 2000.

Ladebauche P: Unit-based family support groups: a reminder, *MCN Am J Matern Child Nurs* 17:18, 1992.

Leininger MM, McFarland MR: *Transcultural nursing: concepts, theories, research and practices,* ed 3, New York, 2002, McGraw-Hill.

Ludwick R, Silva M: Nursing around the world: cultural values and ethical conflicts, *Online J Issues Nurs,* August 14, 2000, available online at http://www.nursingworld.org/ojin/ethcol/ethics_4.htm, accessed June 19, 2003.

Meleis A: *Theoretical nursing,* Philadelphia, 1991, Lippincott.

Melnyk BM: Parental coping with childhood hospitalization: a theoretical framework to guide research and clinical interventions, *Matern Child Nurs J* 23:123, 1995.

Morelli PT, Fong R, Oliveria J: Culturally competent substance abuse treatment for Asian/Pacific Islander women, *J Hum Behav Soc Environ* 3(3/4):263, 2001.

Moynihan P, Nalcerio L, Kiley K: Parent participation, *Nurs Clin North Am* 30:231, 1995.

Niska K, Snyder M, Lia-Hoagberg B: Family ritual facilitates adaptation to parenthood, *Public Health Nurs* 15(5):329, 1998.

Perkins MT: Parent-nurse collaboration: using the caregiver identity emergence phases to assist parents of hospitalized children with disabilities, *J Pediatr Nurs* 8:2, 1993.

Ray LD, Ritchie JA: Caring for chronically ill children at home: factors that influence parents' coping, *J Pediatr Nurs* 8:217, 1993.

Shellabarger SG, Thompson TL: The critical times: meeting parental communication needs throughout the NICU experience, *Neonatal Netw* 12:39, 1993.

Sims SL et al: Decision making in home health care, *West J Nurs Res* 14:186, 1992.

Tak YR, McCubbin M: Family stress, perceived social support and coping following the diagnosis of a child's congenital heart disease, *J Adv Nurs* 39(2):190, 2002.

True RH: Mental health issues of Asian/Pacific island women. In Adams DL, editor: *Health issues for women of color: a cultural diversity perspective,* Thousand Oaks, Calif, 1995, Sage.

• = **Independent;** ▲ = **Collaborative**

Acute Confusion

Kimberly Hickey

NANDA   Definition

Abrupt onset of a cluster of global, transient changes, and disturbances in attention, cognition, psychomotor activity level, consciousness, or sleep-wake cycle

Defining Characteristics

Lack of motivation to initiate and/or follow through with goal-directed or purposeful behavior; fluctuation in psychomotor activity; misperceptions; fluctuation in cognition; increased agitation or restlessness; fluctuation in level of consciousness; fluctuation in sleep-wake cycle; hallucinations

Related Factors (r/t)

Age over 70 years; alcohol abuse; abuse; cognitive impairment; uncontrolled pain; multiple comorbidities; medications; dehydration; infection; sensory deficit; compromised activities of daily living

NOC   (Nursing Outcomes Classification)

Suggested NOC Outcomes

Cognitive Orientation; Distorted Thought Self-Control; Information Processing; Memory; Neurological Status: Consciousness; Sleep

---

Example NOC Outcome with Indicators

Cognitive Orientation as evidenced by the following indicators: Communicates clearly and appropriately for age and ability/Demonstrates control over selected events and situations/Attentiveness/Orientation (Rate each indicator of **Cognitive Orientation:** 1 = extremely compromised, 2 = substantially compromised, 3 = moderately compromised, 4 = mildly compromised, 5 = not compromised [see Section I].)

Client Outcomes

Client Will (Specify Time Frame):

- Demonstrate restoration of cognitive status to baseline
- Obtain adequate amount of sleep
- Demonstrate appropriate motor behavior
- Maintain functional capacity
- Optimize hydration and nutrition

NIC   Interventions (Nursing Interventions Classification)

Suggested NIC Interventions

Delirium Management; Delusion Management

• = Independent; ▲ = Collaborative

Example NIC Activities—Delirium Management
Orient to time, place, and person; Present information in small, concrete portions

Nursing Interventions and Rationales

- Assess the client's behavior and cognition systematically and continually throughout the day and night, as appropriate. **Clinical Research:** *Rapid onset and fluctuating course are hallmarks of delirium (Murphy, 2000). The Confusion Assessment Method is sensitive, specific, reliable, and easy to use (Inouye et al, 1990). Other tools to consider include the Delirium Rating Scale (DRS) and the Neelon/Champagne (NEECHAM) Confusion Scale. Selection depends on the population and reason for assessment (Rapp et al, 2000).* **Nursing and Clinical Research:** *Nurses play a vital role in assessing acute confusion because they provide 24-hour care and see the client in a variety of circumstances (Inouye, 2000; Marr, 1992). Delirium always involves an acute change in mental status; therefore, knowledge of the client's baseline mental status is key in assessing delirium (Flacker and Marcantonio, 1998).*
- Perform an accurate mental status examination that includes the following:
  - Overall appearance, manner, and attitude
  - Behavior characteristics and level of psychomotor behavior
  - Mood and affect (presence of suicidal or homicidal ideation as observed by others and reported by the client)
  - Insight and judgment
  - Cognition as evidenced by level of consciousness, orientation (to time, place, and person), thought process and content (perceptual disturbances such as illusions and hallucinations, paranoia, delusions, abstract thinking)
  - Attention

  Missing a diagnosis of delirium can lead to serious negative consequences. Delirium in adults should be considered a medical emergency (Rosen, 1994). Early intervention in the case of delirium may decrease the severity and length of the delirious episode (Milisen et al, 2001). **Clinical Research:** *Abnormal attention is an important diagnostic feature of delirium (Flacker and Marcantonio, 1998). Delirium is a state of mind, whereas agitation is a behavioral manifestation. Some clients may be delirious without agitation and may actually exhibit withdrawn behavior. This is a hypoactive form of delirium. Some clients present with a mixed hypoactive and hyperactive type of delirium (O'Keefe and Lavan, 1999).*
- ▲ Assess and report possible physiological alterations (e.g., sepsis, hypoglycemia, hypoxia, hypotension, infection, changes in temperature, fluid and electrolyte imbalance, use of medications with known cognitive and psychotropic side effects). **Nursing and Clinical Research:** *Such alterations may be contributing to confusion and must be corrected (Matthiesen et al, 1994). Early attention to these risk factors may prevent delirium (Inouye et al, 2000). Medications are considered the most common cause of delirium in the ICU (Harvey, 1996).*
- ▲ Treat the underlying causes of delirium in collaboration with the health care team:
  - Establish/maintain normal fluid and electrolyte balance; establish/maintain normal nutrition, normal body temperature, normal oxygenation (if the client experiences low oxygen saturation, deliver supplemental oxygen), normal blood glucose levels, normal blood pressure.

- • = **Independent;** ▲ = **Collaborative**

- ■ Communicate client status, cognition, and behavioral manifestations to all necessary providers. Monitor for any trends occurring in these manifestations. **Nursing and Clinical Research:** *Recognize that the client's fluctuating cognition and behavior are the hallmark of delirium and are not to be construed as client preference for certain caregivers (Inouye et al, 1990). Careful monitoring may allow for various symptoms to be related to various causes and interventions (Rapp, Iowa Veterans Affairs Nursing Research Consortium, 1997).*
- ▲ Laboratory results should be closely monitored and physiological support given as appropriate. **Clinical Research:** *Dehydration is a significant risk factor for delirium and should be addressed aggressively (Inouye, 2000).* **Clinical and Nursing Research:** *Once acute confusion has been identified, it is vital to recognize and treat the associated underlying causes (Rapp, Iowa Veterans Affairs Nursing Research Consortium, 1997).*
- • Establish or maintain elimination patterns. **Nursing and Clinical Research:** *Disruption in elimination may be a cause of confusion (Rapp, Iowa Veterans Affairs Nursing Research Consortium, 1997). Changes in elimination patterns may also be a symptom of acute confusion. Prompt response to requests for assistance with elimination in addition to timed voids may assist in maintaining regular elimination, orientation, and patient safety (Rosen, 1994).*
- • Plan care that allows for an appropriate sleep-wake cycle. **Nursing and Clinical Research:** *Disruptions in usual sleep and activity patterns should be minimized because those clients with nocturnal exacerbations experience more complications from delirium (Inouye, 2000).*
- ▲ Conduct a medication review. **Nursing and Clinical Research:** *Medication use is one of the most important modifiable factors that can cause delirium, especially the use of anticholinergics, antipsychotics, and hypnosedatives (Flacker and Marcantonio, 1998; Agostini, Leo-Summers, and Inouye, 2002).*
- • Modulate sensory exposure and establish a calm environment. **Nursing and Clinical Research:** *Extraneous lights and noise can give rise to agitation, especially if misperceived. Sensory overload or sensory deprivation can result in increased confusion (Rosen, 1994). Clients with a hyperactive form of delirium often have increased irritability and startle responses and may be acutely sensitive to light and sound (Casey et al, 1996).*
- • Manipulate the environment to make it as familiar to the client as possible. Use a large clock and calendar. Encourage visits by family and friends. Place familiar objects in sight. **Nursing and Clinical Research:** *An environment that is familiar provides orienting clues, maintains an appropriate balance of sensory stimulation, and secures safety (Rosen, 1994).*
- • Identify yourself by name at each contact; call the client by his or her preferred name. Use appropriate communication techniques for clients at risk for confusion (Inouye, 2000; Rapp, Iowa Veterans Affairs Nursing Research Consortium, 1997).
- • Use orientation techniques. If the client becomes distressed or argumentative about what is real, however, do not argue with the client. Rather, explore the emotion behind the client's non–reality-based statements (Rosen, 1994).
- • Offer reassurance to the client and use therapeutic communication at frequent intervals. **Nursing and Clinical Research:** *Client reassurance and communication are nursing skills that promote trust and orientation and reduce anxiety (Harvey, 1996).*
- • Provide supportive nursing care. **Nursing Research:** *Delirious clients are unable to care for themselves due to their confusion. Their care and safety needs must be anticipated by the nurse (Foreman et al, 1999).*

- • = Independent; ▲ = Collaborative

▲ Identify, evaluate, and treat pain quickly (see **Pain**). **Clinical and Nursing Research:** *Untreated pain is a potential cause of delirium (Inouye, 2000; Milisen et al, 2001).*

▲ Anticipate pain-producing conditions and treat pain with around-the-clock medications. *Clients experiencing delirium often will not report their pain nor be able to request medications prescribed on a prn basis.*

▲ Facilitate appropriate sensory input by having clients use aids (e.g., glasses, hearing aids) as needed. *Sensory impairment contributes to misinterpretation of the environment and significantly contributes to delirium (Inouye, 2000).*

▲ Delirium is frequently treated with an antipsychotic medication. **Clinical Research:** *Be aware of paradoxical effects and side effects such as extrapyramidal symptoms, agitation, sedation, and arrhythmias, because these may exacerbate the delirium (Schwartz and Masand, 2002).*

Geriatric

• Mobilize the client as soon as possible; provide active and passive range of motion. **Nursing and Clinical Research:** *Older clients who had a low level of physical activity before injury are at particular risk for acute confusion (Inouye, 2000; Matthiesen et al, 1994).*

▲ Provide sufficient medication to relieve pain. **Nursing and Clinical Research:** *Older clients may give inaccurate pain histories, underreport symptoms, not want to bother the nurse, or exhibit restlessness, agitation, or increased confusion (Matthiesen et al, 1994).*

• Explain hospital routines and procedures slowly and in simple terms; repeat information as necessary. **Nursing Research:** *Anxiety and sensory impairment decrease the older client's ability to integrate new information (Matthiesen et al, 1994).*

• Provide continuity of care when possible (e.g., provide the same caregivers, avoid room changes). **Nursing Research:** *Continuity of care helps decrease the disorienting effects of hospitalization (Matthiesen et al, 1994).*

• If clients know that they are not thinking clearly, acknowledge the concern. *Fear is frequently experienced by people with delirium.* **Nursing and Clinical Research:** *Confusion is very frightening, and the memory of the delirium can be equally frightening (Breitbart, Gibson, and Tremblay, 2002; Matthiesen et al, 1994).*

• Do not use the intercom to answer a call light. **Nursing Research:** *The intercom may be frightening to an older confused client (Matthiesen et al, 1994).*

• Keep the client's sleep-wake cycle as normal as possible (e.g., avoid letting the client take daytime naps, avoid waking the client at night, give sedatives but not diuretics at bedtime, provide pain relief and back rubs). **Nursing and Clinical Research:** *Acute confusion is accompanied by disruption of the sleep-wake cycle (Inouye, 2000; Matthiesen et al, 1994).*

• Maintain normal sleep-wake patterns (treat with bright light for 2 hours in the early evening). **Nursing Research:** *Light treatment facilitates normal sleep-wake patterns (Rapp, Iowa Veterans Affairs Nursing Research Consortium, 1997).*

Home care

• Some of the interventions described previously may be adapted for home care use.

• Assess and monitor for acute changes in cognition and behavior. **Clinical Research:** *An acute change in cognition and behavior is the classic presentation of delirium. It should be considered a medical emergency (Inouye et al, 1990).*

• Delirium is reversible but can become chronic if untreated, and the client may be discharged from the hospital to home care in state of undiagnosed delirium. **Nursing Re-**

• = Independent; ▲ = Collaborative

search: *Staff should receive training in the assessment of acute confusion; assessment may be complicated by the presence of periods of lucidity (Mentes et al, 1999).*

- Assess for treatable causes of changes in cognition and behavior. *The mnemonic DEMENTIA can be used to remember potential causes of acute or chronic confusion (Smith, 2002):*

  D: Drugs and alcohol—including over-the-counter drugs
  E: Eyes and ears—disorientation due to visual/auditory distortion
  M: Medical disorders—e.g., diabetes, hypothyroidism
  E: Emotional and psychological disturbances—e.g., mood or paranoid disorders
  N: Neurological disorders—e.g., multi-infarct dementia
  T: Tumors and trauma
  I: Infections—e.g., urinary tract or upper respiratory tract
  A: Arteriosclerosis—leading to heart failure, insufficient blood supply to heart and brain, confusion

- Assess fluid intake, dementia status, and occurrence of a fall within the past 30 days in evaluating confusion. **Nursing Research:** *Confusion may be explained by inadequate fluid intake, dementia, or a fall. In the last case, it is unclear if falls are a precipitating event or indicative of frailty (Mentes et al, 1999).*

- Avoid preconceptions about the source of acute confusion; assess each occurrence on the basis of available evidence. *Delirium may not be readily recognized, in part because of its varying presentations and in part because preconceptions interfere with accurate assessment. For example, although delirium may occur in advanced cancer clients prior to death, it also may arise in response to reversible causes that should be identified and treated, depending on the goals of care (Lawlor, 2001).*

- ▲ Institute case management of frail elderly clients to support continued independent living. *Difficulties with acute confusion lead to increasing needs for assistance in using the health care system effectively. Case management combines the nursing activities of client and family assessment, planning and coordination of care among all health care providers, delivery of direct nursing care, and monitoring of care and outcomes. These activities are able to address continuity of care, mutual goal setting, behavior management, and prevention of worsening health problems (Guttman, 1999).*

Client/Family Teaching

- ▲ Teach the family to recognize signs of early confusion and seek medical help. **Nursing Research:** *Early intervention prevents long-term complications (Rapp, Iowa Veterans Affairs Nursing Research Consortium, 1997).*

- Counsel the client and family regarding the symptoms of delirium, its management, and its sequelae. **Clinical Research:** *Families experience a high degree of distress when observing a loved one in delirium. Families should be told that symptoms of delirium may persist for months following a delirious episode so that appropriate plans can be made for continuing care (Marcantonio et al, 2003; Breitbart, Gibson, and Tremblay, 2002).*

REFERENCES

Agostini JV, Leo-Summers LS, Inouye SK: Cognitive and other adverse effects of diphenhydramine use in hospitalized older patients, *Arch Intern Med* 161(17):2091, 2001.

Breitbart W, Gibson C, Tremblay A: The delirium experience: delirium recall and delirium related distress in hospitalized patients with cancer, their spouses/caregivers, and their nurses, *Psychosomatics* 43(3):183, 2002.

• = Independent; ▲ = Collaborative

Casey DA et al: Delirium: quick recognition, careful evaluation, and appropriate treatment. Symposium: fourth of four articles on psychiatric disorders, *Postgrad Med* 100(1):121, 1996.

Flacker JM, Marcantonio ER: Delirium in the elderly: optimal management, *Drugs Aging* 13(2):119, 1998.

Foreman MD et al: Standard of practice protocol: acute confusion/delirium, *Geriatr Nurs* 20:147, 1999.

Guttman R: Case management of the frail elderly in the community, *Clin Nurs Spec* 13(4):174, 1999.

Harvey M: Managing agitation in critically ill patients, *Am J Crit Care* 5:7, 1996.

Inaba-Roland K, Maricle R: Assessing delirium in the acute care setting, *Heart Lung* 21:49, 1992.

Inouye SK: Prevention of delirium in hospitalized older patients: risk factors and targeted intervention strategies, *Ann Med* 32(4):257, 2000.

Inouye SK et al: Clarifying confusion: the Confusion Assessment Method. A new method for detection of delirium, *Ann Intern Med* 113(12):941, 1990.

Inouye SK et al: The Hospitalized Elder Life Program: a model of care to prevent cognitive and functional decline in older hospitalized patients, *J Am Geriatr Soc* 48(12):16797, 2000.

Lawlor PG: Assessment of delirium in patients with advanced cancer, *Home Health Care Consult* 8(9):10, 2001.

Marcantonio ER et al: Delirium symptoms in post-acute care: prevalent, persistent and associated with poor recovery, *J Am Geriatr Soc* 51:4, 2003.

Marr J: Acute confusion, *Nurs Times* 88:16, 1992.

Matthiesen V et al: Acute confusion: nursing interventions in older patients, *Orthop Nurs* 13:25, 1994.

Mentes et al: Acute confusion indicators: risk factors and prevalence using MDS data, *Res Nurs Health* 22:95, 1999.

Milisen K et al: A nurse-led interdisciplinary intervention program for delirium in elderly hip fracture patients, *J Am Geriatr Soc* 49:523, 2001.

Murphy BA: Delirium, *Emerg Med Clin North Am* 18:243, 2000.

O'Keefe ST, Lavan JN: Clinical significance of delirium subtypes in older people, *Age Ageing* 28(2):115, 1999.

Rapp C, Iowa Veterans Affairs Nursing Research Consortium: *Acute confusion/delirium,* Iowa City, 1997, The Consortium, available online at http://www.guideline.gov/VIEWS/summary.asp?guideline=536&summary_type=brief_summary&view=brief_summary&sSearch_string=, accessed Jan 10, 2003.

Rapp CG et al: Acute confusion assessment instruments: clinical versus research usability, *Appl Nurs Res* 13(1):37, 2000.

Rosen SL: Managing delirious older adults in the hospital, *MedSurg Nurs* 3(3):181, 1994.

Schwartz TL, Masand PS: The role of atypical antipsychotics in the treatment of delirium, *Psychosomatics* 43:171, 2002.

Smith GB: Case management guideline: Alzheimer disease and other dementias, *Lippincotts Case Manag* 7:77, 2002.

Chronic Confusion

Kimberly Hickey

NANDA Definition

Irreversible, long-standing, and/or progressive deterioration of intellect and personality characterized by decreased ability to interpret environmental stimuli and decreased capacity for intellectual thought processes, and manifested by disturbances of memory, orientation, and behavior

Defining Characteristics

Altered interpretation and/or response to stimuli; clinical evidence of organic impairment; altered personality; impaired memory (short and long term); impaired socialization; no change in level of consciousness; decreased ability to participate in self-care; decreased ability for meaningful interaction with the environment

• = Independent; ▲ = Collaborative

Related Factors (r/t)

Multi-infarct dementia; Korsakoff's psychosis; brain injury; Alzheimer's disease and related dementias

NOC Outcomes (Nursing Outcomes Classification)

Suggested NOC Outcomes

Cognition; Cognitive Orientation; Distorted Thought Self-Control

---

Example NOC Outcome with Indicators

Cognition as evidenced by the following indicators: Communicates clearly and appropriately for age and ability/Demonstrates control over selected events and situations/Attentiveness/Orientation (Rate each indicator of **Cognition:** 1 = extremely compromised, 2 = substantially compromised, 3 = moderately compromised, 4 = mildly compromised, 5 = not compromised [see Section I].)

Client Outcomes

Client Will (Specify Time Frame):
- Remain content and free from harm
- Function at maximal cognitive level
- Participate in activities of daily living at the maximum of functional ability

NIC Interventions (Nursing Interventions Classification)

Suggested NIC Interventions

Dementia Management; Environmental Management; Reality Orientation; Surveillance: Safety

---

Example NIC Activities—Dementia Management

Use distraction rather than confrontation to manage behavior; Give one simple direction at a time

---

Nursing Interventions and Rationales

- Determine the client's cognitive level using a screening tool such as the Mini-Mental State Exam (MMSE). **Nursing and Clinical Research:** *Use of a standard evaluation tool such as the MMSE can help determine the client's abilities and assist in planning appropriate nursing interventions (Agostinelli et al, 1994; Espino et al, 1998).*
- Gather information about the client's predementia functioning, including social situation, physical condition, and psychological functioning. **Nursing and Clinical Research:** *Knowing the client's background can assist the nurse in identifying agenda behavior and using validation therapy, and will provide guidance for reminiscence. This information may also be useful to the nurse in understanding behavior if the client becomes delusional and hallucinates (Fine and Rouse-Bane, 1995; Cohen-Mansfield, Golander, and Arnheim, 2000).*
- Assess the client for signs of depression: insomnia, poor appetite, flat affect, and withdrawn behavior. **Nursing Research:** *Up to 50% of clients with dementia have depressive symptoms (Cleeland, 1997).*
- Ensure that the client is in a safe environment by removing potential hazards such as

• = Independent; ▲ = Collaborative

sharp objects and harmful liquids. **Clinical Research:** *Clients with dementia lose the ability to make good judgments and can easily harm themselves or others (Painter, 1996).*

- Place an identification bracelet on client. **Clinical Research:** *Clients with dementia wander and can become lost; identification bracelets increase their safety (Painter, 1996).*
- Avoid as much as possible exposing the client to unfamiliar situations and people. Maintain continuity of caregivers. Maintain routines of care by observing established eating, bathing, and sleeping schedules. Send a familiar person with the client when the client goes for diagnostic testing or into unfamiliar environments. **Nursing Research:** *Situational anxiety associated with environmental, interpersonal, or structural change can escalate into agitated behavior (Gerdner and Buckwalter, 1994).*
- Keep the environment quiet and nonstimulating. Avoid or minimize sights and sounds that have a high potential for misinterpretation, such as buzzers, alarms, and overhead paging systems. **Clinical and Nursing Research:** *Sensory overload can result in agitated behavior in a client with dementia. Misinterpretation of the environment can also contribute to agitation (Doody et al, 2001).*
- Begin each interaction with the client by identifying yourself and calling the client by name. Approach the client with a caring, loving, and accepting attitude and speak calmly and slowly. **Nursing Research:** *Dementia clients can sense feelings of compassion; a calm, slow manner projects a feeling of comfort to the client (Stolley, 1994).*
- Give one simple direction at a time and repeat it as necessary. Use verbal and physical prompts, and model the desired action if needed and possible. **Nursing Research:** *People with dementia need time to assimilate and interpret your directions; if you rephrase your question, you give them something new to process, which increases their confusion (Stolley, 1994).*
- Break down self-care tasks into simple steps (e.g., instead of saying, "Take a shower," say to the client, "Please follow me. Sit down on the bed. Take off your shoes. Now take off your socks") **Nursing Research:** *Dementia clients are unable to follow complex commands; breaking down an activity into simple steps makes the activity more feasible (Agostinelli et al, 1994).*
- Keep questions simple; yes or no questions are often preferable. Use positive statements and actions and avoid negative communication. *Negative feedback leads to increased confusion and agitation. It is more effective to go along with the client and then redirect as necessary.*
- If eating in the dining room increases agitation, let the client leave and eat in a quieter environment with a smaller number of people. **Clinical and Nursing Research:** *The noise and confusion in a large dining room can be overwhelming for a dementia client and result in agitated behavior. It is preferable to have dementia clients eat in small groups (Sloane, 1998).*
- Provide finger food if the client has difficulty using eating utensils or is unable to sit to eat. **Clinical Research:** *Feeding oneself is a complex task and may prove challenging for someone with significant dementia (Finley, 1997).*
- Provide boundaries by placing red or yellow tape on the floor or by using a stop sign. *Boundaries help the client identify safe areas; older clients can more easily see red and yellow.*
- Assess the cause of wandering rather than or before attempting to control the wandering. **Nursing Research:** *Wandering indicates a problem and need for intervention; therefore, the reason for the wandering behavior must be determined (Algase, 1999).*
- Write the client's name in large block letters in the room and on the client's clothing and possessions.

- = **Independent;** ▲ = **Collaborative**

- Use symbols rather than words to identify areas such as the bathroom or kitchen.
- Limit visitors to two and provide them with guidelines on what are appropriate topics to discuss with the client and how to best communicate with the client. (See how to converse with a memory-impaired person in the Client/Family Teaching section.)
- Set up scheduled quiet periods in a recliner or room. Use afghans and environmental cues to define rest periods. **Nursing Research:** *Quiet times allow the client's anxiety and building tension levels to decrease (Hall et al, 1995). Fatigue has been associated with the onset of increased confusion and agitation (Stolley, 1994).*
- Provide quiet activities such as listening to music of the client's preference or introduce other cues that promote relaxation in the afternoon or early evening. **Clinical and Nursing Research:** *An increase in confusion and agitation may occur in the late afternoon and early evening and is referred to as "sundowning syndrome." Quiet activities can provide a calming environment (Doody et al, 2001).*
- Provide simple activities for the client, such as folding washcloths and sorting or stacking activities. Avoid misleading and frightening stimuli, which may include the television, mirrors, and pictures of people or animals. **Nursing Research:** *Repetitive activities give clients a positive outlet for behavior (Burgener et al, 1998). They see, hear, and perceive a different world; they may not recognize themselves in the mirror and be afraid of the stranger they see so close to them.*
- If the client becomes increasingly confused and agitated, perform the following steps:
  - Assess the client for physiological causes, including acute hypoxia, pain, medication effects, malnutrition, infections such as urinary tract infection, fatigue, electrolyte disturbances, and constipation. An acute change in behavior is a medical emergency and should be evaluated. **Nursing and Clinical Research:** *Many physiological factors can result in increased agitation of clients with dementia (Gerdner and Buckwalter, 1994; Alexopoulos et al, 1998).*
  - Assess for psychological causes, including changes in the environment, caregiver, and routine; demands to perform beyond capacity; multiple competing stimuli (including discomfort). **Clinical and Nursing Research:** *It is important for the nurse to recognize precipitating events and subsequent behavior to prevent further incidents of agitation (Bair et al, 1999).*
  - Avoid confrontations with the client; allow the client to dissipate energy by performing repetitive tasks or by pacing.
  - If the client is delusional or hallucinating, do not confront him or her with reality. Use validation therapy to verbally reflect back the emotions that the client appears to be feeling. Use statements such as, "It must be frightening to see a fire at the end of your bed," "I can see you are afraid," "I will stay with you," or "Can you tell me more about what is going on right now?" **Clinical and Nursing Research:** *Orienting the client to reality can increase agitation; validation therapy conveys empathy and understanding and can help determine the internal stimulus that is creating the change in behavior (Feil, 1993). Staff training in validation therapy resulted in a decrease in the doses of psychotherapeutic medications used and in incidences of behavior problems in one study (Fine and Rouse-Bane, 1995).*
  - Decrease stimuli in the environment (e.g., turn off the television, take the client to a quiet place). Institute activities associated with pleasant emotions, such as playing soft music the client likes, looking through a photo album, providing favorite food, or using simulated presence therapy. **Nursing and Clinical Research:** *Decreasing stimuli can decrease agitation. Reassuring activities can help bring pleasant emotions to*

• = Independent; ▲ = Collaborative

help soothe the client; these include simulated presence therapy in which the client listens to a tape of a conversation with a loved one (Woods and Ashley, 1995).

■ Avoid using restraints if at all possible. **Nursing and Clinical Research:** *Restraints are not benign interventions and should be used sparingly and judiciously and only when alternatives to manage the behaviors have been tried and have proven unsuccessful. Side effects of restraints include falls, increased confusion, deconditioning, and incontinence (Tinetti, Liu, and Ginter, 1992).*

■ Use prn or low-dose regular dosing of psychotropic or antianxiety drugs only as a last resort. They are effective in managing symptoms of psychosis and aggressive behavior. Start with the lowest possible dose. **Clinical Research:** *Psychotropic drugs such as haloperidol (Haldol) and risperidone (Risperdal) may decrease client function and have side effects that need to be monitored (Katz et al, 1999).*

▲ Avoid the use of anticholinergic medications such as Benadryl. **Clinical Research:** *Anticholinergic medications have a high side-effect profile that includes disorientation, urinary retention, and excessive drowsiness (Nurses Drug Alert, 1995). The anticholinergic side effects outweigh the antihistaminic effects.*

• For predictable difficult times, such as during bathing and grooming, try the following:

■ Massage the client's hands lovingly or use therapeutic touch to relax the client. **Nursing Research:** *Hand massage and therapeutic touch have been shown to induce relaxation that may allow care activities to take place without difficulty (Snyder, Egan, and Burns, 1995).*

■ Use positive behavioral reinforcement for each small step of bathing, such as praising the client for walking toward the shower, sitting in the shower chair, and removing items of clothing. **Nursing Research:** *Positive behavioral reinforcement for desired behavior is effective for clients with dementia (Boehm et al, 1995). Consider a towel bath if shower or tub bathing is too stressful for the client (Hall and Buckwalter, 1999).*

■ Treat the client with the utmost respect and give individualized care. **Nursing Research:** *Treating confused clients with respect and individualizing care can decrease aggression and increase nursing staff satisfaction (Maxfield, Lewis, and Cannon, 1996).*

• For care of early dementia clients with primarily symptoms of memory loss, see the care plan for **Impaired Memory.**

• For care of clients with self-care deficits, see the appropriate care plan **(Feeding Self-care deficit; Dressing Self-care deficit;** and **Toileting Self-care deficit).**

Geriatric

NOTE: Most of the aforementioned interventions apply to the geriatric client.

• Use reminiscence and life review therapeutic interventions; ask questions about the client's work, child raising, or time spent in the service. Ask questions such as, "What was really important to you as you look back?" **Nursing Research:** *Reminiscence and life review can help an older person reframe and accept life events.*

Multicultural

• Assess for the influence of cultural beliefs, norms, and values on the family's or caregiver's understanding of chronic confusion or dementia. **Nursing Research:** *What the family considers normal and abnormal health behavior may be based on cultural percep-*

• = Independent; ▲ = Collaborative

tions (Leininger and McFarland 2002; Cochran, 1998; Doswell and Erlen, 1998; Guarnaccia, 1998).

- Inform the client's family or caregiver of the meaning of and reasons for common behavior observed in clients with dementia. **Nursing Research:** *An understanding of dementia behavior will enable the client's family or caregiver to provide the client with a safe environment.*
- Assist the family or caregiver in identifying barriers that would prevent the use of social services or other supportive services that could help reduce the impact of caregiving. **Nursing Research:** *Expectations of discrimination, lack of knowledge about services, expectations embedded in familism, lack of sense of prevention, lack of health insurance, preference for traditional remedies, and neglect or abuse were barriers identified by researchers studying the low utilization of skilled home care nursing services by elderly Hispanic clients (Crist, 2002). Language may present another barrier to the access of supportive services (McGrath, Vun, and McLeod, 2001).*
- Assess the client for the presence of an instrumental activity of daily living (IADL) disability and chronic health conditions. **Nursing Research:** *African American clients with cognitive impairments had higher IADL disability, poorer self-rated health, higher cognitive errors, and more chronic health conditions (Chumbler et al, 2001).*
- ▲ Refer the family to social services or other supportive services to assist in meeting the demands of caregiving for the client with dementia. **Nursing Research:** *African American caregivers of dementia clients may evidence less desire than others to institutionalize their family members and are more likely to report unmet service needs (Hinrichsen and Ramirez, 1992). Families of dementia clients may report restricted social activity (Haley et al, 1995).*
- ▲ Encourage the family to make use of support groups or other service programs. **Nursing Research:** *Studies indicate that some minority families of clients with dementia may use few support programs even though these programs could have a positive impact on caregiver well-being (Cox, 1999).*
- Validate the family members' feelings with regard to the impact of the client's behavior on family lifestyle. **Nursing Research:** *Validation lets family members know that the nurse has heard and understood what was said, and it promotes the relationship between the nurse and family members (Heineken, 1998).*

Home care

NOTE: Keeping the client as independent as possible is important. Because community-based care is usually less structured than institutional care, however, in the home setting the goal of maintaining safety for the client takes on primary importance.

- The interventions described previously may be adapted for home care use.
- Assess and monitor the client for acute changes in cognition and behavior. *An acute change in cognition and behavior is the classic presentation of delirium. Delirium is reversible, should be considered a medical emergency, and can occur in conjunction with dementia. Delirium can become chronic if untreated, and clients may be discharged from hospitals to home care in states of undiagnosed delirium.*
- Assess for treatable causes of changes in cognition and behavior. *The mnemonic DEMENTIA can be used to remember potential causes (Smith, 2002):*
  D: Drugs and alcohol—including over-the-counter drugs
  E: Eyes and ears—disorientation due to visual/auditory distortion
  M: Medical disorders—e.g., diabetes, hypothyroidism

• = Independent; ▲ = Collaborative

E: Emotional and psychological disturbances—e.g., mood or paranoid disorders

N: Neurological disorders—e.g., multi-infarct dementia

T: Tumors and trauma

I: Infections—e.g., urinary tract or upper respiratory tract

A: Arteriosclerosis—leading to heart failure, insufficient blood supply to heart and brain, and confusion

▲ Before providing any home care, assess the client plan for advance directives (living will and power of attorney). If a plan exists, place a copy in the client file. If no plan exists, offer information on advance directives according to agency policy. Refer for assistance in completing advance directives as necessary. Do not witness a living will. *This is a legal requirement of the Consolidated Omnibus Budget Reconciliation Act (COBRA). The ability of the client to plan advance directives legally depends on the stage of dementia, the degree of certainty of the client's wishes for end-of-life care, and the degree of distress experienced by the client with dementia. Successful completion of advance directives by clients with mild to moderate dementia has been reported (Rempusheski and Hurley, 2000).*

• Assess the client's memory and executive function deficits before assuming the inability to make any medical decisions. *A review of existing research on the decision-making competence of cognitively impaired older adults concluded that many persons with dementia are capable of decision making and that, at least in the early stages of dementia, interventions may improve decisional abilities (Kim, Karlawish, and Caine, 2002).*

▲ Assess the home for safety features and client needs for assistive devices. Explore with the client and family areas of concern. Refer to an occupational therapist for adaptive measures. Problem solve personal and environmental solutions for client protection. *Assistance from an occupational therapist offers sustained benefits in modifying the home environment for optimal adaptation (Gitlin, 2001). A variety of personal items (e.g., shoes, clothing) or environmental aspects (e.g., ready access to stove, loose rugs, flimsy outer door lock) may threaten client safety. Adaptations may include shoes or clothing with Velcro fasteners, stove knob locks, nonskid rugs or removal of rugs, and alarmed doors.*

▲ Evaluate the client's use or history of use of alcohol or drugs; continued use should be halted if the client can be persuaded. Instruct the client and family regarding the influence of substance use on cognition and behavior. Assess for the potential for withdrawal; refer to a physician for withdrawal protocol as indicated. *Continued substance use serves as a barrier to achieving effective outcomes in addressing dementia (Smith, 2002).*

• Provide support to the family of the client with a chronic and disabling condition; be prepared to offer support and information to family members who live at a distance as well. **Clinical Research:** *A study compared primary caregivers of clients having dementia with relatives living more than an hour distant. Both groups sought similar information about the client's disorder and reported similar subjective distress, but the distant relatives were more often dissatisfied with the information received and were less likely to seek out reading materials or lay societies (Thompsell and Lovestone, 2002).*

• Use familiar aspects of the environment (smells, music, foods, pictures) to cue the client, capitalizing on habit to remind the client of activities in which the client can participate (e.g., cooperating with medication administration). **Nursing Research:** *While clients with dementia are probably unable to learn new activities because of deteriorated explicit memory, preserved implicit memory or habit may be useful in maximizing functional ability (Son, Therrien, and Whall, 2002).*

• Instruct the caregiver to provide a balanced activity schedule that neither stresses the

• = **Independent;** ▲ = **Collaborative**

client nor deprives him or her of stimulation; avoid sustained low- or high-stimulation activity. **Nursing Research:** *In one study, imbalances in the pacing of sensory stimulation and sensory calming (i.e., sustained low- and high-stimulation activity) contributed to agitation and functional decline (Kovach and Wells, 2002).*

▲ If the client will require extensive supervision on an ongoing basis, evaluate the client for day care programs. Refer the family to medical social services to assist with this process if necessary. Day care programs provide safe, structured care for the client and respite for the family. *Respite care for caregivers is an essential part of successful long-term care for a confused client.*

• Encourage the family to include the client in family activities when possible. Reinforce the use of therapeutic communication guidelines (see Client/Family Teaching) and sensitivity to the number of people present. *These steps help the client maintain dignity and lead to familial socialization of the client.*

• Assess family caregivers for caregiver stress, loneliness, and depression. *Caring for a loved one with a dementing process is highly stressful. Respite care is a necessary component of the overall care plan.*

• Refer to the care plan for **Caregiver Role Strain. Nursing Research:** *Caregiver loneliness has been associated with depression, relational deprivation, and poorer quality of the current caregiver-client relationship (Beeson et al, 2000).*

• Explore the state of the relationship that existed between the client and caregiver before the onset of dementia, including the strengths and weaknesses of each party. Formulate a plan to assist the couple to deal with the likely worsening of dementia. *Dementia represents a gradual and devastating loss of the marital relationship as it existed formerly. An understanding of the prior relationship is needed before the couple can be helped to anticipate continuing deterioration (Zarit, 2001).*

• Explore with the spouse the process he or she is undergoing to understand the client's behavior; assist with reframing that understanding to be as realistic and positive as possible. **Nursing Research:** *In a qualitative study, wives of clients with Alzheimer's disease described a process of recognizing changes, drawing inferences about their observations, rewriting identities for themselves and their husbands as they took on their husbands' roles and responsibilities, and constructing a new daily life. Reframing interventions can assist caregivers in considering positive aspects of caring along with grief and frustration (Perry, 2002).*

▲ Refer the client to medical social services as necessary to evaluate financial resources and initiate benefits or access to providers. *Limited resources serve as barriers to effective outcomes in addressing dementia (Smith, 2002).*

▲ Institute case management for frail elderly clients to support continued independent living. *Difficulties with chronic confusion lead to increasing needs for assistance in using the health care system effectively. Case management combines the nursing activities of client and family assessment, planning and coordination of care among all health care providers, delivery of direct nursing care, and monitoring of care and outcomes. These activities are able to promote continuity across multiple sites of care, mutual goal setting, behavior management, and prevention of worsening health problems (Guttman, 1999; Tichawa, 2002).*

▲ Refer for homemaker or psychiatric home health care services for respite, client reassurance, and implementation of a therapeutic regimen. *Having responsibility for a person who is chronically confused results in high caregiver stress. Respite decreases caregiver stress. The presence of caring individuals is reassuring to both the client and caregivers, especially during periods of client anxiety. The client who shows chronic confusion, especially if*

• = **Independent;** ▲ = **Collaborative**

it is accompanied by depression, can benefit from the interventions described previously, modified for the home setting.

Client/Family Teaching

- In the early stages of confusion (e.g., initial period following stroke), provide the caregiver with information on illness processes, needed care, and likely trajectory of progress. **Nursing Research:** *In one study, family caregivers of stroke survivors felt abandoned by staff. Caregivers wanted information to ensure that they felt competent, confident, and able safely to provide care; they wanted to understand likely future demands (Brereton and Nolan, 2002).*
- Recommend that the family develop a memory aid wallet or booklet for the client, which contains pictures and text that chronicle the client's life. **Clinical and Nursing Research:** *Using memory aids such as wallets or booklets helps dementia clients make more factual statements and stay on topic, and decreases the number of confused, erroneous, and repetitive statements (Bourgeois, 1992).*
- Teach the family how to converse with a memory-impaired person. Guidelines include the following:
  - Ask the client to have a conversation with you.
  - Guide the conversation to specific, nonthreatening topics and redirect the conversation back on topic when the client begins to ramble.
  - Reassure and help out when the client gets stuck or cannot find the right words.
  - Smile and act interested in what the client is saying even if unsure what it means.
  - Thank the client for talking.
  - Avoid quizzing the client or asking a lot of specific questions.
  - Avoid correcting or contradicting something that was stated even if it is wrong.
  Clinical Research: *These guidelines can help families interact more effectively with clients and decrease frustration levels (Bourgeois, 1992).*
- Teach the family how to set up the environment and use the care techniques/ interventions listed so that cognitive and functional impairments that interact with the client's progressively lowered stress threshold (PLST) will be addressed. Identify stressors and initiate compensatory modifications of the environment. **Nursing Research:** *Alzheimer's clients are unable to deal with stress and have decreased tolerance to stimuli; decreasing stress can decrease confusion and changes in behavior. PLST instruction of caregivers has had a positive influence on response to problem behaviors. A typical PLST care plan includes a structured routine with regular rest periods. Teach the family compensatory modifications of the environment: for example, reduce the temperature on the hot water heater to prevent scalding; replace the toilet seat with one of contrasting color to aid visualization; remove mirrors to reduce misinterpretation of environmental stimuli (Gerdner, Buckwalter, and Reed, 2002).*
- Discuss with the family what to expect as the dementia progresses.
- ▲ Counsel the family about resources available regarding end-of-life-decisions and legal concerns.
- ▲ Inform the family that, as dementia progresses, hospice care may be available in the home in the terminal stages to help the caregiver. **Nursing Research:** *Hospice services in the late stages of dementia can help support the family with nursing services and visitation by the primary care provider, home health aides, social services personnel, volunteer visitors, and a spiritual counselor if desired as the client is dying (Boyd and Vernon, 1998).*

NOTE: The nursing diagnoses **Impaired Environmental interpretation syndrome** and

- **• = Independent; ▲ = Collaborative**

Chronic Confusion are very similar in definition and interventions. **Impaired Environmental interpretation** must be interpreted as a syndrome when other nursing diagnoses would also apply. **Chronic Confusion** may be interpreted as the human response to a situation or situations that require a level of cognition of which the individual is no longer capable. Further research is under way to make this distinction clear to the practicing nurse.

evolve WEBSITES FOR EDUCATION

See the EVOLVE website for World Wide Web resources for client education.

REFERENCES

Agostinelli B et al: Targeted interventions: use of the Mini-Mental State Exam, *J Gerontol Nurs* 20(8):15, 1994.

Alexopoulos GS et al: Treatment of agitation in older persons with dementia, *Postgrad Med* 103(4 suppl):1, 1998.

Algase D: Wandering: a dementia-compromised behavior, *J Gerontol Nurs* 25(9):10, 1999.

Bair B et al: Interventions for disruptive behaviors, *J Gerontol Nurs* 25(1):13, 1999.

Beeson R et al: Loneliness and depression in caregivers of persons with Alzheimer's disease or related disorders, *Issues Ment Health Nurs* 21:779, 2000.

Boehm S et al: Behavioral analysis and nursing interventions for reducing disruptive behaviors of patients with dementia, *Appl Nurs Res* 8(3):118, 1995.

Bourgeois MS: *Conversing with memory impaired individuals using memory aids: a memory aid workbook,* Gaylord, Mich, 1992, Northern Speech Services.

Boyd CO, Vernon GM: Primary care of the older adult with end-stage Alzheimer's disease, *Nurse Pract* 23(4): 63, 1998.

Brereton L, Nolan M: "Seeking": a key activity for new family carers of stroke survivors, *J Clin Nurs* 11:22, 2002.

Buckwalter K et al: A nursing intervention to decrease depression in family caregivers of AD patients, *Gerontologist* 35:792, 1995.

Burgener SC et al: Effective caregiving approaches for patients with Alzheimer's disease, *Geriatr Nurs* 19(3): 121, 1998.

Chumbler NR et al: Differences by race in the health status of rural cognitively impaired Arkansans, *Clin Gerontol* 24(1/2):103, 2001.

Cleeland EA: Depression in people with dementia, *Home Healthc Nurse* 15:781, 1997.

Cochran M: Tears have no color, *Am J Nurs* 98(6):53, 1998.

Cohen-Mansfield J, Golander H, Arnheim G: Self-identity in older persons suffering from dementia: preliminary results, *Soc Sci Med* 51(3):381, 2000.

Cox C: Race and caregiving: patterns of service use by African-American and white caregivers of persons with Alzheimer's, *J Gerontol Soc Work* 32(2):5, 1999.

Crist JD: Mexican American elders' use of skilled home care nursing services, *Public Health Nurs* 19(5):366, 2002.

Doody RS et al: Practice parameter: management of dementia (an evidence-based review), *Neurology* 56:1154, 2001.

Doswell W, Erlen J: Multicultural issues and ethical concerns in the delivery of nursing care interventions, *Nurs Clin North Am* 33(2):353, 1998.

Espino DV et al: Diagnostic approach to the confused elderly patient, *Am Fam Physician* 57(6):1358, 1998.

Feil N: *The validation breakthrough: simple techniques for communicating with people with Alzheimer's-type dementia,* Baltimore, 1993, Health Professions.

Fine J, Rouse-Bane S: Using validation techniques to improve communication with cognitively impaired older adults, *J Gerontol Nurs* 21(6):39, 1995.

Finley B: Nutritional needs of the person with Alzheimer's disease: practical approaches to quality care, *J Am Diet Assoc* 97(10 suppl):S177, 1997.

Gerdner LA, Buckwalter KC: A nursing challenge: assessment and management of agitation in Alzheimer's patients, *J Gerontol Nurs* 20(4):11, 1994.

• = Independent; ▲ = Collaborative

Gerdner LA, Buckwalter KC, Reed D. Impact of a psychoeducational intervention on caregiver response to behavior problems, *Nurs Res* 51(6):363, 2002.

Gitlin LN: Effectiveness of home environmental interventions for individuals with dementia and family caregivers, *Home Health Care Consult* 8(9):22, 2001.

Guarnaccia P: Multicultural experiences of family caregiving: a study of African American, European American, and Hispanic American families, *New Dir Ment Health Serv* 77:45, 1998.

Guttman R: Case management of the frail elderly in the community, *Clin Nurs Spec* 13(4):174, 1999.

Haley WE et al: Psychological, social, and health impact of caregiving: a comparison of black and white dementia family caregivers and noncaregivers, *Psychol Aging* 10(4):540, 1995.

Hall GR et al: Standardized care plan: managing Alzheimer's patients at home, *J Gerontol Nurs* 21(1):37, 1995.

Hall GR, Buckwalter KC: *Bathing persons with dementia*, Iowa City, Ia, 1999, University of Iowa Gerontological Nursing Interventions Research Center.

Heineken J: Patient silence is not necessarily client satisfaction: communication in home care nursing, *Home Healthc Nurse* 16(2):115, 1998.

Hinrichsen GA, Ramirez M: Black and white dementia caregivers: a comparison of their adaptation, *Gerontologist* 32(3):375, 1992.

Katz IR et al: Comparison of Risperidone and placebo for psychosis and behavioral disturbances with dementia: a randomized, double-blind trial, *J Clin Psychiatry* 60(2):107, 1999.

Kim SY, Karlawish JH, Caine ED: Current state of research on decision-making competence of cognitively impaired elderly persons, *Am J Geriatr Psychiatry* 10:151, 2002.

Kovach CR, Wells T: Pacing of activity as a predictor of agitation for persons with dementia in acute care, *J Gerontol Nurs* 22:28, 2002.

Leininger MM, McFarland MR: *Transcultural nursing: concepts, theories, research and practices*, ed 3, New York, 2002, McGraw-Hill.

Maxfield MC, Lewis RE, Cannon S: Training staff to prevent aggressive behavior of cognitively impaired elderly patients during bathing and grooming, *J Gerontol Nurs* 22(1):37, 1996.

McGrath P, Vun M, McLeod L: Needs and experiences of non-English speaking hospice patients and families in an English speaking country, *Am J Hosp Palliat Care* 18(5):305, 2001.

Nurses Drug Alert: Delirium with single dose of diphenhydramine, *Nurses Drug Alert* 19(1):4, 1995.

Painter J: Home environment considerations for people with Alzheimer's disease, *Occup Ther Health Care* 10(3):45, 1996.

Perry J: Wives giving care to husbands with Alzheimer's disease: a process of interpretive caring, *Res Nurs Health* 25:307, 2002.

Rempusheski VF, Hurley AC: Advance directives and dementia, *J Gerontol Nurs* 26(10):27, 2000.

Sloane PD: Advances in the treatment of Alzheimer's disease, *Am Fam Physician* 58(7):1577, 1998.

Smith GB: Case management guideline: Alzheimer disease and other dementias, *Lippincotts Case Manag* 7:77, 2002.

Snyder M, Egan EC, Burns KR: Interventions for decreasing agitation behaviors in persons with dementia, *J Gerontol Nurs* 21(7):34, 1995.

Son G, Therrien B, Whall A: Implicit memory and familiarity among elders with dementia, *J Nurs Sch* 34:263, 2002.

Stolley JM: When your patient has Alzheimer's disease, *Am J Nurs* 94(8):34, 1994.

Thompsell A, Lovestone S: Out of sight out of mind? Support and information given to distant and near relatives of those with dementia, *Int J Geriatr Psychiatry* 17:804, 2002.

Tichawa U: Creating a continuum of care for elderly individuals, *J Gerontol Nurs* 28:46, 2002.

Tinetti ME, Liu WL, Ginter SF: Mechanical restraint use and fall-related injuries among residents of skilled nursing facilities, *Ann Intern Med* 116:369, 1992.

Woods P, Ashley J: Simulated presence therapy: using selected memories to manage problem behaviors in Alzheimer's disease patients, *Geriatr Nurs* 16(1):9, 1995.

Zarit J: A tribute to adaptability: mental illness and dementia in intimate late-life relationships, *Generations* 25(2):70, 2001.

• = **Independent;** ▲ = **Collaborative**

Constipation

Betty J. Ackley

NANDA   Definition

Decrease in normal frequency of defecation, accompanied by difficult or incomplete passage of stool and/or passage of excessively hard, dry stool

Defining Characteristics

Change in bowel pattern; bright red blood with stool; presence of soft, pastelike stool in rectum; distended abdomen; dark, black, or tarry stool; increased abdominal pressure; percussed abdominal dullness; pain with defecation; decreased volume of stool; straining with defecation; decreased frequency of stool; dry, hard, formed stool; palpable rectal mass; feeling of rectal fullness or pressure; abdominal pain; inability to pass stool; anorexia; headache; change in abdominal growling (borborygmi); indigestion; atypical presentation in older adults (e.g., change in mental status, urinary incontinence, unexplained falls, elevated body temperature); severe flatus; generalized fatigue; hypoactive or hyperactive bowel sounds; palpable abdominal mass; abdominal tenderness with or without palpable muscle resistance; nausea and/or vomiting; oozing of liquid stool

Related Factors (r/t)

Functional

Recent environmental changes; habitual denial or ignoring of urge to defecate; insufficient physical activity; irregular defecation habits; inadequate toileting (e.g., timeliness, positioning for defecation, privacy); abdominal muscle weakness

Psychological

Depression; emotional stress; mental confusion

Pharmacological

Antilipemic agents; overdose of laxatives; calcium carbonate; aluminum-containing antacids; nonsteroidal anti-inflammatory drugs (NSAIDs); opiates; anticholinergics; diuretics; iron salts; phenothiazines; sedatives; sympathomimetics; bismuth salts; antidepressants; calcium channel blockers

Mechanical

Rectal abscess or ulcer; pregnancy; rectal anal fissure; tumor; megacolon (Hirschsprung's disease); electrolyte imbalance; rectal prolapse; prostate enlargement; neurological impairment; rectal anal stricture; rectocele; postsurgical obstruction; hemorrhoids; obesity

Physiological

Poor eating habits; decreased motility of gastrointestinal tract; inadequate dentition or oral hygiene; insufficient fiber intake; insufficient fluid intake; change in usual foods and eating patterns; dehydration

• = Independent; ▲ = Collaborative

| NOC | Outcomes (Nursing Outcomes Classification) |

Suggested NOC Outcomes
Bowel Elimination; Hydration

Example NOC Outcome with Indicators

Bowel Elimination as evidenced by the following indicators: Elimination pattern in expected range/Stool soft and formed/Passage of stool without aids/Ease of stool passage (Rate each indicator of **Bowel Elimination:** 1 = extremely compromised, 2 = substantially compromised, 3 = moderately compromised, 4 = mildly compromised, 5 = not compromised [see Section I].)

Client Outcomes

Client Will (Specify Time Frame):
- Maintain passage of soft, formed stool every 1 to 3 days without straining
- State relief from discomfort of constipation
- Identify measures that prevent or treat constipation

| NIC | Interventions (Nursing Interventions Classification) |

Suggested NIC Intervention
Constipation/Impaction Management

Example NIC Activities—Constipation/Impaction Management

Identify factors (e.g., medications, bed rest, and diet) that may cause or contribute to constipation/impaction.

Nursing Interventions and Rationales

- Assess usual pattern of defecation, including time of day, amount and frequency of stool, consistency of stool; history of bowel habits or laxative use; diet including fluid intake; exercise patterns; personal remedies for constipation; obstetrical/gynecological history; surgeries; alterations in perianal sensation; present bowel regimen. *There often are multiple reasons for constipation; the first step is assessment of the usual patterns of bowel elimination.*
- Have the client or family keep a diary of bowel habits using a Management of Constipation Assessment Inventory, including information such as time of day; usual stimulus; consistency, amount, and frequency of stool; fluid consumption; and use of any aids to defecation. **Nursing Research:** *A diary of bowel habits is valuable in treatment of constipation; the use of a diary has proven to be more accurate than client recall in determining the presence of constipation (Karam and Nies, 1994; Hinrichs et al, 2001).*
- ▲ Review the client's current medications. *Many medications affect bowel function, including opiates, antidepressants, antihypertensives, anticholinergics, diuretics, anticonvulsants, NSAIDs, antacids containing aluminum, iron supplements, and muscle relaxants (Wong and Kadakia, 1999).*
- ▲ If the client is receiving opioids, request an order for stool softeners from the primary care practitioner and institute a bowel regimen before the onset of constipation. *The*

• = Independent; ▲ = Collaborative

use of opioids is commonly associated with constipation because of decreased peristalsis, and prevention is the best route of action.

- Palpate for abdominal distention, percuss for dullness, and auscultate bowel sounds. *In clients with constipation the abdomen is often distended, with abdominal rigidity and tenderness and a palpable colon. Bowel sounds will be present (Hinrichs et al, 2001).*

▲ Check for impaction; if present, perform digital removal per physician's order. *If impaction is present, manual removal is necessary before a bowel routine can be instituted (Hinrichs et al, 2001).*

▲ If the client is uncomfortable or in pain due to constipation or has acute or chronic constipation that does not respond to increased fiber, fluid, activity, and appropriate toileting, refer the client to the primary care practitioner for an evaluation of bowel function and health status. *There can be multiple causes of constipation, such as hypothyroidism, depression, somatization, bowel obstruction, and Hirschsprung's disease (Arce, Ermocilla, and Costa, 2002).*

- Provide privacy for defecation. Help the client to the bathroom and close the door if possible. *Toileting is recommended 5 to 15 minutes after meals, especially after breakfast when the gastrocolic reflex is strongest (Hinrichs et al, 2001). Bowel elimination is a very private act, and a lack of privacy can contribute to constipation (Weeks, Hubbartt, and Michaels, 2000).*

- Ask the client to keep a food log of the foods eaten during the last 24 hours. If needed, instruct the client in the need to eat five to nine fruits and vegetables per day, and at least three servings of whole-grain foods. *If the client eats a healthy diet with sufficient fruits and vegetables and sufficient servings of whole-grains foods, the soluble and insoluble fiber that is present in the foods will naturally prevent constipation.*

- Encourage fiber intake of 25 to 30 g/day for adults. Emphasize foods such as fresh fruits, beans, vegetables, and bran cereals. Add fiber to diet gradually with increased intake of fluids. **Nursing Research:** *A daily intake of 25 to 30 g of fiber can increase the frequency of stools in clients with constipation (Brown and Everett, 1990; Cheskin et al, 1995; Gibson et al, 1995; Ouellet et al, 1996). Fiber helps prevent constipation by giving stool bulk. Add fiber to the diet gradually, because a sudden increase can cause bloating, gas, and diarrhea (Doughty, 1996). Dietary supplements of fiber in the form of bran or wheat fiber are helpful for women experiencing constipation during pregnancy (Jewell and Young, 2002).*

- Use a mixture of 1 cup of Kellogg's All-Bran cereal, 1 cup of applesauce, and 1 cup of prune juice; begin administration in small amounts and gradually increase amount. Refer to references for dosing. Keep refrigerated. Always check with the primary care practitioner before initiating this intervention. It is important that the client also ingest sufficient fluids. **Nursing Research:** *This bran mixture has been shown to be effective even with short-term use in elderly clients recovering from acute conditions.* NOTE: *Giving fiber without sufficient fluid has resulted in impaction and bowel obstruction (Gibson et al, 1995). A study involving institutionalized elderly men with chronic constipation demonstrated that, with use of a bran mixture, clients were able to discontinue use of oral laxatives (Howard, West, and Ossip-Klein, 2000). A number of bran mixtures have been shown to effectively decrease constipation (Beverley and Travis, 1992; Gibson et al, 1995), including a mixture known as "power pudding" (Neal, 1995).*

- Encourage a fluid intake of 1.5 to 2 L/day (6 to 8 glasses of liquids per day). If oral intake is low, gradually increase fluid intake. *Fluid intake must be within the cardiac and renal reserve. Adequate fluid intake is necessary to prevent hard, dry stools. Increasing*

- = **Independent;** ▲ = **Collaborative**

fluid intake to 1.5 to 2 L/day while maintaining a fiber intake of 25 g can significantly increase the frequency of stools in clients with constipation (Anti, 1998; Weeks, Hubbartt, and Michaels, 2000).

- Encourage the client to be out of bed as soon as possible and to perform the activities of daily living himself or herself as able. Encourage exercise such as turning and changing positions in bed, lifting the hips off the bed, performing range-of-motion exercises, alternately lifting each knee to the chest, doing wheelchair lifts, doing waist twists, stretching the arms away from the body, and pulling in the abdomen while taking deep breaths. *Activity, even minimal, increases peristalsis, which is necessary to prevent constipation (Weeks, Hubbartt, and Michaels, 2000).*

- Initiate a regular schedule for defecation, using the client's normal evacuation time whenever possible. Offer hot coffee, hot lemon water, or prune juice before breakfast, or while the client sits on the toilet if necessary. An optimal time for many individuals is 30 minutes after breakfast because of the gastrocolic reflex. *Establishing a schedule gives the client a sense of control, but more importantly it promotes evacuation before drying of stool and constipation occur (Doughty, 1992). Ingestion of hot liquids can stimulate peristalsis and result in defecation (Weeks, Hubbartt, and Michaels, 2000).*

- Help the client onto a bedside commode or toilet with the client's hips flexed and feet flat. Have the client deep breathe through the mouth to encourage relaxation of the pelvic floor muscle and use the abdominal muscles to help evacuation. Provide laxatives, suppositories, and enemas only as needed if other more natural interventions are not effective, and as ordered only; establish a client goal of eliminating their use. *Use of laxatives should be avoided because they contribute to further constipation by causing slowed fecal mass intestinal transit time (Evans et al, 1998).*

- Avoid the use of both soapsuds and tap water enemas if possible, or use a low concentration of Castile soap only. If enemas are ordered, measure the amount of fluid given and the amount expelled. *Enema fluid can be retained, and this retained fluid can be harmful for the client prone to fluid overload.* **Nursing Research:** *Soapsuds enemas can damage the colonic mucosa (Schmelzer and Wright, 1993). The use of a soapsuds enema was shown to increase stool output compared with a tap water enema in preoperative liver transplant clients; the amount of mucosal irritation was unknown. Several clients retained large amounts of fluid (Schmelzer et al, 2000).*

- ▲ For the stable neurological client, consider use of a bowel routine of a Therevac enema instead of suppositories every other day. For persistent constipation, refer to a physician for evaluation. **Nursing Research:** *Use of the Therevac SB minienema was found to reduce the time needed for bowel care by as much as 1 hour or more compared with the use of suppositories (Dunn and Galka, 1994).*

Geriatric

- Explain the importance of adequate fiber intake, fluid intake, activity, and established toileting routines to ensure soft, formed stool. *Fiber intake, fluid intake, and activity are often decreased in elderly clients. Increasing fiber and fluids can effectively prevent constipation in the elderly (Rodrigues-Fisher, Bourguignon, and Good, 1993; Hinrichs et al, 2001).* **Nursing Research:** *A study involving institutionalized elderly men with chronic constipation demonstrated that, with use of a bran mixture, clients were able to discontinue use of oral laxatives (Howard, West, and Ossip-Klein, 2000).*

- Determine the client's perception of normal bowel elimination; promote adherence to

• = **Independent;** ▲ = **Collaborative**

a regular schedule. *Misconceptions regarding the frequency of bowel movements can lead to anxiety and overuse of laxatives.*
- Explain Valsalva's maneuver and the reason it should be avoided. *Valsalva's maneuver can cause bradycardia and even death in cardiac clients.*
- Respond quickly to the client's call for help with toileting.
- Avoid regular use of enemas in the elderly. *Enemas can cause fluid and electrolyte imbalances (Yakabowich, 1990) and damage to the colonic mucosa (Schmelzer and Wright, 1993).*
- ▲ Use opioids cautiously. If they are ordered, use stool softeners and bran mixtures to prevent constipation. *Use of opioids can cause constipation (Schaefer and Cheskin, 1998).*
- Position the client on the toilet or commode and place a small footstool under the feet. *Placing a small footstool under the feet increases intra-abdominal pressure and makes defecation easier for an elderly client with weak abdominal muscles.*

Home care
- The interventions described previously may be adapted for home care use.
- Take complaints seriously and evaluate claims of constipation in a matter-of-fact manner. *Continued constipation can lead to bowel obstruction, a medical emergency. Use of a matter-of-fact manner will limit positive reinforcement of the behavior if actual constipation does not exist. Refer to the care plan for* **Perceived Constipation**.
- Assess the self-care management activities the client is already using. **Nursing Research:** *Many older adults seek solutions to constipation, with laxative use a frequent remedy that creates its own problems (Annells and Koch, 2002).*
- The following treatment recommendations have been offered (Annells and Koch, 2002):
  - Acknowledge the client's life-long experience of bowel function; respect beliefs, attitudes, and preferences, and avoid patronizing responses.
  - Make available comprehensive, useful written information about constipation and possible solutions.
  - Make available empathetic and accessible professional care to provide treatment and advice; a multidisciplinary approach (including physician, nurse, and pharmacist) should be used.
  - Institute a bowel management program.
  - Consider affordability when suggesting solutions to constipation; discuss cost-saving strategies.
  - Discuss a range of solutions to constipation and allow the client to choose the preferred options.
  - Have orders in place for a suppository and enema as the need may occur.
  As part of a bowel management program, suppositories or enemas may become necessary.
- Although the use of a bedside commode may be necessitated by the client's condition, allow the client to use the toilet in the bathroom when possible and provide assistance. *Bowel elimination is a very private act, and a lack of privacy can contribute to constipation (Weeks, Hubbartt, and Michaels, 2000).*
- ▲ Carefully monitor the bowel patterns of clients under pain management with opioids. In older clients, routinely advise consumption of fluids, fruits, and vegetables as part of the diet, and ambulation if the client is able. Introduce a bowel management program at the first sign of constipation. *Constipation is a major problem for terminally ill or hospice clients, who may need very high doses of opioids for pain management (Miller and Miller, 2002).*

- = **Independent;** ▲ = **Collaborative**

▲ Refer for consideration of the use of polyethylene glycol 3350 (PEG-3350) for constipation. **Nursing Research:** *In a study of PEG-3350 use for idiopathic constipation, researchers concluded that it appeared to be safe and efficacious when dietary and lifestyle
changes were ineffective. Clients reported increased perceived bowel control, with reduced
complaints of straining, stool hardness, bloating, and gas (Stoltz et al, 2001).*

• Advise the client against attempting to remove impacted feces on his or her own.
Older or confused clients in particular may attempt to remove feces and cause rectal damage.

• Instruct the client and family in appropriate expectations for having bowel movements.
*The client and family may have unrealistic expectations regarding the frequency and type of
bowel movements. Instruction may be required if the client believes that he or she should have
more frequent stools or if the client has gone through an assessment procedure that changes
the stool (e.g., lower gastrointestinal study). Failure to so instruct may result in the client's
and family's acting on expectations and resorting to laxatives inappropriately.*

• When using a bowel program, establish a pattern that is very regular and allows the
client to be part of the family unit. *Regularity of the program promotes psychological
and/or physiological readiness to evacuate stool. Families of home care clients often cannot
proceed with normal daily activities until bowel programs are complete.*

Client/Family Teaching

• Instruct the client on normal bowel function and the need for adequate fluid and fiber
intake, activity, and a defined toileting pattern in a bowel program.

• Encourage the client to heed defecation warning signs and develop a regular schedule
of defecation by using a stimulus such as a warm drink or prune juice. *Most cases of constipation are mechanical and result from habitual neglect of impulses that signal the appropriate time for defecation. The reflex that causes the urge to defecate diminishes after a few
minutes and may remain quiet for several hours; as a result, the stool becomes hardened
and more difficult to expel (Folden, 2002).*

• Encourage the client to avoid long-term use of laxatives and enemas and to gradually
withdraw from their use if they are used regularly. *Use of laxatives should be avoided
because they contribute to further constipation by slowing fecal mass intestinal transit time
(Evans et al, 1998).*

• If not contraindicated, teach the client how to do bent-leg sit-ups to increase abdominal tone; also encourage the client to contract the abdominal muscles frequently
throughout the day. Help the client develop a daily exercise program to increase
peristalsis.

evolve WEBSITES FOR EDUCATION

See the EVOLVE website for World Wide Web resources for client education.

REFERENCES

Annells M, Koch T: Older people seeking solutions to constipation: the laxative mire, *J Clin Nurs* 11:603, 2002.
Anti M: Water supplementation enhances the effect of high-fiber diet on stool frequency and laxative con-
sumption in adult patients with functional constipation, *Hepatogastroenterology* 45(21):727, 1998.
Arce DA, Ermocilla CA, Costa H: Evaluation of constipation, *Am Fam Physician* 65:11, 2002.
Beverley L, Travis I: Constipation: proposed natural laxative mixtures, *J Gerontol Nurs* 18(10):5, 1992.
Brown M, Everett I: Gentler bowel fitness with fiber, *Geriatr Nurs* 11:1, 1990.

• = **Independent;** ▲ = **Collaborative**

Cheskin LJ et al: Mechanisms of constipation in older persons and effects of fiber compared with placebo, *J Am Geriatr Soc* 43:6, 1995.

Doughty D: A step-by-step approach to bowel training, *Progressions* 4:12, 1992.

Doughty D: A physiologic approach to bowel training, *J Wound Ostomy Continence Nurs* 23(1):46, 1996.

Dunn KL, Galka ML: A comparison of the effectiveness of Therevac SB and bisacodyl suppositories in SCI patients' bowel programs, *Rehabil Nurs* 19:334, 1994.

Evans JM et al: Relation of colonic transit to functional bowel disease in older people, *J Am Geriatr Soc* 46:1, 1998.

Folden SL: Practice guidelines for the management of constipation in adults, *Rehabil Nurs* 27(5):169, 2002.

Gibson CJ et al: Effectiveness of bran supplement on the bowel management of elderly rehabilitation patients, *J Gerontol Nurs* 21(10):21, 1995.

Hinrichs M et al: Research-based protocol. Management of constipation, *J Gerontol Nurs* 27(2):17, 2001.

Howard LV, West D, Ossip-Klein DJ: Chronic constipation management for institutionalized older adults, *Geriatr Nurs* 21(2):78, 2000.

Jewell DJ, Young G: Interventions for treating constipation in pregnancy, *Cochrane Library*, CD001142, 2002.

Karam SE, Nies DM: Student/staff collaboration: a pilot bowel management program, *J Gerontol Nurs* 20:3, 1994.

Miller KE, Miller M: Managing common gastrointestinal symptoms at the end of life, *J Hosp Palliat Nurs* 4:1, 2002.

Neal LJ: "Power pudding": natural laxative therapy for the elderly who are homebound, *Home Healthc Nurse* 13(3):66, 1995.

Ouellet LL et al: Dietary fiber and laxation in postop orthopedic patients, *Clin Nurs Res* 5:4, 1996.

Rodrigues-Fisher L, Bourguignon C, Good BV: Dietary fiber nursing intervention: prevention of constipation in older adults, *Clin Nurs Res* 2:464, 1993.

Schaefer DC, Cheskin LJ: Constipation in the elderly, *Am Fam Physician* 58(4):907, 1998.

Schmelzer M et al: Colonic cleansing, fluid absorption, and discomfort following tap water and soapsuds enemas, *Appl Nurs Res* 13(2):83, 2000.

Schmelzer M, Wright K: Working smart, *Am J Nurs* 93:55, 1993.

Stoltz R et al: An efficacy and consumer preference study of polyethylene glycol 3350 for the treatment of constipation in regular laxative users, *Home Health Care Consult* 8(2):21, 2001.

Weeks SK, Hubbartt E, Michaels TK: Keys to bowel success, *Rehabil Nurs* 25(2):66, 2000.

Wong PN, Kadakia S: How to deal with chronic constipation, *Postgrad Med* 106(6):199, 1999.

Yakabowich M: Prescribe with care: the role of laxatives in the treatment of constipation, *J Gerontol Nurs* 16:4, 1990.

Perceived Constipation

Betty J. Ackley

NANDA Definition

State in which individual makes a self-diagnosis of constipation and ensures daily bowel movement through abuse of laxatives, enemas, and suppositories

Defining Characteristics

Expectation of a daily bowel movement that results in overuse of laxatives, enemas, and suppositories; expectation of a bowel movement at same time every day

Related Factors (r/t)

Cultural or family beliefs; faulty appraisals; impaired thought processes

• = Independent; ▲ = Collaborative

| NOC | Outcomes (Nursing Outcomes Classification) |

Suggested NOC Outcomes

Bowel Elimination; Health Beliefs; Health Beliefs: Perceived Threat

---

Example NOC Outcome with Indicators

Bowel Elimination as evidenced by the following indicators: Elimination pattern in expected range/Stool soft and formed/Passage of stool without aids/Ease of stool passage (Rate each indicator of **Bowel Elimination:** 1 = extremely compromised, 2 = substantially compromised, 3 = moderately compromised, 4 = mildly compromised, 5 = not compromised [see Section I].)

Client Outcomes

Client Will (Specify Time Frame):

- Regularly defecate soft, formed stool without using any aids
- Explain the need to decrease or eliminate the use of laxatives, suppositories, and enemas
- Identify alternatives to laxatives, enemas, and suppositories for ensuring defecation
- Explain that defecation does not have to occur every day

| NIC | Interventions (Nursing Interventions Classification) |

Suggested NIC Interventions

Bowel Management; Medication Management

Example NIC Activities—Bowel Management

Note preexistent bowel problems, bowel routine, and use of laxatives

---

Nursing Interventions and Rationales

- Have the client keep a diary of bowel habits using a Management of Constipation Assessment Inventory, including information such as time of day; usual stimulus; consistency, amount, and frequency of stool; fluid consumption; and use of any aids to defecation. **Nursing Research:** *A diary of bowel habits is valuable in the treatment of constipation; the use of a diary has proven to be more accurate than client recall in determining the presence of constipation (Karam and Nies, 1994; Hinrichs et al, 2001).*
- Determine the client's perception of an appropriate defecation pattern. *The client may need to be taught that one bowel movement every 1 to 3 days is normal (Wong and Kadakia, 1999).*
- Monitor the use of laxatives, suppositories, or enemas and suggest replacing them with increased fiber intake along with increased fluids to 2 L/day. *Long-term use of laxatives may result in a cathartic colon, with the inability to have a bowel movement without use of laxatives (Hinrichs et al, 2001). An increase in fiber intake to 25 to 30 g/day along with an increase in fluid intake can help clients with chronic constipation (Anti et al, 1998; Wong and Kadakia, 1999).*
- Ask the client to keep a food log of the foods eaten for the last 24 hours or recall the usual foods eaten. If necessary, teach the client the need to eat five to nine fruits and

• = Independent; ▲ = Collaborative

vegetables per day, and at least three servings of whole-grain foods. *If the client eats a healthy diet with sufficient fruits and vegetables and servings of whole-grains foods, the soluble and insoluble fiber that is present in the foods will naturally prevent constipation.*

- In place of laxatives, use a mixture of 1 cup of Kellogg's All-Bran cereal, 1 cup of applesauce, and 1 cup of prune juice; begin administration in small amounts and gradually increase amount. Refer to references for dosing. Keep refrigerated. Always check with the primary care practitioner before initiating this intervention. It is important that the client also consume sufficient fluids. **Nursing Research:** *This mixture has been shown to be effective even with short-term use in elderly clients recovering from acute conditions.* NOTE: *Giving fiber without sufficient fluid has resulted in impaction and bowel obstruction (Gibson et al, 1995). A study involving institutionalized elderly men with chronic constipation demonstrated that, with use of a bran mixture, clients were able to discontinue use of oral laxatives (Howard, West, and Ossip-Klein, 2000). A number of bran mixtures have been shown to effectively decrease constipation (Beverley and Travis, 1992; Gibson et al, 1995), including a mixture known as "power pudding" (Neal, 1995).*
- Encourage the client to respond promptly to the defecation reflex. *The reflex that causes the urge to defecate diminishes after a few minutes and may remain quiet for several hours; as a result, the stool becomes hardened and more difficult to expel (Folden, 2002).*
- ▲ If the client is uncomfortable or in pain due to constipation or has chronic constipation that does not respond to increased fiber and fluid intake, activity, and appropriate toileting, refer the client to the primary care practitioner for an evaluation of bowel function and health status. *There can be multiple causes of constipation, such as hypothyroidism, depression, somatization, bowel obstruction, and Hirschsprung's disease (Arce, Ermocilla, and Costa, 2002).*
- ▲ Obtain a dietary referral for analysis of the client's diet and input on how to improve the diet to ensure adequate fiber intake and nutrition. Assess for signs of depression, a sedentary lifestyle, a history of sexual abuse, and obesity. Refer for counseling as appropriate. *All of these factors can contribute to constipation (Wong and Kadakia, 1999).*
- Encourage the client to increase activity, walking for at least 30 minutes at least 5 days a week as tolerated. *Increased activity increases bowel motility, which decreases constipation (Wong and Kadakia, 1999; Hinrichs et al, 2001).*
- ▲ Observe for the presence of an eating disorder, the use of laxatives to control or decrease weight; refer for counseling if needed.

Home care

- The interventions described previously may be adapted for home care use.
- Take complaints seriously and evaluate claims of constipation in a matter-of-fact manner. *Continued constipation can lead to bowel obstruction, a medical emergency. Presence of a pattern of perceived constipation does not mean actual constipation cannot occur. However, use of a matter-of-fact manner will limit positive reinforcement of the behavior.*
- Obtain family and client histories of bowel or other patterned behavior problems. *History may reveal a psychological cause for the constipation (e.g., withholding).*
- Observe family cultural patterns related to eating and bowel habits. *Cultural patterns may control bowel habits.*
- Encourage a mindset and program of self-care management. Elicit from the client the self-talk he or she uses to describe body perceptions; correct catastrophizing interpretations. Instruct the client in a healthy lifestyle that supports normal bowel function (e.g., activity, fluid intake, diet) and encourage progressive inclusion of these ele-

• = **Independent;** ▲ = **Collaborative**

ments into daily activities. *A study of cognitive patterns in individuals with somatization syndrome showed that body perceptions were assumed to be a sign of catastrophic occurrence (e.g., "physical complaints are always signs of disease") and concepts of health were very restrictive. Somatizing individuals were acutely aware of bodily sensations that would normally be considered automatic and would seek help immediately to obtain medications or other solutions. They did not participate in other types of health-seeking behavior (Rief, Hiller, and Margraf, 1998).*

- Discuss the client's self image. Help the client to reframe the self-concept as capable. *Somatizing individuals tend to see themselves as weak and therefore avoid exercise (Rief, Hiller, and Margraf, 1998). Developing the ability to see themselves as capable of self-care management may take time, as will making lifestyle changes.*
- Instruct the client and family in appropriate expectations for having bowel movements. Offer instruction and reassurance regarding explanations for variation from the previous pattern of bowel movements. *The client may have unrealistic expectations regarding the frequency or type of bowel movements and may assume that constipation exists when there is a reasonable explanation for deviation from the past pattern. The client may resort to the use of laxatives inappropriately.*
- Contract with the client and/or a responsible family member regarding the use of laxatives. Have the client maintain a bowel pattern diary. Observe for diarrhea or frequent evacuation. *Intermittent care does not allow for 24-hour supervision. Contracting allows guided control of care by the client in partnership with the nurse, and the diary promotes more accurate reporting.*
- ▲ Teach the family to carry out the bowel program per the physician's orders.
- ▲ Refer for home health aide services to assist with personal care, including the bowel program, if appropriate.
- Identify a contingency plan for bowel care if the client is dependent on outside persons for such care.

Client/Family Teaching

- Explain normal bowel function and the necessary ingredients for a regular bowel regimen (e.g., fluid, fiber, activity, and regular schedule for defecation).
- Work with the client and family to develop a diet that fits the client's lifestyle and includes increased fiber.
- Teach the client that it is not necessary to have daily bowel movements and that the passage of anywhere from three stools each day to three stools each week is considered normal.
- Explain to the client the harmful effects of the continual use of defecation aids such as laxatives and enemas.
- Encourage the client to gradually decrease the use of the usual laxatives and enemas and to set a date to have eliminated the use of all defecation aids.
- Determine a method of increasing the client's fluid intake and fit this practice into the client's lifestyle.
- Explain what Valsalva's maneuver is and why it should be avoided.
- Work with the client and family to design a bowel training routine that is based on previous patterns (before laxative or enema abuse) and incorporates the consumption of warm fluids, increased fiber, and increased fluids; privacy; and a predictable routine.

• = Independent; ▲ = Collaborative

Additional Nursing Interventions and Rationales, Client/Family Teaching

See care plan for **Constipation.**

evolve WEBSITES FOR EDUCATION

See the EVOLVE website for World Wide Web resources for client education.

REFERENCES

Anti M et al: Water supplementation enhances the effect of high-fiber diet on stool frequency and laxative consumption in adult patients with functional constipation, *Hepatogastroenterology* 45(21):727, 1998.

Arce DA, Ermocilla CA, Costa H: Evaluation of constipation, *Am Fam Physician* 65:11, 2002.

Beverley L, Travis I: Constipation: proposed natural laxative mixtures, *J Gerontol Nurs* 18(10):5, 1992.

Folden SL: Practice guidelines for the management of constipation in adults, *Rehabil Nurs* 27(5):169, 2002.

Gibson CJ et al: Effectiveness of bran supplement on the bowel management of elderly rehabilitation patients, *J Gerontol Nurs* 21(10):21, 1995.

Hinrichs M et al: Research-based protocol. Management of constipation, *J Gerontol Nurs* 27(2):17, 2001.

Howard LV, West D, Ossip-Klein DJ: Chronic constipation management for institutionalized older adults, *Geriatr Nurs* 21(2):78, 2000.

Karam SE, Nies DM: Student/staff collaboration: a pilot bowel management program, *J Gerontol Nurs* 20(3): 32, 1994.

Neal LJ: "Power pudding": natural laxative therapy for the elderly who are homebound, *Home Healthc Nurse* 13(3):66, 1995.

Rief W, Hiller W, Margraf J: Cognitive aspects of hypochondriasis and somatization syndrome, *J Abnorm Psychol* 107:587, 1998.

Wong PW, Kadakia S: How to deal with chronic constipation: a stepwise method of establishing and treating the source of the problem, *Postgrad Med* 106(6):199, 1999.

Risk for Constipation

Betty J. Ackley

NANDA Definition

At risk for decrease in individual's normal frequency of defecation accompanied by difficult or incomplete passage of stool and/or passage of excessively hard, dry stool

Related Factors (r/t)

Functional

Recent environmental changes; habitual denial or ignoring of urge to defecate; insufficient physical activity; irregular defecation habits; inadequate toileting (e.g., timeliness, positioning for defecation, privacy); abdominal muscle weakness

Psychological

Emotional stress; mental confusion; depression

Physiological

Poor eating habits; decreased motility of gastrointestinal tract; inadequate dentition or oral hygiene; insufficient fiber intake; insufficient fluid intake; change in usual foods and eating patterns; dehydration

• = **Independent;** ▲ = **Collaborative**

Pharmacological
Phenothiazides; antilipemic agents; overuse of laxatives; calcium carbonate; aluminum-containing antacids; nonsteroidal anti-inflammatory agents; opiates; anticholinergics; iron salts; sedatives; sympathomimetics; bismuth salts; antidepressants; calcium channel blockers; anticonvulsants

Mechanical
Rectal abscess or ulcer; pregnancy; postsurgical obstruction; rectal anal fissure; tumor; megacolon (Hirschsprung's disease); electrolyte imbalance; rectal prolapse; prostate enlargement; neurological impairment; rectal anal stricture; rectocele; tumors; hemorrhoids; obesity

NOC   Outcomes (Nursing Outcomes Classification)

Suggested NOC Outcome
Bowel Elimination

> **Example NOC Outcome with Indicators**
>
> **Bowel Elimination** as evidenced by the following indicators: Elimination pattern in expected range/Stool soft and formed/Passage of stool without aids/Ease of stool passage (Rate each indicator of **Bowel Elimination:** 1 = extremely compromised, 2 = substantially compromised, 3 = moderately compromised, 4 = mildly compromised, 5 = not compromised [see Section I].)

Client Outcomes

Client Will (Specify Time Frame):
- Maintain passage of soft, formed stool every 1 to 3 days without straining
- Identify measures that prevent constipation
- Explain rationale for not using laxatives and enemas

NIC   Interventions (Nursing Interventions Classification)

Suggested NIC Intervention
Constipation/Impaction Management

> **Example NIC Activities—Constipation/Impaction Management**
>
> Identify factors (e.g., medications, bed rest, and diet) that may cause or contribute to constipation/impaction; Monitor for signs and symptoms of constipation/impaction

Nursing Interventions and Rationales, Client/Family Teaching
See care plan for **Constipation.**

• = Independent; ▲ = Collaborative

Ineffective Coping

Ann Keeley

NANDA Definition

Inability to form a valid appraisal of internal or external stressors, inadequate choices of practiced responses, and/or inability to access or use available resources

Defining Characteristics

Lack of goal-directed behavior or resolution of problem, including inability to attend; difficulty with organized information; sleep disturbance; abuse of chemical agents; decreased use of social support; use of forms of coping that impede adaptive behavior; poor concentration; fatigue; inadequate problem solving; verbalized inability to cope or ask for help; inability to meet basic needs; destructive behavior toward self or others; inability to meet role expectations; high illness rate; change in usual communication patterns; risk taking

Related Factors (r/t)

Gender differences in coping strategies; inadequate level of confidence in ability to cope; uncertainty; inadequate social support created by characteristics of relationships; inadequate level of perception of control; inadequate resource availability; high degree of threat; situational crises; maturational crises; disturbance in pattern of tension release; inadequate opportunity to prepare for stressor; inability to conserve adaptive energies; disturbance in pattern of appraisal of threat; chronic conditions; alteration in body integrity; cultural variables

NOC   Outcomes (Nursing Outcomes Classification)

Suggested NOC Outcomes

Coping; Decision Making; Impulse Self-Control; Information Processing

> **Example NOC Outcome with Indicators**
>
> **Coping** as evidenced by the following indicator: Identifies effective and ineffective coping patterns and modifies lifestyle (response) as needed (Rate the indicator of **Coping:** 1 = never demonstrated, 2 = rarely demonstrated, 3 = sometimes demonstrated, 4 = often demonstrated, 5 = consistently demonstrated [see Section I].)

Client Outcomes

Client Will (Specify Time Frame):
- Verbalize ability to cope and ask for help when needed
- Demonstrate ability to solve problems related to current needs
- Remain free of destructive behavior toward self or others
- Communicate needs and negotiate with others to meet needs
- Discuss how recent life stressors have overwhelmed normal coping strategies
- Demonstrate new effective coping strategies
- Have illness and accident rates not excessive for age and developmental level

• = Independent; ▲ = Collaborative

| NIC | Interventions (Nursing Interventions Classification) |

Suggested NIC Interventions
Coping Enhancement; Decision-Making Support

Example NIC Activities—Coping Enhancement

Assist the client in developing an objective appraisal of the event; Explore with the client previous methods of dealing with problems

Nursing Interventions and Rationales

- Observe for causes of ineffective coping such as poor self-concept, grief, lack of problem-solving skills, lack of support, or recent change in life situation. **Nursing Research:** *Psychological manifestations of ineffective coping can be understood only after a thorough inquiry into the client's framework for appraisal (Dudley-Brown, 2002).*

- Observe for strengths such as the ability to relate the facts and to recognize the source of stressors. **Nursing Research:** *Successful adaptation requires a coordination of efforts to fit the nursing interventions to the client's perception of the threat, personal values and beliefs, and recognition of personal strengths (Norris and Spelic, 2002).*

- Assess the risk of the client's harming self or others and intervene appropriately. See the care plan for **Risk for Suicide. Nursing Research:** *The value an individual attaches to a stressor will affect the level and type of emotional reaction (Norris and Spelic, 2002).*

- Help the client set realistic goals and identify personal skills and knowledge. **Clinical Research:** *Providing validation of actual stressors and available coping resources and/or strategies aids in a positive adaptation to stress (Pakenham, 2001).* **Nursing Research:** *Efforts to educate regarding possible and/or potential effects of a specific diagnosis and the resources available to assist with coping are a positive factor in successful adaptation (Wassem, Beckham, and Dudley, 2001).*

- Use empathetic communication and encourage the client and family to verbalize fears, express emotions, and set goals. **Nursing Research:** *A nurse's holistic presence with clients is considered to be vital (Cote and Pepler, 2002).*

- Encourage the client to make choices and participate in the planning of care and scheduled activities. **Clinical Research:** *Active involvement in coping plans increases the possibility of a positive adjustment (Pakenham, 2001).*

- Provide mental and physical activities within the client's ability (e.g., reading, television, radio, crafts, outings, movies, dinners out, social gatherings, exercise, sports, games). **Nursing Research:** *Activities that decrease stress and/or increase self-efficacy potentiate a positive approach to perceived stressors (Fisher and Laschinger, 2001).*

- If the client is physically able, encourage moderate aerobic exercise. **Nursing Research:** *Exercise is effective in alleviating anxiety (Blanchard, Courneya, and Laing, 2001).*

- Provide information regarding care before care is given. *Adequate information and training before and after treatment reduces anxiety and fear (Herranz and Gavilan, 1999).*

- Discuss changes with the client before making them. **Nursing Research:** *Nurses are pivotal in communicating to clients the information needed to ensure the best outcome. They are identified by clients as necessary in coordinating all aspects of their care (Hodgkinson and Lester, 2002).*

- **= Independent; ▲ = Collaborative**

- Discuss the client's and family's power to change a situation or the need to accept a situation. **Nursing Research:** *An honest assessment of a particular situation as shared by the nurse is important to the family's sense of what is expected of them in adapting to a health care change (Weiss and Chen, 2002).*
- Use active listening and acceptance to help the client express emotions such as sadness, guilt, and anger (within appropriate limits). **Nursing Research:** *Nurses need to provide an opportunity for clients to address all aspects of the impact of a health status change on their lives (Richer and Ezer, 2002).*
- Encourage the client to describe previous stressors and the coping mechanisms used. **Nursing Research:** *Recounting previous experiences that were perceived by the client as having been dealt with successfully strengthens effective coping and helps eliminate ineffective coping mechanisms (Northouse et al, 2002).*
- Be supportive of coping behaviors; allow the client time to relax. **Nursing Research:** *Sharing of innermost cares and concerns requires that nurses provide opportunities for clients to feel safe enough to share (Richer and Ezer, 2002).*
- Help the client to define what meaning his or her symptoms might have for the client. **Nursing Research:** *Exploring the meaning of health status change and the adjustments required for a successful adaptation within the client's life experience fosters positive growth (Norris and Spelic, 2002; Richer and Ezer, 2002).*
- Encourage the use of cognitive behavioral relaxation (e.g., music therapy, guided imagery). **Nursing Research:** *Relaxation training has been demonstrated to improve overall coping ability (Tyni-Lenne et al, 2002).*
- Use distraction techniques during procedures that cause the client to be fearful. *Distraction is used to direct attention toward a pleasurable experience and block the attention to the feared procedure (DuHamel, Redd, and Johnson-Vickberg, 1999).*
- Use systematic desensitization when introducing new people, places, or procedures that may cause fear and altered coping. *Fear of new things diminishes with repeated exposure (DuHamel, Redd, and Johnson-Vickberg, 1999).*
- Provide the client and/or family with a video of any feared procedure to view before the procedure. Ensure that the video shows a client of similar age and background. *Videos provide the client and/or family with the information necessary to eliminate fear of the unknown (DuHamel, Redd, and Johnson-Vickberg, 1999).*
- ▲ Refer for counseling as needed. **Nursing Research:** *Nurses are perceived as the bridge between the client and all other resources needed to manage an adaptive response to a health care change (Hodgkinson and Lester, 2002).*

Geriatric

- Engage the client in reminiscence. *Reminiscence activates positive memories and evokes well-being (Puentes, 2002).*
- ▲ Assess and report possible physiological alterations (e.g., sepsis, hypoglycemia, hypotension, infection, changes in temperature, fluid and electrolyte imbalances, and use of medications with known cognitive and psychotropic side effects). **Clinical Research:** *Such alterations may be contributing to confusion and must be corrected (Matthiesen et al, 1994). Medications are considered the most common cause of delirium in the ICU (Harvey, 1996).*
- Determine if the individual is displaying a change in personality as a manifestation of difficulty with coping. *An older individual's responses to age-related stress will depend on the balance of personality strengths and weaknesses.* **Nursing Research:** *Negative life*

• = **Independent;** ▲ = **Collaborative**

events will vary in the degree to which they affect the symptoms observed in the elderly (Kraaij, 2001).

- Increase and mobilize the support available to the elderly client. Encourage interaction with family and friends. **Nursing Research:** *Relationships are pivotal in supporting coping in older adults (Cutcliffe and Grant, 2001).*

Multicultural

- Assess for the influence of cultural beliefs, norms, and values on the client's perceptions of effective coping. **Nursing Research:** *The client's coping behavior may be based on cultural perceptions of normal and abnormal coping behavior (Leininger and McFarland, 2002; D'Avanzo et al, 2001; Cochran, 1998; Doswell and Erlen, 1998). Culture influences perceptions of stressors and perceptions of potential coping behaviors as well as resources (Cuellar, 2002).*
- Assess for intergenerational family problems that can overwhelm coping abilities. **Nursing Research:** *Family assessment is integral to nursing care of clients (Northouse et al, 2002).*
- Encourage spirituality as a source of support for coping. **Nursing Research:** *Many African Americans and Latinos identify spirituality, religiousness, prayer, and church-based approaches as coping resources (Samuel-Hodge et al, 2000).*
- Negotiate with the client with regard to the aspects of coping behavior that will need to be modified. **Nursing Research:** *As a part of the assessment of coping behaviors, alternate methods may be introduced and offered to the client as a possible choice in new coping strategies (Wassem, Beckham, and Dudley, 2001).*
- Identify which family members the client can count on for support. **Nursing Research:** *In a variety of different cultures family members are relied on to cope with stress (Donnelly, 2002; White et al, 2002; Aziz and Rowland, 2002; Gleeson-Kreig, Bernal, and Woolley, 2002).*
- Use an empowerment framework to redefine coping strategies. **Nursing Research:** *Use of an empowerment framework will allow individuals to redefine behaviors as coping strategies to confront their environment and connect to natural supports in the community (Dancy et al, 2001).*
- Assess the influence of fatalism on the client's coping behavior. **Nursing Research:** *Fatalistic perspectives, which involve the belief that one cannot control one's own fate, may influence health behaviors in some Asian, African American, and Latino populations (Chen, 2001; Phillips, Cohen, and Moses, 1999; Harmon, Castro, and Coe, 1996).*
- Assess the influence of cultural conflicts that may affect coping abilities. **Nursing Research:** *It may be necessary to help the client to identify and find coping strategies that do not conflict with cultural expectations (Shibusawa and Mui, 2001).*

Home care

- The interventions described previously may be adapted for home care use.
- Observe the family for coping behavior patterns. Obtain family and client history as possible. **Nursing Research:** *Family assessment is necessary to guide interventions (Weiss and Chen, 2002; Northouse et al, 2002).*
- ▲ Assess for suicidal tendencies. Refer for mental health care immediately if indicated. Identify an emergency plan should the client become suicidal. *Ineffective coping can occur in a crisis situation and can lead to suicidal ideation if the client sees no hope for a solu-*

• = Independent; ▲ = Collaborative

tion. A suicidal client is not safe in the home environment unless supported by professional help. Refer to the care plan for **Risk for Suicide**.

- Encourage the client to use self-care management to increase the experience of personal control. Identify with the client all available supports and sense of attachment to others. Refer to the care plan for **Powerlessness. Nursing Research:** *In a study of heart transplantation clients, personal control was positively associated with optimism, well-being, and satisfaction with life, and was negatively associated with anger and depression. Perceived social support helpfulness and attachment were positively associated with better psychological and functional outcomes (Bohachick et al, 2002).*

▲ Refer to medical social services for evaluation and counseling, which will promote adequate coping as part of the medical plan of care. If no primary medical diagnosis has been made, request medical social services to assist with community support contacts. *If the client is involved with the mental health system, actively participate in mental health team planning. Based on knowledge of the home and family, home care nurses can often advocate for clients. These nurses are frequently requested to monitor medication use and therefore need to know the plan of care.*

▲ Refer the client and family to support groups. **Nursing Research:** *Support groups provide an essential resource to clients and their families when adapting to health status change (Fung and Chien, 2002).*

▲ If monitoring medication use, contract with the client or solicit assistance from a responsible caregiver. *Prepouring of medications may be helpful with some clients. Caregivers in the home benefit from interventions that promote self-efficacy and provide a nurse for support (Dibartolo, 2002).*

▲ Institute case management for frail elderly clients to support continued independent living. *Difficulties in coping with changes in health care needs can lead to increasing needs for assistance in using the health care system effectively. Case management combines the nursing activities of client and family assessment, planning and coordination of care among all health care providers, delivery of direct nursing care, and monitoring of care and outcomes. These activities are able to address continuity of care, mutual goal setting, behavior management, and prevention of worsening health problems (Guttman, 1999).*

▲ If the client is homebound, refer for psychiatric home health care services for client reassurance and implementation of a therapeutic regimen. *Psychiatric home care nurses can address issues relating to the client's ability to adjust to changes in health status. Behavioral interventions in the home can help the client to participate more effectively in the treatment plan (Patusky, Rodning, and Martinez-Kratz, 1996).*

NOTE: All of the previously mentioned interventions may be applied in the home setting. Home care may offer psychiatric nursing or the services of a licensed clinical social worker under special programs. Traditionally, insurance does not reimburse for counseling that is not related to a medical plan of care unless it falls under one of the programs just described. Public health agencies generally do not have the clinical support needed to offer psychiatric nursing services to clients. Clients are usually treated in the ambulatory mental health system.

Client/Family Teaching

- Teach the client to problem solve. Have the client define the problem and cause, and list the advantages and disadvantages of the options. **Nursing Research:** *Interventions that support hardiness and self-efficacy facilitate positive adaptation to*

• = Independent; ▲ = Collaborative

stressors (Dibartolo, 2002; Wassem, Beckham, and Dudley, 2001; Fisher and Laschinger, 2001).

- Provide the seriously ill client and his or her family with needed information regarding the condition and treatment. **Clinical Research:** *Clients and families benefit from a sense of trust in health care providers that is based on honest communication regarding their condition and options (Fallowfield, Jenkins, and Beveridge, 2002).*
- Teach relaxation techniques. **Nursing Research:** *Relaxation training has been demonstrated to improve self-efficacy in family caregivers of clients with Alzheimer's disease (Fisher and Laschinger, 2001).*
- Work closely with the client to develop appropriate educational tools that address individualized needs. **Nursing Research:** *Educational level may affect the client's level of concern and ability to process information (Miles et al, 2002).*
- ▲ Teach the client about available community resources (e.g., therapists, ministers, counselors, self-help groups). **Nursing Research:** *Families need assistance in coping with health changes. The nurse is often perceived as the individual who can help them obtain necessary social support (Tak and McCubbin, 2002; Northouse et al, 2002).*

evolve WEBSITES FOR EDUCATION

See the EVOLVE website for World Wide Web resources for client education.

REFERENCES

Aziz N, Rowland JH: Cancer survivorship research among ethnic minority and medically underserved groups, *Oncol Nurs Forum* 29(5):789, 2002.

Blanchard CM, Courneya KS, Laing D: Effects of acute exercise on state anxiety in breast cancer survivors, *Oncol Nurs Forum* 28(10):1617, 2001.

Bohachick P et al: Social support, personal control, and psychological recovery following heart transplant, *Clin Nurs Res* 11:34, 2002.

Chen YC: Chinese values, health and nursing, *J Adv Nurs* 36(2):270, 2001.

Cochran M: Tears have no color, *Am J Nurs* 98(6):53, 1998.

Cote JK, Pepler C: A randomized trial of a cognitive coping intervention for acutely ill HIV-positive men, *Nurs Res* 51(4):237, 2002.

Cuellar NG: A comparison of African American and Caucasian American female caregivers of rural, post-stroke, bedbound older adults, *J Gerontol Nurs* 28(1):36, 2002.

Cutcliffe JR, Grant G: What are the principles and processes of inspiring hope in cognitively impaired older adults within a continuing care environment? *J Psychiatr Ment Health Nurs* 8:427, 2001.

Dancy BL et al: Empowerment: a view of two African American communities, *J Natl Black Nurses Assoc* 12(2): 49, 2001.

D'Avanzo CE et al: Developing culturally informed strategies for substance-related interventions. In Naegle MA, D'Avanzo CE, editors: *Addictions and substance abuse: strategies for advanced practice nursing*, St Louis, 2001, Mosby.

Dibartolo M: Exploring self-efficacy and hardiness in spousal caregivers of individuals with dementia, *J Gerontol Nurs* 28(4):24, 2002.

Dombeck M-TE: Chaos and self-organization as a consequence of spiritual disequilibrium, *Clin Nurse Spec* 16(1):42, 2002.

Donnelly TT: Contextual analysis of coping: implications for immigrants' mental health care, *Issues Ment Health Nurs* 23:715, 2002.

Doswell W, Erlen J: Multicultural issues and ethical concerns in the delivery of nursing care interventions, *Nurs Clin North Am* 33(2):353, 1998.

Dudley-Brown S: Prevention of psychological distress in persons with inflammatory bowel disease, *Issues Ment Health Nurs* 23:403, 2002.

- **= Independent; ▲ = Collaborative**

DuHamel KN, Redd WH, Johnson-Vickberg SM: Behavioral interventions in the diagnosis, treatment and rehabilitation of children with cancer, *Acta Oncol* 38(6):719, 1999.

Fallowfield LJ, Jenkins VA, Beveridge HA: Truth may hurt but deceit hurts more: communication in palliative care, *Palliative Med* 16(4):297, 2002.

Fisher PA, Laschinger HS: A relaxation training program to increase self-efficacy for anxiety control in Alzheimer family caregivers, *Holist Nurs Pract* 15(2):47, 2001.

Fung WY, Chien WT: The effectiveness of a mutual support group for family caregivers of a relative with dementia, *Arch Psychiatr Nurs* 26(3):134, 2002.

Gleeson-Kreig J, Bernal H, Woolley S: The role of social support in the self-management of diabetes mellitus among a Hispanic population, *Public Health Nurs* 19(3):215, 2002.

Guttman R: Case management of the frail elderly in the community, *Clin Nurs Spec* 13(4):174, 1999.

Harmon MP, Castro FG, Coe K: Acculturation and cervical cancer: knowledge, beliefs, and behaviors of Hispanic women, *Women Health* 24(3):37, 1996.

Harvey M: Managing agitation in critically ill patients, *Am J Crit Care* 5:7, 1996.

Herranz J, Gavilan J: Psychosocial adjustment after laryngeal cancer surgery, *Ann Otol Rhinol Laryngol* 108(10):990, 1999.

Hodgkinson R, Lester H: Stresses and coping strategies of mothers living with a child with cystic fibrosis: implications for nursing professionals, *J Adv Nurs* 39(4):370, 2002.

Kraaij V: Negative life events and depressive symptoms in the elderly: a life span perspective, *Aging Ment Health* 5(1):84, 2001.

Leininger MM, McFarland MR: *Transcultural nursing: concepts, theories, research and practices,* ed 3, New York, 2002, McGraw-Hill.

Matthiesen V et al: Acute confusion: nursing interventions in older patients, *Orthop Nurs* 13:25, 1994.

Miles MS et al: Perceptions of stress, worry, and support in black and white mothers of hospitalized, medically fragile infants, *J Pediatr Nurs* 17(2):82, 2002.

Norris J, Spelic SS: Supporting adaptation to body image disruption, *Rehabil Nurs* 27(1):8, 2002.

Northouse L et al: A family-based program of care for women with recurrent breast cancer and their family members, *Oncol Nurs Forum* 29(10):1411, 2002.

Pakenham KI: Application of a stress and coping model to caregiving in multiple sclerosis, *Psychol Health Med* 6(1):13, 2001.

Patusky KL, Rodning C, Martinez-Kratz M: Clinical lessons in psychiatric home care: a case study approach, *J Home Health Case Manag* 9:18, 1996.

Phillips JM, Cohen MZ, Moses G: Breast cancer screening and African-American women: fear, fatalism, and silence, *Oncol Nurs Forum* 26(3):561, 1999.

Puentes WJ: Simple reminiscence: a stress-adaptation model of the phenomenon, *Issues Ment Health Nurs* 23:497, 2002.

Richer MC, Ezer H: Living in it, living with it, and moving on: dimensions of meaning during chemotherapy, *Oncol Nurs Forum* 29(1):113, 2002.

Samuel-Hodge CD et al: Influences on day-to-day self-management of type 2 diabetes among African-American women: spirituality, the multi-caregiver role, and other social context factors, *Diabetes Care* 23(7):928, 2000.

Shibusawa T, Mui AC: Stress, coping and depression among Japanese American elders, *J Gerontol Soc Work* 36(1/2):63, 2001.

Tak YR, McCubbin M: Family stress, perceived social support and coping following the diagnosis of a child's congenital heart disease, *J Adv Nurs* 39(2):190, 2002.

Tyni-Lenne R et al: Beneficial therapeutic effects of physical training and relaxation therapy in women with coronary syndrome X, *Physiother Res Int* 7(1):35, 2002.

Wassem R, Beckham N, Dudley W: Test of a nursing intervention to promote adjustment to fibromyalgia, *Orthop Nurs* 20(3):33, 2001.

Weiss SJ, Chen JL: Factors influencing maternal mental health and family functioning during the low birth-weight infant's first year of life, *J Pediatr Nurs* 17(2):114, 2002.

Wengstrom Y, Haggmark C, Forsberg C: Coping with radiation therapy: effects of a nursing intervention on coping ability for women with breast cancer, *Int J Nurs Pract* 7:8, 2001.

White N et al: A cross-cultural comparison of family resiliency in hemodialysis clients, *J Transcult Nurs* 13(3):218, 2002.

● = **Independent;** ▲ = **Collaborative**

Readiness for enhanced Coping

Gail B. Ladwig

NANDA **Definition**

Pattern of cognitive and behavioral efforts to manage demands that is sufficient for well-being and can be strengthened

Defining Characteristics

Defines stressors as manageable; seeks social support; uses a broad range of problem-oriented and emotion-oriented strategies; uses spiritual resources; acknowledges power; seeks knowledge of new strategies; is aware of possible environmental changes

NOC **Outcomes (Nursing Outcomes Classification)**

Suggested NOC Outcomes

Coping; Decision Making; Social Support

> **Example NOC Outcome with Indicators**
>
> **Coping** as evidenced by the following indicator: Identifies effective coping patterns and uses effective coping strategies (Rate the indicator of **Coping:** 1 = never demonstrated, 2 = rarely demonstrated, 3 = sometimes demonstrated, 4 = often demonstrated, 5 = consistently demonstrated [see Section I].)

Client Outcomes

Client Will (Specify Time Frame):
- Verbalize ability to cope and ask for help when needed
- Demonstrate ability to solve problems related to current needs
- Communicate needs and negotiate with others to meet needs
- State that stressors are manageable
- Demonstrate new effective coping strategies
- Seek social support for problems associated with coping
- Seek spiritual support of personal choice

NIC **Interventions (Nursing Interventions Classification)**

Suggested NIC Interventions

Coping Enhancement; Decision-Making Support

> **Example NIC Activities—Coping Enhancement**
>
> Assist client in developing an objective appraisal of the event; Explore with client previous methods of dealing with problems

Nursing Interventions and Rationales
- Use empathetic communication and encourage the client and family to verbalize fears,

• = Independent; ▲ = Collaborative

express emotions, and set goals. **Nursing Research:** *A nurse's holistic presence with clients is considered to be vital (Cote and Pepler, 2002).*

- Observe for strengths such as the ability to relate the facts and to recognize the source of stressors. **Nursing Research:** *Successful adaptation requires a coordination of efforts to fit the nursing interventions to the client's perception of the threat, personal values and beliefs, and recognition of personal strengths (Norris and Spelic, 2002).*

- Encourage expression of positive thoughts and emotions. **Clinical Research:** *Positive emotions initiate upward spirals toward enhanced emotional well-being (Fredrickson and Joiner, 2002).*

- Encourage the use of cognitive behavioral relaxation (e.g., music therapy, guided imagery). **Nursing Research:** *Relaxation training has been demonstrated to improve overall coping ability (Tyni-Lenne et al, 2002).*

- Encourage the client to use spiritual coping mechanisms such as faith and prayer. **Nursing Research:** *Addressing spiritual needs is acknowledged to be an essential component of holistic nursing care (Narayanasamy, 2002).*

- Help the client set realistic goals and identify personal skills and knowledge. **Nursing and Clinical Research:** *Providing validation of actual stressors and available coping resources and/or strategies aids in a positive adaptation to stress (Pakenham, 2001). Efforts to educate the client regarding possible and/or potential effects of a specific diagnosis and the resources available to assist with coping are a positive factor in successful adaptation (Wassem, Beckham, and Dudley, 2001).*

- Help the client with depression to maintain social support networks or assist in building new ones. **Nursing Research:** *Lay support is vital in restoring the depressed client's health and assisting the client in getting well and resuming his or her place in the public domain. An important task for the nurse is therefore to support the client in maintaining the client's existing social network or in building a new one (Skärsäter et al, 2003).*

- ▲ Consider a workplace stress management program to enhance coping skills. **Clinical Research:** *A work site program that focuses on stress, anxiety, and coping measurement along with small group educational intervention can significantly reduce illness and health care utilization (Rahe et al, 2002).*

- ▲ Refer for cognitive behavioral therapy. **Nursing Research:** *A cognitive behavioral nursing program was effective in increasing adjustment to fibromyalgia. Treatment subjects had improved post-treatment adjustment and symptom severity compared to control subjects (Wassem, Beckham, and Dudley, 2001).*

- ▲ Refer the client with breast cancer to a psychosocial group intervention for coping skills training, stress management, relaxation exercises, and psychosocial support. **Evidence-Based Research:** *In women with primary breast carcinoma, a psychosocial group intervention reduced psychological distress and enhanced coping (Schulz, 2001).*

- Refer to the care plans for **Readiness for enhanced Communication** and **Readiness for enhanced Spiritual well-being.**

Geriatric

- ▲ Refer the client with Alzheimer's disease who is terminally ill to hospice. **Nursing Research:** *Home care and hospice nurses can provide invaluable care in helping families cope with this disease and end-of-life issues (Head, 2003).*

- ▲ Refer the widowed older client to self-help support groups. **Nursing Research:** *Bereaved older clients who attended face-to-face support groups for 20 weeks reported increased*

• = Independent; ▲ = Collaborative

hope, improved skills in developing social relationships, enhanced coping, new role identities, and less loneliness (Stewart et al, 2001).

Multicultural

- Assess for the influence of cultural beliefs, norms, and values on the client's perceptions of effective coping. **Nursing Research:** *The client's coping behavior may be based on cultural perceptions of normal and abnormal coping behavior (Leininger and McFarland, 2002; D'Avanzo et al, 2001; Cochran, 1998; Doswell and Erlen, 1998). Culture influences perceptions of stressors and perception of potential coping behaviors as well as resources (Cuellar, 2002).*
- Encourage spirituality as a source of support for coping. **Nursing Research:** *Many African Americans and Latinos identify spirituality, religiousness, prayer, and church-based approaches as coping resources (Samuel-Hodge et al, 2000).*
- Identify which family members the client can count on for support. **Nursing Research:** *In a variety of different cultures family members are relied on to cope with stress (Donnelly, 2002; White et al, 2002; Aziz and Rowland, 2002; Gleeson-Kreig, Bernal, and Woolley, 2002).*
- Support the inner resources that clients use for coping. **Nursing Research:** *African American women in one study used inner resources to develop self-help strategies to cope with reactions following involuntary pregnancy loss (Van and Meleis, 2003).*
- Use an empowerment framework to redefine coping strategies. **Nursing Research:** *Use of an empowerment framework will allow individuals to redefine behaviors as coping strategies to confront their environment and connect to natural supports in the community (Dancy et al, 2001).*

Home care

- The interventions described previously may be adapted for home care use.
- Observe the family for coping behavior patterns. Obtain family and client history as possible. **Nursing Research:** *Family assessment is necessary to guide interventions (Weiss and Chen, 2002; Northouse et al, 2002).*
- Encourage the client to use self-care management to increase the experience of personal control. Identify with the client all available supports and sense of attachment to others. **Nursing Research:** *In a study of heart transplantation clients, personal control was positively associated with optimism, well-being, and satisfaction with life, and was negatively associated with anger and depression. Perceived social support helpfulness and attachment were positively associated with better psychological and functional outcomes (Bohachick et al, 2002).*
- ▲ Refer the client and family to support groups. **Nursing Research:** *Support groups provide an essential resource to clients and their families when adapting to health status change (Fung and Chien, 2002).*

Client/Family Teaching

- Teach relaxation techniques. **Nursing Research:** *Relaxation training has been demonstrated to improve self-efficacy in family caregivers of clients with Alzheimer's disease (Fisher and Laschinger, 2001).*
- ▲ Teach the client about available community resources (e.g., therapists, ministers, counselors, self-help groups). **Nursing Research:** *Families need assistance in coping with*

• = **Independent;** ▲ = **Collaborative**

health changes. The nurse is often perceived as the individual who can help them obtain necessary social support (Tak and McCubbin, 2002; Northouse et al, 2002).

REFERENCES

Aziz N, Rowland JH: Cancer survivorship research among ethnic minority and medically underserved groups, *Oncol Nurs Forum* 29(5):789, 2002.

Bohachick P et al: Social support, personal control, and psychological recovery following heart transplant, *Clin Nurs Res* 11:34, 2002.

Cochran, M: Tears have no color, *Am J Nurs* 98(6):53, 1998.

Cote JK, Pepler C: A randomized trial of a cognitive coping intervention for acutely ill HIV-positive men, *Nurs Res* 51(4):237, 2002.

Cuellar NG: A comparison of African American and Caucasian American female caregivers of rural, post-stroke, bedbound older adults, *J Gerontol Nurs* 28(1):36, 2002.

Dancy BL et al: Empowerment: a view of two African American communities, *J Natl Black Nurses Assoc* 12(2):49, 2001.

D'Avanzo CE et al: Developing culturally informed strategies for substance-related interventions. In Naegle MA, D'Avanzo CE, editors: *Addictions and substance abuse: strategies for advanced practice nursing*, St Louis, 2001, Mosby.

Donnelly TT: Contextual analysis of coping: implications for immigrants' mental health care, *Issues Ment Health Nurs* 23:715, 2002.

Doswell W, Erlen J: Multicultural issues and ethical concerns in the delivery of nursing care interventions, *Nurs Clin North Am* 33(2):353, 1998.

Fisher PA, Laschinger HS: A relaxation training program to increase self-efficacy for anxiety control in Alzheimer family caregivers, *Holist Nurs Pract* 15(2):47, 2001.

Fredrickson BL, Joiner T: Positive emotions trigger upward spirals toward emotional well-being, *Psychol Sci* 13(2):172, 2002.

Fung WY, Chien WT: The effectiveness of a mutual support group for family caregivers of a relative with dementia, *Arch Psychiatr Nurs* 26(3):134, 2002.

Gleeson-Kreig J, Bernal H, Woolley S: The role of social support in the self-management of diabetes mellitus among a Hispanic population, *Public Health Nurs* 19(3):215, 2002.

Head G: Palliative care for persons with dementia, *Home Healthc Nurse* 21(1):53, 2003.

Leininger MM, McFarland MR: *Transcultural nursing: concepts, theories, research and practices*, ed 3, New York, 2002, McGraw-Hill.

Narayanasamy A: Spiritual coping mechanisms in chronically ill patients, *Br J Nurs* 11(22):1461, 2002.

Norris J, Spelic SS: Supporting adaptation to body image disruption, *Rehabil Nurs* 27(1):8, 2002.

Northouse LL et al: Quality of life of women with recurrent breast cancer and their family members, *J Clin Oncol* 20(19):4050, 2002.

Pakenham KI: Application of a stress and coping model to caregiving in multiple sclerosis, *Psychol Health Med* 6(1):13, 2001.

Rahe RH et al: A novel stress and coping workplace program reduces illness and healthcare utilization, *Psychosom Med* 64(2):278, 2002.

Samuel-Hodge CD et al: Influences on day-to-day self-management of type 2 diabetes among African-American women: spirituality, the multi-caregiver role, and other social context factors, *Diabetes Care* 23(7):928, 2000.

Schulz K: A psychosocial group intervention reduced psychological distress and enhanced coping in primary breast cancer, *Evid Based Ment Health* 4(1):15, 2001.

Skärsäter I et al: A salutogenetic perspective on how men cope with major depression in daily life, with the help of professional and lay support, *Int J Nurs Stud* 40(2):153, 2003.

Stewart M et al: Promoting positive affect and diminishing loneliness of widowed seniors through a support intervention, *Public Health Nurs* 18(1):54, 2001.

Tak YR, McCubbin M: Family stress, perceived social support and coping following the diagnosis of a child's congenital heart disease, *J Adv Nurs* 39(2):190, 2002.

Tyni-Lenne R et al: Beneficial therapeutic effects of physical training and relaxation therapy in women with coronary syndrome X, *Physiother Res Int* 7(1):35, 2002.

Van P, Meleis AI: Coping with grief after involuntary pregnancy loss: perspectives of African American women, *J Obstet Gynecol Neonatal Nurs* 32(1):28, 2003.

● = **Independent**; ▲ = **Collaborative**

Wassem R, Beckham N, Dudley W: Test of a nursing intervention to promote adjustment to fibromyalgia, *Orthop Nurs* 20(3):33, 2001.

Weiss SJ, Chen JL: Factors influencing maternal mental health and family functioning during the low birth-weight infant's first year of life, *J Pediatr Nurs* 17(2):114, 2002.

White N et al: A cross-cultural comparison of family resiliency in hemodialysis clients, *J Transcult Nurs* 13(3): 218, 2002.

Ineffective community Coping

Margaret Lunney

NANDA Definition

Pattern of community activities (for adaptation and problem solving) that is unsatisfactory for meeting the demands or needs of the community

Defining Characteristics

Expressed community powerlessness; failure of community to meet its own expectations; deficits of community participation; deficits in communication methods; excessive community conflicts; expressed difficulty in meeting demands for change; expressed vulnerability; high illness rates; stressors perceived as excessive; increased social problems (e.g., homicides, vandalism, arson, terrorism, robbery, infanticide, abuse, divorce, unemployment, poverty, militancy, mental illness)

Related Factors (r/t)

Natural or manmade disasters; ineffective or nonexistent community systems (e.g., lack of emergency medical, transportation, or disaster planning systems); deficits in community social support services and resources; inadequate resources for problem solving

NOC Outcomes (Nursing Outcomes Classification)

Suggested NOC Outcomes

Community Competence; Community Health Status

Example NOC Outcome with Indicators

Community Competence (select the level of achievement on the scale: 1 = poor demonstration, 2 = fair demonstration, 3 = average demonstration, 4 = good demonstration, 5 = excellent demonstration [see Section I]) as evidenced by the following indicators: Prevalence of health promotion programs/Health status of infants, children, adolescents, adults, elders/Attendance at programs for healthy states (Rate each indicator of **Community Competence** on the same five-point scale.)

Community Outcomes

Community Will (Specify Time Frame):
- Participate in community actions to improve power resources
- Develop improved communication among community members
- Participate in problem solving
- Demonstrate cohesiveness in problem solving

• = Independent; ▲ = Collaborative

- Develop new strategies for problem solving
- Express power to deal with change and manage problems

NIC   Interventions (Nursing Interventions Classification)

Suggested NIC Interventions

Environmental Management: Community; Health Policy Monitoring
    NIC Interventions developed for use with individuals can be adapted for use with communities: Coping Enhancement; Culture Brokerage; Mutual Goal Setting; Support System Enhancement

---

Example NIC Activities—Coping Enhancement

Explore with community members previous methods of dealing with life problems; Assist community to solve problems in a constructive manner

---

Nursing Interventions and Rationales

NOTE: The diagnosis of **Ineffective Coping** does not apply and should not be used when stress is being imposed by external sources or circumstance. If the community is a victim of circumstances, using the nursing diagnosis **Ineffective Coping** is equivalent to blaming the victim. See the care plans for **Ineffective community Therapeutic regimen management** and **Readiness for enhanced community Coping.**

- Establish a collaborative partnership with the community (see the care plan for **Ineffective community Therapeutic regimen management** for references). **Clinical Research:** *In studies conducted at the Center for Urban Epidemiological Studies in Harlem, NY, collaborative partnerships between the community and providers/researchers were effective in solving community problems and improving community health (Galea et al, 2001).*
- Participate with community members in the identification of stressors and assessment of distress; for example, observe and participate in community meetings and task forces. **Clinical Research:** *It may be possible to reduce or eliminate some of the stressors. Not all stressors produce distress. Based on data analyses of the National Examination Survey I, it was determined that a cycle of decline exists between distress and perceived health (Farmer and Ferraro, 1997). From nurses' stories related to community health nursing (N = 25), it was suggested that attendance at community meetings helps nurses to gain a community/population perspective (Diekemper, Smithbattle, and Drake, 1999).*
- Identify community strengths with community members and avoid defining the community in objective terms. **Nursing Research:** *In a qualitative study of clinic users (N = 13) and clinic board members and staff (N = 13) in a community health center, the community was objectified by staff members at the same time that clinic users described the strengths of the community. These differences "translated into disparate expectations" of services (Drevdahl, 1999).*
- Determine the extent of stress proliferation (i.e., primary stressors associated with contextual circumstances such as poverty) and the presence of secondary stressors related to the primary stressors (e.g., poor nutrition and housing conditions). **Theoretical Rationale:** *Stress proliferation contributes to inability to manage the excessive stressors (Pearlin, Aneshensel, and Leblanc, 1997). Nurses can help communities prevent primary stressors from leading to secondary stressors.*

- = Independent; ▲ = Collaborative

- Work with community members to increase awareness of ineffective coping behaviors (e.g., conflicts that prevent community members from working together, anger and hate that paralyze the community). **Theoretical Rationale:** *Problem solving is essential for effective coping. Community members in partnership with providers can modify behaviors that interfere with problem solving (Anderson and McFarlane, 2000; Chinn, 2001; Wallerstein, 2000).*
- Provide support to the community and help community members to identify and mobilize additional supports. **Nursing Research:** *In a 13-month three-group randomized clinical trial involving 125 women diagnosed with early-stage breast cancer, women in the two groups that received regular social support reported more positive outcomes, such as less mood disturbance and less loneliness, in the three phases of data collection (Samarel, Tulman, and Fawcett, 2002). Often people need help in mobilizing supports that are available (Pender, Murdaugh, and Parsons, 2002).*
- Use focus group methods to evaluate and strengthen interventions. **Nursing Research:** *Focus group methodology strengthened population interventions in a Medicaid managed care population in Nebraska (Kaiser, Barry, and Kaiser, 2002).*
- Use mentoring strategies for community members. **Nursing Research:** *In a focus group study of 43 African American teens and adults on the community problem of teenage pregnancy, the participants selected mentoring as a strategy to teach, counsel, and provide information (Tabi, 2002).*
- Advocate for the community in multiple arenas (e.g., television, newspapers, and governmental agencies). **Theoretical Rationale:** *Advocacy is a specific form of caring that enhances power resources for community coping (Chinn, 2001). Power resources include knowledge, motivation, belief system (hope), physical strength and reserve, psychological stamina and support network, positive self-concept, and energy (Miller, 2000).*
- Write grant proposals to help community members obtain funds for programs that reduce stress or improve coping. (See Coley and Scheinberg, 2000, for program proposal-writing methods.) **Theoretical Rationale:** *The programs that are necessary may be expensive, and often funds may not be available without the assistance of public or privately funded grants (Anderson and McFarland, 2000).*
- Work with members of the community to identify and develop coping strategies that promote a sense of power (e.g., obtaining sources for funding, collaborating with other communities). **Nursing Research:** *In a study of 39 blind subjects, those experiencing power as defined by Barrett's theory of power (power is being aware of what one is choosing to do, feeling free to do it, and doing it intentionally) reported better emotional and general health than individuals lacking power (Leksell et al, 2001). A first step in power enhancement is for the community to identify and develop its own coping strategies (Chinn, 2001).*
- Obtain police support for community partnerships aimed at healthy coping. **Clinical Research:** *Police programs have led to innovative programs that contribute to community health (Frommer and Papouchado, 2000).*
- Support positive attitudes and feelings as a basis for change. **Nursing Research:** *In a qualitative study using key informants from a South African community characterized by violence, community members described positive as well as negative experiences from living with violence. Positive experiences included feelings of solidarity, bravery, and increased appreciation (Madela and Poggenpoel, 1993).*

- = **Independent;** ▲ = **Collaborative**

Multicultural

- Acknowledge the stressors unique to racial/ethnic communities. **Nursing Research:** *Targeted alcohol and tobacco marketing, high levels of unemployment, lack of health insurance, and racism are stressors unique to culturally diverse communities (D'Avanzo et al, 2001).*
- Identify the health services and information resources that are currently available in the community. **Theoretical Rationale:** *Helping a community to cope requires an understanding of the contextual nature of coping, including social, cultural, political, economic, and historical conditions (Donnelly, 2002).*
- Work with members of the community to prioritize and target health goals specific to the community. **Theoretical Rationale:** *Such prioritization and targeting will increase feelings of control over and sense of ownership of programs (Anderson and McFarlane, 2000; Chinn, 2001; National Institutes of Health, 1998).*
- Approach community leaders and members of color with respect, warmth, and professional courtesy. **Theoretical Rationale:** *Instances of disrespect and lack of caring have special significance for individuals of color (D'Avanzo et al, 2001).*
- Establish and sustain partnerships with key individuals within communities when developing and implementing programs. **Theoretical Rationale:** *Local leaders are excellent sources of information and their participation will enhance the credibility of programs (National Institutes of Health, 1998).*
- Use community church settings as a forum for advocacy, teaching, and program implementation. **Nursing Research:** *Evaluation of a faith-based program supplied to 125 people from 18 congregations showed an increase in health promotion knowledge, rise in consumer satisfaction, and improvement in health (Kotecki, 2002). A literature review of church-based health promotion programs showed that they are successful in helping people to adopt health-promoting behaviors (Peterson, Atwood, and Yates, 2002). Church-based programs are especially effective in communities of color.*
- Ask political leaders to become part of the partnership process. **Theoretical Rationale:** *The Carnegie Commission on Preventing Deadly Conflict established the importance of political leaders' working to prevent community conflicts and violence (Hamburg, George, and Ballentine, 1999).*
- Protect children from exposure to community conflicts. **Clinical Research:** *In a 15-month study of 97 urban 6- to 10-year-old boys who had witnessed community violence and antisocial behavior, reports of witnessing community conflicts were associated with antisocial behavior by children, including children from families with low family conflict (Miller et al, 1999).*

Community Teaching

- Teach strategies for stress management.
- Explain the relationship between enhancing power resources and coping.

evolve **WEBSITES FOR EDUCATION**

See the EVOLVE website for World Wide Web resources for client education.

• = Independent; ▲ = Collaborative

REFERENCES

Anderson ET, McFarlane J: *Community as partner: theory and practice in nursing,* ed 3, Philadelphia, 2000, Lippincott Williams & Wilkins.

Chinn PL: *Peace and power: building communities for the future,* ed 5, Boston, 2001, Jones & Bartlett.

Coley SM, Scheinberg CA: *Proposal writing,* ed 2, Thousand Oaks, Calif, 2000, Sage.

D'Avanzo CE et al: Developing culturally informed strategies for substance-related interventions. In Naegle MA, D'Avanzo CE, editors: *Addictions and substance abuse: strategies for advanced practice nursing,* St Louis, 2001, Mosby.

Diekemper M, Smithbattle L, Drake MA: Bringing the population into focus: a natural development in community health nursing practice, part I, *Public Health Nurs* 16(1):3, 1999.

Donnelly TT: Contextual analysis of coping: implications for immigrants' mental health care, *Issues Ment Health Nurs* 23(7):715, 2002.

Drevdahl D: Meanings of community in a community health center, *Public Health Nurs* 16(6):417, 1999.

Farmer MM, Ferraro KF: Distress and perceived health: mechanisms of health decline, *J Health Soc Behav* 39: 298, 1997.

Frommer P, Papouchado K: Police as contributors to healthy communities, Aiken, South Carolina, *Public Health Rep* 115(2-3):249, 2000.

Galea S et al: Collaboration among community members, local health service providers, and researchers in an urban research center in Harlem New York, *Public Health Rep* 116(6):530, 2001.

Hamburg DA, George A, Ballentine K: Preventing deadly conflict: the critical role of leadership, *Arch Gen Psychiatry* 56(11):971, 1999.

Kaiser MM, Barry TL, Kaiser KL: Using focus groups to evaluate and strengthen public health nursing population-focused interventions, *J Transcult Nurs* 13(4):303, 2002.

Kotecki CN: Developing a health promotion program for faith-based communities, *Holist Nurs Pract* 16(3):61, 2002.

Leksell JK et al: Power and self-perceived health in blind diabetic and nondiabetic individuals, *J Adv Nurs* 34(4), 511, 2001.

Madela EN, Poggenpoel M: The experience of a community characterized by violence: implications for nursing, *J Adv Nurs* 18(5):691, 1993.

Miller JF: *Coping with chronic illness: overcoming powerlessness,* ed 3, Philadelphia, 2000, FA Davis.

Miller LS et al: Witnessed community violence and anti-social behavior in high risk, urban boys, *J Clin Child Psychol* 28(1):2, 1999.

National Institutes of Health: *Salud para su corazón: bringing heart health to Latinos—a guide for building community programs,* DHHS Pub No 98-3796, Washington, DC, 1998, US Government Printing Office.

Pearlin L, Aneshensel CS, Leblanc AJ: The forms and mechanisms of stress proliferation: the case of AIDS caregivers, *J Health Soc Behav* 38(3):223, 1997.

Pender NJ, Murdaugh CL, Parsons MA: *Health promotion in nursing practice,* ed 4, Upper Saddle River, NJ, Prentice Hall, 2002.

Peterson J, Atwood JR, Yates B: Key elements for church-based health promotion programs: outcome-based literature review, *Public Health Nurs* 19(6):401, 2002.

Samarel N, Tulman L, Fawcett J: Effects of two types of social support and education on adaptation to early-stage breast cancer, *Res Nurs Health* 25(6):459, 2002.

Tabi MM: Community perspective on a model to reduce teenage pregnancy, *J Adv Nurs* 40(3):275, 2002.

Wallerstein N: A participatory evaluation model for healthier communities: developing indicators for New Mexico, *Public Health Rep* 115(2-3):199, 2000.

Readiness for enhanced community Coping

Margaret Lunney

NANDA Definition

Pattern of community activities for adaptation and problem solving that is satisfactory for meeting the demands or needs of the community but that can also be improved for management of current and future problems and stressors

- • = **Independent; ▲ = Collaborative**

Defining Characteristics

One or more of the following characteristics that indicate effective coping: positive communication between community/aggregates and larger community; availability of programs for recreation and relaxation; sufficiency of resources for managing stressors; agreement that community is responsible for stress management; active planning by community for predicted stressors; active problem solving by community when faced with issues; positive communication among community members

NOC Outcomes (Nursing Outcomes Classification)

Suggested NOC Outcomes

Community Competence; Community Health Status

> ### Example NOC Outcome with Indicators
>
> **Community Competence** (select the level of achievement on the following scale: 1 = poor demonstration, 2 = fair demonstration, 3 = average demonstration, 4 = good demonstration, 5 = excellent demonstration [see Section I]) as evidenced by the following indicators: Prevalence of health promotion programs/ Health status of infants, children, adolescents, adults, elders/Attendance at programs for healthy states (Rate each indicator of **Community Competence** on the same five-point scale.)

Community Outcomes

Community Will (Specify Time Frame):

- Develop enhanced coping strategies
- Maintain effective coping strategies for management of stress

NIC Interventions (Nursing Interventions Classification)

Suggested NIC Interventions

Environmental Management: Community; Health Policy Monitoring
    NIC Interventions developed for use with individuals can be adapted for use with communities: Coping Enhancement; Culture Brokerage; Mutual Goal Setting; Support System Enhancement

> ### Example NIC Activities—Coping Enhancement
>
> Explore with community members previous methods of dealing with life problems; Assist the community to solve problems in a constructive manner

Nursing Interventions and Rationales

NOTE: Interventions depend on the specific aspects of community coping that can be enhanced (e.g., planning for stress management, communication, development of community power, community perceptions of stress, community coping strategies). Nursing interventions are conducted in collaboration with key members of the community, community/public health nurses, and members of other disciplines (Anderson and McFarlane, 2000; Bolton et al, 1998; Chinn, 2001).

- = Independent; ▲ = Collaborative

- Describe the role of the community/public health nurse in working with healthy communities (Stanhope, 2001). **Theoretical Rationale:** *Members of society are not familiar with nurses' roles in public health.*
- Help the community to obtain funds for additional programs. (See Coley and Scheinberg, 2000, for proposal-writing methods.) **Theoretical Rationale:** *Healthy communities may need additional funding sources to strengthen community resources.*
- Encourage positive attitudes toward the community through the media and other sources. **Clinical Research:** *Negative attitudes or stigmas create additional stress and deficits in social support (Lubkin and Larsen, 2002).*
- Help community members to collaborate with one another for power enhancement and coping skills. **Theoretical Rationale:** *Community members may not have sufficient skills to collaborate for enhanced coping. Effective collaboration skills can be promoted by health care providers (Courtney et al, 1996; Chinn, 2001).*
- Encourage critical thinking. **Nursing Research:** *Critical thinking supports problem-solving ability (Scheffer and Rubenfeld, 2000).*
- Demonstrate optimum use of the power resources of knowledge, motivation, belief system (hope), physical strength and reserve, psychological stamina and support network, positive self-concept, and energy. **Nursing Research:** *Optimum use of power resources supports coping (Miller, 2000). Community members benefit from observations of nurses' use of resources.*
- Collaborate with community members to improve educational levels within the community. **Nursing Research:** *In a study of 18 randomly selected communities and 900 elders living in those communities, higher educational levels were associated with less stress pertaining to health, and fewer helpers were needed by the educated elderly (Preston and Bucher, 1996). Higher educational levels are associated with lower levels of emotional and physical distress (Ross and Van Willigen, 1997).*

Multicultural

- Acknowledge the stresses unique to racial/ethnic communities. *Targeted alcohol and tobacco marketing, high levels of unemployment, lack of health insurance, and racism are stressors unique to culturally diverse communities (D'Avanzo et al, 2001).*
- Identify what health services and information are currently available in the community. *This will assist with focusing efforts and promote wise use of valuable resources (National Institutes of Health, 1998).*
- Work with members of the community to prioritize and target health goals specific to the community. *This will increase feelings of control over and sense of ownership of programs (National Institutes of Health, 1998).*
- Approach community leaders and members of color with respect, warmth, and professional courtesy. **Theoretical Rationale:** *Instances of disrespect and lack of caring have special significance for individuals of color (D'Avanzo et al, 2001).*
- Establish and sustain partnerships with key individuals within communities when developing and implementing programs. **Clinical Research:** *Local leaders are excellent sources of information and their participation will enhance the credibility of programs (National Institutes of Health, 1998).*
- Use community church settings as a forum for advocacy, teaching, and program implementation. **Nursing Research:** *Evaluation of a faith-based program supplied to 125 people from 18 congregations showed an increase in health promotion knowledge, rise in consumer satisfaction, and improvement in health (Kotecki, 2002). A literature review of*

• = Independent; ▲ = Collaborative

church-based health promotion programs showed that they are successful in helping people to adopt health-promoting behaviors (Peterson, Atwood, and Yates, 2002). Church-based programs are especially effective in communities of color.

Community Teaching

- Review coping skills, power for coping, and the use of power resources.

evolve WEBSITES FOR EDUCATION

See the EVOLVE website for World Wide Web resources for client education.

REFERENCES

Anderson ET, McFarlane J: *Community as partner: theory and practice in nursing,* ed 3, Philadelphia, 2000, Lippincott Williams & Wilkins.

Bolton LB et al: Community health collaboration models for the 21st century, *Nurs Admin Q* 22(3):6, 1998.

Chinn PL: *Peace and power: building communities for the future,* ed 5, Boston, 2001, Jones & Bartlett.

Coley SM, Scheinberg CA: *Proposal writing,* ed 2, Thousand Oaks, Calif, 2000, Sage.

Courtney R et al: The partnership model: working with individuals, families, and communities toward a new vision of health, *Public Health Nurs* 13:177, 1996.

D'Avanzo CE et al: Developing culturally informed strategies for substance-related interventions. In Naegle MA, D'Avanzo CE, editors: *Addictions and substance abuse: strategies for advanced practice nursing,* St Louis, 2001, Mosby.

Kotecki CN: Developing a health promotion program for faith-based communities, *Holist Nurs Pract* 16(3):61, 2002.

Lubkin IM, Larsen PD: *Chronic illness: impact and interventions,* ed 5, Boston, Mass, 2002, Jones & Bartlett.

Miller JF: *Coping with chronic illness: overcoming powerlessness,* ed 3, Philadelphia, 2000, FA Davis.

National Institutes of Health: *Salud para su corazón: bringing heart health to Latinos—a guide for building community programs,* DHHS Pub No 98-3796, Washington, DC, 1998, US Government Printing Office.

Peterson J, Atwood JR, Yates B: Key elements for church-based health promotion programs: outcome-based literature review, *Public Health Nurs* 19(6):401, 2002.

Preston DB, Bucher JA: The effects of community differences on health status, health stress, and helping networks in a sample of 900 elderly, *Public Health Nurs* 13:72, 1996.

Ross CE, Van Willigen M: Education and subjective quality of life, *J Health Soc Behav* 38:275, 1997.

Scheffer BK, Rubenfeld MG: A consensus statement on critical thinking, *J Nurs Educ* 15:350, 2000.

Stanhope M: *Foundations of community and public health nursing practice,* ed 5, St Louis, 2001, Mosby.

Defensive Coping

Ann Keeley

NANDA Definition

Repeated projection of falsely positive self-evaluations based on self-protective pattern that defends against underlying perceived threats to positive self-regard

Defining Characteristics

Grandiosity; rationalization of failures; hypersensitivity to slight/criticism; denial of obvious problems/weaknesses; projection of blame/responsibility; lack of follow-through or participation in treatment or therapy; superior attitude toward others; hostile laughter or ridicule of others; difficulty in perception of reality, reality testing; difficulty

- • = Independent; ▲ = Collaborative

establishing/maintaining relationships, occurs when a specific pattern of ineffective (defensive) coping is sustained over time

Related Factors (r/t)

Situational crises; psychological impairment; substance abuse; HIV infection

NOC   Outcomes (Nursing Outcomes Classification)

Suggested NOC Outcomes

Coping; Decision Making; Impulse Self-Control; Information Processing

Example NOC Outcome with Indicators

Coping as evidenced by the following indicators: Identifies effective and ineffective coping patterns/Modifies lifestyle as needed (Rate each indicator of **Coping:** 1 = never demonstrated, 2 = rarely demonstrated, 3 = sometimes demonstrated, 4 = often demonstrated, 5 = consistently demonstrated [see Section I].)

Client Outcomes

Client Will (Specify Time Frame):

- Acknowledge need for change in coping style
- Accept responsibility for own behavior
- Establish realistic goals with validation from caregivers
- Solicit caregiver validation in decision making

NIC   Interventions (Nursing Interventions Classification)

Suggested NIC Intervention

Self-Awareness Enhancement

Example NIC Activities—Self-Awareness Enhancement

Encourage client to recognize and discuss thoughts and feelings; Assist client in identifying behaviors that are self-destructive

Nursing Interventions and Rationales

- Assess for the presence of denial as a coping mechanism. *Denial is a defensive avoidance of emotion. It can be beneficial as a coping mechanism, but total denial can be detrimental (Robinson, 1999).*
- Do not confront denial if its consequences are not a significant threat to health. **Nursing Research:** *A period of denial may be necessary for the client to develop a construct within which the given information has meaning and can be appraised as not being a threat to survival (Norris and Spelic, 2002).*
- Determine whether the client has a positive or negative overall appraisal of a given event. **Clinical Research:** *A negative appraisal of the event can lead to anxiety, depression, and other symptoms (Mazur et al, 1999).*
- Develop a trusting, therapeutic relationship with the client and family. *A genuine connection can ease defensiveness or uneasiness (Robinson, 1999).*

• = Independent; ▲ = Collaborative

- Ask appropriate questions using an assessment tool such as Fast Alcohol Screening Test (FAST) to assess whether denial is being used in association with alcoholism. For each question, the client is asked to circle the appropriate response: Less than monthly, Monthly, Weekly, Daily, or Almost Daily
  1. MEN: How often do you have EIGHT or more drinks on one occasion: WOMEN: How often do you have SIX or more drinks on one occasion?
  2. How often during the last year have you been unable to remember what happened the night before because you had been drinking?
  3. How often during the last year have you failed to do what was normally expected of you because of drinking?
  4. In the last year has a relative or friend, or a doctor or other health worker been concerned about your drinking or suggested you cut down?

  Clinical Research: *The four-item FAST alcohol questionnaire had good sensitivity and specificity across a range of settings when the Alcohol Use Disorders Identification Test (AUDIT) alcohol assessment score was used as the gold standard. The FAST questionnaire is quick to administer, since more than 50% of clients are categorized using just one question (Hodgson et al, 2002). Include drug use in addition to drinking in the questionnaire (Hinkin et al, 2001). T-ACE and TWEAK are modified to be used with women.* **Nursing Research:** *Alcoholism rates are increasing in women, and women may have distinct assessment risk factors (Becker and Walton-Moss, 2001). Brief addiction screening tools are available (Gorski, 2002).*

- Determine the client's perception of the problem and then provide reality-based examples of the true situation (e.g., witnesses to an accident, blood alcohol levels, problems caused by alcohol). **Nursing Research:** *Psychological manifestations of defensive coping can be understood only after a thorough inquiry into the client's framework for appraisal (Dudley-Brown, 2002).*

- Help the client identify patterns of response in life that may be maladaptive. *A clear, honest recounting of life incidents and their consequences in a trusting relationship may provide the motivation necessary to seek a change in behavior (Faltz and Skinner, 2002).*

▲ Promote the client's feelings of self-worth by using group or individual therapy, role playing, one-to-one interactions, and role modeling. **Nursing Research:** *A variety of methods may be used to assist clients in their attempts to assimilate the implications of a health status change (Whittemore et al, 2002).*

- Support strengths and normal observations with "I note that" or "I want you to notice." Tell clients when they do something well. **Nursing Research:** *Nurses effectively support adaptation to a change in health status by actively listening to the client at all stages and encouraging reflection and self-understanding throughout the process (Whittemore et al, 2002).*

- Teach the client to use positive thinking by blocking negative thoughts with the word "Stop!" and inserting positive thoughts (e.g., "I'm a good [person, friend, student]"). *Interventions that encourage the cognitive reframing of a change in health status within a more positive framework support adaptation to a change in health status (Dudley-Brown, 2002).*

- Provide feedback regarding others' perceptions of the client's behavior through group or milieu therapy or one-to-one interactions. **Nursing Research:** *Group therapy is an effective component of treatment in women with a dual diagnosis (Moser, Sowell, and Phillips, 2001).*

- Encourage the client to use "I" statements and to accept responsibility for and conse-

• = **Independent;** ▲ = **Collaborative**

quences of actions. **Clinical Research:** *Interventions that support self-efficacy and a building of the sense of self as an individual who can control his or her own response facilitate the client's meeting of his or her goals (Brun and Rapp, 2001).*
- Refer to the care plans for **Ineffective Denial** and **Dysfunctional Family processes: alcoholism.**

Geriatric
- Assess the client for anger and identify previous outlets for anger. *Nurses can help individuals to cope effectively with a change in health status by teaching them alternative methods of coping (Reynaud and Meeker, 2002).*
- Explore new outlets for anger, including physical activities within the client's capabilities (e.g., hitting a pillow, woodworking, sanding, scrubbing floors). **Clinical Research:** *Stress, along with the client's method of coping with it, is a risk factor for substance abuse behavior. Instruction in effective stress-reducing strategies may lower the risk (Brady and Sonne, 1999).*
- Utilize the CAGE tool with this population and include drug use along with drinking. An affirmative answer to two or more of the following questions is considered a basis for suspicion of alcohol abuse:
  C: Have you ever felt you ought to **Cut down** on drinking?
  A: Have people **Annoyed** you by criticizing your drinking?
  G: Have you ever felt bad or **Guilty** about your drinking?
  E: Have you ever had a drink the first thing in the morning to steady your nerves or get rid of a hangover **(Eye opener)**?
  Nursing Research: *Alcoholism and drug abuse are present in the geriatric population, and the CAGE tool is effective in identifying individuals at risk (Hinkin et al, 2001). Individuals with these problems are more likely to be found in health care settings that are not substance abuse specific (Weisner, 2001).*
- Assess the client for dementia or depression. *A thorough assessment must be conducted to determine if the aberrant behavior has an organic origin (Green, 2002). Clients may not readily admit to psychological or substance abuse symptoms (Boyd and Stanley, 2002).*
- If a traumatic event has occurred, support positive religious coping behaviors. **Nursing Research:** *Religious coping behaviors, when positive, can facilitate a more constructive health outcome (Bell Meisenhelder, 2002).*

Multicultural
- Assess for the influence of cultural beliefs, norms, and values on the client's feelings of defensiveness. **Nursing Research:** *The "denial" perceived by the nurse may be an expected behavior within the culture of the client (Lindenberg et al, 2002).*
- Acknowledge racial/ethnic differences at the onset of care. **Nursing Research:** *Acknowledgment of race/ethnicity issues will enhance communication, establish rapport, and promote treatment outcomes (D'Avanzo et al, 2001).*
- Use therapeutic communication techniques that emphasize acceptance, offer the self, validate the client's concerns, and convey respect. **Nursing Research:** *Open communication by the nurse will facilitate the use of health care resources by immigrant populations. Care needs to be taken to incorporate the concept of health and healing prevalent in the client's culture (Chen and Rankin, 2002; White et al, 2002; Donnelly, 2002).*
- Give a rationale when assessing ethnically diverse clients for alcohol use/misuse or other sensitive behaviors. **Nursing Research:** *Depending on the culture, aspects of*

• = Independent; ▲ = Collaborative

responsibility may have different values than in the Western health care system (Rungre-angkulkij et al, 2002; White et al, 2002; Shin, 2002). African Americans and other people of color may expect white caregivers to hold negative and preconceived ideas about people of color. Giving a rationale for questions asked will help reduce this perception (D'Avanzo et al, 2001).

Home care

- The interventions described previously may be adapted for home care use.
- Include in the initial assessment client and family histories of mental health problems. **Nursing Research:** *A thorough understanding of the family history of mental health problems, the attempts made to seek help, and the cultural context of the behavior will facilitate a successful intervention by the nurse (Rungreangkulkij et al, 2002; Shin, 2002; Donnelly, 2002; Aziz and Rowland, 2002).*
- Observe family dynamics for dysfunctional and supportive communication. **Nursing Research:** *An understanding of the family structure, patterns of communication, health care history, and cultural influences will facilitate effective interventions on the part of the nurse. In the context of some family patterns of communication, defensive coping may be a learned behavior (Hellemann, Lee, and Kury, 2002).*
- ▲ Refer to a mental health professional for possible psychodrama therapy, especially if the client experiences difficulty in coping with a traumatic event. **Clinical Research:** *Psychodrama has been shown to help people begin to reframe their feelings of victimization as feelings of survival and begin to see the future as hopeful (Carbonell, Parteleno-Barehmi, 1999).*
- ▲ In the absence of primary medical diagnoses, refer to medical social services for assistance in contacting appropriate community services. **Nursing Research:** *The nurse is often perceived as the "constant" in a client's relationship with the health care system and as such can help bridge the gap between the client and available resources (Tak and McCubbin, 2002; Northouse et al, 2002).*
- ▲ If medical diagnoses coexist with defensive coping, confirm and validate the client's mental health plan and progress. **Nursing Research:** *The nurse is often perceived as the "constant" in a client's relationship with the health care system and as such can help bridge the gap between the client and available resources (Tak and McCubbin, 2002; Northouse et al, 2002).*
- ▲ Refer to a therapist for debriefing if a traumatic or critical event has occurred. *Critical incident debriefing has decreased the number of psychological problems caused by traumatic events (Johal and Bennett, 1999).* **Clinical Research:** *A review of psychological debriefing, however, has concluded that there is little evidence for its use. Early intervention recommendations are to assess the need for sustained treatment, to provide psychological first aid, and to supply education about trauma and information about treatment resources. Recommendations for secondary prevention of post-traumatic stress disorder include education, anxiety management, cognitive restructuring, exposure, and relapse prevention (Litz et al, 2002).*
- ▲ Refer for psychiatric home health care services for client reassurance and implementation of a therapeutic regimen. **Nursing Research:** *Psychiatric home care nurses can address issues relating to the client's ability to adjust to changes in health status. Behavioral interventions and reality orientation in the home can help the client to participate more effectively in the treatment plan (Patusky, Rodning, and Martinez-Kratz, 1996).*

• = **Independent;** ▲ = **Collaborative**

Client/Family Teaching

▲ Teach the client the actions and side effects of medications and the importance of taking them as prescribed, even when the client is feeling good. **Nursing Research:** *Education about the desired effects and potential side effects increases the knowledge and effective decision-making ability of the client (Moser, Sowell, and Phillips, 2001).*

▲ Work with the client's support group to identify harmful behaviors and to seek help for the client if he or she is unable to control behavior. **Nursing Research:** *When possible, the client's family system should be a component of the treatment (Cook, 2001). Families need assistance in identifying resources and therapeutic responses as they adapt to the individual client's behaviors (Faltz and Skinner, 2002).*

• When a traumatic event has occurred, encourage the use of written disclosure. Instruct the person to write about the event over a period of days. *Written disclosure has been found to decrease the number of office visits and complaints of physical and psychological symptoms following the event (Johal and Bennett, 1999).*

• Support family efforts using religious coping behaviors. **Nursing Research:** *Interventions to enhance positive religious coping facilitate recovery (Bell Meisenhelder, 2002; Newlin, Knafl, and Meldus, 2002).*

evolve WEBSITES FOR EDUCATION

See the EVOLVE website for World Wide Web resources for client education.

REFERENCES

Aziz N, Rowland JH: Cancer survivorship research among ethnic minority and medically underserved groups, *Oncol Nurs Forum* 29(5):789, 2002.

Becker K, Walton-Moss B: Detecting and addressing alcohol abuse in women, *Nurse Pract* 26(10):13, 2001.

Bell Meisenhelder J: Terrorism, posttraumatic stress, and religious coping, *Issues Ment Health Nurs* 23(8):771, 2002.

Boyd MA, Stanley M: Mental health assessment of the elderly. In Boyd MA: *Psychiatric nursing in contemporary practice,* ed 2, Philadelphia, 2002, Lippincott.

Brady KT, Sonne SC: The role of stress in alcohol use, alcoholism treatment, and relapse, *Alcohol Res Health* 23(4):263, 1999.

Brun C, Rapp RC: Strengths-based case management: individual's perspectives on strengths and the case manager relationship, *Soc Work* 46(3):278, 2001.

Carbonell DM, Parteleno-Barehmi C: Psychodrama groups for girls coping with trauma, *Int J Group Psychother* 49(3):285, 1999.

Chen J-L, Rankin SH: Using the resiliency model to deliver culturally sensitive care to Chinese families, *J Pediatr Nurs* 17(3):157, 2002.

Cook LS: Adolescent addiction and delinquency in the family system, *Issues Ment Health Nurs* 22:151, 2001.

D'Avanzo CE et al: Developing culturally informed strategies for substance-related interventions. In Naegle MA, D'Avanzo CE, editors: *Addictions and substance abuse: strategies for advanced practice nursing,* St Louis, 2001, Mosby.

Donnelly TT: Contextual analysis of coping: implications for immigrants' mental health care, *Issues Ment Health Nurs* 23:715, 2002.

Dudley-Brown S: Prevention of psychological distress in persons with inflammatory bowel disease, *Issues Ment Health Nurs* 23:403, 2002.

Faltz BG, Skinner MK: Substance abuse disorders. In Boyd MA, editor: *Psychiatric nursing in contemporary practice,* ed 2, Philadelphia, 2002, Lippincott.

Gorski T: *Women at risk: brief screening tools,* 2002, available online at http://www.tgorski.com/clin_mod/atp/women_at_risk-brief_screening_tools.htm#TWEAK, accessed Feb 19, 2003.

Green GC: Guidelines for assessing and diagnosing acute psychosis: a primer, *J Emerg Nurs* 28:S1, 2002.

• = **Independent;** ▲ = **Collaborative**

Hellemann MV, Lee KA, Kury FS: Strengths and vulnerabilities of women of Mexican descent in relation to depressive symptoms, *Nurs Res* 51(3):175, 2002.

Hinkin CH et al: Screening for drug and alcohol abuse among older adults using a modified version of the CAGE, *Am J Addict* 10:319, 2001.

Hodgson R et al: The FAST alcohol screening test, *Alcohol Alcohol* 37(1):61, 2002.

Johal SS, Bennett P: Written disclosure: a way of coping with traumatic stress, *Nurs Stand* 13(37):43, 1999.

Lindenberg CS et al: Reducing substance use and risky sexual behavior among young, low-income, Mexican-American women: comparison of two interventions, *Appl Nurs Res* 16(2):137, 2002.

Litz BT et al: Early intervention for trauma: current status and future direction, *Clin Psychol Sci Pract* 9:112, 2002.

Mazur E et al: Cognitive moderators of children's adjustment to stressful divorce events: the role of negative cognitive errors and positive illusions, *Child Dev* 70(1):231, 1999.

Moser KM, Sowell RL, Phillips KD: Issues of women dually diagnosed with HIV infection and substance use problems in the Carolinas, *Issues Ment Health Nurs* 22:23, 2001.

Newlin K, Knafi K, Meldus GD: African-American spirituality: a concept analysis, *ANS Adv Nurs Sci* 25(2):57, 2002.

Norris J, Spelic SS: Supporting adaptation to body image disruption, *Rehabil Nurs* 27(1):8, 2002.

Northouse L et al: A family-based program of care for women with recurrent breast cancer and their family members, *Oncol Nurs Forum* 29(10):1411, 2002.

Patusky KL, Rodning C, Martinez-Kratz M: Clinical lessons in psychiatric home care: a case study approach, *J Home Health Case Manag* 9:18, 1996.

Reynaud SN, Meeker BJ: Coping styles of older adults with ostomies, *J Gerontol Nurs* 28(5):30, 2002.

Robinson AW: Getting to the heart of denial, *Am J Nurs* 99(5):38, 1999.

Rungreangkulkij S et al: Psychological morbidity of Thai families of a person with schizophrenia, *Int J Nurs Stud* 39:35, 2002.

Shin JK: Help-seeking behaviors by Korean immigrants for depression, *Issues Ment Health Nurs* 23:461, 2002.

Tak YR, McCubbin M: Family stress, perceived social support and coping following the diagnosis of a child's congenital heart disease, *J Adv Nurs* 39(2):190, 2002.

Weisner C: The provision of services for alcohol problems: a community perspective for understanding access, *J Behav Health Serv Res* 28(2):130, 2001.

White N et al: A cross-cultural comparison of family resiliency in hemodialysis clients, *J Transcult Nurs* 13(3):218, 2002.

Whittemore R et al: Lifestyle change in type 2 diabetes, *Nurs Res* 51(1):18, 2002.

Compromised family Coping

T. Heather Herdman, Beverly Pickett, Gail B. Ladwig, and Mary Markle

NANDA   Definition

Situation in which usually supportive primary person (family member or close friend) provides insufficient, ineffective, or compromised support, comfort, assistance, or encouragement that may be needed by client to manage or master adaptive tasks related to health challenge

Defining Characteristics

Objective

Significant person attempts assistive or supportive behaviors with less than satisfactory results; significant person displays protective behavior disproportionate (too little or too much) to client's abilities or need for autonomy; significant person withdraws or enters into limited or temporary personal communication with client at time of need

Subjective

Client expresses or confirms a concern or complaint about significant other's response to his or her health problem; significant person describes or confirms an inadequate un-

• = **Independent**; ▲ = **Collaborative**

derstanding or knowledge base, which interferes with effective assistance or supportive behaviors; significant person describes preoccupation with personal reaction (e.g., fear, anticipatory grief, guilt, or anxiety) to client's illness, disability, or other situational or developmental crisis

Related Factors (r/t)

Temporary preoccupation of a significant person who tries to manage emotional conflicts and personal suffering and is unable to perceive or act effectively with regard to client's needs; temporary family disorganization and role changes; prolonged disease or disability progression that exhausts supportive capacity of significant person; other situational or developmental crises or problems significant person may be facing; inadequate or incorrect information or understanding by primary person; lack of support given by client to significant person

NOC   Outcomes (Nursing Outcomes Classification)

Suggested NOC Outcomes

Anxiety Self-Control; Caregiver Emotional Health; Caregiver-Patient Relationship; Caregiver Well-Being; Family Coping; Hope; Knowledge: Health Behavior, Health Resources; Participation in Health Care Decisions; Social Support

> **Example NOC Outcome with Indicators**
>
> **Family Coping** as evidenced by the following indicators: Reports decrease in stress/Verbalizes sense of control/Modifies lifestyle as needed/Employs behaviors to reduce stress/Verbalizes need for assistance (Rate each indicator of **Family Coping:** 1 = never demonstrated, 2 = rarely demonstrated, 3 = sometimes demonstrated, 4 = often demonstrated, 5 = consistently demonstrated [see Section I].)

Client Outcomes

Family/Significant Person Will (Specify Time Frame):
- Verbalize internal resources to help deal with the situation
- Verbalize knowledge and understanding of illness, disability, or disease
- Provide support and assistance as needed
- Identify need for and seek outside support

NIC   Interventions (Nursing Interventions Classification)

Suggested NIC Interventions

Anticipatory Guidance; Caregiver Support; Coping Enhancement; Emotional Support; Family Integrity Promotion; Family Involvement Promotion; Family Mobilization; Family Support; Hope Instillation; Mutual Goal Setting; Normalization Promotion; Support System Enhancement

> **Example NIC Activities—Family Support**
>
> Appraise family's emotional reaction to client's condition; Promote trusting relationship with family

• = Independent; ▲ = Collaborative

Nursing Interventions and Rationales

- Assess the strengths and deficiencies of the family system. *Assessments allow for anticipatory care and guidance to help members acquire and maintain supports and coping strategies (Ducharmes and Rowat, 1992; Thomas, 2000).*
- Consider the use of family theory as a framework to help guide interventions (e.g., family stress theory, social exchange theory). *Theory helps to identify the focus, means, and goals of nursing practice. It enhances communication and increases autonomy and accountability for care (Gillis et al, 1989; Meleis, 1991).*
- Assess the adolescent's perception of support from family and friends during crisis. *Some teens find parents and friends burdensome during a time of grief, while others find their support critical for coping with crises. Recognition of individual perception can assist families in negotiating times of crisis (Rask, Kaunonen, and Paunonen-Ilmonen, 2002).*
- Observe for the cause of family problems. *Ongoing assessment provides clues about underlying feelings (Barry, 1989).*
- Assist the significant person in expanding the repertoire of coping skills. *Coping skills can decrease the family's vulnerability to stress and can strengthen and maintain family resources that protect the family.*
- Help family members recognize the need for help and teach them how to ask for it. *Recognizing the need for help and knowing how to ask for it enables family members to maintain control (Szabo and Strang, 1999).*
- Assess how family members interact with each other; observe verbal and nonverbal communication and individual and group responses to stress. *Understanding how families cope with stress is important. One person's problems affect the entire family (Mears, 1990).* **Nursing Research:** *Family cohesion, presence of a partner, emotional support, and a mother's satisfaction with her family all contributed to her better mental health in a research study focusing on mothers of low-birth-weight infants (Weiss and Chen, 2002).*
- Help family members identify strengths and make a list that each member can refer to for positive reinforcement. *Positive feedback from one family member reinforces a particular action or behavior of another member.*
- Encourage family members to verbalize feelings. Spend time with them, sit down and make eye contact, and offer coffee and other nourishment. *The expression of feelings helps family caregivers to regain and maintain control (Szabo and Strang, 1999). Acceptance of nourishment indicates a beginning acceptance of the situation.*
- Talk with the family about the importance of sharing feelings and ways to do so (e.g., role playing, writing a letter to a significant other). *Sharing feelings allows the family an opportunity to communicate in an effective yet nonthreatening manner.*
- Mothers may require additional support in their role of caring for chronically ill children. *Mothers exhibit greater efforts than fathers in coping patterns, including strategies to acquire social support outside the family, increase self-worth, and decrease psychological tensions (Brazil and Krueger, 2002).*
- Involve the client and family in the planning of care as much as possible. *Involving the client and family in the care plan or treatment regimen encourages compliance with treatment and enhances the client's feeling of control (Barry, 1989).*
- Provide privacy during family visits. If possible, maintain flexible visiting hours to accommodate more frequent family visits. If possible, arrange staff assignments so the same staff members have contact with the family. Familiarize other staff members with the situation in the absence of the usual staff member. *Providing privacy, main-*

• = Independent; ▲ = Collaborative

taining flexible hours, and arranging consistent staff assignments will reduce stress, enhance communication, and facilitate the building of trust.

- Determine whether the family is suffering from additional stressors (e.g., child care issues, financial problems). **Nursing Research:** *One study found that, in mothers of low-birth-weight infants, the presence of other life stressors and the family's use of internally focused coping strategies contributed to worse mental health outcomes for the mother (Weiss and Chen, 2002).*

- ▲ Refer the family to appropriate resources for assistance as indicated (e.g., counseling, psychotherapy, financial or spiritual support). *If family members do not know whom to contact, many helpful services may be underused (Mears, 1990).*

- Encourage family-centered care of clients during and after discharge. *Family-centered care supports families by building on their strengths and respecting their different coping methods (Ahmann, 1994).*

Geriatric

- Assess the physical, emotional, and spiritual needs of the significant person and meet needs while visiting (e.g., ensure that a person with diabetes eats meals). *Meeting the needs of the significant person will optimize individual health and well-being and thus enhance the health and well-being of the family.*

- Assist in finding transportation to enable family members to visit. *If a family member is homebound and unable to visit, encourage alternative contact (e.g., telephone, cards and letters, e-mail) to provide ongoing scheduled progress reports. Reducing loneliness and isolation has many positive psychosocial and physical health benefits (Bulechek and McCloskey, 1992).*

Multicultural

- Acknowledge racial/ethnic differences at the onset of care. **Nursing Research:** *Acknowledgment of race/ethnicity issues will enhance communication, establish rapport, and promote treatment outcomes (D'Avanzo et al, 2001; Ludwick and Silva, 2000; Vontress and Epp, 1997).*

- Approach families of color with respect, warmth, and professional courtesy. **Nursing Research:** *Instances of disrespect and lack of caring have special significance for families of color (D'Avanzo et al, 2001; Vontress and Epp, 1997).*

- Assess for the influence of cultural beliefs, norms, and values on the family's perceptions of coping. **Nursing Research:** *What the family considers normal and abnormal coping behavior may be based on cultural perceptions (Leininger and McFarland, 2002; Cochran, 1998; Doswell and Erlen, 1998).*

- Give a rationale when assessing families with regard to sensitive issues. **Nursing Research:** *African Americans and other people of color may expect white caregivers to hold negative and preconceived ideas about them. Giving a rationale for questions asked will help reduce this perception (D'Avanzo et al, 2001; Vontress and Epp, 1997).*

- Use a family-centered approach when working with Latino, Asian, African American, and Native American clients. **Nursing Research:** *Latinos may perceive the family as a source of support, solver of problems, and source of pride. Asian Americans may regard the family as the primary decision maker and influence on individual family members (D'Avanzo et al, 2001; Guarnaccia, 1998). Elders may play a key role in decision making for some Asian populations (Davis, 2000). Native American families may have extended structures and exert powerful influences over functioning (Seiderman et al, 1996).*

- = **Independent;** ▲ = **Collaborative**

- Facilitate modeling and role playing for family regarding healthy ways to communicate and interact. **Nursing Research:** *It is helpful for families and the client to practice communication skills in a safe environment before trying them in a real-life situation (Rivera-Andino and Lopez, 2000).*
- Validate the family's feelings regarding the impact of the client's illness on the family's lifestyle. **Nursing Research:** *Validation lets family members know that the nurse has heard and understood what was said, and it promotes the relationship between nurse and family members (Heineken, 1998).*
- Work to provide caregivers who understand the importance of cultural beliefs and values the family may hold. **Nursing Research:** *There are differences in some cultures regarding health beliefs, practices, and values (Camphinha-Bacote and Narayan, 2000).*

Home care
- The interventions described previously may be adapted for home care use.
- Assess the reason behind the breakdown of family coping. *Knowledge of the reasons behind compromised coping will assist in identification of appropriate interventions. Are family members physically able to aid client? Is there a lack of resources? Do past relationship issues interfere with motivation? Are family members feeling stressed dealing with client's care needs? Refer to the care plan for* **Caregiver role strain.**
- During the time of compromised coping, increase visits to ensure the safety of the client, support of the family, and assistance with coping strategies. Provide reassurance regarding expectations for prognosis as appropriate. *Increased time for expressions of support, active listening, and empathy can nurture the client and family and move them toward more effective coping.* **Nursing Research:** *A study identified the need for support of the spouses of heart transplantation clients (Bohachick et al, 2001).*
- ▲ Assess the needs of the caregiver in the home. Intervene to meet needs as appropriate to total case management and explore all available resources that may be used to provide adequate home care (e.g., parish nursing as an effective adjunct, home health aide services to relieve caregiver's fatigue). Encourage caregivers not to neglect their own physical, mental, and spiritual health and give more specific information about the client's needs and ways to meet them. *Meeting the needs of caregivers supports their ability to meet the needs of the client. Assess the client and caregiver separately and in interaction. Do not assume that the client and his or her spouse experience similar patterns of distress or psychological adjustment.* **Nursing Research:** *In one study, the highest level of distress in heart transplantation clients related to effects on their ability to work, while spouses felt higher levels of psychological distress (Bohachick et al, 2001).*
- ▲ Refer the family to medical social services for evaluation and supportive counseling. *Dedicating time for nurturing the caregivers and reassuring the client allows them to express feelings and feel hope.*
- ▲ Serve as an advocate, mentor, and role model for caregiving. Write down or contract for the care needed by the client. *Therapeutic use of self by the nurse and concrete task definition and assignment reinforce positive coping strategies and allow caregivers to feel less guilty when tasks are delegated to multiple caregivers.*
- ▲ When a terminal illness is the precipitating factor for ineffective coping, offer hospice services and support groups as possible resources. *Nonjudgmental support from helpers with no agenda allows verbalization of feelings. The hospice paradigm addresses the physical, emotional, and spiritual needs of the dying and their loved ones.*
- With a cancer client, encourage family discussion of stressors (including the meaning

- **= Independent; ▲ = Collaborative**

of the illness, fear of recurrence, the client's employment status) and resources (family social support). **Nursing Research:** *Stressors and resources have been shown to play an important role in determining family quality of life among cancer survivors (Mellon and Northouse, 2001).*

- Encourage the client and family to discuss changes in daily functioning and routines created by the client's illness. Validate discomfort resulting from changes. *Individuals who live together for a long period tend to become entrained to each others' patterns: meals are expected at certain times, a spouse becomes accustomed to the client's sleep habits. Changes in these patterns may result in a vague discomfort that may be relieved when its source is known.*
- Support positive individual and family coping efforts. *Positive feedback reinforces desired behaviors and supports the family unit.*
▲ If compromised family coping interferes with the ability to support the client's treatment plan, refer for psychiatric home health care services for family counseling and implementation of a therapeutic regimen. *Psychiatric home care nurses can address issues relating to family members' ability to adjust to changes in the client's health status. Behavioral interventions in the home can help the family to participate more effectively in the treatment plan (Patusky, Rodning, and Martinez-Kratz, 1996).*

Client/Family Teaching

- Provide truthful information for the family and significant people regarding the client's specific illness or condition, including anticipatory guidance for expected outcomes. **Nursing Research:** *Research on the family needs identified as most important by all family members pointed to the need to receive information (Daly et al, 1994).*
- Promote individual and family relaxation and stress-reduction strategies. *The immune system weakens in response to stress; relaxation elicits the opposite, healthful response (Bulechek and McCloskey, 1992).*
- Involve the client and family in the planning of care as often as possible; mutual goal setting is often an effective strategy. *Family members of any trauma client admitted to the level I trauma center of one hospital are invited by the trauma staff to attend weekly multidisciplinary meetings. Through these meetings, family concerns can become a positive care factor, and the tasks of nurses, doctors, and social workers are made easier (Boettcher and Schiller, 1990).*

~~evolve~~ WEBSITES FOR EDUCATION

See the EVOLVE website for World Wide Web resources for client education.

REFERENCES

Ahmann E: Family centered care: the time has come, *Pediatr Nurs* 20(6), 1994.
Barry P: *Psychosocial nursing assessment and intervention,* Philadelphia, 1989, Lippincott.
Boettcher M, Schiller W: The use of a multidisciplinary group meeting for families of critically ill trauma patients, *Intensive Care Nurs* 6(3):129, 1990.
Bohachick P et al: Psychosocial impact of heart transplantation on spouses, *Clin Nurs Res* 10:6, 2001.
Brazil K, Krueger P: Patterns of family adaptation to childhood asthma, *J Pediatr Nurs* 17(3):167, 2002.
Bulechek G, McCloskey J: *Advanced nursing interventions,* Philadelphia, 1992, WB Saunders.
Camphinha-Bacote J, Narayan M: Culturally competent health care at home, *Home Care Provid* 5(6):213, 2000.
Cochran M: Tears have no color, *Am J Nurs* 98(6):53, 1998.

- **• = Independent; ▲ = Collaborative**

Daly K et al: The effect of two nursing interventions on families of ICU patients, *Clin Nurs Res* 3(4):414, 1994.

D'Avanzo CE et al: Developing culturally informed strategies for substance-related interventions. In Naegle MA, D'Avanzo CE, editors: *Addictions and substance abuse: strategies for advanced practice nursing,* St Louis, 2001, Mosby.

Davis RE: The convergence of health and family in the Vietnamese culture, *J Fam Nurs* 6(2):136, 2000.

Doswell W, Erlen J: Multicultural issues and ethical concerns in the delivery of nursing care interventions, *Nurs Clin North Am* 33(2):353, 1998.

Ducharmes F, Rowat K: Conjugal support, family coping behaviors and the well-being of elderly couples, *Can J Nurs Res* 24:5, 1992.

Gillis C et al: *Toward a science of family nursing,* Menlo Park, Calif, 1989, Addison-Wesley.

Guarnaccia P: Multicultural experiences of family caregiving: a study of African American, European American, and Hispanic American families, *New Dir Ment Health Serv* 77:45, 1998.

Heineken, J: Patient silence is not necessarily client satisfaction: communication in home care nursing, *Home Healthc Nurse* 16(2):115, 1998.

Leininger MM, McFarland MR: *Transcultural nursing: concepts, theories, research and practices,* ed 3, New York, 2002, McGraw-Hill.

Ludwick R, Silva M: Nursing around the world: cultural values and ethical conflicts, *Online J Issues Nurs,* 2000, available online at http://www.nursingworld.org/ojin/ethcol/ethics_4.htm, accessed Jan 10, 2003.

Mears D: Enhancing family coping skills, *Nurs Homes* 39:32, 1990.

Meleis A: *Theoretical nursing,* Philadelphia, 1991, Lippincott.

Mellon S, Northouse LL: Family survivorship and quality of life following a cancer diagnosis, *Res Nurs Health* 24:446, 2001.

Patusky KL, Rodning C, Martinez-Kratz M: Clinical lessons in psychiatric home care: a case study approach, *J Home Health Case Manag* 9:18, 1996.

Rask K, Kaunonen MM, Paunonen-Ilmonen M: Adolescent coping with grief after the death of a loved one, *Int J Nurs Pract* 8(3):137, 2002.

Rivera-Andino J, Lopez L: When culture complicates care, *RN* 63(7):47, 2000.

Seiderman RY et al: Assessing American Indian families, *MCN Am J Matern Child Nurs* 21(6):274, 1996.

Szabo V, Strang V: Experiencing control in caregiving, *Image J Nurs Sch* 31(1):71, 1999.

Thomas D et al: Parish nursing assessment—what should you know? *Home Healthc Nurs Manag* 4(5):11, 2000.

Vontress CE, Epp LR: Historical hostility in the African American client: implications for counseling, *J Multicult Counseling Dev,* 25:170, 1997.

Weiss S, Chen J: Factors influencing maternal mental health and family functioning during the low birthweight infant's first year of life, *J Pediatr Nurs* 17(2):114, 2002.

Disabled family Coping

T. Heather Herdman, Beverly Pickett, Gail B. Ladwig, and Mary Markle

NANDA DEFINITION

Behavior of significant person (family member or other primary person) that disables his or her capacity and client's capacity to effectively address tasks essential to either person's adaptation to the health challenge

Defining Characteristics

Intolerance; agitation; depression; aggression; hostility; taking on of illness signs of client; rejection; psychosomaticism; neglectful relationships with other family members; neglectful care of client with regard to basic human needs and/or illness treatment; distortion of reality regarding client's health problem, including extreme denial about its existence or severity; impaired restructuring of meaningful life for self; impaired individualization; prolonged overconcern for client; desertion; decisions and actions that are detrimental to economic or social well-being; continuation of usual routines, disregard

• = Independent; ▲ = Collaborative

of client's needs; abandonment; client's development of helpless, inactive dependence; disregard of needs

Related Factors (r/t)

Chronically unexpressed feelings of guilt, anxiety, hostility, despair, etc., in significant person; arbitrary handling of family's resistance to treatment, which tends to solidify defensiveness by dealing inadequately with underlying anxiety; dissonant or discrepant coping styles for dealing with adaptive tasks by significant person and client or among significant people; highly ambivalent family relationships

NOC Outcomes (Nursing Outcomes Classification)

Suggested NOC Outcomes

Abuse Protection; Abusive Behavior Self-Restraint; Anxiety Self-Control; Caregiver Emotional Health; Caregiver-Patient Relationship; Caregiver Performance: Direct Care, Indirect Care; Caregiver Stressors; Caregiver Well-Being; Family Coping; Hope; Knowledge: Health Behaviors, Health Resources; Participation in Health Care Decisions; Social Support

> ### Example NOC Outcome with Indicators
>
> **Caregiver Performance: Direct Care** as evidenced by the following indicators: Provision of emotional support to care recipient/Knowledge of treatment plan/Performance of treatments/Anticipation of care recipient's needs/Demonstration of unconditional positive regard for care recipient/Confidence in performing needed tasks (Rate each indicator of **Caregiver Performance: Direct Care:** 1 = Not adequate, 2 = Slightly adequate, 3 = Moderately adequate, 4 = Substantially adequate, 5 = Totally adequate [see Section I].)

Client Outcomes

Family/Significant Person Will (Specify Time Frame):

- Express realistic understanding and expectations of the client
- Participate positively in the client's care within the limits of his or her abilities
- Identify responses that are harmful
- Acknowledge and accept the need for assistance with circumstances
- Express feelings openly, honestly, and appropriately

NIC Interventions (Nursing Interventions Classification)

Suggested NIC Interventions

Abuse Protection Support; Anticipatory Guidance; Anxiety Reduction; Caregiver Support; Coping Enhancement; Counseling; Crisis Intervention; Emotional Support; Family Integrity Promotion; Family Involvement Promotion; Family Mobilization; Family Support; Family Therapy; Guilt Work Facilitation; Mutual Goal Setting; Normalization Promotion; Support System Enhancement

> ### Example NIC Activities—Family Therapy
>
> Determine the client's usual roles within the family system; Monitor for adverse therapeutic responses

• = Independent; ▲ = Collaborative

Nursing Interventions and Rationales

- Observe for causative and contributing factors. *Ongoing assessments provide clues about underlying feelings (Barry, 1989).*
- Review the client's background. *The client's background is largely responsible for the reactions seen (Lipkin and Cohen, 1992).*
- Identify patterns of family behaviors and interactions before the illness occurred. *Most family members have certain roles that are disrupted by illnesses and hospitalizations; this disruption results in shifts in family functioning.*
- Consider the use of family theory as a framework to help guide interventions (e.g., family stress theory, social exchange theory). *Theory helps to identify the focus, means, and goals of nursing practice. It enhances communication and increases autonomy and accountability for care (Gillis et al, 1989; Meleis, 1991).*
- Identify current behaviors of family members, such as withdrawal (e.g., not visiting, briefly visiting, ignoring client when visiting), anger and hostility toward the client and others, or expression of guilt. *Many of these behaviors are defense mechanisms used by the ego to protect itself until it can fully accept the implications of the illness.* **Nursing Research:** *Family cohesion, presence of a partner, emotional support, and a mother's satisfaction with her family all contributed to her better mental health in a research study focusing on mothers of low-birth-weight infants (Weiss and Chen, 2002).*
- Note other stressors in the family (e.g., financial, job related). *This information allows the nurse to develop an appropriate plan of care.* **Nursing Research:** *One study found that, in mothers of low-birth-weight infants, the presence of other life stressors and the family's use of internally focused coping strategies contributed to worse mental health outcomes for the mother (Weiss and Chen, 2002).*
- Encourage family members to verbalize feelings by discussing ways to solve problems associated with the client's condition. *Many families find it difficult to maintain open and empathetic communication during times of acute stress. Interventions that help mobilize family strengths, such as problem-solving communication, may effectively promote the adaptation of families of critically injured clients (Leske and Jiricka, 1998).*
- Assess the adolescent's perception of support from family and friends during crisis. *Some teens find parents or friends burdensome during time of grief, while others find their support critical for coping with crises. Recognition of individual perception can assist families in negotiating times of crisis (Rask, Kaunonen, and Paunonen-Ilmonen, 2002).*
- Serve as a role model for interpersonal skills that will help the family members improve their verbal interactions. *Interpersonal skills such as active listening, warmth, employing friendliness, empathy, consideration, and competence are essential for promoting a therapeutic relationship.*
- Provide consistent structure for family interactions (e.g., length of visits, number of visitors, content of interactions). *Consistency and structure provide stability during times of stress and crisis.*
- Help the family identify its personal strengths. *Individual coping skills assist in adjusting to life crises.*
- Mothers may require additional support in their role of caring for chronically ill children. *Mothers exhibit greater efforts than fathers in coping patterns, including strategies to acquire social support outside the family, increase self-worth, and decrease psychological tensions (Brazil and Krueger, 2002).*
- ▲ Encourage family members to participate in appropriate support programs (e.g., chronic obstructive pulmonary disease [COPD] support groups, Arthritis I Can Cope

• = Independent; ▲ = Collaborative

groups, Alzheimer's support groups). *Support group participation develops coping skills, enhances communication skills, and facilitates exchange of useful information (Northouse and Peters-Golden, 1993).*

▲ Evaluate the family's perceived strength of its social support system. Encourage the family to use social support to increase its resiliency and to moderate stress. *Perceived social support is a factor influencing resiliency and ability to cope with stress (Tak and McCubbin, 2002).*

▲ Provide continuity of care by maintaining effective communication among staff members. Initiate regular multidisciplinary client-care conferences that involve the client and family in problem solving. *Continuity of care enhances health status. Involvement of the client and family in case conferences is proactive and empowering.*

▲ Serve as case manager to explore and use all available resources appropriate for the situation (e.g., community mental health services, reimbursement options). *Resources will provide the family with information and assistance if necessary and appropriate.*

▲ Observe for any symptoms of elder or child abuse or neglect. *Abuse can take several forms, such as physical assaults that may or may not result in injury, verbal attacks, isolation, and social and emotional neglect. Prompt reporting of abuse according to local and state law is necessary. In most states, reporting of abuse is mandated by law.*

Geriatric

▲ Refer the family to appropriate senior community resources (e.g., senior centers, Medicare assistance, meal programs, parish nursing services, charitable organizations). *Many federal, state, and local community-based resources for seniors are underused.*

▲ If actual or potential abuse or neglect is an issue, report it to the appropriate agency. *The purpose of protective services is to preserve the family.*

▲ Encourage the family member to participate in appropriate support groups (e.g., COPD support groups, Arthritis I Can Cope groups, Alzheimer's support groups). *Support groups provide people with a setting in which they can discuss their illness-related problems with others who have the same problems.*

• Work with the family to manage common challenges related to normal aging. *Having knowledge of the normal developmental challenges of aging can reduce the stress such challenges place on families.*

Multicultural

• Work to provide caregivers who understand the importance of cultural beliefs and values the family may hold. **Nursing Research:** *Cultures can differ with regard to health beliefs, practices, and values (Camphinha-Bacote, Narayan, 2000; Guarnaccia, 1998).*

• Acknowledge racial/ethnic differences at the onset of care. **Nursing Research:** *Acknowledgment of race/ethnicity issues will enhance communication, establish rapport, and promote treatment outcomes (D'Avanzo et al, 2001; Ludwick and Silva, 2000; Vontress and Epp, 1997).*

• Approach families of color with respect, warmth, and professional courtesy. **Nursing Research:** *Instances of disrespect and lack of caring have special significance for families of color (D'Avanzo et al, 2001; Vontress and Epp, 1997).*

• Assess for the influence of cultural beliefs, norms, and values on the family's perceptions of coping. **Nursing Research:** *What the family considers normal and abnormal coping behavior may be based on cultural perceptions (Leininger and McFarland, 2002; Cochran, 1998; Doswell and Erlen, 1998).*

• = **Independent;** ▲ = **Collaborative**

- Give a rationale when assessing families with regard to sensitive issues. **Nursing Research:** *African Americans and other people of color may expect white caregivers to hold negative and preconceived ideas about people of color. Giving a rationale for questions asked will help reduce this perception (D'Avanzo et al, 2001; Vontress and Epp, 1997).*
- Use a family-centered approach when working with Latino, Asian, African American, and Native American clients. **Nursing Research:** *Latinos may perceive the family as a source of support, solver of problems, and source of pride. Asian Americans may regard the family as the primary decision maker and influence on individual family members (D'Avanzo et al, 2001). Native American families may have extended structures and exert powerful influences over functioning (Seiderman et al, 1996).*
- Facilitate modeling and role playing for the family regarding healthy ways to communicate and interact. **Nursing Research:** *It is helpful for family members and the client to practice communication skills in a safe environment before trying them in a real-life situation (Rivera-Andino and Lopez, 2000).*
- Validate the feelings of family members or significant caregivers regarding the impact of the client's illness on family lifestyle. **Nursing Research:** *Validation is a therapeutic communication technique that lets the individual know that the nurse has heard and understood what was said and promotes the relationship between the nurse and that individual (Heineken, 1998).*

Home care
NOTE: This diagnosis presents the complex and difficult problem of securing an appropriate response by the family to a client's illness and caregiving needs. The same problem in the home setting creates an unusually high risk for abuse of the client. The nurse is cautioned that the margin of time for planning and effectively supporting the family unit to avoid abuse may be minimal or even negligible. Suspected or actual abuse should be reported to adult protective services.
- The interventions described previously may be adapted for home care use.
- If the client has been in an institution, establish empathetic contact with the client and family before discharge. *Contact with the family in a nonthreatening manner helps establish a trusting relationship, easing the transition to home.*
- Assess the family member's ability and willingness to assist in client care. Determine if the family member is an appropriate source of support for the client. *Knowledge of the reasons behind disabled coping will assist in identification of appropriate interventions. Is the family member's response consistent with the previous relationship with the client or have illness or other factors influenced the relationship? Is there a history of psychiatric disorder that is being exacerbated? Is there a lack of resources that places additional stress on the caregiver? Is the family member feeling stressed in dealing with the client's care needs? Refer to the care plan for* **Caregiver role strain.** Alter expectations of the family member's assistance to the client, depending on assessment findings.
- Assess the family member's understanding of the client's illness and behavior. Instruct in appropriate expectations of the client and correct any misconceptions. *The family member may be proceeding from false assumptions about the client's illness or behavior. For example, in the absence of comprehension of dementia, the family member may assume that the client's illness-related behaviors are signs of stubbornness, laziness, or willful acting out.*
- During the time of compromised coping, increase visits to assess the safety of the client and family, provide assistance with coping strategies, identify dysfunctional coping

• = Independent; ▲ = Collaborative

mechanisms, and intervene as necessary. *Increased opportunity for interaction and appropriate intervention will enhance the safety and health status of the client and family. Frequent assessment of the client's health status promotes early detection and treatment of problems. Changes in the client's health status (especially any deterioration in status) can precipitate more problems with the family or caregiver and place the client at greater risk.*

- Identify any changes in skills needed for client care and support caregiving efforts. Assess the needs of the caregiver in the home. Intervene to meet needs as appropriate to total case management and explore all available resources that may be used to provide adequate home care (e.g., add home health aide services; coordinate services with mental health agencies; encourage caregivers not to neglect their own physical, mental, and spiritual health; and give more specific information about the client's needs and ways to meet them). *Support from the nurse through teaching and positive feedback helps caregivers to have a realistic perception of what can be expected of the client and shows them they are valued for the efforts made; meeting the needs of caregivers supports their ability to meet the needs of the client; home health aides may be used as role models for caregiving and can observe the status of the client and family. Caution the home health aide to document objectively.*

▲ Serve as an advocate, mentor, and role model for appropriate behavior. Write down or contract for the care needed by the client. *Therapeutic use of self by the nurse and concrete task definition and assignment reinforce positive coping strategies.*

▲ When a terminal illness is the precipitating factor for ineffective coping, offer hospice services and support groups as possible resources. *Nonjudgmental support from helpers with no agenda allows verbalization of feelings. The hospice paradigm addresses the physical, emotional, and spiritual needs of the dying and their loved ones.*

- Support positive individual and family coping efforts. *Positive feedback reinforces desired behaviors and supports the family unit.*

▲ If disabled family coping interferes with the family member's ability to support the client's treatment plan, refer for psychiatric home health care services for family and client counseling and implementation of a therapeutic regimen. *Psychiatric home care nurses can address issues relating to the family member's and client's ability to adjust to changes in health status. Behavioral interventions in the home can help the family member and client to participate more effectively in the treatment plan (Patusky, Rodning, and Martinez-Kratz, 1996).*

Client/Family Teaching

- Encourage family members to ask for a break in caregiving and to spend time away from the client. *Caregivers who were able to maintain control recognized when they were losing control and needed a break from caregiving (Szabo and Strang, 1999).*

- Provide truthful information regarding the client's illness to the family; use anticipatory guidance to prepare for expected outcomes. *Information is an important need of the families of critically ill clients. Meeting this need requires a multidisciplinary approach and an environment that values the delivery of humanistic care (Henneman and Cardin, 1992). Families need a framework that can serve as a standard against which they can measure progress (Northouse and Peters-Golden, 1993).*

- Involve the client and family in the planning of care as often as possible; mutual goal setting is often an effective strategy. *Family members of any trauma client admitted to the level I trauma center are invited by the trauma staff to attend weekly multidisciplinary*

• = **Independent;** ▲ = **Collaborative**

meetings. In this way family concerns can become a positive care factor, and the tasks of nurses, doctors, and social workers are made easier (Boettcher and Schiller, 1990).

- Discuss with the family appropriate ways to demonstrate feelings. *Learning basic components of therapeutic communication helps family members to express feelings appropriately.*
- Help the family identify the health care needs of the client and family; teach the skills necessary to address health care needs. *Once needs are identified, skill mastery by the family will optimize health status. Skill mastery is an empowering and positive coping mechanism.*
- Promote individual and family relaxation and stress-reduction strategies. *The immune system weakens in response to stress; relaxation elicits the opposite, healthful response (Bulechek and McCloskey, 1992).*

evolve WEBSITES FOR EDUCATION

See the EVOLVE website for World Wide Web resources for client education.

REFERENCES

Barry P: *Psychosocial nursing assessment and intervention,* Philadelphia, 1989, Lippincott.

Boettcher M, Schiller W: The use of a multidisciplinary group meeting for families of critically ill trauma patients, *Intensive Care Nurs* 6(3):129, 1990.

Brazil K, Krueger P: Patterns of family adaptation to childhood asthma. *J Pediatr Nurs* 17(3):167, 2002.

Bulechek G, McCloskey J: *Advanced nursing interventions,* Philadelphia, 1992, WB Saunders.

Camphinha-Bacote J, Narayan M: Culturally competent health care at home, *Home Care Provid* 5(6):213, 2000.

Cochran M: Tears have no color, *Am J Nurs* 98(6):53, 1998.

D'Avanzo CE et al: Developing culturally informed strategies for substance-related interventions. In Naegle MA, D'Avanzo CE, editors: *Addictions and substance abuse: strategies for advanced practice nursing,* St Louis, 2001, Mosby.

Doswell W, Erlen J: Multicultural issues and ethical concerns in the delivery of nursing care interventions, *Nurs Clin North Am* 33(2):353, 1998.

Gillis C et al: *Toward a science of family nursing,* Menlo Park, Calif, 1989, Addison-Wesley.

Guarnaccia P: Multicultural experiences of family caregiving: a study of African American, European American, and Hispanic American families, *New Dir Ment Health Serv* 77:45, 1998.

Heineken J: Patient silence is not necessarily client satisfaction: communication in home care nursing, *Home Healthc Nurse* 16(2):115, 1998.

Henneman EA, Cardin S: Need for information: interventions for practice, *Crit Care Nurs Clin North Am* 4(4): 615, 1992.

Leininger MM, McFarland MR: *Transcultural nursing: concepts, theories, research and practices,* ed 3, New York, 2002, McGraw-Hill.

Leske J, Jiricka M: Impact of family demands and family strengths and capabilities on family well-being and adaptation after critical injury, *Am J Crit Care* 7(5):383, 1998.

Lipkin G, Cohen R: *Effective approaches to patients' behavior,* New York, 1992, Springer.

Ludwick R, Silva M: Nursing around the world: cultural values and ethical conflicts, *Online J Issues Nurs,* August 14, 2000, available online at http://www.nursingworld.org/ojin/ethcol/ethics_4.htm, accessed June 19, 2003.

Meleis A: *Theoretical nursing,* Philadelphia, 1991, Lippincott.

Northouse L, Peters-Golden H: Cancer and the family: strategies to assist spouses, *Semin Oncol Nurs* 9:74, 1993.

Patusky KL, Rodning C, Martinez-Kratz M: Clinical lessons in psychiatric home care: a case study approach, *J Home Health Case Manag* 9:18, 1996.

Rask K, Kaunonen M, Paunonen-Ilmonen M: Adolescent coping with grief after the death of a loved one, *Int J Nurs Pract* 8(3):137, 2002.

Rivera-Andino J, Lopez L: When culture complicates care, *RN* 63(7):47, 2000.

Seiderman RY et al: Assessing American Indian families, *MCN Am J Matern Child Nurs* 21(6):274, 1996.

Szabo V, Strang V: Experiencing control in caregiving, *Image J Nurs Sch* 31(1):71, 1999.

- = Independent; ▲ = Collaborative

Tak YR, McCubbin M: Family stress, perceived social support and coping following the diagnosis of a child's congenital heart disease, *J Adv Nurs* 39(2):190, 2002.

Vontress CE, Epp LR: Historical hostility in the African American client: implications for counseling, *J Multicul Counseling Dev* 25:170, 1997.

Weiss S, Chen J: Factors influencing maternal mental health and family functioning during the low birthweight infant's first year of life, *J Pediatr Nurs* 17(2):114, 2002.

Readiness for enhanced family Coping

T. Heather Herdman, Beverly Pickett, Gail B. Ladwig, and Mary Markle

NANDA Definition

Effective management of adaptive tasks by family member involved with client's health challenge, who now exhibits desire and readiness for enhanced health and growth with regard to self and in relation to client

Defining Characteristics

Individual expresses interest in making contact on a one-to-one basis or through mutual aid group with another person who has experienced a similar situation; attempts to describe growth impact of the crisis on his or her own values, priorities, goals, or relationships; moves in the direction of health promotion and health-enriching lifestyle that supports and monitors maturational processes; audits and negotiates treatment programs and generally chooses experiences that optimize wellness

Related Factors (r/t)

Needs sufficiently gratified and adaptive tasks effectively addressed to enable goals of self-actualization to surface

NOC   Outcomes (Nursing Outcomes Classification)

Suggested NOC Outcomes

Anxiety Self-Control; Caregiver Emotional Health; Caregiver-Patient Relationship; Caregiver Well-Being; Family Coping; Hope; Knowledge: Health Behavior, Health Resources; Participation in Health Care Decisions; Social Support

> **Example NOC Outcome with Indicators**
>
> **Family Coping** as evidenced by the following indicators: Identifies effective coping patterns/Verbalizes sense of control/Seeks information concerning illness and treatment/Uses available social support/Identifies multiple coping strategies (Rate each indicator of **Family Coping:** 1 = never demonstrated, 2 = rarely demonstrated, 3 = sometimes demonstrated, 4 = often demonstrated, 5 = consistently demonstrated [see Section I].)

Client Outcomes

Family Will (Specify Time Frame):
- State a plan for growth
- Perform tasks needed for change
- State positive effects of changes made

- = **Independent; ▲ = Collaborative**

| NIC | Interventions (Nursing Interventions Classification) |

Suggested NIC Interventions

Anticipatory Guidance; Caregiver Support; Coping Enhancement; Emotional Support; Family Integrity Promotion; Family Involvement Promotion; Family Mobilization; Family Support; Hope Instillation; Mutual Goal Setting; Normalization Promotion; Support System Enhancement

---

Example NIC Activities—Family Support

Facilitate communication of concerns and feelings between client and family or among family members; Identify and respect family's coping mechanisms

---

Nursing Interventions and Rationales

- Observe the traits the family possesses that will help initiate change, such as having a positive attitude or stating that change is possible. *The nurse can then identify the strengths on which the family may rely and build, and the weaknesses from which the family needs protection.*
- Consider the use of family theory as a framework to help guide interventions (e.g., family stress theory, social exchange theory). *Theory helps to identify the focus, means, and goals of nursing practice. It enhances communication and increases autonomy and accountability for care (Gillis et al, 1989; Meleis, 1991).*
- Allow family members time to verbalize their concerns; provide one-to-one interaction with the family. *Interactions allow the family to gather and impart information, decrease anxiety, and provide input for the plan of care.*
- Provide truthful information and constructive advice about the client's illness and treatment. *Having knowledge about the illness helps family members to develop their coping strategies (Van Hammond and Deans, 1995).*
- Evaluate the family's perceived strength of its social support system. Encourage the family to use social support to increase its resiliency and to moderate stress. *Perceived social support is a factor influencing resiliency and ability to cope with stress (Tak and McCubbin, 2002).*
- When a client is having surgery, give the family a 5- to 10-minute progress report about halfway through the surgical procedure. **Nursing Research:** *Family members who were given progress reports during an intraoperative waiting period experienced lower anxiety scores and had significantly lower mean arterial pressures and heart rates than those who did not receive the reports (Leske, 1995).*
- Allow the family to be present during invasive procedures and resuscitation efforts. *This facilitates effective coping of family members during the crisis of critical illness (Twibell, 1998).*
- Have family members share the responsibility for change and encourage all to have input. *It is important to view the entire family as a system and also as individual stakeholders when trying to promote positive change.*
- Encourage family members to write down their goals. *The more involved the family is in goal development, the greater the probability that the goals will be achieved.*
- Explore with the family members ways to attain their goals (e.g., adult education classes; enrichment courses; family activities such as sports, cooking, or reading; sharing of time together).

- = Independent; ▲ = Collaborative

- Educate the client and family regarding illness and take time to answer questions. *Empowerment of family members through education increases the family's knowledge and understanding and ability to deal with the illness (Van Hammond and Deans, 1995).*
- Encourage setting aside leisure time free of obligatory tasks for family members to enjoy each other's company; because everyone is busy, family members may need to set up a schedule for leisure time. *Help family members communicate with each other using techniques they are comfortable with, such as role playing, letter writing, or tape recording messages. These techniques give the family an opportunity to communicate in an effective yet nonthreatening manner.*
- ▲ Identify support groups that discuss problems and concerns similar to those of the family (e.g., Al-Anon, Arthritis I Can Cope). Such groups allow family members to discuss issues and concerns with others who share the same lived experience.

Geriatric
- Encourage family members to reminisce with the older family member.
- Start and maintain a log of anecdotal stories about the older family member.
- Encourage children in the family to spend time with and share activities with the older family member. *These activities allow for knowledge of and respect for one another; they support the normal developmental tasks of aging.*
- ▲ Refer the family to parenting classes and classes for coping with the needs of older parents. *Such groups allow family members to discuss the challenges of aging parents with others who share the same experience.*

Multicultural
- Acknowledge racial/ethnic differences at the onset of care. *Acknowledgment of race/ethnicity issues will enhance communication, establish rapport, and promote treatment outcomes (D'Avanzo et al, 2001).*
- Approach families of color with respect, warmth, and professional courtesy. *Instances of disrespect and lack of caring have special significance for families of color (D'Avanzo et al, 2001).*
- Assess for the influence of cultural beliefs, norms, and values on the family's perceptions of coping. *What the family considers normal and abnormal coping behavior may be based on cultural perceptions (Leininger, 1996).*
- Use a family-centered approach when working with Latino, Asian, African American, and Native American clients. *Latinos may perceive the family as a source of support, solver of problems, and source of pride. Asian Americans may regard the family as the primary decision maker and influence on individual family members (D'Avanzo et al, 2001). Native American families may have extended structures and exert powerful influences over functioning (Seiderman et al, 1996).*
- Facilitate modeling and role playing for family with regard to healthy ways to communicate and interact. *It is helpful for family members and the client to practice communication skills in a safe environment before trying them in a real-life situation (Rivera-Andino and Lopez, 2000).*
- Validate family members' feelings regarding the impact of the client's illness on family lifestyle. *Validation lets the individual know that the nurse has heard and understood what was said, and it promotes the relationship between the nurse and the individual (Stuart and Laraia, 2001; Giger and Davidhizar, 1995).*

- = **Independent**; ▲ = **Collaborative**

Home care

- The nursing interventions described previously in the care plan for **Compromised family Coping** should be used in the home environment with adaptations as necessary.

Client/Family Teaching

- Teach that it is normal for changes in family relationships to occur. Work with the family to manage common challenges related to family dynamics. *Having knowledge of normal family dynamics promotes growth and self-actualization and supports effective coping.*
- Promote individual and family relaxation and stress-reduction strategies. *The immune system weakens in response to stress; relaxation elicits the opposite, healthful response (Bulechek and McCloskey, 1992).*

evolve WEBSITES FOR EDUCATION

See the EVOLVE website for World Wide Web resources for client education.

REFERENCES

Bulechek G, McCloskey J: *Advanced nursing interventions,* Philadelphia, 1992, WB Saunders.

D'Avanzo CE et al: Developing culturally informed strategies for substance-related interventions. In Naegle MA, D'Avanzo CE, editors: *Addictions and substance abuse: strategies for advanced practice nursing,* St Louis, 2001, Mosby.

Giger JN, Davidhizar RE: *Transcultural nursing,* ed 2, St Louis, 1995, Mosby.

Gillis C et al: *Toward a science of family nursing,* Menlo Park, Calif, 1989, Addison-Wesley.

Leininger MM: *Transcultural nursing: theories, research and practices,* ed 2, Hilliard, Ohio, 1996, McGraw-Hill.

Leske JS: Effects of intraoperative progress reports on anxiety levels of surgical patients' family members, *Appl Nurs Res* 8(4):169, 1995.

Meleis A: *Theoretical nursing,* Philadelphia, 1991, Lippincott.

Rivera-Andino J, Lopez L: When culture complicates care, *RN* 63(7):47, 2000.

Seiderman RY et al: Assessing American Indian families, *MCN Am J Matern Child Nurs* 21(6):274, 1996.

Stuart GW, Laraia MT: Therapeutic nurse-patient relationship. In Stuart GW, Laraia MT, editors: *Principles and practice of psychiatric nursing,* St Louis, 2001, Mosby.

Tak YR, McCubbin M: Family stress, perceived social support and coping following the diagnosis of a child's congenital heart disease, *J Adv Nurs* 39(2):190, 2002.

Twibell RS: Family coping during critical illness, *Dimens Crit Care Nurs* 17(2):100, 1998.

Van Hammond T, Deans C: A phenomenological study of families and psychoeducation support groups, *J Psychosoc Nurs Ment Health Serv* 33(10):7, 1995.

Risk for sudden infant Death syndrome

Betty J. Ackley

NANDA Definition

Presence of risk factors for sudden death of an infant under 1 year of age

• = Independent; ▲ = Collaborative

Risk Factors

Modifiable: Infants placed to sleep in the prone or side-lying position; Prenatal and/or postnatal infant smoke exposure; Infant overheating/overwrapping; Soft underlayment/loose articles in the sleep environment; Delayed or nonattendance of prenatal care

Potentially Modifiable: Low birth weight; Prematurity; Young maternal age

Nonmodifiable: Male gender; Ethnicity (e.g., African American, Native American race of mother); Seasonality of sudden infant death syndrome (SIDS) deaths (higher in winter and fall months); SIDS mortality peaks between infant age of 2 to 4 months

Related Factors (r/t)

See Risk Factors

NOC   Outcomes (Nursing Outcomes Classification)

Suggested NOC Outcomes

Knowledge: Child Physical Safety; Parenting Performance; Safe Home Environment

> #### Example NOC Outcome with Indicators
>
> **Knowledge: Child Physical Safety** as evidenced by the following indicators: Description of methods to prevent SIDS/Demonstration of first aid techniques (Rate each indicator of **Knowledge: Child Physical Safety:** 1 = None, 2 = Limited, 3 = Moderate, 4 = Substantial, 5 = Extensive [see Section I].)

Client Outcomes

Client Will (Specify Time Frame):

- Explain appropriate measures to prevent SIDS
- Demonstrate correct techniques for positioning the infant, protecting the infant from harm

NIC   Interventions (Nursing Interventions Classification)

Suggested NIC Interventions

Infant Care; Teaching: Infant Safety

> #### Example NIC Activities—Teaching: Infant Safety
>
> Place infant on back to sleep and keep loose bedding, pillows, and toys out of crib; Avoid holding infant while smoking or drinking

Nursing Interventions and Rationales

- Position infant on their back to sleep, do not position in the prone position. **Clinical Research:** *Research has demonstrated that the prone position for sleeping infants is a risk factor for SIDS (Dwyer et al, 1991; Mitchell et al, 1991; Taylor et al, 1996). Population studies have demonstrated a striking trend in decreased incidence of SIDS since parents have been taught to **not** place infants in the prone position (Ponsonby et al, 2002). The introduction of the "Back to Sleep" program has not brought about an increase in the inci-*

- = Independent; ▲ = Collaborative

dences of aspiration-related deaths. The rate of infant death related to SIDS has declined (Malloy, 2002).

- Avoid use of loose bedding such as blankets and sheets for sleeping. If blankets are used, they should be tucked in around the crib mattress so the infant's face is less likely to become covered by bedding. "One strategy is to make up the bedding so that the infant's feet are able to reach the foot of the crib (feet to foot), with the blankets tucked in around the crib mattress and reaching only the level of the infant's chest. Another strategy is to use sleep clothing with no other covering over the infant" (American Academy of Pediatrics, 2000, p 654). **Clinical Research:** *Epidemiological studies have identified soft surfaces as a significant risk factor for SIDS, especially when these items are placed under the sleeping infant (Brooke et al, 1997; Mitchell et al, 1998; Ponsonby et al, 1998).*

- Avoid overheating the infant by lightly clothing the child for sleep, and avoiding over-bundling. The infant should not feel hot to touch. **Clinical Research:** *Overheating the infant has been associated with increased risk of SIDS (Gilbert et al, 1992; Ponsonby et al, 1992).*

- Provide the infant a certain amount of time in prone position or "tummy time" while the infant is awake and observed. *A period of time on their tummy is recommended for developmental reasons and to help prevent flat spots on the back of the head" (American Academy of Pediatrics, 2000).*

- Use electronic respiratory or cardiac monitors to detect cardiorespiratory arrest only if ordered. **Clinical Research:** *There is no evidence that infants prone to SIDS can be identified by monitoring of respiratory or cardiac function in the hospital (Malloy and Hoffman, 1996).*

Home care
- Most of the interventions above are relevant.
- Evaluate home for potential safety hazards such as inappropriate cribs, cradles, or strollers.
- Determine where and how the child sleeps.

Multicultural
- Discuss cultural norms with families in order to provide care that is appropriate for promoting safety for the infant in sleeping arrangements and care. **Nursing Research:** *Misinterpretation of parenting behaviors can occur when the nurse and parent are from different cultures (Guarnaccia, 1998).*

- Encourage American Indian mothers to avoid drinking and to avoid wrapping infants in excessive blankets or clothing. **Clinical Research:** *In one study an association was shown between binge drinking during pregnancy and having two or more layers of clothing on the infant in the American Indian population (Iyasu et al, 2002).*

- Encourage African American mothers to find alternatives to bed sharing and to avoid placing pillows, soft toys, and soft bedding in the sleep environment. **Clinical Research:** *Studies have demonstrated a higher incidence of SIDS in African American infants. In one study the infants in death were commonly found in the supine position, but they were more likely to be sharing a bed with another person (Unger et al, 2003). Another study indicated that the greatest impact for SIDS reduction in the African American population was the need to change behaviors regarding sleep locations by reducing placing infants for sleep on adult beds, sofas, or cots (Rasinski et al, 2003).*

- = Independent; ▲ = Collaborative

Client/Family Teaching

- Teach families to not place the infant in the prone position and to instead position the infant on his or her back for sleep. **Clinical Research:** *Research has demonstrated that the prone position for sleeping infants is a risk factor for SIDS (Dwyer et al, 1991; Mitchell et al, 1991; Taylor et al, 1996). Population studies have demonstrated a striking trend in decreased incidence of SIDS since parents have been taught to **not** place infants in the prone position (Ponsonby et al, 2002). The introduction of the "Back to Sleep" program has not brought about an increase in the incidences of aspiration-related deaths. The rate of infant death related to SIDS has declined (Malloy, 2002.)*
- Teach the parents to place the infant supine to sleep with the head rotated to one side for a week, and then to the other side for a week. Parents should also change the orientation of the crib at intervals so the infant turns the head in alternate directions. *This is necessary to prevent the infant from developing a flat area on the back of the head (American Academy of Pediatrics, 2000).*
- Teach parents that the supine position (wholly on the back) confers the lowest risk of SIDS and is preferred. However, while side sleeping is not as safe as supine, it also has a significantly lower risk than prone. If the side position is used, bring the dependent arm forward to lessen the likelihood of the infant rolling to the prone position" (American Academy of Pediatrics, 2000, p 654).
- Recommend the following infant care practices to parents:
  - Infants should not be put to sleep on soft surfaces such as waterbeds, sofas, or soft mattresses
  - Avoid placing soft materials in the infant's sleeping environment such as pillows, quilts, and comforters. Do not use sheepskins under a sleeping infant.
  - Avoid placing soft objects such as stuffed toys and other gas-trapping objects in an infant's sleeping environment.
  - Avoid the use of loose bedding, such as blankets and sheets. If blankets are to be used, they should be tucked in around the crib mattress so the infant's face is less likely to become covered by bedding. "One strategy is to make up the bedding so that the infant's feet are able to reach the foot of the crib (feet to foot), with the blankets tucked in around the crib mattress and reaching only the level of the infant's chest. Another strategy is to use sleep clothing with no other covering over the infant" (American Academy of Pediatrics, 2000, p 654).

  Clinical Research: *Epidemiological studies have identified soft surfaces as a significant risk factor for SIDS, especially when these items are placed under the sleeping infant (Brook et al, 1997; Mitchell et al, 1998; Ponsonby et al, 1998).*
- Teach parents the need to obtain a crib that conforms to the safety standards of the Consumer Product Safety Commission. Although many cradles and bassinets also may provide safe sleeping enclosures, safety standards have not been established for these items (American Academy of Pediatrics, 2000).
- Teach parents that sleeping with an infant may be hazardous under certain conditions, especially if alcohol or medications/illicit drugs are used by the parents or the sleep surface is not appropriate. *Sleep surfaces designed for adults may have the risk of entrapment between the mattress and the structure of the bed (e.g., the headboard, footboard, side rails, and frame), the wall, or adjacent furniture, as well as between railings in the headboard or footboard (American Academy of Pediatrics, 2000).* **Clinical Research:** *In one study of SIDS deaths, over half of the infants were sleeping in the same bed as an adult, which suggests that some of the deaths were due to unintentional suffocation from the adult or*

• = Independent; ▲ = Collaborative

from compressible bedding (Person et al, 2002). Another study demonstrated that parents who were under the influence of alcohol or illicit drugs or were smoking were more likely to have a SIDS result (James et al, 2003).

- Recommend an alternative to sleeping with an infant; parents might consider placing the infant's crib near their bed to allow for more convenient breastfeeding and parent contact.
- Recommend that adults (other than the parents), children, or other siblings avoid sharing a bed with an infant.
- Teach parents to avoid overheating the infant by lightly clothing the child for sleep and avoiding overbundling. The infant should not feel hot to touch. The bedroom temperature should be comfortable to an adult wearing light bedclothing. **Clinical Research:** *Overheating the infant has been associated with an increased risk of SIDS (Gilbert et al, 1992; Ponsonby et al, 1992).*
- Question parents regarding following recommendations for the prevention of SIDS at each well-baby visit or visit with health care practitioner for illness. Strongly encourage compliance with precautions to prevent SIDS. **Clinical Research:** *A survey of moms in Britain demonstrated that while the majority of the moms knew the precautions, 25% of the moms were not following the recommended practice (Roberts and Upton, 2000).*
- Teach the need to stop smoking during pregnancy and to not smoke around the infant, that smoking is a risk factor for SIDS. **Nursing Research:** *A study demonstrated that newborns whose mothers smoked have a limited ability to maximize and vary their heart rate, which can result in the infant being unable to maximize cardiac output during stress, which puts the infant at an increased risk for morbidity and possibly mortality (Sherman et al, 2002).* **Clinical Research:** *Research has demonstrated that smoking during pregnancy is a risk factor for SIDS (Alm et al, 1998; Pollack, 2001; Schoendorf and Kiely, 1992). Smoke in the environment after birth is considered a risk factor in several studies (Mitchell et al, 1993; Schoendorf and Kiely, 1992).*
- Recommend parents with infants in child care make it very clear to the employees that the infant must be placed in the supine position *only* to sleep, not prone or side-lying. **Clinical Research:** *A survey of licensed child care facilities demonstrated that only 14.3% were in compliance with the recommendation that infants be placed in the supine position to sleep (Ford and Linker, 2002).*
- ▲ Teach parents living in deprived areas of precautions to prevent SIDS. **Clinical Research:** *A study in New Zealand demonstrated that SIDS is more common in infants living in deprived areas, although SIDS can occur in infants living in any situation (Mitchell et al, 2000).*
- ▲ Involve family members in learning and practicing rescue techniques, including treatment of choking, breathing, and CPR. Initiate referral to formal training classes. Family members need adequate preparation to deal with emergency situations and should take part in the AHA Basic Lifesaving Course or the American Red Cross Infant/Child CPR Course (Gotsch et al, 2002). **Nursing Research:** *A study demonstrated that learning CPR did not reduce anxiety in the parents regarding SIDS but did increase their confidence in dealing with emergencies (Clarke, 1998).*

• = Independent; ▲ = Collaborative

evolve WEBSITES FOR EDUCATION

See the EVOLVE website for World Wide Web resources for client education.

REFERENCES

Alm B et al: A case-control study of smoking and sudden infant death syndrome in the Scandinavian countries 1992 to 1995. The Nordic Epidemiological SIDS Study, *Arch Dis Child*, 78:329, 1998.

American Academy of Pediatrics, Task Force on Infant Sleep Position and Sudden Infant Death Syndrome: Changing concepts of sudden infant death syndrome: implications for infant sleeping environment and sleep position (RE9946), *Pediatrics* 105(3):650, 2000.

Brooke H et al: Case-control study of sudden infant death syndrome in Scotland, *BMJ* 314:1516, 1997.

Clarke K: Research. Infant CPR: the effect on parental anxiety regarding SIDS, *Br J Midwifery*, 6(11):710, 1998.

Dwyer T et al: Prospective cohort study of prone sleeping position and sudden infant death syndrome, *Lancet* 337:1244, 1991.

Ford KM, Linker LA: Compliance of licensed child care centers with the American Academy of Pediatrics' recommendations for infant sleep positions, *J Community Health Nurs* 19(2):83, 2002.

Gilbert R et al: Combined effect of infection and heavy wrapping on the risk of sudden unexpected infant death, *Arch Dis Child* 67:171, 1992.

Gotsch K, Annest JL, Holmgreen P: Nonfatal choking-related episodes among children—United States, 2001, *MMWR Morb Mortal Wkly Rep* 51(42):945, 2002.

Guarnaccia P: Multicultural experiences of family caregiving: a Study of African American, European American, and Hispanic American families, *New Direct Ment Health Serv* 77:45, 1998.

Iyasu S et al: Risk factors for sudden infant death syndrome among northern plains Indians, *JAMA* 288(21):2717, 2002.

James C, Klenka H, Manning D: Sudden infant death syndrome: bed sharing with mothers who smoke, *Arch Dis Child* 88(2):112, 2003.

Malloy MH, Hoffman H: Home apnea monitoring and sudden infant death syndrome, *Prev Med* 25:645, 1996.

Malloy MS: Trends in postneonatal aspiration deaths and reclassification of sudden infant death syndrome: impact of the "Back to Sleep" program, *Pediatrics* 109(4):661, 2002.

Mitchell EA, Stewart AW, Crampton P: Deprivation and sudden infant death syndrome, *Soc Sci Med* 51(1):147, 2000.

Mitchell EA et al: Results from the first year of the New Zealand cot death study, *N Z Med J* 104:71, 1991.

Mitchell EA et al: Smoking and the sudden infant death syndrome, *Pediatrics* 91:893, 1993.

Mitchell EA et al: Sheepskin bedding and the sudden infant death syndrome, *J Pediatr* 133:701, 1998.

Person TL, Lavezzi WA, Wolf BC: Cosleeping and sudden unexpected death in infancy, *Arch Pathol Lab Med* 126(3):343, 2002.

Pollack HA: Sudden infant death syndrome, maternal smoking during pregnancy, and the cost-effectiveness of smoking cessation intervention, *Am J Public Health* 91(3):432, 2001.

Ponsonby A, Dwyer T, Cochrane J: Population trends in sudden infant death syndrome, *Semin Perinatol* 26(4):296, 2002.

Ponsonby AL et al: Thermal environment and SIDS: case-control study, *BMJ* 304:277, 1992.

Ponsonby AL et al: Association between use of a quilt and sudden infant death syndrome: case-control study, *BMJ* 316:195, 1998.

Rasinski KA et al: Effect of a sudden infant death syndrome risk reduction education program on risk factor compliance and information sources in primarily black urban communities, *Pediatrics* 11(4 pt 1):e347, 2003.

Roberts H, Upton D: Research. New mother's knowledge of sudden infant death syndrome, *Br J Midwifery* 8(3):147, 2000.

Schoendorf KC, Kiely JL: Relationship of sudden infant death syndrome to maternal smoking during and after pregnancy, *Pediatrics* 90:905, 1992.

Taylor JA et al: Prone sleep position and the sudden infant death syndrome in King County Washington: a case-control study, *J Pediatr* 128:626, 1996.

Unger B et al: Racial disparity and modifiable risk factors among infants dying suddenly and unexpectedly, *Pediatrics* 111(2):E127, 2003.

• = Independent; ▲ = Collaborative

Ineffective Denial

Ann Keeley

NANDA Definition

The conscious or unconscious attempt to reduce anxiety or fear by disavowing the knowledge or meaning of an event, leading to the detriment of health

Defining Characteristics

Delays seeking or refuses health care attention to the detriment of health; does not perceive personal relevance of symptoms or danger; displaces source of symptoms to other organs; displays inappropriate affect; does not admit fear of death or invalidism; makes dismissive gestures or comments when speaking of distressing events; minimizes symptoms; unable to admit impact of disease on life pattern; uses home remedies (self-treatment) to relieve symptoms; displaces fear of impact of condition

Related Factors (r/t)

Fear of consequences; chronic or terminal illness; actual or perceived fear of possible losses (e.g., job, significant other); refusal to acknowledge substance abuse problem; fear of the social stigma associated with disease

NOC   Outcomes (Nursing Outcomes Classification)

Suggested NOC Outcomes

Acceptance: Health Status; Anxiety Self-Control; Health Beliefs: Perceived Threat; Symptom Control

> #### Example NOC Outcome with Indicators
>
> **Anxiety Self-Control** as evidenced by the following indicators: Eliminates precursors of anxiety/Reports absence of physical manifestations of anxiety/Controls anxiety response (Rate each indicator of **Anxiety Self-Control:** 1 = never demonstrated, 2 = rarely demonstrated, 3 = sometimes demonstrated, 4 = often demonstrated, 5 = consistently demonstrated [see Section I].)

Client Outcomes

Client Will (Specify Time Frame):

- Seek out appropriate health care attention when needed
- Use home remedies only when appropriate
- Display appropriate affect and verbalize fears
- Remain substance free
- Actively engage in treatment program related to identified "substance" of abuse
- Demonstrate alternate adaptive coping mechanism

NIC   Interventions (Nursing Interventions Classification)

Suggested NIC Intervention

Anxiety Reduction

• = Independent; ▲ = Collaborative

> ### Example NIC Activities—Anxiety Reduction
>
> Use a calm, reassuring approach; Stay with the patient to promote safety and reduce fear

Nursing Interventions and Rationales

- Assess the client's understanding of symptoms and illness. **Nursing Research:** *Negative responses to a need for change in behavior related to an alteration in health status can only be understood following a thorough assessment of the client's appraisal framework (Dudley-Brown, 2002).*
- Spend time with the client, allow time for responses. *Nursing presence, one-on-one interaction, connecting with the client's experience, going beyond the scientific data, and knowing what will work and when to act all support the nurse-client relationship and affirm their respective selves. As a result, the client grows in awareness of his or her own being (Doona et al, 1999).*
- Assess whether the use of denial is helping or hindering the patient's care. *Denial can allow coping in the face of stress; however, total denial can be life-threatening (Robinson, 1999).*
- Allow the client to express and use denial as a coping mechanism. **Nursing Research:** *This time period of denial may be necessary for the client to develop a construct within which the information has meaning and can be appraised as not a threat to survival (Norris and Spelic, 2002).*
- Assess for subtle signs of denial (e.g., unrealistic display of optimism, downplaying of symptoms, inability to admit one's own fear). *Minimization and denial are part of the alcoholism pathophysiology (Becke and Walton-Moss, 2001).*
- Avoid confrontation. *Challenging a patient's denial may cause an increase in anxiety (Robinson, 1999). Rather than direct confrontation, informing of the reality of consequences of a specific behavior may be more therapeutically assimilated into the client's appraisal framework. Assess individual spiritual coping style (Faltz and Skinner, 2002).*
- Support the client's spiritual coping measures. **Nursing Research:** *Most religious coping is considered positive (Meisenhelder, 2002). Physical and mental health are interrelated with spiritual health (Taylor, 2002).*
- Develop a trusting, therapeutic relationship with the client/family. *A genuine connection can ease defensiveness or uneasiness (Robinson, 1999).*
- Encourage individual family members to share their concerns and worries. **Nursing Research:** *This may help reframe the experience in a way that is acceptable. Allows the nurse to identify possible misperceptions and/or questions (Mellon, 2002).*
- Ask appropriate questions using an assessment tool such as FAST to assess whether denial is being used in association with alcoholism or drug use. The client is asked to circle the appropriate response for each question: Less than monthly; Monthly; Weekly; Daily; Almost Daily.
  1. MEN: How often do you have EIGHT or more drinks on one occasion; WOMEN: How often do you have SIX or more drinks on one occasion?
  2. How often during the last year have you been unable to remember what happened the night before because you had been drinking?
  3. How often during the last year have you failed to do what was normally expected of you because of drinking?

- **● = Independent; ▲ = Collaborative**

4. In the last year has a relative or friend, or a doctor or other health worker been concerned about your drinking or suggested you cut down?

Clinical Research: *The four-item FAST alcohol questionnaire had good sensitivity and specificity, across a range of settings, when the AUDIT alcohol assessment score was used as the gold standard. The FAST questionnaire is quick to administer, because more than 50% of clients are categorized using just one question (Hodgson et al, 2002). Include in questionnaire drug use in addition to drinking (Hinkin et al, 2001). T-ACE and TWEAK are modified to be used with women.* **Nursing Research:** *Alcoholism rates are increasing in women and women may have distinct assessment risk factors (Becker and Walton-Moss, 2001). Brief addiction screening tools (Gorski retrieved from www on February 19, 2003: http://www.tgorski.com/clin_mod/atp/women_at_risk-brief_screening_tools.htm#TWEAK).*

- Sit at eye level. *Honest caring behaviors on the part of the nurse facilitate acceptance of reality on the part of the client (Haltz and Skinner, 2002).*
- Use touch if appropriate and with permission. Touch the client's hand or arm. *Appropriate expression of caring on the part of the nurse facilitates therapeutic client response (Haltz and Skinner, 2002).*
- Explain signs and symptoms of illness; as necessary, reinforce use of prescribed treatment plan. *A straightforward education on the effects of an abused substance is integral to motivation on the part of the client (Becker and Walton-Moss, 2001).*
- Have the client make choices regarding treatment and actively involve him or her in the decision-making process. **Clinical Research:** *Interventions that increase the self-efficacy of clients support maintenance of abstinence (Vielva and Iraurgi, 2001).*
- Help the client recognize existing and additional sources of support; allow time for adjustment. *The influence of environment on a positive adaptation is significant (Moser et al, 2001).*
- Encourage the client/family to describe prior crises and methods of coping. **Nursing Research:** *Allows the nurse to identify the family's communication style and adapt his or her interventions. Provides the nurse an opportunity to point out family strengths that may be used (Mellon, 2002).*
- ▲ If appropriate, refer family to a skilled mental health counselor for help in planning an intervention to observe whether denial has been or is being used as a coping mechanism in other areas of life. *Referral may be necessary to provide the most thorough assessment and treatment choices for the client (Becker and Walton-Moss, 2001).*
- Refer to care plans **Defensive Coping** and **Dysfunctional Family processes: alcoholism**

Geriatric
- Identify recent losses of the client, because grieving may prolong denial. Encourage the client to take one day at a time. *Elderly clients often have experienced significant, multiple losses in a variety of domains. This may complicate adaptation to an individual change in health status as the resources formerly used for successful adaptation are no longer available (Boyd and Stanley, 2002).*
- Encourage the client to verbalize feelings. *Verbalization allows the client to release emotions and develop a sense of control.*
- Encourage communication among family members. *Communication problems within families are pivotal in the development of family adjustment to a change in health status and or adaptation to a life change (Hanson, 2002).*

- **= Independent; ▲ = Collaborative**

- Recognize denial. *Denial is a defensive avoidance of emotion. It can be beneficial as a coping mechanism, but total denial can be detrimental (Robinson, 1999).*
- Use reality-focusing techniques. Wherever possible, provide realistic feedback, allowing the client to validate his or her perceptions. *Providing validation of actual stressors and available resources aids in a positive adaptation (Pakenham, 2001).*

Multicultural

- Assess for the influence of cultural beliefs, norms, and values on the client's understanding of and ability to acknowledge health status. **Nursing Research:** *Willingness to acknowledge health status may be based on cultural perceptions (Cochran, 1998; Doswell and Erlen, 1998; Leininger and McFarland, 2002).*
- Discuss with the client those aspects of his or her health behavior/lifestyle that will remain unchanged by health status. **Nursing Research:** *Aspects of the client's life that are meaningful and valuable to him or her should be understood and preserved without change (Leininger and McFarland, 2002).*
- Negotiate with the client regarding the aspects of health behavior that will need to be modified as a result of health status. **Nursing Research:** *Give and take with the client will lead to culturally congruent care (Leininger and McFarland, 2002).*
- Assess the role of fatalism on the client's ability to acknowledge health status. **Nursing Research:** *Fatalistic perspectives, which involve the belief that you cannot control your own fate, may influence health behaviors in some Asian, African American, and Latino populations (Chen, 2001; Harmon et al, 1996; Phillips et al, 1999).*
- Validate the client's feelings of anxiety and fear related to health status. **Nursing Research:** *Validation is the therapeutic communication technique that lets the client know that the nurse has heard and understands what was said, and it promotes the nurse-client relationship (Heineken, 1998).*

Home care

- Observe family interaction and roles. Assess whether denial is being used to meet the needs of another family member. *Communication problems within families are pivotal in the development of family adjustment to a change in health status and or adaptation to a life change (Hanson, 2002).*
- ▲ Refer the client and family to psychiatric clinical nurse specialist or medical social services for evaluation and treatment as indicated per physician order. *It may be necessary to involve the entire family to effectively treat the client.*
- ▲ Refer the client/family for follow-up if prolonged denial is a risk. *Prolonged denial almost always interferes with successful treatment. Only when denial subsides does the patient regain control (Robinson, 1999).*
- ▲ Identify an emergency plan, including how to contact hotlines and receive emergency services. *Denial may be abandoned when the need for emergency care is perceived by the client or the family.*
- Encourage communication between family members, particularly when dealing with the loss of a significant person. *Communication problems within families are pivotal in the development of family adjustment to a change in health status and or adaptation to a life change (Hanson, 2002).* **Nursing Research:** *An understanding of the family structure, patterns of communication, health care history, and cultural influences will facilitate effective interventions on the part of the nurse. In the context of some family patterns of communication, defensive coping may be a learned behavior (Hellemann et al, 2002).*

- **= Independent; ▲ = Collaborative**

Client/Family Teaching

- Teach signs and symptoms of illness and appropriate responses (e.g., taking medication, going to the emergency department, calling the physician). Provide a list of names and numbers. *Family members should be involved at all points of care to ensure that the necessary care will be provided in a safe, accurate manner (Harmon, 2001).*
- Teach family members that denial may continue throughout the adjustment to home and not to be confrontational. *Denial is normal especially during phases of adjustment, and reprimanding can lead to increased frustration and further denial (Robinson, 1999).*
- ▲ If the problem is substance abuse, refer to an appropriate community agency (e.g., Alcoholics Anonymous). **Nursing Research:** *Families need assistance in coping with health changes. The nurse is often perceived as the individual who can help them obtain necessary social support (Northouse et al, 2002; Tak and McCubbin, 2002).*
- Teach families of clients with brain injuries that denial has been associated with damage to the right hemisphere. *The client may exhibit inappropriate affect and anxiety.*
- ▲ Inform family of available community support resources. *Mutual support groups can have a positive effect not only in Western cultures but also in the Eastern cultures (Fung and Chien, 2002).*

evolve WEBSITES FOR EDUCATION

See the EVOLVE website for World Wide Web resources for client education.

REFERENCES

Becker KL, Walton-Moss B: Detecting and addressing alcohol abuse in women, *Nurse Pract* 26(10):13, 2001.

Boyd MA, Stanley M: Mental health assessment of the elderly. In Boyd MA, editor: *Psychiatric nursing in contemporary practice,* ed 2, Philadelphia, 2002, Lippincott.

Chen YC: Chinese values, health and nursing, *J Adv Nurs* 36(2):270, 2001.

Cochran M: Tears have no color, *Am J Nurs* 98(6):53, 1998.

Davidhizar R, Newman-Giger J: Patients' use of denial: coping with the unacceptable, *Nurs Stand* 12(43):44, 1998.

Doona M, Chase S, Haggerty L: Nursing presence, *J Holist Nurs* 17(1):54, 1999.

Doswell W, Erlen J: Multicultural issues and ethical concerns in the delivery of revising care interventions, *Nurs Clin North Am* 33(2):353, 1998.

Faltz BG, Skinner MK: Substance abuse disorders. In Boyd MA, editor: *Psychiatric nursing in contemporary practice,* ed 2, Philadelphia, 2002, Lippincott.

Fung WY, Chien WT: The effectiveness of a mutual support group for family caregivers of a relative with dementia, *Arch Psychiatr Nurs* 16(3):134, 2002.

Gorski T: Women at risk: brief screening tools, available on-line at http://www.tgorski.com/clin_mod/atp/women_at_risk-brief_sceening_tools.htm#TWEAK, accessed February 19, 2003.

Harmon MP, Castro FG, Coe K: Acculturation and cervical cancer: knowledge, beliefs, and behaviors of Hispanic women, *Women Health* 24(3):37, 1996.

Harmon SMH: *Family health care nursing,* Philadelphia, 2001, FA Davis.

Heineken J: Patient silence is not necessarily client satisfaction: communication in home care nursing, *Home Healthc Nurse* 16(2):115, 1998.

Hellemann MS V, Lee KA, Kary FS: Strengths and vulnerabilities of women of Mexican descent in relation to depressive symptoms, *Nurs Res* 51(3):175, 2002.

Hinkin CH et al: Screening for drug and alcohol abuse among older adults using a modified version of the CAGE, *Am J Addict* 10:319, 2001.

Hodgson R et al: The FAST alcohol screening test, *Alcohol Alcohol* 37(1):61, 2002.

Leininger MM, McFarland MR: *Transcultural nursing: concepts, theories, research and practices,* ed 3, New York, 2002, McGraw-Hill.

• = Independent; ▲ = Collaborative

Meisenhelder JB: Terrorism, posttraumatic stress, and religious coping, *Issues Ment Health Nurs* 23:771, 2002.

Mellon S: Comparisons between cancer survivors and family members on meaning of the illness and family quality of life, *Oncol Nurs Forum* 29(7):1117, 2002.

Moser KM, Sowell RL, Phillips KD: Issues of women dually diagnosed with HIV infection and substance use problems in the Carolinas, *Issues Ment Health Nurs* 22:23, 2001.

Norris J, Spelic SS: Supporting adaption to body image disruption, *Rehabil Nurs* 27(1):8, 2002.

Pakenham KI: Application of a stress and coping model to caregiving in multiple sclerosis, *Psychol Health Med* 6(1):13, 2001.

Phillips JM, Cohen MZ, Moses G: Breast cancer screening and African American women: fear, fatalism, and silence, *Oncol Nurs Forum* 26(3):561, 1999.

Russell GC: The role of denial in clinical practice, *J Adv Nurs* 18:938, 1993.

Taylor EJ: *Spiritual care: nursing theory, research and practice,* Upper Saddle River, NJ, 2002, Prentice-Hall.

Vielva I, Iraurgi I: Cognitive and behavioural factors as predictors of abstinence following treatment for alcohol dependence, *Addiction* 96:297, 2001.

Impaired Dentition

Gail B. Ladwig and Betty J. Ackley

NANDA Definition

Disruption in tooth development/eruption patterns or structural integrity of individual teeth

Defining Characteristics

Excessive plaque; crown or root caries; halitosis; tooth enamel discoloration; toothache; loose teeth; excessive calculus; incomplete eruption for age (may be primary or permanent teeth); malocclusion or tooth misalignment; premature loss of primary teeth; worn down or abraded teeth; tooth fracture(s); missing teeth or complete absence; erosion of enamel; asymmetrical facial expression

Related Factors (r/t)

Ineffective oral hygiene; sensitivity to heat or cold; barriers to self-care; nutritional deficits; dietary habits; genetic predisposition; selected prescription medications; premature loss of primary teeth; excessive intake of fluorides; chronic vomiting; chronic use of tobacco, coffee, tea, red wine; lack of knowledge regarding dental health; excessive use of abrasive cleaning agents; bruxism

NOC Outcomes (Nursing Outcomes Classification)

Suggested NOC Outcomes

Oral Hygiene; Self-Care: Oral Hygiene

> **Example NOC Outcome with Indicators**
>
> **Oral Hygiene** as evidenced by the following indicators: Cleanliness of teeth/Cleanliness of gums/Cleanliness of dentures/Tooth integrity/Gum integrity (Rate each indicator of **Oral Hygiene:** 1 = extremely compromised, 2 = substantially compromised, 3 = moderately compromised, 4 = mildly compromised, 5 = not compromised [see Section I].)

• = Independent; ▲ = Collaborative

Client Outcomes

Client Will (Specify Time Frame):

- Have clean teeth, gums healthy pink color, mouth with pleasant odor
- Demonstrate ability to masticate foods without difficulty
- State no pain originating from teeth
- Demonstrate measures can take to improve dental hygiene

NIC	Interventions (Nursing Interventions Classification)

Suggested NIC Interventions

Oral Health Maintenance; Oral Health Promotion: Oral Health Restoration

---

Example NIC Activities—Oral Health Maintenance

Establish a mouth care routine; Arrange for dental check-ups as needed

---

Nursing Interventions and Rationales

- ▲ Inspect oral cavity/teeth at least once daily and note any discoloration, presence of debris, amount of plaque buildup, presence of lesions, edema, or bleeding, intactness of teeth. Refer to a dentist or periodontist as appropriate. *Systematic inspection can identify impending problems (Walton et al, 2001).*
- Monitor the client's nutritional and fluid status to determine if adequate. *Malnutrition predisposes clients to dental disease.*
- Assess the client for underlying medical condition that may be causing halitosis. **Clinical Research:** *Extraoral halitosis can be subdivided into: halitosis from the upper respiratory tract including the nose; halitosis from the lower respiratory tract; blood-borne halitosis. In blood-borne halitosis, malodorant compounds in the bloodstream are carried to the lungs where they volatilize and enter the breath. Potential sources of blood-borne halitosis are some systemic diseases, metabolic disorders, medication, and certain foods (Tangreman, 2002).* **Clinical Research:** *Patients who believe they have oral malodor often have a dry mouth condition instead (Kleinberg et al, 2002).*
- Determine the client's mental status and manual dexterity; if the client is unable to care for self, dental hygiene must be provided by nursing personnel. The nursing diagnosis **Bathing/hygiene Self-care deficit** is then also applicable.
- Determine the client's usual method of oral care. Whenever possible, build on the client's existing knowledge base and current practices to develop an individualized plan of care.
- If the client is unable to brush own teeth, follow this procedure:
  1. Use a soft bristle baby toothbrush.
  2. Use tap water or saline as a solution.
  3. Brush teeth in an up-and-down manner.
  4. Suction as needed.
  Avoid using foam sticks to clean teeth; use only to swab out the oral cavity. *Use of this nursing protocol results in improved oral hygiene in a vulnerable population (Stiefel et al, 2000).* **Nursing Research:** *Foam sticks are not effective for removing plaque; the toothbrush is much more effective (DeWalt, 1975; Pearson and Hutton, 2002).*
- If the client is free of bleeding disorders and is able to swallow, encourage the client to brush teeth with a soft toothbrush using fluoride-containing toothpaste after every

• = Independent; ▲ = Collaborative

meal and to floss teeth daily. *The toothbrush is the most important tool for oral care; tooth-brushing is the most effective method of reducing plaque and controlling periodontal disease (Stiefel et al, 2000).*

- Direct the toothbrush vertically toward the tooth surfaces. **Clinical Research:** *One study demonstrated that brushing with the toothbrush bristles perpendicular to the surface of the teeth has a high efficacy of plaque removal and maintains good gingival condition (Sasahara and Kawamura, 2000).*
- The tongue must also be cleaned when performing oral hygiene maintenance. Brush tongue with soft toothbrush and follow with a mouth rinse. Use tap water or saline only for a mouth rinse. Avoid the use of hydrogen peroxide, lemon-glycerin swabs, or alcohol-based mouthwashes. *Tongue brushing and mouth rinsing are basic treatment measures for halitosis (Yaegaki et al, 2002).* **Nursing Research:** *Hydrogen peroxide can cause mucosal damage and is extremely foul tasting to clients (Tombes and Gallucci, 1993). Lemon-glycerin swabs can result in decreased salivary amylase and oral moisture, as well as erosion of tooth enamel (Foss-Durant and McAffee, 1997; Poland, 1987).*
- If the client does not have a bleeding disorder, encourage the client to floss daily with approximately 18 inches of floss using a gentle rubbing up and down motion. *Floss is useful to remove plaque buildup between the teeth (Brown and Yoder, 2002).*
- If platelet numbers are decreased, or if the client is edentulous, use moistened toothettes for oral care. *A toothbrush can cause soft tissue injury and bleeding in clients with low numbers of platelets (Armstrong, 1994).*
- Provide scrupulous dental care to critically ill clients. *Cultures of the teeth of critically ill clients have yielded significant bacterial colonization, which can cause nosocomial pneumonia (Scannapieco et al, 1992).*
- If teeth are nonfunctional for chewing, modification of oral intake (e.g., edentulous diet, soft diet) may be necessary. The nursing diagnosis **Imbalanced Nutrition: less than body requirements** may apply.
- If the client is unable to swallow, keep suction nearby when providing oral care.
- See care plan for **Impaired Oral mucous membrane.**

Geriatric
- Consider recommending use of an ultrasonic toothbrush if any impairment of manual dexterity exists. *Use of an ultrasonic toothbrush was shown to reduce plaque and bleeding in a study of 12 patients more than 65 years old (Whitmyer et al, 1998).*
- Carefully observe oral cavity and lips for abnormal lesions when providing dental care. *Malignant lesions in the mouth are common in the elderly, especially if there is a history of smoking or alcohol use. The elderly are least likely to see a dentist, and often lesions are pain-less until they invade other structures (Aubertin, 1997).*
- ▲ Consider professional oral health care for the elderly in nursing homes. **Clinical Research:** *POHC administered by dental hygienists to a group of elderly patients needing daily nursing care was associated with a reduction in prevalence of fever and fatal pneumonia (Adachi, 2002).*
- Ensure that dentures are removed and cleaned regularly, preferably after every meal and before bedtime; select appropriate adhesives to improve breath. Dentures left in the mouth at night impede circulation to the palate and predispose the client to oral lesions. **Clinical Research:** *Fixodent denture adhesives provide the denture wearer with a noticeable improvement in breath (Myatt et al, 2002).*
- ▲ Recognize that halitosis in older adults is a common condition that may have oral or

• = **Independent;** ▲ = **Collaborative**

nonoral sources. *Bad breath may reflect serious local or systemic conditions, including gingivitis, periodontal disease, diabetic acidosis, hepatic failure, or respiratory infection. Nonoral sources require treatment of the underlying cause, whereas suspected oral sources require referral for a dental evaluation (Durham et al, 1993).*

Infants/children

- Expectant mothers should eat a healthy, balanced diet that is rich in calcium. A set of teeth is in place when the baby is born. The teeth usually start to form in the gums during the second trimester of pregnancy. To encourage the development of good, strong teeth, expectant mothers should eat a healthy, balanced diet that is rich in calcium (Koop, 2003).

Infant oral hygiene

- Gently wipe baby's gums with a washcloth or sterile gauze at least once a day. *Wiping gums prevents bacterial buildup in the mouth (Koop, 2003).* **Evidence-Based Research:** *Infants of breastfeeding mothers need early and consistent mouth care when the teeth erupt. This study was not able to determine a definite time when breastfed infants should be weaned after eruption of teeth to prevent caries; therefore early and consistent mouth care is imperative (Valaitis et al, 2000).*
- Never allow child to fall asleep with a bottle containing milk, formula, fruit juice, or sweetened liquids. If child needs a comforter between regular feedings, at night, or during naps, fill a bottle with cool water or give the child a clean pacifier recommended by your dentist or physician. Never give child a pacifier dipped in any sweet liquid. Avoid filling child's bottle with liquids such as sugar water and soft drinks. *Decay in infants and children is referred to as baby bottle tooth decay. It can destroy the teeth and most often occurs in the upper front teeth, but other teeth may also be affected. Decay occurs when sweetened liquids are given and are left clinging to an infant's teeth for long periods. Many sweet liquids cause problems, including milk, formula, and fruit juice. Bacteria in the mouth use these sugars as food. They then produce acids that attack the teeth. Each time your child drinks these liquids, acids attack for 20 minutes or longer. After many attacks, the teeth can decay. It is not just what is put in the child's bottle that causes decay, but how often—and for how long (American Dental Association, 2003).*
- When multiple teeth appear, brush with small toothbrush with small (pea-sized) amount of fluoride toothpaste. Recommend that child receive a fluoride gel treatment topically. **Clinical Research:** *Fluoride gels can inhibit caries formation in the teeth of children (Marinho et al, 2002; MMWR, 2001).*

Older children

- ▲ Talk with your dentist about dental sealants. *They can help prevent cavities in permanent teeth.* **Clinical Research:** *Sealants should be available to all children regardless of socioeconomic status. In this study, children of low socioeconomic status in this study had a higher rate of caries in primary and permanent teeth than children of higher socioeconomic status (Gillcrist et al, 2001).*
- Use dental floss to help prevent gum disease. Talk with your dentist about when to start. Do not permit your child to smoke or chew tobacco. Set a good example—do not use tobacco products yourself. If a permanent tooth is knocked out, rinse it gently and put it back into the socket or in a glass of cold milk or water. See a dentist immediately (Consumer Information, 2001).

- • = Independent; ▲ = Collaborative

- Drink fluoridated water when possible. **Clinical Research:** *Drinking water fluoridation is associated with an increase in the percentage of 5-year-old children with no experience of tooth decay (Gray and Davies-Slowik, 2001).*
▲ Parasitosis should be considered as a possible cause of halitosis in the pediatric patient population. **Clinical Research:** *Among those children who had evidence of parasites in stool samples at the beginning of the trial, 18 of 28 who were treated with mebendazole recovered from halitosis. Mebendazole therapy seems to offer benefit to those children with parasites as a potential cause of their halitosis (Ermis, 2002).*

Multicultural

- Assess for the influence of cultural beliefs, norms, and values on the client's understanding of dental care. **Nursing Research:** *What the client considers normal and abnormal dental care may be based on cultural perceptions (Cochran, 1998; Doswell and Erlen, 1998; Leininger and McFarland, 2002).*
- Assess for access to dental care insurance. **Nursing Research:** *Poverty and lack of dental care insurance may prevent the obtainment of dental care (Woolfolk et al, 1999).*
- Instruct mothers on the danger of feeding infants bottles filled with soda, juice, or milk when the infant goes to sleep. **Nursing Research:** *Studies have shown that Navajo, African American, Latino, and some other cultural groups engage in this feeding practice, which is known to cause dental caries in children (Andrews, 2003).*
- Assess for dental anxiety. **Nursing Research:** *Anxiety is a major reason for infrequent dental checkups (Woolfolk et al, 1999).*
- Validate the client's feelings with regard to dental health and access to dental care. **Nursing Research:** *Validation is the therapeutic communication technique that lets the client know that the nurse has heard and understands what was said, and it promotes the nurse-client relationship (Heineken, 1998).*

Home care

- Assess client patterns for daily and professional dental care and related patterns (e.g., smoking, nail biting). Assess for environmental influences on dental status (e.g., fluoride). **Clinical Research:** *Many dental problems are preventable with good dental hygiene and care. Behaviors to preserve oral health in old age are essential (Barmes, 2000).*
- Assess client facilities and financial resources for providing dental care. *Lack of appropriate facilities or financial resources is a barrier to positive dental care patterns. Provision for dental care may be missing from health care plans or unavailable to the uninsured.*
- Request dietary log from the client, adding column for type of food (i.e., soft, pureed, regular).
- Observe typical meal to assess first-hand the impact of impaired dentition on nutrition. *Clients, especially the elderly, are often hesitant to admit nutritional changes that may be embarrassing.*
- Identify mechanical needs for food preparation and ease of ingestion/digestion to meet the client's dental/nutritional needs.
- Assist the client with accessing financial or other resources to support optimum dental and nutritional status.

Client/Family Teaching

- Teach how to inspect the oral cavity and monitor for problems with the teeth and gums.

- **= Independent; ▲ = Collaborative**

- Teach how to implement a personal plan of dental hygiene, including appropriate brushing of teeth and tongue and use of dental floss. **Clinical Research:** *Toothbrushing and flossing appropriately used and in conjunction with regular professional care, are capable of virtually preventing caries and most periodontal disease and maintaining oral health (Choo et al, 2001).*
- Teach the client the value of having an optimal fluoride concentration in drinking water, and to brush teeth twice daily with fluoride toothpaste. *This recommendation helps achieve maximum protection against dental caries (MMWR, 2001).*
- Teach clients of all ages the need to decrease intake of sugary foods and to brush teeth regularly. **Clinical Research:** *One study demonstrated that intake of foods such as caramel, toffees, and sugar lumps increased the number of organisms on the teeth significantly. Just 1 day of withdrawal of normal oral hygiene resulted in an approximately 10-fold increase in the number of microorganisms on the teeth (Beighton et al, 1999).*
- Suggest chewing gum with sugar to reduce oral malodor. *Sugarless chewing gum increased methyl mercaptan, one of the principal components of oral malodor (Yaegaki, 2002).*
- Inform individuals who are considering tongue piercing of the potential complications such as chipping and cracking of teeth and possible trauma to the gingiva. If piercing is done, teach the client how to care for the wound, and prevent complications. *These are examples of possible complication, often clients are not informed of appropriate care following piercing (De Moor et al, 2000; Knox, 2002).* **Clinical Research:** *Complications identified in the literature: postoperative swelling, infection, and bleeding, damage to the dentition, and trauma to the soft tissues (Knox, 2002).*

evolve WEBSITES FOR EDUCATION

See the EVOLVE website for World Wide Web resources for client education.

REFERENCES

Adachi M et al: Effect of professional oral health care on the elderly living in nursing homes, *Oral Surg Oral Med Oral Pathol Oral Radiol Endod* 94(2):191, 2002.

American Dental Association: Preventing baby bottle tooth decay, available on-line at http:www.ada.org/public/faq/bottle.html#decay, accessed February 25, 2003.

Andrews MM: Transcultural perspectives in the nursing care of children. In Andrews MM, Boyle J, editors: *Transcultural concepts in nursing practice*, Philadelphia, 2003, Lippincott.

Aubertin MA: Oral cancer screening in the elderly: the home healthcare nurse's role, *Home Healthc Nurse* 15(9): 595, 1997.

Barmes DE: Public policy on oral health and old age: a global view, *J Public Health Dent* 60(4):335, 2000.

Beighton D et al: The influence of specific foods and oral hygiene on the microflora of fissures and smooth surfaces of molar teeth: a 5-day study, *Caries Res* 33(5):349, 1999.

Brown CG, Yoder LH: Stomatitis: an overview, *Am J Nurs* 102(suppl 4):20, 2002

Choo A, Delac DM, Messer LB: Oral hygiene measures and promotion: review and considerations, *Aust Dent J* 46(3):166, 2001.

Cochran M: Tears have no color, *Am J Nurs* 98(6):53, 1998.

Consumer information: *Child health guide: put prevention into practice*, Rockville, Md, Agency for Health Care Policy and Research, available on-line at www.ahcpr.gov/ppip/ppchild.htm#dental, accessed May 26, 2001.

De Moor RJ, De Witte AM, De Bruyne MA: Tongue piercing and associated oral and dental complications, *Endod Dent Traumatol* 16(5):232, 2000.

DeWalt EM: Effect of timed hygienic measures on oral mucosa in a group of elderly subjects, *Nurs Res* 24(2): 104, 1975.

- = Independent; ▲ = Collaborative

Doswell W, Erlen J: Multicultural issues and ethical concerns in the delivery of revising care interventions, *Nurs Clin North Am* 33(2):353, 1998.

Durham TM, Malloy T, Hodges ED: Halitosis: knowing when "bad breath" signals systemic disease, *Geriatrics* 48(8):55, 1993.

Ermis B et al: A randomized placebo-controlled trial of mebendazole for halitosis, *Arch Pediatr Adolesc Med* 156(10):995, 2002.

Gillcrist JA, Brumley DE, Blackford JU: Community socioeconomic status and children's dental health, *J Am Dent Assoc* 132(2):216, 2001.

Gray MM, Davies-Slowik J: Changes in the percentage of 5-year-old children with no experience of decay in Dudley towns since the implementation of fluoridation schemes in 1987, *Br Dent J* 190(1):30, 2001.

Heineken J: Patient silence is not necessarily client satisfaction: communication in home care nursing, *Home Healthc Nurse* 16(2):115, 1998.

Kleinberg I, Wolff MS, Codipilly DM: Role of saliva in oral dryness, oral feel and oral malodour, *Int Dent J* 52(suppl 3):236, 2002.

Knox KT: The potential complications of intra-oral and peri-oral piercing, *Dent Health* 41:3, 2002.

Koop CE: Kids' dental health, available on-line at http://www.drkoop.com/template.asp?page=newsdetailandap=93andid=508508, accessed February 25, 2003.

Leininger MM, McFarland MR: *Transcultural nursing: concepts, theories, research and practices,* ed 3, New York, 2002, McGraw-Hill.

Marinho VC et al: Fluoride gels for preventing dental caries in children and adolescents, *Cochrane Library* 3(CD002280), 2002.

MMWR: Recommendations for using fluoride to prevent and control dental caries in the United States, *MMWR Recomm Rep* 50(RR-14):1, 2001

Myatt GJ et al: A clinical study to assess the breath protection efficacy of denture adhesive, *J Contemp Dent Pract* 3(4):1, 2002.

Pearson LS, Hutton JL: A controlled trial to compare the ability of foam swabs and toothbrushes to remove dental plaque, *J Adv Nurs* 39(5):480, 2002.

Roberts J: Developing an oral assessment and intervention tool for older people, *Br J Nurs* 9(18):2033, 2000.

Sasahara H, Kawamura M: Behavioral dental science: the relationship between tooth-brushing angle and plaque removal at the lingual surfaces of the posterior teeth in the mandible, *J Oral Sci* 42(2):79, 2000.

Scannapieco FA, Stewart EM, Mylotte JM: Colonization of dental plaque by respiratory pathogens in medical intensive care patients, *Crit Care Med* 20:740, 1992.

Stiefel KA et al: Improving oral hygiene for the seriously ill patient: implementing research-based practice, *Medsurg Nurs* 9(1):40, 2000.

Tombes MB, Gallucci B: The effects of hydrogen peroxide rinses on the normal oral mucosa, *Nurs Res* 42:332, 1993.

Valaitis R et al: A systematic review of the relationship between breastfeeding and early childhood caries, *Can J Public Health* 91(6):411, 2000.

Walton JC, Miller J, Tordecilla L: Elder oral assessment and care, *Medsurg Nurs* 10:1, 2001.

Whitmyer CC et al: Clinical evaluation of the efficacy and safety of an ultrasonic toothbrush system in an elderly patient population, *Geriatr Nurs* 19(1):29, 1998.

Winslow EH: Research for practice: don't use H_2O_2 for oral care, *Am J Nurs* 94(3):19, 1994.

Woolfolk MW et al: Determining dental checkup frequency, *J Am Dental Assoc* 130(5):715, 1999.

Yaegaki K et al: Tongue brushing and mouth rinsing as basic treatment measures for halitosis, *Int Dent J* 52(suppl 3):192, 2002.

Risk for delayed Development

T. Heather Herdman, Gail B. Ladwig, and Mary Markle

NANDA Definition

At risk for delay of 25% or more in one or more of the areas of social or self-regulatory behavior or cognitive, language, gross, or fine motor skills.

• = Independent; ▲ = Collaborative

Risk Factors

Prenatal
Maternal age younger than 15 or older than 35 years; substance abuse; infections; genetic or endocrine disorders; unplanned or unwanted pregnancy; lack of, late, or poor prenatal care; inadequate nutrition; illiteracy; poverty; depression or other mental disorders; lack of knowledge; domestic abuse

Individual
Prematurity; seizures; congenital or genetic disorders; positive drug screening test; brain damage (e.g., hemorrhage in postnatal period, shaken baby, abuse, accident); vision impairment; hearing impairment or frequent otitis media; chronic illness; technology dependence; failure to thrive; inadequate nutrition; foster or adopted child; lead poisoning; chemotherapy; radiation therapy; natural disaster; behavior disorders; substance abuse

Environmental
Poverty; violence

Caregiver
Abuse; mental illness; mental retardation or severe learning disability

NOC　Outcomes (Nursing Outcomes Classification)

Suggested NOC Outcomes
Child Development: 2 Months, 4 Months, 6 Months, 12 Months, 2 Years, 3 Years, 4 Years, Middle Childhood, Adolescence; Mobility; Neurological Status; Physical Maturation: Female, Male; Self-Care: Activities of Daily Living (ADL), Bathing, Dressing, Eating, Hygiene, Instrumental Activities of Daily Living (IADL), Toileting

---

Example NOC Outcome with Indicators

Child Development as evidenced by the following indicators: Appropriate milestones of physical, cognitive, and psychosocial age appropriate progression (Rate each indicator of **Child Development:** 1 = extreme delay from expected range, 2 = substantial delay from expected range, 3 = moderate delay from expected range, 4 = mild delay from expected range, 5 = no delay from expected range [see Section I].)

Client Outcomes

Parents/Primary Caregiver Will (Specify Time Frame):
- Describe realistic, age-appropriate patterns of development
- Promote activities and interactions that support age-related developmental tasks

NIC　Interventions (Nursing Interventions Classification)

Suggested NIC Interventions
Active Listening; Developmental Enhancement: Child; Emotional Support; Kangaroo Care; Self-Care Assistance; Self-Responsibility Facilitation

• = Independent; ▲ = Collaborative

> **Example NIC Activities—Developmental Enhancement: Child**
>
> Teach caregivers about normal developmental milestones and associated behaviors; Enhance parental effectiveness

Nursing Interventions and Rationales

- Refer to care plan for **Delayed Growth and development**.

NOTE: Determination of the etiology for delayed development is critical because it will direct the selection of interventions for treating the diagnosis. Parenting skill deficits, lack of consistency between caregivers, and hospitalization versus a chronic medical condition/developmental disability will necessitate different strategies. A hospitalization experience with regressive behaviors can be a transient occurrence as opposed to a chronic situation, which may have more severe and longer delays requiring more in-depth intervention. Parenting skills and consistent expectations between multiple caregivers can be addressed by more intensive education efforts (Seideman and Kleine, 1995; Stutts, 1994).

Multicultural

- Acknowledge racial/ethnic differences at the onset of care. **Nursing Research:** *Acknowledgment of race/ethnicity issues will enhance communication, establish rapport, and promote treatment outcomes (D'Avanzo et al, 2001; Ludwick and Silva, 2000; Vontress and Epp, 1997).*
- Assess for the influence of cultural beliefs, norms, and values on the client's perceptions of child development. **Nursing Research:** *What the client considers normal and abnormal child development may be based on cultural perceptions (Cochran, 1998; Doswell and Erlen, 1998; Leininger and McFarland, 2002).*
- Use a neutral, indirect style when addressing areas in which improvement is needed (such as a need for verbal stimulation) when working with clients. **Nursing Research:** *Using indirect statements such as "Other mothers have tried" or "I had a client who tried 'X' and it seemed to work very well" will assist in avoiding resentment from the parent (Seiderman et al, 1996).*
- Assess whether exposure to community violence is contributing to developmental problems. **Nursing Research:** *Exposure to community violence has been associated with increases in aggressive behavior and depression (Gorman-Smith and Tolan, 1998).*
- Validate the client's feelings and concerns related to child's development. **Nursing Research:** *Validation is the therapeutic communication technique that lets the client know that the nurse has heard and understands what was said, and it promotes the nurse-client relationship (Heineken, 1998).*

Home care

- Assess for the presence of substances that could cause developmental delay. *Children's access to substances that cause neurological deficits (e.g., lead-based paints) should be identified and removed.*
- Assist family to identify appropriate skill-building activities for child. *Exposure to age-appropriate or lower age games, toys, activities can provide essential stimuli for development. Family members may need to adjust expectations of child's behaviors to be appropriate not only for age but also for any developmental limitations.*

• = **Independent;** ▲ = **Collaborative**

- Provide emotional support for family members' reactions to evidence of developmental delay. *Parents may be distressed by the potential for developmental delay in a child.*
- ▲ If possible, refer family to a program of animal-assisted therapy. **Nursing Research:** *Research suggests that interactions with dogs may assist clients with pervasive developmental disorders (PDDs) to establish bonds with their social environment. Children with PDD were more playful, more focused, and more aware of their social environment in the presence of a therapy dog as opposed to a toy or a stuffed dog (Martin and Farnum, 2002).*

Client/Family Teaching

- ▲ Encourage mothers to abstain from alcohol and cocaine use during pregnancy; refer to treatment programs for substance abuse. **Clinical Research:** *Findings indicate that deficiencies in motor development remain detectable at 2 years of age in children exposed to drugs prenatally. Although other environmental variables may influence motor development, children exposed to cocaine and to alcohol in utero may encounter developmental challenges that impede later achievement (Arendt et al, 1999).*
- ▲ Provide support groups and education on human immunodeficiency virus (HIV) and caring for infants with this diagnosis. *Developmental delay has been well documented in HIV-infected infants (Potterton and Eales, 2001).*
- Provide developmental care interventions to preterm infants to improve neurodevelopmental outcomes. **Clinical Research:** *Developmental care is effective to improve outcomes (Symington and Pinelli, 2002).*
- Provide neonatal positioning procedures for preterm infants to prevent extremity malalignment, skull deformities, and gross motor delay. *Alignment and shaping of the musculoskeletal system occur with each body position change in an NICU—use of proper positioning strategies promotes skeletal integrity, postural control, and sensorimotor organization (Sweeney and Gutierrez, 2002).*
- Encourage adequate antepartum and postpartum care for both mother and child. *Access to prenatal and postnatal health care promotes optimal growth and development (Bland, 2000; Starfield, 1992).*
- Counsel parents, siblings, and caregivers about the importance of smoking cessation and the necessity of eliminating all secondhand smoke exposure. *Cigarette smoke is a well-known carcinogen that also contributes to chronic respiratory infections in children (Gergen et al, 1998).*
- Teach caregivers of children appropriate developmental interactions; use anticipatory guidance to facilitate preparation for developmental milestones. **Clinical Research:** *Children with IQ scores of 90 or higher had more developmentally appropriate interaction by caregivers (P = 0.043) and higher scores on six of eight subscales and Total HOME (P = 0.05) than the group of children with IQ scores of less than 90. Conclusions: Two postnatal factors—home environment and caregiver-child interaction—were associated with full-scale IQ scores of 90 or higher, whereas prenatal and natal factors were not. These potentially malleable postnatal factors can be targeted for change to improve cognitive outcome of inner-city children (Hurt et al, 1998).*

evolve WEBSITES FOR EDUCATION

See the EVOLVE website for World Wide Web resources for client education.

• = Independent; ▲ = Collaborative

REFERENCES

Arendt R et al: Motor development of cocaine-exposed children at age two years, *Pediatrics* 103(1):86, 1999.

Bland M et al: Late third trimester treatment of rectovaginal group B streptococci with benzathine penicillin G, *Am J Obstet Gynecol* 183(2):372, 2000.

Cochran M: Tears have no color, *Am J Nurs* 98(6):53, 1998.

D'Avanzo CE et al: Developing culturally informed strategies for substance-related interventions. In Naegle MA, D'Avanzo CE, editors: *Addictions and substance abuse: strategies for advanced practice nursing,* St Louis, 2001, Mosby.

Doswell W, Erlen J: Multicultural issues and ethical concerns in the delivery of revising care interventions, *Nurs Clin North Am* 33(2):353, 1998.

Gergen PJ et al: The burden of environmental tobacco smoke exposure on the respiratory health of children 2 months through 5 years of age in the United States, *Pediatrics* 101(2):E8, 1998.

Giger JN, Davidhizar RE: *Transcultural nursing,* ed 2, St Louis, 1995, Mosby.

Gorman-Smith D, Tolan P: The role of exposure to community violence and developmental problems among inner city youth, *Dev Psychopathol* 10(1):101, 1998.

Heineken J: Patient silence is not necessarily client satisfaction: communication in home care nursing, *Home Healthc Nurse* 16(2):115, 1998.

Hurt H et al: Inner-city achievers: who are they? *Arch Pediatr Adolesc Med* 152(10):993, 1998.

Leininger MM, McFarland MR: *Transcultural nursing: concepts, theories, research and practices,* ed 3, New York, 2002, McGraw-Hill.

Ludwick R, Silva M: Nursing around the world: cultural values and ethical conflicts, *Online J Issues Nurs,* available on-line at http://www.nursingworld.org/ojin/ethcol/ethics_4.htm.

Martin F, Farnum J: Animal-assisted therapy for children with pervasive developmental disorders, *West J Nurs Res* 24:657, 2002.

Potterton J, Eales C: Prevalence of developmental delay in infants who are HIV positive, *S Afr J Physiother* 57(3):11, 2001.

Seideman RJ, Kleine PF: Theory of transformed parenting: parenting a child with developmental delay/mental retardation, *Nurs Res* 44:38, 1995.

Seiderman RY et al: Assessing American Indian families, *MCN Am J Matern Child Nurs* 21(6):274, 1996.

Starfield B: *Primary care,* New York, 1992, Oxford University Press.

Stuart GW, Laraia MT: Therapeutic nurse-patient relationship. In Stuart GW, Laraia MT, editors: *Principles and practice of psychiatric nursing,* St Louis, 2001, Mosby.

Stutts AL: Selected outcomes of technology dependent children receiving home care and prescribed child care services, *Pediatr Nurs* 20:501, 1994.

Sweeney J, Gutierrez T: Musculoskeletal implications of preterm infant positioning in the NICU, *J Perinat Neonat Nurs* 16(1):58, 2002.

Symington A, Pinelli J: Developmental care for promoting development and preventing morbidity in preterm infants, *Cochrane Library* 3(CD001814), 2002.

Vontress CE, Epp LR: Historical hostility in the African American client: implications for counseling, *J Multicult Counseling Dev* 25:170, 1997.

Diarrhea

Betty J. Ackley

NANDA   Definition

Passage of loose, unformed stools

Defining Characteristics

Hyperactive bowel sounds; at least three loose liquid stools per day; urgency; abdominal pain; cramping

• = Independent; ▲ = Collaborative

Related Factors (r/t)

Psychological
High stress levels and anxiety

Situational
Alcohol abuse; toxins; laxative abuse; radiation; tube feedings; adverse effects of medications; contaminants; travel

Physiological
Inflammation; malabsorption; infectious processes; irritation; parasites

NOC   Outcomes (Nursing Outcomes Classification)

Suggested NOC Outcomes
Bowel Elimination; Electrolyte and Acid-Base Balance; Fluid Balance; Hydration; Treatment Behavior: Illness or Injury

---

Example NOC Outcome with Indicators

Bowel Elimination as evidenced by the following indicators: Elimination pattern in expected range/Stool soft and formed/Diarrhea not present/Control of bowel movements/Comfort of stool passage/Painful cramps not present (Rate each indicator of **Bowel Elimination:** 1 = extremely compromised, 2 = substantially compromised, 3 = moderately compromised, 4 = mildly compromised, 5 = not compromised [see Section I].)

Client Outcomes

Client Will (Specify Time Frame):
- Defecate formed, soft stool every day to every third day
- Maintain a rectal area free of irritation
- State relief from cramping and less or no diarrhea
- Explain cause of diarrhea and rationale for treatment
- Maintain good skin turgor and weight at usual level
- Contain stool appropriately (if previously incontinent)

NIC   Interventions (Nursing Interventions Classification)

Suggested NIC Intervention
Diarrhea Management

Example NIC Activities—Diarrhea Management

Evaluate medication profile for gastrointestinal side effects; Suggest trial elimination of foods containing lactose

---

Nursing Interventions and Rationales

- Assess pattern of defecation or have the client keep a diary that includes the following: time of day defecation occurs; usual stimulus for defecation; consistency, amount, and frequency of stool; type of, amount of, and time food consumed; fluid intake; history of bowel habits and laxative use; diet; exercise patterns; obstetrical/gynecological, medical, and surgical histories; medications; alterations in perianal sensations; and

- = Independent; ▲ = Collaborative

present bowel regimen. *Assessment of defecation pattern will help direct treatment (Hogan, 1998; Mertz et al, 1995).*

- Identify cause of diarrhea if possible (e.g., viral, rotavirus, HIV); food; medication effect; radiation therapy; protein malnutrition; laxative abuse; stress). See Related Factors (r/t). *Identification of the underlying cause is imperative because the treatment and expected outcome depend on it. If the onset of diarrhea is sudden with no obvious cause, a colonoscopy is recommended to rule out colon cancer. When reviewing medication, assess for medications that increase peristalsis, such as metoclopramide (Reglan). HIV infection is also commonly associated with diarrhea (Anastasi, 1993).*
- If the client has watery diarrhea, a low-grade fever, abdominal cramps, and a history of antibiotic therapy, consider possibility of *Clostridium difficile* infection. C. difficile *infection and pseudomembranous colitis have become increasingly common because of the frequent use of broad-spectrum antibiotics (Gantz et al, 1998; Vogel, 1995).*
- ▲ If the client has diarrhea associated with antibiotic therapy, consult with primary care practitioner regarding the use of probiotics such as yogurt with active cultures to treat diarrhea (Van Niel et al, 2002) or also use probiotics to prevent diarrhea when first beginning antibiotic therapy. **Clinical Research:** *A study demonstrated that ingestion of Lactobacillus could be helpful to treat children with acute infectious diarrhea caused by a virus (Van Niel et al, 2002). Probiotics have been shown to be helpful to prevent antibiotic-associated diarrhea (D'Souza et al, 2002; Teitelbaum and Walker, 2002).*
- ▲ Use Standard Precautions when caring for clients with diarrhea to prevent spread of infectious diarrhea; use gloves and hand washing. *C. difficile has been shown to be contagious and at times epidemic. C. difficile is spread by direct or indirect contact, placing other clients at risk for infection (Miller et al, 1998).*
- ▲ Obtain stool specimens as ordered to either rule out or diagnose an infectious process (e.g., ova and parasites, *C. difficile* infection, bacterial cultures). **Clinical Research:** *One study of medical patients demonstrated that more than 30% developed nosocomial diarrhea after admission to a nursing unit, and the majority of cases were caused by C. difficile (McFarland, 1995). If the client has infectious diarrhea, avoid using medications that slow peristalsis. If an infectious process is occurring, such as C. difficile infection or food poisoning, medication to slow down peristalsis should generally not be given (Bliss et al, 2000). The increase in gut motility helps eliminate the causative factor, and use of antidiarrheal medication could result in a toxic megacolon (Gantz et al, 1998).*
- Observe and record number and consistency of stools per day; if desired, use a fecal incontinence collector for accurate measurement of output. *Documentation of output provides a baseline and helps direct replacement fluid therapy.*
- Inspect, palpate, percuss, and auscultate abdomen; note whether bowel sounds are frequent.
- Assess for dehydration by observing skin turgor over sternum and inspecting for longitudinal furrows of the tongue. Watch for excessive thirst, fever, dizziness, lightheadedness, palpitations, excessive cramping, bloody stools, hypotension, and symptoms of shock. *Severe diarrhea can cause deficient fluid volume with extreme weakness (Hogan, 1998) and cause death in the very young, the chronically ill, and the elderly.*
- Observe for symptoms of sodium and potassium loss (e.g., weakness, abdominal or leg cramping, dysrhythmia). Note results of electrolyte laboratory studies. *Stool contains electrolytes; excessive diarrhea causes electrolyte abnormalities that can be especially harmful to clients with existing medical conditions.*
- Monitor and record intake and output; note oliguria and dark, concentrated urine.

- **● = Independent; ▲ = Collaborative**

Measure specific gravity of urine if possible. *Dark, concentrated urine, along with a high specific gravity of urine, is an indication of deficient fluid volume.*

- Weigh the client daily and note decreased weight. *An accurate daily weight is an important indicator of fluid balance in the body (Metheny, 2000).*
- Give clear fluids as tolerated (e.g., clear soda, Jell-O), serving at lukewarm temperature. For children with diarrhea, give reduced osmolarity oral rehydration therapy liquids (Pedialyte) as directed by physician. **Nursing and Clinical Research:** *Oral rehydration therapy is effective for treating mild to moderate dehydration in children with diarrhea and may help prevent the need for hospitalization with administration of intravenous fluids (Larson, 2000). Reduced osmolarity oral rehydration fluid compared with standard rehydration fluid resulted in lower stool volume, less need for intravenous fluids, and less vomiting (Hahnn et al, 2002).*
- ▲ If diarrhea is associated with cancer or cancer treatment, once infectious cause of diarrhea is ruled out, provide medications as ordered to stop diarrhea. *The loss of proteins, electrolytes, and water from diarrhea in a cancer client can lead to rapid deterioration and possibly fatal dehydration (Kornblau et al, 2000).*
- ▲ If the client has chronic diarrhea causing fecal incontinence at intervals, consider suggesting use of dietary fiber from psyllium or gum Arabic after consultation with primary practitioner. **Nursing and Clinical Research:** *A study demonstrated that use of a fiber supplement decreased the number of incontinent stools and improved stool consistency in a group of adults (Bliss et al, 2001). The use of soluble dietary fiber is useful for controlling diarrhea and normalizing the intestinal flora (Nakao et al, 2002).*
- ▲ If diarrhea is chronic and there is evidence of malnutrition, consult with primary care practitioner for a dietary consult and possible use of a hydrolyzed formula (a clear liquid supplement containing increased protein) to maintain nutrition while the gastrointestinal system heals. *A hydrolyzed formula contains protein that is partially broken down to small peptides or amino acids for people who cannot digest nutrients (Cataldo et al, 1999).*
- Encourage the client to eat small, frequent meals and to consume foods that normally cause constipation and are easy to digest (e.g., bananas, crackers, pretzels, rice, potatoes, applesauce). Encourage the client to avoid milk products, foods high in fiber, and caffeine (dark sodas, tea, coffee, chocolate). *Bland, starchy foods are initially recommended when starting to eat solid food again (Rice, 1994).*
- Provide a readily available bedpan, commode, or bathroom. If the client has diarrhea and incontinence, consider use of a Perineal Assessment Tool to measure the risk for perineal skin injury. **Nursing Research:** *An instrument entitled the Perineal Assessment Tool has been developed to determine the risk of perineal skin injury. The initial results of the study are encouraging, and further studies are needed (Nix, 2002).*
- Maintain perirectal skin integrity. Cleanse with a mild cleansing agent (perineal skin cleanser). Apply protective ointment prn (Haisfield-Wolfe and Rund, 2000). If skin is still excoriated and desquamated, apply a wound hydrogel. Avoid the use of rectal Foley catheters. *Moisture-barrier ointments protect the skin from excoriation. Rectal Foley catheters can cause rectal necrosis, sphincter damage, or rupture, and the nursing staff may not have the time to properly follow the necessary and very time-consuming steps of their care (Bosley, 1994; Fiers, 1996).*
- If the client is receiving a tube feeding, do not assume it is the cause of diarrhea. Perform a complete assessment to rule out other causes such as medication effects, sorbitol in medications, or an infection. *Research has shown that tube feedings do not usually*

- = Independent; ▲ = Collaborative

cause diarrhea (Campbell, 1994). However, sorbitol in medication has been linked to diarrhea (Drug Watch, 1994).

- If the client is receiving a tube feeding, note rate of infusion, and prevent contamination of feeding by rinsing container every 8 hours and replacing it every 24 hours. *Rapid administration of tube feeding and contaminated feedings have been associated with diarrhea.*
- If the client is receiving a tube feeding, suggest formulas that contain a bulking agent such as Jevity, or add soluble dietary fiber to the feeding per physicians/dietitians order. **Clinical Research:** *Bulking agents including soluble fiber are useful in tube feedings to prevent or treat diarrhea in the tube-fed client (Nakao et al, 2002).*

Geriatric

▲ Evaluate medications the client is taking. Recognize that many medications can result in diarrhea, including digitalis, propranolol, angiotensin-converting enzyme (ACE) inhibitors, histamine-receptor antagonists, NSAIDs, anticholinergic agents, oral hypoglycemia agents, antibiotics, and others. *A drug-associated cause should always be considered when treating diarrhea in the older person; many drugs can result in diarrhea (Ratnaike, 2000).*

▲ Monitor the client closely to detect whether an impaction is causing diarrhea; remove impaction as ordered. *Impactions are more common in the elderly than in younger clients. It is very important that the client be checked for impaction before being given any antidiarrheal medication (Carnaveli and Patrick, 1993).*

▲ Seek medical attention if diarrhea is severe or persists for more than 24 hours, or if the client has symptoms of dehydration or electrolyte disturbances such as lassitude, weakness, or prostration. *Elderly clients can dehydrate rapidly. The greatest concern for elderly clients with severe diarrhea is hypokalemia. Hypokalemia is treatable but when missed can be fatal (Carnaveli and Patrick, 1993).*

- Provide emotional support for clients who are having trouble controlling unpredictable episodes of diarrhea. *Diarrhea can be a great source of embarrassment to the elderly and can lead to social isolation and a feeling of powerlessness (Carnaveli and Patrick, 1993).*

Home care

- Above interventions may be adapted for home care use.
- Assess the home for general sanitation and methods of food preparation. Reinforce principles of sanitation for food handling. *Poor sanitation or mishandling of food may cause bacterial infection or transmission of dangerous organisms from utensils to food.*
- Assess for methods of handling soiled laundry if the client is bed bound or has been incontinent. Instruct or reinforce Universal Precautions with family and blood-borne pathogen precautions with agency caregivers. *The Bloodborne Pathogen Regulations of the Occupational Safety and Health Administration (OSHA) identify legal guidelines for caregivers.*

▲ When assessing medication history, include over-the-counter drugs, both general and those currently being used to treat the diarrhea. Instruct clients not to mix over-the-counter medications when self-treating. *Mixing over-the-counter medications can further irritate the gastrointestinal system, intensifying the diarrhea or causing nausea and vomiting.*

▲ Evaluate current medications for indication that specific interventions are warranted.

- **= Independent;** ▲ **= Collaborative**

Blood levels of medications may increase during prolonged episodes of diarrhea, indicating the need for close monitoring of the client or direct intervention.

▲ Consult with physician regarding need for blood work or stool specimens. *Laboratory tests may be needed to identify presence of a bacterial pathogen or assess for electrolyte imbalance.*

▲ Evaluate need for home health aide or homemaker service referral. *Caregiver may need support for maintaining client cleanliness to prevent skin breakdown (e.g., may benefit from assistance with washing bedclothes).*

▲ Evaluate need for durable medical equipment in the home. *The client may need bedside commode, call bell, or raised toilet seat to facilitate prompt toileting.*

Client/Family Teaching

• Encourage avoidance of coffee, spices, milk products, and foods that irritate or stimulate the gastrointestinal tract.
• Teach appropriate method of taking ordered antidiarrheal medications; explain side effects.
• Explain how to prevent the spread of infectious diarrhea (e.g., careful hand washing, appropriate handling and storage of food).
• Help the client to determine stressors and set up an appropriate stress reduction plan.
• Teach signs and symptoms of dehydration and electrolyte imbalance.
• Teach perirectal skin care.

evolve WEBSITES FOR EDUCATION

See the EVOLVE website for World Wide Web resources for client education.

REFERENCES

Anastasi J: Diarrhea in acquired immune deficiency syndrome (AIDS), *Ostomy Wound Manage* 39:14, 1993.

Bliss D et al: Supplementation with dietary fiber improves fecal incontinence, *Nurs Res* 50(4):203, 2001.

Bliss DZ et al: Fecal incontinence in hospitalized patients who are acutely ill, *Nurs Res* 49(2):101, 2000.

Bockus S: When your patient needs tube feeding: making the right decision, *Nursing* 93:34, 1993.

Bosley C: Three methods of stool management for patients with diarrhea, *Ostomy Wound Manage* 40:52, 1994.

Campbell C: Research for practice: diarrhea not always linked to tube feedings, *Am J Nurs* 94(4):59, 1994.

Carnaveli DL, Patrick M: *Nursing management for the elderly,* ed 3, Philadelphia, 1993, Lippincott.

Cataldo CB, DeBruyne LK, Whitney EN: *Nutrition and diet therapy,* Belmont, Calif, 1999, Wadsworth.

Doughty D: Maintaining normal bowel function in the patient with cancer, *J Enterostomal Nurs* 18:90, 1991.

Drug Watch: Sorbitol: missing link to diarrhea, *Am J Nurs* 10:50, 1994.

D'Souza AL et al: Probiotics in prevention of antibioitic associated diarrhea: meta-analysis, *BMJ* 324(7350), 2002.

Fiers S: Breaking the cycle: the etiology of incontinence dermatitis and evaluating and using skin care products, *Ostomy Wound Manage* 42:32, 1996.

Gantz NM, Gerding DN, Johnson PC: Managing and containing *Clostridium difficile* disease, *Patient Care* April 15:171, 1998.

Hahn S, Kim S, Garner P: Reduced osmolarity oral rehydration solution for treating dehydration caused by acute diarrhea in children, *Cochrane Database Syst Rev* 1(CD002847), 2000.

Haisfield-Wolfe ME, Rund C: A nursing protocol for the management of perineal-rectal skin alterations, *Clin J Oncol Nurs* 4(1):15, 2000.

Hogan CM: The nurse's role in diarrhea management, *Oncol Nurs Forum* 25(5):879, 1998.

Kornblau S et al: Management of cancer treatment-related diarrhea: issues and therapeutic strategies, *J Pain Symptom Manage* 19(2):118, 2000.

• = Independent; ▲ = Collaborative

Larson CE: Evidence-based practice: safety and efficacy of oral rehydration therapy for the treatment of diarrhea and gastroenteritis in pediatrics, *Pediatr Nurs* 26(2):177, 2000.

McFarland LV: Epidemiology of infectious and iatrogenic nosocomial diarrhea in a cohort of general medicine patients, *Am J Infect Control* 23:295, 1995.

Mertz HR et al: Validation of a new measure of diarrhea, *Dig Dis Sci* 40:1873, 1995.

Metheny N: *Fluid and electrolyte balance: nursing considerations,* ed 4, Philadelphia, 2000, Lippincott.

Miller JM, Walton JC, Tordecilla LL: Recognizing and managing Clostridium difficile-associated diarrhea, *Medsurg Nurs* 7(6):348, 1998.

Nakao M et al: Usefulness of soluble dietary fiber for the treatment of diarrhea during general nutrition in elderly patients, *Nutrition* 18(1):35, 2002.

Nix DH: Validity and reliability of the Perineal Assessment Tool, *Ostomy Wound Manage* 48:2, 2002.

Ratnaike RN: Drug-induced diarrhea in older persons, *Clin Geriatr* 8(1):67, 2000.

Rice KH: Oral rehydration therapy: a simple, effective solution, *J Pediatr Nurs* 9:349, 1994.

Teitelbaum JE, Walker WA: Nutritional impact of pre-and probiotics as protective gastrointestinal organisms, *Annu Rev Nutr* 22:107, 2002.

Van Niel CW et al: Lactobacillus therapy for acute infectious diarrhea in children: a meta-analysis, *Pediatrics* 109(4):678, 2002.

Vogel LC: Antibiotic-induced diarrhea, *Orthop Nurs* 14:38, 1995.

Risk for Disuse syndrome

Betty J. Ackley

NANDA Definition

At risk for a deterioration of body systems as the result of prescribed or unavoidable musculoskeletal inactivity

Risk Factors

Paralysis; altered level of consciousness; mechanical immobilization; prescribed immobilization; severe pain (NOTE: complications from immobility can include pressure ulcer, constipation, stasis of pulmonary secretions, thrombosis, urinary tract infection and/or retention, decreased strength or endurance, orthostatic hypotension, decreased range of joint motion, disorientation, disturbed body image, and powerlessness.)

Related Factors (r/t)

See Risk Factors

NOC Outcomes (Nursing Outcomes Classification)

Suggested NOC Outcomes

Endurance; Immobility Consequences: Physiological; Mobility; Neurological Status: Consciousness; Pain Level

> **Example NOC Outcome with Indicators**
>
> **Immobility Consequences: Physiological** as evidenced by the following indicators: Pressure ulcers/Constipation/Decreased nutrition status/Urinary calculi/Decreased muscle strength (Rate each indicator of **Immobility Consequences: Physiological:** 1 = severe, 2 = substantial, 3 = moderate, 4 = slight, 5 = none [see Section I].)

• = Independent; ▲ = Collaborative

Client Outcomes

Client Will (Specify Time Frame):
- Maintain full range of motion in joints
- Maintain intact skin, good peripheral blood flow, and normal pulmonary function
- Maintain normal bowel and bladder function
- Express feelings about imposed immobility
- Explain methods to prevent complications of immobility

NIC Interventions (Nursing Interventions Classification)

Suggested NIC Interventions
Energy Management; Exercise Therapy: Joint Mobility, Muscle Control

> ### Example NIC Activities—Energy Management
>
> Determine the client's physical limitations; Determine the client's significant other's perception of causes of fatigue

Nursing Interventions and Rationales

- Use a functional assessment instrument to evaluate abilities including instruments such as the Barthel Index, the Katz Index of activities of Daily Living, or the FIM instrument. *There are many instruments available to measure client function, and a baseline measurement of function should be done to determine appropriate level of care and services (Quigly, 2001).*
- Have the client do exercises in bed if not contraindicated (e.g., flexing and extending feet and quadriceps, performing gluteal and abdominal sitting exercises, lifting small weights to maintain muscle strength). *Unused muscles lose 1% to 3% of their strength per day, even in healthy persons. A person who is immobilized for 3 weeks may lose half of his or her muscle strength (Fried and Fried, 2001). In-bed exercises help maintain muscle strength and tone (Kasper and Talbor, 2002; Metzlar and Harr, 1996).* **Clinical Research:** *Strength improvement in response to resisted exercise is possible even in the very elderly, extremely sedentary client with multiple chronic diseases and functional disabilities. Increased strength can help prevent falls (Connelly, 2000).*
- ▲ If not contraindicated by the client's condition, obtain referral to physical therapy for use of tilt table to provide weight bearing on long bones. *The upright position helps maintain bone strength, increase circulation, and prevent postural hypotension. The best way to prevent osteoporosis is to begin weight-bearing exercises as soon as possible (Jiricka, 1994).*
- Perform range of motion exercises for all possible joints at least twice daily; perform passive or active range of motion exercises as appropriate. *If not used, muscles weaken and shorten and are predisposed to contractures; if nonuse continues, the contracture eventually involves the tendons, ligaments, and joint capsules and limits the range of motion (Jiricka, 1994).*
- Use high-top sneakers or specialized boots from the occupational therapy department to prevent footdrop; remove shoes twice daily to provide foot care. *Sneakers or boots help keep the foot in normal anatomical alignment; footdrop can make it difficult or impossible to walk after bed rest.*
- Position the client so that joints are in normal anatomical alignment at all times. *Im-*

• = Independent; ▲ = Collaborative

proper positioning can damage peripheral nerves and blood vessels, as well as cause joint deformities (Fried and Fried, 2001).

- Get the client up in a chair as soon as appropriate; use a stretcher-chair if necessary. Assist the client to walk as soon as medically possible. **Clinical Research:** *Almost all clients can get out of bed now with use of the stretcher-chair, which converts from a stretcher to a chair. Bed rest is almost always harmful to clients; early mobilization is better than bed rest for most health conditions (Allen et al, 1999).*

- Consider use of a continuous lateral rotation therapy bed. *Continuous lateral rotation therapy has been shown to be effective for prevention of deep vein thrombosis (DVT) in spinal cord injury clients (Von Rueden and Harris, 1995).* **Clinical Research:** Continuous lateral rotation therapy has been shown to be effective for the prevention of pneumonia in transplant clients (Whiteman et al, 1995).

▲ If at all possible, help the client begin a walking program, using a physical therapist as needed. **Clinical Research:** *Early mobilization has been shown to improve the outcome for clients after treatment of medical conditions and procedures (Allen et al, 1999).*

- Be very careful when helping the client into a chair and when transferring. Be sure to lock beds and wheelchairs. Recognize that there is a high probability for falls. **Clinical Research:** *Nonambulatory clients have a substantially greater number of serious falls than their ambulatory peers: 87% of falls with injuries involved equipment misuse such as not locking beds and wheelchairs, 82% occurred while seated or transferring, and 54% occurred at chair or bed height only (Thapa et al, 1996).*

- Minimize cardiovascular deconditioning by positioning clients as close to the upright position as possible several times daily. *The hazards of bed rest in the elderly are multiple, serious, quick to develop, and slow to reverse. Decondition of the cardiovascular system occurs within days and involves fluid shifts, fluid loss, decreased cardiac output, decreased peak oxygen uptake, and increased resting heart rate (Fried and Fried, 2001; Resnick, 1998a).*

- When getting the client up after bed rest, do so slowly and watch for signs of postural hypotension, tachycardia, nausea, diaphoresis, or syncope. Take the blood pressure lying, sitting, and standing, waiting 2 minutes between each reading. *Sitting or standing after 3 or 4 days of bed rest results in postural hypotension because of cardiovascular reflex dysfunction (Jiricka, 1994; Metzlar and Harr, 1996).*

- Obtain assistive devices such as braces, crutches, or canes to help the client reach and maintain as much mobility as possible. Turn the client at least every 2 hours and carefully observe skin condition, especially bony prominences. *Turning clients is of paramount importance to prevent all of the complications of bed rest (Metzlar and Harr, 1996). Routine turning has been demonstrated to reduce the length of stay of critical care patients (Von Reuden and Harris, 1995).*

- Provide the client with a pressure-relieving horizontal support surface. *Support surfaces can help to relieve pressure. If foam is used, it must be 4 inches thick, or use a static air mattress or low–air-loss surface as appropriate (Maklebust and Sieggreen, 1996). More research is needed to set definitive guidelines with regard to which pressure-relieving horizontal support surfaces are most effective (Maklebust, 1999).*

▲ Request a physical therapy referral to help the client learn how to move self in bed including bridging and also how to transfer out of bed (Fried and Fried, 2001).

▲ Apply graduated compression stockings as ordered. Ensure proper fit by measuring, remove at least twice, in the morning with bath and in the evening to assess condition of extremity, then reapply. **Nursing and Clinical Research:** *A meta-analysis of 11*

• = Independent; ▲ = Collaborative

studies with 1752 subjects demonstrated that graduated compression stockings reduced the incidence of DVT in a high-risk orthopedic surgical population and that additional anti-thrombotic measures along with stockings decreased the incidence even further (Joanna Briggs Institute, 2001). Graduated compression stockings, alone or used in conjunction with other prevention modalities, prevent deep venous thrombosis in hospitalized patients (Amarigiri and Lees, 2000).

- Monitor peripheral circulation and especially note color, pulse, and calf or thigh swelling; check Homans' sign, but recognize that it is an unreliable sign of DVT. *Because of venous stasis, pressure of mattress against veins, and hypercoagulability of blood, bed rest predisposes the client to deep vein thrombosis (Fried and Fried, 2001; Harper and Lyles, 1988). DVT may result in pulmonary embolism in an immobilized client (Metzlar and Harr, 1996).*

- Have the client cough and deep breathe or use incentive spirometry every 2 hours while awake. Bed rest compromises breathing because of decreased chest expansion and decreased size of thoracic compartment; deep breathing helps prevent complications (Jiricka, 1994).

- Monitor respiratory functions, noting breath sounds and respiratory rate. Percuss for new onset of dullness in lungs. *Immobility results in hypoventilation, which predisposes the client to atelectasis, the pooling of respiratory secretions, and thus pneumonia (Fried and Fried, 2001; Tempkin et al, 1997).*

- Note bowel function daily. Provide increased fluids, fiber, and natural laxatives such as prune juice as needed. *Constipation is common in immobilized clients because of decreased activity and fluid and food intake.*

- Increase fluid intake to 2000 ml/day within the client's cardiac and renal reserve. *Adequate fluids help prevent kidney stones and constipation and help counteract dehydration associated with bed rest (Rubin, 1988).*

- Encourage intake of a balanced diet with adequate amounts of fiber and protein. *Reduced muscular activity and lowered metabolism generally reduce the appetite of a client on bed rest (Rubin, 1988).*

Geriatric

- Recognize the importance of keeping elderly clients active if possible. *In the elderly, 10% to 15% of muscle strength can be lost for every week that muscles are resting completely (Mobily and Kelley, 1991).*

▲ If geriatric, the client is scheduled for an elective surgery that will result in admission into ICU and immobility, or recovery from a knee replacement, initiate a prehabilitation program that includes a warm-up, aerobic strength, flexibility, and functional task work. **Nursing Research:** *By increasing the functional capacity of the individual prior to the stressor of inactivity, the predictable declines in physical activity can be prevented or alleviated (Topp et al, 2002). In a study, clients who performed strength activities preoperatively walked significantly greater distances postoperatively after total hip replacement (Whitney and Parkman, 2002).*

▲ Refer to physical therapy for an individualized strength training program. Monitor for signs of depression: flat affect, poor appetite, insomnia, many somatic complaints. *Depression can commonly accompany decreased mobility and function in the elderly (Resnick, 1998b).*

- Keep careful track of bowel function in the elderly; do not allow the client to become constipated. *The elderly can easily develop impactions as a result of immobility.*

- = **Independent**; ▲ = **Collaborative**

Home care

NOTE: Care for all body systems because the immobilized or otherwise at risk client must continue in the home as stated in the previously mentioned interventions. The primary nurse monitors and adjusts the plan of care accordingly per physician orders.

- • Some of the above interventions may be adapted for home care use.
- ▲ Begin discharge planning as soon as possible with case manager or social worker to assess need for home support systems and community or home health services.
- ▲ Become oriented to all programs of care for the client before discharge from institutional care.
- ▲ Confirm the immediate availability of all necessary assistive devices for home.
- ▲ Continuity in management of care promotes success in meeting client-centered goals.
- • Perform complete physical assessment and recent history at initial visit. *A complete assessment validates the status of the client upon discharge and defines client problems needing immediate intervention. Presence of decubitus may indicate need for additional treatment measures.*
- ▲ Refer to physical and occupational therapies for immediate evaluations of the client's potential for independence and functioning in the home setting and for follow-up care. *Early identification of client needs allows for early intervention and prevention of secondary problems.*
- • Allow the client to have as much input and control of the plan of care as possible. *Client perception of control increases self-esteem and motivation to follow medical plan of care.*
- • Assess knowledge of all care with caregivers. Review as necessary. *Having the necessary knowledge and skills to perform care decreases caregiver role strain and supports safety of the client.*
- ▲ Support the family of the client in assumption of caregiver activities. Refer for home health aide services for assistance and respite as appropriate. Refer to medical social services as appropriate.
- ▲ Institute case management of frail elderly to support continued independent living. *Disuse syndrome represents and can lead to increasing needs for assistance in using the health care system effectively. Case management combines nursing activities of the client and family assessment, planning and coordination of care among all health care providers, delivery of direct nursing care, and monitoring of care and outcomes. These activities are able to address continuity of care, mutual goal setting, behavior management, and prevention of worsening health problems (Guttman, 1999).*

Client/Family Teaching

- • Teach how to perform range of motion exercises in bed if not contraindicated.
- • Teach the family how to turn and position the client and provide all care necessary.

NOTE: Nursing diagnoses that are commonly relevant when the client is on bed rest include **Constipation, Risk for impaired Skin integrity, Disturbed Sensory perception; Disturbed Sleep pattern, Adult Failure to thrive,** and **Powerlessness.**

evolve WEBSITES FOR EDUCATION

See the EVOLVE website for World Wide Web resources for client education.

• = Independent; ▲ = Collaborative

REFERENCES

Allen C, Glasziou P, Del Mar C: Bed rest: a potentially harmful treatment needing more careful attention, *Lancet* 354(9186):1229, 1999.

Amarigiri SV, Lees TA: Elastic compression stockings for prevention of deep vein thrombosis, *Cochrane Database Syst Rev* 3(CD001484), 2000.

Connelly DM: Resisted exercise training of institutionalized older adults for improved strength and functional mobility: a review, *Top Geriatr Rehabil* 15(3):6, 2000.

Corcoran PJ: Use it or lose it: the hazards of bed rest and inactivity, *West J Med* 154:536, 1991.

Fried KM, Fried GW: Immobility. In Derstine JB, Hargrove SD, editors: *Comprehensive rehabilitation nursing*, Philadelphia, 2001, WB Saunders.

Guttman R: Case management of the frail elderly in the community, *Clin Nurs Spec* 13(4):174, 1999.

Harper CM, Lyles YM: Physiology and complications of bed rest, *J Am Geriatr Soc* 36:1047, 1988.

Jiricka MK: Alterations in activity intolerance. In Porth CM, editor: *Pathophysiology: concepts of altered health states*, Philadelphia, 1994, Lippincott.

Joanna Briggs Institute: Best practice: graduated compression stockings for the prevention of post-operative venous thromboembolism, *Evidenced Based Practice Information Sheets for Health Professions* 5:2, 2001.

Kasper CE, Talbor LA: Skeletal muscle damage and recovery, *AACN Clin Issues* 13(2):237, 2002.

Maklebust JA: An update on horizontal patient support surfaces, *Ostomy Wound Manage* 45(1A):70S, 1999.

Maklebust JA, Sieggreen M: *Pressure ulcers: guidelines for prevention and nursing management*, ed 2, 1996, Springhouse.

Metzlar DJ, Harr J: Positioning your patient properly, *Am J Nurs* 96:33, 1996.

Mobily PR, Kelley LS: Iatrogenesis in the elderly: factors of immobility, *J Gerontol Nurs* 17:5, 1991.

Quigley P: Functional assessment. In Derstine JB, Hargrove SD, editors: *Comprehensive rehabilitation nursing*, Philadelphia, 2001, WB Saunders.

Resnick B: Predictors of functional ability in geriatric rehabilitation patients, *Rehabil Nurs* 23(1):21, 1998a.

Resnick N: *Geriatric medicine in current medical diagnosis and treatment*, ed 37, Stamford, Conn, 1998b, Appleton and Lange.

Rubin M: The physiology of bed rest, *Am J Nurs* 88:50, 1988.

Tempkin T, Tempkin A, Goodman H: Geriatric rehabilitation, *Nurs Pract Forum* 8(2):59, 1997.

Thapa P et al: Injurious falls in nonambulatory nursing home residents: a comparative study of circumstances, incidence, and risk factors, *J Am Geriatr Soc* 44:273, 1996.

Topp R, Ditmyer M, King K: The effect of bedrest and potential of prehabilitation on patients in the intensive care unit, *AACN Clin Issues* 13(2):263, 2002.

Von Rueden KT, Harris JR: Pulmonary dysfunction related to immobility in the trauma patient, *AACN Clin Issues* 6:212, 1995.

Whiteman K et al: Effects of continuous lateral rotation therapy on pulmonary complications in liver transplant patients, *Am J Crit Care* 4:133, 1995.

Whitney JA, Parkman S: Preoperative physical activity, anesthesia, and analgesia: effects on early postoperative walking after total hip replacement, *Appl Nurs Res* 15(1):19, 2002.

Deficient Diversional activity

Betty J. Ackley

NANDA   Definition

Decreased stimulation from or interest or engagement in recreational or leisure activities

Defining Characteristics

Usual hobbies cannot be undertaken in hospital; patient's statements regarding boredom and the wish for something to do, to read, etc.

Related Factors (r/t)

Environmental lack of diversional activity as a result of long-term hospitalization or frequent or lengthy treatments

• = Independent; ▲ = Collaborative

| NOC | Outcomes (Nursing Outcomes Classification) |

Suggested NOC Outcomes

Leisure Participation; Play Participation; Social Involvement

Example NOC Outcome with Indicators

Leisure Participation as evidenced by the following indicators: Expression of satisfaction with leisure activities/Reports of relaxation from leisure activities/Reports of restfulness of leisure activities (Rate each indicator of **Leisure Participation:** 1 = not adequate, 2 = slightly adequate, 3 = moderately adequate, 4 = substantially adequate, 5 = totally adequate [see Section I].)

Client Outcomes

Client Will (Specify Time Frame):

- Engage in personally satisfying diversional activities

| NIC | Interventions (Nursing Interventions Classification) |

Suggested NIC Interventions

Recreation Therapy; Self-Responsibility Facilitation

Example NIC Activities—Recreation Therapy

Assist the client to identify meaningful recreational activities; Provide safe recreational equipment

Nursing Interventions and Rationales

- Observe for symptoms of deficient diversional activity: yawning, restlessness, flat facial expression, and statements of boredom (Radziewicz, 1992).
- Observe ability to engage in activities that require good vision and use of hands. *Diversional activities must be tailored to the client's capabilities.*
- Discuss activities with clients that are interesting and feasible in the present environment. *Encourage the client to share feelings about situation of inactivity away from usual life activities. Work and hobbies provide structure and continuity to life; the client can feel a sense of loss when unable to engage in usual activities.*
- Encourage a mix of physical and mental activities (e.g., crafts, videotapes). Provide activities that are entertaining, such as videotapes, joke books, or a "humor room." *Humor can help clients reduce anxiety and survive in a high technology environment (Radziewicz, 1992).*
- Use "bread therapy"—have clients bake bread with a bread maker two times per day or prn. *Assembling the ingredients is a group activity can be therapeutic. The smell of bread baking gives a homelike, loving atmosphere to a health care environment.*
- ▲ Arrange animal-assisted therapy, with a dog or cat for the client to interact with and care for. *Studies have demonstrated increased feelings of self-worth, reduced anxiety, reduced blood pressure and triglycerides, and increased relaxation and social functioning in clients involved in animal-assisted therapy (Stanley-Hermans and Miller, 2002).*
- Encourage the client to schedule visitors so that they are not all present at once or at

• = Independent; ▲ = Collaborative

inconvenient times. *A schedule prevents the client from becoming exhausted from frequent company.*

- Provide reading material, television, radio, and books on tape. Provide virtual reality experiences for children, which can be used as distraction techniques during chemotherapy treatments. Recommend programs such as Magic Carpet, Sherlock Holmes Mystery, and Seventh Guest. *Virtual reality experiences as a distraction technique can be effective and result in positive clinical outcomes (Schneider and Workman, 2000).*
- If clients are able to write, have them keep journals; if clients are unable to write, have them record thoughts on tape. *Keeping a journal is diversional and can also help the client deal with the many feelings that result from hospitalization or confinement. A journal can also help the client gain perspective on the situation.*
- ▲ Request recreational or art therapist to assist with providing diversional activities. *Recreational therapists specialize in helping people have fun. Art therapy can be effective for helping people express emotions, as well as provide diversion (Shaw and Wilkinson, 1996).*
- ▲ Request an order for a child life specialist or, if not available, a play therapist for children. Encourage activities such as video projects, use of computer-based support groups for children, such as Starbright World, a computer network where children interact virtually, sharing their experiences and escaping hospital routines. *Therapeutic play is extremely important for children, especially children isolated after bone marrow transplantation (Kuntz et al, 1996). A child life specialist can provide psychosocial assessment and care and therapeutic activities to help children progress developmentally when hospitalized or isolated (Rode et al, 1998).*
- Provide a change in scenery; get the client out of the room as much as possible. *A lack of sensory stimulation and diversity have significantly adverse effects on clients (Hamilton, 1992).*
- Help the client to experience nature through looking at a nature scene from a window, or walking through a park or garden if possible. **Nursing Research:** *Exposure to a natural environment can be helpful to promote relaxation, stress recovery, and mental restoration (Cimprich, 1993, Jones and Haight, 2002).*
- Structure the environment as needed to promote optimal comfort and sensory diversity (e.g., have family bring in posters, banners, or a sound system; change lighting; change direction bed faces). *Modification of the environment is sometimes necessary for the well-being of the client (Williams, 1988).*
- Recommend activities in which the client can watch movement of animals and develop involvement (e.g., bird-watching, keeping a fish tank).
- Work with family to provide music that is enjoyable to the client. **Nursing Research:** *Research has shown that music can help decrease anxiety in hospitalized clients (Evans, 2002; Smolen et al, 2002).*
- Structure the client's schedule around personal wishes for time of care, relaxation, and participation in fun activities. *Increased client control fosters increased client self-esteem.*
- Spend time with the client when possible or arrange for a friendly visitor. *Simply being available for the client as a fellow human being is important and helpful (Gardner, 1992).*

Geriatric

- If the client is able, arrange for him or her to attend a group senior citizen exercise session for progressive strength training, even if exercise can only be done while seated. *Strength training can help seniors improve balance, coordination, range of motion, flexibility, and spatial awareness while receiving social support and having fun (Brill, 1999).*

● = Independent; ▲ = Collaborative

- Encourage involvement in senior citizen activities (e.g., AARP, YMCA, church groups, Gray Panthers). Arrange transportation to activities as needed.
- Encourage clients to use their ability to help others by volunteering. *Assisting others can help the client grow as a generative human being.*
- Provide an environment that promotes activity (e.g., one that has adequate lighting for crafts, large-print books); allow periods of solitude and privacy. *Periods of solitude are important for emotional well-being in the elderly.*
- Use reminiscence therapy either individually or in groups. **Nursing Research:** *Reminiscence therapy can increase social interaction, self-esteem, and well-being (Burnside, 1990; Jonsdottir et al, 2001; Taylor-Price, 1995) and also decrease symptoms of depression (Jones and Beck-Little, 2002).*
- ▲ Use the Eden Alternative with the elderly; bring in appropriate plants for the elderly client to care for, animals such as birds, fish, dogs and cats as appropriate for the client, and children to visit. *The Eden Alternative offers a more natural human habitat where the quality of life is improved resulting in less loneliness, helplessness, and boredom (Barba et al, 2002).*

Multicultural

- ▲ Assess for the influence of cultural beliefs, norms, and values on the client's leisure activity interests. **Nursing Research:** *Leisure interests or hobbies may be based on cultural preferences (Cochran, 1998; Doswell and Erlen, 1998; Leininger and McFarland, 2002).*
- ▲ Validate the client's feelings and concerns related to lack of stimulation or interest in leisure activities. **Nursing Research:** *Validation is a therapeutic communication technique that lets the client know that the nurse has heard and understands what was said and promotes the nurse-client relationship (Heineken, 1998).*

Home care

NOTE: Many of the previously listed interventions should be administered in the home setting (e.g., modifying the environment to stimulate the client, scheduling visitors to allow for rest and activity). Some adaptations will be necessary.

- ▲ Explore with the client previous interests; consider related activities that are within the client's capabilities. *New activities that build on past interests may attract the client's attention and broaden perception of available activities (e.g., a client who enjoyed gardening but is now immobilized may be tempted by landscaping books to plan next season's garden).*
- ▲ Assess the client for depression. Refer for mental health services as indicated. *Anhedonia, or lack of interest in previously enjoyed activities, is part of the syndrome of depression. Increase in diversional activities is unlikely unless the underlying depression is treated.*
- Assess the family's ability to respond to the client's psychosocial needs for stimulation. Assist as able. *Individuals and caregivers provide care through the context of their own cultural experiences.*
- ▲ Refer to occupational therapy to assist the client and family with identifying diversional activities within the capability of the client and family. *Some services require the consultation of specialty prepared professionals.*
- ▲ Introduce (or continue) friendly volunteer visitors if the client is willing and able to have the company. If transportation is an issue or if the client does not want visitors in the home, consider alternatives (e.g., telephone contacts, computer messaging). *Sim-*

- = **Independent;** ▲ = **Collaborative**

ply being available for the client as a fellow human being is important and helpful (Gardner, 1992).

▲ In the presence of a psychiatric disorder, refer for psychiatric home health care services for client reassurance and implementation of therapeutic regimen. *Psychiatric home care nurses can address issues relating to the client's depression and its interference with ability to adjust to changes in health status. Behavioral interventions in the home can assist the client to participate more effectively in treatment plan (Patusky et al, 1996).*

Client/Family Teaching

• Work with the client and family on learning diversional activities that the client is interested in (e.g., knitting, hooking rugs, writing memoirs).

• If the client is in isolation, give the client complete information on why isolation is needed and how it should be accomplished, especially guidelines for visitors. **Nursing Research:** *In one study, 21 clients who were in isolation identified their greatest needs, which were for more information about the isolation regulations and the need for guidelines for visitors so that visitors would be comfortable and continue to visit (Ward, 2000).*

evolve WEBSITES FOR EDUCATION

See the EVOLVE website for World Wide Web resources for client education.

REFERENCES

Barba BE, Tesh AS, Courts NF: Promoting thriving in nursing homes, the Eden alternative, *J Gerontol Nurs* 28(3):7 2002.

Brill PA: Effective approach toward prevention and rehabilitation in geriatrics, *Activities Adaptation Aging* 23(4):21, 1999.

Burnside IM: *The effect of reminiscence groups on fatigue, affect, and life satisfaction in older women*, Austin, 1990, University of Texas at Austin (PhD dissertation).

Cimprich B: Development of an intervention to restore attention in cancer patients, *Cancer Nurs* 16(2):83, 1993.

Cochran M: Tears have no color, *Am J Nurs* 98(6):53, 1998.

Doswell W, Erlen J: Multicultural issues and ethical concerns in the delivery of revising care interventions, *Nurs Clin North Am* 33(2):353, 1998.

Evans D: The effectiveness of music as an intervention for hospital patients: a systematic review, *J Adv Nurs* 37(1):8, 2002.

Gardner DL: Presence. In Bulechek GM, McCloskey JC, editors: *Nursing interventions: essential nursing treatments*, Philadelphia, 1992, WB Saunders.

Giger JN, Davidhizar RE: *Transcultural nursing*, ed 2, St Louis, 1995, Mosby.

Hamilton DB: Reminiscence therapy. In Bulechek GM, McCloskey JC, editors: *Nursing interventions: essential nursing treatments*, Philadelphia, 1992, WB Saunders.

Heineken J: Patient silence is not necessarily client satisfaction: communication in home care nursing, *Home Healthc Nurse* 16(2):115, 1998.

Jones ED, Beck-Litle R: The use of reminiscence therapy for the treatment of depression in rural-dwelling older adults, *Issues Ment Health Nurs* 23:3, 2002.

Jones MM, Haight BK: Environmental transformations: an integrative review, *J Gerontol Nurs* 28(3):23, 2002.

Jonsdottir H et al: Group reminiscence among people with end-stage chronic lung diseases, *J Adv Nurs* 35(1):79, 2001.

Kuntz N et al: Therapeutic play and bone marrow transplantation, *J Pediatr Nurs* 11(6):359, 1996.

Leininger MM, McFarland MR: *Transcultural nursing: concepts, theories, research and practices*, ed 3, New York, 2002, McGraw-Hill.

Patusky KL, Rodning C, Martinez-Kratz M: Clinical lessons in psychiatric home care: a case study approach, *J Home Healthc Manag* 9:18, 1996.

• = Independent; ▲ = Collaborative

Radziewicz RM: Using diversional activities to enhance coping, *Cancer Nurs* 15(4):293, 1992.

Rode D et al: Therapeutic use of technology, *Am J Nurs* 98(12):32, 1998.

Schneider SM, Workman ML: Virtual reality as a distraction intervention for older children receiving chemotherapy, *Pediatr Nurs* 26(6):593, 2000.

Shaw R, Wilkinson W: Therapy and rehabilitation: building the pyramids—palliative care patients' perceptions of making art, *Int J Palliat Nurs* 2(4):217, 1996.

Smolen D, Topp R, Singer L: The effect of self-selected music during colonoscopy on anxiety, heart rate, and blood pressure, *Appl Nurs Res* 15(3):126, 2002.

Stanley-Hermanns M, Miller J: Animal-assisted therapy, *Am J Nurs* 102(10):69, 2002.

Stuart GW, Laraia MT: Therapeutic nurse-patient relationship. In Stuart GW, Laraia MT, editors: *Principles and practice of psychiatric nursing,* St Louis, 2001, Mosby.

Taylor-Price C: *The efficacy of structured reminiscence group psychotherapy as an intervention to decrease depression and increase psychological well-being in female nursing home residents,* Mississippi State, Miss, 1995, Mississippi State University (PhD dissertation).

Ward D: Infection control: reducing the psychological effects of isolation, *Br J Nurs* 9(3):162, 2000.

Williams MA: The physical environment and patient care, *Am Rev Nurs Res* 6:61, 1988.

Disturbed Energy field

Gail B. Ladwig

NANDA Definition

A disruption of the flow of energy surrounding a person's being, which results in a disharmony of mind and spirit

Defining Characteristics

Temperature change (warmth/coolness); visual changes (image/color); disruption of the field (vacant/hold/spike/bulge), movement (wave/spike/tingling/dense/flowing), sounds (tone/words)

NOC Outcomes (Nursing Outcomes Classification)

Suggested NOC Outcomes

Comfort Level; Spiritual Health

> ### Example NOC Outcome with Indicators
>
> **Comfort Level** as evidenced by the following indicators: Reported physical well-being/Reported satisfaction with symptom control (Rate each indicator of **Comfort Level:** 1 = none, 2 = limited, 3 = moderate, 4 = substantial, 5 = extensive [see Section I].)

Client Outcomes

Client Will (Specify Time Frame):

- State sense of well-being
- State feeling of relaxation
- State decreased pain
- State decreased tension
- Demonstrate evidence of physical relaxation (e.g., decreased blood pressure, pulse, respiration rate, muscle tension)

• = Independent; ▲ = Collaborative

| NIC | Interventions (Nursing Interventions Classification) |

Suggested NIC Intervention
Therapeutic Touch

> ### Example NIC Activities—Therapeutic Touch
>
> Focuses awareness on inner self; Focuses awareness on the intention to facilitate wholeness and healing at all levels of consciousness

Nursing Interventions and Rationales

- Refer to care plans for **Anxiety, Acute Pain,** and **Chronic Pain**
- Administer therapeutic touch (TT) as described in following discussion (may also include healing touch and Reiki practice). **Nursing Research:** *Meta-analytic techniques were used to integrate the research-based literature with scientific evidence supporting TT as a nursing intervention in the past decade. The results seem to indicate that TT has a positive, medium effect on physiological and psychological variables (Peters, 1999).* **Nursing Research***: TT relieves discomfort and distress and facilitates healing. For some patients, TT may serve as a beneficial adjuvant nursing intervention (Meehan, 1998). TT has been shown to induce relaxation, decrease anxiety, and speed healing (Dalglish, 1999).* **Clinical Research:** *In this random sample of female volunteers receiving TT, the experimental group participants showed significant reductions in tension, confusion, and anxiety and a significant increase in vigor across sessions (Lafreniere et al, 1999).* **Nursing Research***: In this qualitative study of five postpartum women who participated in TT for 2 months during home visits, TT seemed to add a dimension of mutual caring that added a special and unique quality to the home visit (Kiernan, 2002).*
- Guidelines for Therapeutic Touch
  - TT may be practiced by anyone with the requisite preparation, desire, and commitment. Required preparation is the completion of a minimum 12 contact hour basic workshop by a TT practitioner who meets the criteria as a "NH-PAI, Inc (Nurse Healer–Professional Associates International) qualified TT teacher." Health care professionals need to have practiced TT on a consistent basis for at least 1 year under the direction of a mentor (during the mentorship year, at the discretion and under the supervision of a mentor, the health care professional can begin utilizing TT in a health care/hospital setting). A further requirement of the practitioner is the completion of a 14 contact hour intermediate level course of instruction by a qualified TT teacher.
  - Those who are not licensed health care professionals may practice TT within their families, religious or spiritual community, and friends. Investigation of state licensing laws and regulations is necessary prior to accepting fees for practicing TT to ensure lawful practices. Those who are licensed to perform specific or general health-related services, including counseling or massage therapy, need to clarify roles and scope of practice parameters with their respective state regulatory entity or board or an attorney.
  - TT practitioners adhere to a code of ethics in the practice of TT. Keeping client information confidential, using TT only with permission of the client, charging rea-

• = Independent; ▲ = Collaborative

sonable fees for services, and practicing responsible use of other interventions in conjunction with the TT process are important elements of that code.
- TT is conducted according to the standards for its practice developed by Dr. Dolores Krieger and Dora Kunz and in accordance with the above guidelines (Nurse Healers-Professional Associates International Inc., 2000).
• Administer TT by performing the following steps:
  - Centering in the present moment: Shift awareness from the physical environment to an inner focus on the center within self, a center of calm and balance through which nurses perceive themselves and the client as a unitary whole. *The point of entry into the TT process is the act of centering (Krieger, 1997).* **Nursing Research:** *This study suggests that TT, when provided by the nurse in the clinical setting, can promote feelings of comfort, peace, calm, and security among patients (Hayes and Cox, 1999).*
  - Assessment: Pass palmar surface of hands 2 to 4 inches over the client's body from head to toe. **Nursing Research:** *The key constructs that emerged in this study are associated with feelings such as tingling, warmth, coolness, comfort, peace, calm, and security. The results emphasized the relationship associated with what is known by the mind and instinctively felt by the body (Hayes and Cox, 1999). Validation study cues include heat, decreased or disrupted energy flow, cold, tingling, pulsating, congestion, heaviness, unbalance, decreased flow, and field symmetry (Mornhinweg et al, 1996).*
  - Treatment (unruffling): Use hands to brush or smooth out the energy flow. Sweep the hands downward and out of the field from head to toe, and concentrate on the areas of disturbance that were identified during the assessment. *Unruffling facilitates the vital energy flows that are already in the healee's system (Krieger, 1997).*
  - Direction and modulation of energy: Rest hands on or near the body area where a block of congestion is detected or in other areas of energy imbalance. Facilitate transfer of energy to these areas. *This step corrects energy imbalances (Krieger, 1997).*
  - Stop: Stop procedure when there are no longer any clues or when the client indicates it is time to stop. Place hands over the solar plexus (just above the waist) and focus specifically on facilitating the flow of healing energy to the client. *This final phase allows for rest and evaluation (Jurgens et al, 1987).*

Multicultural
• Assess for the influence of cultural beliefs, norms, and values on the client's sense of disharmony of mind and spirit. **Nursing Research:** *The client's sense of disharmony may have cultural roots (Cochran, 1998; Doswell and Erlen, 1998; Leininger and McFarland, 2002).*
• Assess for the presence of specific culture-bound syndromes that may manifest as disturbances in energy or spirit. **Nursing Research:** *Voodoo death, evil eye, and trance dissociation are some of the culture-bound syndromes that have symptoms of disharmony of mind and spirit (Arnault, 1998).*
• Validate the client's feelings and concerns related to sense of disharmony or energy disturbance. **Nursing Research:** *Validation is a therapeutic communication technique that lets the client know that the nurse has heard and understands what was said, and it promotes the nurse-client relationship (Heineken, 1998).*

Home care
• See Guidelines for Therapeutic Touch.
▲ Help the client and family accept TT as a healing intervention. Consultation and col-

• = **Independent;** ▲ = **Collaborative**

laboration with a specialist may be the best approach to nursing care. Numerous studies have reported positive outcomes of Healing Touch as a noninvasive complementary therapy (Umbreit, 2000).

- Assist the family with providing an appropriate space in which TT can be administered.
▲ Assess clients with bipolar disorder for the occurrence of social rhythm disruption, particularly during periods of stressful life events. Refer for mental health treatment. *Stressful life events, particularly those involving social rhythm disruption, appear to play a role in initiating manic episodes (Malkoff-Schwartz et al, 2000).*
▲ In the presence of a psychiatric disorder, refer for psychiatric home health care services for client reassurance and implementation of therapeutic regimen. *Psychiatric home care nurses can address issues relating to the client's bipolar disorder and its interference with ability to adjust to changes in health status. Behavioral interventions in the home can assist the client to participate more effectively in treatment plan (Patusky et al, 1996).*

Client/Family Teaching

- Teach the TT process to family members. TT enables caregivers to embrace their compassion and to touch people with effect (Dalglish, 1999).
- Teach that when working with the very young, old, or ill, or in the head area, TT should be gentle and used only for short periods. Exercise caution when using TT with patients who may exhibit an extreme sensitivity to the process (e.g., premature infants, frail elderly, psychotic clients) (Sayer-Adams, 1994).
- Teach the client how to use guided imagery. The nurse can facilitate healing by helping the client recontact and reclaim parts of the self (resolve energy disturbance) through guided imagery (Rancour, 1994).
- Teach the client to use deep breathing to relax. Ask the client to have the disease, affected organ, or symptom assume an image. After the image has been identified, ask the client to speak with the image to address an unresolved issue. By describing a previously unacknowledged part of the self, liberated energy can transform resistance, defenses, and disease into self-acceptance, peace, and wholeness (Remen, 1994).

evolve WEBSITES FOR EDUCATION

See the EVOLVE website for World Wide Web resources for client education.

REFERENCES

Arnault DS: Framework for culturally relevant psychiatric nursing. In Varcarolis EM, editor: *Foundations of psychiatric mental health nursing,* ed 3, Philadelphia, 1998, WB Saunders.
Cochran M: Tears have no color, *Am J Nurs* 98(6):53, 1998.
Dalglish S: Worklife. Therapeutic touch in an acute care community hospital, *Can Nurse* 95(3):57, 1999.
Doswell W, Erlen J: Multicultural issues and ethical concerns in the delivery of revising care interventions, *Nurs Clin North Am* 33(2):353, 1998.
Giger JN, Davidhizar RE: *Transcultural nursing,* ed 2, St Louis, 1995, Mosby.
Hayes J, Cox C: The experience of therapeutic touch from a nursing perspective, *Br J Nurs* 8(18):1249, 1999.
Heineken J: Patient silence is not necessarily client satisfaction: communication in home care nursing, *Home Healthc Nurse* 16(2):115, 1998.
Jurgens A, Meehan T, Wilson H: Therapeutic touch as a nursing intervention, *Holist Nurse Pract* 2:1, 1987.
Kiernan J: The experience of Therapeutic Touch in the lives of five postpartum women, *MCN Am J Matern Child Nurs* 27(1):47, 2002.

• = Independent; ▲ = Collaborative

Krieger D: *Therapeutic Touch inner workbook,* Santa Fe, NM, 1997, Bear and Company.

Lafreniere KD et al: Effects of therapeutic touch on biochemical and mood indicators in women, *J Altern Complement Med* 5(4):367, 1999.

Leininger MM, McFarland MR: *Transcultural nursing: concepts, theories, research and practices,* ed 3, New York, 2002, McGraw-Hill.

Malkoff-Schwartz S et al: Social rhythm disruption and stressful life events in the onset of bipolar and unipolar episodes, *Psychol Med* 30:1005, 2000.

Meehan T: Therapeutic touch as a nursing intervention, *J Adv Nurs* 28(1):117, 1998.

Mornhinweg G: Energy field disturbance validation study, *Healing Touch Newsletter* 6:11, 1996.

Nurse Healers-Professional Associates International: *Guidelines of recommended standards and scope of practice for Therapeutic Touch,* available on-line at http://www.therapeutic-touch.org/content/guidelines.asp, accessed February 22, 2003.

Patusky KL, Rodning C, Martinez-Kratz M: Clinical lessons in psychiatric home care: a case study approach, *J Home Healthc Manage* 9:18, 1996.

Peters RM: The effectiveness of therapeutic touch: a meta-analytic review, *Nurs Sci Q* 12(1):52, 1999.

Rancour P: Interactive guided imagery with oncology patients, *J Holist Nurs* 12:149, 1994.

Remen N: Psychosynthesis and healing, *J Holist Nurs* 12:150, 1994.

Sayer-Adams J: Complementary therapies: therapeutic touch nursing function, *Nurs Stand* 8:25, 1994.

Umbreit AW: Healing touch: applications in the acute care setting, *AACN Clin Issues* 11(1):105, 2000.

Impaired Environmental interpretation syndrome

Betty J. Ackley and Nancy English

NANDA   Definition

Consistent lack of orientation to person, place, and time, or circumstances for more than 3 to 6 months, necessitating a protective environment

Defining Characteristics

Chronic confusional states; consistent disorientation in known and unknown environments; loss of occupation or social functioning resulting from memory decline; slow to respond to questions; inability to follow simple directions/instructions, concentrate, or reason

Related Factors (r/t)

Depression; dementia (e.g., Alzheimer's, multi-infarct, Pick's disease, AIDS, Parkinson's disease, alcoholism)

NOC   Outcomes (Nursing Outcomes Classification)

Suggested NOC Outcomes

Cognitive Orientation; Concentration; Information Processing; Memory; Neurological Status: Consciousness

• = Independent; ▲ = Collaborative

> ### Example NOC Outcome with Indicators
>
> **Concentration** as evidenced by the following indicators: Maintains focus without being distracted/Responds appropriately to visual cues/Responds appropriately to language cues/Draws a circle (on command)/Draws a pentagon (on command) (Rate each indicator of **Concentration:** 1 = never demonstrated, 2 = rarely demonstrated, 3 = sometimes demonstrated, 4 = often demonstrated, 5 = consistently demonstrated [see Section I].)

Client Outcomes

Client Will (Specify Time Frame):
- Remain content and free from harm
- Function at maximal cognitive level
- Independently participate in ADLs at the maximum of functional ability

NIC   Interventions (Nursing Interventions Classification)

Suggested NIC Interventions
Dementia Management; Environmental Management; Reality Orientation; Surveillance: Safety

> ### Example NIC Activities—Dementia Management
>
> Encourage the client to verbalize memories of loss, both past and current; Help the client to identify personal coping strategies

Nursing Interventions and Rationales, Client/Family Teaching

See care plan for **Chronic Confusion.**

evolve WEBSITES FOR EDUCATION

See the EVOLVE website for World Wide Web resources for client education.

Adult Failure to thrive

Gail B. Ladwig

NANDA   Definition

Progressive functional deterioration of a physical and cognitive nature with remarkably diminished ability to live with multisystem diseases, cope with ensuing problems, and manage care

Defining Characteristics

Anorexia—does not eat meals when offered; states does not have an appetite, is not hungry, or "I don't want to eat"; inadequate nutritional intake—eating less than body re-

• = Independent; ▲ = Collaborative

quirements; consumption of minimal to no food at most meals (i.e., consumes less than 75% of normal requirements); weight loss (from baseline weight)—5% unintentional weight loss in 1 month or 10% unintentional weight loss in 6 months; physical decline (decline in bodily function)—evidence of fatigue, dehydration, incontinence of bowel and bladder; frequent exacerbations of chronic health problems (e.g., pneumonia, urinary tract infections); cognitive decline (decline in mental processing) as evidenced by problems with responding appropriately to environmental stimuli, demonstrated difficulty in reasoning, decision making, judgment, memory, and concentration; decreased perception; decreased social skills; social withdrawal—noticeable decrease from usual past behavior in attempts to form or participate in cooperative and interdependent relationships (e.g., decreased verbal communication with staff, family, friends); decreased participation in ADLs that the older person once enjoyed; self-care deficit—no longer looks after or takes charge of physical cleanliness or appearance; difficulty performing simple self-care tasks; neglect of home environment and/or financial responsibilities; apathy as evidenced by lack of observable feeling or emotion in terms of normal ADLs and environment; altered mood state—expresses feelings of sadness, being low in spirit; expresses loss of interest in pleasurable outlets such as food, sex, work, friends, family, hobbies, or entertainment; verbalizes desire for death

Related Factors (r/t)

Depression; apathy; fatigue

NOC   Outcomes (Nursing Outcomes Classification)

Suggested NOC Outcomes

Physical Aging; Psychosocial Adjustment: Life Change; Will to Live

---

Example NOC Outcome with Indicators

Will to Live as evidenced by the following indicators: Expression of determination to live/Expression of hope/Use of strategies to compensate for problems associated with disease (Rate each indicator of **Will to Live:** 1 = Severe, 2 = Substantial, 3 = Moderate, 4 = Slight, 5 = None [see Section I].)

Client Outcomes

Client Will (Specify Time Frame):

- Resume highest level of functioning possible
- Consume adequate dietary intake for weight and height
- Maintain usual weight
- Have adequate fluid intake with no signs of dehydration
- Participate in ADLs
- Participate in social interactions
- Maintain clean personal and home environment
- Express feelings associated with losses

NIC   Interventions (Nursing Interventions Classification)

Suggested NIC Interventions

Hope Instillation; Mood Management; Self-Care Assistance

• = Independent; ▲ = Collaborative

Example NIC Activities—Hope Installation
Help the client/family to identify areas of hope in life; Involve the client actively in own care

Nursing Interventions and Rationales

- Elderly clients who have failure to thrive (FTT) should be evaluated by review of the patient's ADLs, cognitive function, and mood; a targeted history and physical examination; and selected laboratory studies. *Early recognition of dementia is an important factor in obtaining timely and appropriate care (Insel and Badger, 2002).* **Clinical Research:** *This retrospective review of the medical record of patients with altered mental status indicated that the patient history and physical examination were most useful in diagnostic terms (Kanich et al, 2002).*

▲ Assess possible causes for adult FTT and treat any underlying problems such as depression, malnutrition, diarrhea, renal failure, and illnesses that are caused by physical and cognitive changes. **Clinical Research:** *Malnutrition is a frequent condition; both widely represented in the geriatric population and underestimated in diagnostic and therapeutic work-up, and is known to affect health status and life expectancy of elderly people (Vetta et al, 1999). An initial clinical assessment that combines multiple and varied sources of information is recommended to evaluate patients with suspected dementia (U.S. Department of Health and Human Services, 1996).* **Clinical Research:** *Physicians who care for elderly patients should be alert to the possible presence of diarrhea and malabsorption if there is unexplained weight loss and FTT. Older patients may not admit to having chronic diarrhea, particularly if they also are incontinent (Holt, 2001).* **Clinical Research:** *Retrospective chart review indicated that renal failure was found in 26.4% of the oldest-old admitted to an acute geriatric department. The elderly client with renal failure is more often admitted for failure to thrive (Van den Noortgate et al, 2001).*

▲ Carefully assess for elder abuse and refer for treatment. **Clinical Research:** *Elderly men and women of all socioeconomic and ethnic backgrounds are vulnerable to mistreatment, and most often it goes undetected (Kahan and Paris, 2003).*

- Assess for signs of fatigue and sensory changes that may indicate an infection is present that may be related to undetected diabetes mellitus or HIV. **Clinical Research:** *In this multicenter study a group of care home residents not known to have diabetes and able to undergo testing, a substantial proportion had undetected diabetes based on a 2-hour postglucose load (Sinclair et al 2001).* **Clinical Research:** *Many older adults are sexually active and often demonstrate risky sexual behavior, such as dispensing with the use of condoms; and the isolation that frequently accompanies old age can lead to alcoholism and injectable drug use (Lieberman, 2000).*

- Assess for all etiologies including depression using a geriatric depression scale. Be alert for depression in clients newly admitted to nursing homes. **Clinical Research:** *New depression may be the first sign of impending cognitive dysfunction (Sarkisian and Lachs, 1996). The geriatric depressions scale is recommended to determine the presence of depression (Jamison, 1997). Depression in newly admitted nursing home residents is a frequently overlooked area of nursing concern (Ryden et al, 1998).*

- Note changes in the elderly client's appetite and assess for depression. *Depression can lead to FTT by two routes: a direct path of decreased appetite as a symptom of depression and*

• = Independent; ▲ = Collaborative

an indirect path of increasing disability as an effect of depression (Katz and DiFilippo, 1997).

- Note if the client is irritable and is blaming others. **Nursing Research:** *Recent findings support the presence of these behaviors as symptomatic of depression (Proffitt et al, 1996).*

- Screen for depression in persons with adult macular degeneration (AMD) and low vision or vision loss. **Clinical Research:** *This study of 114 elderly AMD clients indicated that 49 patients met DSM-IV criteria for syndromal depression and that visual acuity was the only variable significantly associated with vision-specific function. Although there are no effective treatments for restoring vision in AMD, depression is treatable. Both psychotherapy and antidepressants are efficacious and may indirectly improve function among older people with vision loss (Casten et al, 2002).*

- Provide cognitive therapy for clients who are identified as depressed. Reinforce their value as a person and provide reality as to "who they really are." *Clients who are depressed can be helped by examining "who they are" compared with "who they believe they are" (Drake et al, 1996).*

- ▲ Consider the use of "light therapy." **Clinical Research:** *The results of this placebo-controlled study suggest that bright light treatment may be effective among institutionalized older adults, providing nonpharmacological intervention in the treatment of depression (Sumaya et al, 2001).*

- Instill hope and encourage the expression of positive thoughts. **Clinical Research:** *The findings from this study of 1002 older disabled women suggest that positive emotions can protect older persons against adverse health outcomes (Penninx et al, 2000).* **Clinical Research:** *The data from this study confirm the argument that hopefulness appears to be central to a family's coping with the impact of mental illness. Nurses should be mindful of their capacity to sustain or diminish the hopes of family members (Bland and Darlington, 2002).*

- Monitor weight loss, leaving 25% or more of food uneaten at most meals, psychiatric/mood diagnoses, and deteriorated ability to participate in activities of daily living. **Nursing Research:** *This study demonstrated the above criteria as significant predictors of protein calorie malnutrition (Crogan et al, 2002). Diagnosis and intervention of malnutrition can prevent loss of function and independence and decrease morbidity and mortality in the elderly (Ennis et al, 2001).*

- Offer nutrient-dense foods: dairy and fruit products, such as vanilla custard, strawberry yogurt, vanilla/apple yogurt, orange/peach juice, apple/berry/grape juice, and applesauce. (These suggested foods were used in the research below in the Netherlands; adopt appropriate foods for the individual tastes of the elderly client.) **Clinical Research:** *A randomized intervention study of 161 frail elderly in the Netherlands demonstrated that the group receiving nutrient-dense foods had increased blood nutrient values and decreased homocysteine levels. The results also suggest a beneficial effect on bone mass and density for those consuming enriched foods compared with controls, although this needs further clinical confirmation (De Jong, 2001).*

- Play soothing music during mealtimes to increase the amount of food eaten. **Clinical Research:** *One study suggested that dinner music, particularly soothing music, can reduce irritability, fear, panic, and depressed mood and can stimulate the appetite of demented patients in a nursing home. In this study the patients were less irritable, anxious, and depressed during the periods when music was playing (Ragneskog et al, 1996).*

- Decrease noise and increase lighting in the dining area. **Clinical Research:** *This case study indicates that lighting enhancement and noise reduction may further improve die-*

• = Independent; ▲ = Collaborative

tary intake, which, in turn, may promote improved nutritional status (McDaniel et al, 2001).

- Offer comfort foods and happy hour: foods associated with bygone years, intended to trigger recollections of pleasant childhood experiences and feelings of caring and healing, and a "happy hour" beverage, presented in a social milieu. *These are two approaches that have demonstrated effectiveness in stimulating oral intake in the FTT client (Wood and Vogen, 1998).*
- Provide appropriate nutrition for the client whose obesity may be affecting physical performance and thus has limited ability to perform ADLs, which leads to functional dependence. **Clinical Research:** *Malnutrition includes obesity (overnutrition); obesity among older persons is defined as being at least 30% above ideal body weight. Obesity may contribute to the previously mentioned problems (Still et al, 1997).*
- Provide opportunities for interaction with the natural environments. **Clinical Research:** *This demonstrates evidence to support the intuitive belief that interaction with the natural world is a vital part of biopsychosocial-spiritual well-being (Irvine and Warber, 2002).*
- Provide opportunities for visitation from animals. **Nursing Research:** *Animal visitation programs have been used in a wide variety of clinical settings with predominantly positive outcomes reported anecdotally (Johnson et al, 2002).* **Clinical Research:** *Pets play a central role in the lives of many elderly people (Ebenstein and Worthan, 2001).*
- Encourage clients to reminiscence about past experiences. *Reminiscing helps to foster social relatedness (Jamison, 1997).*
- Encourage clients to pray if they wish. **Nursing Research:** *Various studies have discovered that various groups of people have used prayer for managing their symptoms of aging or illness (Meraviglia, 1999).*
- Encourage elderly clients to interact with others on a regular basis. Have them participate in activities for seniors in their community. **Clinical Research:** *FTT of an elderly client is usually accompanied by social withdrawal (Palmer and Foley, 1990).*
- Help clients to participate in activities by assessing motivation and helping them to identify reasons to participate such as better mobility, more independence, feelings of well-being. **Nursing Research:** *Motivation has been identified as an important factor in the older adult's ability to perform functional activities (Resnick, 1998).*
- Frail elderly clients should also participate in carefully supervised group exercise programs accompanied by music. (The exercise program used in the research below was a twice-weekly 45-minute group session. Subjects performed exercises such as walking, stooping, and chair stands under the supervision of skilled trainers. Exercises were moderate but gradually increased in intensity and included different materials, such as balls, ropes, weights, and elastic bands.) (Another treatment used a wheelchair bicycle in a recreation therapy protocol, which combined small group activity therapy and one-on-one bike rides with a staff member.) **Clinical Research:** *This intervention study of 161 frail elderly clients in the Netherlands indicated that exercise preserved lean body mass and energy intake, it helped to improve or maintain physical fitness and the functioning vital for independent living (De Jong, 2001).* **Research Clinical Trial:** *In long-term care residents with dementia using wheelchair bicycle riding, depression levels were significantly reduced. Improvements were also found in sleep and levels of activity engagement (Buettne and Fitzsimmons, 2002).* **Nursing Research:** *Subjects in this study reported significantly enhanced mood while exercising to music compared with subjects exercising without music (Murrock, 2002).*

- ● = Independent; ▲ = Collaborative

- Provide physical touch for clients. Touch their hand or arm when speaking with them; offer hugs with permission. *Touch helps with integration and fosters social relatedness. Tactile stimulation benefits the older adult's psychological well-being (Jamison, 1997).*
- Administer TT. **Clinical Research:** *Results of this clinical trial of (n = 16) patients in the advanced stages of dementia of the Alzheimer's type (DAT), showed that discomfort levels decreased significantly after five TT sessions, becoming significantly lower than levels in the control group (n = 10) (Giasson et al, 1999).*
- Refer to care plans for **Imbalanced Nutrition: less than body requirements, Hopelessness,** and **Disturbed Energy field**.

Multicultural

- Assess for the influence of cultural beliefs, norms, and values on the family's or caregiver's understanding of FTT. **Nursing Research:** *What the family considers normal and abnormal health behavior may be based on cultural perceptions (Cochran, 1998; Doswell and Erlen, 1998; Guaranccia, 1998; Leininger and McFarland, 2002).*
- Validate the family's feelings and concerns related to the FTT symptoms. **Nursing Research:** *Validation is therapeutic communication technique that lets the family know that the nurse has heard and understands what was said, and it promotes the nurse-client relationship (Heineken, 1998).*

Home care

- Above interventions may be adapted for home care use.
- ▲ Begin discharge planning as soon as possible with case manager or social worker to assess need for home support systems, assistive devices, and community or home health services.
- ▲ Assess and track areas of decreased functioning resulting from failure to thrive. Ensure that all symptomatology is considered for necessary action. *Clients may change response to stressors/needs with changes in environment or interventions.*
- Give permission for role activity changes. Negotiate and clarify role expectations and reevaluate as necessary. *Failure to thrive may require an extended period of recovery. Chronic illness often requires role changes to preserve a functional unit. Comfort level with role activities supports continued recovery.*
- Provide support for family/caregivers. *Support for caregivers decreases caregiver burden.*
- If FTT is due to a dementing illness, refer to care plan for **Chronic Confusion**.
- ▲ Refer to medical social services or mental health counseling, resource identification, and/or community support groups. If necessary, contract with the client to attend sessions. *Counseling support can increase coping ability; group participation provides support and offers new problem-solving strategies to the client.*
- ▲ Refer to home health aide services for assistance with ADLs throughout the duration of decreased participation. *Maintaining ADLs and the integrity of the environment prevents further decline in status of those areas and decreases frustration as the client recovers and resumes responsibility for them.*
- ▲ Institute case management of frail elderly to support continued independent living. *Failure to thrive represents and can lead to increasing needs for assistance in using the health care system effectively. Case management combines nursing activities of the client and family assessment, planning and coordination of care among all health care providers, delivery of direct nursing care, and monitoring of care and outcomes. These activities are able to ad-*

• = **Independent;** ▲ = **Collaborative**

dress continuity of care, mutual goal setting, behavior management, and prevention of worsening health problems (Guttman, 1999).

▲ Refer for homemaker or psychiatric home health care services for respite, client reassurance, and implementation of therapeutic regimen. *Responsibility for a person at high risk for adult failure to thrive may provide high caregiver stress. Respite decreases caregiver stress. The presence of caring individuals is reassuring to both the client and caregivers, especially during periods of client anxiety or inability to follow treatment regimen. Failure to thrive behavior, especially if accompanied by depression, can make use of the interventions described above, modified for the home setting. Psychiatric home care nurses can address issues relating to the client's depression and its interference with ability to adjust to changes in health status. Behavioral interventions in the home can assist the client to participate more effectively in treatment plan (Patusky et al, 1996).*

Client/Family Teaching

• If adult FTT is related to dementia, help the caregiver to understand the diagnosis and help to identify needs that the caregiver will have to assist the client with, such as nutrition, maintenance of adequate fluid intake, toileting, self-care, and safety. *When the etiology of adult FTT is dementia, the caregiver needs to be educated on how to handle it (Jamison, 1997).*

• Instruct the family on the use of verbal cues to encourage eating, such as "Pick up your spoon; use the spoon to scoop up the pudding; now put the spoon with the pudding in your mouth." *Verbal cueing is effective for improving nutritional status (Jamison, 1997).*

▲ Discuss the possibility with the physician of a drug holiday when the etiology is delirium. *Delirium may resolve with a drug holiday (Jamison, 1997).*

▲ Provide referral for evaluation of hearing and appropriate hearing aids. **Clinical Research:** *This study of 60 subjects older than 65 years (mean age, 79 years) living in nursing homes demonstrated that hearing loss affects the communication, sociability, and psychological aspects of quality of life (Tsuruoka et al, 2001).*

▲ Refer for psychotherapy and possible medication if the etiology is depression. *Treatment of the etiology is necessary; the previously mentioned are treatments that may be used for depression (Jamison, 1997).*

▲ Refer for possible medication therapy when the diagnosis is dementia. **Clinical Research:** *In this retrospective cohort study of residents with dementia in nursing homes, there were 1449 users of tacrine and 6119 nonusers of tacrine. Tacrine was associated with lower mortality (Ott and Lapane, 2002).*

evolve WEBSITES FOR EDUCATION

See the EVOLVE website for World Wide Web resources for client education.

REFERENCES

Bland R, Darlington Y: The nature and sources of hope: perspectives of family caregivers of people with serious mental illness, *Perspect Psychiatr Care* 38(2):61, 2002.

Buettner LL, Fitzsimmons S: AD-venture program: therapeutic biking for the treatment of depression in long-term care residents with dementia, *Am J Alzheimers Dis Other Demen* 17(2):121, 2002.

Casten RJ, Rovner BW, Edmonds SE: The impact of depression in older adults with age-related macular degeneration, *J Vis Impair Blindness* 96(6):399, 2002.

Cochran M: Tears have no color, *Am J Nurs* 98(6):53, 1998.

• = Independent; ▲ = Collaborative

Crogan NL, Corbett CF, Short RA: The minimum data set: predicting malnutrition in newly admitted nursing home residents, *Clin Nurs Res* 11(3):341, 2002.

De Jong N: Sensible aging: using nutrient-dense foods an physical exercise with the frail elderly, *Nutr Today* 36(4):202, 2001.

Doswell W, Erlen J: Multicultural issues and ethical concerns in the delivery of revising care interventions, *Nurs Clin North Am* 33(2):353, 1998.

Drake RE, Price JL, Drake RE: Helping depressed clients discover personal power, *Perspect Psychiatr Care* 32(4):30, 1996.

Ebenstein H, Worthan J: The value of pets in geriatric practice: a program example, *J Gerontol Soc Work* 35(2), 2001.

Ennis BW, Saffel-Shrier S, Verson H: Diagnosing malnutrition in the elderly, *Nurse Pract* 26(3):52, 2001.

Giasson M et al: Therapeutic Touch, *Infirm Que* 6(6):38, 1999.

Guarnaccia P: Multicultural experiences of family caregiving: a Study of African American, European American, and Hispanic American families, *New Direct Ment Health Serv* 77:45, 1998.

Heineken J: Patient silence is not necessarily client satisfaction: communication in home care nursing, *Home Healthc Nurse* 16(2):115, 1998.

Holt PR: Diarrhea and malabsorption in the elderly, *Gastroenterol Clin North Am* 30(2):427, 2001.

Insel KC, Badger TA: Deciphering the 4 D's: cognitive decline, delirium, depression and dementia—a review, *J Adv Nurs* 38(4):360, 2002.

Irvine KN, Warber SL: Greening healthcare: practicing as if the natural environment really mattered, *Altern Ther Health Med* 8(5):76, 2002.

Jamison M: Failure to thrive in older adults, *J Gerontol Nurs* 23(2):13, 1997.

Johnson RA, Odendaal JS, Meadows RL: Animal-assisted interventions research: issues and answers, *West J Nurs Res* 24(4):422, 2002.

Kahan FS, Paris BE: Why elder abuse continues to elude the health care system, *Mt Sinai J Med* 70(1):62, 2003.

Kanich W et al: Altered mental status: evaluation and etiology in the ED, *Am J Emerg Med* 20(7):613, 2002.

Katz IR, DiFilippo S: Neuropsychiatric aspects of failure to thrive in late life, *Clin Geriatr Med* 13:4, 1997.

Leininger MM, McFarland MR: *Transcultural nursing: concepts, theories, research and practices*, ed 3, New York, 2002, McGraw-Hill.

Lieberman R: HIV in older Americans: an epidemiologic perspective, *J Midwifery Women's Health* 45(2):176, 2000.

McDaniel JH et al: Impact of dining room environment on nutritional intake of Alzheimer's residents: a case study, *Am J Alzheimers Dis Other Demen* 16(5):297, 2001.

Meraviglia M: Critical analysis of spirituality and its empirical indicators, prayer and meaning in life, *J Holist Nurs* 17(1):18, 1999.

Murrock CJ: The effects of music on the rate of perceived exertion and general mood among coronary artery bypass graft patients enrolled in cardiac rehabilitation phase II, *Rehabil Nurs* 27(6):227, 2002 (Including commentary by Miller ET).

Ott BR, Lapane KL: Tacrine therapy is associated with reduced mortality in nursing home residents with dementia, *J Am Geriatr Soc* 50(1):35, 2002.

Palmer RM, Foley JM: Failure to thrive in the elderly: diagnosis and management, *Geriatrics* 45:9, 1990.

Patusky KL, Rodning C, Martinez-Kratz M: Clinical lessons in psychiatric home care: a case study approach, *J Home Healthc Manag* 9:18, 1996.

Penninx BW et al: The protective effect of emotional vitality on adverse health outcomes in disabled older women, *J Am Geriatr Soc* 48(11):1359, 2000.

Proffitt C, Augspurger P, Byrne M: Geriatric depression: a survey of nurses' knowledge and assessment practices, *Issues Ment Health Nurs* 17(2):123, 1996.

Ragneskog H et al: Influence of dinner music on food intake and symptoms common in dementia, *Scand J Caring Sci* 10(1):11, 1996.

Resnick B: Functional performance of older adults in a long-term care setting, *Clin Nurs Res* 7(3):230, 1998.

Ryden MB et al: Assessment of depression in a population at risk newly admitted nursing home residents, *J Gerontol Nurs* 24(2):21, 1998.

Sarkisian C, Lachs M: "Failure to thrive" in older adults, *Ann Intern Med* 124(12):1072, 1996.

Sinclair AJ et al: Prevalence of diabetes in care home residents, *Diabetes Care* 24(6):1066, 2001.

Still C, Apovian C, Jensen G: Failure to thrive in older adults, *Ann Intern Med* 126(8):668, 1997.

Sumaya IC et al: Bright light treatment decreases depression in institutionalized older adults: a placebo-controlled crossover study, *J Gerontol A Biol Sci Med Sci* 56(6):M356, 2001.

• = Independent; ▲ = Collaborative

Tsuruoka H et al: Hearing impairment and quality of life for the elderly in nursing homes, *Auris Nasus Larynx* 28(1):45, 2001.

U.S. Department of Health and Human Services: *Recognition and initial assessment of Alzheimer's disease and related dementia, Clinical practice guideline No. 19 [302],* Rockville, Md, 1996, Public Health Service, AHCPR.

Van den Noortgate NJ et al: Renal function in the oldest-old on an acute geriatric ward, *Int Urol Nephrol* 32(4): 531, 2001.

Vetta F et al: The impact of malnutrition on the quality of life in the elderly, *Clin Nutr* 18(5):259, 1999.

Wood P, Vogen BD: Feeding the anorectic client: comfort foods and happy hour, *Geriatr Nurs* 19(4):192, 1998.

Risk for Falls

Betty J. Ackley and Teepa Snow

NANDA Definition

Increased susceptibility to falling that may cause physical harm

Risk Factors

Adults

History of falls; wheelchair use; 65 years of age or older; female (if elderly); lives alone; lower limb prosthesis; use of assistive devices (e.g., walker, cane)

Physiological

Presence of acute illness; postoperative conditions; visual difficulties; hearing difficulties; arthritis; orthostatic hypotension; sleeplessness; faintness when turning or extending neck; anemias; vascular disease; neoplasms (i.e., fatigue/limited mobility, urgency and/or incontinence, diarrhea, decreased lower extremity strength, postprandial blood sugar changes, foot problems, impaired physical mobility, impaired balance, difficulty with gait, unilateral neglect, proprioceptive deficits, neuropathy)

Diminished mental status (e.g., confusion, delirium, dementia, impaired reality testing)

Medication

Antihypertensive agents; ACE inhibitors; diuretics; tricyclic antidepressants; alcohol use; antianxiety agents; opiates; hypnotics or tranquilizers

Environment

Restraints; weather conditions (e.g., wet floors/ice); throw/scatter rugs; cluttered environment; unfamiliar, dimly lit room; no antislip material in bath and/or shower

Children (<2 Years of Age)

Male gender when younger than 1 year; lack of autorestraints; lack of gate on stairs; lack of window guard; bed located near window; unattended infant on bed/changing table/sofa; lack of parental supervision

Related Factors (r/t)

See Risk Factors.

• = Independent; ▲ = Collaborative

NOC   Outcomes (Nursing Outcomes Classification)

Suggested NOC Outcomes

Fall Prevention Behavior; Knowledge: Child Physical Safety

> #### Example NOC Outcome with Indicators
>
> **Fall Prevention Behavior** as evidenced by the following indicators: Correct use of assistive devices/ Elimination of clutter, spills, glare from floors/Use of safe transfer procedures (Rate each indicator of **Fall Prevention Behavior:** 1 = not adequate, 2 = slightly adequate, 3 = moderately adequate, 4 = substantially adequate, 5 = totally adequate [see Section I].)

Client Outcomes

Client Will (Specify Time Frame):

- Remain free of falls
- Change environment to minimize the incidence of falls
- Explain methods to prevent injury

NIC   Interventions (Nursing Interventions Classification)

Suggested NIC Interventions

Dementia Management; Fall Prevention; Surveillance: Safety

> #### Example NIC Activities—Fall Prevention
>
> Assist unsteady individual with ambulation; Monitor gait, balance, and fatigue level with ambulation

Nursing Interventions and Rationales

- Determine risk of falling by using an evaluation tool such as the Fall Risk Assessment (Farmer, 2000), The Conley Scale (Conley et al, 1999), or the FRAINT Tool for fall risk assessment (Parker, 2000). *Risk factors for falling include recent history of falls, confusion, depression, altered elimination patterns, cardiovascular/respiratory disease impairing perfusion or oxygenation, postural hypotension, dizziness or vertigo, primary cancer diagnosis, and altered mobility (Farmer, 2000; Hendrich et al, 1995; Wilson, 1998). Predictors of fall risk in the community included atrial fibrillation, neurological problems, living alone, and not adhering to a regular exercise program (Resnick, 1999).*
- Screen all clients for stability and mobility skills (supine to sit, sitting supported and unsupported, sit to stand, standing, walking and turning around, transferring, stooping to floor and recovering, and sitting down). Use tools such as the Balance Scale by Tinetti or the Get Up and Go Scale by Mathais. *It is helpful to determine the client's functional abilities and then plan for ways to improve problem areas or determine methods to ensure safety (Lewis et al, 1994; MacKnight and Rockwood, 1996; Tinetti, 2003).*
- Recognize that when people attend to another task while walking, such as carrying a cup of water, clothing, or supplies, they are more likely to fall. **Clinical Research:** *Those who slow down when given a carrying task are at a higher risk for subsequent falls (Lundin-Olsson et al, 1998).*
- Be careful when getting a mostly immobile the client up. Be sure to lock the bed and

• = **Independent;** ▲ = **Collaborative**

wheelchair and have sufficient personnel to protect the client from falls. *The most important preventative measure to reduce the risk of injurious falls for nonambulatory residents involves increasing safety measures while transferring, including careful locking of equipment such as wheelchairs and beds before moves (Thapa et al, 1996). These immobile clients commonly sustain the most serious injuries when they fall.*

- Identify clients likely to fall by placing a "Fall Precautions" sign on the doorway and by keying the Kardex and chart. Use a "high-risk fall" arm band and room marker to alert staff for increased vigilance and mobility assistance. *These steps alert the nursing staff of the increased risk of falls (Cohen and Guin, 1991).*
- If necessary to place the client in a wrist or vest restraint, use increased vigilance and watch for falls. *The risk of falling is highest soon after a client has been placed in a mechanical restraint (Arbesman and Wright, 1999).*
- ▲ Evaluate the client's medications to determine whether medications increase the risk of falling; consult with physician regarding the client's need for medication if appropriate. *Polypharmacy, or taking more than four medications, has been associated with increased falls. Medications increasing the risk of falls include diuretics, hypnotics, sedatives, opiates, antidepressants, and psychotropic and antihypertensive agents (Wilson, 1998). Medications such as benzodiazepines and antipsychotic and antidepressant medications given to promote sleep actually increase the rate of falls (Capezuti, 1999b).* **Clinical Research:** *Use of selective serotonin reuptake inhibitors and tricyclic antidepressants resulted in increased incidences of falls (Leipzig et al, 1999; Liu et al, 1998; Thapa et al, 1998).*
- Thoroughly orient the client to environment. Place the call light within reach and show how to call for assistance; answer call light promptly.
- Use 1/4- to 1/2-length side rails only, and maintain bed in a low position. Ensure that wheels are locked on bed and commode. Keep dim light in room at night. *Use of full side rails can result in the client climbing over the rails, leading with the head, and sustaining a head injury. Side rails with widely spaced vertical bars and side rails not situated flush with the mattress have been associated with asphyxiation deaths because of rail and in-bed entrapment and should not be used (Capezuti, 1999a; Hanger et al, 1999; Todd et al, 1997).*
- Routinely assist the client with toileting on his or her own schedule. Always take the client to bathroom on awakening, before bedtime, and before administering sedatives (Wilson, 1998). Keep the path to the bathroom clear, label the bathroom, and leave the door open. *The majority of falls are related to toileting. It is more acceptable to fall than to "wet yourself." Studies have indicated that falls are often linked to the need to eliminate in a hurry (Cohen, Guin, 1991; Wilson, 1998).*
- ▲ Avoid use of restraints; obtain a physician's order if restraints are necessary. If elderly clients are restrained and fall, they can sustain severe injuries, including strangulation, asphyxiation, or head injury from leading with their heads to get out of the bed (DiMaio et al, 1986; Evans and Strumpf, 1990). *Restraint-free extended care facilities were shown to have fewer residents with ADL deficiencies and fewer residents with bowel or bladder incontinence than were facilities that use restraints (Castle and Fogel, 1998). Restraint use can lead to depression, anger, infection, pressure ulcers, deconditioning, and sometimes death (Rogers and Bocchino, 1999). The risk of falling is highest soon after a client is placed in a mechanical restraint (Arbesman and Wright, 1999).* **Nursing Research:** *No differences in nighttime fall rates was shown between a group of severely impaired nursing home residents who were restrained versus a similar group who were not restrained (Capezuti et al, 1999b).* **Clinical Research:** *Restrained elderly clients often ex-*

• = Independent; ▲ = Collaborative

perience an increased number of falls, possibly as a result of muscle deconditioning or loss of coordination (Tinetti et al, 1992).

- In place of restraints, use the following:
  - Alarm systems with ankle, above the knee, or wrist sensors
  - Bed or wheelchair alarms
  - Increased observation of the client
  - Locked doors to unit
  - Low or very low height beds
  - Border-defining pillow/mattress to remind the client to stay in bed

  These alternatives to restraints can be helpful to prevent falls (Capezuti et al, 1999a; Wilson, 1998; Commodore, 1995).
- If the client is extremely agitated, consider using a special safety bed that surrounds the client. If the client has a traumatic brain injury, use the Emory cubicle bed. *Special beds can be an effective alternative to restraints and can help keep the client safe during periods of agitation (Williams et al, 1990).*
- If the client has a new onset of confusion (delirium), provide reality orientation when interacting. Have family bring in familiar items, clocks, and watches from home to maintain orientation. *Reality orientation can help prevent or decrease the confusion that increases risk of falling for clients with delirium.* See interventions for **Acute Confusion**.
- If the client has chronic confusion with dementia, use validation therapy that reinforces feelings but does not confront reality. *Validation therapy is effective for clients with dementia (Fine and Rouse-Bane, 1995).* See interventions for **Chronic Confusion.**
- Ask family to stay with the client to prevent the client from accidentally falling or pulling out tubes.
- If the client is unsteady on feet, use a walking belt or two nursing staff members when ambulating the client. *The client can walk independently with a walking belt, but the nurse can rapidly ensure safety if the knees buckle.*
- Place a fall-prone client in a room that is near the nurses' station. *Such placement allows more frequent observation of the client.*
- Help clients sit in a stable chair with arm rests. Avoid use of wheelchairs and geri-chairs except for transportation as needed. *Clients are likely to fall when left in a wheelchair or geri-chair because they may stand up without locking the wheels or removing the footrests. Wheelchairs do not increase mobility; people just sit in them the majority of the time (Lipson and Braun, 1993; Simmons et al, 1995).*
- Ensure that the chair or wheelchair fits the build, abilities, and needs of the client to ensure propulsion with legs or arms and ability to reach the floor, eliminating footrests and minimizing problems with shearing. *The seating system should fit the needs of the client so that the client can move the wheels, stand up from the chair without falling, and not be harmed by the chair. Footrests can cause skin tears and bruising, as well as postural alignment and sitting posture problems (Lipson and Braun, 1993; Rader et al, 2000).*
- Avoid use of wheelchairs as much as possible because they can serve as a restraint device. Most people in wheelchairs do not move. *Wheelchairs unfortunately serve as a restraint device. A study has shown that only 4% of residents in wheelchairs were observed to propel them independently and only 45% could propel them, even with cues and prompts. Another study showed that no residents could unlock wheelchairs without help, the wheelchairs were not fitted to residents, and residents were not trained in propulsion (Simmons et al, 1995).*
- ▲ Refer to physical therapy for strengthening exercises, gait training, and help with bal-

• = **Independent**; ▲ = **Collaborative**

ance to increase mobility. **Clinical Research:** *Balance, gait training and strengthening exercises in physical therapy have been shown to be effective for preventing falls (Gillespie et al, 2001; Robertson et al, 2001).*

Geriatric

- Encourage the client to wear glasses and use walking aids when ambulating.
- Help the client obtain and wear a specially designed hip protector when ambulating. Hip protectors are worn in a specially designed stretchy undergarment containing a pocket on each side for placement of the protector. **Clinical Research:** *The risk of a hip fracture in the elderly can be reduced by use of an anatomically designed external hip protector when ambulating (Kannus et al, 2000). After a meta-analysis of thousands of participants, hip protectors appear to reduce the risk of hip fractures (Parker et al).*
- Consider use of a "Merri-walker" adult walker that surrounds body if the client is mobile but unsafe because of wobbling.
- If the client experiences dizziness because of orthostatic hypotension when getting up, teach methods to decrease dizziness, such as rising slowly, remaining seated several minutes before standing, flexing feet upward several times while sitting, sitting down immediately if feeling dizzy, and trying to have someone present when standing. *The elderly develop decreased baroreceptor sensitivity and decreased ability of compensatory mechanisms to maintain blood pressure when standing up, resulting in postural hypotension (Aaronson et al, 1991; Matteson et al, 1997).*
- ▲ If the client is experiencing syncope, determine symptoms that occur before syncope, and note medications that the client is taking. Refer for medical care. *The circumstances surrounding syncope often suggest the cause. Use of many medications, including diuretics, antihypertensives, digoxin, beta-blockers, and calcium channel blockers can cause syncope. Use of the tilt table can be diagnostic in incidences of syncope (Cox, 2000).*
- ▲ Refer to physical therapy for strength training, using free weights or machines. *Strength improvement in response to resisted exercise is possible even in the very elderly, extremely sedentary client, with multiple chronic diseases and functional disabilities. Increased strength can help prevent falls (Connelly, 2000).*
- ▲ If an elderly woman has symptoms of urge incontinence, refer to a urologist for evaluation and ensure the path to the bathroom is well light and free of obstructions. *Urge urinary incontinence was associated with an increased incidence of falls in older women (Brown et al, 2000).*

Home care

- Some of the above interventions may be adapted for home care use.
- If the client was identified as a fall risk in the hospital, recognize that there is a high incidence of falls after discharge, and use all measures possible to reduce the incidence of falls. **Nursing Research:** *The rate of falls is substantially increased in the geriatric client who has been recently hospitalized, especially during the first month after discharge (Mahoney et al, 2000).*
- Assess and monitor for acute changes in cognition and behavior. *An acute change in cognition and behavior is the classic presentation of delirium. Delirium is reversible and should be considered a medical emergency. Delirium can become chronic if untreated, and clients may be discharged from hospitals to home care in states of undiagnosed delirium.* **Nursing Research:** *Falls may be a precipitating event or an indication of frailty consistent with acute confusion (Mentes et al, 1999).*

• = Independent; ▲ = Collaborative

- Assess home environment for threats to safety: clutter, slippery floors, scatter rugs, unsafe stairs and stairwells, blocked entries, extension cords (across pathway), high beds, pets, and pet excrement. Use antiskid acrylic floor wax, nonskid rugs, use of stair rails, and skid-proof strips near the bed to prevent slippage. Evaluate need for safety devices in bathing area (e.g., hand grip, shower chair, hand-held showerhead). *Clients suffering from impaired mobility, impaired visual acuity, and neurological dysfunction, including dementia and other cognitive functional deficits, are all at risk for injury from common hazards. These recommendations were shown to be effective to reduce falls (Tinetti, 2003).*

▲ Institute a home-based, nurse-delivered exercise program to reduce falls or refer to physical therapy services for client and family education of safe transfers and ambulation and for strengthening exercises (for the client). *A home-based, nurse-delivered exercise program was effective in reducing the number of falls, especially in clients over 80 years of age (Robertson et al, 2001).* **Nursing Research:** *A meta-analysis of studies demonstrated a 4% reduction in the rate of falls in individuals who received fall prevention programs (Hill-Westmoreland et al, 2002).*

▲ Instruct the client and family or caregivers on how to correct identified hazards. Refer to occupational therapy services for assistance if needed. **Clinical Research:** *Home visits by an occupational therapist to assess and modify the home environment have been shown to be effective to reduce the number of falls (Cummings et al, 1999).*

▲ Use a multifactorial assessment along with interventions targeted to the identified risk factors. Key components of the interventions include evaluating need for all medications, balance, gait and strength training, use of strategies to deal with postural hypotension if present, home safety evaluation with needed modifications, and any needed cardiovascular treatment. **Clinical Research:** *The use of a multifactorial assessment along with interventions identified has been shown to be very effective in reducing the number of falls (Close et al, 1999; Tinetti et al, 1994).*

- Encourage balanced diet, with particular inclusion of vitamin D and calcium. *Hypovitaminosis D and hypocalcemia are common in older adults, contributing to falls, musculoskeletal complaints, and functional and mobility deficits (Dharmarajan et al, 2001).*

- If the client lives alone or spends a lot of time alone, teach the client what to do if he or she falls and cannot get up, and make sure he or she has a personal emergency response system or a cellular phone that is available from the floor (Tinetti, 2003). If the client is at risk for falls, use gait belt and additional persons when ambulating. *Gait belts decrease the risk of falls during ambulation.*

- Ensure appropriate nonglare lighting in the home. Ask the client to install indoor strip or "runway" type of lighting to baseboards to help clients balance. Install motion sensitive lighting that turns on automatically when the client gets out of bed to go to the bathroom. *Up to 79% of the elderly have inadequate lighting in their homes predisposing them to falls (Slay, 2002). The disorientation of waking in the dark could affect the client's balance. Caregiver may be alerted by light that the client is awake and out of bed.*

- Have the client wear supportive low-heeled shoes with good traction when ambulating. *Supportive shoes provide the client with better balance and protect the client from instability on uneven surfaces.*

▲ Refer to physical therapy services for the client and family education of safe transfers and ambulation and for strengthening/balance exercises (for the client) for ambulation and transfers.

- Provide a signaling device for clients who wander or are at risk for falls. *Orienting a*

• = **Independent;** ▲ = **Collaborative**

vulnerable client to a safety net relieves anxiety of the client and caregiver and allows for rapid response to a crisis situation.

- Provide medical identification bracelet for clients at risk for injury from dementia, seizures, or other medical disorders.
- Suggest a T'ai chi class designed for the elderly to selected clients who have sufficient balance to participate. **Clinical Research:** *One study demonstrated that elderly who participated in a T'ai chi class had half the number of falls as elderly clients who did not (Wolf et al, 1996).*

Client/Family Teaching

- Teach the client how to safely ambulate at home, including using safety measures such as hand rails in bathroom, and need to avoid carrying things or performing other tasks while walking *In the frail elderly, multitasking results in decreased motor performance, and may lead to falls (Hauer et al, 2002).*
- Teach the client the importance of maintaining a regular exercise program such as walking. *Lack of a consistent exercise program was one of the variables associated with a higher incidence of falls (Resnick, 1999).*

ᵉᵛᵒˡᵛᵉ **WEBSITES FOR EDUCATION**

See the EVOLVE website for World Wide Web resources for client education.

REFERENCES

Aaronson L, Carlon-Wolfe W, Schoener S: Pressures that fall on rising, *Geriatr Nurs* 12:67, 1991.

Arbesman MD, Wright C: Mechanical restraints, rehabilitation therapies, and staffing adequacy as risk factors for falls in an elderly hospitalized population, *Rehabil Nurs* 24(3):122, 1999.

Brown JS et al: Urinary incontinence: does it increase risk for falls in fractures? *J Am Geriatr Soc* 48(7):721, 2000.

Capezuti E et al: Individualized interventions to prevent bed-related falls and reduce siderail use, *J Gerontol Nurs* 25(11):26, 1999a.

Capezuti E et al: Outcomes of nighttime physical restraint removal for severely impaired nursing home residents, *Am J Alzheimers Dis* 14(3):157, 1999b.

Castle NG, Fogel B: Characteristics of nursing homes that are restraint free, *Gerontologist* 38(2):181, 1998.

Close J et al: Prevention of falls in the elderly trial (Profet): a randomized controlled trial, *Lancet* 353:93, 1999.

Cohen L, Guin P: Implementation of a patient fall prevention program, *J Neurosci Nurs* 23:315, 1991.

Commodore DI: Falls in the elderly population: a look at incidence, risks, healthcare costs, and preventive strategies, *Rehabil Nurs* 20:84, 1995.

Conley D, Schultz AA, Selvin R: The challenge of predicting patients at risk for falling: development of the Conley Scale, *Medsurg Nurs* 8(6):348, 1999.

Connelly DM: Resisted exercise training of institutionalized older adults for improved strength and functional mobility: a review, *Top Geriatr Rehabil* 15(3):6, 2000.

Cox MM: Uncovering the cause of syncope, *Patient Care* 30:39, 2000.

Dharmarajan TS, Ahmed S, Russell RO: Recurrent falls from hypocalcemia due to vitamin D deficiency: a preventable problem in home care, *Home Healthc Consult* 8(8):8, 2001.

DiMaio V, Dana S, Bix R: Death caused by restraint vests, *JAMA* 255:905, 1986.

Evans L, Strumpf N: Myths about elder restraint, *Image J Nurs Sch* 22:124, 1990.

Farmer BC: Try this: fall risk assessment, *J Gerontol Nurs* 26(7):6, 2000.

Fine JI, Rouse-Bane S: Using validating techniques to improve communication with cognitively impaired older adults, *J Gerontol Nurs* 21:39, 1995.

Gillespie LD et al: Interventions for preventing falls in elderly people, *Cochrane Database Syst Rev* 3(L CD00340), 2001.

• = **Independent;** ▲ = **Collaborative**

Hanger HC, Ball MC, Wood LA: An analysis of falls in the hospital: can we do without bedrails? *J Am Geriatr Soc* 47(5):529, 1999.

Hauer K, Marburger C, Oster P: Motor performance deteriorates with simultaneously performed cognitive tasks in geriatric patients, *Arch Phys Med Rehabil* 83(2):217, 2002.

Hendrich A et al: Hospital falls: development of a predictive model for clinical practice, *Appl Nurs Res* 8:129, 1995.

Hill-Westmoreland EE, Soeken K, Spellbring AM: A meta-analysis of fall prevention programs for the elderly: how effective are they? *Nurs Res* 51(1):1, 2002.

Kannus P et al: Prevention of hip fracture in elderly people with use of a hip protector, *New Engl J Med* 343(21):1506, 2000.

Lewis BJ et al: *The functional tool book,* Washington, DC, 1994, Learn.

Lipson J, Braun S: *Toward a restraint-free environment: reducing the use of physical and chemical restraint in long-term care and acute settings,* Baltimore, 1993, Health Professions Press.

Liu et al: Use of selective serotonin-reuptake inhibitors of tricyclic antidepressants and risk for hip fractures in elderly people, *Lancet* 351, 1998.

Lundin-Olsson L, Nysberg L, Gustafson Y: Attention, frailty, and falls: the effect of a manual task on basic mobility, *J Am Geriatr Soc* 46:758, 1998.

MacKnight C, Rockwood K: Mobility and balance in the elderly: a guide to bedside assessment, *Postgrad Med* 99(3):269, 1996.

Mahoney JE et al: Temporal association between hospitalization and rate of falls after discharge, *Arch Intern Med* 160(18):2788, 2000.

Matteson MA, McConnell ES, Linton AD: *Gerontological nursing,* ed 2, Philadelphia, 1997, WB Saunders.

Mentes et al: Acute confusion indicators: risk factors and prevalence using MDS data, *Res Nurs Health* 22:95, 1999.

Parker MJ, Gillespie LD, Gillespie WJ: Hip protectors for preventing hip fractures in the elderly, *Cochrane Library* CD001255, 2001.

Parker R: Assessing the risk of falls among older inpatients, *Prof Nurse* 15(8):511, 2000.

Rader J, Jones D, Miller L: The importance of individualized wheelchair seating for frail older adults, *J Gerontol Nurs* 26(11):24, 2000.

Resnick B: Falls in a community of older adults, *Clin Nurs Res* 8(3):251, 1999.

Robertson MC et al: Effectiveness and economic evaluation of a nurse delivered home exercise programme to prevent falls, *BMJ* 322(7288):697, 2001.

Rogers PD, Bocchino NL: Restraint free care—is it possible? *Am J Nurs* 99(10):27, 1999.

Simmons S et al: Wheelchairs as mobility restraints: predictors of wheelchair activity in nonambulatory nursing home residents, *J Am Geriatr Soc* 43:384, 1995.

Slay DH: Home-based environmental lighting assessments for people who are visually impaired: developing techniques and tools, *J Vis Impair Blindness* 96(2):109, 2002.

Thapa P et al: Injurious falls in nonambulatory nursing home residents: a comparative study of circumstances, incidence, and risk factors, *J Am Geriatr Soc* 44:273, 1996.

Thapa P et al: Antidepressants and the risk of falls among nursing home residents, *N Engl J Med* 339(13):875, 1998.

Tinetti ME: Preventing falls in elderly persons, *N Engl J Med* 348(1):42, 2003.

Tinetti ME, Liu WL, Ginter SF: Mechanical restraint use and fall-related injuries among residents of skilled nursing facilities, *Ann Intern Med* 116:369, 1992.

Tinetti ME et al: A multifactorial intervention to reduce the risk of falling among elderly people living in the community, *N Engl J Med* 331:821, 1994.

Todd JF, Ruhl CE, Gross TP: Injury and death associated with hospital bed side-rails: reports of the US Food and Drug Administration from 1985 to 1995, *Am J Public Health* 87(10):1675, 1997.

Williams LM, Morton GA, Patrick CH: The Emory cubicle bed: an alternative to restraints for agitated traumatically brain injured clients, *Rehabil Nurs* 15:30, 1990.

Wilson EB: Preventing patient falls, *AACN Clin Issues* 9(1):100, 1998.

Wolf SL et al: Reducing frailty and falls in older persons: an investigation of tai chi and computerized balance training, *J Am Geriatr Soc* 44:489, 1996.

• = **Independent; ▲ = Collaborative**

Dysfunctional Family processes: alcoholism

Gail Ladwig

NANDA Definition

The state in which the psychosocial, spiritual, and physiological functions of the family unit are chronically disorganized, leading to conflict, denial of problems, resistance to change, ineffective problem solving, and a series of self-perpetuating crises

Defining Characteristics

Roles and Relationships

Inconsistent parenting/low perception of parental support; ineffective spouse communication/marital problems; intimacy dysfunction; deterioration in family relationships/disturbed family dynamics; altered role function/disruption of family roles; closed communication systems; chronic family problems; family denial; lack of cohesiveness; neglected obligations; lack of skills necessary for relationships; reduced ability of family members to relate to each other for mutual growth and maturation; family unable to meet security needs of its members; disrupted family rituals; economic problems; family does not demonstrate respect for individuality and autonomy of its members; triangulating family relationships; pattern of rejection

Behavioral

Refusal to get help/inability to accept and receive help appropriately; inadequate understanding or knowledge of alcoholism; ineffective problem-solving skills; loss of control of drinking; manipulation; rationalization/denial of problems; blaming; inability to meet emotional needs of its members; alcohol abuse; broken promises; criticizing; dependency; impaired communication; difficulty with intimate relationships; enabling to maintain drinking; expression of anger inappropriately; isolation; inability to meet spiritual needs of its members; inability to express or accept wide ranges of feelings; inability to deal with traumatic experiences constructively; inability to adapt to change; immaturity; harsh self-judgment; lying; lack of dealing with conflict; lack of reliability; nicotine addiction; orientation toward tension relief rather than achievement of goals; seeking approval and affirmation; difficulty having fun; agitation; chaos; contradictory, paradoxical communication; diminished physical contact; disturbances in academic performance in children; disturbances in concentration; escalating conflict; failure to accomplish current or past developmental tasks/difficulty with life cycle transitions; family special occasions are alcohol centered; controlling communication/power struggles; self-blaming; stress-related physical illnesses; substance abuse other than alcohol; unresolved grief; verbal abuse of spouse or parent

Feelings

Insecurity; lingering resentment; mistrust; vulnerability; rejection; repressed emotions; responsibility for alcoholic's behavior; shame/embarrassment; unhappiness; powerlessness; anger/suppressed rage; anxiety, tension, or distress; emotional isolation/loneliness; frustration; guilt; hopelessness; hurt; decreased self-esteem/worthlessness; hostility; lack of identity; fear; loss; emotional control by others; misunderstood; moodiness; aban-

• = Independent; ▲ = Collaborative

donment; being different from other people; being unloved; confused love and pity; confusion; failure; depression; dissatisfaction

Related Factors (r/t)

Abuse of alcohol; genetic predisposition; lack of problem-solving skills; family history of alcoholism; resistance to treatment; biochemical influences; addictive personality

NOC Outcomes (Nursing Outcomes Classification)

Suggested NOC Outcomes

Family Coping; Family Functioning; Family Health Status; Substance Addiction Consequences

> **Example NOC Outcome with Indicators**
>
> **Family Coping** as evidenced by the following indicators: Confronts problems/Regulates behavior of members/Absence of substance abuse (Rate each indicator of **Family Coping**: 1 = never demonstrated, 2 = rarely demonstrated, 3 = sometimes demonstrated, 4 = often demonstrated, 5 = consistently demonstrated [see Section I].)

Client Outcomes

Family Will (Specify Time Frame):

- Develop relationship with nurse that demonstrates at least minimal level of trust
- Demonstrate an understanding of alcoholism as a family illness and the severity of the threat to emotional and physical health of family members
- Develop and state a belief in feasibility and effectiveness of efforts to address alcoholism
- Demonstrate change from dysfunctional patterns by moving from inappropriate to appropriate role relationships, improving cohesion among family members, decreasing conflict and social isolation, and improving coping behaviors
- Maintain improvements

NIC Interventions (Nursing Interventions Classification)

Suggested NIC Interventions

Family Process Maintenance; Substance Use Treatment

> **Example Activities—Family Process Maintenance**
>
> Identify effects of role changes on family processes; Assist family members to use existing support measures

Nursing Interventions and Rationales

- Demonstrate high levels of empathy and expectancy of positive outcomes in interactions with family members. *A Swiss campaign used a short intervention approach that focused on an empathic and open discussion of drinking habits. This approach is efficient; takes little time; and, for nondependent patients, can considerably reduce the quantity of alcohol consumed (Stoll and Wick, 2000).*
- When completing a family assessment, assess behaviors of alcohol abuse, loss of con-

• = Independent; ▲ = Collaborative

trol of drinking, denial, nicotine addiction, impaired communication, inappropriate expression of anger, and enabling behaviors. **Nursing Research:** *This study clinically validated the defining characteristics for altered family process alcoholism using subjects (n = 150) who completed Fehring's (1987) Clinical Diagnostic Validation (CDV) (Bartek et al, 1999).* **Nursing Research:** *Assessment factors are included under interventions because it has been noted that assessment questions initiate a family process of self-examination and family problem solving and also provide assessment data (Craft and Willadsen, 1992).*

- Screen clients for at-risk drinking during routine primary care visits. At-risk drinking is defined as consuming an average of two or more drinks per day (chronic drinking), or two or more occasions of consuming five or more drinks in the past month (binge drinking), or, in the past month, one or more occasion of driving after consuming three or more drinks (drinking and driving). **Clinical Research:** *At least 1 in 10 patients making routine primary care visits have drinking practices that place them at risk for negative consequences from drinking. In this study, 3439 patients with advance appointments in 23 primary care practices completed a health survey before their visit (Curry et al, 2000).*

- Ask appropriate questions using an assessment tool such as FAST to assess whether denial is being used in association with alcoholism or drug use. The client is asked to circle the appropriate response for each question: Less than monthly; Monthly; Weekly; Daily; Almost Daily
  1. MEN: How often do you have EIGHT or more drinks on one occasion; WOMEN: How often do you have SIX or more drinks on one occasion?
  2. How often during the last year have you been unable to remember what happened the night before because you had been drinking?
  3. How often during the last year have you failed to do what was normally expected of you because of drinking?
  4. In the last year has a relative or friend, or a doctor or other health worker been concerned about your drinking or suggested you cut down?

  Clinical Research: *The four-item FAST alcohol questionnaire had good sensitivity and specificity, across a range of settings, when the AUDIT alcohol assessment score was used as the gold standard. The FAST questionnaire is quick to administer, since more than 50% of clients are categorized using just one question (Hodgson et al, 2002): Include drug use in addition to drinking in questionnaire (Hinkin et al, 2001). T-ACE and TWEAK are modified to be used with women.* **Nursing Research:** *Alcoholism rates are increasing in women and women may have distinct assessment risk factors (Becker and Walton-Moss, 2001). Brief addiction screening tools (Gorski, 2003).*

- Educate family members about alcoholism, being careful not to label or stigmatize them. *Children of alcoholics frequently build up defenses, shame, guilt, and loneliness. They need to be reassured that they did not cause the alcoholism and are not responsible for solving the problem (SAMHSA's National Clearinghouse for Alcohol and Drug Information, 1996).*

- ▲ Educate family members about available educational and support programs. **Clinical Research:** *A program aimed at early intervention and problem behaviors in preschool children in alcoholic families indicates that prevention programming is more appropriately family based rather than aimed at individuals (Nye et al, 1999).*

- Stress individual self-focus as a first step in problem resolution. **Nursing Research:** *Health Beliefs Model Research confirms that client understanding of the severity of the threat*

• = Independent; ▲ = Collaborative

to personal and family health and a belief in the feasibility and effectiveness of treatment are important motivating factors in changing health-related behavior (Damrosch, 1991; Giuffra, 1993).

- Help family to restructure family patterns of interaction and function to support the development of consistency, a predictable environment, emotional nurturance, and positive modeling. **Clinical Research:** *Studies indicate that consistency, a predictable environment, emotional nurturance, and positive social modeling may act as ameliorating factors in the dysfunctional environment (Seilhamer et al, 1993).*
- Assist with stabilization and maintenance of positive change in the family. Instruct the alcoholic's family members before the client's discharge to give verbal messages that convey concern about the alcoholic's problem drinking, their observations of the alcoholic's past episodes of drinking, and wishes and support for abstinence. **Clinical Research:** *This intervention method can help the alcoholic face the reality of his or her drinking problem and alcohol dependence and thus remain longer in long-range rehabilitation programs, which is a prerequisite for successful recovery from alcohol dependence. Patients' maintenance of abstinence was significantly better only when both they and their family members attended hospital outpatient follow-up sessions and/or self-help group meetings (Ino and Hayasida, 2000).*
- Instill hope and encourage the expression of positive thoughts. **Clinical Research:** *The data from this multicenter study confirm the argument that hopefulness appears to be central to a family's coping with the impact of mental illness. Nurses should be mindful of their capacity to sustain or diminish the hopes of family members (Bland and Darlington, 2002).*
- ▲ Provide school-based prevention programs using peer leaders at an early age. **Clinical Research:** *The results of this study suggest that targeting middle school-aged children and designing programs that can be delivered primarily by peer leaders will increase the effectiveness of school-based substance use prevention programs (Gottfredson et al, 2003).*
- Monitor family closely for return to old patterns of behavior. **Nursing Research:** *This report indicated the presence of family feelings of unhappiness, hurt, frustration, guilt, moodiness, powerlessness, loneliness, mistrust, anger, anxiety, and hopelessness (Bartek et al, 1999).*
- Provide activities that are physical in nature, such as adventure therapy and therapeutic camping, as part of a substance abuse treatment program. **Clinical Research:** *The results of this study add to the limited body of research supporting outdoor adventure and therapeutic camping experiences integrated with traditional relapse prevention activities as an adjunct to substance abuse treatment (Bennett et al, 1998).*
- ▲ Consider alternative therapies such as acupuncture. *Acupuncture may be helpful in detoxification and is valuable when used in combination with counseling (Serrano, 2003).*
- ▲ Refer for possible use of medications such as naltrexone and acamprosate to control problem drinking. **Clinical Research:** *The results of this randomized, double-blind, placebo-controlled protocol study support the efficacy of pharmacotherapeutic strategies in the relapse prevention of alcoholism. Naltrexone and acamprosate, especially in combination, considerably enhance the potential of relapse prevention (Kiefer et al, 2003).*
- Refer to care plans **Ineffective Denial** and **Defensive Coping.**

Geriatric

- Include assessment of possible alcohol abuse when assessing elderly family members. **Clinical Research:** *Alcohol abuse and alcoholism are common but underrecognized problems among older adults. One third of older alcoholic persons develop a problem with alcohol in*

- = **Independent;** ▲ = **Collaborative**

later life, whereas the other two thirds grow older with the medical and psychosocial sequelae of early-onset alcoholism (Rigler, 2000).
• Use CAGE tool with this population and include drug use along with drinking. An affirmative answer to two or more of the following questions is considered a basis for suspicion of alcohol abuse:
  C: Have you ever felt you ought to **Cut down** on drinking?
  A: Have people **Annoyed** you by criticizing your drinking?
  G: Have you ever felt bad or **Guilty** about your drinking?
  E: Have you ever had a drink first thing in the morning to steady your nerves or get rid of a hangover (**Eye opener**)?
  Nursing Research: *Alcoholism and drug abuse are present in the geriatric population and the CAGE tool is effective in identifying individuals at risk (Hinkin et al, 2001). Individuals with these problems are more likely to be found in health care settings that are not substance abuse specific (Weisner, 2001).*

Multicultural

• Acknowledge racial/ethnic differences at the onset of care. **Nursing Research:** *Acknowledgment of race/ethnicity issues will enhance communication, establish rapport, and promote treatment outcomes (D'Avanzo et al, 2001; Ludwick and Silva, 2000; Vontress and Epp, 1997).*
• Approach families of color with respect, warmth, and professional courtesy. **Nursing Research:** *Instances of disrespect and lack of caring have special significance for families of color (D'Avanzo, 2001; Vontress and Epp, 1997).*
• Give rationale when assessing black families about alcohol use and misuse. **Nursing Research:** *Many blacks may expect white caregivers to hold negative and preconceived ideas. Giving a rationale for questions asked will help alleviate this perception (D'Avanzo et al, 2001; Vontress and Epp, 1997).*
• Use a family-centered approach when working with Latino, Asian American, African American, and Native American clients. **Nursing Research:** *Latinos may perceive family as a source of support, solver of problems, and source of pride. Asian Americans may regard the family as the primary decision-maker and influence on individual family members (D'Avanzo et al, 2001). Native American families may be extended structures that could exert powerful influences over functioning (Seiderman et al, 1996).*
• When working with Asian American clients, provide opportunities for the family to save face. **Nursing Research:** *This will allow the family to not have to own the shame of the alcohol problem. Asian American families may avoid situations that bring shame on the family unit (Chen, 2001; D'Avanzo et al, 2001).*

Home care

NOTE: In the community setting, alcoholism as an etiology for dysfunctional family processes must be considered in two categories. The first is when the client suffers personally from the illness; the second is when a significant other suffers from the illness, that is, the client is not the active alcoholic but may be dependent on the alcoholic for caregiving. The listed considerations apply to both situations with appropriate adaptation for the circumstances.
• Above interventions may be adapted for home care use.
• Identify client/family expectations of the home care nurse and nurse expectations of the client/family by use of a well-defined contract. Be specific and realistic. Adjust the

• = Independent; ▲ = Collaborative

contract only with clear consent and understanding of the client/family. *A well-defined contract supports success in meeting goals and encourages positive family dynamics. A contract defines conditions under which care can be safely provided and under which care cannot continue. Safety of the staff should never be jeopardized.*

▲ Work with family members to support a sense of valued fit on their part; include them in treatment planning, and identify the importance of their roles in the client's care. At the same time, encourage their pursuit of positive outside activities that enhance their sense of belonging. **Nursing Research:** *Sense of belonging (valued fit) has been identified as a buffer to depression among both depressed and nondepressed individuals with a family history of alcoholism. A buffering effect was not found for individuals with a family history of drug abuse (Sargent et al, 2002).*

▲ Establish well-defined contingency and emergency plans for the care of the client. **Clinical Research:** *Safety of the client between visits is a primary goal of the home care nurse (Stanhope and Lancaster, 1996).*

• Request concrete, measurable tasks of the client and family for caregiving and provide concrete, nonjudgmental instruction to the client/family regarding the interactions of alcohol use with medications, therapeutic regimen. *The client/family will exercise ultimate control over whether or not to continue alcohol use. Clear information, delivered without judgment of the person, may provide the client/family with motivation to modify, if not discontinue, alcohol use.*

▲ Observe for abuse of other medications. Notify physician of problems noted. *Cross-addiction is a concern. Clients may substitute the use of other psychoactive medications for alcohol, or may be already addicted to hypnotics and/or pain medications. The presence of other addictions may raise issues with regard to withdrawal and synergistic effects.*

▲ If the client is a recovering alcoholic, extreme care must be taken in the use of psychoactive or pain medications. Notify physician if inappropriate medications have been inadvertently ordered. *Addiction to alcohol increases the potential for readdiction, especially if strong pain medications are introduced. In many instances, it is policy to prescribe nothing stronger than Extra-Strength Tylenol for recovering alcoholics in need of pain medication. Sleep medications should be avoided.*

▲ Refer for medical social work services at outset of care. *The social worker can help identify, set the structure for, and guide appropriate client/family and client/family/nurse interactions that will promote the plan of care throughout the length of the stay.*

▲ Provide information regarding available substance use treatment programs and support groups. *A variety of program types are available, from Alcoholics Anonymous to intensive inpatient treatment, with specialty units available in some areas for older adults.*

• Acknowledge without judging when resolution of alcoholism is not a goal of care. *It is usually not appropriate for terminally ill or hospice clients or their families to change family life patterns. Recognizing this fact nonjudgmentally helps the client or family use remaining energy to complete other end-of-life work.*

▲ Refer for psychiatric home health care services for client reassurance and implementation of therapeutic regimen. *Psychiatric home care nurses can address issues relating to the client's or family member's alcoholism and its interference with ability to adjust to changes in health status. Behavioral interventions in the home can assist the client to participate more effectively in treatment plan (Patusky et al, 1996).*

• = Independent; ▲ = Collaborative

evolve WEBSITES FOR EDUCATION

See the EVOLVE website for World Wide Web resources for client education.

REFERENCES

AHCPR (Agency for Healthcare Research and Quality): *Evidence report/technology assessment number 3: Pharmacotherapy for alcohol dependence,* AHCPR Pub No 99-E004, available on-line at www.ahcpr.gov/clinic/index.html#evidence, accessed Jan 16, 2000.

Bartek JK, Lindeman M, Hawks JH: Clinical validation of characteristics of the alcoholic family, *Nurs Diagn* 10(4):158, 1999.

Becker KL, Walton-Moss B: Detecting and addressing alcohol abuse in women, *Nurse Pract* 26(10):13, 2001.

Bennett LW, Cardone S, Jarczyk J: Effects of therapeutic camping program on addiction recovery, *J Subst Abuse Treat* 15(5):469, 1998.

Bland R, Darlington Y: The nature and sources of hope: perspectives of family caregivers of people with serious mental illness, *Perspect Psychiatr Care* 38(2):61, 2002.

Chen YC: Chinese values, health and nursing, *J Adv Nurs* 36(2):270, 2001.

Craft MJ, Willadsen JA: Interventions related to family, *Nurs Clin North Am* 27:517, 1992.

Curry SJ et al: At-risk drinking among patients making routine primary care visits, *Prev Med* 31(5):595, 2000.

Damrosch S: General strategies for motivating people to change their behavior, *Nurs Clin North Am* 26:833, 1991.

D'Avanzo CE et al: Developing culturally informed strategies for substance-related interventions. In Naegle MA, D'Avanzo CE, editors: *Addictions and substance abuse: strategies for advanced practice nursing,* St Louis, 2001, Mosby.

Giuffra MJ: Nursing strategies with alcohol and drug problems in the family. In Naegle MA, editor: *Substance abuse in education in nursing,* vol III, Pub No 15-2464, New York, 1993, National League for Nursing Press.

Gorski T: *Women at risk brief screening tools,* available on-line at http://www.tgorski.com/clin_mod/atp/women_at_risk-brief_sceening_tools.htm#TWEAK, accessed February 19, 2003.

Gottfredson DC, Wilson DB: Characteristics of effective school-based substance abuse prevention, *Prev Sci* 4(1):27, 2003.

Hinkin CH et al: Screening for drug and alcohol abuse among older adults using a modified version of the CAGE, *Am J Addict* 10:319, 2001.

Hodgson R et al: The FAST alcohol screening test, *Alcohol Alcohol* 37(1):61, 2002.

Ino A, Hayasida M: Before-discharge intervention method in the treatment of alcohol dependence, *Alcohol Clin Exp Res* 24(3):373, 2000.

Kiefer F et al: Comparing and combining naltrexone and acamprosate in relapse prevention of alcoholism: a double-blind, placebo-controlled study, *Arch Gen Psychiatry* 60(1):92, 2003.

Ludwick R, Silva M: Nursing around the world: cultural values and ethical conflicts, *Online J Issues Nurs,* available on-line at http://www.nursingworld.org/ojin/ethcol/ethics_4.htm.

Nye CL, Zucker RA, Fitzgerald HE: Early family-based intervention in the path to alcohol problems: rationale and relationship between treatment process characteristics and child and parenting outcomes, *J Stud Alcohol Suppl* 13:10, 1999.

Patusky KL, Rodning C, Martinez-Kratz M: Clinical lessons in psychiatric home care: a case study approach, *J Home Healthc Manag* 9:188, 1996.

Rigler SK: Alcoholism in the elderly, *Am Fam Physician* 61(6):1710, 2000.

SAMHSA (Substance Abuse and Mental Health Services Administration), National Clearinghouse on Alcohol and Drug Information: *Children of substance abusers,* available on-line at www.samhsa.gov, accessed June 19, 2003.

Sargent J et al: Sense of belonging as a buffer against depressive symptoms, *J Am Psychiatr Nurs Assoc* 8:120, 2002.

Seiderman RY et al: Assessing American Indian families, *MCN Am J Matern Child Nurs* 21(6):274, 1996.

Seilhamer RA, Jacob T, Dunn NJ: The impact of alcohol consumption on parent-child relationships in families of alcoholics, *J Stud Alcohol* 54:189, 1993.

Serrano R: *Solution focused addictions counseling, acupuncture treatment for substance abuse,* available on-line at http://www.holisticwebs.com/solution/sfac4.html, accessed January 18, 2003.

Stanhope M, Lancaster J, editors: *Community health nursing: promoting health of aggregates, families, and individuals,* ed 4, St Louis, 1996, Mosby.

• = Independent; ▲ = Collaborative

Stoll B, Wick HD: Short intervention approach: one-way of reducing excessive alcohol consumption, *Abhangigkeiten* Feb 2000.

Vontress CE, Epp LR: Historical hostility in the African American client: Implications for counseling, *J Multicult Counseling Dev* 25:170, 1997.

Weisner C: The provision of services for alcohol problems: a community perspective for understanding access, *J Behav Health Serv Res* 28(2):130, 2001.

Readiness for enhanced Family processes

Gail B. Ladwig

NANDA Definition

A pattern of family functioning that is sufficient to support the well-being of family members and can be strengthened

Defining Characteristics

Expresses willingness to enhance family dynamics; Family functioning meets physical, social, and psychological needs of family members; Activities support the safety and growth of family members; Communication is adequate; Relationships are generally positive; interdependent with community; family task are accomplished; Family roles are flexible and appropriate for developmental stages; Respect for family members is evident; Family adapts to change; Boundaries of family members are maintained; Energy level of family supports activities of daily living; Family resilience is evident; Balance exists between autonomy and cohesiveness

NOC   Outcomes (Nursing Outcomes Classification)

Suggested NOC Outcomes

Family Coping; Family Physical Environment; Health Orientation; Health Promoting Behavior; Health Seeking Behavior; Leisure Participation; Parent-Infant Attachment; Parenting Performance; Psychosocial Adjustment: Life Change; Risk Control; Role Performance; Social Support; Spiritual Health

> **Example NOC Outcome with Indicators**
>
> **Family Coping** as evidenced by the following indicators: Confronts problems/Manages problems/Involves family members in decision making (Rate each indicator of **Family Coping:** 1 = never demonstrated, 2 = rarely demonstrated, 3 = sometimes demonstrated, 4 = often demonstrated, 5 = consistently demonstrated [see Section I].)

Client Outcomes

Client Will (Specify Time Frame):

- Identify ways to cope effectively and use appropriate support systems (family)
- Meet physical, psychosocial, and spiritual needs of members or seeks appropriate assistance (family)
- Demonstrate knowledge of potential environmental, lifestyle, and genetic risks to health and use appropriate measures to decrease possibility of risk (family)
- Focus on wellness, disease prevention, and maintenance (family and individual)

- = **Independent;** ▲ = **Collaborative**

- Seek balance among exercise, work, leisure, rest, and nutrition (family and individual)

NIC   Interventions (Nursing Interventions Classification)

Suggested NIC Interventions

Active Listening; Anticipatory Guidance; Attachment Promotion; Coping Enhancement; Decision-Making Support; Environmental Management: Attachment Process; Exercise Promotion; Family Integrity Promotion; Family Involvement Promotion; Family Mobilization; Family Process Maintenance; Health Screening; Mutual Goal Setting; Parent Education: Adolescent, Childrearing Family; Risk Identification; Role Enhancement

---

Example NIC Activities—Risk Identification

Determine community support systems; Determine presence and quality of family support

---

Nursing Interventions and Rationales

- Assess the family's stress level and coping abilities during the initial nursing assessment. **Nursing Research:** *Nurses need to assess the family's baseline stress level and effectiveness of coping responses and assist the family as a whole as well as individual members in meeting their varying needs. Families differ in their ability to cope with multiple stressors (Rutledge et al, 2000a).*
- Use family-centered care, and role modeling for holistic care of families. **Nursing Research:** *Specific techniques of role modeling and reflective practice are suggested as effective approaches to teach family sensitive care in clinical settings where families are part of the care environment (Tomlinson et al, 2002).*
- Discuss with the family members how they have handled previous crises. *Such a discussion gives the nurse clues and information that can help in plan of care. Families that have a broad and diverse array of coping behaviors are more likely than others to meet needs and to have a good outcome (Coleman and Taylor, 1995).*
- Support family empowerment; strength and resourcefulness. **Nursing Research:** *The family can empower itself but it is also possible to empower the family from the outside, such as in child health clinics (Pelkonen, 2002).*
- Provide a parenting class series based on individual and couple changes in meaning/identity, roles, and relationship/interaction during the transition to parenthood. Address mother/father roles, infant communication abilities, and patterns of the first 3 months of life in a mutually enjoyable, possibility-focused way. **Nursing Research:** *This study demonstrated that interventions that enhance mutual parent-child interaction through increased sensitivity to cues and responsiveness to infant needs or signals are important avenues for facilitating secure attachment, father and mother involvement, optimal development, and prevention of child abuse and neglect (Bryan, 2000).*
- Spend time with family members; allow them to verbalize their feelings. **Nursing Research:** *Interactions help the client and family feel relieved and allow anxiety levels to decrease. Critical care nurses can provide support for families after the death of a loved one (Coolican and Politoski, 1994).*
- Encourage family members to find meaning in a serious illness like cancer. **Nursing Research:** *The positive dimensions of survivorship in meaning of the illness and family*

- = Independent; ▲ = Collaborative

quality of life (QOL) were seen for patients and family members with cancer (Mellon, 2002).

- Have family members participate in client conferences that involve all members of the health care team. *Conferences allow for distribution of information, input by all members at one time, and a decrease in anxiety levels of family members.*
- ▲ Provide family-centered care to explore and use all available resources appropriate for situation (e.g., counseling, social services, self-help groups, pastoral care). **Nursing Research:** *Meeting the need of families involves various kinds of interventions including those that offer reassurance and provide information. Family-centered care is a philosophical approach to meeting these needs (Rutledge et al, 2000b). Families are profoundly affected by the social contexts of mental illnesses (Rose et al, 2002).*

Geriatric

- Carefully listen to residents and family members in the long-term care facility. **Nursing Research:** *This study suggests that by listening to residents and family members nurses can improve life for residents and dignify them as individuals (Iwasiw et al, 2002).*
- Support caregivers' awareness of the positive effects of their contribution to the well-being of parents **Nursing Research:** *This study indicates that family satisfaction of caregivers of elderly parents may be influenced by reciprocity, emotional well-being, and family functioning (Carruth et al, 1997).*
- Teach family members about impact of developmental events (e.g., retirement, death, change in health status, and household composition). *Knowledge regarding normative developmental challenges of aging can reduce the stress such challenges place on families.*
- Encourage social networks, social integration, and social engagement with friends, children and relatives for the elderly **Clinical Research:** *This longitudinal study indicates that few social ties, poor integration, and social disengagement are risk factors for cognitive decline among community-dwelling elderly persons (Zunzunegui, 2003).*

Multicultural

- Assess for the influence of cultural beliefs, norms, and values on the family's perceptions of normal functioning. **Nursing Research:** *What the family considers normal and abnormal family functioning may be based on cultural perceptions (Leininger, 2002).*
- With the client's consent, facilitate a group meeting for family members to discuss how the family is functioning. **Nursing Research:** *A family meeting opens communication and lets each family member know it is okay to talk about what is happening (Rivera-Andino and Lopez, 2000).*
- Facilitate modeling and role-playing for the client and family regarding healthy ways to start a discussion about the client's prognosis. **Nursing Research:** *It is helpful for families and the client to practice communication skills in a safe environment before trying them in a real-life situation (Rivera-Andino and Lopez, 2000).*
- Identify and acknowledge the stresses unique to racial/ethnic families. **Nursing Research:** *Financial difficulties and maintaining cultural values are two of the most common family stressors cited by women of color (Majumdar and Ladak, 1998). In this study, women in Turkey perceive themselves as wives sharing everything within the family. Women's decision-making rate was lower than that of men, except for selecting clothes (Erci, 2003).*
- Offer frequent gestures of support to family members. **Nursing Research:** *Black mothers of seriously ill children identified support from the health care team as their highest source of satisfaction (Miles et al, 1999).*

- • = Independent; ▲ = Collaborative

- Encourage the family members to demonstrate and offer caring and support to each other. **Nursing Research:** *The familial characteristics of care and support have been associated with fostering resiliency. Resilience is the ability to experience adverse conditions and successfully overcome them (Calvert, 1997).*
- Validate the family's feelings regarding concerns about family functioning. **Nursing Research:** *Validation lets the client know that the nurse has heard and understands what was said, and it promotes the nurse-client relationship (Giger and Davidhizar, 1995; Stuart and Laraia, 2001).*
- Provide post partum home care for immigrant women who have a longer than usual post partum hospital stay, of more than 36 hours, and whose health and social concerns have not been documented as resolved. **Nursing Research:** *This study suggests that immigrant women may be receiving suboptimal care in the postpartum period (Katz and Gagnon, 2002).*

Home care

- The nursing interventions described previously for **Readiness for enhanced Family processes** should be used in the home environment with adaptations as necessary.
- Provide a videophone network for peer support for frail elderly people living at home. **Clinical Research:** *A videophone network appears to be helpful for elderly people in their peer support relationships. It supports and improves the functional independence of frail elderly people at home (Ezumi et al, 2003).*
- Encourage families to assist women caring for husbands with chronic obstructive pulmonary disease (COPD) to provide respite care so the women may have recreation time. **Nursing Research:** *Women caregivers of husbands with COPD were dissatisfied with their lack of recreation, as well as support from friends, families, and health care providers (Bergs, 2002).*

Client/Family Teaching

- Refer to Client/Family Teaching in **Readiness for enhanced family Coping** for suggestions that may be used with minor adaptations.

evolve WEBSITES FOR EDUCATION

See the EVOLVE website for World Wide Web resources for client education.

REFERENCES

Bergs D: "The hidden client"—women caring for husbands with COPD: their experience of quality of life, *J Clin Nurs* 11(5):613, 2002.

Bryan AA: Enhancing parent-child interaction with a prenatal couple intervention, *MCN Am J Matern Child Nurs* 25(3):139, 2000.

Calvert WJ: Protective factors within the family, and their role in fostering resiliency in African American adolescents, *J Cult Divers* 4(4):110, 1997.

Carruth AK et al: Reciprocity, emotional well-being, and family functioning as determinants of family satisfaction in caregivers of elderly parents, *Nurs Res* 46(2):93, 1997.

Coleman W, Taylor E: Family-focused pediatrics: issues, challenges, and clinical methods, *Pediatr Clin North Am* 42(1):119, 1995.

Coolican MB, Politoski G: Donor family programs, *Crit Care Nurs Clin North Am* 6(3):613, 1994.

Erci B: Women's efficiency in decision making and their perception of their status in the family, *Public Health Nurs* 20(1):65, 2003.

- = Independent; ▲ = Collaborative

Ezumi H et al: Peer support via video-telephony among frail elderly people living at home, *J Telemed Telecare* 9(1):30, 2003.

Giger JN, Davidhizar RE: *Transcultural nursing*, ed 2, St Louis, 1995, Mosby.

Iwasiw C et al: Resident and family perspectives: the first year in a long-term care facility, *J Gerontol Nurs* 29(1): 45, 2003.

Katz D, Gagnon AJ: Evidence of adequacy of postpartum care for immigrant women, *Can J Nurs Res* 34(4):71, 2002.

Leininger MM, McFarland MR: *Transcultural nursing: concepts, theories, research and practices*, ed 3, New York, 2002, McGraw-Hill.

Majumdar B, Ladak S: Management of family and workplace stress experienced by women of color from various cultural backgrounds, *Can J Public Health* 89(1):48, 1998.

Mellon S: Comparisons between cancer survivors and family members on meaning of the illness and family quality of life, *Oncol Nurs Forum* 29(7):1117, 2002.

Pilkonen M, Hakulinen T: An empowerment model for family nursing, *Hoitotiede* 14(5):202, 2002 (in Finnish).

Rivera-Andino J, Lopez L: When culture complicates care, *RN* 63(7):47, 2000.

Rose L, Mallinson RK, Walton-Moss B: A grounded theory of families responding to mental illness, *Nurs Res* 24(5):516, 2002.

Rutledge DN, Donaldson NE, Pravikoff DS: Caring for families of patients in acute or chronic health care settings: Part I—Principles, *Online J Clin Innovat* 3(3):1, 2000a.

Rutledge DN, Donaldson NE, Pravikoff DS: Caring for families of patients in acute or chronic care settings: Part II—Interventions, *Online J Clin Innovat* 3(3):1, 2000b.

Stuart GW, Laraia MT: Therapeutic nurse-patient relationship. In Stuart GW, Laraia MT, editors: *Principles and practice of psychiatric nursing*, St Louis, 2001, Mosby.

Tomlinson PS et al: Clinical innovation for promoting family care in paediatric intensive care: demonstration, role modelling and reflective practice, *J Adv Nurs* 38(2):161, 2002.

Zunzunegui MV et al: Social networks, social integration, and social engagement determine cognitive decline in community-dwelling Spanish older adults, *Gerontol B Psychol Sci Soc Sci* 58(2):S93, 2003.

Interrupted Family processes

Gail B. Ladwig

NANDA Definition

Change in family relationships and/or functioning

Defining Characteristics

Changes in power alliances; assigned tasks; effectiveness in completing assigned tasks; mutual support; availability for affective responsiveness and intimacy; patterns and rituals, participation in problem solving; participation in decision making; communication patterns; availability for emotional support; satisfaction with family; stress-reduction behaviors; expressions of conflict with and/or isolation from community resources; somatic complaints; expressions of conflict within family

Related Factors (r/t)

Power shift of family members; family roles shift; shift in health status of a family member; developmental transition and/or crisis; situational transition and/or crisis; informal or formal interaction with community; modification in family social status; modification in family finances

• = Independent; ▲ = Collaborative

| **NOC** | **Outcomes (Nursing Outcomes Classification)** |

Suggested NOC Outcomes

Family Coping; Family Social Climate; Family Functioning; Family Normalization; Parenting Performance; Psychosocial Adjustment: Life Change; Role Performance

> #### Example NOC Outcome with Indicators
>
> **Family Coping** as evidenced by the following indicators: Confronts problems/Manages problems/Involves family members in decision making (Rate each indicator of **Family Coping**: 1 = never demonstrated, 2 = rarely demonstrated, 3 = sometimes demonstrated, 4 = often demonstrated, 5 = consistently demonstrated [see Section I].)

Client Outcomes

Client Will (Specify Time Frame):

- Express feelings (family)
- Identify ways to cope effectively and use appropriate support systems (family)
- Treat impaired family member as normally as possible to avoid overdependence (family)
- Meet physical, psychosocial, and spiritual needs of members or seeks appropriate assistance (family)
- Demonstrate knowledge of illness or injury, treatment modalities, and prognosis (family)
- Participate in the development of the plan of care to the best of ability (significant person)

| **NIC** | **Interventions (Nursing Interventions Classification)** |

Suggested NIC Interventions

Family Integrity Promotion; Family Process Maintenance; Family Therapy; Normalization Promotion; Role Enhancement; Support System Enhancement

> #### Example NIC Activities—Normalization Promotion
>
> Collaborate with family in problem solving; Assist family in altering prescribed therapeutic regimen to fit normal schedule, when appropriate

Nursing Interventions and Rationales

- Assess the family's stress level and coping abilities during the initial nursing assessment. **Nursing Research:** *Nurses need to assess the family's baseline stress level and effectiveness of coping responses and to assist the family as a whole as well as individual members in meeting their varying needs. Families differ in their ability to cope with multiple stressors (Rutledge et al, 2000a).*
- Use family-centered care and role modeling for holistic care of families. **Nursing Research:** *Specific techniques of role modeling and reflective practice are suggested as effective approaches to teach family-sensitive care in clinical settings where families are part of the care environment (Tomlinson et al, 2002).*

• = Independent; ▲ = Collaborative

- Spend time with family members; allow them to verbalize their feelings. **Nursing Research:** *Interactions help the client and family feel relieved and allow anxiety levels to decrease. Critical care nurses can provide support for families after the death of a loved one (Coolican and Politoski, 1994).*
- Acknowledge the range of emotions and feelings that may be experienced when there is a change of health status in a family member; counsel family members that it is normal to be angry, afraid, etc. **Nursing Research:** *This study describes the experiences of the patient's family's experiences after the death of patients in the ICU. The experiences of the family members resembled a vortex: a downward spiral of prognoses, difficult decisions, feelings of inadequacy, and eventual loss despite the members' best efforts, and perhaps no good-byes (Kirchoff et al, 2002).*
- Encourage family members to list their personal strengths. *A list of strengths provides information that family members can refer to for positive feedback.*
- Involve family members in the care and information/patient teaching sessions with the client. *Family-focused activities can help families cope better with the hospital experience (Worthington, 1995).*
- Encourage family to visit the client; adjust visiting hours to accommodate family's schedule (e.g., schedule around work, school, babysitting needs). Assist with sleeping arrangements if family is spending the night; provide a place to lie down, pillows, and blankets.
- Allow and encourage family to assist in the client's care. Allow family presence during invasive procedures and resuscitation. *Assisting with the client's care helps maintain the family's connectedness. Strategies to facilitate effective coping of family members during the crisis of critical illness include family attendance during invasive procedures and resuscitation efforts (Twibell, 1998).* **Nursing Research:** *Families of hospitalized children may wish to participate more actively in the actual physical care of the patient than family members of an adult patient (Rutledge et al, 2000b).*
- ▲ Consider use of video home training as a method of early support in problems of family life control. *Video home training is a method in supporting family life control that consists of goal-orientated reflection by parents on videotaped episodes of their everyday family life under the guidance of a family counselor.* **Nursing Research:** *The findings show that video home training helped the families to gain better control over their family life. The process of videotaping family life, in-depth analysis of the videotapes, recognition of instances of successful interaction, and search for new alternatives gave participants a feeling that it would be possible for them to make their everyday life fluent and functional (Häggman-Laitila et al, 2003).*
- ▲ Provide family-centered care to explore and use all available resources appropriate for situation (e.g., counseling, social services, self-help groups, pastoral care). **Nursing Research:** *Meeting the need of families involves various kinds of interventions including those that offer reassurance and provide information. Family-centered care is a philosophical approach to meeting these needs (Rutledge et al, 2000b).*

Geriatric
- Teach family members about the impact of developmental events (e.g., retirement, death, change in health status, and household composition). *Knowledge regarding normative developmental challenges of aging can reduce the stress that such challenges place on families.*
- Encourage family members to be involved in the care of relatives who are in residential

• = **Independent;** ▲ = **Collaborative**

care settings. **Nursing Research:** *In this study it was demonstrated that family members continue to provide care to their relatives within the long-term care facility, and establish a role for themselves within the formal care system (Janzen, 2000).*

- Support group problem solving among family members and include the older member. *Problem solving is an effective method to manage stressors for family members of all ages.*
▲ Refer family for counseling with a psychotherapist who is knowledgeable about gerontology.
- Refer to care plan for **Readiness for enhanced family Coping**.

Multicultural

- Assess for the influence of cultural beliefs, norms, and values on the family's perceptions of normal functioning. **Nursing Research:** *What the family considers normal and abnormal family functioning may be based on cultural perceptions (Cochran, 1998; Doswell and Erlen, 1998; Guaranccia, 1998; Leininger and McFarland, 2002).*
- With the client's consent, facilitate a group meeting for family members to discuss how the family is functioning. **Nursing Research:** *A family meeting opens communication and lets each family member know it is okay to talk about what is happening (Rivera-Andino and Lopez, 2000).*
- Facilitate modeling and role-playing for the client and family regarding healthy ways to start a discussion about the client's prognosis. **Nursing Research:** *It is helpful for families and the client to practice communication skills in a safe environment before trying them in a real-life situation (Rivera-Andino and Lopez, 2000).*
- Identify and acknowledge the stresses unique to racial/ethnic families. **Nursing Research:** *Financial difficulties and maintaining cultural values are two of the most common family stressors cited by women of color (Ludwick and Silva, 2000; Majumdar and Ladak, 1998; Vontress and Epp, 1997).*
- Offer frequent gestures of support to family members. **Nursing Research:** *Black mothers of seriously ill children identified support from the health care team as their highest source of satisfaction (Miles et al, 1999).*
- Encourage the family members to demonstrate and offer caring and support to each other. **Nursing Research:** *The familial characteristics of care and support are associated with fostering resiliency in black families. Resilience is the ability to experience adverse conditions and to successfully overcome them (Calvert, 1997).*
- Validate the family's feelings regarding concerns about current crisis and family functioning. **Nursing Research:** *Validation is a therapeutic communication technique that lets the client know that the nurse has heard and understands what was said, and it promotes the nurse-client relationship (Heineken, 1998).*

Home care

- The nursing interventions described previously for **Compromised family Coping** should be used in the home environment with adaptations as necessary.
- Assist help from the family when communicating with clients in advanced stages of cancer who are no longer able to communicate their illness and symptom needs. **Nursing Research:** *Next of kin (NOK) play an integral role in fostering optimal quality of life in symptomatic patients who are coping with cancer in the home setting (Lobchuk and Degner, 2002).*

• = **Independent;** ▲ = **Collaborative**

Client/Family Teaching

- Refer to Client/Family Teaching in **Compromised family Coping** and **Readiness for enhanced family Coping** for suggestions that may be used with minor adaptations.

evolve WEBSITES FOR EDUCATION

See the MERLIN website for World Wide Web resources for client education.

REFERENCES

Calvert WJ: Protective factors within the family, and their role in fostering resiliency in African American adolescents, *J Cult Divers* 4(4):110, 1997.

Cochran M: Tears have no color, *Am J Nurs* 98(6):53, 1998.

Coolican MB, Politoski G: Donor family programs, *Crit Care Nurs Clin North Am* 6(3):613, 1994.

Doswell W, Erlen J: Multicultural issues and ethical concerns in the delivery of revising care interventions, *Nurs Clin North Am* 33(2):353, 1998.

Guarnaccia P: Multicultural experiences of family caregiving: A Study of African American, European American, and Hispanic American families, *New Direct Ment Health Serv* 77:45, 1998.

Häggman-Laitila A et al: Video home training as a method of supporting family life control, *J Clin Nurs* 12(1): 93, 2003.

Heineken J: Patient silence is not necessarily client satisfaction: communication in home care nursing, *Home Healthc Nurse* 16(2):115, 1998.

Janzen WM: *Family members caring for relatives with Alzheimer disease in long-term care facilities,* Edmonton, Alberta, Canada, 2000, University of Alberta (doctoral dissertation).

Kirchhoff KT et al: The vortex: families' experiences with death in the intensive care unit, *Am J Crit Care* 11(3): 200, 2002.

Leininger MM, McFarland MR: *Transcultural nursing: concepts, theories, research and practices,* ed 3, New York, 2002, McGraw-Hill.

Lobchuk MM, Degner LF: Patients with cancer and next-of-kin response comparability on physical and psychological symptom well-being: trends and measurement issues, *Cancer Nurs* 25(5):358, 2002.

Ludwick R, Silva M: Nursing around the world: cultural values and ethical conflicts, *Online J Issues Nurs,* available on-line at http://www.nursingworld.org/ojin/ethcol/ethics_4.htm.

Majumdar B, Ladak S: Management of family and workplace stress experienced by women of color from various cultural backgrounds, *Can J Public Health* 89(1):48, 1998.

Miles MS, Wilson SM, Docherty SL: African American mothers' responses to hospitalization of an infant with serious health problems, *Neonatal Netw* 18(8):17, 1999.

Rivera-Andino J, Lopez L: When culture complicates care, *RN* 63(7):47, 2000.

Rutledge DN, Donaldson NE, Pravikoff DS: Caring for families of patients in acute or chronic health care settings: Part I—Principles, *Online J Clin Innovat* 3(3):1, 2000a.

Rutledge DN, Donaldson NE, Pravikoff DS: Caring for families of patients in acute or chronic care settings: Part II—Interventions, *Online J Clin Innovat* 3(3):1, 2000b.

Stuart GW, Laraia MT: Therapeutic nurse-patient relationship. In Stuart GW, Laraia MT, editors: *Principles and practice of psychiatric nursing,* St Louis, 2001, Mosby.

Tomlinson PS et al: Clinical innovation for promoting family care in paediatric intensive care: demonstration, role modelling and reflective practice, *J Adv Nurs* 38(2):161, 2002.

Twibell RS: Family coping during critical illness, *Dimens Crit Care Nurs* 17(2):100, 1998.

Vontress CE, Epp LR: Historical hostility in the African American client: Implications for counseling, *J Multicult Counseling Dev* 25:170, 1997.

Worthington R: Effective transitions for families: life beyond the hospital, *Pediatr Nurs* 21:8, 1995.

• = **Independent;** ▲ = **Collaborative**

Fatigue

Betty J. Ackley and Gail B. Ladwig

NANDA Definition

An overwhelming, sustained sense of exhaustion and decreased capacity for physical and mental work at usual level

Defining Characteristics

Inability to restore energy even after sleep; lack of energy or inability to maintain usual level of physical activity; increase in rest requirements; tired; inability to maintain usual routines; verbalization of an unremitting and overwhelming lack of energy; lethargic or listless; perceived need for additional energy to accomplish routine tasks; increase in physical complaints; compromised concentration; disinterest in surroundings, introspection; decreased performance; compromised libido; drowsy; feelings of guilt for not keeping up with responsibilities

Related Factors (r/t)

Psychological

Boring lifestyle; stress; anxiety; depression

Environmental

Humidity; lights; noise; temperature

Situational

Negative life events; occupation

Physiological

Sleep deprivation; pregnancy; poor physical condition; disease states (cancer, HIV, multiple sclerosis); increased physical exertion; malnutrition; anemia

NOC Outcomes (Nursing Outcomes Classification)

Suggested NOC Outcomes

Concentration; Endurance; Energy Conservation; Nutritional Status: Energy

---

Example NOC Outcome with Indicators

Endurance as evidenced by the following indicators: Performance of usual routine/Activity/Rested appearance/Blood oxygen level within normal limits/Expresses feelings about loss/Verbalizes acceptance of loss/Describes meaning of the loss or death/Reports decreased preoccupation with loss/Expresses positive expectations about the future (Rate each indicator of **Endurance:** I = extremely compromised, 2 = substantially compromised, 3 = moderately compromised, 4 = mildly compromised, 5 = not compromised [see Section I].)

Client Outcomes

Client Will (Specify Time Frame):
• Verbalize increased energy and improved well-being

• = Independent; ▲ = Collaborative

- Explain energy conservation plan to offset fatigue

NIC   Interventions (Nursing Interventions Classification)

Suggested NIC Intervention
Energy Management

> **Example NIC Activities—Energy Management**
>
> Determine patient's physical limitations; Determine patient's significant other's perception of causes of fatigue

Nursing Interventions and Rationales

- Assess severity of fatigue on a scale of 0 to 10; assess frequency of fatigue, activities associated with increased fatigue, ability to perform activities of daily living (ADLs), times of increased energy, ability to concentrate, mood, and usual pattern of activity. Consider use of an instrument such as the Profile of Mood State Short Form Fatigue Subscale, the Multidimensional Assessment of Fatigue, the Lee Fatigue Scale, the Multidimensional Fatigue Inventory, the HIV-Related Fatigue Scale, or the Dutch Fatigue Scale to accurately assess fatigue. *These assessments have all shown to have good internal reliability. The Profile of Mood State Short Form Fatigue Scale was the strongest performer in one study (Meek et al, 2000).* **Nursing Research:** *The Dutch Fatigue Scale, which is based on NANDA's defining characteristics, is a reliable and valid measurement tool for assessment of fatigue (Tiesing et al, 2001). The HIV-Related Fatigue Nursing Research Scale is valuable for measuring fatigue in HIV-positive clients (Barroso and Lynn, 2002).*
- Evaluate adequacy of nutrition and sleep. Encourage the client to get adequate rest. Refer to **Imbalanced Nutrition: less than body requirements** or **Disturbed Sleep pattern** if appropriate. NOTE: *Sometimes clients with chronic fatigue syndrome can sleep excessively and need support to limit sleeping. The most commonly suggested treatment for fatigue is rest (Nail and Winningham, 1995). Inadequate nutrition or poor sleep can contribute to fatigue.*
- ▲ Determine with help from the primary care practitioner whether there is a physiological or psychological cause of fatigue that could be treated, such as anemia, electrolyte imbalance, hypothyroidism, depression, or medication effect. *The presence of fatigue is associated with biological, psychological, social, and personal factors (Belza et al, 1993). Fatigue should not be tolerated if it can be readily reversed with treatment.*
- ▲ Work with the physician to determine if the client has chronic fatigue syndrome. The Centers for Disease Control and Prevention defines chronic fatigue syndrome as "Clinically evaluated, unexplained, persistent, or relapsing chronic fatigue (over 6 months' duration) that is of new or definite onset (has not been lifelong); is not the result of ongoing exertion; is not alleviated by rest; and results in substantial reduction in previous levels of occupational, educational, social, or personal activities. In addition, four or more the following symptoms must concurrently be present for over 6 months: impaired memory or concentration, sore throat, tender cervical or axial lymph nodes, muscle pain, multijoint pain, new headaches, unrefreshing sleep, and postexertion malaise lasting more than 24 hours" (Walker, 1999).
- Encourage the client to express feelings about fatigue; use active listening techniques and help identify sources of hope. **Clinical Research:** *Chronic fatigue is a disabling*

- = **Independent;** ▲ = **Collaborative**

illness characterized by persistent fatigue accompanied by rheumatologic, cognitive, and infectious appearing symptoms (Craig and Kakumanu, 2002).

- Encourage the client to keep a journal of activities, symptoms of fatigue, and feelings. *The journal helps the client monitor progress toward resolving or coping with fatigue and express feelings, which helps with adjustment (Jones, 1992).*
- Assist the client with ADLs as necessary; encourage independence without causing exhaustion.
- Help the client set small, easily achieved short-term goals such as writing two sentences in a journal daily or walking to the end of the hallway twice daily.
- Encourage walking exercise. **Nursing Research:** *Women undergoing treatment for cancer exercised 90 minutes per week on 3 or more days and reported significantly less fatigue and emotional distress as well as higher functional ability and quality of life than did women who were less active during treatment (Mock et al, 2002).*
- ▲ With the physician's approval, refer to physical therapy for carefully monitored aerobic exercise program. **Nursing Research:** *Aerobic exercise and physical therapy can reduce fatigue in some oncology clients (Stone, 2002, 2000).* **Research Review:** *An exercise program for patients receiving radiation treatments for cancer of the breast also helped improve emotional health and increased sleep (Mock et al, 1997). A customized exercise program can be helpful to the client with chronic fatigue syndrome (Jain and DeLisa, 1998).* **Evidence-Based Research:** *Supervised aerobic exercise training has beneficial effects on physical capacity and fibromyalgia symptoms (Busch et al, 2002).*
- ▲ Refer the client to diagnosis-appropriate support groups such as National Chronic Fatigue Syndrome Association or Multiple Sclerosis Association. *Support groups can help clients deal with body changes and cope with the frequent depression that accompanies fatigue (Jain and DeLisa, 1998; Jones, 1992).*
- Help the client identify essential and nonessential tasks and determine which can be delegated. Give the client permission to limit social and role demands if needed (e.g., switch to part-time employment, hire cleaning service). *The nurse can help the client look at life realistically to balance available energy and energy demands.*
- ▲ For a cardiac client, recognize that fatigue is common following a myocardial infarction (Lee et al, 2000). Refer to cardiac rehabilitation for carefully prescribed and monitored exercise program. *Carefully monitored exercise is thought to decrease symptoms of fatigue in heart patients (Friedman and King, 1995).*
- For fatigue with multiple sclerosis, encourage energy conservation, "recharging efforts," excellent self-care, and consider use of a cooling suit for clients with multiple sclerosis whose fatigue increases in a warm environment. **Nursing Research:** *Results of this study indicate that use of a cooling suit by individuals with multiple sclerosis may decrease their sense of fatigue (Flensner and Lindencrona, 2002).*
- For attentional fatigue, suggest restorative activities such as sitting outside, birdwatching, and gardening (Erickson, 1996). *Being outside and enjoying nature can help people recover their strength and think more clearly.*
- ▲ If not coping well, refer for cognitive therapy to help deal with symptoms of fatigue and help change negative thought patterns. *Cognitive therapy can be effective for clients with chronic fatigue syndrome (Fisher, 1997; Walker, 1999), also for clients with HIV (Rose et al, 1998).* **Evidence-Based Research:** *Cognitive behavior therapy significantly benefits physical functioning in adult outpatients with chronic fatigue syndrome (Price and Couper, 2002).*

• = **Independent;** ▲ = **Collaborative**

▲ If fatigue is associated with chemotherapy, be sure to treat nausea, vomiting, and pain effectively and prevent mouth sores if possible. **Clinical Research:** *Increased fatigue was seen in breast cancer clients receiving chemotherapy if they were also experiencing unrelieved pain, had nausea with vomiting, or developed mouth sores (Jacobsen et al, 1999).*

▲ Refer the client to occupational therapy to learn new energy-conserving ways to perform tasks. *Occupational therapy can help clients learn energy-conserving techniques so that clients can perform ADLs without exhaustion.*

▲ If the client is very weak, refer to physical therapy for prescription and use of a mobility aid such as a walker.

Geriatric

• Identify recent losses; monitor for depression as a possible contributing factor to fatigue. **Nursing Research:** *Thirty elderly women with depression identified symptoms of fatigue and weakness (Ugarriza, 2002).*

▲ Review medications for side effects. *Certain medications (e.g., beta-blockers, antihistamines, pain medications) may cause fatigue in the elderly.*

Home care

• Above interventions may be adapted for home care use.

• Assess the client's history and current patterns of fatigue as they relate to the home environment; environmental and behavioral triggers of increased fatigue. *Fatigue may be more pronounced in specific settings for physical, environmental (e.g., stairs required to reach bathroom, patterns of movement around home, cleaning activities that require high energy), or psychological (e.g., rooms associated with loss of loved ones) reasons.*

▲ Refer to occupational therapy if substantial intervention is needed to assist the client in adapting to home and daily patterns.

• Assist the client with identifying or creating a safe, restful place within the home that can be used routinely (e.g., a room with familiar, nonthreatening, or nonfrightening belongings). *Withdrawal to a secluded area can allow the client to rest and regain strength.*

▲ For clients receiving chemotherapy, intervene to:
  ■ Relieve symptom distress (negative mood, nausea, difficulty sleeping)
  ■ Encourage as much physical activity as possible
  ■ Support a positive attitude for the future
  ■ Support adequate recovery time between treatments.
  Nursing Research: *The above factors have been identified as contributing to fatigue, particularly during early stages of chemotherapy (Berger and Walker, 2001).*

▲ Refer cancer clients to a community-based pain and fatigue management program, such as the I Feel Better program, if available. **Clinical Research:** *A program such as I Feel Better was received with enthusiasm and rapid enrollment by cancer clients (Grant et al, 2000).*

• Teach the client/family the importance of and methods for setting priorities for activities, especially those having a high energy demand (e.g., home/family events). Instruct in realistic expectations and behavioral pacing. **Nursing Research:** *The client and/or family may assume a more rapid rate of energy recovery than actually occurs. Assistance may be needed to insure accuracy of expectations for the client. Unrealistic expectations provoke guilt feelings in the client, leading to efforts that can exceed the client's energy capacity (Patusky, 2002).*

• = **Independent**; ▲ = **Collaborative**

- Assess effect of fatigue on the client's relatedness; recognize that the client's fatigue affects the whole family. Initiate the following interventions:
  - Avoid dismissing reports of fatigue; validate the client's experience and foster hope for eventual treatment, if not resolution, of the fatigue.
  - Identify with the client ways in which he or she continues to be a valued part of his or her social environment.
  - Identify with the client ways in which he or she continues to participate in equitable exchange with others.
  - Encourage the client to maintain regular family routines (e.g., meals, sleep patterns) as much as possible.
  - Initiate cognitive restructuring to refute the client's guilt-producing and negative thought patterns.
  - Assess and intervene with family/friend's contributions to guilt-inducing self-talk.
  - Work with the client to inoculate against the negative thinking of others.
  - Explore family life and demands to identify accommodations.
  - Support the client's efforts at limit setting on the demands of others.
  - Assist the client to move toward a state of parallelism by working to identify and relieve sources of physical or emotional discomfort. Degree of involvement, limited by fatigue, need not be changed.
  - **Nursing Research:** *Based on reports of fatigued women, the above interventions have been suggested as addressing problem areas. Parallelism is a state of comfortable noninvolvement, and was described by some fatigued women as achievable and relatively positive state, given their fatigue (Patusky, 2002). Closeness and acceptance in relationships may decrease the psychological burden and modify the fatigue of chemotherapy recipients (Berger and Walker, 2001).*
- ▲ Refer for family therapy in the event the client's fatigue interferes with normal family functioning. *Family therapy may be necessary to address underlying problems that may be magnified by the influence of fatigue (Patusky, 2002).*
- ▲ If fatigue has affected the client's ability to participate in relationships effectively, refer for psychiatric home health care services for client reassurance and implementation of therapeutic regimen. *Psychiatric home care nurses can address issues relating to the client's ability to adjust to changes in health status. Behavioral interventions in the home can assist the client to participate more effectively in the treatment plan (Patusk et al, 1996).*

Client/Family Teaching

- Share information about fatigue and how to live with it, including need for positive self-talk. *Client education legitimizes fatigue and enhances the client's control through self-care and positive self-talk (Fisher, 1997).*
- Teach strategies for energy conservation (e.g., sitting instead of standing during showering, storing items at waist level). *These strategies decrease the amount of energy used (Johnson and Coward, 2001).*
- Teach the client to carry a pocket calendar, make lists of required activities, and post reminders around the house. *Chronic fatigue is often associated with memory loss and sometimes difficulty thinking (Jain and DeLisa, 1998).*
- Teach the importance of following a healthy lifestyle with adequate nutrition and rest, pain relief, and appropriate exercise to decrease fatigue.

• = Independent; ▲ = Collaborative

- Teach stress-reduction techniques such as controlled breathing, imagery, and use of music.
- See **Anxiety** care plan if appropriate; anxiety is correlated with increased fatigue.

evolve **WEBSITES FOR EDUCATION**

See the MERLIN website for World Wide Web resources for client education.

REFERENCES

Barroso J, Lynn MR: Psychometric properties of the HIV-Related Fatigue Scale, *J Assoc Nurses AIDS Care* 13(1):66, 2002.

Belza BL et al: Correlates of fatigue in older adults with rheumatoid arthritis, *Nurs Res* 42(2):93, 1993.

Berger AM, Walker SN: An explanatory model of fatigue in women receiving adjuvant breast cancer chemotherapy, *Nurs Res* 50:42, 2001.

Busch A et al: Exercise for treating fibromyalgia syndrome, *Cochrane Database Syst Rev* 3(CD003786), 2002.

Craig T, Kakumanu S: Chronic fatigue syndrome: evaluation and treatment, *Am Fam Physician* 65(5):1083, 2002.

Erickson JM: Anemia, *Semin Oncol Nurs* 12(1):2, 1996.

Fisher L: Chronic fatigue syndrome, *Prof Nurse* 12(8):578, 1997.

Flensner G, Lindencrona C: The cooling-suit: case studies of its influence on fatigue among eight individuals with multiple sclerosis, *J Adv Nurs* 37(6):541, 2002.

Friedman MM, King KK: Correlates of fatigue in older women with heart failure, *Heart Lung* 24(6):512, 1995.

Grant M et al: Developing a community program on cancer pain and fatigue, *Cancer Pract* 8(4):187, 2000.

Jacobsen PB et al: Fatigue in women receiving adjuvant chemotherapy for breast cancer: characteristics, course, and correlates, *J Pain Symptom Manage* 18(4):233, 1999.

Jain SS, DeLisa JA: Chronic fatigue syndrome: a literature review from a physiatric perspective, *Am J Phys Med Rehabil* 77(2):160, 1998.

Johnson M, Dickerson Coward D: Cancer related fatigue: nursing assessment and management, *Am J Nurs* April(suppl):19, 2001.

Jones CA: These patients truly need our help, *RN* 55:46, 1992.

Lee H et al: Fatigue, mood, and hemodynamic patterns after myocardial infarction, *Appl Nurs Res* 13(2):60, 2000.

Meek PM et al: Psychometric testing of fatigue instruments for use with cancer patients, *Nurs Res* 49(4):181, 2000.

Mock V et al: Effects of exercise on fatigue, physical functioning, and emotional distress during radiation therapy for breast cancer, *Oncol Nurs Forum* 24(6):991, 1997.

Mock V et al: Fatigue and quality of life outcomes of exercise during cancer treatment, *Cancer Pract* 9(3):119, 2001.

Nail LM, Winningham ML: Fatigue and weakness in cancer patients: the symptom experience, *Semin Oncol Nurs* 11(4):272, 1995.

Patusky KL: Relatedness theory as a framework for the treatment of fatigued women, *Arch Psychiatr Nurs* 5:224, 2002.

Patusky KL, Rodning C, Martinez-Kratz M: Clinical lessons in psychiatric home care: a case study approach, *J Home Healthc Manag* 9:18, 1996.

Price JR, Couper J: Cognitive behavior therapy for chronic fatigue syndrome in adults, *Cochrane Library* 3(CDO01027), 2002.

Rose L et al: The fatigue experience: persons with HIV infection, *J Adv Nurs* 28(2):295, 1998.

Schwartz AL: Daily fatigue patterns and effect of exercise in women with breast cancer, *Cancer Pract* 8(1):16, 2000.

Stone P: The measurement, causes and effective management of cancer-related fatigue, *Int J Palliative Nurs* 8(3):120, 2002.

Tiesinga LJ et al: Sensitivity, specificity and usefulness of the Dutch Fatigue Scale, *Nurs Diagn* 12(3):93, 2001.

Ugarriza DN: Elderly women's explanation of depression, *J Gerontol Nurs* 28(5):22, 2002.

Walker TL: Chronic fatigue syndrome. Do you know what it means? *Am J Nurs* 99(3):70, 1999.

- **= Independent; ▲ = Collaborative**

Fear

Michele Walters and Gail Ladwig

NANDA Definition

Response to perceived threat that is consciously recognized as a danger

Defining Characteristics

Report of apprehension; increased tension; decreased self-assurance; excitement; being scared; jitteriness; dread; alarm; terror; panic

Cognitive

Identifies object of fear; stimulus believed to be a threat; diminished productivity, learning ability, problem-solving ability

Behaviors

Increased alertness; avoidance or attack behaviors; impulsiveness; narrowed focus on "it" (i.e., the focus of the fear)

Physiological

Increased pulse; anorexia; nausea; vomiting; diarrhea; muscle tightness; fatigue; increased respiratory rate and shortness of breath; pallor; increased perspiration; increased systolic blood pressure; pupil dilation; dry mouth

Related Factors (r/t)

Natural/innate origin (e.g., sudden noise, height, pain, loss of physical support); learned response (e.g., conditioning, modeling from or identification with others); separation from support system in potentially stressful situation (e.g., hospitalization, hospital procedures); unfamiliarity with environmental experience(s); language barrier; sensory impairment; innate releasers (neurotransmitters); phobic stimulus

NOC Outcomes (Nursing Outcomes Classification)

Suggested NOC Outcome

Fear Self-Control

Example NOC Outcome with Indicators

Fear Self-Control as evidenced by the following indicators: Eliminates precursors of fear/Seeks information to reduce fear/Plans coping strategies for fearful situations (Rate each indicator of **Fear Self-Control:** 1 = never demonstrated, 2 = rarely demonstrated, 3 = sometimes demonstrated, 4 = often demonstrated, 5 = consistently demonstrated [see Section I].)

Client Outcomes

Client Will (Specify Time Frame):
- Verbalize known fears
- State accurate information about the situation

• = **Independent; ▲ = Collaborative**

- Identify, verbalize, and demonstrate those coping behaviors that reduce own fear
- Report and demonstrate reduced fear

NIC   Interventions (Nursing Interventions Classification)

Suggested NIC Interventions
Anxiety Reduction; Coping Enhancement; Security Enhancement

> **Example NIC Activities—Anxiety Reduction**
>
> Use a calm reassuring approach; Stay with the patient to promote safety and reduce fear

Nursing Interventions and Rationales

- Assess source of fear with the client. **Clinical Research:** *The capacity to experience fear is adaptive, enabling rapid and energetic response to imminent threat or danger (Poulton and Menzies, 2002).*
- Have the client draw the object of their fear. *This is a reliable assessment tool for children. Because human figure drawings are reliable tools for assessing anxiety and fears in children, practitioners should incorporate these drawings as part of their routine assessments of fearful children (Carroll and Ryan-Wenger, 1999).*
- Discuss situation with the client and help distinguish between real and imagined threats to well-being. **Clinical Research:** *Fear activation occurs before conscious cognitive analysis of the stimulus can occur (Mineka and Ohman, 2002).*
- If the client's fear is a reasonable response, empathize with the client. Avoid false reassurances and be truthful. Reassure clients that seeking help is both a sign of strength and a step toward resolution of the problem (Bailey and Bailey, 1993).
- If possible, remove the source of the client's fear with accurate and appropriate amounts of information. **Nursing Research:** *Clients' uncertainty regarding the outcomes can lead to feelings of distress. In one study, the major strategy used to reduce distress was information management, in which the amount and type of incoming information was controlled (Shaw et al, 1994).*
- If possible, help the client confront the fear. *Self-discovery enhances feelings of control.*
- Stay with clients when they express fear; provide verbal and nonverbal (touch and hug with permission and if culturally acceptable) reassurances of safety if safety is within control. *The nurse's presence and touch demonstrate caring and diminish the intensity of feelings such as fear (Olson and Sneed, 1995).* **Clinical Research:** *Of 376 patients surveyed in 20 family practices throughout Ontario, Canada, 66% believe touch is comforting and healing and view distal touches (on the hand and shoulder) as comforting (Osmun et al, 2000).*
- Explain all activities, procedures (in advance when possible), and issues that involve the client; use nonmedical terms and calm, slow speech; and verify the client's understanding. **Nursing Research:** *Deficient knowledge or unfamiliarity is one factor associated with fear (Garvin et al, 1992; Whitney, 1992).*
- Explore coping skills used previously by the client to deal with fear; reinforce these skills and explore other outlets. **Nursing Research:** *Recounting previous experiences that were perceived by the client as having been dealt with successfully strengthens effective coping and helps eliminate ineffective coping mechanisms (Northouse et al, 2002).*
- Provide backrubs and massage for clients to decrease anxiety. **Nursing Research:** *The*

• = **Independent;** ▲ = **Collaborative**

dependent variable, anxiety, was measured before back massage, immediately following, and 10 minutes later on four consecutive evenings. There was a statistically significant difference in the mean anxiety (STAI) score between the back massage group and the no-intervention group (Fraser and Kerr, 1993). **Clinical Research:** *Massage was done by parents before venous puncture of hospitalized preschoolers and school-aged children. The results obtained indicated that massage had a significant effect on nonverbal reactions, especially those related to muscular relaxation (Garcia et al, 1997).*

- Use TT and Healing Touch techniques. **Nursing Research:** *Anxiety was reduced significantly in a TT group but was unchanged in a TT placebo group. Healing Touch may be one of the most useful nursing interventions available to reduce anxiety (Fishel, 1998).*
▲ Refer for cognitive behavioral group therapy. **Clinical Research:** *In this study of 253 persons with neck or back pain, the experimental group who received the standardized six-session cognitive behavioral group sessions had significantly better results with regard to fear avoidance beliefs than the comparison group (Linton and Ryberg, 2001).*
▲ Animal-assisted therapy can be incorporated into the care of perioperative patients. **Nursing Research:** *In a study done on perioperative clients, interaction with animals was shown to reduce blood pressure and cholesterol, decrease anxiety, and improve a person's sense of well-being (Miller and Ingram, 2000).*
- Encourage clients to express their fears in narrative form. **Clinical Research:** *One of the main ways in which people adjust to threats associated with serious illness is through the use of narrative, which helps to make sense of illness (Crossley, 2003).*
- Refer to care plans for **Anxiety** and **Death Anxiety**

Geriatric

- Establish a trusting relationship so that all fears can be identified. *An elderly client's response to a real fear may be immobilizing.*
- Monitor for dementia and use appropriate interventions. *Fear may be an early indicator of disorientation or impaired reality testing in elderly clients.*
- Note if the client is irritable and is blaming others. **Nursing Research:** *The presence of these other behaviors are symptoms of depression (Proffitt et al, 1996).*
- Provide a protective and safe environment, use consistent caregivers, and maintain the accustomed environmental structure. *Elderly clients tend to have more perceptual impairments and adapt to changes with more difficulty than younger clients, especially during an illness.*
- Observe for untoward changes if antianxiety drugs are taken. *Advancing age renders clients more sensitive to both the clinical and toxic effects of many agents.*
- Assess for fear of falls in hospitalized patients with hip fractures to determine risk of poor health outcomes. **Nursing Research:** *Fear of falls correlated with poor health outcomes and has a major impact on function, especially with regard to walking (Mckee et al, 2002; Resnick, 1999).*
- Encourage exercises to improve physical skills and levels of mobility to decrease fear of falling. *Improving physical skills and levels of mobility counteract excessive fear during activity performance (Li et al, 2002).*

Pediatric

- Instruct parents that nighttime fear is common in children. *Nighttime fears are relatively common in normal children with fear of intruders being the most common (Muris et al, 2001).*

- = **Independent;** ▲ = **Collaborative**

- Explore coping skills used previously by the client to deal with fear. Children generally rate their coping behaviors as helpful. *A variety of coping behaviors reported were seeking support from parents, avoidance, distraction, trying to sleep, and clinging to stuffed animals (Muris et al, 2001).*
- Teach parents to use cognitive-behavioral strategies such as positive coping statements ("I am a brave girl [boy]. I can take care of myself in the dark.") and rewards of bravery tokens for appropriate behavior. *Cognitive-behavioral strategies appear to be effective interventions, but more research is indicated due to methodological limitations (Gordon and King, 2002).*
- Screen for depression in clients who report social/school fears. *Evidence corroborates a significant relationship between depression and childhood social/school fears (Neal et al, 2002).*

Multicultural

- Assess for the presence of culture-bound anxiety/fear states. **Nursing Research:** *The context in which anxiety/fear is experienced, its meaning, and responses to it are culturally mediated (Charron, 1998; Kavanagh, 1999).*
- Assess for the influence of cultural beliefs, norms, and values on the client's perspective of a stressful situation. **Nursing Research:** *What the client considers stressful may be based on cultural perceptions (Cochran, 1998; Doswell and Erlen, 1998; Leininger and McFarland, 2002).*
- Identify what triggers fear response. **Nursing Research:** *Arab Muslim clients may express a high correlation between fear and pain (Sheets and El-Azhary, 1998).*
- Identify how the client expresses fear. **Nursing Research:** *Research indicates that the expression of fear may be culturally mediated (Shore and Rapport, 1998).*
- Validate the client's feelings regarding fear. **Nursing Research:** *Validation is therapeutic communication technique that lets the client know that the nurse has heard and understands what was said, and it promotes the nurse-client relationship (Heineken, 1998).*

Home care

- Above interventions may be adapted for home care use.
- Assess to differentiate the presence of fear versus anxiety.
- Refer to care plan for **Anxiety.**
- During initial assessment, determine whether current or previous episodes of fear relate to the home environment (e.g., perception of danger in home or neighborhood or of relationships that have a history in the home). *Investigating the source of the fear allows the client to verbalize feelings and the nurse to determine appropriate interventions.*
- Identify with the client what steps may be taken to make the home a "safe" place to be. *Identifying a given area as a safe place reduces fear and anxiety when the client is in that area.*
- ▲ Encourage the client to seek or continue appropriate counseling to reduce fear associated with stress or to resolve alterations in irrational thought processes. *Correcting mistaken beliefs reduces anxiety.*
- ▲ Encourage the client to have a trusted companion, family member, or caregiver present in the home for periods when fear is most prominent. Pending other medical diagnoses, a referral to homemaker/home health aide services may meet this need. *Creating periods when fear and anxiety can be reduced allows the client periods of rest and supports positive coping.*

- = Independent; ▲ = Collaborative

▲ Offer to sit with a terminally ill client quietly as needed by the client or family, or provide hospice volunteers to do the same. *Terminally ill clients and their families often fear the dying process. The presence of a nurse or volunteer lets clients know they are not alone. Fears are reduced, and the dying process becomes more easily tolerated.*

Client/Family Teaching

- Teach the client the difference between warranted and excessive fear. *Different interventions are indicted for rational and irrational fears.*
- Teach stress management interventions to clients who experience emotions of fear. *Acute stress caused by strong emotions such as fear can sometimes cause sudden death in people with underlying coronary artery disease (Pashkow, 1999).*
- Teach families to share personal stories about an illness using the computer-based psychoeducational application experience journal. *The educational journal was reported to be useful for increasing understanding of familial feelings for families facing pediatric illness (DeMaso et al, 2000).*
- Teach the client to visualize or fantasize absence of the fear or threat and successful resolution of the conflict or outcome of the procedure.
- Teach the client to identify and use distraction or diversion tactics when possible. *Early interruption of the anxious response prevents escalation (Pope, 1995).*
- Teach clients to use guided imagery when they are fearful: have them use all senses to visualize a place that is "comfortable and safe" for them. *Results from this study showed that the psychological intervention of guided imagery significantly improved subjects' perceived quality of life and decreased fears (Moody et al, 1993).*
- Teach the client to allow fearful thoughts and feelings to be present until they dissipate. *Purposefully and repetitively allowing and even devoting time and energy to a thought reduces associated anxiety (Beck and Emery, 1985).*
- ▲ Teach use of appropriate community resources in emergency situations (e.g., hotlines, emergency departments, law enforcement, judicial systems). *Serious emergencies need immediate assistance to ensure the client's safety.*
- ▲ Encourage use of appropriate community resources in nonemergency situations (e.g., family, friends, neighbors, self-help and support groups, volunteer agencies, churches, recreation clubs and centers, seniors, youths, others with similar interests).
- ▲ Teach the client appropriate use of ordered medications.
- ▲ In event of bioterrorism provide accurate information ensure that health care personal have appropriate training and preparation. **Clinical Research:** *Clear, consistent, accessible, reliable, and redundant information (received from trusted sources) will diminish public uncertainty about the cause of symptoms that might otherwise prompt persons to seek unnecessary treatment. Training for providers is essential.*

𝐞𝐯𝐨𝐥𝐯𝐞 WEBSITES FOR EDUCATION

See the EVOLVE website for World Wide Web resources for client education.

REFERENCES

Bailey DS, Bailey DR: *Therapeutic approaches to the care of the mentally ill*, ed 3, Philadelphia, 1993, FA Davis.
Beck AT, Emery G: *Anxiety disorder and phobias: a cognitive perspective*, New York, 1985, Basic Books.

• = Independent; ▲ = Collaborative

Benedek DM; Holloway HC; Becker SM: Emergency mental health management in bioterrorism events, *Emerg Med Clin North Am* 20(2):393, 2002.

Carroll M, Ryan-Wenger N: School-age children's fears, anxiety, and human figure drawings, *J Pediatr Health Care* 13(1):24, 1999.

Charron HS: Anxiety disorders. In Varcarolis EM, editor: *Foundations of psychiatric mental health nursing*, ed 3, Philadelphia, 1998, WB Saunders.

Cochran M: Tears have no color, *Am J Nurs* 98(6):53, 1998.

Crossley ML: 'Let me explain': narrative employment and one patient's experience of oral cancer, *Soc Sci Med* 56(3):439, 2003.

DeMaso DR et al: The experience journal: a computer-based intervention for families facing congenital heart disease, *Am Acad Child Adolesc Psychiatr* 39(6):727, 2000.

Doswell W, Erlen J: Multicultural issues and ethical concerns in the delivery of revising care interventions, *Nurs Clin North Am* 33(2):353, 1998.

Fishel A: Nursing management of anxiety and panic, *Nurs Clin North Am* 33(1):135, 1998.

Fraser J, Kerr JR: Psychophysiological effects of back massage on elderly institutionalized patients, *J Adv Nurs* 18(2):238, 1993.

Garcia RM, Horta AL, Farias F: The effect of massage before venipuncture on the reaction of pre-school and school children, *Rev Esc Enferm USP* 31(1):119, 1997.

Garvin BJ, Huston GP, Baker CF: Information used by nurses to prepare patients for a stressful event, *Appl Nurs Res* 5:158, 1992.

Gordon J, King N: Children's night-time fears: an overview, *Counselling Psychology Q* 15(2):121, 2002.

Heineken J: Patient silence is not necessarily client satisfaction: communication in home care nursing, *Home Healthc Nurs* 16(2):115, 1998.

Kavanagh KH: The role of cultural diversity in mental health nursing. In Fontaine KL, Fletcher JS, editors: *Mental health nursing*, ed 4, Menlo Park, Calif, 1999, Addison-Wesley.

Leininger MM, McFarland MR: *Transcultural nursing: concepts, theories, research and practices*, ed 3, New York, 2002, McGraw-Hill.

Li F et al: Self-efficacy as a mediator between fear of falling and functional ability in the elderly, *J Aging Health* 14(4):452, 2002.

Linton SJ, Ryberg M: A cognitive-behavioral group intervention as prevention for persistent neck and back pain in a non-patient population: a randomized controlled trial, *Pain* 90(1-2):83, 2001.

Mckee K et al: Fear of falling, falls efficacy, and health outcomes in older people following hip fracture, *Disabil Rehabil* 24(6):327, 2002.

Miller J, Ingram L: Perioperative nursing and animal-assisted therapy, *AORN J* 72(3):477, 2000.

Mineka S, Ohman A: Phobias and preparedness: the selective, automatic, and encapsulated nature of fear, *Biol Psychiatry* 15:52(10), 2002.

Moody L, Fraser M, Yarandi H: Effects of guided imagery in patients with chronic bronchitis and emphysema, *Clin Nurs Res* 2(4):478, 1993.

Muris P et al: Children's night-time fears: parent-child ratings of frequency, content, origins, coping behaviors and severity, *Behav Res Ther* 39:13, 2001.

Neal J, Edelmann R, Glachan M: Behavioural inhibition and symptoms of anxiety and depression: is there a specific relationship with social phobia? *Br J Clin Psychol* 41:361, 2002.

Northouse L et al: A family-based program of care for women with recurrent breast cancer and their family members, *Oncol Nurs Forum* 29(10):1411, 2002.

Olson M, Sneed N: Anxiety and therapeutic touch, *Issues Ment Health Nurs* 16(2):97, 1995.

Osmun WE et al: Patients' attitudes to comforting touch in family practice, *Can Fam Physician* 46(12):2411, 2000.

Pashkow F: Is stress linked to heart disease? the evidence grows stronger, *Cleve Clin J Med* 66(2):75, 1999.

Pope DS: Music noise and the human voice in the nurse-patient environment, *Image J Nurs Sch* 27:291, 1995.

Poulton R, Menzies RG: Non-associative fear acquisition: a review of the evidence from retrospective and longitudinal research, *Behav Res Ther* 40(2):127, 2002.

Proffitt C, Augspurger P, Byrne M: Geriatric depression: a survey of nurses' knowledge and assessment practices, *Issues Ment Health Nurs* 17(2):123, 1996.

Resnick B: Motivation to perform activities of daily living in the institutionalized older adult: can a leopard change its spots? *J Adv Nurs* 29(4):792, 1999.

Shaw C, Wilson S, O'Brien M: Information needs prior to breast biopsy, *Clin Nurs Res* 3(2):119, 1994.

Sheets DL, El-Azhary RA: The Arab Muslim client: implications for anesthesia, *AANA J* 66(3):304, 1998.

• = **Independent; ▲ = Collaborative**

Shore GN, Rapport MD: The fear survey schedule for children-revised (FSSC-HI): ethnocultural variations in children's fearfulness, *J Anxiety Disord* 12(5):437, 1998.

Whitney G: Concept analysis of fear, *Nurs Diag* 3:159, 1992.

Readiness for enhanced Fluid balance

Betty J. Ackley

NANDA Definition

A pattern of equilibrium between fluid volume and chemical composition of body fluids that is sufficient for meeting physical needs and can be strengthened

Defining Characteristics

Expresses willingness to enhance fluid balance; Stable weight; Moist mucous membranes; Food and fluid intake adequate for daily needs; Straw-colored urine with specific gravity within normal limits; Good tissue turgor; No excessive thirst; Urine output appropriate for intake; No evidence of edema or dehydration

Related Factors (r/t)

Motivation to improve hydration status

NOC Outcomes (Nursing Outcomes Classification)

Suggested NOC Outcomes

Fluid Balance; Hydration; Nutritional Status: Food and Fluid Intake

> **Example NOC Outcome with Indicators**
>
> **Fluid Balance** as evidenced by the following indicators: Skin hydration/Moist mucous membranes/Orthostatic hypotension not present/24-hour intake and output balanced/Urine specific gravity WNL (Rate each indicator of **Fluid Balance:** 1 = extremely compromised, 2 = substantially compromised, 3 = moderately compromised, 4 = mildly compromised, 5 = not compromised [see Section I].)

WNL, Within normal limits.

Client Outcomes

Client Will (Specify Time Frame):

- Maintain light yellow urine output
- Maintain elastic skin turgor, moist tongue, and mucous membranes
- Explain measures that can be taken to improve fluid intake.

NIC Interventions (Nursing Interventions Classification)

Suggested NIC Intervention

Fluid Management

• = Independent; ▲ = Collaborative

Example NIC Activities—Fluid Management

Monitor hydration status (e.g., moist mucous membranes, adequacy of pulses, and orthostatic blood pressure) as appropriate; Monitor food/fluid ingested and calculate daily caloric intake, if appropriate

---

Nursing Interventions and Rationales

- Discuss normal fluid requirements. A guideline is 1 ml of fluid per each calories needed, so an average intake would be between 2000 and 3000 ml/day, or 8 to 12 cups of fluid (Cataldo et al, 2003).
- Recommend mainly intake of water, but milk or fruit juice can also be effective in maintaining good fluid balance (Cataldo et al, 2003).
- Recommend the client avoid the use of alcoholic beverages and beverages containing caffeine to provide fluid to the body. *Both alcohol and caffeine act as a diuretic, causing increased loss of fluid in the urine (Kleiner, 1999).*
- Recommend the client avoid intake of carbonated beverages, instead suggest the client drink water. *Most carbonated beverages contain large amounts of sugar, 10 or more teaspoons of sugar, and are a significant source of empty calories.*

Geriatric

- Encourage the elderly client to develop a pattern of drinking water regularly. *Thirst sensations diminish with aging, dehydration can threaten elderly clients (Cataldo et al, 2003).* **Clinical Research:** *A study demonstrated that healthy men aged 67-75 years were less thirsty and replaced less fluid than did young people during fluid deprivation (Philips et al, 1984).*

Client/Family Teaching

- Teach the client to drink water before and during engaging in activities that can result in dehydration quickly such as the distance runner or the gardener in hot weather. Following is a hydration schedule for physical activity*:

When to drink	Approximate amount of fluid
2 Hours before activity	2 to 3 cups
15 Minutes before activity	1 to 2 cups
Every 15 minutes during activity	$1/2$ to 1 cup
After activity	At least 2 cups for every pound of body weight lost

*Source: (Murray, 2000).

Thirst lags behind loss of fluid volume, and in situations with rapid loss of fluid, dehydration can happen quickly (Cataldo et al, 2003). **Clinical Research:** *A study demonstrated that there was a decrease in long-term memory when exercising in a hot environment and not replacing lost fluids, which did not occur if the subject ingested fluids to restore fluid balance (Clan et al, 2001). A study demonstrated that drinking fluids earlier resulted in a faster rate of plasma and fluid balance restoration, even though similar amounts of fluid were ingested (Kovacs et al, 2002).*

• **= Independent; ▲ = Collaborative**

- Teach clients who work in hot environments or exercise in hot environments to increase intake of both water and use of electrolyte-carbohydrate beverages, the sports drinks are needed when exercise exceeds 1 hour or during prolonged competitive games that require repeated intermittent activity (Welsh et al, 2002). *A review of the literature demonstrated that drinks containing low to moderate levels of electrolytes and carbohydrates may provide significant advantages in industrial situations (Clap et al, 2002).* **Clinical Research:** *A study demonstrated that drinking flavored drinks during sports athletic activity compared with water enhanced fluid balance (Minehan et al, 2002).*
- Ask the client to monitor the color of urine to tell if adequately hydrated. *In a hydrated person the urine should be light yellow—the color of lemonade. Urine the color of apple juice indicates slight dehydration (Cataldo et al, 2003).* **Nursing Research:** *A research study on elderly veterans demonstrated that urine color correlated significantly with urine osmolality, serum sodium, and blood urea nitrogen (BUN)/creatinine ratio (Wakefield et al, 2002).*

REFERENCES

Cataldo CB, DeBruyne LK, Whitney EN: *Nutrition and diet therapy,* ed 6, Belmont, Calif, 2003, Thomson Wadsworth.

Clan C et al: Effects of fluid ingestion on cognitive function after heat stress or exercise-induced dehydration, *Int J Psychophysiol* 42(3):243, 2001.

Clap AJ et al: A review of fluid replacement for workers in hot jobs, *AIHA J* 63:2, 2002.

Kleiner SM: Water: An essential but overlooked nutrient, *J Am Diet Assoc* 99(2):200, 1999.

Kovacs EM et al: Effect of high and low rates of fluid intake on post-exercise rehydration, *Int J Sport Nutr Exerc Metab* 12(1):14, 2002.

Minehan MR, Riley MD, Burke LM: Effect of flavor and awareness of kilojoule content of drinks on preference and fluid balance in team sports, *Int J Sport Nutr Exerc Metab* 12(1):81, 2002.

Murray R: Fluid and electrolytes. In Rosenbloom CA, editor: *Sports nutrition: a guide for the professional working with active people,* ed 3, Chicago, 2000, American Dietetic Association.

Philips PA et al: Reduced thirst after water deprivation in healthy elderly men, *N Engl J Med* 311:753, 1984.

Wakefield B et al: Monitoring hydration status in elderly veterans, *West J Nurs Res* 24(2):132, 2002.

Welsh RS et al: Carbohydrates and physical/mental performance during intermittent exercise to fatigue, *Med Sci Sports Exerc* 34:723, 2002.

Deficient Fluid volume

Betty J. Ackley

NANDA   Definition

Decreased intravascular, interstitial, and/or intracellular fluid (refers to dehydration, water loss alone without change in sodium level)

Defining Characteristics

Decreased urine output; increased urine concentration; weakness; sudden weight loss (except in third-spacing); decreased venous filling; increased body temperature; decreased pulse volume/pressure; change in mental state; elevated hematocrit; decreased skin/tongue turgor; dry skin/mucous membranes; thirst; increased pulse rate; decreased blood pressure

Related Factors (r/t)

Active fluid volume loss; failure of regulatory mechanisms

- • = **Independent;** ▲ = **Collaborative**

Outcomes (Nursing Outcomes Classification)

Suggested NOC Outcomes

Electrolyte and Acid-Base Balance; Fluid Balance; Hydration; Nutritional Status: Food and Fluid Intake

---

Example NOC Outcome with Indicators

Maintains **Fluid Balance** as evidenced by the following indicators: Skin hydration/Moist mucous membranes/ Orthostatic hypotension not present/24-hour intake and output balanced/Urine specific gravity WNL (Rate each indicator of **Fluid Balance:** 1 = extremely compromised, 2 = substantially compromised, 3 = moderately compromised, 4 = mildly compromised, 5 = not compromised [see Section I].)

WNL, Within normal limits.

Client Outcomes

Client Will (Specify Time Frame):

- Maintain urine output more than 1300 ml/day (or at least 30 ml/hr)
- Maintain normal blood pressure, pulse, and body temperature
- Maintain elastic skin turgor; moist tongue and mucous membranes; and orientation to person, place, and time
- Explain measures that can be taken to treat or prevent fluid volume loss
- Describe symptoms that indicate the need to consult with health care provider

Interventions (Nursing Interventions Classification)

Suggested NIC Interventions

Fluid Management; Hypovolemia Management; Shock Management: Volume

---

Example NIC Activities—Fluid Management

Monitor hydration status (e.g., moist mucous membranes, adequacy of pulses, and orthostatic blood pressure) as appropriate; Administer intravenous fluids at room temperature

---

Nursing Interventions and Rationales

- Monitor for the existence of factors causing deficient fluid volume (e.g., vomiting, diarrhea, difficulty maintaining oral intake, fever, uncontrolled type 2 diabetes, diuretic therapy). *Early identification of risk factors and early intervention can decrease the occurrence and severity of complications from deficient fluid volume. The gastrointestinal system is a common site of abnormal fluid loss (Metheny, 2000).*
- Watch for early signs of hypovolemia, including restlessness, weakness, muscle cramps, and postural hypotension. *Late signs include oliguria, abdominal or chest pain, cyanosis, cold clammy skin, and confusion (Fauci et al, 1998).*
- Monitor total fluid intake and output every 8 hours (or every hour for the unstable client). Recognize that urine output is not always an accurate indicator of fluid balance. *A urine output of less than 30 ml/hr is insufficient for normal renal function and indicates hypovolemia or onset of renal damage (Metheny, 2000). Urine output can be unreliable to indicate fluid balance because if the client is hypothermic or elderly or has renal dysfunc-*

• = **Independent;** ▲ = **Collaborative**

tion, the client may be unable to concentrate urine leading to falsely high urine output (Schulman, 2002).

- Watch trends in output for 3 days; include all routes of intake and output and note color and specific gravity of urine. *Monitoring for trends for 2 to 3 days gives a more valid picture of the client's hydration status than monitoring for a shorter period (Metheny, 2000). Dark-colored urine with increasing specific gravity reflects increased urine concentration.*
- Monitor daily weight for sudden decreases, especially in the presence of decreasing urine output or active fluid loss. Weigh the client on the same scale with the same type of clothing at same time of day, preferably before breakfast. *Body weight changes reflect changes in body fluid volume (Suhayda and Walton, 2002). A 1-pound weight loss reflects a fluid loss of about 500 ml (Metheny, 2000).*
- Monitor vital signs of clients with deficient fluid volume every 15 minutes to 1 hour for the unstable client (every 4 hours for the stable client). Observe for tachycardia, tachypnea, decreased pulse pressure first, then hypotension, decreased pulse volume, and increased or decreased body temperature. *A decreased pulse pressure is an earlier indicator of shock than is the systolic blood pressure (Mikhail, 1999). Decreased intravascular volume results in hypotension and decreased tissue oxygenation. The temperature will be decreased as a result of decreased metabolism, or it may be increased if there is infection or hypernatremia present (Metheny, 2000).*
- Check orthostatic blood pressures with the client lying, sitting, and standing. *A 15 mm Hg drop when upright or an increase of 15 beats/min in the pulse rate are seen with deficient fluid volume (Metheny, 2000).*
- Monitor for inelastic skin turgor, thirst, dry tongue and mucous membranes, longitudinal tongue furrows, speech difficulty, dry skin, sunken eyeballs, weakness (especially of upper body), and confusion. *Tongue dryness, longitudinal tongue furrows, dryness of the mucous membranes of the mouth, upper body muscle weakness, thirst, confusion, speech difficulty, and sunkenness of eyes are symptoms of deficient fluid volume (Metheny 2000).*
- Provide frequent oral hygiene, at least twice a day (if mouth is dry and painful, provide hourly while awake). *Oral hygiene decreases unpleasant tastes in the mouth and allows the client to respond to the sensation of thirst.*
- Provide fresh water and oral fluids preferred by the client (distribute over 24 hours [e.g., 1200 ml on days, 800 ml on evenings, and 200 ml on nights]); provide prescribed diet; offer snacks (e.g., frequent drinks, fresh fruits, fruit juice); instruct significant other to assist the client with feedings as appropriate. *The oral route is preferred for maintaining fluid balance (Metheny, 2000). Distributing the intake over the entire 24-hour period and providing snacks and preferred beverages increases the likelihood that the client will maintain the prescribed oral intake.*
- Provide free water with tube feedings as appropriate (50 to 100 ml every 4 hours) or 30 ml/kg of body weight (Suhayda and Walton, 2002). *This provides water for replacement of intravascular or intracellular volume as necessary. Tube feeding has been found to increase the risk for dehydration (Lavizzo-Mourey et al, 1988; Sheehy et al, 1999).*
- Institute measures to rest the bowel when the client is vomiting or has diarrhea (e.g., restrict food or fluid intake when appropriate, decrease intake of milk products). Hydrate the client with ordered intravenous solutions if prescribed. *The most common cause of deficient fluid volume is gastrointestinal loss of fluid. At times it is preferable to allow the gastrointestinal system to rest before resuming oral intake. Hydration should be maintained (see care plan for* **Diarrhea** *or* **Nausea**).

- **= Independent; ▲ = Collaborative**

- Provide oral replacement therapy as ordered and tolerated with a hypotonic glucose-electrolyte solution when the client has acute diarrhea or nausea/vomiting. Provide small, frequent quantities of slightly chilled solutions. *Maintenance of oral intake stabilizes the ability of the intestines to digest and absorb nutrients; glucose-electrolyte solutions increase net fluid absorption while correcting deficient fluid volume (Cohen et al, 1995). Use carbohydrate-electrolyte solutions such as sports replacement drinks, cola, and ginger ale, which are often tolerated better than other solutions, sometimes even with vomiting and diarrhea (Suhayda and Walton, 2002).* **Clinical Research:** *A study demonstrated that decreasing the osmolality of standard glucose-electrolyte oral replacement solutions improves the absorption of water, and stool volume (Farthing, 2002).*
▲ Administer antidiarrheals and antiemetics as appropriate. *The goal is to stop the loss that results from vomiting or diarrhea.*
▲ If the client requires intravenous fluid replacement, maintain patent intravenous access, set an appropriate intravenous infusion flow rate, and administer at a constant flow rate as ordered. *Isotonic intravenous fluids such as 0.9% normal saline or lactated Ringer's allow replacement of intravascular volume (Metheny, 2000).*
- Assist with ambulation if the client has postural hypotension. *Postural hypotension can cause dizziness, which places the client at higher risk for injury.*
- Promote skin integrity (e.g., monitor areas for breakdown, ensure frequent weight shifts, prevent shearing, promote adequate nutrition). *Deficient fluid volume decreases tissue oxygenation, which makes the skin more vulnerable to breakdown.*

Critically ill
- Monitor central venous pressure, right atrial pressure, and pulmonary wedge pressure for decreases. *Hemodynamic parameters are sensitive indicators of intravascular fluid volume, and hemodynamic measurements are especially needed in the client with cardiac or renal problems (Metheny, 2000).*
- Monitor serum and urine osmolality, serum sodium, BUN/creatinine ratio, and hematocrit for elevations. *These are all measures of concentration and will be elevated with decreased intravascular volume (Fauci et al, 1998).*
▲ When ordered, initiate a fluid challenge of crystalloids (0.9% normal saline or lactated Ringer's) for replacement of intravascular volume; monitor the client's response to prescribed fluid therapy and fluid challenge, especially noting central venous pressure and pulmonary capillary wedge pressure readings, vital signs, urine output, blood lactate concentrations, and lung sounds. *A fluid challenge can help the client with deficient fluid volume regain intravascular volume quickly, but the client must be carefully observed to ensure that he or she does not go into fluid volume overload (Kruse et al, 2003). In trauma clients, if there is no clinical improvement after 2 L of crystalloids, then generally a blood transfusion should be initiated (Jordan, 2000).*
- Position the client flat with legs elevated when hypotensive, if not contraindicated. *This position enhances venous return, thus contributing to the maintenance of cardiac output.*
- If the client is critically ill, monitor trends in serum lactic acid levels and base deficit obtained from blood gasses as ordered. *A trend of increasing lactic acid levels and increasing base deficit can help identify occult hypoperfusion, which results in decreased survival and increased incidence of organ failure (Schulman, 2002).*
▲ Consult physician if signs and symptoms of deficient fluid volume persist or worsen. *Prolonged deficient fluid volume increases the risk for development of complications, including shock, multiple organ failure, and death.*

- = **Independent;** ▲ = **Collaborative**

Geriatric

- Monitor elderly clients for deficient fluid volume carefully, noting new onset of weakness, dizziness, or dry mouth with longitudinal furrows. *The elderly are predisposed to deficient fluid volume because of decreased fluid in body, decreased thirst sensation, and decreased ability to concentrate urine (Bennett, 2000; Sheehy et al, 1999; Suhayda and Walton, 2002).*
- Check skin turgor of elderly client on the forehead, sternum or inner thigh; also look for the presence of longitudinal furrows on the tongue and dry mucous membranes. *Elderly people commonly have decreased skin turgor from normal age-related loss of elasticity; therefore checking skin turgor on the arm is not reflective of fluid volume (Bennett, 2000; Suhayda and Walton, 2002). The presence of longitudinal furrows or dry mucous membranes is a good indication of dehydration in the elderly (Bennett, 2000; Sheehy et al, 1999).*
- Encourage fluid intake by offering fluids regularly to cognitively impaired clients. *The elderly have a decreased thirst sensation (Metheny, 2000), and short-term memory loss may impede the client's memory of fluid intake.*
- Incorporate regular hydration into daily routines (e.g., extra glass of fluid with medication or social activities). Consider use of a beverage cart and a hydration assistant to routinely offer increased beverages to clients in extended care. **Nursing and Clinical Research:** *A nursing study demonstrated that institution of a beverage cart with a trained hydration assistant resulted in increased number of bowel movements, less use of laxatives, decreased number of falls, less urinary tract infections, respiratory infections and skin breakdown (Robinson and Rosher, 2002). A study demonstrated that verbal prompting and offering preference fluids resulted in increased fluid intake among nursing home residents (Simmons et al, 2001).*
- Note the color of urine and compare against a urine color chart to monitor adequate fluid intake. **Nursing Research:** *A research study on elderly veterans demonstrated that urine color correlated significantly with urine osmolality, serum sodium, and BUN/creatinine ratio (Wakefield et al, 2002).*
- Monitor elderly clients for excess fluid volume during the treatment of deficient fluid volume: listen to lung sounds, watch for edema, and note vital signs. *The elderly client has a decreased ability to adapt to rapid increases in intravascular volume and can quickly develop heart failure.*

Home care

- Determine if it is appropriate to intervene for deficient fluid volume or to allow the client to die comfortably without fluids as desired. *Deficient fluid volume may be a symptom of impending death in terminally ill clients. The deficit may result in a mild euphoria and a more comfortable death (Bennett, 2000).*
- Teach family members how to monitor output in the home (e.g., use of commode "hat" in the toilet, urinal, or bedpan, or use of catheter and closed drainage). Instruct them to monitor both intake and output. *An accurate measure of fluid intake and output is an important indicator of client fluid status (Metheny, 2000).*
- When weighing the client, use same scale each day. Be sure scale is on a flat (not cushioned) surface. Do not weigh the client with scale placed on any kind of rug. Use bed or chair scales for clients who are unable to stand. *An accurate daily weight is an excellent reflection of fluid balance (Metheny, 2000).*
- ▲ Teach family about complications of deficient fluid volume and when to call physician.
- ▲ If the client is receiving intravenous fluids, there must be a responsible caregiver in the

• = **Independent;** ▲ = **Collaborative**

home. Teach caregiver about administration of fluids, complications of intravenous administration (e.g., fluid volume overload, speed of medication reactions), and when to call for assistance. Assist caregiver with administration for as long as necessary to maintain client safety. *Administration of intravenous fluids in the home is a high-technology procedure and requires sufficient professional support to ensure safety of the client.*

▲ Identify an emergency plan, including when to call 911. *Some complications of deficient fluid volume cannot be reversed in the home and are life threatening. Clients progressing toward hypovolemic shock will need emergency care.*

Client/Family Teaching

- Instruct the client to avoid rapid position changes, especially from supine to sitting or standing.
- Teach the client and family about appropriate diet and fluid intake.
- Teach the client and family how to measure and record intake and output accurately.
- Teach the client and family about measures instituted to treat hypovolemia and to prevent or treat fluid volume loss.
- Instruct the client and family about signs of deficient fluid volume that indicate they should contact health care provider.

evolve WEBSITES FOR EDUCATION

See the EVOLVE website for World Wide Web resources for client education.

REFERENCES

Bennett JA: Dehydration: hazards and benefits, *Geriatr Nurs* 21(2):84, 2000.

Blow O et al: The golden hours and the silver day: detection and correction of occult hypoperfusion within 24 hours improves outcome from major trauma, *J Trauma* 47(5):964, 1999.

Cohen M et al: Use of a single solution for oral rehydration and maintenance therapy of infants with diarrhea and mild to moderate dehydration, *Pediatrics* 95:639, 1995.

Farthing MJ: Oral rehydration: an evolving solution, *J Pediatr Gastroenterol Nutr* 34(suppl 1):S64, 2002.

Fauci AS et al, editors: *Harrison's principles of internal medicine,* ed 14, New York, 1998, McGraw-Hill.

Jordan KS: Fluid resuscitation in acutely injured patients, *J Intravenous Nurs* 23(2):81, 2000.

Kruse JA, Fink MP, Carlson RW: *Saunders manual of critical care,* Philadelphia, 2003, WB Saunders.

Lavizzo-Mourey RM, Johnson J, Stolley P: Risk factors for dehydration among elderly nursing home residents, *J Am Geriatr Soc* 36(3):213, 1988.

Metheny N: *Fluid and electrolyte balance: nursing considerations,* ed 4 Philadelphia, 2000, Lippincott.

Mikhail J: Resuscitation endpoints in trauma, *AACN Clin Issues* 10(1):10, 1999.

Schulman C: End points of resuscitation: choosing the right parameters to monitor, *Dimens Crit Care Nurs* 21:1, 2002.

Sheehy CM, Perry PA, Cromwell SL: Dehydration: biological considerations, age-related changes, and risk factors in older adults, *Biol Res Nurs* 1(1):30, 1999.

Simmons SF, Alessi C, Schnelle JF: An intervention to increase fluid intake in nursing home residents: prompting and preference compliance, *J Am Geriatr Soc* 49(7):926, 2001.

Suhayda R, Walton JC: Preventing and managing dehydration, *Medsurg Nurs* 11(6):267, 2002.

Wakefield B et al: Monitoring hydration status in elderly veterans, *West J Nurs Res* 24(2):132, 2002.

• = Independent; ▲ = Collaborative

Excess Fluid volume

Betty J. Ackley and Martha A. Spies

NANDA Definition

Increased isotonic fluid retention

Defining Characteristics

Jugular vein distention; decreased hemoglobin and hematocrit; weight gain over short period; changes in respiratory pattern, dyspnea or shortness of breath; orthopnea; abnormal breath sounds (rales or crackles); pulmonary congestion; pleural effusion; intake exceeds output; S3 heart sound; change in mental status; restlessness; anxiety; blood pressure changes; pulmonary artery pressure changes; increased central venous pressure; oliguria; azotemia; specific gravity changes; altered electrolytes; edema, may progress to anasarca; positive hepatojugular reflex

Related Factors (r/t)

Compromised regulatory mechanism; excess fluid intake; excess sodium intake

NOC Outcomes (Nursing Outcomes Classification)

Suggested NOC Outcomes

Electrolyte and Acid-Base Balance; Fluid Balance; Hydration

Example NOC Outcome with Indicators

Fluid Balance as evidenced by the following indicators: Peripheral edema not present/Neck vein distention not present/Body weight stable/24-hour intake and output balanced/Urine specific gravity WNL/Adventitious breath sounds not present (Rate each indicator of **Fluid Balance:** 1 = extremely compromised, 2 = substantially compromised, 3 = moderately compromised, 4 = mildly compromised, 5 = not compromised [see Section I].)

WNL, Within normal limits.

Client Outcomes

Client Will (Specify Time Frame):

- Remain free of edema, effusion, anasarca; weight appropriate for the client
- Maintain clear lung sounds; no evidence of dyspnea or orthopnea
- Remain free of jugular vein distention, positive hepatojugular reflex, and gallop heart rhythm
- Maintain normal central venous pressure, pulmonary capillary wedge pressure, cardiac output, and vital signs
- Maintain urine output within 500 ml of intake and normal urine osmolality and specific gravity
- Remain free of restlessness, anxiety, or confusion
- Explain measures that can be taken to treat or prevent excess fluid volume, especially fluid and dietary restrictions and medications
- Describe symptoms that indicate the need to consult with health care provider

• = Independent; ▲ = Collaborative

NIC   Interventions (Nursing Interventions Classification)

Suggested NIC Interventions
Fluid Management; Fluid Monitoring

Example NIC Activities—Fluid Monitoring

Weigh daily and monitor trends; Maintain accurate intake and output record

Nursing Interventions and Rationales

- Monitor location and extent of edema; use a millimeter tape in the same area at the same time each day to measure edema in extremities. *Generalized edema (e.g., in the upper extremities and eyelids) is associated with decreased oncotic pressure as a result of nephrotic syndrome. Measuring the extremity with a millimeter tape is more accurate than using the 1+ to 4+ scale (Metheny, 2000). Heart failure and renal failure are usually associated with dependent edema because of increased hydrostatic pressure; dependent edema will cause swelling in the legs and feet of ambulatory clients and the presacral region of clients on bed rest.* **Nursing Research:** *Dependent edema was found to demonstrate the greatest sensitivity as a defining characteristic for excess fluid volume (Rios et al, 1991).*
- Monitor daily weight for sudden increases; use same scale and type of clothing at same time each day, preferably before breakfast. *Body weight changes reflect changes in body fluid volume. Clinically it is extremely important to get an accurate body weight of a client with fluid imbalance (Metheny, 2000).*
- Monitor lung sounds for crackles, monitor respirations for effort, and determine the presence and severity of orthopnea. *Pulmonary edema results from excessive shifting of fluid from the vascular space into the pulmonary interstitial space and alveoli. Pulmonary edema can interfere with the oxygen/carbon dioxide exchange at the alveolar-capillary membrane (Metheny, 2000), resulting in dyspnea and orthopnea.*
- With head of bed elevated 30 to 45 degrees, monitor jugular veins for distention in the upright position; assess for positive hepatojugular reflex. *Increased intravascular volume results in jugular vein distention, even in a client in the upright position, and also a positive hepatojugular reflex.*
- Monitor central venous pressure, mean arterial pressure, pulmonary artery pressure, pulmonary capillary wedge pressure, and cardiac output; note and report trends indicating increasing pressures over time. *Increased vascular volume with decreased cardiac contractility increases intravascular pressures, which are reflected in hemodynamic parameters. Over time, this increased pressure can result in uncompensated heart failure.*
- Monitor vital signs; note decreasing blood pressure, tachycardia, and tachypnea. Monitor for gallop rhythms. If signs of heart failure are present, see nursing care plan for **Decreased Cardiac output.** *Heart failure results in decreased cardiac output and decreased blood pressure. Tissue hypoxia stimulates increased heart and respiratory rates.*
- Monitor serum osmolality, serum sodium, BUN/creatinine ratio, and hematocrit for decreases. *These are all measures of concentration and will decrease (except in the presence of renal failure) with increased intravascular volume. In clients with renal failure, the BUN will increase because of decreased renal excretion.*
- Monitor intake and output; note trends reflecting decreasing urine output in relation

• = Independent; ▲ = Collaborative

to fluid intake. *Accurately measuring intake and output is very important for the client with fluid volume overload.*

- Monitor the client's behavior for restlessness, anxiety, or confusion; use safety precautions if symptoms are present. *When excess fluid volume compromises cardiac output, the client will experience cerebral tissue hypoxia, and the client may demonstrate restlessness and anxiety before any physiological alterations occur (Fauci et al, 1998). When the excess fluid volume results in hyponatremia, symptoms such as agitation, irritability, inappropriate behavior, confusion, and seizures may occur (Kruse et al, 2003).*

- Monitor for the development of conditions that increase the client's risk for excess fluid volume. *Common causes are heart failure, renal failure, and liver failure, all of which result in decreased glomerular filtration rate and fluid retention. Other causes are increased intake of oral or intravenous fluids in excess of the client's cardiac and renal reserve levels, increased levels of antidiuretic hormone, or movement of fluid from the interstitial space to the intravascular space (Fauci et al, 1998). Early detection allows the institution of specific treatment measures before the client develops pulmonary edema.*

- ▲ Assist with CRRT (continuous renal replacement therapy) as ordered if the client is critically ill and excessive fluid must be removed. *CRRT is indicated for severe volume overload, oliguric renal failure, metabolic acidosis, and azotemia with uremic symptoms (Kruse et al, 2003).*

- ▲ Provide a restricted-sodium diet as appropriate if ordered. *Restricting the sodium in the diet will favor the renal excretion of excess fluid. Take care to avoid hyponatremia. Decreasing sodium can be more important that restricting fluid intake (Fauci et al, 1998).*

- ▲ Monitor serum albumin level and provide protein intake as appropriate. *Serum albumin is the main contributor to serum oncotic pressure, which favors the movement of fluid from the interstitial space into the intravascular space. When serum albumin is low, peripheral edema may be severe.*

- ▲ Administer prescribed loop, thiazide, and/or potassium-sparing diuretics as appropriate; these may be given intravenously or orally. *Therapeutic responses to diuretic therapy include natriuresis, diuresis, elimination of edema, vasodilation, reduction of cardiac filling pressures, decreased renal vasculature resistance, and increased renal blood flow (Cody et al, 1994; DePriest, 1997).*

- ▲ Monitor for side effects of diuretic therapy: orthostatic hypotension (especially if the client is also receiving ACE inhibitors) and electrolyte and metabolic imbalances (hyponatremia, hypocalcemia, hypomagnesemia, hyperuricemia, and metabolic alkalosis). In clients receiving loop or thiazide diuretics, observe for hypokalemia. Observe for hyperkalemia in clients receiving a potassium-sparing diuretic, especially with the concurrent administration of an ACE inhibitor. *The blood pressure reduction in response to ACE inhibitors is greater in the presence of sodium depletion and diuretic therapy. The incidence of electrolyte and metabolic imbalances ranges from 14% to 60%; the most common is hypokalemia (Cody et al, 1994).*

- ▲ Implement fluid restriction as ordered, especially when serum sodium is low; include all routes of intake. Schedule fluids around the clock, and include the type of fluids preferred by the client. *Fluid restriction may decrease intravascular volume and myocardial workload. Overzealous fluid restriction should not be used because hypovolemia can worsen heart failure. In one study, instituting fluid restriction, distributing fluids over a 24-hour period, and using a fluid restriction when the client had hyponatremia all had high intervention content validity scores for the fluid management intervention label (Cullen,*

• = Independent; ▲ = Collaborative

1992). Client involvement in planning will enhance participation in the necessary fluid restriction.

- Maintain the rate of all intravenous infusions carefully. *This is done to prevent inadvertent exacerbation of excess fluid volume.*
- Turn clients with dependent edema frequently (i.e., at least every 2 hours). *Edematous tissue is vulnerable to ischemia and pressure ulcers (Cullen, 1992).*
- Provide for scheduled rest periods. *Bed rest can induce diuresis related to diminished peripheral venous pooling, resulting in increased intravascular volume and glomerular filtration rate (Metheny, 2000).*
- Promote a positive body image and good self-esteem. *Visible edema may alter the client's body image (Cullen, 1992).* See the care plan for **Disturbed Body image**.
- ▲ Consult with physician if signs and symptoms of excess fluid volume persist or worsen. *Because excess fluid volume can result in pulmonary edema, it must be treated promptly and aggressively (Fauci et al, 1998).*

Geriatric
- Recognize that the presence of risk factors for excess fluid volume is particularly serious in the elderly. *Decreased cardiac output and stroke volume are normal aging changes that increase the risk for excess fluid volume (Metheny, 2000).*

Home care
- Assess client and family knowledge of disease process causing excess fluid volume. Teach about disease process and complications of excess fluid volume, including when to contact physician. *Knowledge of disease and complications promotes early detection of and intervention for pending problems.*
- Assess client and family knowledge and compliance with medical regimen, including medications, diet, rest, and exercise. Assist family with integrating restrictions into daily living. *Knowledge promotes compliance. Assistance with integration of cultural values, especially those related to foods, with medical regimen promotes compliance and decreased risk of complications.*
- If the client is confined to bed rest or has difficulty reclining, follow previously mentioned positioning recommendations.
- ▲ Teach and reinforce knowledge of medications. Instruct the client not to use over-the-counter medications (e.g., diet medications) without first consulting the physician. Instruct the client to make primary physician aware of medications ordered by other physicians. *There is potential for undesirable interaction among multiple medications, especially when use of over-the-counter and other prescribed medications is not monitored.*
- ▲ Identify emergency plan for rapidly developing or critical levels of excess fluid volume when diuresing is not safe at home. *When out of control, excess fluid volume can be life threatening.*
- ▲ Teach about signs and symptoms of both excess and deficient fluid volume and when to call physician. *Fluid volume balance can change rapidly with aggressive treatment.*

Client/Family Teaching
- Describe signs and symptoms of excess fluid volume and actions to take if they occur.
- Teach the importance of fluid and sodium restrictions. Help the client and family to devise a schedule for intake of fluids throughout entire day. Refer to dietitian concerning implementation of low-sodium diet.

- **= Independent; ▲ = Collaborative**

- Teach how to take diuretics correctly: take one dose in the morning and second dose (if taken) no later than 4 PM. Adjust potassium intake as appropriate for potassium-losing or potassium-sparing diuretics. Note the appearance of side effects such as weakness, dizziness, muscle cramps, numbness and tingling, confusion, hearing impairment, palpitations or irregular heartbeat, and postural hypotension.
- For the client undergoing hemodialysis, spend time with the client to detect any factors that may interfere with the client's compliance with the fluid restriction or restrictive diet. **Nursing Research:** *The nurse who knows the client well is able to develop individualized interventions to help the client adhere to the restriction (Morgan, 2001).*
- ▲ Emphasize the need to consult with health care provider before taking over-the-counter medications (Byers and Goshorn, 1995; Dunbar et al, 1998).

🅴🆅🅾🅻🆅🅴 WEBSITES FOR EDUCATION

See the EVOLVE website for World Wide Web resources for client education.

REFERENCES

Byers J, Goshorn J: How to manage diuretic therapy, *Am J Nurs* 95(2):38, 1995.
Cody R, Kubo S, Pickworth K: Diuretic treatment for the sodium retention of congestive heart failure, *Arch Intern Med* 154:1905, 1994.
Cullen L: Interventions related to fluid and electrolyte imbalance, *Nurs Clin North Am* 27:569, 1992.
DePriest J: Reversing oliguria in critically ill patients, *Postgrad Med* 102(3):245, 1997.
Dunbar SB, Jacobson LH, Deaton C: Heart failure: strategies to enhance patient self-management, *AACN Clin Issues* 9(2):244, 1998.
Fauci AS et al, editors: *Harrison's principles of internal medicine,* ed 14, New York, 1998, McGraw-Hill.
Kruse JA, Finnk MP, Carlson RW: *Saunders manual of critical care,* Philadelphia, 2003, WB Saunders.
Metheny N: *Fluid and electrolyte balance: nursing considerations,* ed 4, Philadelphia, 2000, Lippincott.
Rios H et al: Validation of defining characteristics of four nursing diagnoses using a computerized data base, *J Prof Nurs* 7:293, 1991.

Risk for deficient Fluid volume

Betty J. Ackley

NANDA   Definition

At risk for experiencing vascular, cellular, or intracellular dehydration

Risk Factors

Factors influencing fluid needs (e.g., hypermetabolic state); extremes of age; extremes of weight; excessive losses of fluid through normal routes (e.g., diarrhea); loss of fluids through abnormal routes (e.g., indwelling tubes); deviations affecting access, intake, or absorption of fluids (e.g., physical immobility); knowledge deficiency regarding fluid volume; medication (e.g., diuretics)

Related Factors (r/t)

See Risk Factors

- = Independent; ▲ = Collaborative

| **NOC** | Outcomes (Nursing Outcomes Classification) |

Suggested NOC Outcomes
Fluid Balance; Hydration; Knowledge: Treatment Regimen

Example NOC Outcome with Indicators

Fluid Balance as evidenced by the following indicators: Skin hydration/Moist mucous membranes/Orthostatic hypotension not present/24-hour intake and output balanced/Urine specific gravity WNL (Rate each indicator of **Fluid Balance:** 1 = extremely compromised, 2 = substantially compromised, 3 = moderately compromised, 4 = mildly compromised, 5 = not compromised [see Section I].)

WNL, Within normal limits.

Client Outcomes

Client Will (Specify Time Frame):
- Maintain urine output of more than 1300 ml/day (or at least 30 ml/hr)
- Maintain normal blood pressure, pulse, and body temperature
- Maintain elastic skin turgor; moist tongue and mucous membranes; and orientation to person, place, and time
- Explain measures that can be taken to treat or prevent fluid volume loss
- Describe symptoms that indicate the need to consult with health care provider

| **NIC** | Interventions (Nursing Interventions Classification) |

Suggested NIC Interventions
Fluid Management; Fluid Monitoring, Hypovolemia Management

Example NIC Activities—Fluid Management

Monitor hydration status (e.g., moist mucous membranes, adequacy of pulses, and orthostatic blood pressure) as appropriate

---

Nursing Interventions and Rationales

- Use appropriate preoperative fasting guidelines as ordered: "allow the consumption of clear liquids up to two hours before elective surgery, a light breakfast (tea and toast, for example) six hours before the procedure, and a heavier meal eight hours beforehand" (Crenshaw and Winslow, 2002, p 36). **Nursing and Clinical Research:** *Research has demonstrated that pulmonary aspiration is a rare complication of anesthesia, and prolonged fasting before surgery can lead to dehydration, headache, and hypoglycemia (Hung, 1992; Smith et al, 1997). A study demonstrated that most patients received instructions of NPO after midnight for preoperative fasting, resulting in some patients with afternoon surgeries fasting up to 20 hours from liquids, and 37 hours from solids (Crehshaw and Winslow, 2002).*
- See care plan for **Deficient Fluid volume.**

• = Independent; ▲ = Collaborative

Geriatric

- Aim for 1500 ml of oral liquids per day unless contraindicated by a medical condition such as congestive heart failure.
- Allow adequate time for eating and drinking at meals. *Meals can provide two thirds of daily fluids if clients are encouraged to consume liquids and have sufficient time to do so (Bennett, 2000).*
- Provide water that is freely available on the bedside or beside the chair.
- Incorporate regular hydration into daily routines (e.g., extra glass of fluid with medication or social activities). Consider use of a beverage cart and a hydration assistant to routinely offer increased beverages to clients in extended care. **Nursing Research:** *A study demonstrated that institution of a beverage cart with a trained hydration assistant resulted in increased number of bowel movements, less use of laxatives, decreased number of falls, less urinary tract infections, respiratory infections, and skin breakdown (Robinson and Rosher, 2002).*
- Note the color of urine and compare against a urine color chart to monitor adequate fluid intake. **Nursing Research:** *A research study on elderly veterans demonstrated that urine color correlated significantly with urine osmolality, serum sodium, and blood urea nitrogen to creatinine ratios (Wakefield et al, 2002).*
- Encourage consumption of fluids with medications. **Clinical Research:** *In one study it was shown that liquids consumed with medication made the difference between adequate and inadequate fluid intake for some clients (Lavizzo-Mourey et al, 1988).*
- Ensure that clients who are immobile or restrained get adequate fluids. *These are methods to increase fluid intake in the elderly and prevent deficient fluid volume (Bennett, 2000).*

Client/Family Teaching

- Teach clients who work in hot environments or exercise in hot environments to increase intake of both water and use of electrolyte-carbohydrate beverages. *A review of the literature demonstrated that drinks containing low to moderate levels of electrolytes and carbohydrates may provide significant advantages in industrial situations (Clap et al, 2002).*

evolve WEBSITES FOR EDUCATION

See the EVOLVE website for World Wide Web resources for client education.

REFERENCES

Bennett JA: Dehydration: hazards and benefits, *Geriatr Nurs* 21(2):84, 2000.
Clap AJ et al: A review of fluid replacement for workers in hot jobs, *AIHA J* 63:2, 2002.
Crenshaw JT, Winslow EH: Preoperative fasting: old habits die hard, *Am J Nurs* 102(5):36, 2002.
Hung P: Preoperative fasting, *Nurs Times* 88:48, 1992.
Lavizzo-Mourey RJ, Johnson J, Stolley P: Risk factors for dehydration among elderly nursing home residents, *J Am Geriatr Soc* 36(3):213, 1988.
Robinson SB, Rosher RB: Can a beverage cart help improve hydration? *Geriatr Nurs* 23:4, 2002.
Smith AF et al: Shorter preoperative fluid fasts reduce postoperative emesis, *BMJ* 314:7092, 1997.
Wakefield B et al: Monitoring hydration status in elderly veterans, *West J Nurs Res* 24(2):132, 2002.

• = Independent; ▲ = Collaborative

Risk for imbalanced Fluid volume

Terri Foster and Betty J. Ackley

NANDA **Definition**

At risk for decrease, increase, or rapid shift from one to the other of intravascular, interstitial, and/or intracellular fluid (refers to body fluid loss, gain, or both)

Risk Factors

Major invasive procedures

NOC **Outcomes (Nursing Outcomes Classification)**

Suggested NOC Outcomes

Electrolyte and Acid-Base Balance; Fluid Balance; Hydration

Example NOC Outcome with Indicators

Fluid Balance as evidenced by the following indicators: Blood pressure IER [Section I]/Peripheral pulses palpable/Skin hydrated/Mucous membranes moist/Serum electrolytes/Hematocrit WNL/Peripheral edema not present/Neck vein distention not present/Body weight stable/24-hour intake and output balanced/Urine specific gravity WNL/Adventitious breath sounds not present (Rate each indicator of **Fluid Balance:** 1 = extremely compromised, 2 = substantially compromised, 3 = moderately compromised, 4 = mildly compromised, 5 = not compromised [see Section I].)

IER, In expected range; *WNL,* within normal limits.

Client Outcomes

Client Will (Specify Time Frame):

- Have clear lung sounds, show respiratory rate of 12 to 20 breaths/min, and be free of dyspnea postoperatively
- Maintain urine output of at least 30 to 50 ml/hr, 1300 ml/24 hr
- Have blood pressure, pulse rate, and pulse oximetry within preoperative limits
- Have laboratory values within expected range
- Have nonedematous extremities and dependent areas
- Have mental orientation unchanged from preoperative status

NIC **Interventions (Nursing Interventions Classification)**

Suggested NIC Interventions

Acid-Base Management; Acid-Base Monitoring; Autotransfusion; Bleeding Precautions; Bleeding Reduction: Wound; Electrolyte Management; Fluid Management; Fluid Monitoring; Hemodynamic Regulation; Hypervolemia Management; Hypovolemia Management; Intravenous Therapy; Invasive Hemodynamic Monitoring; Shock Management: Volume; Vital Signs Monitoring.

• = Independent; ▲ = Collaborative

```
┌─────────────────────────────────────────────────────────────────────┐
│ Example NIC Activities—Fluid Management                               │
├─────────────────────────────────────────────────────────────────────┤
│ Maintain accurate intake and output record; Monitor vital signs       │
└─────────────────────────────────────────────────────────────────────┘
```

Nursing Interventions and Rationales

- Carefully assess the client's preoperative status and history. *Use of aspirin or other non-steroidal anti-inflammatory or anticoagulant therapy can affect bleeding, as can hemophilia, von Willebrand's disease, or disseminated intravascular coagulation. Use of laxatives, preoperative dehydration, infection, abnormal drainage, or hemorrhage can lead to hypotension during anesthesia induction if not corrected preoperatively.*

▲ Use appropriate preoperative fasting guidelines as ordered: "allow the consumption of clear liquids up to two hours before elective surgery, a light breakfast (tea and toast, for example) six hours before the procedure, and a heavier meal eight hours beforehand" (Crenshaw and Winslow, 2002, p 36). **Nursing and Clinical Research:** *Research has demonstrated that pulmonary aspiration is a rare complication of anesthesia, and prolonged fasting before surgery can lead to dehydration, headache, and hypoglycemia (Hung, 1992; Smith et al, 1997). A study demonstrated that most clients received instructions to take nothing by mouth (NPO) after midnight for preoperative fasting; as a result, some clients with afternoon surgeries fasted up to 20 hours from liquids and 37 hours from solids (Crenshaw and Winslow, 2002).*

▲ Monitor vital signs, noting especially pulse rate and blood pressure. If systolic blood pressure is less than 100, notify the anesthesiologist. *Blood pressure and pulse rate are an indication of fluid volume. Low pressures and increased pulse rate are seen in hypovolemia, which can be dangerous in the surgical client. A blood pressure lower than 90 mm Hg for more than 1 hour can result in acute renal failure postoperatively in the cardiac surgery client (Suen et al, 1998).*

- Monitor for signs of hypovolemia. *Hypovolemia can occur in the surgical client due to NPO status, hemorrhage, or third spacing. Signs include decreased urinary output, decreased central venous pressure, hypotension, and increased pulse and respiration rate. Hypovolemia can lead to decreased cardiac output, inadequate organ perfusion, and renal failure (Litwack, 1999). When large amounts of fluid are removed from the body, the possibility of hypovolemia exists (Trott et al, 1998).* **Nursing Research:** *In a study of 100 clients who underwent major elective surgery with an anticipated blood loss of more than 500 ml, it was concluded that goal-directed fluid administration leads to an earlier return of bowel function, a lower incidence of postoperative nausea and vomiting, and a decrease in length of postoperative hospital stay (Gan et al, 2002).*

- Monitor for signs of hypervolemia. *Surgical clients with preexisting chronic kidney or liver disease or congestive heart failure may be prone to hypervolemia. Increased fluid intake, especially of sodium-containing fluid via the intravenous route, can predispose the surgical client to hypervolemia. Signs of hypervolemia include peripheral edema, puffy eyelids, pleural effusion, pulmonary edema, increased central venous pressure, and increased pulmonary artery pressure (Litwack, 1999).*

- Monitor for signs of third spacing. *Third spacing can occur due to surgery itself. It may be necessary to replace fluid intraoperatively. Treatment is sometimes controversial and includes colloid replacement (albumin, plasma, Hespan, dextran) and crystalloid replacement*

- = Independent; ▲ = Collaborative

(dextrose 5% in normal saline, dextrose 5% in lactated Ringer's solution) in varying combinations (Litwack, 1999).

▲ In the critically ill surgical client with a pulmonary artery catheter, monitor pressures, especially wedge pressure. *Pulmonary artery pressures are helpful for determining fluid balance, including preload and afterload, and they can help to guide fluid administration and administration of vasoactive IV drips such as dopamine.*

▲ If hypotension develops, administer fluid challenge as ordered, giving a specified amount of IV fluid, such as rapidly delivered IV 0.9% normal saline, and monitoring response by observing vital signs, lung sounds, and urine output. *A fluid challenge can help reverse deficient fluid volume rapidly.*

• Keep all IV fluids on a volumetric pump. *This is done to ensure that IV fluids do not "run in" and overload the client and that the client receives sufficient fluids.*

• Carefully keep track of input and output of fluids during surgery. *Assessment, accurate documentation of intake and output, and management of fluid and electrolyte imbalances is crucial to prevent serious problems. The main goal of fluid management should be to ensure adequate oxygen delivery through the optimization of blood oxygenation, perfusion pressure, and circulating volume (Kreimeier, 2000).* **Nursing Research:** *Fluid absorption was evident in a study of 148 clients undergoing percutaneous nephrolithotomy. This could be clinically significant in clients with compromised cardiorespiratory or renal status and in pediatric clients, and could lead to fluid overload (Kukreja et al, 2002).*

▲ Measure urine output hourly. If urine output is less than 30 ml/hr or 0.5 ml/kg/hr, notify the anesthesiologist. *Urine output is an indicator of fluid balance in the body. An output below 30 ml/hr may indicate deficient fluid volume, which can result in systemic hypoperfusion, decreased oxygen delivery, and organ system failure (Rothrock, 1996; Weissman, 1994). Assessment, accurate documentation of intake and output, and management of fluid and electrolyte imbalances is crucial to prevent serious problems.*

• Monitor for electrolyte imbalance. *When large amounts of tissue and fluids are removed from the body, the possibility of hypovolemia exists (Trott et al, 1998). Removing large amounts of fluids during surgery increases renal flow (Meeker and Rothrock, 1999). Surgery itself, gastrointestinal (GI) loss of potassium from preoperative bowel preparations, stress, diuretic use, and nasogastric suction intraoperatively can all contribute to the development of hypokalemia (Litwack, 1999). Hypokalemia can cause EKG changes and cardiac dysrhythmias (Litwack, 1999). For safe correction of hypokalemia, IV potassium is given slowly and urine output is measured (Litwack, 1999). Surgeries that involve the use of large amounts of hypotonic irrigating solution can cause an increased loss of salt that lowers the salt/water ratio (hyponatremia) (Litwack, 1999). To prevent or correct hyponatremia, it is recommended that normal saline solutions be used for surgical irrigation and that input and output be monitored (Litwack, 1999).* **Nursing Research:** *In a study of 12 clients who underwent surgical procedures lasting over 4 hours, metabolic acidosis was found to occur in relation to chloride administration; this was probably due to the normal saline IV, because there was no increase in plasma volume (Waters et al, 1999).*

• If large amounts of hypotonic irrigation solution (e.g., glycine) are used during surgery, carefully keep track of fluid inflow and outflow. *If there is a deficit of 1000 ml or more in outflow, request an order for testing of serum sodium level (Kriplani et al, 1998) and also serum osmolality (Metheny, 2000).* **Nursing Research:** *In a study of 697 women who underwent a hysteroscopy, 5% experienced excessive hypotonic fluid absorption (Belloni, 2001). Research has shown that, when a fluid deficit of 1000 ml occurs and the procedure is halted, serious sequelae are seen only rarely (Belloni, 2001).*

• = Independent; ▲ = Collaborative

- Transurethral resection of the prostate syndrome: Watch for symptoms of headache, visual changes, agitation, lethargy, vomiting, muscle twitching, bradycardia, diminished pupillary reflexes, hypertension, and respiratory distress (Metheny, 2000).
- Endometrial ablation: If the client is undergoing general anesthesia, watch for symptoms of decreased body temperature, decreased oxygen saturation, dilated pupils, and tremulousness (Metheny, 2000). *Serious fluid overload and dilutional hyponatremia can develop in surgeries such as transurethral resection of the prostate, transcervical resection of the endometrium, or hysteroscopy as a result of absorption of large amounts of irrigation solution into the vascular system and can cause permanent morbidity or death (Indman et al, 1998; Kriplani et al, 1998; Meeker and Rothrock, 1999). Saline cannot be used for irrigation in these cases because it conducts electrical current, and electrosurgical cautery is used during the procedure (Meeker and Rothrock, 1999).*
- Observe the surgical client for signs of hyperkalemia: cardiac dysrhythmias, heart block, asystole, abdominal distention, and weakness. *Massive blood transfusions and tissue breakdown from surgery, crush injuries, or burns can lead to hyperkalemia (Meeker and Rothrock, 1999). Clients who have undergone bilateral thyroid surgery should be observed for hypocalcemia (Metheny, 2000).*
- Observe closely for signs of hypokalemia in a client who has been under prolonged stress or has lost GI fluids. *Hypokalemia commonly causes dysrhythmias. Stress and/or GI fluid loss in surgical clients make them susceptible to hypokalemia.*
- Recognize that the surgical client may develop hyponatremia related to inappropriate antidiuretic hormone (ADH) secretion, which can be caused by trauma, thrombosis, abscesses, hemorrhages, or hematomas (Leite, 2001). *ADH, which acts on the kidneys to control water loss and retention, has an important effect in surgical clients under stress (Metheny, 2000). ADH regulates water absorption in the renal tubules and collecting ducts. ADH production is stimulated by stress, surgery, pain, trauma, anesthetics, and mechanical ventilation. An increase in ADH production can cause increased plasma osmolality and decreased circulating blood volume (Litwack, 1999).*
- Accurately measure blood loss intraoperatively. *Weighing sponges is a reliable means of estimating blood loss and gauging replacement needs (Meeker and Rothrock, 1999). Estimates of intraoperative blood loss can be inaccurate, which can lead to inappropriate fluid management (Kreimeier, 2000).*

Geriatric
- Be especially vigilant when monitoring vital signs and fluids in elderly surgical clients. *During surgery, homeostatic mechanisms to regulate fluid balance are depressed in the elderly, and many elderly clients have renal insufficiency or heart failure, which can result in increased morbidity and sometimes mortality postoperatively (Metheny, 2000).*
- Assess for preoperative dehydration. *NPO status, diuretic therapy, poor nutritional status, preexisting cardiopulmonary disease, and vomiting can all predispose the geriatric client to fluid and electrolyte imbalance (Litwack, 1999).*

Pediatric
- Monitor the pediatric surgical client closely for signs of fluid loss. *Small losses can be life-threatening to pediatric clients (Metheny, 2000).*

• = Independent; ▲ = Collaborative

evolve WEBSITES FOR EDUCATION

See the EVOLVE website for World Wide Web resources for client education.

REFERENCES

Belloni C: Intraoperative complications of 697 consecutive operative hysteroscopies, *Minerva Ginecol* 53:1, 2001.

Crenshaw JT, Winslow EH: Preoperative fasting: old habits die hard, *Am J Nurs* 102:36, 2002.

Gan TJ et al: Goal-directed intraoperative fluid administration reduces length of hospital stay after major surgery, *Anesthesiology* 97:4, 2002.

Hung P: Preoperative fasting, *Nurs Times* 88(48):57, 1992.

Indman PD et al: Complications of fluid overload from resectoscopic surgery, *J Am Assoc Gynecol Laparosc* 5:1, 1998.

Kreimeier U: Pathophysiology of fluid imbalance, *Crit Care* 4(suppl 2):S3, 2000.

Kriplani A et al: Biochemical, hemodynamic and hematological changes during transcervical resection of the endometrium using a 1.5% glycine as the irrigation solution, *Eur J Obstet Gynecol Reprod Biol* 80(1):99, 1998.

Kukreja RA et al: Fluid absorption during percutaneous nephrolithotomy: does it matter? *J Endourol* 16:4, 2002.

Leite W: *Fluid and electrolyte disorders—part I: disorders of sodium balance*, available online at http://www.medstudents.com.br/cirur/cirur1.htm, accessed March 5, 2001.

Litwack K: *Core curriculum for perianesthesia nursing practice*, ed 4, Philadelphia, 1999, WB Saunders.

Meeker MH, Rothrock JC: *Alexander's care of the patient in surgery*, ed 11, St Louis, 1999, Mosby.

Metheny NM: *Fluid and electrolyte balance: nursing considerations*, ed 4, Philadelphia, 2000, Lippincott.

Rothrock JC: *Perioperative nursing care plans*, ed 2, St Louis, 1996, Mosby.

Smith AF et al: Shorter preoperative fluid fasts reduce postoperative emesis, *BMJ* 314(7092):1486, 1997.

Suen WS et al: Risk factors for development of acute renal failure requiring dialysis in patients undergoing cardiac surgery, *Angiology* 49(10):789, 1998.

Trott WA et al: Safety considerations and fluid resuscitation in liposuction: an analysis of 53 consecutive patients, *Plast Reconstr Surg* 102(6):220, 1998.

Waters JH et al: Causes of metabolic acidosis in prolonged surgery, *Crit Care Med* 27(10):2142, 1999.

Weissman C: Ensuring perioperative fluid homeostasis in critically ill patients, *J Crit Illness* 9(12):183, 1994.

Impaired Gas exchange

Betty J. Ackley

NANDA Definition

Excess or deficit in oxygenation and/or carbon dioxide elimination at the alveolar-capillary membrane

Defining Characteristics

Visual disturbances; decreased carbon dioxide; dyspnea; abnormal arterial blood gas levels; hypoxia; irritability; somnolence; restlessness; hypercapnia; tachycardia; cyanosis; abnormal skin color (pale, dusky); hypoxemia; hypercarbia; headache on awakening; abnormal rate, rhythm, depth of breathing; diaphoresis; abnormal arterial pH; nasal flaring

Related Factors (r/t)

Ventilation-perfusion imbalance; alveolar-capillary membrane changes

• = Independent; ▲ = Collaborative

| NOC | Outcomes (Nursing Outcomes Classification) |

Suggested NOC Outcomes

Respiratory Status: Gas Exchange, Ventilation

Example NOC Outcome with Indicators

Achieves appropriate **Respiratory Status: Gas Exchange** as evidenced by the following indicators: Mental status IER/Restlessness not present/Cyanosis not present/Somnolence not present/Pao_2 WNL/$Paco_2$ WNL/ Arterial pH WNL/O_2 saturation WNL/End-tidal CO_2 IER (Rate each indicator of **Respiratory Status:** 1 = extremely compromised, 2 = substantially compromised, 3 = moderately compromised, 4 = mildly compromised, 5 = not compromised [see Section I].)

IER, In expected range; *WNL*, within normal limits.

Client Outcomes

Client Will (Specify Time Frame):

- Demonstrate improved ventilation and adequate oxygenation as evidenced by blood gas levels within normal parameters for that client
- Maintain clear lung fields and remain free of signs of respiratory distress
- Verbalize understanding of oxygen supplementation and other therapeutic interventions

| NIC | Interventions (Nursing Interventions Classification) |

Suggested NIC Interventions

Acid-Base Management; Airway Management

Example NIC Activities—Acid-Base Management

Monitor for symptoms of respiratory failure (e.g., low Pao_2 and elevated $Paco_2$ levels and respiratory muscle fatigue); Monitor determinants of tissue oxygen delivery (e.g., Pao_2, Sao_2, and hemoglobin levels, and cardiac output) if available

---

Nursing Interventions and Rationales

- Monitor respiratory rate, depth, and effort, including use of accessory muscles, nasal flaring, and abnormal breathing patterns. *Increased respiratory rate, use of accessory muscles, nasal flaring, abdominal breathing, and a look of panic in the client's eyes may be seen with hypoxia.*
- Auscultate breath sounds every 1 to 2 hours. *The presence of crackles and wheezes may alert the nurse to airway obstruction, which may lead to or exacerbate existing hypoxia. In severe exacerbations of chronic obstructive pulmonary disease (COPD), lung sounds may be diminished or distant with air trapping (Zampella, 2003).*
- Monitor the client's behavior and mental status for the onset of restlessness, agitation, confusion, and (in the late stages) extreme lethargy. *Changes in behavior and mental status can be early signs of impaired gas exchange (Misasi and Keyes, 1994). In the late stages the client becomes lethargic and somnolent.*
- Monitor oxygen saturation continuously using pulse oximetry. Note blood gas results

• = **Independent;** ▲ = **Collaborative**

as available. *An oxygen saturation of less than 90% (normal: 95% to 100%) or a partial pressure of oxygen of less than 80 mm Hg (normal: 80 to 100 mm Hg) indicates significant oxygenation problems (Berry and Pinard, 2002; Grap, 2002).*

- Observe for cyanosis of the skin; especially note color of the tongue and oral mucous membranes. *Central cyanosis of the tongue and oral mucosa is indicative of serious hypoxia and is a medical emergency. Peripheral cyanosis in the extremities may or may not be serious (Carpenter, 1993).*

- If the client has unilateral lung disease, alternate semi-Fowler's position with a lateral position (with 10- to 15-degree elevation and "good lung down" for 60 to 90 minutes). This method is contraindicated for clients with pulmonary abscess or hemorrhage or interstitial emphysema. *Gravity and hydrostatic pressure cause the dependent lung to become better ventilated and perfused, which increases oxygenation (Lasater-Erhard, 1995; Yeaw, 1992).*

- If the client has bilateral lung disease, position the client in either semi-Fowler's or a side-lying position, which increases oxygenation as indicated by pulse oximetry (or, if the client has a pulmonary catheter, venous oxygen saturation). Turn the client every 2 hours. Monitor mixed venous oxygen saturation closely after turning. If it drops below 10% or fails to return to baseline promptly, turn the client back into the supine position and evaluate oxygen status. **Nursing Research:** *Turning is important to prevent complications of immobility, but in critically ill clients with low hemoglobin levels or decreased cardiac output, turning on either side can result in desaturation (Winslow, 1992). Critically ill clients should be turned carefully and watched closely (Gawlinksi and Dracup, 1998).*

- If the client is obese or has ascites, consider positioning the client in reverse Trendelenburg's position at 45 degrees for periods as tolerated. **Nursing Research:** *A study demonstrated that use of reverse Trendelenburg's position at 45 degrees resulted in increased tidal volumes and decreased respiratory rates in a group of intubated clients with obesity, abdominal distention, and ascites (Burns et al, 1994).*

▲ If the client has adult respiratory distress syndrome, or difficulty maintaining oxygenation, consider positioning the client prone with the upper thorax and pelvis supported, allowing the abdomen to protrude. Monitor oxygen saturation and turn back to supine position if desaturation occurs. **Nursing and Clinical Research:** *Oxygenation levels have been shown to improve in the prone position, probably due to decreased shunting and better perfusion of the lungs (Curley, Thompson, and Arnold, 2000; Mure et al, 1997; Vollman and Bander, 1996).*

- If the client is acutely dyspneic, consider having the client lean forward over a bedside table, if tolerated. *Leaning forward can help decrease dyspnea, possibly because gastric pressure allows better contraction of the diaphragm (Celli, 1998). This is called the tripod position and is used during times of distress (Zampella, 2003).*

- Help the client to deep breathe and perform controlled coughing. Have the client inhale deeply, hold the breath for several seconds, and cough two or three times with the mouth open while tightening the upper abdominal muscles as tolerated. *This technique can help increase sputum clearance and decrease cough spasms (Celli, 1998). Controlled coughing uses the diaphragmatic muscles, which makes the cough more forceful and effective.*

NOTE: If the client has excessive fluid in the respiratory system, see the interventions for **Ineffective Airway clearance.**

▲ Monitor the effects of sedation and analgesics on the client's respiratory pattern; use judiciously. *Both analgesics and medications that cause sedation can depress respiration*

• = **Independent;** ▲ = **Collaborative**

at times. However, these medications can be very helpful for decreasing the sympathetic nervous system discharge that accompanies hypoxia.

- Schedule nursing care to provide rest and minimize fatigue. *The hypoxic client has limited reserves; inappropriate activity can increase hypoxia.*
- ▲ Administer humidified oxygen through an appropriate device (e.g., nasal cannula or face mask per the physician's order); watch for onset of hypoventilation as evidenced by increased somnolence after initiating or increasing oxygen therapy. *A client with chronic lung disease may need a hypoxic drive to breathe and may hypoventilate during oxygen therapy.*
- Provide adequate fluids, within the client's cardiac and renal reserve, to liquefy secretions.
- If the client is severely debilitated from chronic respiratory disease, consider the use of a wheeled walker to help in ambulation. **Clinical Research:** *Use of a wheeled walker has been shown to result in significant decrease in disability, hypoxemia, and breathlessness during a 6-minute walk test (Honeyman, Barr, and Stubbing, 1996).*
- ▲ Monitor nutritional status. Refer the client for a dietary consultation if needed. **Clinical Research:** *Many clients with emphysema are malnourished. Improved nutrition can help increase muscle aerobic capacity and exercise tolerance (Palange et al, 1995).*
- ▲ Refer the COPD client to a pulmonary rehabilitation program. **Clinical Research:** *Pulmonary rehabilitation has been shown to relieve dyspnea and fatigue, and enhance clients' sense of control over their disease. Rehabilitation is an important component of the management of COPD (Lacasse et al, 2002).*

NOTE: If the client becomes ventilator dependent, see the care plan for **Impaired spontaneous ventilation.**

Geriatric

- ▲ Use central nervous system depressants carefully to avoid decreasing respiration rate. *An elderly client is prone to respiratory depression.*
- ▲ Maintain low-flow oxygen therapy. *An elderly client is susceptible to oxygen-induced respiratory depression.*
- Encourage the client to stop smoking. *Elderly clients who stop smoking experience substantial health benefits (Foyt, 1992).*

Home care

- Assess the home environment for irritants that impair gas exchange. Help the client to adjust the home environment as necessary (e.g., install an air filter to decrease the level of dust).
- ▲ Refer the client to occupational therapy as necessary to assist the client in adaptation to the home and environment and in energy conservation.
- Assist the client with identifying and avoiding situations that exacerbate impairment of gas exchange (e.g., stress-related situations, exposure to pollution of any kind, proximity to noxious gas fumes such as chlorine bleach). *Irritants in the environment decrease the client's effectiveness in accessing oxygen during breathing.*
- Instruct the client to keep the home temperature above 20° C (68° F) and to avoid cold weather. *Cold air temperatures cause constriction of the blood vessels and increased moisture, which impairs the client's ability to absorb oxygen.*
- Instruct the client to limit exposure to persons with respiratory infections.

- • = Independent; ▲ = Collaborative

- Instruct the family in the complications of the disease and the importance of maintaining the medical regimen, including when to call a physician.
- Assess nutritional status. Instruct the client to eat several small meals and use dietary supplements as necessary. For some clients, drinking 30 ml of a supplement such as Ensure or Pulmocare every hour while awake can be helpful. *Weight loss in a client with COPD has a negative effect on the course of the disease; it can result in loss of muscle mass in the respiratory muscles, including the diaphragm, which can lead to respiratory failure (Berry and Baum, 2001).*
- ▲ Refer the client for home health aide services as necessary for assistance with activities of daily living. *Clients with decreased oxygenation have decreased energy to carry out personal and role-related activities.*
- ▲ Assess family role changes and coping ability. Refer the client to medical social services as appropriate for assistance in adjusting to chronic illness. *Inability to maintain the level of social involvement experienced before illness leads to frustration and anger in the client and may create a threat to the family unit.* **Nursing Research:** *Clients with chronic lung problems were described as negative, helpless, confused, and socially obstreperous by family members in one study (Leidy and Traver, 1996).*
- Support the family of the client with chronic illness. *Severely compromised respiratory functioning causes fear and anxiety in clients and their families. Reassurance from the nurse can be helpful.*

Client/Family Teaching

- Teach the client how to perform pursed-lip breathing and controlled diaphragmatic breathing, and how to use the tripod position. Have the client watch the pulse oximeter to note improvement in oxygenation with these breathing techniques. *Controlled-breathing techniques can help reduce anxiety and decrease panic and dyspnea (Celli, 1998).*
- Teach the client energy conservation techniques and the importance of alternating rest periods with activity. See nursing interventions for **Fatigue.**
- ▲ Teach the importance of not smoking; be aggressive in approach, and ask the client to set a date for smoking cessation. Recommend nicotine replacement therapy (nicotine patch or gum). Refer the client to smoking-cessation programs. Encourage clients who relapse to keep trying to quit. *All health care clinicians should be aggressive in helping smokers quit (Agency for Health Care Policy Research, 1996).* **Clinical Research:** *Giving up smoking can slow the course of disease, and some clients may even regain some lung function (Anthonisen et al, 1994).*
- ▲ Instruct the family regarding home oxygen therapy if ordered (e.g., delivery system, liter flow, safety precautions).
- Teach the client relaxation techniques to help reduce stress responses and panic attacks resulting from dyspnea. **Nursing Research:** *Relaxation therapy can help reduce dyspnea and anxiety (Gift, Moore, and Soeken, 1992).*

evolve WEBSITES FOR EDUCATION

See the EVOLVE website for World Wide Web resources for client education.

• = **Independent;** ▲ = **Collaborative**

REFERENCES

Agency for Health Care Policy Research: *Smoking cessation,* Clinical Practice Guideline No. 18, US Government Printing No. 017-026-00159-0, Washington, DC, 1996, The Agency.

Anthonisen NR et al: Effects of smoking intervention and the use of an inhaled anticholinergic bronchodilator on the rate of decline of FEV_1. The Lung Health Study, *JAMA* 272:1497, 1994.

Berry BE, Pinard AE: Assessing tissue oxygenation, *Crit Care Nurse* 22(3):22, 2002.

Berry JK, Baum CL: Malnutrition in chronic obstructive pulmonary disease: adding insult to injury, *AACN Clin Issues* 12(2):210, 2001.

Burns SM et al: Effect of body position on spontaneous respiratory rate and tidal volume in patients with obesity, abdominal distention and ascites, *Am J Crit Care* 3:102, 1994.

Carpenter KD: A comprehensive review of cyanosis, *Crit Care Nurse* 13:66, 1993.

Celli BR: Pulmonary rehabilitation for COPD, *Postgrad Med* 103(4):159, 1998.

Curley MA, Thompson JE, Arnold JH: The effects of early and repeated prone positioning in pediatric patients with acute lung injury, *Chest* 118(1):156, 2000.

Foyt MM: Impaired gas exchange in the elderly, *Geriatr Nurs* 13:262, 1992.

Gawlinski A, Dracup K. Effect of positioning on Svo_2 in the critically ill patient with a low ejection fraction, *Nurs Res* 47(5):293, 1998.

Gift AG, Moore T, Soeken K: Relaxation to reduce dyspnea and anxiety in COPD patients, *Nurs Res* 41(4): 242, 1992.

Grap MJ. Protocols for practice: applying research at the bedside: pulse oximetry, *Crit Care Nurse* 22(3):69, 2002.

Honeyman P, Barr P, Stubbing DG: Effect of a walking aid on disability, oxygenation, and breathlessness in patients with chronic airflow limitation, *J Cardiopulm Rehabil* 16:63, 1996.

Lacasse Y et al: Pulmonary rehabilitation for chronic obstructive pulmonary disease, *Cochrane Library* (CD003793), 2002.

Lasater-Erhard M: The effect of patient position on arterial oxygen saturation, *Crit Care Nurse* 15(5):31, 1995.

Leidy NK, Traver GA: Adjustment and social behavior in older adults with chronic obstructive pulmonary disease: the family's perspective, *J Adv Nurs* 23:252, 1996.

Misasi RS, Keyes JL: The pathophysiology of hypoxia, *Crit Care Nurse* 14:55, 1994.

Mure M et al: Dramatic effect on oxygenation in patients with severe acute lung insufficiency treated in the prone position, *Crit Care Med* 25(9):1539, 1997.

Palange P et al: Nutritional state and exercise tolerance in patients with COPD, *Chest* 107:1206, 1995.

Vollman KM, Bander JJ: Improved oxygenation utilizing a prone positioner in patients with acute respiratory distress syndrome, *Intensive Care Med* 22:10, 1105.

Winslow EH: Turn for the worse, *Am J Nurs* 92:16C, 1992.

Winslow EH: High Fowler's won't always ease breathing, *Am J Nurs* 96:59, 1996.

Yeaw P: Good lung down, *Am J Nurs* 92:27, 1992.

Zampella MA. COPD: managing flare-ups, *RN* 14:14, 2003.

Grieving

Betty J. Ackley and Gail B. Ladwig

NANDA Definition

State in which an individual or group of individuals reacts to an actual or perceived loss, which may be loss of a person, object, function, status, relationship, or body part

NOTE: Grieving is not an official NANDA nursing diagnosis, but it is included because the authors believe that grieving is part of the normal human response to loss and that nurses can use interventions to help the client grieve. Grieving is a wellness-oriented nursing diagnosis (Arnold, 1996).

Defining Characteristics

Verbal expression of distress at loss; anger; sadness; crying; difficulty in expressing loss; alterations in eating habits, sleep patterns, dream patterns, activity levels, or libido; reliv-

• = **Independent; ▲ = Collaborative**

ing of past experiences; interference with life function; alterations in concentration or pursuit of tasks

Related Factors (r/t)

Actual or perceived object loss, which may include loss of people, possessions, job, status, home, ideals, or parts and processes of the body

NOC   Outcomes (Nursing Outcomes Classification)

Suggested NOC Outcomes

Grief Resolution; Hope; Mood Equilibrium; Psychosocial Adjustment: Life Change

---

Example NOC Outcome with Indicators

Grief Resolution with plans for a positive future as evidenced by the following indicators: Expresses feelings about loss/Verbalizes acceptance of loss/Describes meaning of loss or death/Reports decreased preoccupation with loss/Expresses positive expectations about the future (Rate each indicator of **Grief Resolution:** 1 = never demonstrated, 2 = rarely demonstrated, 3 = sometimes demonstrated, 4 = often demonstrated, 5 = consistently demonstrated [see Section I].)

Client Outcomes

Client Will (Specify Time Frame):

- Express feelings of guilt, fear, anger, or sadness
- Identify problems associated with grief (e.g., changes in appetite, insomnia, loss of libido, decreased energy, alteration in activity level)
- Plan for the future one day at a time
- Function at normal developmental level and perform activities of daily living

NIC   Interventions (Nursing Interventions Classification)

Suggested NIC Interventions

Grief Work Facilitation; Grief Work Facilitation: Perinatal Death

---

Example NIC Activities—Grief Work Facilitation

Encourage client to verbalize memories of the loss, both past and current; Assist client to identify personal coping strategies

---

Nursing Interventions and Rationales

- Use a grief instrument such as the Hogan Grief Reaction Checklist (HGRC) to evaluate the client with regard to the six factors in the normal trajectory of the grieving process: Despair, Panic Behavior, Blame and Anger, Detachment, Disorganization, and Personal Growth. **Clinical Research:** *The HGRC was developed empirically from data collected from bereaved adults who had experienced the death of a loved one (Hogan, Greenfield, and Schmidt, 2001).*
- Allow family members to participate in care of the body of the deceased if desired. Help survivors say goodbye in the most loving and caring way possible. **Nursing Research:** *One study revealed a theme of a need to remember and to hold onto the memory.*

- • = **Independent;** ▲ = **Collaborative**

Participants in this study found comfort in knowing they were not alone (Hentz, 2002).

- Allow the family "holding" behaviors, including taking photographs of the deceased or clipping a piece of hair. *Memory keepsakes facilitate the grief process (Buxbaum and Brant, 2001).*

- Help the bereaved client survive during times of acute grief. Ensure that the client maintains sufficient nutrition and help the client determine a routine to make it through each day. *A newly bereaved person can be stunned and helpless (Gifford and Cleary, 1990). It is common for a newly bereaved person to eat minimally for several days (Rodebaugh, Schwindt, and Valentine, 1999), but after that it is important that the person eat to maintain health.* **Clinical Research:** *One study indicated that bereaved individuals, whether they had counseling for grief resolution or not, had a moderate risk for poor nutrition. The implication is that food issues need to be included in grief resolution interventions (Johnson, 2002).*

- Encourage the client to share memories and tell stories of the person or object of loss by making comments such as, "Tell me about your wife [husband, parent]." Conduct an in-depth personal interview to learn about the client and loved one or loss. *A personal history can help a nurse understand the unique loss that the person has experienced, the meaning of the loss to the individual, and the strengths the person brings to the situation (Solari-Twadell et al, 1995).* **Clinical Research:** *The goal in the aftermath of September 11, 2001, was to allow the victims to tell their stories. By sharing their stories, individuals start the process of moving from helpless victim to proactive survivor (Pessin et al, 2002).*

- Consider the use of a "grief map." This allows the individual to conceptualize each phenomenon of grief and to visualize progress through the issues associated with the feelings. **Clinical Research:** *The grief map provides a constructive multidimensional framework for dealing with the phenomena of the grieving process and for rebuilding life following major loss. It provides individuals with a means of describing their experiences (Clark, 2001).*

- Actively listen to the client's expression of grief; do not interrupt, do not tell your own story, and do not offer meaningless platitudes such as, "It will be better this way." *These behaviors do not help and can often hurt (Gifford and Cleary, 1990; Hoffman, 1997).*

- Encourage the client to "cry out" his or her grief and express feelings, including sadness and anger. **Clinical Research:** *In a content analysis of the narratives of 85 mourners, nine unique meaning constructs emerged, the most prominent of which spoke to the theme of feeling the absence of the deceased (Gamino, Hogan, and Sewell, 2002).*

- If the client or family members are expressing anger, try not to react in anger. Instead, allow feelings to be expressed, listen to the expressions of anger, and accept their right to those feelings. Try lowering your voice and slowing your rate of speech as you respond to the client and/or family. *It is not therapeutic to respond to anger with anger. Instead, strive to be therapeutic, helping the client and/or family express the anger and gain control of themselves by modeling calm behavior (Rueth and Hall, 1999).*

- Help the client identify previous successful personal coping strategies. Use music if appropriate. **Nursing Research:** *One study revealed the theme of a need to remember and to hold onto the memory (Hentz, 2002). Four case studies demonstrated the usefulness of music therapy in assisting palliative care clients and families to cope with grief and loss (Hilliard, 2001b).* **Clinical Research:** *The investigator concluded that participation of grieving children in music therapy–based bereavement groups served to reduce grief symptoms among the subjects as evaluated in the home (Hilliard, 2001a).*

- ▲ Refer the client for spiritual counseling if desired. **Clinical Research:** *A prospective cohort study included people about to be bereaved, with follow-up continuing for 14 months*

- = **Independent;** ▲ = **Collaborative**

after the death. Those who professed stronger spiritual beliefs seemed to resolve their grief more rapidly and completely after the death of a close person than did people with no spiritual beliefs (Walsh et al, 2002).

- Provide information about the grief process, including the stages of grieving: denial, anger, bargaining, and acceptance (Kubler-Ross, 1969), or reeling, feeling, dealing, and healing (Rodebaugh, Schwindt, and Valentine, 1999). Help the client realize that spasms of grief can come at any time, that most people don't go through the stages in a predictable fashion, and that the grieving process takes time and is painful. *This information helps normalize the grief experience and provides clients with hope that they can survive (Gifford and Cleary, 1990; Rodebaugh, Schwindt, and Valentine, 1999).*

- Help the client determine the best way and place to find social support. Encourage the client to continue to use supports for 1 to 2 years. *Social support has been identified as an important predictor of a positive bereavement experience (Steen, 1998).* **Clinical Research:** *Social support has been shown to help bereaved individuals as they reconstruct their lives and find new meaning in life (Hogan and Schmidt, 2002).* **Nursing Research:** *In a study of adolescents dealing with the death of a loved one, the most important factors that helped adolescents cope with the grief were self-help and support from parents, relatives, and friends (Rask, Kaunonen, and Paunonen-Ilmonen, 2002).*

- ▲ Assess for causes of dysfunctional grieving (e.g., sudden death, highly dependent or ambivalent relationship with the deceased, lack of coping skills, lack of social support, previous physical or mental health problems, death of a child, death of a wife, death of a loved one by suicide). Refer for counseling, starting 2 to 8 weeks after the loss and for up to 3 months following bereavement (Steen, 1998). Refer to the care plan for **Dysfunctional Grieving.** *Life circumstances can interfere with normal grieving (Steen, 1998).*

- Assess for signs of depression: feelings of worthlessness, inability to eat or sleep, sleeping all the time. *Depression can occur in nearly half of all grieving people, and 10% of people who are grieving suffer major depression (Steen, 1998).*

- Encourage family members to set aside time to talk with one another about the loss without criticizing or belittling one another's feelings. *Help families to grieve as a system, not just as individual mourners (Steen, 1998).* **Nursing Research:** *A study analyzing the grief and coping of mothers who had lost children under the age of 7 years found that the spouse, remaining children, grandparents, next of kin, friends, and colleagues were the main sources of support (Laakso and Paunonen-Ilmonen, 2002).*

- ▲ Identify available community resources, including bereavement groups at local hospitals and hospice centers. Volunteers who provide bereavement support can also be effective. *Support groups can have positive effects on bereavement outcomes (Hoffman, 1997). Group counseling is an effective intervention because it addresses the issue of disenfranchised grief (Barlow and Morrison, 2002).*

- ▲ Recognize times when you as a nurse are affected by loss and need grief resolution. Attend a grief resolution group, ask for help from pastoral services, speak with a kind friend who is supportive, or seek counseling. *Nursing staff can experience unresolved grief from the death of a client or may suffer other losses that require grief resolution so that they can function effectively and be able to give to others (Hittle, 1995).*

Geriatric

- Use reminiscence therapy in conjunction with the expression of emotions. *Reminiscence therapy can help the client look back at past experiences and use coping techniques that were effective in the past (Puentes, 1998).*

• = Independent; ▲ = Collaborative

- Identify previous losses and assess the client for depression. *Losses and changes associated with aging often occur in rapid succession without adequate recovery time (Hegge and Fischer, 2000).* **Nursing Research:** *Having more than two concurrent losses increases the incidence of unresolved grief (Herth, 1990). The grieving elderly widow may develop depression that results in poor nutrition, noncompliance with medication regimens, decreasing cognition, and multiple health problems (Fischer and Hegge, 2000).*
- Monitor an older adult who has been treated for bereavement-related depression for relapse or recurrence. **Clinical Research:** *In a 2-year study, 36% of older adults treated for bereavement-related depression experienced relapse or recurrence (Pasternak et al, 1997).*
- Evaluate the social support system of the elderly client. If the support system is minimal, help the client determine how to increase available support. **Nursing Research:** *The elderly who have poor grieving outcomes often do not live with family members and have a minimal support system. The support of family (especially children) and friends is a common way for elderly widows to cope with a loss (Hegge and Fischer, 2000).*
- Provide support for the family when the loss is associated with dementia of the family member. *Psychosocial death is a significant dimension of the dementia of the Alzheimer's-type disease process. One article explored daughters' chronic grieving throughout the illness of a parent. The daughters' narratives revealed that witnessing the deterioration of a mind was a burdensome, grave learning process that encompassed many losses (Furlini, 2001).*

Multicultural

- Assess for the influence of cultural beliefs, norms, and values on the client's grief and mourning practices. **Nursing Research:** *Grief and mourning practices may be based on cultural conventions (Cochran, 1998; Doswell and Erlen, 1998; Leininger and McFarland, 2002). Some African Americans place great emphasis on attendance at funerals; many Native American tribes hold long, somber wakes during which food and memorial gifts are distributed; Chinese and Japanese families may have specific funeral rituals that must be followed precisely to ensure safe passage of their loved ones into the next world; Latinos may hold wakes, use prayer during a novena, and light candles in honor of the dead; in West Indian/Caribbean cultures death arrangements may be made by a kinsman of the deceased (McQuay, 1995).*
- Assess for the influence of cultural beliefs, norms, and values on the client's expressions of grief. **Nursing Research:** *African Americans may be expected to act "strong" and go about the business of life after a death; Native Americans may not talk about the death because of beliefs that such talk will detract from spirituality and bring bad luck; Latinos may wear black and act subdued during their* luto *(mourning) period; Southeast Asian families may wear white when mourning (McQuay, 1995).*
- Identify whether the client had been notified of the deceased's health status and was able to be present at the deathbed. **Nursing Research:** *Not being present during terminal illness and death can disrupt the grieving process (McQuay, 1995).*
- Validate the client's feelings regarding the loss. **Nursing Research:** *Validation is a therapeutic communication technique that lets the client know that the nurse has heard and understood what was said, and it promotes the nurse-client relationship (Heineken, 1998).*

Home care

NOTE: Grieving may be encountered as the client comes to terms with his or her own loss or death, or as the family reacts to the client's death.

- The interventions described previously may be adapted for home care use.

- **= Independent; ▲ = Collaborative**

- Listen actively as the client grieves his or her own death, or real or perceived loss. Normalize the client's expressions of grief for himself or herself. *Active listening supports the client without intrusive advice giving. Normalizing lets the client know that his or her responses are appropriate ways of preparing for death.*
- If the agency has served the deceased as a client, allow the primary caregivers to attend the services. *Families experiencing the loss of a loved one perceive staff attendance at services as a significant statement of caring and support.*
- Plan the first home visit within 10 days after the loss by the client; be guided by the type of loss and the family's schedule following the loss. *Support is a contributing factor to completion of grief work. The nurse can provide support and guidance.*
- If the loss is of a loved one, allow the client to express feelings about the loss through interaction with the home environment (e.g., looking at pictures, keeping special chairs or clothing). Symbols of the lost loved one can be comforting and allow the bereaved to accept the loss in stages. *Support and normalize the family grieving process.*
- A wide range of behaviors and perceptions occurs during the grieving response. Do not react with shock or disbelief at family members' reports (e.g., feeling like the deceased is still there).
- ▲ Refer the client to medical social services as necessary for losses not related to death. *Support is helpful to grief work for all types of losses. Social workers can assist the client with planning for financial changes as a result of job losses and help with community referrals as appropriate.*
- ▲ Refer the bereaved to hospice bereavement programs. *Relief of the suffering of clients and families—physical, emotional, and spiritual—is the goal of hospice care (Krisman-Scott and McCorkle, 2002).*
- ▲ Refer the bereaved spouse to an Internet self-help group if desired. **Nursing Research:** *An Internet-based self-help group can assist the bereaved spouse in coping, receiving support, developing a sense of family, sharing information, and helping others (Bacon, Condon, and Fernsler, 2000).*
- Modify expectations of the client's response according to the degree of anticipation of the loved one's death. *If the loved one died at an old age or of a natural cause, the client may have experienced anticipatory grieving; the current reaction may be less than expected. If the loved one died of accidental or criminal causes, the grief reaction may be magnified. Grief may be prolonged, and a referral for supportive counseling is more likely to be needed.*
- ▲ After loss of a pregnancy, encourage the client to follow through on a counseling referral. **Nursing and Clinical Research:** *Parents with a history of perinatal loss are at higher risk for depressive symptoms and pregnancy-specific anxiety during subsequent pregnancies, particularly before the third trimester. Mothers had a higher level of symptoms than fathers (Armstrong, 2002; Franche and Mikail, 1999).*

evolve WEBSITES FOR EDUCATION

See the EVOLVE website for World Wide Web resources for client education.

REFERENCES

Armstrong DS: Emotional distress and prenatal attachment in pregnancy after perinatal loss, *J Nurs Scholarsh* 34:339, 2002.
Arnold J: Rethinking grief: nursing implications for health promotion, *Home Healthc Nurse* 14(10):777, 1996.

- • = Independent; ▲ = Collaborative

Bacon ES, Condon EH, Fernsler JI: Young widows' experience with an internet self-help group, *J Psychosoc Nurs Ment Health Serv* 38(7):24, 2000.

Barlow CA, Morrison H: Survivors of suicide. Emerging counseling strategies, *J Psychosoc Nurs Ment Health Serv* 40(1):28, 2002.

Buxbaum L, Brant JM: When a parent dies from cancer, *Clin J Oncol Nurs* 5(4):135, 2001.

Clark S: Mapping grief: an active approach to grief resolution, *Death Stud* 25(6):531, 2001.

Cochran, M: Tears have no color, *Am J Nurs* 98(6):53, 1998.

Doswell W, Erlen J: Multicultural issues and ethical concerns in the delivery of nursing care interventions, *Nurs Clin North Am* 33(2):353, 1998.

Fischer C, Hegge M: The elderly woman at risk, *Am J Nurs* 100(6):54, 2000.

Franche R, Mikail S: The impact of perinatal loss on adjustment to subsequent pregnancy, *Soc Sci Med* 48:1613, 1999.

Furlini L: The parent they knew and the "new" parent: daughters' perceptions of dementia of the Alzheimer's Type, *Home Health Care Serv Q* 20(1):21, 2001.

Gamino LA, Hogan NS, Sewell KW: Feeling the absence: a content analysis from the Scott and White grief study, *Death Stud* 26(10):793, 2002.

Gifford BJ, Cleary BB: Supporting the bereaved, *Am J Nurs* 90(2):49, 1990.

Hegge M, Fischer C: Grief responses of senior and elderly widows: practice implications, *J Gerontol Nurs* 26(2): 35, 2000.

Heineken J: Patient silence is not necessarily client satisfaction: communication in home care nursing, *Home Healthc Nurse* 16(2):115, 1998.

Hentz P: The body remembers: grieving and a circle of time, *Qual Health Res* 12(2):161, 2002.

Herth K: Relationship of hope, coping styles, concurrent losses, and setting to grief resolution in the elderly widow(er), *Res Nurs Health* 13:109, 1990.

Hilliard RE: The effects of music therapy–based bereavement groups on mood and behavior of grieving children: a pilot study, *J Music Ther* 38(4):291, 2001a.

Hilliard RE: The use of music therapy in meeting the multidimensional needs of hospice patients and families, *J Palliat Care* 17(3):161, 2001b.

Hittle JM: Grieving together, *Am J Nurs* 95(7):55, 1995.

Hoffman C: Volunteers providing bereavement support, *Caring* 16(11):48, 1997.

Hogan NS, Greenfield DB, Schmidt LA: Development and validation of the Hogan Grief Reaction Checklist, *Death Stud* 25(1):1, 2001.

Hogan NS, Schmidt LA: Testing the grief to personal growth model using structural equation modeling, *Death Stud* 26(8):615, 2002.

Johnson CS: Nutritional considerations for bereavement and coping with grief, *J Nutr Health Aging* 6(3):171, 2002.

Krisman-Scott MA, McCorkle R: The tapestry of hospice, *Holist Nurs Pract* 16(2):32, 2002.

Kubler-Ross E: *On death and dying*, New York, 1969, Macmillan.

Laakso H, Paunonen-Ilmonen M: Mothers' experience of social support following the death of a child, *J Clin Nurs* 11(2):176, 2002.

Leininger MM, McFarland MR: *Transcultural nursing: concepts, theories, research and practices*, ed 3, New York, 2002, McGraw-Hill.

McQuay JE: Cross-cultural customs and beliefs related to health crises, death, and organ donation/transplantation: a guide to assist health care professionals understand different responses and provide cross-cultural assistance, *Crit Care Nurs Clin North Am* 7(3):581, 1995.

Pasternak RE et al: The posttreatment illness course of depression in bereaved elders, *Am J Geriatr Psychiatry* 5:54, 1997.

Pessin N et al: Sharing stories, healing shattered lives, *Caring* 21(1):6, 2002.

Puentes WJ: Incorporating simple reminiscence techniques into acute care nursing practice, *J Gerontol Nurs* 24(2):15, 1998.

Rask K, Kaunonen M, Paunonen-Ilmonen M: Adolescent coping with grief after the death of a loved one, *Int J Nurs Pract* 8(3):137, 2002.

Rodebaugh LS, Schwindt RG, Valentine FM: How to handle grief, *Nursing* 29(10):52, 1999.

Rueth TW, Hall SE: Dealing with the anger and hostility of those who grieve, *Am J Hosp Palliat Care* 16(6): 743, 1999.

Solari-Twadell PA et al: The pinwheel model of bereavement, *Image* 27(4):323, 1995.

• = Independent; ▲ = Collaborative

Steen KF: A comprehensive approach to bereavement, *Nurse Pract* 23(3):54, 1998.

Walsh K et al: Spiritual beliefs may affect outcome of bereavement: prospective study, *BMJ* 324(7353):1551, 2002.

Anticipatory Grieving

Betty J. Ackley and Gail B. Ladwig

NANDA Definition

Intellectual and emotional responses and behaviors by which individuals, families, and communities work through the process of modifying self-concept based on the perception of potential loss

Defining Characteristics

Expression of distress at potential loss; sorrow; guilt; denial of potential loss; anger; altered communication patterns; potential loss of significant object (e.g., people, possessions, job, status, home, ideals, parts and processes of the body); denial of significance of the loss; bargaining; alteration in eating habits, sleep patterns, dream patterns, activity level, or libido; difficulty taking on new or different roles; resolution of grief before the reality of loss

Related Factors (r/t)

Perceived or actual impending loss of people, objects, possessions, job, status, home, ideals, or parts and processes of the body (Carpenito, 1993)

NOC Outcomes (Nursing Outcomes Classification)

Suggested NOC Outcomes

Coping; Family Coping; Grief Resolution; Psychosocial Adjustment: Life Change

> #### Example NOC Outcome with Indicators
>
> **Grief Resolution** with plans for a positive future as evidenced by the following indicators: Expresses feelings about loss/Verbalizes acceptance of loss/Describes meaning of loss or death/Reports decreased preoccupation with loss/Expresses positive expectations about the future (Rate each indicator of **Grief Resolution:** 1 = never demonstrated, 2 = rarely demonstrated, 3 = sometimes demonstrated, 4 = often demonstrated, 5 = consistently demonstrated [see Section I].)

Client Outcomes

Client Will (Specify Time Frame):

- Express feelings of guilt, anger, or sorrow
- Identify problems associated with anticipatory grief (e.g., changes in activity, eating, or libido)
- Seek help in dealing with anticipated problems
- Plan for the future one day at a time

• = Independent; ▲ = Collaborative

| NIC | Interventions (Nursing Interventions Classification) |

Suggested NIC Interventions

Grief Work Facilitation; Grief Work Facilitation: Perinatal Death

Example NIC Activities—Grief Work Facilitation

Encourage client to verbalize memories of the loss, both past and current; Assist client to identify personal coping strategies

Nursing Interventions and Rationales

- If grief results from the impending death of a loved one, allow family members to stay with the loved one during the dying process if desired and help them determine appropriate times to take breaks. *Families often feel disorganized and helpless; they need support from nurses to be with the dying person (Walters, 1995).*
- Encourage family members to touch the dying client if they are comfortable with doing so. *Sharing personal space with touch can help establish connectedness and help with grieving (Walters, 1995).*
- Encourage family members to listen carefully to messages given by the dying loved one; they may hear symbolic or obscure language referring to the dying process. *As people approach death, they develop an understanding of how their death will unfold, and they communicate this awareness in symbolic language (Callanan, 1994).*
- If the dying client is denying the seriousness of his or her condition, do not negate the denial. *Denial protects clients from hopelessness and may be their coping mechanism to deal with reality. Not everyone needs to go through all the stages of grieving (McClement and Degner, 1995).*
- Help the dying client to maintain hope by focusing on the moment, reviewing his or her assets, and maintaining important relationships. *Hope is not a cure for the dying; hope maintains a connection to the world (McClement and Degner, 1995).*
- Help family members to let the loved one go if appropriate; give the loved one permission to die. *Sometimes dying people wait until they know their family members are strong enough to accept the loss before they allow themselves to die (Callanan, 1994).*
- Use therapeutic communication with open-ended questions such as, "What are your thoughts and fears?" **Clinical Research:** *In a retrospective cohort study, individuals who had experienced the death of a family member were asked to rate the quality of the dying experience after the family member's death (Curtis et al, 2002).*
- Keep family members informed about the client's condition. **Nursing Research:** *Lack of communication from health care providers contributes to the anxiety and distress reported by families. A qualitative study of the experience of clients' families after a client's death in the intensive care unit demonstrated that families' information about the client is often lacking or inadequate. The best antidote for families' uncertainty is effective communication (Kirchhoff et al, 2002).*
- Actively listen to the client's and/or family's expression of grief; do not interrupt, do not tell your own story, and do not offer meaningless platitudes such as, "It will be better this way." *Just being with the client and/or family and listening can be the most helpful thing the nurse does (Furman, 2000). Behaviors such as telling one's own story and reciting meaningless platitudes do not help and can often hurt (Gifford and Cleary, 1990).*

• = **Independent;** ▲ = **Collaborative**

- Encourage the client to "cry out" grief and express feelings, including sadness or anger. *Grief is work and is best treated as an active process in which the grieving client expresses and feels the grief.*
- Encourage the client to take care of any unfinished business if appropriate. Have the client make an advance directive with support. *A large number of Americans would prefer to rely more on family and friends rather than their physicians with regard to end-of-life care and decisions (Foster and McLellan, 2002).* **Clinical Research:** *In one qualitative study of dying clients and their families and caregivers, respondents from all groups showed consensus on the importance of naming someone to make decisions, knowing what to expect about one's physical condition, having financial affairs in order, having treatment preferences in writing, and knowing that one's physician is comfortable talking about death and dying (Steinhauser et al, 2001).*
- Help the client build memories. This can be done a number of ways, including the following:
  - Writing love letters—letters to be opened on family birthdays or other special days after death
  - Making audiotape or videotape recordings—to share memories and say goodbye
  - Writing a journal—an autobiography to be read by children and loved ones
  - Planning his or her own funeral
  - Writing his or her own obituary
  - Leaving a legacy—designating money for favorite causes
  These are creative ways to nurture family relationships by leaving mementos for loved ones (Brant, 1998).
- ▲ Assess for spiritual distress and refer the client for spiritual counseling if desired and appropriate. *Spiritual support can help clients; the nurse should approach the client with a nonjudgmental, listening ear and refer to the appropriate spiritual leader (Brant, 1998).*
- Help the client and/or family determine how best to obtain social support. *Social support has been identified as an important predictor of a positive bereavement experience (Cooley, 1992; Costello, 1999).* **Clinical Research:** *Social support is shown to assist the bereaved individuals as they reconstruct their lives and find new meaning in life (Hogan and Schmidt, 2002).* **Nursing Research:** *In a study of adolescents dealing with the death of a loved one, the most important factors that helped adolescents cope with the grief were self-help and support from parents, relatives, and friends (Rask, Kaunonen, and Paunonen-Ilmonen, 2002).*
- Identify problems with eating or sleeping, and intervene with suggestions as appropriate. *A grieving client can feel stunned and helpless and may be unable to consume food for a period (Gifford and Cleary, 1990).* **Clinical Research:** *One study indicated that bereaved individuals, irrespective of whether they had counseling for grief resolution or not, had a moderate risk for poor nutrition. The implication is that food issues need to be included in grief resolution interventions (Johnson, 2002).*
- Encourage the caregiver of a dying person to live one day at a time and recognize that mourning is occurring while caring for the loved one. Help the caregiver express feelings of loss and encourage the caregiver to practice self-care. Refer to the care plan for **Caregiver role strain** if appropriate. **Nursing Research:** *Caregivers grieve as they care for the dying person. They can develop an increased intimacy and involvement in the relationship, which can help them have a positive bereavement outcome (Brown and Powell-Cope, 1993; Costello, 1999).*

• = **Independent;** ▲ = **Collaborative**

Geriatric

- Assist the client with end-of-life decisions and advance directives. **Clinical Research:** *One descriptive study exploring the attitudes of older adults with medical illness about the end of life found that older adults should be asked not only questions about general values, but also specific questions about their end-of-life choices and the reasons for these choices. A thorough understanding of an individual's end-of-life preferences may help health professionals working with older adults develop client-centered care plans for the end of life (Vig, Davenport, and Pearlman, 2002).*

Multicultural

- Assess for the influence of cultural beliefs, norms, and values on the client's grief and mourning practices. **Nursing Research:** *Grief and mourning practices may be based on cultural conventions (Cochran, 1998; Doswell and Erlen, 1998; Leininger and McFarland, 2002). Some African Americans may place great emphasis on attendance at funerals; many Native American tribes hold long, somber wakes during which food and memorial gifts are distributed; Chinese and Japanese families may have specific funeral rituals that must be followed precisely to ensure safe passage of their loved one to the next world; Latinos may hold wakes, use prayer during a novena, and light candles in honor of the dead; in West Indian/Caribbean cultures death arrangements may be made by a kinsman of the deceased (McQuay, 1995).*
- Assess for the influence of cultural beliefs, norms, and values on the client's expressions of grief. **Nursing Research:** *African Americans may be expected to act "strong" and go about the business of life after a death; Native Americans may not talk about the death because of beliefs that such talk will detract from spirituality and bring bad luck; Latinos may wear black and act subdued during their* luto *(mourning) period; Southeast Asian families may wear white when mourning (McQuay, 1995).*

Home care

NOTE: Hospice care encourages clients and families to experience the client's final days in the setting of choice. All of the previously mentioned interventions can and should be applied in the home setting when that is the setting selected.

- Listen actively; normalize the client's and family's expressions of grief for a loved one who is expected to die. *Active listening supports the client and family without intrusive advice giving. Normalizing lets the client and family know that their responses are appropriate ways of preparing for death.*
- When the potential loss is of a loved one, refer the grieving client to hospice volunteer services for support. *Social support has been identified as the most important predictor of a positive bereavement experience (Cooley, 1992). Relief of suffering of clients and families—physical, emotional, and spiritual—is the goal of hospice care (Krisman-Scott and McCorkle, 2002).*
- ▲ When the client has a history of loss of a pregnancy, assess the client's need for a counseling referral during subsequent pregnancies. **Nursing and Clinical Research:** *Parents with a history of perinatal loss are at higher risk for depressive symptoms and pregnancy-specific anxiety during subsequent pregnancies, particularly before the third trimester. Mothers had a higher level of symptoms than fathers (Armstrong, 2002; Franche and Mikail, 1999).*

• = **Independent;** ▲ = **Collaborative**

Client/Family Teaching

- Teach caregivers that they are doing anticipatory grieving as they care for their loved ones, which is part of the reason care can be so difficult. The grief can become more acute as death approaches. *Anticipatory grieving allows adaptation to the loss to begin before the loved one's death (Costello, 1999).*

evolve WEBSITES FOR EDUCATION

See the EVOLVE website for World Wide Web resources for client education.

REFERENCES

Armstrong DS: Emotional distress and prenatal attachment in pregnancy after perinatal loss, *J Nurs Scholarsh* 34:339, 2002.

Brant JM: The art of palliative care: living with hope, dying with dignity, *Oncol Nurs Forum* 25(6):995, 1998.

Brown MA, Powell-Cope G: Themes of loss and dying in caring for a family member with AIDS, *Res Nurs Health* 16:179, 1993.

Callanan M: Farewell messages: dealing with death, *Am J Nurs* 94(5):19, 1994.

Carpenito JL: *Nursing diagnosis: applications to clinical practice,* ed 5, Philadelphia, 1993, Lippincott.

Cochran M: Tears have no color, *Am J Nurs* 98(6):53, 1998.

Cooley ME: Bereavement care: a role for nurses, *Cancer Nurs* 15:125, 1992.

Costello J: Anticipatory grief: coping with the impending death of a partner, *Int J Palliat Nurs* 5(5):223, 1999.

Curtis JR et al: A measure of the quality of dying and death. Initial validation using after-death interviews with family members, *J Pain Symptom Manage* 24(1):17, 2002.

Doswell W, Erlen J: Multicultural issues and ethical concerns in the delivery of nursing care interventions, *Nurs Clin North Am* 33(2):353, 1998.

Foster LW, McLellan LJ: Translating psychosocial insight into ethical discussions supportive of families in end-of-life decision-making, *Soc Work Health Care* 35(3):37, 2002.

Franche R, Mikail S: The impact of perinatal loss on adjustment to subsequent pregnancy, *Soc Sci Med* 48:1613, 1999.

Furman J: Taking a holistic approach to the dying time, *Nursing* 30(6):46, 2000.

Gifford BJ, Cleary BB: Supporting the bereaved, *Am J Nurs* 90:49, 1990.

Hogan NS, Schmidt LA: Testing the grief to personal growth model using structural equation modeling, *Death Stud* 26(8):615, 2002.

Johnson CS: Nutritional considerations for bereavement and coping with grief, *J Nutr Health Aging* 6(3):171, 2002.

Kirchhoff KT et al: The vortex: families' experiences with death in the intensive care unit, *Am J Crit Care* 11(3): 200, 2002.

Krisman-Scott MA, McCorkle R: The tapestry of hospice, *Holist Nurs Pract* 16(2):32, 2002.

Leininger MM, McFarland MR: *Transcultural nursing: concepts, theories, research and practices,* ed 3, New York, 2002, McGraw-Hill.

McClement SE, Degner LF: Expert nursing behaviors in care of the dying adult in the intensive care unit, *Heart Lung* 24(5):408, 1995.

McQuay JE: Cross-cultural customs and beliefs related to health crises, death, and organ donation/transplantation: a guide to assist health care professionals understand different responses and provide cross-cultural assistance, *Crit Care Nurs Clin North Am* 7(3):581, 1995.

Rask K, Kaunonen M, Paunonen-Ilmonen M: Adolescent coping with grief after the death of a loved one, *Int J Nurs Pract* 8(3):137, 2002.

Steinhauser KE et al: Preparing for the end of life: preferences of patients, families, physicians, and other care providers, *J Pain Symptom Manage* 22(3):727, 2001.

Vig EK, Davenport NA, Pearlman RA: Good deaths, bad deaths, and preferences for the end of life: a qualitative study of geriatric outpatients, *J Am Geriatr Soc* 50(9):1541, 2002.

Walters AJ: A hermeneutic study of the experiences of relatives of critically ill patients, *J Adv Nurs* 22:998, 1995.

• = Independent; ▲ = Collaborative

Dysfunctional Grieving

Betty J. Ackley and Gail B. Ladwig

NANDA Definition

Extended unsuccessful use of intellectual and emotional responses by which individuals, families, and communities attempt to work through the process of modifying self-concept based on the perception of loss

NOTE: It is now recognized that sometimes what was previously diagnosed as **Dysfunctional Grieving** might instead be **Chronic Sorrow**, in which grief lingers and is reactivated at intervals (Eakes, Burke, and Hainsworth, 1998). Refer to the nursing diagnosis **Chronic Sorrow** if appropriate.

Defining Characteristics

Repetitive use of ineffectual behaviors associated with attempts to reinvest in relationships; crying; sadness; reliving of past experiences with little or no reduction (diminishment) of intensity of grief; labile affect; expression of unresolved issues; interference with life functioning; verbal expression of distress at loss; idealization of lost object (e.g., people, possessions, job, status, home, ideals, parts and processes of the body); difficulty in expressing loss; denial of loss; anger; alterations in eating habits, sleep patterns, dream patterns, activity level, libido, concentration, and/or pursuit of tasks; developmental regression; expression of guilt; prolonged interference with life functioning; onset or exacerbation of somatic or psychosomatic responses

Related Factors (r/t)

Actual or perceived object loss (e.g., of people, possessions, job, status, home, ideals, parts and processes of the body)

NOC Outcomes (Nursing Outcomes Classification)

Suggested NOC Outcomes

Coping; Family Coping; Grief Resolution; Psychosocial Adjustment: Life Change

---

Example NOC Outcome with Indicators

Grief Resolution with plans for a positive future as evidenced by the following indicators: Expresses feelings about loss/Verbalizes acceptance of loss/Describes meaning of loss or death/Reports decreased preoccupation with loss/Expresses positive expectations about the future (Rate each indicator of **Grief Resolution:** 1 = never demonstrated, 2 = rarely demonstrated, 3 = sometimes demonstrated, 4 = Often demonstrated, 5 = consistently demonstrated [see Section I].)

• = Independent; ▲ = Collaborative

Client Outcomes

Client Will (Specify Time Frame):

- Express appropriate feelings of guilt, fear, anger, or sadness
- Identify problems associated with grief (e.g., changes in appetite, insomnia, night-mares, loss of libido, decreased energy, alteration in activity levels)
- Seek help in dealing with grief-associated problems
- Plan for the future one day at a time
- Identify personal strengths
- Function at a normal developmental level and perform activities of daily living after an appropriate length of time

NIC Interventions (Nursing Interventions Classification)

Suggested NIC Interventions

Grief Work Facilitation; Grief Work Facilitation: Perinatal Death; Guilt Work Facilitation

Example NIC Activities—Grief Work Facilitation

Encourage client to verbalize memories of the loss, both past and current; Assist client to identify personal coping strategies

Nursing Interventions and Rationales

- Assess the client's state of grieving. Use a tool such as the Hogan Grief to Personal Growth Model or the Grief Experience Inventory. **Clinical Research:** *These are commonly used measures of grief that have been shown to measure grief effectively (Gamino, Sewell, and Easterling, 2000; Hogan and Schmidt, 2002).*
- Assess for the causes of dysfunctional grieving (e.g., sudden bereavement [less than 2 weeks to prepare for the oncoming loss], highly dependent or ambivalent relationship with the deceased, inadequate coping skills, lack of social support, previous physical or mental health problems, death of a child, loss of a spouse). **Clinical Research:** *Life circumstances can interfere with normal grieving and can be risk factors for dysfunctional grieving (Gamino, Sewell, and Easterling, 2000; Steele, 1992; Stewart, 1995).*
- Observe for the following reactions to loss, which predispose a client to dysfunctional grieving:
  - Delayed grieving: the bereaved exhibits little emotion and continues with a busy life
  - Inhibited grieving: the bereaved exhibits various physical conditions and does not feel grief
  - Chronic grieving: the behaviors of the normal grief period continue beyond a reasonable time

    These maladaptive grief reactions indicate that the client needs help with grief work (Gifford and Cleary, 1990).
- Identify problems of eating and sleeping; ensure that basic human needs are being met. *Losses often interrupt appetite and sleep (Bateman et al, 1992).* **Clinical Research:** *One study indicated that bereaved individuals, irrespective of whether they had counseling for grief resolution or not, had a moderate risk for poor nutrition. The implication is that food issues need to be included in grief resolution interventions (Johnson, 2002).*
- Develop a trusting relationship with the client by using therapeutic communication

• = Independent; ▲ = Collaborative

techniques. **Clinical Research:** *In a study of fathers who had lost infants before birth, fathers sought understanding from both the hospital personnel and their partners, as well as from relatives. Being able to protect their partner and to grieve in their own way was important to the fathers (Samuelsson, Radestad, and Segesten, 2001).*

• Establish a defined time to meet and discuss feelings about the loss and to perform grief work.

• Encourage the client to "cry out" grief and to talk about feelings of anger, sadness, and guilt. *Grief is work and is best treated as an active process in which the bereaved expresses and feels the grief. Expression of guilt or anger is necessary to progress through the grieving process and feel better (Bateman et al, 1992).*

▲ Assess for spiritual distress and refer the client to the appropriate spiritual leader. *Intrinsic spirituality can help the client grieve (Gamino, Sewell, and Easterling, 2000).* **Nursing Research:** *The nurse should approach the client with a nonjudgmental, listening ear and refer the client to the appropriate spiritual leader (Brant, 1998).*

• Help the client recognize that, although sadness will occur at intervals for the rest of his or her life, it will become bearable. *The sadness associated with chronic sorrow is permanent, but as the grief resolves, there can be times of satisfaction and even happiness (Grainger, 1990; Teel, 1991).* **Nursing Research:** *Grief has a lasting nature; it changes and softens but never ends (Carter, 1989).*

• Help the client complete the following "guilt work" exercises:
  ▪ Identify "if onlys" and put them into perspective
  ▪ Deal with "I didn't do" by looking at what was accomplished
  ▪ Forgive himself or herself; say to the client, "You are being awfully hard on yourself; try not to hurt yourself over something you could not have controlled"
  The client may need to resolve guilt before successfully grieving and moving on with life.

• Help the client review past experiences, role changes, and coping skills. **Nursing Research:** *In one study, getting over the loss was not a focus for many of the participants. The theme of a need to remember and to hold onto the memory was evident (Hentz, 2002).*

• Encourage the client to keep a journal and write about the bereavement experience. **Clinical Research:** *Writing projects can be helpful for clients who are grieving, especially for those experiencing the unique bereavement of suicidal death (Range, Kovac, and Marion, 2000).*

• Help the client to identify his or her own strengths to use in dealing with loss; reinforce these strengths; consider the use of music. **Clinical Research:** *In a clinical controlled trial, single-session music therapy interventions with hospice clients demonstrated significant results in three client problem areas: pain control, physical comfort, and relaxation (Krout, 2001).*

• If the client or family members are expressing anger, try not to react in anger. Instead, allow feelings to be expressed, listen to the expressions of anger, and accept their right to those feelings. Try lowering your voice and slowing your rate of speech as you respond to the client and/or family. *It is not therapeutic to respond to anger with anger. Instead, strive to be therapeutic, helping the client and/or family members express the anger and gain control of themselves by modeling calm behavior (Rueth and Hall, 1999).*

• Expect the client to meet responsibilities; give positive reinforcement. *Help the client to identify areas of hope in life and to determine their purposes if possible.* **Nursing Research:** *A significant positive relationship has been found between the level of grief resolution and the level of hope (Herth, 1990). Grieving people who have little purpose in life often experience more anger than individuals with more purpose.*

• = Independent; ▲ = Collaborative

- Encourage the client to make time to talk to family members about the loss with the help of professional support as needed and without criticism or belittling of one another's feelings about the loss. *Once these feelings are shared, family members can begin to accept the unacceptable (Gifford and Cleary, 1990).*
▲ Identify available community resources, including bereavement groups at local hospitals and hospice centers. *Support groups can have positive effects on bereavement for both children and adults (Cooley, 1992; Heiney, Dunaway, and Webster, 1995; Stewart, 1995).*
▲ Determine whether the client is experiencing depression, suicidal tendencies, or other emotional disorders. Refer the client for counseling as appropriate. **Clinical Research:** *Counseling, including the use of relaxation therapy, desensitization, and biofeedback in addition to traditional psychotherapy, has been shown to be helpful (Arnette, 1996). Depression syndromes occur in almost one half of all grieving people, and 10% suffer major depression (Steen, 1998). Cognitive behavior therapy can be helpful for traumatic grief (Jacobs and Prigerson, 2000).*

Geriatric

- Use reminiscence therapy in conjunction with the expression of emotions (Puentes, 1998).
- Identify previous losses and assess the client for depression. Signs of depression are often masked by somatic complaints. **Nursing Research:** *Losses and changes associated with older age often occur in rapid succession without adequate recovery time. Having more than two concurrent losses increases the incidence of unresolved grief (Herth, 1990). The elderly often express grief in the form of somatic complaints (Steen, 1998).*
- Evaluate the social support system of the elderly client. If the support system is minimal, help the client determine how to increase available support. *The elderly who have poor grieving outcomes often do not live with family members and have a minimal support system.*

Multicultural

- Assess for the influence of cultural beliefs, norms, and values on the client's grief and mourning practices. **Nursing Research:** *Grief and mourning practices may be based on cultural conventions (Cochran, 1998; Doswell and Erlen, 1998; Leininger and McFarland. 2002). Some African Americans may place great emphasis on attendance at funerals; many Native American tribes hold long, somber wakes during which food and memorial gifts are distributed; Chinese and Japanese families may have specific funeral rituals that must be followed precisely to ensure safe passage of their loved ones into the next world; Latinos may hold wakes, use prayer during a novena, and light candles in honor of the dead; in West Indian/Caribbean cultures death arrangements might be made by a kinsman of the deceased (McQuay, 1995).*
- Assess for the influence of cultural beliefs, norms, and values on the client's expressions of grief. **Nursing Research:** *African Americans may be expected to act "strong" and go about the business of life after a death; Native Americans may not talk about the death because of beliefs that such talk will detract from spirituality and bring bad luck; Latinos may wear black and act subdued during their* luto *(mourning) period; Southeast Asian families may wear white when mourning (McQuay, 1995).*
- Identify whether the client had been notified of the health status of the deceased and was able to be present during illness and death. **Nursing Research:** *Not being present during terminal illness and death can disrupt the grieving process (McQuay, 1995).*

- = **Independent;** ▲ = **Collaborative**

- Validate the client's feelings regarding the loss. **Nursing Research:** *Validation is a therapeutic communication technique that lets the client know that the nurse has heard and understood what was said, and it promotes the nurse-client relationship (Heineken, 1998).*

Home care
- The interventions described previously may be adapted for home care use.
- Encourage the client to make choices about daily living and the home environment that acknowledge the loss. *Helping with grief work allows the client to accept the reality of the loss and realize that grieving is a healthy response.*
- Evaluate the long-term support system of the bereaved client. Encourage the client to interact with the support system at defined intervals. **Nursing Research:** *Participants in one study found comfort in knowing that they were not alone (Hentz, 2002).*
- Discourage the client from making any drastic life changes immediately. *Dysfunctional grief may leave the client vulnerable to making irrational choices or to being influenced by others.*
▲ Refer the client to or encourage continued interaction with hospice volunteers and bereavement programs as continuing forms of support. **Nursing Research:** *In a study of group interventions for widowed survivors of suicide victims, participants experienced a significant reduction in overall depression, psychological distress, and grief, as well as an increase in social adjustment (Constantino, Sekula, and Rubinstein, 2001).*
▲ Refer the client to medical social services, especially the hospice program social worker, for assistance with grief work. *Consulting with or referring to specialty services is sometimes the best way to provide care.*
▲ Evaluate the need for psychiatric referral. *Dysfunctional grief may be classified as a major depressive episode if the client expresses guilt about things other than reactions concerning the loved one's death; thoughts of death other than feeling that he or she would be better off dead or should have died in place of the loved one; morbid preoccupation with worthlessness; psychomotor retardation; marked and prolonged functional impairment; or hallucinations other than thinking that he or she is seeing or hearing the deceased person (American Psychiatric Association, 2000).*
▲ After loss of a pregnancy, encourage the client to follow through with a counseling referral. **Nursing and Clinical Research:** *Parents with a history of perinatal loss are at higher risk for depressive symptoms and pregnancy-specific anxiety during subsequent pregnancies, particularly before the third trimester. Mothers had a higher level of symptoms than fathers (Armstrong, 2002; Franche and Mikail, 1999).*
▲ If the client is identified as having a psychiatric disorder, refer for psychiatric home health care services or "interapy" (online therapy) for client reassurance and implementation of a therapeutic regimen. *Psychiatric home care nurses can address issues relating to the client's dysfunctional grieving. Behavioral interventions in the home can help the client to participate more effectively in the treatment plan, resolve grief issues, and receive the appropriate level of care (Patusky, Rodning, and Martinez-Kratz, 1996).* **Clinical Research:** *In a controlled trial of "interapy," 80% of the treated participants who had posttraumatic stress and grief showed clinically significant improvement after therapy (Lange et al, 2001).*

• = Independent; ▲ = Collaborative

evolve WEBSITES FOR EDUCATION

See the EVOLVE website for World Wide Web resources for client education.

REFERENCES

American Psychiatric Association: *Diagnostic and statistical manual of mental disorders,* ed 4, Washington, DC, 2000, The Association.

Armstrong DS: Emotional distress and prenatal attachment in pregnancy after perinatal loss, *J Nurs Scholarsh* 34:339, 2002.

Arnette JD: Physiological effects of chronic grief: a biofeedback treatment approach, *Death Stud* 20:59, 1996.

Bateman A et al: Dysfunctional grieving, *J Psychosoc Nurs* 30(12):5, 1992.

Brant JM: The art of palliative care: living with hope, dying with dignity, *Oncol Nurs Forum* 25(6):995, 1998.

Carter SL: Themes of grief, *Nurs Res* 38(6):354, 1989.

Cochran M: Tears have no color, *Am J Nurs* 98(6):53, 1998.

Constantino RE, Sekula LK, Rubinstein EN: Group intervention for widowed survivors of suicide, *Suicide Life Threat Behav* 31(4):428, 2001.

Cooley ME: Bereavement care: a role for nurses, *Cancer Nurs* 15:125, 1992.

Doswell W, Erlen J: Multicultural issues and ethical concerns in the delivery of nursing care interventions, *Nurs Clin North Am* 33(2):353, 1998.

Eakes GG, Burke ML, Hainsworth MA: Theory: middle-range theory of chronic sorrow, *Image J Nurs Sch* 30:179, 1998.

Franche R, Mikail S: The impact of perinatal loss on adjustment to subsequent pregnancy, *Soc Sci Med* 48:1613, 1999.

Gamino LA, Sewell KW, Easterling LW: Scott and White Grief Study—phase 2: toward an adaptive model of grief, *Death Stud* 24:633, 2000.

Gifford BJ, Cleary B: Supporting the bereaved, *Am J Nurs* 90:49, 1990.

Grainger RD: Successful grieving, *Am J Nurs* 90:12, 1990.

Heineken J: Patient silence is not necessarily client satisfaction: communication in home care nursing, *Home Healthc Nurse* 16(2):115, 1998.

Heiney SP, Dunaway NC, Webster J: Good grieving: an intervention program for grieving children, *Oncol Nurs Forum* 22(4):649, 1995.

Hentz P: The body remembers: grieving and a circle of time, *Qual Health Res* 12(2):161, 2002.

Herth K: Relationship of hope, coping styles, concurrent losses, and setting to grief resolution in the elderly widow(er), *Res Nurs Health* 13:109, 1990.

Hogan NS, Schmidt LA: Testing the grief to personal growth model using structural equation modeling, *Death Stud* 26(8):615, 2002.

Jacobs S, Prigerson H: Psychotherapy of traumatic grief: a review of evidence for psychotherapeutic treatments, *Death Stud* 24:479, 2000.

Johnson CS: Nutritional considerations for bereavement and coping with grief, *J Nutr Health Aging* 6(3):171, 2002.

Krout RE: The effects of single-session music therapy interventions on the observed and self-reported levels of pain control, physical comfort, and relaxation of hospice patients, *Am J Hosp Palliat Care* 18(6):383, 2001.

Lange A et al: Interapy, treatment of posttraumatic stress through the Internet: a controlled trial, *J Behav Ther Exp Psychiatry* 32(2):73, 2001.

Leininger MM, McFarland MR: *Transcultural nursing: concepts, theories, research and practices,* ed 3, New York, 2002, McGraw-Hill.

McQuay JE: Cross-cultural customs and beliefs related to health crises, death, and organ donation/transplantation: a guide to assist health care professionals understand different responses and provide cross-cultural assistance, *Crit Care Nurs Clin North Am* 7(3):581, 1995.

Patusky KL, Rodning C, Martinez-Kratz M: Clinical lessons in psychiatric home care: a case study approach, *J Home Health Case Manage* 9:18, 1996.

Puentes WJ: Incorporating simple reminiscence techniques into acute care nursing practice, *J Gerontol Nurs* 24(2):15, 1998.

Range LM, Kovac SH, Marion MS: Does writing about the bereavement lessen grief following sudden, unintentional death? *Death Stud* 24:115, 2000.

• = **Independent;** ▲ = **Collaborative**

Rueth TW, Hall SE: Dealing with the anger and hostility of those who grieve, *Am J Hosp Palliat Care* 16(6): 743, 1999.

Samuelsson M, Radestad I, Segesten K: A waste of life: fathers' experience of losing a child before birth, *Birth* 28(2):124, 2001.

Steele L: Risk factor profile for bereaved spouses, *Death Stud* 16:387, 1992.

Steen KF: A comprehensive approach to bereavement, *Nurse Pract* 23(3):54, 1998.

Stewart ES: Family-centered care for the bereaved, *Pediatr Nurs* 21:181, 1995.

Teel CS: Chronic sorrow: analysis of the concept, *J Adv Nurs* 16:1311, 1991.

Delayed Growth and development

T. Heather Herdman and Gail B. Ladwig

NANDA Definition

Deviations from age-group norms

Defining Characteristics

Altered physical growth; delay or difficulty in exercising skills (motor, social, expressive) typical of age group; inability to perform self-care or self-control activities appropriate for age; flat affect; listlessness; decreased responses

Related Factors (r/t)

Prescribed dependence; indifference; separation from significant others; environmental and stimulation deficiencies; effects of physical disability; inadequate caretaking; inconsistent responsiveness; multiple caretakers

NOC Outcomes (Nursing Outcomes Classification)

Suggested NOC Outcomes

Child Development: 2 Months, 4 Months, 6 Months, 12 Months, 2 Years, 3 Years, 4 Years, Preschool, Middle Childhood, Adolescence; Growth; Mobility; Neurological Status; Physical Maturation: Female, Male; Self-Care: Activities of Daily Living (ADL), Bathing, Dressing, Eating, Hygiene, Instrumental Activities of Daily Living (IADL), Toileting; Personal Well-Being

---

Example NOC Outcome with Indicators

Growth as evidenced by indicators of normal increase in body size and weight (Rate each indicator of **Growth:** 1 = extreme deviation from expected range, 2 = substantial deviation from expected range, 3 = moderate deviation from expected range, 4 = mild deviation from expected range, 5 = no deviation from expected range [see Section I].)

Client Outcomes

Client/Parents/Caregiver Will (Specify Time Frame)
- Describe realistic, age-appropriate patterns of growth and development
- Promote activities and interactions that support age-related developmental tasks

• = Independent; ▲ = Collaborative

- Display consistent, sustained achievement of age-appropriate behaviors (social, interpersonal, and/or cognitive) and/or motor skills
- Achieve realistic developmental and/or growth milestones based on existing abilities, extent of disability, and functional age
- Exhibit limited temporary behavioral regression that reverses shortly after episode of illness or hospitalization
- Attain steady gains in growth patterns

NIC   Interventions (Nursing Interventions Classification)

Suggested NIC Interventions
Active Listening; Body Image Enhancement; Developmental Enhancement: Adolescent, Child; Emotional Support; Kangaroo Care; Nutrition Therapy; Nutritional Monitoring; Positioning; Self-Care Assistance; Self-Responsibility Facilitation

> **Example NIC Activities—Nutritional Monitoring**
>
> Monitor trends in weight loss and gain; Monitor food preferences and choices

Nursing Interventions and Rationales

NOTE: Determination of the etiological basis for delayed growth and development is critical because it will direct the selection of interventions for treating the client. Parenting skill deficits, lack of consistency between caregivers, hospitalization, and a chronic medical condition or developmental disability will necessitate different strategies. A hospitalization experience with regressive behaviors can be a transient occurrence, whereas a chronic situation may result in more severe and longer delays requiring more in-depth intervention. Parenting skills and consistent expectations by multiple caregivers can be addressed by more intensive education efforts (Seideman and Kleine, 1995; Stutts, 1994).

▲ To determine risk for or actual deviations in normal development, consider the use of a screening tool. One such tool is the Family Protective-Risk Index, which was developed by examining eight factors—mother's education, father's education, family income sufficiency, type of family, family relations, stressful life events in the family, child rearing, and the physical environment at home—that were found to be related to child development in any age group (1 to 2 years, 3 to 5 years, and 6 to 12 years). Other tools are the Brigance Infant and Toddler Screens. **Clinical Research:** *The Family Protective-Risk Index is a suitable measure to use in identifying families that need close assistance to prevent the slow growth and development of children (Isaranurug, Nanthamongkolchai, and Kaewsiri, 2002).* **Clinical Research:** *The Brigance Infant and Toddler Screens are shown to be accurate, valid, and reliable tools that can be administered by a range of professionals using either parental interview or direct elicitation and observation, or both (Glascoe, 2002).* **Nursing Research:** *Children in foster care have significantly higher rates of all health problems than the general population of children, including acute and chronic illnesses, growth and developmental problems, serious mental health problems, and difficulties accessing health services (Kools and Kennedy, 2003).*

- Note and emphasize the positive attributes of the parents and family. *Accepting the family's value system with respect will support and encourage the parents and family to increase their involvement (Reis, 1993).*

• = Independent; ▲ = Collaborative

- Regularly compare height and weight measurements for the child or adolescent with established age-appropriate norms and previous measurements. *This process identifies delayed growth patterns and deviations from the norm (US Public Health Service, 1995).*
▲ Initiate referrals for a more comprehensive growth and/or development evaluation if indicated. *Presence of a risk factor alone does not always obviate the need for referrals. The number and weight of risk factors and normal differences of each child must be considered (Curry and Duby, 1994).*
▲ Identify coexisting health or medical conditions that may be contributing to the alteration in growth and/or development, and refer the client to a specialist in the appropriate health care discipline for management. **Evidence-Based Research:** *A specific cause can be determined in the majority of children with global developmental delay. Certain routine screening tests are indicated and, depending on history and examination findings, additional specific testing may be performed (Shevell et al, 2003).*
- Examine parental/caregiver expectations of future learning, ability, and developmental achievements of children with developmental disabilities. **Nursing Research:** *Initiation of measures to support or enhance family and child motivation and ability increases achievement (Edwards-Beckett, 1994).*
- Assist the family in discerning the child's regressive responses to illness, hospitalization, or chronic health conditions. Explain the manifestations of regression, magical thinking, separation anxiety, and fears. **Nursing Research:** *A child may regress to earlier developmental levels. Children's responses differ from those of adults depending on the child's stage of cognitive development and previous encounters. When parents are able to understand their child's reactions to stress and illness, they are better able to support the child (Ziegler and Prior, 1994).*
- Provide support groups and education on HIV and caring for infants with this diagnosis. *Developmental delay has been well documented in HIV-infected infants (Potterton and Eales, 2001).*
- Provide meaningful stimulation for hospitalized infants and children. *Stimulation is essential to the development of gross and fine motor adaptive skills, language, and personal-social functioning in infants and children. Disruption of this process for infants, even those without preexisting developmental delays, can occur in the absence of intervention. Hospitalized infants are often subjected to understimulation or an overabundance of meaningless stimulation (Slusher and McClure, 1995).*
- Provide opportunities for mother-infant skin-to-skin contact (kangaroo care or KC) for preterm infants. **Clinical Research:** *One study showed that the neurodevelopmental profile was more mature for infants receiving KC. Results underscore the role of early skin-to-skin contact in the maturation of the autonomic and circadian systems in preterm infants (Feldman and Eidelman, 2003).*
- Engage the child in appropriate play activities. Refer the child to a play/recreational therapist (if available) for supplemental strategies. **Clinical Research:** *Play is essential for learning in children. Toys should be safe, affordable, and developmentally appropriate. Children do not need expensive toys (Glassy and Romano, 2003).*
- Enlist and encourage involvement of the parents and/or family as participants in care, particularly for hospitalized infants, toddlers, preschoolers, or school-aged children, whenever possible without exceeding the parent's/family's emotional and physical limits. *Frequent and consistent parent/family contact and care diminish normal separation*

• = Independent; ▲ = Collaborative

anxiety. Most infants and toddlers find this presence comforting and as a result are better able to cope with the situation and stress (Craft and Willadsen, 1992).

- Model age-appropriate and cognitively appropriate caregiver skills by doing the following:
  - Communicating with the child in a manner appropriate to cognitive level of development
  - Giving the child tasks and responsibilities appropriate to age or functional age level
  - Instituting the use of safety devices such as assistive equipment
  - Encouraging the child to perform ADLs as appropriate

  These actions illustrate parenting and child-rearing skills and behaviors for parents and family members (McCloskey and Bulechek, 1992).
- Furnish an environment that promotes additional sleep and rest opportunities. **Nursing Research:** *A balance of sleep, rest, and activity is essential for sustained progression of growth and development (White et al, 1990).*
- Provide developmental care interventions to preterm infants to improve neurodevelopmental outcomes (Symington and Pinelli, 2002).
- Provide neonatal positioning procedures for preterm infants to prevent extremity malalignment, skull deformities, and gross motor delay. *Alignment and shaping of the musculoskeletal system occur with each body position change in an NICU—use of proper positioning strategies promotes skeletal integrity, postural control, and sensorimotor organization (Sweeney and Gutierrez, 2002).*

Multicultural
- Acknowledge racial/ethnic differences at the onset of care. **Nursing Research:** *Acknowledgment of race/ethnicity issues will enhance communication, establish rapport, and promote treatment outcomes (D'Avanzo et al, 2001; Ludwick and Silva, 2000; Vontress and Epp, 1997).*
- Assess for the influence of cultural beliefs, norms, and values on the client's perceptions of child development. **Nursing Research:** *What the client considers normal and abnormal child development may be based on cultural perceptions (Cochran, 1998; Doswell and Erlen, 1998; Leininger and McFarland, 2002).*
- Use a neutral, indirect style in addressing areas in which improvement is needed (such as a need for verbal stimulation) when working with Native American clients. **Nursing Research:** *Using indirect statements such as "Other mothers have tried . . ." or "I had a client who tried 'X' and it seemed to work very well" will assist in avoiding resentment of the parent (Seiderman et al, 1996).*
- Assess whether exposure to community violence is contributing to developmental problems. **Nursing Research:** *Exposure to community violence has been associated with increases in aggressive behavior and depression in children (Gorman-Smith and Tolan, 1998).*
- Validate the client's feelings and concerns related to the child's development. **Nursing Research:** *Validation is a therapeutic communication technique that lets the client know that the nurse has heard and understood what was said, and it promotes the nurse-client relationship (Heineken, 1998).*

Home care
- The interventions described previously may be adapted for home care use.
- Assess for the presence of substances that could cause developmental delay. *Children's*

• = Independent; ▲ = Collaborative

access to substances that cause neurological deficits (e.g., lead-based paints) should be identified and eliminated.

▲ Refer maternal drug users to home intervention programs. **Clinical Research:** *Ongoing maternal drug use was associated with worse developmental outcomes among a group of drug-exposed infants. A home intervention led to higher scores on the Bayley Scales of Infant Development among drug-exposed infants (Schuler, Nair, and Kettinger, 2003).*

• Help the family to identify appropriate skill-building activities for the child. *Exposure to age-appropriate or lower-age games, toys, and activities can provide essential stimuli for development. Family members may need to adjust their expectations of the child's behaviors to be appropriate not only for age but also for any developmental limitations.*

• Provide emotional support for family members in their reactions to evidence of developmental delay. *Parents may be distressed by the potential for developmental delay in a child.*

▲ If possible, refer the family to a program of animal-assisted therapy. **Nursing Research:** *Research suggests that interactions with dogs may assist clients with pervasive developmental disorders (PDDs) to establish bonds with their social environment. Children with PDD were more playful, more focused, and more aware of their social environment in the presence of a therapy dog than in the presence of a toy or a stuffed dog (Martin and Farnum, 2002).*

Client/Family Teaching

• Provide anticipatory guidance for parents and/or caregivers regarding realistic expectations for attainment of growth and development milestones. Clarify expectations and correct misconceptions. *Parents/caregivers who understand both what is normal and what is realistic for their child are better equipped to provide a nurturing, supportive environment (Denehy, 1990).*

• Have parents and/or caregivers rehearse coping strategies for approaching developmental milestones and acknowledge positive actions and behaviors. *As children progress to another developmental stage, such as adolescence, families are challenged to master developmental tasks that seem enigmatic. Anticipating and preparing can strengthen their ability to deal with situations and enhance achievement (Reisch and Forsyth, 1992).*

• Teach methods of providing meaningful stimulation for infants and children. *Stimulation is essential to the development of gross and fine motor adaptive skills, language, and personal-social functioning in infants and children (Slusher and McClure, 1995).*

• Instruct the client with regard to age-appropriate activities and play, nutrition, discipline, and safety, and support growth and development. *Parents are then better equipped to promote the growth and development of the child (McCloskey and Bulechek, 1992).* **Evidence-Based Nursing Research:** *The use of baby walkers is controversial. Some studies suggested that they may delay walking by 11 to 26 days; other studies were inconclusive. There was no support that they aided walking. Further work is required to determine if they are an independent causal factor in accidents (Burrows and Griffiths, 2002).*

▲ Elicit the involvement of parents and caregivers in social support groups and parenting classes.

▲ Furnish information about community resources. *Support groups and other opportunities to obtain guidance serve to empower parents and clarify and reinforce knowledge and parenting skills (Kinney, Mannetter, and Carpenter, 1992; McCloskey and Bulechek, 1992).*

• = Independent; ▲ = Collaborative

REFERENCES

Burrows P, Griffiths P: Do baby walkers delay onset of walking in young children? *Br J Community Nurs* 7(11): 581, 2002.

Cochran M: Tears have no color, *Am J Nurs* 98(6):53, 1998.

Craft MJ, Willadsen JA: Interventions related to family. In Bulechek GM, McCloskey JC, editors: Symposium on nursing interventions, *Nurs Clin North Am* 27:517, 1992.

Curry DM, Duby JC: Developmental surveillance by pediatric nurses, *Pediatr Nurs* 20:40, 1994.

D'Avanzo CE et al: Developing culturally informed strategies for substance-related interventions. In Naegle MA, D'Avanzo CE, editors: *Addictions and substance abuse: strategies for advanced practice nursing,* St Louis, 2001, Mosby.

Denehy JA: Anticipatory guidance. In Craft MJ, Denehy JA, editors: *Nursing interventions for infants and children,* Philadelphia, 1990, WB Saunders.

Doswell W, Erlen J: Multicultural issues and ethical concerns in the delivery of nursing care interventions, *Nurs Clin North Am* 33(2):353, 1998.

Edwards-Beckett J: Caregivers' expectations of future learning of dependents with a developmental disability, *J Pediatr Nurs* 9:27, 1994.

Feldman R, Eidelman A: Skin-to-skin contact (kangaroo care) accelerates autonomic and neurobehavioural maturation in preterm infants, *Dev Med Child Neurol* 45(4):274, 2003.

Glascoe FP: The Brigance Infant and Toddler Screen: standardization and validation, *J Dev Behav Pediatr* 23(3):145, 2002.

Glassy D, Romano J: Selecting appropriate toys for young children: the pediatrician's role, *Pediatrics* 111(4 pt 1):911, 2003.

Gorman-Smith D, Tolan P: The role of exposure to community violence and developmental problems among inner city youth, *Dev Psychopathol* 10(1):101, 1998.

Heineken J: Patient silence is not necessarily client satisfaction: communication in home care nursing, *Home Healthc Nurse* 16(2):115, 1998.

Isaranurug S, Nanthamongkolchai S, Kaewsiri D: Family protective-risk index and its implications, *J Med Assoc Thai* 85(11):1198, 2002.

Kinney CK, Mannetter R, Carpenter MA: Support groups. In Bulechek GM, McCloskey JC, editors: *Nursing interventions: essential nursing treatment,* Philadelphia, 1992, WB Saunders.

Kools S, Kennedy C: Foster child health and development: implications for primary care, *Pediatr Nurs* 29(1):39, 2003.

Leininger MM, McFarland MR: *Transcultural nursing: concepts, theories, research and practices,* ed 3, New York, 2002, McGraw-Hill.

Ludwick R, Silva M: Nursing around the world: cultural values and ethical conflicts, *Online J Issues Nurs,* August 14, 2000, available on-line at http://www.nursingworld.org/ojin/ethicol/ethics_4.htm, accessed June 19, 2003.

Martin F, Farnum J: Animal-assisted therapy for children with pervasive developmental disorders, *West J Nurs Res* 24:657, 2002.

McCloskey JC, Bulechek GM, editors: *Nursing interventions classification (NIC),* St Louis, 1992, Mosby.

Potterton J, Eales C: Prevalence of developmental delay in infants who are HIV positive, *S Afr J Physiother* 57(3):11, 2001.

Reis M: The neglected preschooler, *Can Nurse* 89:42, 1993.

Reisch SK, Forsyth DM: Preparing to parent the adolescent: a theoretical overview, *J Child Adolesc Psychiatr Ment Health Nurs* 5:31, 1992.

Schuler ME, Nair P, Kettinger L: Drug-exposed infants and developmental outcome: effects of a home intervention and ongoing maternal drug use, *Arch Pediatr Adolesc Med* 157(2):133, 2003.

Seideman RJ, Kleine PF: A theory of transformed parenting: parenting a child with developmental delay/mental retardation, *Nurs Res* 44:38, 1995.

Seiderman RY et al: Assessing American Indian families, *MCN Am J Matern Child Nurs* 21(6):274, 1996.

• = Independent; ▲ = Collaborative

Shevell M et al: Practice parameter: evaluation of the child with global developmental delay: report of the Quality Standards Subcommittee of the American Academy of Neurology and the Practice Committee of the Child Neurology Society, *Neurology* 60(3):367, 2003.

Slusher IL, McClure MJ: Infant stimulation during hospitalization, *J Pediatr Nurs* 7:276, 1995.

Stutts AL: Selected outcomes of technology-dependent children receiving home care and prescribed child care services, *J Pediatr Nurs* 20:501, 1994.

Sweeney J, Gutierrez T: Musculoskeletal implications of preterm infant positioning in the NICU, *J Perinat Neonatal Nurs* 16(1):58, 2002.

Symington A, Pinelli J: Developmental care for promoting development and preventing morbidity in preterm infants, *Cochrane Library* 3(CD001814), 2002.

US Public Health Service: Body measurement, *J Am Acad Nurs Pediatr* 7:339, 1995.

Vontress CE, Epp LR: Historical hostility in the African American client: implications for counseling, *J Multicult Counseling Dev* 25:170, 1997.

White MA et al: Sleep onset latency and distress in hospitalized children, *Nurs Res* 39:134, 1990.

Ziegler DB, Prior MM: Preparation for surgery and adjustment to hospitalization, *Nurs Clin North Am* 29:655, 1994.

Risk for disproportionate Growth

Gail B. Ladwig

NANDA Definition

At risk for growth above the 97th percentile or below the 3rd percentile for age, crossing two percentile channels; disproportionate growth

Risk Factors

Prenatal

Congenital/genetic disorders; maternal malnutrition; multiple gestation; teratogen exposure; substance use/abuse

Individual

Infection; prematurity; malnutrition; organic and inorganic factors; caregiver and/or individual maladaptive feeding behaviors; anorexia; insatiable appetite; infection; chronic illness; substance abuse

Environmental

Deprivation; teratogen exposure; lead poisoning; poverty; violence; natural disasters

Caregiver

Abuse; mental illness; mental retardation or severe learning disability

NOC Outcomes (Nursing Outcomes Classification)

Suggested NOC Outcomes

Body Image; Child Development: 2 Months, 4 Months, 6 Months, 12 Months, 2 Years, 3 Years, 4 Years, Preschool, Middle Childhood, Adolescence; Coping; Growth; Impulse Self-Control; Knowledge: Diet; Nutritional Status: Nutrient Intake; Physical Maturation: Female, Male; Self-Esteem; Weight: Body Mass

• = Independent; ▲ = Collaborative

Client Outcomes

Client Will (Specify Time Frame):
- State information related to possible teratogenic agents
- State information related to adequate nutrition
- Seek help from appropriate professionals for nutritional needs

NIC   Interventions (Nursing Interventions Classification)

Suggested NIC Interventions
Behavior Management; Behavior Modification; Counseling; Developmental Enhancement: Adolescent, Child; Impulse Control Training; Nutrition Therapy; Nutritional Monitoring; Teaching: Infant Nutrition, Toddler Nutrition

Nursing Interventions and Rationales
NOTE: Management of a risk diagnosis necessitates the use of approaches incorporating primary and secondary prevention. Primary prevention interventions, which include activities such as nutrition counseling, focus on thwarting the development of a disease or condition. Secondary prevention is achieved through screening, monitoring, and surveillance (Shortridge and Valanis, 1992).

▲ Assess and limit exposure to all drugs (prescription, "recreational," and over the counter) and give the mother information on known teratogenic agents (Table III-1).
   Clinical Research: *No drug can be considered safe during pregnancy. Consequently, a pregnant woman should never take a medication that has not been prescribed for her own benefit or that of her fetus. It should be emphasized that any drug has the potential for causing a birth defect, so no listing of known teratogens is ever complete (refer to Polifka and Friedman, 1999, for a good clinically oriented review) (Florida Birth Defects Registry, 2003).*

• = **Independent;** ▲ = **Collaborative**

TABLE III-1

Teratogenic Agents

Drug	Risk/Effect
ACE inhibitors (captopril, enalapril, etc.)	Appear to be teratogenic when used in the 2nd and 3rd trimesters, causing fetal calvarial hypoplasia, oligohydramnios, and renal anomalies.
Alcohol	Risk is for FAS, alcohol-related birth defects, or alcohol-related neurodevelopmental abnormalities. FAS may be characterized by microcephaly, IUGR, and/or developmental delay. Chronic alcoholism is considered most harmful. Binge drinking may also confer significant risk. No safe limit for prenatal alcohol consumption has been established.
Anticonvulsants (hydantoin, valproic acid, carbamazepine, and primidone [Mysoline])	Effects may include cardiac defects, microcephaly, IUGR, hypoplastic nails, depressed nasal bridge, cleft lip, hip dislocation, hypoplastic nose, low-set ears, small mandible; risk increases with number of anticonvulsants used concurrently.
Antineoplastics (alkylating agents)	Case reports show 10-50% of cases were malformed for different drugs in this class, including busulfan, chlorambucil, cyclophosphamide, and mechlorethamine. The malformation rate for first trimester exposure is quoted at 11.6%. Problems seen include IUGR, cleft palate, agenesis of kidney, malformations of digits, cardiac anomalies, and cloudy corneas.
Antineoplastics (antimetabolites)	Only case reports are available, but an average of 40% of cases were malformed. This class includes aminopterin, 5-fluorouracil, methotrexate, and methylaminopterin, which are strong folic acid antagonists. First trimester exposure produces risk for cleft lip and palate, low-set ears, cranial anomalies, and anencephaly. Fetal abnormalities with cyclophosphamide and vinblastine have also been noted.
Cocaine	Can cause vascular disruption anomalies (e.g., intestinal atresia, limb reductions), IUGR, microcephaly, genitourinary tract defects, irritability, and muscular rigidity in the newborn.
Fluconazole	Fetal anomalies have been observed only when high-dose parenteral therapy is used (e.g., treatment of the mother for coccidiomycosis meningitis).
Diethylstilbestrol	In female offspring, increases risk for cancer, uterine and cervical malformations, reduced fertility, preterm deliveries, perinatal mortality, and SABs; in male offspring, may cause cysts of epididymis, cryptorchidism, hypogonadism, and diminished spermatogenesis.
Lithium	Small increase in risk for cardiac defects (Ebstein's anomaly in particular). Important in this drug to consider benefits and risk potentials.
Methimazole	Antithyroid drug that may increase the risk for prematurity, small-for-gestational-age infants, and scalp defects.
Methylene blue	Reported to cause intestinal atresias when injected into amniotic fluid during amniocentesis.
Penicillamine	Increases risk for connective tissue defects, cerebral palsy, and hydrocephalus.

• = Independent; ▲ = Collaborative

Drug	Risk/Effect
Retinoids (isotretinoin, etretinate, acitretin)	Use of systemic retinoids increases risk for SAB; deformities of cranium, ears, face, limbs, and liver; hydrocephalus; microcephalus; heart defects; and cognitive defects without dysmorphology. Quoted risk for adverse outcome with use of isotretinoin is 38%. These agents have a prolonged teratogen risk because they are stored in adipose tissue and can persist for months.
Tetracyclines	Use from the 20th gestational week on causes dental staining.
Thalidomide	High risk for limb defects, facial hemangiomas, microtia, and ocular and renal anomalies. Now back on the market.
Warfarin (Coumadin) and indandiones (Anisindione) anticoagulants	Increased risk for SAB, stillbirth, and prematurity as well as fetal warfarin syndrome (CNS defects, nasal hypoplasia, skull defects, abnormal ears, malformed eyes, microcephaly, skeletal deformities, mental retardation, etc.). Malformations are reported in 16% of exposed fetuses, hemorrhages in 3%, and stillbirths in 8%.

CNS, Central nervous system; *FAS,* fetal alcohol syndrome; *IUGR,* intrauterine growth retardation; *SAB,* spontaneous abortion.

▲ Reduce the risk of TORCH infections (toxoplasmosis, other infections, rubella, cytomegalovirus [CMV] infection, and herpes simplex):
  ■ Varicella-zoster and rubella viruses: vaccinate nonimmune women prior to conception.
  ■ CMV: practice meticulous hand washing and secretion control and limit exposure to large numbers of infants and children.
  ■ *Toxoplasma gondii:* avoid exposure to cat litter and avoid work in garden or areas where cat feces may be present; do not feed undercooked meats to cats.
  ■ Parvovirus: limit contact with persons with known fifth disease.
  ■ Herpes virus: practice meticulous hand washing and secretion control, especially in contact with young infants.
  Clinical Research: *Infection with any of the aforementioned agents can cause fetal harm resulting in serious damage to the central nervous system and other organs (Florida Birth Defects Registry, 2003).*
▲ Promote a team approach toward preconception and pregnancy glucose control for women with diabetes. **Clinical Research:** *Offspring of women with diabetes mellitus type 1 or type 2 have a two- to fourfold increased risk of birth defects. Available data suggest that excellent preconception and first trimester glucose control in the mother can greatly reduce, if not eliminate, this risk. The increased risk for fetal structural birth defects in women with gestational diabetes is of lesser magnitude, but fetal morbidity may still be high in the second and third trimesters if gestational diabetes is not under good control. Programs with a team approach have been the most successful (Florida Birth Defects Registry, 2003).*
▲ Women with phenylketonuria (PKU) should be referred to a nutritionist experienced in the dietary implications of phenylalanine restriction. Since 40% of all pregnancies are unplanned, women with PKU are urged to maintain phenylalanine restriction throughout their childbearing years. **Clinical Research:** *Women with PKU (in whom the disorder was identified first at birth but who have become adults) who do not maintain strict dietary control may have blood phenylalanine levels above 20 mg/dl. Phenylalanine crosses the placenta at this high level and causes direct fetal damage, although the ac-*

• = Independent; ▲ = Collaborative

tivity of the enzyme phenylalanine hydroxylase may be normal in the fetus. Phenylalanine has been found to be one of the most potent teratogens, with over 90% of fetuses affected with microcephaly and developmental delay when maternal serum levels are above 25 mg/dl. Dietary restriction of phenylalanine should thus be started before conception, and birth outcomes can be normal with such restriction. Initiation of phenylalanine restriction in the first trimester improves developmental outcome, but this is often too late to avoid structural birth defects and brain damage in the fetus (Florida Birth Defects Registry, 2003).

- Provide for adequate nutrition and nutritional monitoring in clients with developmental disorders. **Clinical Research:** *When nutrition therapy is given in the early stages of diagnosis and treatment of cerebral palsy, growth delays may be prevented or remediated (Sanders et al, 1990). Nutrient needs may be altered as a result of long-term medication for conditions such as epilepsy, recurrent urinary or respiratory tract infections, chronic constipation, and behavioral problems (American Dietetic Association, 2003).*

▲ Adequate intake of vitamin D is set at 200 IU/day by the National Academy of Sciences. Because adequate sunlight exposure is difficult to determine, a supplement of 200 IU/day is recommended for the following groups to prevent rickets and vitamin D deficiency in healthy infants and children:

  ■ All breastfed infants unless they are weaned to at least 500 mL/day of vitamin D–fortified formula or milk
  ■ All nonbreastfed infants who are ingesting less than 500 mL/day of vitamin D–fortified formula or milk
  ■ Children and adolescents who do not receive regular sunlight exposure, do not ingest at least 500 mL/day of vitamin D–fortified milk, or do not take a daily multivitamin supplement containing at least 200 IU of vitamin D.

  Clinical Research: *Cases of rickets in infants attributable to inadequate vitamin D intake and decreased exposure to sunlight continue to be reported in the United States. Rickets is an example of extreme vitamin D deficiency. A state of deficiency occurs months before rickets is obvious on physical examination. The new recommendation by the National Academy of Sciences for adequate intake of vitamin D to prevent vitamin D deficiency in normal infants, children, and adolescents is 200 IU/day (Gartner and Greer, 2003).*

▲ All women of childbearing age who are capable of becoming pregnant should take 400 µg of folic acid daily. **Evidence-Based Research:** *Periconceptional use of folic acid reduces the incidence of neural tube defects (NTDs). In fact, up to 70 percent of NTDs could be prevented if all women who can become pregnant consumed 400 µg of folic acid from at least a month prior to conception through the first trimester of pregnancy (Florida Birth Defects Registry, 2003).*

▲ Provide for adequate nutrition for clients with active intestinal inflammation. **Clinical research:** *Nutrition is clearly disturbed by active intestinal inflammation. Appetite is reduced, yet energy substrates are diverted into the inflammatory process; thus weight loss is characteristic. The nutritional disturbance represents part of a profound defect of somatic function. Linear growth and pubertal development in children are notably retarded, body composition is altered, and significant psychosocial disturbance may be present. Increasing evidence shows that an aggressive nutritional program may in itself be sufficient to reduce the mucosal inflammatory response. Recent research suggests that enteral nutrition alone may reduce the levels of many proinflammatory cytokines to normal values and allow mucosal healing (Murch and Walker-Smith, 1998).*

▲ Provide for adequate nutrition for pediatric and adolescent clients on long-term oral glucocorticoid therapy (e.g., those treated for chronic severe asthma). **Clinical Re-**

- **= Independent;** ▲ **= Collaborative**

search: *Growth may be inhibited by long-term use of these agents; however, recent studies suggest that use of the inhaled form of such agents does not affect long-term growth (Prescriber's Letter, 2000).*

▲ Provide tube feedings per physician's orders when appropriate for clients with neuromuscular impairment. **Clinical Research:** *Infants with isolated neonatal swallowing dysfunction have a good long-term prognosis. Nasogastric feedings followed by a gastrostomy is recommended in those without gastroesophageal reflux. Jejunal feedings are necessary in some. Although most infants improve over time, they may need nutritional support for 3 years or more (Heuschkel et al, 2003).*

• Refer to the care plan for **Delayed Growth and development.**

Multicultural

• Assess for the influence of cultural beliefs, norms, values, and expectations on parents' perceptions of normal growth and development. **Nursing Research:** *How the parent views normal growth and development may be based on cultural perceptions (Cochran, 1998; Doswell and Erlen, 1998; Leininger and McFarland, 2002).*

• Negotiate with clients regarding which aspects of healthy nutrition can be modified while still honoring cultural beliefs. **Nursing Research:** *Give and take with clients will lead to culturally congruent care (Leininger and McFarland, 2002).*

• Assess whether the parents are concerned about the amount of food eaten. **Nursing Research:** *Some cultures may add semisolid food within the first month of life because of concerns that the infant is not getting enough to eat and the perception that "big is healthy" (Bentley et al, 1999; Higgins, 2000).*

• Assess the influence of family support on patterns of nutritional intake. **Nursing Research:** *Women are the keepers and transmitters of culture in families. Female family members can play a dominant role in how children and infants are fed (Cesario, 2001; Pillitteri, 1999).*

Home care

• The interventions described previously may be adapted for home care use.

• Provide aids to assist in compliance with the care plan (e.g., prepare medication schedules and put a week's medication in daily containers).

• Provide sufficient outside supports (e.g., written notices, calendars, planned ride shares) to assist with follow-through of the agreed-upon actions. *Cues play a significant role in stimulating completion of desired health actions.*

▲ Include a health promotion focus for clients with disabilities, with the goals of reducing secondary conditions (e.g., obesity, hypertension, pressure sores), maintaining functional independence, providing opportunities for leisure and enjoyment, and enhancing overall quality of life. *Greater emphasis on health promotion for persons with disabilities must take place in the community to accomplish the listed goals (Rimmer, 1999). New enablement models and functional assessment measures are available to evaluate rehabilitation and forecast future needs (Chiriboga, Ottenbacher, and Haber, 1999).*

• Encourage a mind-set and program of self-care management. **Nursing Research:** *Partnership based on respect and caring can focus the older adult on fostering health while aging. An exploration of the beliefs held by the older adult about aging provide an opportunity to introduce positive role models and images of aging, alternative ways of dealing with adversity, and new views of the self as reasonably healthy. Actions such as scheduled so-*

• = **Independent;** ▲ = **Collaborative**

cialization can be introduced to build a repertoire of skills that support the self-concept (Leenerts, Teel, and Pendleton, 2002).

- Establish a written contract with the client to follow the agreed-upon health care regimen. *Written agreements reinforce the verbal agreement and serve as a reference.*
- Meet with the client following completion of the proposed actions to review the contract and determine the next course of action. Do this until the client is able to initiate and follow through independently. *Successful completion of contracts promotes improved self-esteem and positive coping.*
- Using self-care management precepts, instruct the client in the multiple possible situations to which he or she may need to respond; include the use of role playing. Instruct the client in generating hypotheses from available evidence rather than solely from experience. **Nursing Research:** *A study of people with long-standing type 1 diabetes found that the need to react to unanticipated blood glucose levels could be frequent. When the situation contained familiar elements, clients were able to respond rapidly and expertly. When the situation was unfamiliar, decision making could be less accurate; clients would formulate a guess based on past experience and seek clues to confirm that guess, rather than generate a decision based on available evidence (Paterson and Thorne, 2000).*

Client/Family Teaching

- Provide anticipatory guidance for parents and caregivers regarding expectations for normal patterns of growth. Clarify expectations and correct misconceptions. *Parents and caregivers with this knowledge will be able to recognize and report early deviations in normal growth, which allows for more timely intervention.*
- ▲ Refer clients to a registered dietitian for nutritional counseling. *Help from qualified professionals is often needed to meet the nutritional needs of clients with deviations in normal growth.*
- ▲ Teach families the importance of taking measures to prevent lead poisoning: Wash the hands before preparing the child's food. Wash the child's hands before serving food. Wash bottle nipples and pacifiers frequently, especially if they fall on the floor. Wash the child's toys frequently. Stomp the feet before coming into the house to clean shoes of outside soil that may carry lead from exterior house paint. Damp mop frequently along baseboards, around door frames, under windowsills, and around iron radiators. Wash windowsills and window wells frequently. (The window well is the depression behind the windowsill into which the window fits when it is closed.) Move the crib away from window wells. Always damp mop before sweeping or vacuuming. Home vacuum cleaners do not trap lead dust; they blow it into the air. *The child's exposure to ingested lead can be lowered by following these instructions (Stapleton, 2003).*

evolve WEBSITES FOR EDUCATION

See the EVOLVE website for World Wide Web resources for client education.

REFERENCES

American Dietetic Association: Nutrition in comprehensive program planning for persons with developmental disabilities (1996-1999), *J Am Diet Assoc* 97:189, 1997, available online at http://www.eatright.org/adap0297b.html, accessed April 18, 2003.

• = Independent; ▲ = Collaborative

Bentley M et al: Infant feeding practices of low-income, African-American, adolescent mothers: an ecological, multigenerational perspective, *Soc Sci Med* 49(8):1085, 1999.

Cesario S: Care of the Native American woman: strategies for practice, education, and research, *J Gynecol Neonat Nurs* 30(1):13, 2001.

Chiriboga DA, Ottenbacher K, Haber DA: Disability in older adults. 3. Policy implications, *Behav Med* 24: 171, 1999.

Cochran M: Tears have no color, *Am J Nurs* 98(6):53, 1998.

Doswell W, Erlen J: Multicultural issues and ethical concerns in the delivery of nursing care interventions, *Nurs Clin North Am* 33(2):353, 1998.

Florida Birth Defects Registry (Professional): *Prevention strategies index: strategies to prevent birth defects: limit all drug exposures (prescriptions, "recreational," and over-the-counter),* available online at http://fbdr.hsc.usf.edu/ professional/prevention/drugabuse.html, accessed April 18, 2003.

Gartner M, Greer F: Prevention of rickets and vitamin D deficiency: new guidelines for vitamin D intake, *Pediatrics* 111(4):908, 2003, available online at http://www.aap.org/policy/s010116.html, accessed April 18, 2003.

Heuschkel RB et al: Isolated neonatal swallowing dysfunction: a case series and review of the literature, *Dig Dis Sci* 48(1):30, 2003.

Higgins B: Puerto Rican cultural beliefs: influence on infant feeding practices in western New York, *J Transcult Nurs* 11(1):19, 2000.

Leenerts MH, Teel CS, Pendleton MK: Building a model of self-care for health promotion in aging, *J Nurs Scholarsh* 34:355, 2002.

Leininger MM, McFarland MR: *Transcultural nursing: concepts, theories, research and practices,* ed 3, New York, 2002, McGraw-Hill.

Murch SH, Walker-Smith JA: Nutrition in inflammatory bowel disease, *Baillieres Clin Gastroenterol* 12(4):719, 1998.

Paterson B, Thorne S: Expert decision making in relation to unanticipated blood glucose levels, *Res Nurs Health* 23:147, 2000.

Pillitteri A: Nutritional needs of the newborn. In Pillitteri A, editor: *Maternal and child health nursing: care of the childbearing and childrearing family,* Philadelphia, 1999, Lippincott Williams & Wilkins.

Polifka JE, Friedman JM: Clinical teratology: identifying teratogenic risks in humans, *Clin Genet* 56:409, 1999.

Prescriber's Letter, National Institutes of Health: Childhood Asthma Management Program (CAMP), *N Engl J Med* 7(11):62, 2000.

Rimmer JH: Health promotion for people with disabilities: the emerging paradigm shift from disability prevention to prevention of secondary conditions, *Phys Ther* 79:495, 1999.

Sanders K et al: Growth response to enteral feeding by children with cerebral palsy, *JPEN J Parenter Enteral Nutr* 14:23, 1990.

Shortridge L, Valanis B: The epidemiological model applied in community health nursing. In Stanhope M, Lancaster J, editors: *Community health nursing: process and practice for promoting health,* ed 3, St Louis, 1992, Mosby.

Stapleton R: *Help prevent childhood lead poisoning: a resource for parents,* available online at http:// nolead.home.mindspring.com/whatcani.htm#what%20can%20i%20do, accessed April 18, 2003.

Ineffective Health maintenance

Gail B. Ladwig

NANDA Definition

Inability to identify, manage, or seek out help to maintain health

Defining Characteristics

History of lack of health-seeking behavior; reported or observed lack of equipment, financial, and/or other resources; reported or observed impairment of personal support systems; expressed interest in improving health behaviors; demonstrated lack of knowledge regarding basic health practices; demonstrated lack of adaptive behaviors to internal and

• = **Independent; ▲ = Collaborative**

external environmental changes; reported or observed inability to take responsibility for following basic health practices in any or all functional pattern areas

Related Factors (r/t)

Disabled family coping; perceptual-cognitive impairment (complete or partial lack of gross or fine motor skills); lack of or significant alteration in communication skills (written, verbal, or gestural); unachieved developmental tasks; lack of material resources; dysfunctional grieving; disabling spiritual distress; inability to make deliberate and thoughtful judgments; ineffective coping

NOC Outcomes (Nursing Outcomes Classification)

Suggested NOC Outcomes
Health Beliefs: Perceived Resources; Health-Promoting Behavior; Health-Seeking Behavior

---
Example NOC Outcome with Indicators

Health-Seeking Behavior as evidenced by the following indicators: Completes health-related tasks/ Performs self-screening when indicated/Contacts health professionals when indicated (Rate each indicator of **Health-Seeking Behavior:** 1 = never demonstrated, 2 = rarely demonstrated, 3 = sometimes demonstrated, 4 = often demonstrated, 5 = consistently demonstrated [see Section I].)

Client Outcomes

Client Will (Specify Time Frame):
- Discuss fear of or blocks to implementing health regimen
- Follow mutually agreed upon health care maintenance plan
- Meet goals for health care maintenance

NIC Interventions (Nursing Interventions Classification)

Suggested NIC Interventions
Health Education; Health System Guidance; Support System Enhancement

---
Example NIC Activities—Health Education

Prioritize identified learner needs based on client preference, skills of nurse, resources available, and likelihood of successful goal attainment; Emphasize immediate or short-term positive health benefits to be gained from positive lifestyle behaviors rather than long-term benefits or negative effects of noncompliance

---

Nursing Interventions and Rationales

- Assess the client's feelings, values, and reasons for not following the prescribed plan of care. See Related Factors. *A factor to assess when examining client responsibility is the level of dissatisfaction with current lifestyle and readiness for change (Clark, 1996).*
- Assess for family patterns, economic issues, and cultural patterns that influence compliance with a given medical regimen. *Responsiveness to clients enables the nurse to gain an understanding of clients' lives and to cultivate their connections to a responsive community, encouraging clients to avoid getting into "receiving" behaviors (Smith-Battle, 1997).*

- = **Independent;** ▲ = **Collaborative**

- Help the client determine how to arrange a daily schedule that incorporates the new health care regimen (e.g., taking pills before meals).
- ▲ Refer the client to social services for financial assistance if needed. **Clinical Research:** *Information-seeking behavior is a strategy that many people use as a means of dealing with and reducing stress when coping with an illness such as cancer (van der Molen, 1999).*
- ▲ Identify support groups related to the disease process (e.g., Reach to Recovery for a woman who has had a mastectomy).
- Help the client to choose a healthy lifestyle and to have appropriate diagnostic screening tests. **Nursing Research:** *One study found that women who adopt a healthy lifestyle and practice preventive healthy behaviors can reduce the risks of some cancers and other diseases such as heart disease and sexually transmitted infections (Furniss, 2000).*
- Assist the client in reducing stress. **Nursing Research:** *In a convenience sample of 24 men and women who were admitted to a regional hospital in Victoria, Australia, with a provisional diagnosis of myocardial infarction, stress was the most commonly cited cause of illness (King, 2002).*
- Identify complementary healing modalities such as herbal remedies, acupuncture, healing touch, yoga, or cultural shamans that the client uses in addition to or instead of the prescribed allopathic regimen. **Clinical Research:** *Expenditures for alternative medicine professional services increased by 45% from 1990 to 1997. Total visits to alternative medical practitioners exceeded total visits to all U.S. primary care practitioners (Eisenberg et al, 1998). A widening recognition of the mind-body-spirit connection in Western medicine has resulted in a growing interest in ancient health practices such as yoga (Herrick and Ainsworth, 2000).*
- ▲ Refer the client to community agencies for appropriate follow-up care (e.g., day treatment or adult day health program). **Nursing Research:** *Increased social support has been related to a reduction in mortality rates and incidence of physical and mental illness (Callaghan and Morrissey, 1993).* **Clinical Research:** *One study showed a positive response when a community youth setting, such as the Girl Scouts, was used for interventions to prevent disordered eating behaviors (Neumark-Sztainer et al, 2000).*
- Obtain or design educational material that is appropriate for the client; use pictures if possible. **Nursing Research:** *Verbal reinforcement of personalized written instructions appears to be the best intervention. In one study, compliance was better with the use of computer-generated, personalized instructions than with the use of handwritten instructions (Hayes, 1998).*
- Ensure that follow-up appointments are scheduled before the client is discharged; discuss a way to ensure that appointments are kept. **Nursing Research:** *The client brings to the learning situation a unique personality, established social interaction patterns, cultural norms and values, and environmental influences (Bohny, 1997).*

Geriatric
- Assess sensory deficits and psychomotor skills in terms of the client's ability to comply with a health program. **Nursing Research:** *Barriers to health promotion in people with chronic illness were fatigue, time, inadequate safety measures, and lack of accessible facilities (Stuifbergen, 1997).*
- Discuss "symptoms of daily living" in addition to the major illness. **Nursing Research:** *Older adults are unlikely to report day-to-day symptoms such as headaches because they do not view them as illnesses. However, these day-to-day complaints may foretell more serious problems (Musil et al, 1988).*

- = **Independent**; ▲ = **Collaborative**

- Recognize resistance to change in lifelong patterns of personal health care. **Nursing Research:** The client brings to the learning situation a unique personality, established social interaction patterns, cultural norms and values, and environmental influences (Bohny, 1997).
- Discuss with the client realistic goals for changes in health maintenance. **Clinical Research:** *The focus of a chronic illness may be care rather than cure. A study of 86 people found that the oldest old may have increased optimism but decreased satisfaction. They have a sense of realism about the tasks of aging and have a present-focused orientation (Lennings, 2000).*
- Instruct the client in the symptoms of myocardial infarction and the need for timeliness in seeking care. **Nursing Research:** *Women, especially those of advanced age, delay longer before seeking treatment for signs and symptoms of acute myocardial infarction. Effective treatment is time dependent; mortality and morbidity rise with increased prehospital delay (Lefler, 2002).*
- Consider the age of the client when suggesting screening for disease. **Clinical Research:** *Even if one assumes that the mortality reduction with screening persists in the elderly, 80% of the benefit is achieved before 80 years of age for colon cancer, before 75 years of age for breast cancer, and before 65 years of age for cervical cancer. The small benefit of screening in the elderly may be outweighed by the harms: anxiety, additional testing, and unnecessary treatment (Rich and Black, 2000).*

Multicultural

- Assess for the influence of cultural beliefs, norms, and values on the client's ability to modify health behavior. **Nursing Research:** *What the client considers normal and abnormal health behavior may be based on cultural perceptions (Cochran, 1998; Doswell and Erlen, 1998; Leininger and McFarland, 2002).*
- Discuss with the client those aspects of health behavior and lifestyle that will remain unchanged by health status. **Nursing Research:** *Aspects of the client's life that are meaningful and valuable to him or her should be understood and preserved without change (Leininger and McFarland, 2002).*
- Negotiate with the client regarding the aspects of health behavior that will need to be modified. **Nursing Research:** *Give and take with the client will lead to culturally congruent care (Leininger and McFarland, 2002).*
- Assess the effect of fatalism on the client's ability to modify health behavior. **Nursing Research:** *Fatalistic perspectives, which involve the belief that one cannot control one's own fate, may influence health behaviors in some Asian, African American, and Latino populations (Chen, 2001; Harmon, Castro, and Coe, 1996; Phillips, Cohen, and Moses, 1999).*
- Validate the client's feelings regarding the impact of health status on current lifestyle. **Nursing Research:** *Validation is a therapeutic communication technique that lets the client know that the nurse has heard and understood what was said, and it promotes the nurse-client relationship (Heineken, 1998).*

Home care

- The interventions described previously may be adapted for home care use.
- ▲ Provide aids to assist in compliance with the plan of care (e.g., prepare medication schedules and put a week's medication in daily containers).

- = Independent; ▲ = Collaborative

- Provide sufficient outside supports (e.g., written notices, calendars, planned ride shares) to assist with follow-through on the agreed-upon actions. *Cues play a significant role in stimulating completion of desired health actions.*
- ▲ Include a health promotion focus for the client with disabilities, with the goals of reducing secondary conditions (e.g., obesity, hypertension, pressure sores), maintaining functional independence, providing opportunities for leisure and enjoyment, and enhancing overall quality of life. **Clinical Research:** *Greater emphasis on health promotion for persons with disabilities must take place in the community to accomplish the listed goals (Rimmer, 1999).* **Clinical Research:** *New enablement models and functional assessment measures are available to evaluate rehabilitation and forecast future needs (Chiriboga, Ottenbacher, and Haber, 1999).*
- Encourage a mind-set and program of self-care management. **Nursing Research:** *Partnership based on respect and caring can help the older adult to foster health while aging. An exploration of the beliefs held by the older adult about aging provides an opportunity to introduce positive role models. Actions such as scheduled socialization can be introduced to build a repertoire of skills that support the self-concept (Leenerts, Teel, and Pendleton, 2002).*
- Establish a written contract with the client to follow the agreed-upon health care regimen. *Written agreements reinforce the verbal agreement and serve as a reference.*
- Meet with the client following completion of the proposed actions to review the contract and determine the next course of action. Do this until the client is able to initiate and follow through independently. Successful completion of contracts promotes improved self-esteem and positive coping.
- Using self-care management precepts, instruct the client about multiple possible situations to which he or she may need to respond; include the use of role playing. Instruct in generating hypotheses from available evidence rather than solely from experience. **Nursing Research:** *A study of people with long-standing type 1 diabetes found that the need to react to unanticipated blood glucose levels could be frequent. When the situation contained familiar elements, clients were able to respond rapidly and expertly. When the situation was unfamiliar, decision making could be less accurate; clients would formulate a guess based on past experience and seek clues to confirm that guess, rather than generate a decision based on available evidence (Paterson and Thorne, 2000).*

Client/Family Teaching

- Provide the family with lists of addresses where information can be obtained from the Internet. (Most libraries have Internet access with printing capabilities.) *Internet-based technologies have emerged as potentially powerful tools to enable meaningful communication and proactive partnership in care for various medical conditions (Patel, 2001).* **Nursing Research:** *A study of 469 Internet postings of clients with implantable defibrillators showed that the clients used the Internet for practical information seeking and support in coping (Dickerson, Flaig, and Kennedy, 2000).*
- Have the client and family demonstrate at least twice any procedures to be done at home. *Practicing a procedure exposes problems, enhances skill level, and promotes confidence in performing new behaviors.*
- Teach the client about the symptoms associated with discontinuation of a selective serotonin reuptake inhibitor (SSRI) and consider dosage tapering. **Nursing Research:** *Based on emerging research findings, nurses are urged to become more aware of SSRI discontinuation syndrome. To ameliorate or avoid the associated symptoms, client education is recommended, and dosage tapering is encouraged whenever possible (Finfgeld, 2002).*

- ● = **Independent;** ▲ = **Collaborative**

- Explain nonthreatening aspects before introducing more anxiety-producing possible side effects of the disease or medical regimen. *An individual's perception of barriers and benefits has consistently been most predictive of subsequent behavior (Fenn, 1998).*
- Treat tobacco use as a chronic problem. Acknowledge the pleasure associated with smoking. Encourage the client to work towards a goal of permanent abstinence. Advise the client about possible relapse. **Nursing Research:** *In a convenience sample of 20 pregnant women, the women were able to abstain from smoking during pregnancy but relapsed after the birth of the baby. Recognition of the chronic nature of the problem and the development of long-term care delivery systems are needed to assist clients in achieving the goals of permanent abstinence and better personal and family health (Buchanan, 2002).* **Clinical Research:** *This study suggested that an acknowledgment of the attractive, pleasurable aspects of smoking may be seen as unacceptable and irresponsible but this could well provide an opportunity to relate to the everyday and multiple practices of smoking and encourage cessation (McKie et al, 2003).*

evolve WEBSITES FOR EDUCATION

See the EVOLVE website for World Wide Web resources for client education.

REFERENCES

Bohny B: A time for self-care: role of the home healthcare nurse, *Home Healthc Nurse* 15(4):281, 1997.

Buchanan L: Implementing a smoking cessation program for pregnant women based on current clinical practice guidelines, *J Am Acad Nurse Pract* 14(6):243, 2002.

Callaghan P, Morrissey G: Social support and health: a review, *J Adv Nurs* 203:18, 1993.

Chen YC: Chinese values, health and nursing, *J Adv Nurs* 36(2):270, 2001.

Chiriboga DA, Ottenbacher K, Haber DA: Disability in older adults. 3. Policy implications, *Behav Med* 24: 171, 1999.

Clark C: *Wellness practitioner: concepts, research and strategies,* New York, 1996, Springer.

Cochran M: Tears have no color, *Am J Nurs* 98(6):53, 1998.

Dickerson SS, Flaig DM, Kennedy MC: Therapeutic connection: help seeking on the Internet for persons with implantable cardioverter defibrillators, *Heart Lung* 29(4):248, 2000.

Doswell W, Erlen J: Multicultural issues and ethical concerns in the delivery of nursing care interventions, *Nurs Clin North Am* 33(2):353, 1998.

Eisenberg M et al: Trends in alternative medicine use in the United States 1990-1997, *JAMA* 280(18):1569, 1998.

Fenn M: Health promotion: theoretical perspectives and clinical applications, *Holist Nurs Pract* 12(2):1, 1998.

Finfgeld DL: Selective serotonin reuptake inhibitor. Discontinuation syndrome, *J Psychosoc Nurs Ment Health Serv* 40(12):8, 2002.

Furniss K: Tomatoes, Pap smears, and tea? Adopting behaviors that may prevent reproductive cancers and improve health, *J Obstet Gynecol Neonatal Nurs* 29(6):641, 2000.

Harmon MP, Castro FG, Coe K: Acculturation and cervical cancer: knowledge, beliefs, and behaviors of Hispanic women, *Women Health* 24(3):37, 1996.

Hayes K: Randomized trial of geragogy-based medication instruction in the emergency department, *Nurs Res* 47(4):211, 1998.

Heineken J: Patient silence is not necessarily client satisfaction: communication in home care nursing, *Home Healthc Nurse* 16(2):115, 1998.

Herrick CM, Ainsworth AD: Invest in yourself: yoga as a self-care strategy, *Nurs Forum* 35(2):32, 2000.

King R: Illness attributions and myocardial infarction: the influence of gender and socio-economic circumstances on illness beliefs, *J Adv Nurs* 37(5):431, 2002.

Leenerts MH, Teel CS, Pendleton MK: Building a model of self-care for health promotion in aging, *J Nurs Scholarsh* 34:355, 2002.

Lefler L: The advanced practice nurse's role regarding women's delay in seeking treatment with myocardial infarction, *J Am Acad Nurse Pract* 14(10):449, 2002.

- = Independent; ▲ = Collaborative

Leininger MM, McFarland MR: *Transcultural nursing: concepts, theories, research and practices*, ed 3, New York, 2002, McGraw-Hill.

Lennings CJ: Optimism, satisfaction and time perspective in the elderly, *Int J Aging Hum Dev* 51(3):167, 2000.

McKie L et al: Eliciting the smoker's agenda: implications for policy and practice, *Soc Sci Med* 56(1):83, 2003.

Musil CM et al: Health problems and health actions among community-dwelling older adults: results of a health diary study, *Appl Nurs Res* 11(3):138, 1988.

Neumark-Sztainer D et al: Primary prevention of disordered eating among preadolescent girls: feasibility and short-term effect of a community-based intervention, *J Am Diet Assoc* 100(12):1466, 2000.

Patel AM: Using the Internet in the management of asthma, *Curr Opin Pulm Med* 7(1):39, 2001.

Paterson B, Thorne S: Expert decision making in relation to unanticipated blood glucose levels, *Res Nurs Health* 23:147, 2000.

Phillips JM, Cohen MZ, Moses G: Breast cancer screening and African American women: fear, fatalism, and silence, *Oncol Nurs Forum* 26(3):561, 1999.

Rich JS, Black WC: When should we stop screening? *Eff Clin Pract* 3(2):78, 2000.

Rimmer JH: Health promotion for people with disabilities: the emerging paradigm shift from disability prevention to prevention of secondary conditions, *Phys Ther* 79:495, 1999.

Smith-Battle L: The responsive use of self in community health nursing practice, *ANS Adv Nurs Sci* 10(2):75, 1997.

Stuifbergen A: Health promotion: an essential component of rehabilitation for persons with chronic disabling conditions, *ANS Adv Nurs Sci* 19(4):138, 1997.

van der Molen B: Relating information needs to the cancer experience. 1: Information as a key coping strategy, *Eur J Cancer Care (Engl)* 8(4):238, 1999.

Health-seeking behaviors

Gail B. Ladwig

NANDA Definition

Active seeking (by individual in stable health) of ways to alter personal health habits and/or environment to move toward higher level of health

NOTE: Stable health is defined as the achievement of age-appropriate illness-prevention measures; report of good or excellent health from the client; and control of signs and symptoms of disease, if present.

Defining Characteristics

Expressed or observed desire to seek higher level of wellness for self or family; demonstrated or observed lack of knowledge of health-promoting behaviors; stated or observed unfamiliarity with wellness community resources; expressed concern about effect of current environmental conditions on health status; expressed or observed desire for increased control of health practice

Related Factors (r/t)

Role change; change in developmental level (e.g., marriage, parenthood, empty-nest status, retirement); lack of knowledge regarding need for preventive health behaviors, appropriate health screenings, optimal nutrition, weight control, regular exercise program, stress management, supportive social network, and responsible role participation

NOC Outcomes (Nursing Outcomes Classification)

Suggested NOC Outcomes

Adherence Behavior; Health Beliefs; Health Orientation; Health-Promoting Behavior; Health-Seeking Behavior

• = Independent; ▲ = Collaborative

> **Example NOC Outcome with Indicators**
>
> **Health-Seeking Behavior** as evidenced by the following indicators: Completes health-related tasks/ Performs self-screening when indicated/Contacts health professionals when indicated (Rate each indicator of **Health-Seeking Behavior:** 1 = never demonstrated, 2 = rarely demonstrated, 3 = sometimes demonstrated, 4 = often demonstrated, 5 = consistently demonstrated [see Section I].)

Client Outcomes

Client Will (Specify Time Frame):
- Maintain ideal weight and be knowledgeable about nutritious diet
- Demonstrate ways to fit newly prescribed change in health habits into lifestyle
- List community resources available for assistance with achieving wellness
- List ways to include wellness behaviors in current lifestyle

NIC   Interventions (Nursing Interventions Classification)

Suggested NIC Interventions
Health Education; Health System Guidance; Support System Enhancement

> **Example NIC Activities—Health Education**
>
> Prioritize identified learner needs based on client preference, skills of nurse, resources available, and likelihood of successful goal attainment; Emphasize immediate or short-term positive health benefits to be gained by positive lifestyle behaviors rather than long-term benefits or negative effects of noncompliance

Nursing Interventions and Rationales
- Discuss the client's beliefs about health and his or her ability to maintain health. **Nursing Research:** *One study indicated that understanding the transitions of women with chronic illness will enable nurses to move beyond the biomedically orientated concepts of nursing practice toward a holistic approach (Kralik, 2002).*
- Identify barriers and benefits to being healthy. *An individual's perception of barriers and benefits has consistently been most predictive of behavior changes (Fenn, 1998).*
- Identify environmental and social factors that the client perceives as health promoting. **Nursing Research:** *Exposure to a health-promoting environment had statistically significant direct and indirect effects (Conrad et al, 1996).*

Nutritional
- Determine the client's height and weight. Compare results with the standard weight for age and height.
- Encourage the client to eat a diet that contains fresh foods, is low in saturated (visible) fat, and contains no added salt. *Consumption of high levels of saturated fats and cholesterol is strongly associated with cardiovascular disease, obesity, diabetes, and hypertension (Clark, 1996).*
- Assess the role that stress plays in overeating and weight-cycling. *Women who weight-cycle are triggered to overeat by unpleasant feelings or stress, whereas normal-weight subjects tend to overeat in social situations (Smith-Battle, 1997).*

• = Independent; ▲ = Collaborative

Exercise

▲ Advise the client to consult with a physician for testing to determine the ability to tolerate a specific regimen. *Previous bone injuries or inflammatory disease may rule out jogging and aerobic exercises.*

• Explore with the client weightlifting options to increase muscle strength and stamina.

• Help the client focus on the enjoyment of exercise. Set up a support and reward system. *An individual's perception of barriers and benefits has consistently been most predictive of subsequent behavior (Fenn, 1998).*

• Consider using music with exercise. **Nursing Research:** *In a study of 30 coronary artery bypass clients, one group reported a significantly enhanced mood while exercising to music and another group reported a significantly decreased mood without music. Enhancement of mood might lead to increased compliance with a regular exercise routine (Murrock, 2002).*

• Encourage aerobic exercises that increase heart rate within the prescribed limit. Encourage the client to exercise at least three times per week for 20 or more minutes using exercises that the client prefers (e.g., walking, jogging, aerobics, swimming, bicycling, yoga, Tai Chi). *Brisk walking is superior to jogging or running because walking causes fewer injuries and has been shown to be more effective for weight loss (Clark, 1996, p 175).* **Nursing Research:** *Yoga and Tai Chi are stretching exercises that promote energy and muscle balance. A widening recognition of the mind-body-spirit connection in Western medicine has resulted in a growing interest in ancient health practices such as yoga (Herrick and Ainsworth, 2000).* **Clinical Research:** *Regular exercise such as brisk walking resulted in reduction of body weight and body fat among overweight and obese postmenopausal women (Irwin et al, 2003).*

Stress management

• Ask the client to define stress in terms of lifestyle events and assign events a value on a scale from 1 to 5. *This exercise helps to distinguish between anxiety as a personality trait and anxiety as a coping response to threatening events.*

• Determine ways in which the client relieves stress and evaluate their effectiveness. *Stress management techniques are of two types, those that focus on body systems and those that focus on handling stress differently through behavioral responses (Clark, 1996, p 69).*

• Determine the client's social support network. **Nursing Research:** *Exposure to a health-promoting environment had statistically significant direct and indirect effects (Conrad et al, 1996).*

• Teach stress-relieving techniques (e.g., deep and slow breathing, progressive muscle relaxation, meditation, imagery, problem solving). **Clinical Research:** *Body-mind training resulted in an improved capability for physical and mental relaxation as indicated from lower-amplitude electromyograph traces, higher-amplitude alpha brain waves, and decrease in state anxiety in individuals with chronic toxic encephalopathy (Engel and Andersen, 2000).*

Smoking, drinking, self-medication

• Discuss the risk-taking behaviors of smoking, drinking, and self-medication.

• Discuss the frequency of risk-taking habits. *People move through a series of behaviors—precontemplation, preparation, action, and maintenance—in their effort to change or adopt a new behavior (Fenn, 1998, p 5).*

• = Independent; ▲ = Collaborative

▲ Refer a client who smokes to Smoke Enders or a similar community-based program. Discuss ways in which the client can deal with a change in behavior. **Clinical Research:** *Although complete cessation of smoking is preferred, sustained reduction is likely to decrease the risk of disease and is a valuable public health outcome (Wakefield et al, 1992).*

▲ Refer a client who drinks alcohol excessively to Alcoholics Anonymous. Identify a support person to help the client into the organization. **Nursing Research:** *The period after treatment for alcohol abuse is a major life transition that requires extensive coping efforts, social support, and environmental control (Murphy, 1993).*

▲ Identify patterns of self-medication with over-the-counter medications and herbal remedies, and excessive use of prescribed medications. *Medications and herbal preparations are most effective when taken as intended. Combining remedies predisposes the client to unwanted side effects.*

• Refer to the care plans for **Dysfunctional Family processes: alcoholism, Ineffective Denial,** and **Defensive Coping.**

Health-seeking behaviors

• Teach stress-relieving techniques (e.g., deep and slow breathing, progressive muscle relaxation, exercise, meditation, power strategies, problem solving, imagery, verbalization of feelings, spiritual practice [prayer]). *Stress management addresses the sources of tension through physical performance, emotional expression, transcendent spiritual experiences, social relationships, and the surrounding environment.*

• Recognize and allow the client to discuss the choice of complementary therapies available, such as spiritual practice, relaxation, imagery, exercise, lifestyle, diet (e.g., macrobiotic, vegetarian), and nutritional supplementation. **Nursing Research:** *A study of cancer clients found that the clients unanimously believed that complementary therapies helped to improve their quality of life by assisting them in coping more effectively with stress, decreasing the discomforts of treatment and illness, and giving them a sense of control (Sparber et al, 2000).* **Clinical Research:** *One study demonstrated that the use of complementary/alternative medicine for cancer care is widespread. There is a clearly expressed need for complementary/alternative medical treatments by clients and a willingness to pay for them (Lewith, Broomfield, and Prescott, 2002).*

Health screening, appropriate health care

• Assess the frequency of illness-preventing practices, such as routine physical examinations, dental examinations, influenza immunization, breast self-examinations (and mammograms as recommended) for women, testicular self-examinations and prostate examinations for men, and screening for familial diseases such as glaucoma and elevated cholesterol level. See the care plan for **Ineffective Health maintenance. Clinical Research:** *Immunization against influenza is an effective intervention that reduces serologically confirmed cases by 60% to 70% (Hull et al, 2002). Reducing uncertainty about how to perform breast self-examination is seen as a key to promoting self-examination (Babrow and Kline, 2000).*

• Provide a phone call to remind the client of appointments. **Clinical Research:** *At an adolescent clinic in Australia the use of telephone reminders (intention-to-treat analysis) significantly reduced the nonattendance rate from 20% to 8% (Sawyer, Zalan, and Bond, 2002).*

• = **Independent;** ▲ = **Collaborative**

Geriatric

- Assess the client's awareness of deficits that may result from normal aging (e.g., changes in sleep patterns or frequency of urination, loss of visual acuity in night driving, loss of hearing, dietary changes, memory changes, loss of significant others). **Nursing Research:** *If symptoms of health problems are not viewed as an illness, older adults are unlikely to report them to the health care provider. Annual checkups focusing on disease symptoms may fail to uncover day-to-day complaints that foretell more serious problems (Musil, 1998).*

- Identify coping mechanisms that promote wellness and place control of life choices back with the client. Discuss ways to prepare for retirement security. *An active sense of accountability for one's own well-being provides the necessary motivation to pursue a health-enhancing lifestyle (Walker, 1993).*

- ▲ Find suitable housing that provides support, safety, protection, meals, and social events. *Only 5% of older adults live in an institution at any one time. The risk of institutionalization increases with age (Walker, 1993).*

- ▲ Give the client information about community resources for the elderly (e.g., services providing transportation to appointments, Meals-on-Wheels, home visitation services, pets, American Association of Retired Persons, Elder Hostel, Internet addresses). *The aging process occurs throughout the life span. The elderly client hopes to be independent and useful for as long as possible without being a burden on others. The website http:// www.healthfinder.org/justforyou/justforyou.asp?KeyWordID=172&branch=1 offers health information for seniors on a variety of topics.*

- ▲ Assess the environment for signs of elder abuse and report as appropriate. **Nursing Research:** *Activities categorized as mistreatment include force feeding; overmedication/undermedication; withholding of care or needed therapies; and failure to provide health devices such as dentures, glasses, or ambulatory support devices (Rosenblatt, 1997).*

- ▲ Teach health-protecting behaviors to the elderly: monitoring cholesterol intake, exercising, having the stool checked for occult blood, or undergoing a mammogram, Papanicolaou test, or prostate or skin evaluation. **Nursing Research:** *Because common reasons given for not engaging in health screenings are advanced age, absence of direction by primary health care providers, and lack of interest in following up abnormal findings, consider hosting a wellness day in a continuing care retirement community (Resnick, 2000).*

- Teach the importance of exercise. **Clinical Research:** *One study suggested that educating older adults about the benefits of exercise increases the likelihood of their initiating and adhering to an exercise program (Boyette et al, 2002). In a study of 16 senior citizens who participated in 50-minute movement therapy sessions, these individuals improved in their functional motion as measured by the Tinetti scale, and specifically the gait scale; their leg strength increased; and their leg pain significantly decreased (Hartshorn et al, 2002).*

- ▲ Form collaborative multidisciplinary partnerships with nurse-managed clinics for health promotion and chronic disease care management for community-residing older adults. **Nursing Research:** *In one study, senior citizens who participated in a community-based health promotion program reported better general health, performance of roles, and social functioning. Participants required 4.2 doctor visits per year compared with 7.1 office visits for a national comparison group, and 1.6 hospital days per year compared with 2.1 hospital days for the same reference population (Nuñez et al, 2003).*

- Consider the age of the client when suggesting screening for disease. **Clinical Research:** *Even if one assumes that the mortality reduction with screening persists in the el-*

• = Independent; ▲ = Collaborative

derly, 80% of the benefit is achieved before 80 years of age for colon cancer, before 75 years of age for breast cancer, and before 65 years of age for cervical cancer. The small benefit of screening in the elderly may be outweighed by the harms: anxiety, additional testing, and unnecessary treatment (Rich and Black, 2000).

Multicultural

- Assess for the influence of cultural beliefs, norms, and values on the client's beliefs about health behavior. **Nursing Research:** *What the client considers normal and abnormal health behavior may be based on cultural perceptions (Cochran, 1998; Doswell and Erlen, 1998; Leininger and McFarland, 2002).*
- Acknowledge and praise those aspects of the client's behavior and lifestyle that are health promoting. **Nursing Research:** *Aspects of the client's life that are meaningful and valuable to him or her should be understood and preserved without change (Leininger and McFarland, 2002).*
- Negotiate with the client the aspects of health behavior that will require further modification. **Nursing Research:** *Give and take with the client will lead to culturally congruent care (Leininger and McFarland, 2002).*
- Validate the client's feelings regarding the impact of health behavior on current lifestyle. **Nursing Research:** *Validation is a therapeutic communication technique that lets the client know that the nurse has heard and understood what was said, and it promotes the nurse-client relationship (Heineken, 1998).*

Home care

NOTE: All the previously listed nursing interventions are applicable to the home care setting. For more information, see Home Care interventions in the care plan for **Ineffective Health maintenance.**

Client/Family Teaching

- Discuss the role of environmental and social factors in supporting a healthy family life. *The people are the community. Reciprocal relationships to build community education with a view to prevention is key to enhancing health (Davis, 1998).*
- Use videos and written material to provide information. **Nursing Research:** *In a study using an intervention including an educational video and written instructions designed to reduce prehospital delays in clients with chest pain, a significant increase was seen in the use of ambulances in the intervention group but not in the control group (Blank and Smithline, 2002).*
- ▲ Provide and review pamphlets about health-seeking opportunities and wellness and provide the family with lists of addresses where information can be found on the Internet. (Most libraries have Internet access with printing capabilities.) **Clinical Research:** *Internet-based technologies have emerged as potentially powerful tools to enable meaningful communication and proactive partnership in care for various medical conditions (Patel, 2001).* **Nursing Research:** *In a study involving a convenience sample of 32 consumers, subjects found that the websites generated from a list of approximately 90 relevant Internet documents under the broad heading of quality health care were easy to use, and they indicated that the Internet resources would help them assess the quality of care they receive from physicians, nurses, and others (Oermann, Lesley, and Kuefler, 2002).*
- Identify physical and emotional threats to family security (e.g., domestic violence, child abuse, school violence). *According to Maslow's Hierarchy of Needs, wellness and*

• = **Independent;** ▲ = **Collaborative**

health–promoting behaviors can be undertaken only when personal and social safety and security issues are resolved.

evolve WEBSITES FOR EDUCATION

See the EVOLVE website for World Wide Web resources for client education.

REFERENCES

Babrow AS, Kline KN: From "reducing" to "coping with" uncertainty: reconceptualizing the central challenge in breast self-exams, *Soc Sci Med* 51(12):1805, 2000.

Blank FS, Smithline HA: Evaluation of an educational video for cardiac patients, *Clin Nurs Res* 11(4):403, 2002.

Boyette LW et al: Personal characteristics that influence exercise behavior of older adults, *J Rehabil Res Dev* 39(1):95, 2002.

Clark C: *Wellness practitioner: concepts, research and strategies,* New York, 1996, Springer.

Cochran M: Tears have no color, *Am J Nurs* 98(6):53, 1998.

Conrad KM et al: The work site environment as a cue to smoking reduction, *Res Nurs Health* 19(1):21, 1996.

Davis R: Community caring: an ethnographic study within an organizational culture, *Public Health Nurs* 14(2):92, 1998.

Doswell W, Erlen J: Multicultural issues and ethical concerns in the delivery of nursing care interventions, *Nurs Clin North Am* 33(2):353, 1998.

Engel L, Andersen L: Effects of body-mind training and relaxation stretching on persons with chronic toxic encephalopathy, *Patient Educ Couns* 39(2-3):155, 2000.

Fenn M: Health promotion: theoretical perspectives and clinical applications, *Holist Nurs Pract* 12(2):1, 1998.

Hartshorn K et al: Senior citizens benefit from movement therapy, *J Bodywork Movement Ther* 6(1), 2002.

Heineken J: Patient silence is not necessarily client satisfaction: communication in home care nursing, *Home Healthc Nurse* 16(2):115, 1998.

Herrick CM, Ainsworth AD: Invest in yourself: yoga as a self-care strategy, *Nurs Forum* 35(2):32, 2000.

Hull S et al: Boosting uptake of influenza immunisation: a randomised controlled trial of telephone appointing in general practice, *Br J Gen Pract* 52(482):712, 2002.

Irwin ML et al: Effect of exercise on total and intra-abdominal body fat in postmenopausal women: a randomized controlled trial, *JAMA* 289(3):323, 2003.

Kralik D: The quest for ordinariness: transition experienced by midlife women living with chronic illness, *J Adv Nurs* 39(2):146, 2002.

Leininger MM, McFarland MR: *Transcultural nursing: concepts, theories, research and practices,* ed 3, New York, 2002, McGraw-Hill.

Lewith GT, Broomfield J, Prescott P: Complementary cancer care in Southampton: a survey of staff and patients, *Complement Ther Med* 10(2):100, 2002.

Murphy S: Coping strategies of abstainers from alcohol up to 3 years post treatment, *Image J Nurs Sch* 25:32, 1993.

Murrock CJ: The effects of music on the rate of perceived exertion and general mood among coronary artery bypass graft clients enrolled in cardiac rehabilitation phase II [includes commentary by ET Miller], *Rehabil Nurs* 27(6):227, 2002.

Musil C: Health problems and health actions among community dwelling older adults: results of a health diary study, *Appl Nurs Res* 11(3):138, 1998.

Nuñez DE et al: Community-based senior health promotion program using a collaborative practice model: the Escalante Health Partnerships, *Public Health Nurs* 20(1):25, 2003.

Oermann MH, Lesley M, Kuefler SF: Using the Internet to teach consumers about quality care, *Jt Comm J Qual Improv* 28(2):83, 2002.

Patel AM: Using the Internet in the management of asthma, *Curr Opin Pulm Med* 7(1):39, 2001.

Resnick B: Hosting a wellness day: promoting health in the old-old, *Clin Excell Nurse Pract* 4(6):326, 2000.

Rich JS, Black WC: When should we stop screening? *Eff Clin Pract* 3(2):78, 2000.

Rosenblatt D: Elder mistreatment, *Crit Care Nurs Clin North Am* 9(2):183, 1997.

• = **Independent;** ▲ = **Collaborative**

Sawyer SM, Zalan A, Bond LM: Telephone reminders improve adolescent clinic attendance: a randomized controlled trial, *J Paediatr Child Health* 38(1):79, 2002.

Smith-Battle L: The responsive use of self in community health nursing practice, *Adv Nurs Sci* 10(2):75, 1997.

Sparber A et al: Use of complementary medicine by adult patients participating in cancer clinical trials, *Oncol Nurs Forum* 27(4):623, 2000.

Wakefield M et al: Workplace smoking restrictions, occupational status and reduced cigarette consumption, *J Occup Med* 34:693, 1992.

Walker S: Wellness for elders, *Holist Nurs Pract* 38:7, 1993.

Impaired Home maintenance

Gail B. Ladwig

NANDA Definition

Inability to independently maintain a safe and growth-promoting immediate environment

Defining Characteristics

Subjective

Household members express difficulty in maintaining their home in a comfortable fashion; household members describe outstanding debts or financial crises; household requests assistance with home maintenance

Objective

Disorderly surroundings; unwashed or unavailable cooking equipment, clothes, or linen; accumulation of dirt, food wastes, or hygienic wastes; offensive odors; inappropriate household temperature; overtaxed family members (e.g., exhausted, anxious); lack of necessary equipment or aids; presence of vermin or rodents; repeated hygienic disorders, infestations, or infections

Related Factors (r/t)

Client/family member with disease or injury; unfamiliarity with neighborhood resources; lack of role modeling; lack of knowledge; insufficient family organization or planning; inadequate support systems; impaired cognitive or emotional functioning; insufficient finances

NOC Outcomes (Nursing Outcomes Classification)

Suggested NOC Outcomes

Family Functioning; Parenting: Psychosocial Safety; Parenting Performance; Role Performance; Self-Care: Instrumental Activities of Daily Living (IADL)

Example NOC Outcome with Indicators

Family Functioning as evidenced by the following indicators: Regulates behavior of members/Obtains adequate resources to meet needs of family members (Rate each indicator of **Family Functioning:** 1 = never demonstrated, 2 = rarely demonstrated, 3 = sometimes demonstrated, 4 = often demonstrated, 5 = consistently demonstrated [see Section I].)

• = Independent; ▲ = Collaborative

Client Outcomes

Client Will (Specify Time Frame):

- Wear clean clothing, eat nutritious meals, and have a sanitary and safe home
- Have the resources to cope physically and emotionally with the chronic illness process
- Use community resources to assist with treatment needs

NIC	Interventions (Nursing Interventions Classification)

Suggested NIC Intervention

Home Maintenance Assistance

Example NIC Activities—Home Maintenance Assistance

Provide information on how to make home safe and clean; Help family use social support network

Nursing Interventions and Rationales

- Establish a plan of care with the client and family based on the client's needs and the caregiver's capabilities. **Nursing Research:** *Broad categories of health promotion identified in a study of persons with chronic illness were physical activity, nutritional strategies, life adjustment, maintenance of a positive attitude, and interpersonal support (Stuifbergen, 1997). Health care workers need to provide support when the client and family are facing difficult decisions (Hurley and Volicer, 2002).*
- Assess the concerns of family members, especially the primary caregiver, about long-term home care. **Clinical Research:** *Caregiver characteristics significantly associated with yielding up care to another included older age, greater use of respite services, fewer social activities, poorer mental health, and greater depression. Dementia severity was the key predictor of the decision to relinquish care (Bond and Clark, 2002.).*
- Set up a system of relief for the main caregiver in the home and plan for sharing of household duties. **Clinical Research:** *The level of burden was affected directly by behavioral problems in the care receiver, frequency of getting a break, caregiver self-esteem, and caring for the client at odd hours (Chappell and Reid, 2002).*
- Encourage social relationships with family and friends, even if by phone. **Clinical Research:** *Telephone support was considered important by caregivers of elderly persons (Colantonio et al, 2001).*
- ▲ Initiate referral to community agencies as needed, including housekeeping services, Meals-on-Wheels, wheelchair-compatible transportation services, and oxygen therapy services. **Nursing Research:** *Barriers to health promotion in people with chronic illness are fatigue, time, inadequate safety measures, and lack of accessible facilities (Stuifbergen, 1997, p 14).*
- ▲ Obtain adaptive equipment and telemedical equipment, as appropriate, to help family members continue to maintain the home environment. **Nursing Research:** *Telemedical equipment available for the home includes infusion pumps, pulse oximeters, 12-lead EKG machines, and telestethoscopes (McNeal, 1998).*
- Consider the use of permethrin-impregnated mattress liners to control dust mites. **Clinical Research:** *A trial of permethrin-impregnated bedding significantly reduced house dust mites in mattresses for at least 27 months. Allergen concentrations were significantly*

• = Independent; ▲ = Collaborative

lowered at 15 months after intervention. No adverse side effects were reported (Cameron and Hill, 2002).

▲ Refer the client to social services to help with debt consolidation or financial concerns. *Financial help ranges from Medicaid and private insurance to aid from specific foundations such as the Shriners Burn Center for Children. Hospital discharge planners are an important resource for coordinating agencies.*

▲ Ask the family to identify support people who can help with home maintenance. *Churches, nursing home health agencies, and hospice organizations are sources for reliable in-home support. Community health agencies can evaluate whether the home is safe enough for providing health care to a chronically ill person, can provide direct care, and can assist with resource coordination. Consider supportive housing for clients with mental illness.* **Clinical Research:** *Supportive housing programs, which provide independent housing along with health and social services, hold great promise for mentally ill individuals who are homeless (Culhane, Metreaux, and Hadley, 2002).*

Geriatric

▲ Explore community resources to assist with home care (e.g., senior centers, Department of Aging, hospital discharge planners, the Internet, or church parish nurse). *Promoting the health of the population has always required an organic relationship to the community and knowledge of specific subpopulations (Smith-Battle, 1997). An Internet resource is the website of geriatrician Dr. Robert S. Stall: http://www.acsu.buffalo.edu/~drstall.*

• Visit the client's home to assess safety features (e.g., no throw rugs, safety bars in the bathroom, stair borders that distinguish each step, adequate nonglare lighting). **Clinical Research:** *The eye retina changes with age, which makes it easier to perceive red and yellow tones. With age, some glare occurs in bright light, and contrast and shadows blur. A 5-year study documented that increasing age was a strong predictor of visual impairment in an older Australian population (Foran, Mitchell, and Wang, 2003).* **Nursing Research:** *Bath grab bars can minimize the effects of many age-related deficits that may contribute to bath-related falls. One study indicated that they are underutilized and their use needs to be supported (Lockett, Aminzadeh, and Edwards, 2002).*

• Encourage regular eye examinations. *Early detection of eye changes is imperative to prevent irreversible damage (Age Net, 2003).*

• The following interventions should be considered for those with low or failing sight:

• Reduce glare.
   ▪ Use nonglare light bulbs.
   ▪ Remove wax from floors to reduce glare.
   ▪ Encourage the client to wear sunglasses.
   ▪ Use sheer curtains or blinds.

• Use proper lighting.
   ▪ Use night lights in the bedroom, bathroom, and hallways.
   ▪ Use dimmer switches and three-way bulbs to control light.
   ▪ Put bright lights at the top and bottom of a staircase.
   ▪ Use consistent lighting to minimize shadows.

• Enhance color contrast.
   ▪ Use colored tape to define steps.
   ▪ Paint walls and staircase to contrast with floor.
   ▪ Put glow-in-the-dark tape on light switches and door knobs.
   ▪ Use colored dishes.

• = **Independent;** ▲ = **Collaborative**

- Encourage the client to use low-vision aids.
  - Use magnifiers to improve near vision.
  - Hang magnifiers around the neck for convenience when sewing, doing crafts, or reading.
  - Request large-print medication labels, books, and phones.
  - Use handrails on stairs.
  - Keep flashlights in a convenient location.
  Vision loss can cause less hardship if adaptive strategies and aids are used. Use of aids increases safety and promotes a sense of independence (Age Net, 2003).
- ▲ During the home visit, be alert for signs of elder abuse. Report any findings. **Nursing Research:** *Activities categorized as mistreatment include force feeding; overmedication/undermedication; withholding care or needed therapies; failure to provide safety precautions; and failure to provide health devices such as dentures, glasses, or ambulatory devices (Rosenblatt, 1997).*
- See the care plan for **Risk for Injury.**

Multicultural

- Acknowledge the stresses unique to racial/ethnic communities. **Nursing Research:** *Targeted alcohol and tobacco marketing, high levels of unemployment, lack of health insurance, and racism are stresses unique to culturally diverse communities and often accompany poor housing (D'Avanzo et al, 2001; Ludwick and Silva, 2000; Zambrana, Dorrington, and Hayes-Bautista, 1995). One in 10 Latino children lives in a "severely distressed neighborhood," compared with 1 in 63 non-Hispanic white children (Annie E. Casey Foundation, 1994).*
- ▲ Identify what services and information are currently available in the community to assist with housing needs. **Nursing Research:** *This identification will assist in focusing efforts and promote the wise use of valuable resources (National Heart, Lung, and Blood Institute, 1998).*
- Approach families of color with respect, warmth, and professional courtesy. **Nursing Research:** *Instances of disrespect and lack of caring have special significance for individuals of color (D'Avanzo et al, 2001; Vontress and Epp, 1997).*

Home care

NOTE: By definition, this nursing diagnosis consists of primarily community-based interventions. Home care and public health nursing are two community resources that can help the family to restore or improve home management. The previous interventions incorporate these resources.

Client/Family Teaching

- Teach the caregiver the need to set aside some personal time every day to meet his or her own needs. **Nursing Research:** *The most prominent needs were found to be the need for security and the need to provide security to the child. Family needs and need for relief were also identified. (Hallström, Runesson, and Elander, 2002).*
- Encourage family members to perform home maintenance activities (e.g., cooking, cleaning, fire prevention). *When one family member becomes ill and requires home care, the roles of other family members may change.*

- = Independent; ▲ = Collaborative

▲ Identify support groups within the community to assist families in the caregiver role. **Nursing Research:** *Caregivers' participation in support groups provides effective assistance to caregivers of clients with schizophrenia (Chou, Liu, and Chu, 2002).*

• Provide support when the family must move their family member to an assisted living facility (ALF). **Nursing Research:** *Secondary data analysis in one study showed that all elements of a crisis were evident among caregivers in the process of moving their relative to an ALF. Perceived lack of family support in conjunction with physical and psychological exhaustion were crisis mediators (Liken, 2001).*

▲ Provide written instructions for medication management and side effects, written instructions for equipment brought to the home, and resource phone numbers for emergency needs. **Nursing Research:** *Verbal reinforcement of personalized written instructions appears to be the best intervention. In one study, the use of computer-generated, personalized instructions improved adherence compared with the use of handwritten instructions (Hayes, 1998).*

𝑒𝑣𝑜𝑙𝑣𝑒 **WEBSITES FOR EDUCATION**

See the EVOLVE website for World Wide Web resources for client education.

REFERENCES

Age Net: *Visual changes,* available online at http://agenet.agenet.com/?Url = link.asp?DOC/36, accessed Feb 25, 2003.

The Annie E. Casey Foundation: *Kids count data book: state profiles of child well-being,* ed 5, Baltimore, 1994, The Foundation.

Bond MJ, Clark MS: Predictors of the decision to yield care of a person with dementia, *Australas J Ageing* 21(2): 86, 2002.

Cameron MM, Hill N: Permethrin-impregnated mattress liners: a novel and effective intervention against house dust mites (Acari: Pyroglyphididae), *J Med Entomol* 39(5):755, 2002.

Chappell NL, Reid RC: Burden and well-being among caregivers: examining the distinction, *Gerontologist* 42(6):772, 2002.

Chou K, Liu S, Chu H: The effects of support groups on caregivers of patients with schizophrenia, *Int J Nurs Stud* 39(7):713, 2002.

Colantonio A et al: What support do caregivers of elderly want? Results from the Canadian Study of Health and Aging, *Can J Public Health* 92(5):376, 2001.

Culhane DP, Metreaux S, Hadley T: Supportive housing for homeless people with severe mental illness, *LDI Issue Brief* 7(5):1, 2002.

D'Avanzo CE et al: Developing culturally informed strategies for substance-related interventions. In Naegle MA, D'Avanzo CE, editors: *Addictions and substance abuse: strategies for advanced practice nursing,* St Louis, 2001, Mosby.

Foran S, Mitchell P, Wang JJ: Five-year change in visual acuity and incidence of visual impairment: the Blue Mountains Eye Study, *Ophthalmology* 110(1):41, 2003.

Hallström I, Runesson I, Elander G: International pediatric nursing. Observed parental needs during their child's hospitalization, *J Pediatr Nurs* 17(2):140, 2002.

Hayes K: Randomized trial of geragogy-based medication instruction in the emergency department, *Nurs Res* 47(4):211, 1998.

Hurley AC, Volicer L: Alzheimer disease: "It's okay, Mama, if you want to go, it's okay," *JAMA* 288(18):2324, 2002.

Liken MA: Caregivers in crisis: moving a relative with Alzheimer's to assisted living, *Clin Nurs Res* 10(1):52, 2001.

Lockett D, Aminzadeh F, Edwards N: Development and evaluation of an instrument to measure seniors' attitudes toward the use of bathroom grab bars, *Public Health Nurs* 19(5):390, 2002.

• = **Independent;** ▲ = **Collaborative**

Ludwick R, Silva M: Nursing around the world: cultural values and ethical conflicts, *Online J Issues Nurs*, August 14, 2000, available online at http://www.nursingworld.org/ojin/ethcol/ethics_4.htm, accessed June 19, 2003.

McNeal G: Telecommunication techniques in high-tech home care, *Adv Pract Nurse* 10(3):279, 1998.

National Heart, Lung, and Blood Institute of the National Institutes of Health: *Salud para su corazón: bringing heart health to Latinos—a guide for building community programs*, NIH Pub No. 98-3796, Washington, DC, 1998, US Department of Health and Human Services.

Rosenblatt D: Elder mistreatment, *Crit Care Nurs Clin North Am* 9(2):183, 1997.

Smith-Battle L: The responsive use of self in community health nursing practice, *ANS Adv Nurs Sci* 10(2):75, 1997.

Stuifbergen A: Health promotion: an essential component of rehabilitation for persons with chronic disabling conditions, *ANS Adv Nurs Sci* 19(4):1, 1997.

Vontress CE, Epp LR: Historical hostility in the African American client: implications for counseling, *J Multicult Counseling Dev* 25:170, 1997.

Zambrana RE, Dorrington C, Hayes-Bautista D: Family and child health: a neglected vision. In Zambrana RE, editor: *Understanding Latino families*, Thousand Oaks, Calif, 1995, Sage.

Hopelessness

Ann Keeley

NANDA Definition

Subjective state in which individual sees limited or unavailable alternatives or personal choices and is unable to mobilize energy for problem solving on his or her own behalf

Defining Characteristics

Passivity; decreased verbalization; blunted or flat affect; verbal cues (e.g., saying "I can't," sighing); closing of eyes; anorexia; decreased response to stimuli; increased/decreased sleep; lack of initiative; lack of involvement in care; passively allowing care; shrugging in response to speaker; turning away from speaker

Related Factors (r/t)

Abandonment; prolonged activity restriction creating isolation; loss of beliefs in transcendent values/God; long-term stress; failing or deteriorating chronic physiological and/or psychological condition; negative life review; perception of demands that overwhelm personal resources

NOC Outcomes (Nursing Outcomes Classification)

Suggested NOC Outcomes

Decision Making; Hope; Mood Equilibrium; Nutritional Status: Food and Fluid Intake; Quality of Life; Sleep

> **Example NOC Outcome with Indicators**
>
> Has a presence of **Hope** as evidenced by the expression of a positive orientation, faith, and will to live (Rate indicator of **Hope:** 1 = no expression, 2 = limited expression, 3 = moderate expression, 4 = substantial expression, 5 = extensive expression [see Section I].)

• = Independent; ▲ = Collaborative

Client Outcomes

Client Will (Specify Time Frame):
- Verbalize feelings, participate in care
- Make positive statements (e.g., "I can" or "I will try")
- Set goals
- Make eye contact, focus on speaker
- Maintain appropriate appetite for age and physical health
- Sleep appropriate length of time for age and physical health
- Express concern for another
- Initiate activity

NIC Interventions (Nursing Interventions Classification)

Suggested NIC Intervention
Hope Instillation

> #### Example NIC Activities—Hope Instillation
>
> Assist client/family to identify areas of hope in life; Demonstrate hope by recognizing client's intrinsic worth and viewing client's illness as only one facet of the individual; Expand client's repertoire of coping mechanisms

Nursing Interventions and Rationales

▲ Monitor and document the potential for suicide. (Refer the client for appropriate treatment if a potential for suicide is identified.) See the care plan for **Risk for Suicide** for specific interventions. *Hopelessness is directly associated with suicidal behavior and also with a variety of other dysfunctional personal characteristics (Fritsch et al, 2000). Previous suicide attempts and hopelessness are the most powerful clinical predictors of future completed suicide (Malone et al, 2000).*

- Explore the client's definition of hope. **Nursing Research:** *As individuals experience the effects of a life event or illness, their definition of hope may change. It is important for the nurse to be clear what the client's current definition includes. This intervention needs to occur with each encounter (Kylma, Vehvilainen-Julkunen, and Lahdevirta, 2001).*

- Assist in identifying sources of hope. **Nursing Research:** *Depending on the population being served, there may be specific interventions more helpful in promoting hope (Cutcliffe and Grant, 2001).*

- Assist the client in identifying reasons for living. *Interventions that increase the awareness of reasons for living may decrease hopelessness and decrease risk for suicide (Malone et al, 2000).*

- Provide realistic feedback. **Nursing Research:** *Accurate information allows the nurse-client relationship to redefine hope in the present (Kylma, Vehvilainen-Julkunen, and Lahdevirta, 2001).*

- Assess for pain and respond with appropriate measures for pain relief. *Fear of pain and ability to cope with pain are significant risk factors for hopelessness (Duggleby, 2001).*

- Assist with problem solving and decision making. *Impaired problem-solving ability and dysfunctional attitude have been shown to correlate with hopelessness (Cannon et al, 1999).*

- Determine appropriate approaches based on the underlying condition or situation that is contributing to feelings of hopelessness. *Understanding the source of the hopelessness,*

• = Independent; ▲ = Collaborative

be it a victimizing relationship or a physical alteration, will indicate the approaches that may be most beneficial to the client (Schreiber, 2001).

- Assist the client in looking at alternatives and setting goals that are important to him or her. *Use of the nurse's knowledge along with the client's experience within the context of a supportive relationship stimulates an unfolding of possibilities (Kylma, Vehvilainen-Julkunen, and Lahdevirta, 2001).*
- In dealing with possible long-term deficits, work with the client to set small, attainable goals. *Working on mutually agreed upon goals that are meaningful to the client will support hopefulness (Duggleby, 2001).*
- Spend one-on-one time with the client. Use empathy; try to understand what the client is saying and communicate this understanding to the client. *Hope is constructed in exploring the possibilities. As a person experiences the understanding of another, he or she may explore with that person (the nurse) the possibilities in his or her life (Wang, 2000). Experiencing warmth, empathy, genuineness, and unconditional positive regard can inspire hope (Cutcliffe, 1998). Physical presence and active listening inspire hope in the client (Duggleby, 2001).*
- Encourage decision making in the daily schedule. *Hopelessness may be an outgrowth of a perceived loss of control and/or self-efficacy. As changes occur, the nurse interacts with the client to evaluate their impact on life goals and assists in making adaptations that support hopefulness (Kylma, Vehvilainen-Julkunen, and Lahdevirta, 2001).*
- Encourage expression of feelings and acknowledge acceptance of them. *Hope is ultimately dependent on external validation in the form of positive interpersonal relationships (Cutcliffe and Grant, 2001).*
- Give the client time to initiate interactions. After an appropriate amount of time is allowed, approach the client in an accepting and nonjudgmental manner. *The establishing of new relationships and control over events within them is constructive within the context of nurturing hopefulness (Kylma, Vehvilainen-Julkunen, and Lahdevirta, 2001).*
- Encourage the client to participate in group activities. *Group activities provide social support and help the client to identify alternative ways to problem solve. Group experiences allow the opportunity to care for others and to be cared for (Kylma, Vehvilainen-Julkunen, and Lahdevirta, 2001).*
- Encourage exercise of the mind to alleviate boredom. Watching or listening to the news, listening to music, reminiscing, and writing letters help to relieve the monotony of hospitalization. *Activities that include discussions of happy events in the past will foster hope (Duggleby, 2001).*
- Review the client's strengths with the client. Have the client list his or her own strengths on a note card and carry this list for future reference. *Working with the client to identify positive experiences and personal strengths facilitates the development of hopefulness (Kylma, Vehvilainen-Julkunen, and Lahdevirta, 2001).*
- Communicate clearly what the illness trajectory and/or course of treatment will involve. *Efforts must be taken to eliminate as much uncertainty as possible (Kylma, Vehvilainen-Julkunen, and Lahdevirta, 2001).*
- Use humor as appropriate. *Humor is an effective intervention for hopelessness (Duggleby, 2001).*
- Involve family and significant others in the plan of care. *Significant caring relationships foster hope (Duggleby, 2001). Social support is a significant variable related to hope (Ehrenberger et al, 2002).*

- = **Independent**; ▲ = **Collaborative**

- Encourage the family and significant others to express care, hope, and love for the client. *Caring relationships have a positive influence on the presence of hope (Cutcliffe and Grant, 2001; Duggleby, 2001).*
- Assess for signs and symptoms of depression. *Hopelessness is one symptom of depression.*
- Use touch to demonstrate caring, if culturally appropriate and with the client's permission, and encourage the family to do the same. *Human touch and human presence may in some way directly and/or indirectly restore the human-centered dignity and affirmation of being that is necessary for the emergence of hope (Cutcliffe, 1998).*
- Facilitate access to resources to support a positive spirituality. *Spiritual beliefs and practices that are practiced within a positive framework facilitate hope (Duggleby, 2001).*
- For additional interventions, see the care plans for **Spiritual distress, Readiness for enhanced Spiritual well-being,** and **Disturbed Sleep pattern.**

Geriatric

- Assess for clinical signs and symptoms of depression; differentiate depression from organic dementia. *In the elderly, the differentiation of depression and dementia is critical prior to establishing a plan of care.*
- ▲ If depression is suspected, confer with the primary physician regarding referral for mental health services. *In older adults, hopelessness and suicidal wishes are present with high levels of depressive symptoms suggestive of treatable pathology (Uncapher et al, 1998).*
- Take threats of self-harm or suicide seriously. *The elderly have the highest rate of completed suicide of all age groups (Uncapher et al, 1998). Hopelessness is often linked to depression and suicidal ideation in the elderly. Elderly people who are depressed or have experienced recent losses and live alone are at the highest risk (Uncapher et al, 1998).*
- Identify significant losses that may be leading to feelings of hopelessness. *Helping clients to cope with grief and make more psychological energy available to them will support their hopefulness.*
- Discuss stages of emotional responses to multiple losses.
- Use reminiscence and life-review therapies to identify past coping skills. *Help the client acknowledge positive accomplishments and review survival of past illnesses to promote hope for dealing with the current illness (Johnson, Dahlen, and Roberts, 1997).*
- Express hope to the client and give positive feedback whenever appropriate. *The nurse's communication of caring for the client facilitates movement in the direction of hope (Cutcliffe and Grant, 2001).*
- Identify the client's past and current sources of spirituality. Help the client explore life and identify those experiences that are noteworthy. The client may want to read the Bible or other religious text or have it read to him or her. *Spirituality is often identified by clients as a bridge between hopelessness and a sense of meaning (Fryback and Reinert, 1999).*
- Encourage visits from children. *Children stimulate a sense of hope in many older adults (Gaskins and Forte, 1995). Social relationships foster hopefulness (Dugglesby, 2001).*
- ▲ Administer medications as ordered and evaluate for possible drug interactions that may produce and/or exacerbate observed symptoms. *The elderly have compromised ability to metabolize medications and are often taking a variety of drugs with side effects that may produce observed symptoms.*
- Position the client by a window, take the client outside, or encourage activities such as gardening (if ability allows). *Environmental changes can foster hope (Cutcliffe and Grant, 2001).*

- **= Independent; ▲ = Collaborative**

- If possible, have the client perform daily regular exercise adapted to his or her abilities. *Exercise has been demonstrated to be an effective treatment for depression.*

Multicultural

- Assess for the influence of cultural beliefs, norms, and values on the client's feelings of hopelessness. **Nursing Research:** *The client's expressions of hopelessness may be based on cultural perceptions (Cochran, 1998; Doswell and Erlen, 1998; Leininger and McFarland, 2002).*
- Assess the effect of fatalism on the client's expression of hopelessness. **Nursing Research:** *Fatalistic perspectives, which involve the belief that one cannot control one's own fate, may influence health behaviors in some Asian, African American, and Latino populations (Chen, 2001; Harmon, Castro, and Coe, 1996; Phillips, Cohen, and Moses, 1999).*
- Encourage spirituality as a source of support for hopelessness. **Nursing Research:** *African Americans and Latinos may identify spirituality, religiousness, prayer, and church-based approaches as coping resources (Bourjolly, 1998; Mapp and Hudson, 1997; Samuel-Hodge et al, 2000).*
- Validate the client's feelings regarding the impact of health status on current lifestyle. **Nursing Research:** *Validation is a therapeutic communication technique that lets the client know that the nurse has heard and understood what was said, and it promotes the nurse-client relationship (Heineken, 1998).*

Home care

- Assess for isolation within the family unit. Encourage the client to participate in family activities. If the client cannot participate, encourage him or her to be in the same area and watch family activities. If possible, move the client's bed or primary sitting place to an active household area. *Significant caring relationships foster hope (Duggleby, 2001). Participation in events increases energy and promotes a sense of belonging. Hope is facilitated by meaningful interpersonal relationships (Cutcliffe and Grant, 2001).*
- ▲ If depression is suspected, confer with the primary health care provider regarding referral for mental health services. *In older adults, hopelessness and suicidal wishes are present with high levels of depressive symptoms suggestive of treatable pathology (Uncapher et al, 1998).*
- Reminisce with the client about his or her life. *The process of remembering past pleasant activities and sharing them in a supportive environment inspires hope (Duggleby, 2001). Use of the self in the context of an interpersonal relationship with the client will facilitate hope (Cutcliffe and Grant, 2001).*
- Identify areas in which the client can have control. Allow the client to set achievable goals in these areas. Assist the client when necessary to negotiate desirable outcomes. *Mobilization of resources to promote self-efficacy promotes hope (Kylma, Vehvilainen-Julkenen, Lahdevirta, 2001).*
- Clearly explain potential benefits and risks of a proposed intervention. *Clear, direct communication of the potential of an intervention to overcome a threat, along with honest discussion of negative aspects, empowers the client and promotes hope (Pinikahana and Happell, 2002).*
- If illness precipitated the hopelessness, discuss knowledge of and previous experience with the disease. Help the client to identify past coping strengths. *Uncertainty is a danger when it results in pessimism. Knowledge of the disease and previous positive coping experience with the illness potentiate hope (Richer and Ezer, 2002).*

- • = **Independent;** ▲ = **Collaborative**

▲ Provide plant or pet therapy if possible. *Caring for pets or plants helps to redefine the client's identity and makes him or her feel needed and loved.*

▲ Provide a safe environment so that the client cannot harm himself or herself. (See also the no-suicide contract in the following section). Provide one-to-one contact when necessary. Refer the client for immediate mental health treatment if needed. *Hopelessness is an accurate indicator of suicidal risk. A safe environment reassures the client.*

▲ If it is consistent with the client's religious beliefs, refer for spiritual counseling by clergy of the client's choice.

▲ In the presence of a psychiatric disorder, refer for psychiatric home health care services for client reassurance and implementation of a therapeutic regimen. *Psychiatric home care nurses can address issues relating to the client's depression and hopelessness, and the interference of these factors with the ability to adjust to changes in health status. Behavioral interventions in the home can help the client to participate more effectively in the treatment plan (Patusky, Rodning, and Martinez-Kratz, 1996).*

Client/Family Teaching

• Provide information regarding the client's condition, treatment plan, and progress. *Clear, direct communication of the potential of an intervention to overcome a threat along with honest discussion of negative aspects empowers the client and promotes hope (Pinikahana and Happell, 2002).*

• Provide positive reinforcement, praise, and acknowledgment of the challenges of caregiving to family members. *Nurses provide much-needed support and encouragement to caregivers (Dibartolo, 2002).*

• Teach the use of stress-reduction techniques, relaxation, and imagery. Many cassette tapes on relaxation and meditation are available. Assist the client and caregivers with relaxation based on their preference from the initial assessment. *Stress management techniques are effective interventions for clients and their caregivers (Ducharme and Trudeau, 2002).*

• Encourage families to express love, concern, and encouragement, and allow the client to verbalize feelings.

▲ Refer the client to self-help groups such as I Can Cope and Make Today Count. **Nursing Research:** *Self-help and/or professionally led curriculum-based support programs for families are effective in reducing stress and facilitating coping and hope (Northouse et al, 2002).*

▲ Refer the family to community support groups targeted to the specific needs of the family caregivers. *Support groups provide validation of feelings, information, and an opportunity for sharing of creative strategies among participants (Fung and Chien, 2002).*

▲ Supply a crisis phone number and negotiate a no-suicide contract with the client stating that the crisis number will be used if thoughts of self-harm occur. *A no-suicide contract is one type of intervention used with clients who have suicidal thoughts (Valente, 1989).*

evolve WEBSITES FOR EDUCATION

See the EVOLVE website for World Wide Web resources for client education.

• = Independent; ▲ = Collaborative

REFERENCES

Bourjolly JN: Differences in religiousness among black and white women with breast cancer, *Soc Work Health Care* 28(1):21, 1998.

Cannon B et al: Dysfunctional attitudes and poor problem solving skills predict hopelessness in major depression, *J Affect Disord* 55(1):45, 1999.

Chen YC: Chinese values, health and nursing, *J Adv Nurs* 36(2):270, 2001.

Cochran M: Tears have no color, *Am J Nurs* 98(6):53, 1998.

Cutliffe JR: Hope, counseling and complicated bereavement reactions, *J Adv Nurs* 28(4):754, 1998.

Cutcliffe JR, Grant G: What are the principles and processes of inspiring hope in cognitively impaired older adults within a continuing care environment? *J Psychiatr Ment Health Nurs* 8:427, 2001.

Dibartolo MC: Exploring self-efficacy and hardiness in spousal caregivers of individuals with dementia, *J Gerontol Nurs* 28(4):24, 2002.

Doswell W, Erlen J: Multicultural issues and ethical concerns in the delivery of nursing care interventions, *Nurs Clin North Am* 33(2):353, 1998.

Ducharme F, Trudeau D: Qualitative evaluation of a stress management intervention for elderly caregivers at home: a constructivist approach, *Issues Ment Health Nurs* 23:691, 2002.

Duggleby W: Hope at the end of life, *J Hospice Palliat Nurs* 3(2):51, 2001.

Ehrenberger HE et al: Testing a theory of decision-making derived from King's systems framework in women eligible for a cancer clinical trial, *Nurs Sci Q* 15(2):156, 2002.

Fritsch S et al: Personality characteristics of adolescent suicide attempters, *Child Psychiatry Hum Dev* 30(4):219, 2000.

Fryback PB, Reinert BR: Spirituality and people with potentially fatal diagnoses, *Nurs Forum* 34(1):13, 1999.

Fung W, Chien W: The effectiveness of a mutual support group for family caregivers of a relative with dementia, *Arch Psychiatr Nurs* 16(3):134, 2002.

Gaskins S, Forte L: The meaning of hope: implications for nursing practice and research, *J Gerontol Nurs* 21:17, 1995.

Harmon MP, Castro FG, Coe K: Acculturation and cervical cancer: knowledge, beliefs, and behaviors of Hispanic women, *Women Health* 24(3):37, 1996.

Heineken J: Patient silence is not necessarily client satisfaction: communication in home care nursing, *Home Healthc Nurse* 16(2):11, 1998.

Kylma J, Vehvilainen-Julkunen K, Lahdevirta J: Hope, despair and hopelessness in living with HIV/AIDS: a grounded theory study, *J Adv Nurs* 33(6):764, 2001.

Johnson LH, Dahlen R, Roberts SL: Supporting hope in congestive hearty failure patients, *Dimens Crit Care Nurs* 16(2):65, 1997.

Leininger MM, McFarland MR: *Transcultural nursing: concepts, theories, research and practices,* ed 3, New York, 2002, McGraw-Hill.

Malone KM et al: Protective factors against suicidal acts in major depression: reasons for living, *Am J Psychiatry* 157(7):1084, 2000.

Mapp I, Hudson R: Stress and coping among African American and Hispanic parents of deaf children, *Am Ann Deaf* 142(1):48, 1997.

Northouse L et al: A family-based program of care for women with recurrent breast cancer and their family members, *Oncol Nurs Forum* 29(10):1411, 2002.

Patusky KL, Rodning C, Martinez-Kratz M: Clinical lessons in psychiatric home care: a case study approach, *J Home Health Case Manag* 9:18, 1996.

Phillips JM, Cohen MZ, Moses G: Breast cancer screening and African American women: fear, fatalism, and silence, *Oncol Nurs Forum* 26(3):561, 1999.

Pinikahana J, Happell B: Exploring the complexity of compliance in schizophrenia, *Issues Ment Health Nurs* 23: 513, 2002.

Richer MC, Ezer H: Living in it, living with it, and moving on: dimensions of meaning during chemotherapy, *Oncol Nurs Forum* 29(1):113, 2002.

Samuel-Hodge CD et al: Influences on day-to-day self-management of type 2 diabetes among African-American women: spirituality, the multi-caregiver role, and other social context factors, *Diabetes Care* 23(7): 928, 2000.

Schreiber R: Wandering in the dark: women's experiences with depression, *Health Care Women Int* 22(1/2):85, 2001.

Uncapher H et al: Hopelessness and suicidal ideation in older adults, *Gerontologist* 38(1):62, 1998.

• = **Independent;** ▲ = **Collaborative**

Valente SM: Adolescent suicide: assessment and intervention, *J Child Adolesc Psychiatr Ment Health Nurs* 2:34, 1989.

Wang CH: Developing a concept of hope from a human science perspective, *Nurs Sci Q* 13(3):248, 2000.

Hyperthermia

Marcia LaHaie and Terry VandenBosch

NANDA | Definition

Body temperature elevated above normal range

NOTE: Elevated body temperature can be either fever or hyperthermia. Fever is a normal response in which the core body temperature increases at least 0.8° to 1.1° C (1.5° to 2.0° F) above an individual's normal temperature (>38° C [>100.5° F]). This elevation is in response to a chemical signal (endogenous pyrogen) released as part of an inflammatory response, such as in infection or tissue injury. Because there is a proportional enhancement of the immune system for each degree of temperature elevation, fever is believed to be adaptive to 40° C (104° F) (Kluger, 1991; Kluger et al, 1996). Hyperthermia is an abnormal increase in core body temperature, usually above 40° C (104° F), that occurs as a result of disorders of temperature control. Causes include brain trauma, heat stroke, drugs (e.g., cocaine, "ecstasy"), or malignant hyperthermia of anesthesia. Hyperthermia is not adaptive (Holtzclaw, 1992) and should be treated as a medical emergency.

Defining Characteristics

- Fever: core body temperature elevated at least 0.8° to 1.1° C (1.5° to 2.0° F) above individual's normal temperature (>38° C [>100.5° F])
- Hyperthermia: body temperature above 40° C (104° F) with flushed or hot skin, increased respiratory rate, and tachycardia

Related Factors (r/t)

- Fever: Infection; tissue injury; illness or trauma; dehydration; blood transfusion; medication; neoplasm; increased metabolic rate
- Hyperthermia: Exposure to hot environment; vigorous activity; inappropriate clothing; inability or decreased ability to perspire; brain injury; medication; anesthesia; severe illness; trauma

NOC | Outcomes (Nursing Outcomes Classification)

Suggested NOC Outcomes

Thermoregulation; Thermoregulation: Newborn

> #### Example NOC Outcome with Indicators
>
> **Thermoregulation** as evidenced by the following indicators: Body temperature WNL/Skin temperature IER/No skin color changes/Hydration adequate/Reported thermal comfort (Rate each indicator of **Thermoregulation:** 1 = extremely compromised, 2 = substantially compromised, 3 = moderately compromised, 4 = mildly compromised, 5 = not compromised [see Section I].)

IER, In expected range; *WNL,* within normal limits.

- = Independent; ▲ = Collaborative

Client Outcomes

Client Will (Specify Time Frame):
- Maintain oral temperature within adaptive levels (below 40° C [104° F]) or lower, depending on the presence of cardiopulmonary illness and client comfort
- Remain free of dehydration

NIC   Interventions (Nursing Interventions Classification)

Suggested NIC Interventions
Fever Treatment; Malignant Hyperthermia Precautions; Temperature Regulation

> **Example NIC Activities—Fever Treatment**
>
> Institute use of a continuous core temperature–monitoring device as appropriate; Monitor for decreasing levels of consciousness

Nursing Interventions and Rationales

▲ Assess an afebrile hospitalized client's temperature per institutional policy if the client exhibits signs or symptoms of infection, if the client has chills, or at least once a day between 5 PM and 7 PM. *Temperature screening of afebrile clients can be based on daily circadian rhythm patterns (Beaudry, VandenBosch, and Anderson, 1995). Shivering indicates a rising body temperature.*

• Measure and record a febrile client's temperature at least every 4 to 6 hours or whenever a change in condition occurs (e.g., chills, change in mental status). *Recognizing the pattern of a fever can help determine the source (Cunha, 1996; Holtzclaw, 1992).*

• Temperature can be measured with acceptable accuracy using an electronic probe in the mouth or via the external auditory canal (tympanic membrane) (Smitz et al, 2000). Although inconvenient, rectal temperature measurement is highly accurate (Schmitz et al, 1995; Varney et al, 2002). Use of a glass (mercury) thermometer is also highly accurate (Latman et al, 2001) but involves increased time (6 to 7 minutes), risk of mercury contamination, and risk of rectal perforation, although the occurrence is rare. Where equipment is available in ICU settings, temperature measurement by intravascular or bladder thermistor is a highly accurate method (Nierman, 1991). Axillary measurements should not be used (Schmitz et al, 1995). **Nursing Research:** *There was no significant difference between average oral and average tympanic temperatures in adult surgical clients (Gilbert, Barton, and Counsell, 2002).*

• Use the same site and method (device) for temperature measurement for a given client so that temperature trends are assessed accurately. **Nursing Research:** *A difference in the site (oral, rectal, axillary, pulmonary) of temperature measurement results in a significant difference in temperature reading (Schmitz et al, 1995).*

▲ Notify the physician of temperature according to institutional standards or written orders, or when temperature reaches 38° C (100.5° F). Also notify the physician of the presence of a change in mental status. *A change in mental status may indicate the onset of septic shock.*

▲ Administer antipyretic medication per physician orders, when infection-induced fever is above 40° C (104° F), and when the client cannot tolerate the increase in metabolic demand (Mackowiak and Plaisance, 1998). *The antipyretic acetaminophen is preferred over aspirin. Elimination of fever will interfere with its enhancement of the im-*

• = **Independent;** ▲ = **Collaborative**

mune response *(Klein and Cunha, 1996). Acetaminophen was better than aspirin for reducing fever in endotoxemia and did not affect the humoral response of the subjects (Pernerstorfer et al, 1999). Nonsteroidal antipyretic drugs can cause gastrointestinal toxicity (Plaisance, 2000).*

▲ Assess fluid loss and facilitate oral intake or administer intravenous fluids to accomplish fluid replacement. *Increased metabolic rate and diaphoresis associated with fever cause loss of body fluids.*

• When diaphoresis is present, assist the client with bathing and changing into dry clothing. *Bathing and clothing changes increase comfort and decrease the possibility of continued shivering caused by water evaporation from the skin.*

• Do not use external cooling measures such as ice packs, tepid water baths, or removal of blankets and clothing for fever management; these measures cause shivering and are ineffective. *External cooling induces both cutaneous vasoconstriction and shivering (Kurz et al, 1995). If the client's temperature drops in response to external cooling measures, the hypothalamus resets the body temperature at a higher level, which results in more shivering (Klein and Cunha, 1996). Shivering leads to significantly increased oxygen consumption (Holtzclaw, 1993).*

▲ Cooling blanket use is indicated for temperature reduction if the client's fever is above 40.6° C (105° F) and/or if a high body temperature is related to hyperthermia, a disorder of temperature regulation. *Cooling blankets are used when the client's oral temperature exceeds 40.6° C (105° F) and cannot be controlled by antipyretics (Styrt and Sugarman, 1990) and when the fever is caused by a heat-related illness (Morgan, 1990).*

▲ When using a cooling blanket, choose a convective airflow system, set the temperature regulator to 0.6° to 1.1° C (1° to 2° F) below the client's current temperature, and wrap the client's extremities with towels to prevent shivering. **Nursing Research:** *Blankets that use convective airflow for cooling may be more effective than those that cool by conductive water flow (Creechan, Vollman, and Kravutske, 2001). Higher blanket temperatures are as effective as lower temperatures in reducing fever and cause less discomfort (Caruso et al, 1992). To prevent shivering when a hypothermia blanket is used for fever reduction, wrap the client's extremities in towels (Caruso et al, 1992).*

Geriatric

• An oral temperature of 0.8° to 1.1° C (1.5° to 2.0° F) above baseline or above 37.2° C (99° F) (37.5° C [99.5° F] rectal temperature) should be considered a fever in the elderly. *Baseline temperature is lower in the elderly (Downton, Andrews, and Puxty, 1987). The upward limit for normal temperature in the elderly is 37.2° C (99° F) (Darowski, Weinbert, and Guz, 1991). Febrile response to infection was found to be reduced with increasing age, and baseline temperatures were generally lower in older clients (Roghmann, Warner, and Mackowiak, 2001).*

• Rectal temperature may be useful to diagnose fever. Nursing judgment must be used to determine if rectal temperature measurement is acceptable to the client, especially a client with mental changes or dementia. **Nursing Research:** *Rectal thermometry identified fevers in elderly clients that were missed by the oral and tympanic routes (Varney et al, 2002).*

• Assess for other signs and symptoms of infection in addition to or in the absence of fever in the elderly. *The temperature response is blunted in the elderly because of changes in physiology resulting from aging (Norman and Yoshikawa, 1996). In elderly clients with*

• = **Independent;** ▲ = **Collaborative**

a serious bacterial infection, 20% to 30% had a blunted or absent fever response (Norman, Grahn, and Yoshikawa, 1985). The onset of pyrexia in the elderly with infections can be delayed several hours; the delay was more than 12 hours for 12% of clients (McAlpine et al, 1986).

▲ Help the client seek medical attention immediately if fever is present. To diagnose the fever source, assess for possible precipitating factors, including changes in medication, environmental changes, and recent medical interventions or infectious exposures. *Fever in the elderly, especially the very old, is much more likely than in younger persons to be an indication of a serious bacterial infection (Norman and Yoshikawa, 1996). Hyperthermia can be precipitated by many medications prescribed for the elderly (Harchelroad, 1993).*

• In hot weather, encourage elderly clients to drink 8 to 10 glasses of fluid per day (within their cardiac and renal reserves) regardless of whether they are thirsty. Assess for the need for and presence of fans or air conditioning. *The elderly are more susceptible to a hot environment than are younger adults because of a decreased sensitivity to heat, decreased sweat gland function, and decreased thirst (Brody, 1994). The number of geriatric deaths rises as environmental temperatures increase in the hot summer months (Bull and Morton, 1978; Worfolk, 2000).*

▲ In hot weather, monitor the elderly client for signs of heat exhaustion: temperature of 37.8° C (100° F) to 38.9° C (102° F), orthostatic blood pressure signs, weakness, restlessness, mental status changes, faintness, thirst, nausea, and vomiting. If signs are present, move the client to a cool place, have the client lie down, give sips of water, check orthostatic blood pressure, sponge with tepid water, and notify the physician. *The elderly are predisposed to heat exhaustion and should be watched carefully for its occurrence; if it is present, it should be treated promptly (Worfolk, 2000).*

Home care

• Some of the interventions described previously may be adapted for home care use.
• Assess whether the client or family has a thermometer. Instruct as needed in the type of thermometer (non–mercury containing preferred; sublingual or tympanic location rather than skin patches) and how to use and read it accurately. *An accurate temperature reading is one indicator of the client's condition.*
▲ Teach the client and family to use acetaminophen rather than aspirin or ibuprofen for fever reduction at home to prevent possible adverse effects. (NOTE: Acetaminophen may be harmful if the client has liver or kidney dysfunction.)
• Help the client prevent and monitor for heat stroke/hyperthermia during times of high outdoor temperatures.
▲ In the event of temperature elevation above the adaptive range, institute measures to decrease temperature (e.g., get the client out of the sun and into a cool place, remove excess clothing, have the client drink fluids). Keep the physician informed if temperature does not stabilize below 40° C (104° F). Use an emergency plan as directed by a physician or when temperature indicators approach the level of hyperthermia. *Hyperthermia is an acute and possibly life-threatening symptom. The client cannot stay at home safely.*
▲ If the client is in hospice or is terminally ill, follow the client's wishes and the physician's orders in determining the management of fever. Keep the client comfortable and free of pain. *The goal of terminal care is to provide comfort and dignity during the dying process.*

• = **Independent**; ▲ = **Collaborative**

Client/Family Teaching

- Teach that infection-induced fever enhances the immune system (the beneficial effect occurs at oral temperatures of less than 40° C [104° F]), so the client can participate in the decision of whether to treat the fever. If treatment is elected or appropriate, instruct in the use of acetaminophen as the most effective means for fever reduction with fewer potential side effects than other antipyretics. *Fevers of less than 40° C (104° F) enhance immune system functioning (Roberts, 1991). Acetaminophen effectively reduces fever (Koch-Weser, 1976) and has less potential for detrimental effects (Aronoff and Neilson, 2001).*
- Teach the client that shivering with infection-induced fever has detrimental effects and that activities that can cause shivering (e.g., blanket removal, lowering of room temperature, tepid water baths, ice packs) should be avoided. *External cooling measures result in shivering and discomfort (Styrt and Sugarman, 1990).*
- Recommend a liberal intake of fluids to prevent heat-induced hyperthermia and dehydration in the presence of fever, but avoidance of liquids that contain alcohol, caffeine, or large amounts of sugar. *Liberal fluid intake replaces fluid lost through perspiration and respiration. The presence of alcohol, caffeine, and sugar in fluids can promote diuresis, unless the client regularly consumes that type of beverage.*
- Teach the client to stay in a cooler environment during periods of excessive outdoor heat or, if the client does go out, to avoid vigorous physical activity, wear lightweight, loose-fitting clothing, and wear a hat to minimize sun exposure. *Such methods reduce exposure to high environmental temperatures, which can cause heat stroke and hyperthermia.*

evolve WEBSITES FOR EDUCATION

See the EVOLVE website for World Wide Web resources for client education.

REFERENCES

Aronoff DM, Neilson EG: Antipyretics: mechanisms of action and clinical use in fever suppression, *Am J Med* 111:304, 2001.

Beaudry M, VandenBosch T, Anderson J: Research utilization: once a day temperatures for afebrile patients, *Clin Nurs Spec* 10:21, 1995.

Brody GM: Hyperthermia and hypothermia in the elderly, *Clin Geriatr Med* 10:213, 1994.

Bull G, Morton J: Environment, temperature, and death rates, *Age Ageing* 7:210, 1978.

Caruso CC et al: Cooling effects and comfort of four cooling blanket temperatures in humans with fever, *Nurs Res* 41(2):68, 1992.

Creechan T, Vollman K, Kravutske ME: Cooling by convection vs cooling by conduction for treatment of fever in critically ill adults, *Am J Crit Care* 10(1):52, 2001.

Cunha BA: The clinical significance of fever patterns, *Infect Dis Clin North Am* 10:33, 1996.

Darowski A, Weinbert JR, Guz A: Normal rectal, auditory, sublingual, and axillary temperature in febrile patients in a warm environment, *Age Ageing* 20:113, 1991.

Downton JH, Andrews K, Puxty JAH: Silent pyrexia in the elderly, *Age Ageing* 16:41, 1987.

Gilbert M, Barton AJ, Counsell CM: Comparison of oral and tympanic temperatures in adult surgical patients, *Appl Nurs Res* 15:42, 2002.

Harchelroad F: Acute thermoregulatory disorders, *Clin Geriatr Med* 9:621, 1993.

Holtzclaw BJ: The febrile response in critical care: state of the science, *Heart Lung* 21(5):482, 1992.

Klein NC, Cunha BA: Treatment of fever, *Infect Dis Clin North Am* 10:211, 1996.

Kluger MJ: Fever: role of pyrogens and cryogens, *Physiol Rev* 71:93, 1991.

Kluger MJ et al: The adaptive value of fever, *Infect Dis Clin North Am* 10:1, 1996.

• = Independent; ▲ = Collaborative

Koch-Weser J: Drug therapy. Acetaminophen, *N Engl J Med* 295:1297, 1976.

Kurz A et al: Heat balance and distribution during core-temperature plateau in anesthetized humans, *Anesthesiology* 83:491, 1995.

Latman NS et al: Evaluation of clinical thermometers for accuracy and reliability, *Biomed Instrum Technol* 35: 259, 2001.

Mackowiak P, Plaisance KI: Benefits and risks of antipyretic therapy, *Ann N Y Acad Sci* 856:214, 1998.

McAlpine CH et al: Pyrexia in infection in the elderly, *Age Ageing* 15:230, 1986.

Morgan SP: A comparison of three methods of managing fever in the neurologic patient, *J Neurosci Nurs* 22:19, 1990.

Nierman D: Core temperature measurement in the intensive care unit, *Crit Care Med* 19:818, 1991.

Norman DC, Grahn D, Yoshikawa TT: Fever and aging, *J Am Geriatr Soc* 33:859, 1985.

Norman DC, Yoshikawa TT: Fever in the elderly, *Infect Dis Clin North Am* 10:93, 1996.

Pernerstorfer T et al: Acetaminophen has greater antipyretic efficacy in endotoxemia: a randomized, double-blind, placebo-controlled trial, *Clin Pharmacol Ther* 66:51, 1999.

Plaisance KI: Toxicities of drugs used in the management of fever, *Clin Infect Dis* 31(suppl 5):S219, 2000.

Roberts NJ: The immunological consequences of fever. In Mackowiak PA, editor: *Fever: basic mechanisms and management*, New York, 1991, Raven Press.

Roghmann MC, Warner J, Mackowiak PA: The relationship between age and fever magnitude, *Am J Med Sci* 322:68, 2001.

Schmitz T et al: A comparison of five methods of temperature measurement in febrile intensive care patients, *Am J Crit Care* 4:286, 1995.

Smitz S et al: Comparison of rectal and infrared ear temperatures in older hospital inpatients, *J Am Geriatr Soc* 48(1):63, 2000.

Styrt B, Sugarman B: Antipyresis and fever, *Arch Intern Med* 150:1589, 1990.

Varney SM et al: A comparison of oral, tympanic, and rectal temperature measurement in the elderly, *J Emerg Med* 22:153, 2002.

Worfolk JB: Heat waves: their impact on the health of elders, *Geriatr Nurs* 21:70, 2000.

Hypothermia

Betty J. Ackley

NANDA Definition

Body temperature below normal range

Defining Characteristics

Pallor; reduction in body temperature below normal range; shivering; cool skin; cyanotic nailbeds; hypertension and then hypotension; piloerection; slow capillary refill; tachycardia

Related Factors (r/t)

Exposure to cool or cold environment; use of medications causing vasodilation; malnutrition; inadequate clothing; illness or trauma; evaporation from skin in cool environment; decreased metabolic rate; damage to hypothalamus; consumption of alcohol; aging; inability or decreased ability to shiver; inactivity

NOC Outcomes (Nursing Outcomes Classification)

Suggested NOC Outcomes

Thermoregulation; Thermoregulation: Newborn

• = Independent; ▲ = Collaborative

> **Example NOC Outcome with Indicators**
>
> **Thermoregulation** as evidenced by the following indicators: Body temperature WNL/Skin temperature IER/No skin color changes /Hydration adequate/Reported thermal comfort (Rate each indicator of **Thermo-regulation:** 1 = extremely compromised, 2 = substantially compromised, 3 = moderately compromised, 4 = mildly compromised, 5 = not compromised [see Section I].)

IER, In expected range; *WNL,* within normal limits.

Client Outcomes

Client Will (Specify Time Frame):
- Maintain body temperature within normal range
- Identify risk factors of hypothermia
- State measures to prevent hypothermia
- Identify symptoms of hypothermia and actions to take when hypothermia is present

NIC   Interventions (Nursing Interventions Classification)

Suggested NIC Interventions
Hypothermia Treatment; Temperature Regulation; Temperature Regulation: Intraoperative; Vital Signs Monitoring

> **Example NIC Activities—Temperature Regulation**
>
> Institute use of a continuous core temperature–monitoring device, as appropriate; Promote adequate fluid and nutritional intake

Nursing Interventions and Rationales

- Remove the client from the cause of the hypothermic episode (e.g., cold environment, cold or wet clothing). Ensure that the client is in a warm environment. *The goal is to eliminate the causative or contributing factor and begin the warming process.*
- Cover the client with warm blankets and apply a covering to the head and neck to conserve body heat. *Most heat is lost from the head and back; these areas should be warmly covered (Edwards, 1999).*
- Take the temperature at least hourly; if more than mild hypothermia is present (temperature lower than 35° C [95° F]), use a continuous temperature-monitoring device.
- ▲ Use a pulmonary artery catheter temperature-measuring device if available; if not, consider using a bladder catheter that measures temperature. **Nursing Research:** *Measurement of the pulmonary artery temperature is considered the gold standard in assessing core body temperature. If a pulmonary artery catheter is not appropriate for the client, temperature measurement with a temperature-sensitive indwelling urinary catheter can be effective and provide a reliable indication of core temperature (Erickson and Meyer, 1994; Fallis, 2002).*
- If the client is awake, measure the oral temperature, instead of the tympanic or axillary temperature. **Nursing Research:** *Oral temperature measurement provides a more accurate temperature than tympanic measurement (Fisk and Arcona, 2001; Giuliano et al, 2000; Lee, McKenzie, and Cathcart, 1999). Axillary temperatures are often inaccurate*

• = Independent; ▲ = Collaborative

(Fulbrook, 1997). The oral temperature is usually accurate even in an intubated client (Fallis, 2002).

- Monitor the client's vital signs every hour and as appropriate. Note changes associated with hypothermia, such as initially increased pulse rate, respiratory rate, and blood pressure with mild hypothermia, and then decreased pulse rate, respiratory rate, and blood pressure with moderate to severe hypothermia. *With mild hypothermia, there is activation of the sympathetic nervous system, which can increase the values of vital signs. As hypothermia progresses, decreased circulating volume develops, which results in decreased cardiac output and depressed oxygen delivery. Hypoxia, metabolic acidosis, and intrinsic irritability of a cold myocardium result in various dysrhythmias (Edwards, 1999; Ruffolo, 2002; Smith and Yamat, 2000).*

- Attach electrodes and a cardiac monitor. Watch for dysrhythmias. *With hypothermia the client is prone to dysrhythmias because of the cold myocardium; dysrhythmias may include atrial fibrillation, ventricular fibrillation, or asystole (Andreoni and Massey, 2001; Ruffolo, 2002).*

- Monitor for signs of hypothermia (e.g., shivering, cool skin, piloerection, pallor, slow capillary refill, cyanotic nailbeds, decreased mentation, coma). *Such monitoring indicates the client's response to interventions and provides evidence of persistent hypothermia.*

- Monitor for signs of coagulopathy (e.g., oozing of blood from any open areas or from intravascular catheter sites or mucous membranes). Also note results of clotting studies as available. *Coagulopathy is a common occurrence during hypothermia in trauma clients (Eddy, Morris, and Cullinane, 2000; Ruffolo, 2002).*

▲ For mild hypothermia (core temperature of 35° C [95° F]), rewarm client passively:
  - Set room temperature to 21° to 24° C (70° to 75° F).
  - Layer clothing and blankets and cover the client's head; use insulated metallic blankets.
  - Keep the client dry.
  - Offer warm fluid if the physician has ordered it.

- For mild hypothermia, allow the client to rewarm at his or her own pace. Heat is regained through the body's ability to generate heat. *Passive rewarming is not encouraged for clients with temperatures lower than 28° C (82.4° F) because it is a slow process and may increase the risk of cardiac arrest in these circumstances (Cochrane, 2001; Edwards, 1999).*

▲ For moderate hypothermia (core temperature 32° to 28° C [89.6° to 82.4° F]) use active external rewarming methods. The rewarming rate should not exceed 1° C (1.8° F) per hour. Methods include the following:
  - Carbon-fiber resistive heating blanket
  - Electric blankets
  - Radiant heat lights

  Clinical Research: *Resistive heating using a carbon-fiber blanket was shown to be much more effective to rewarm hypothermic subjects than use of metallic-foil blankets (Greif et al, 2000). The carbon-fiber resistive heating blanket was shown to be more effective than regular blankets to maintain the client's core body temperatures during transport (Kober et al, 2001).*

▲ For severe hypothermia (core temperature below 28° C [82.4° F]) use active core-rewarming techniques:
  - Administer heated and humidified oxygen through the ventilator as ordered.
  - Administer heated IV fluids at prescribed temperature.

- **• = Independent; ▲ = Collaborative**

■ Perform peritoneal lavage, bladder irrigations, or continuous arteriovenous extracorporeal blood rewarming, per physician's order.

■ Recognize that the client may need cardiopulmonary bypass to maintain life. *Severe hypothermia is associated with acidosis, coma, ventricular fibrillation, apnea, thrombocytopenia, platelet dysfunction, impaired clotting, and increased mortality in trauma clients and requires prompt core body rewarming (Eddy, Morris, and Cullinane, 2000; Ruffolo, 2002).*

• Check blood pressure frequently when rewarming; watch for hypotension. *As the body warms, formerly vasoconstricted vessels dilate, which results in hypotension (Edwards, 1999).*

▲ Administer IV fluids, using a rapid infuser IV fluid warmer as ordered. *Fluids are often needed to maintain adequate fluid volume. If the client develops untreated fluid depletion, hypotension with decreased cardiac output and acute renal failure can result (Edwards, 1999). A rapid infuser warmer is needed to keep IV fluids warmed sufficiently to be effective in raising the body temperature (Ruffolo, 2002).*

• Determine the factors leading to the hypothermic episode; see Related Factors. *It is important to assess risk factors and precipitating events to prevent another incident of hypothermia and to direct treatment.*

▲ Request a social service referral to help the client obtain the heat, shelter, and food needed to maintain body temperature. *A preventive approach that includes adequate food and fluid intake, shelter, heat, and clothing decreases the risk of hypothermia.*

▲ Encourage proper nutrition and hydration. Request a referral to a dietitian to identify appropriate dietary needs. *Insufficient calorie and fluid intake predispose the client to hypothermia.*

Geriatric

• Assess neurological signs frequently, watching for confusion and decreased level of consciousness. *Older adults are less likely to shiver or complain of feeling cold. Early signs of hypothermia are subtle (Florez-Duquet and McDonald, 1998).*

• Warm a hypothermic elderly client slowly, at a rate of 0.6° C (1° F) per hour. *Slow warming avoids overheating and allows the body to accommodate, which decreases the risk of complications (Miller, 1995).*

Home care

NOTE: Hypothermia is not a symptom that appears in the normal course of home care. When it occurs, it is a clinical emergency and the client/family should access emergency medical services immediately.

• Some of the interventions described earlier may be adapted for home care use.

• Before a medical crisis occurs, confirm that the client or family has a thermometer and can read it. Instruct as needed. Verify that the thermometer registers accurately. *An accurate temperature is one indicator of the client's condition.*

• Instruct the client or family to take the temperature when the client displays cyanosis, pallor, or shivering.

▲ Monitor temperature every hour, as noted previously. *If the temperature of the client begins dropping below the normal range, apply layers of clothing or blankets, or adjust environmental heat to the comfort level. Do not overheat. Contact a physician. Passive rewarming is the only method of rewarming that is appropriate for home care under normal circumstances.*

• = Independent; ▲ = Collaborative

▲ If temperature continues to drop, activate the emergency system and notify a physician. *Hypothermia is a clinically acute condition that cannot be managed safely in the home.*

▲ If the client is in hospice care or is terminally ill, follow advance directives, client wishes, and the physician's orders. Keep the client free of pain. *The goal of terminal care is to provide dignity and comfort during the dying process.*

Client/Family Teaching

• Teach the client and family signs of hypothermia and the method of taking the temperature (age-appropriate).

• Teach the client methods to prevent hypothermia: wearing adequate clothing, including a hat and mittens; heating the environment to a minimum of 20° C (68° F); and ingesting adequate food and fluid. *Simple measures such as layering clothes, wearing a hat, and avoiding extremes in temperature prevent significant heat loss (Laskowski-Jones, 2000).*

▲ Teach the client and family about medications such as sedatives, opioids, and anxiolytics that predispose the client to hypothermia (as appropriate). *If the client has had hypothermia in the past, using alternative medications is an option if there is no contraindication (Miller, 1995).*

evolve WEBSITES FOR EDUCATION

See the EVOLVE website for World Wide Web resources for client education.

REFERENCES

Anderoni C, Massey D: Continuous arteriovenous rewarming: rapid restoration of normothermia in the emergency department, *J Emerg Nurs* 27(6):533, 2001.

Cochrane DA: Hypothermia: a cold influence on trauma, *Int J Trauma Nurs* 7(1):8, 2001.

Eddy VA, Morris JA, Cullinane DC: Hypothermia, coagulopathy, and acidosis, *Surg Clin North Am* 80(3):845, 2000.

Edwards S: Hypothermia, *Prof Nurse* 14(4):253, 1999.

Erickson RS, Meyer LT: Accuracy of infrared ear thermometry and other temperature methods in adults, *Am J Crit Care* 3(1):40, 1994.

Fallis WM: Monitoring urinary bladder temperature in the intensive care unit: state of the science, *Am J Crit Care* 11(1):38, 2002.

Fisk J, Arcona S: Comparing tympanic membrane and pulmonary artery catheter temperatures, *Dimens Crit Care Nurs* 20(2):44, 2001.

Florez-Duquet M, McDonald RB: Cold-induced thermoregulation and biological aging, *Physiol Rev* 78(2):339, 1998.

Fulbrook P: Core body temperature measurement: a comparison of axilla, tympanic membrane and pulmonary artery blood temperature, *Intensive Crit Care Nurs* 13(5):266, 1997.

Giuliano KK et al: Temperature measurement in critically ill adults: a comparison of tympanic and oral methods, *Am J Crit Care* 9(4):254, 2000.

Greif R et al: Resistive heating is more effective than metallic-foil insulation in an experimental model of accidental hypothermia: a randomized controlled trial, *Ann Emerg Med* 35(4):337, 2000.

Kober A et al: Effectiveness of resistive heating compared with passive warming in treating hypothermia associated with minor trauma: a randomized trial, *Mayo Clin Proc* 76(4):369, 2001.

Laskowski-Jones L: Responding to winter emergencies, *Nursing* 30(1):34, 2000.

Lee VK, McKenzie NE, Cathcart M: Ear and oral temperatures under usual practice conditions, *Res Nurs Pract* 1(1):8, 1999.

Miller CA: *Nursing care of older adults,* ed 2, Glenview, Ill, 1995, Scott Foresman/Little, Brown.

Ruffolo DC: Hypothermia in trauma: the cold, hard facts, *RN* 65(2):46, 2002.

Smith CE, Yamat RA: Avoiding hypothermia in the trauma patient, *Curr Opin Anaesthesiol* 13:167, 2000.

• = **Independent**; ▲ = **Collaborative**

Disturbed personal Identity

Gail B. Ladwig

NANDA   **Definition**

Inability to distinguish between self and nonself

Defining Characteristics

Withdrawal from social contact; change in ability to determine relationship of the body to the environment; inappropriate or grandiose behavior (Carpenito, 1993)

Related Factors (r/t)

Situational crisis; psychological impairment; chronic illness; pain

NOC   **Outcomes (Nursing Outcomes Classification)**

Suggested NOC Outcomes

Identity; Personal Autonomy

> **Example NOC Outcome with Indicators**
>
> **Identity:** Verbalizes affirmations of personal identity/Exhibits congruent verbal and nonverbal behavior/ Distinguishes self from environment and other human beings (Rate each indicator of **Identity:** 1 = never demonstrated, 2 = rarely demonstrated, 3 = sometimes demonstrated, 4 = often demonstrated, 5 = consistently demonstrated [see Section I].)

Client Outcomes

Client Will (Specify Time Frame):
- Show interest in surroundings
- Respond to stimuli with appropriate affect
- Perform self-care and self-control activities appropriate for age
- Acknowledge personal strengths
- Engage in interpersonal relationships
- Verbalize willingness to change lifestyle and use appropriate community resources

NIC   **Interventions (Nursing Interventions Classification)**

Suggested NIC Interventions

Decision-Making Support; Self-Esteem Enhancement

> **Example NIC Activities—Decision-Making Support**
>
> Inform client of alternative views or solutions; Facilitate client's articulation of goals for care

Nursing Interventions and Rationales

- Assess carefully for a history of abuse. **Clinical Research:** *In one series of clients fulfilling diagnostic criteria for dissociative identity disorder, otherwise known as multiple person-*

• = **Independent;** ▲ = **Collaborative**

ality disorder, the disorder represented a significant component of a complex syndrome associated with a history of severe ongoing developmental trauma dating from early childhood (Middleton and Butler, 1998).

- Assess for any history of seizure disorder; adhere to the diagnostic criteria for dissociative disorder in the *Diagnostic and Statistical Manual of Mental Disorders,* fourth edition *(DSM-IV)* and conduct a structured clinical interview. **Clinical Research:** *Misdiagnosis of persons with seizures and dissociative symptoms can be avoided by careful adherence to DSM-IV dissociative disorder criteria, the use of video-electroencephalographic monitoring, and systematic assessment of dissociative symptoms with the Structured Clinical Interview for DSM-IV (SCID-D) (Bowman and Coons, 2000).*

- Avoid labeling the client with terms such as multiple personality disorder (MPD). **Clinical Research:** *In one study more clients attempted suicide after being diagnosed with MPD than before diagnosis; the reverse was true for other clients hospitalized with a mood disorder (Fetkewicz, Sharma, and Merskey, 2000).*

- Offer reassurance to the client and use therapeutic communication at frequent intervals. **Clinical Research:** *Reassurance of the client and communication are nursing skills that promote trust and orientation and reduce anxiety (Harvey, 1996).*

- Work with the client on setting personal goals. *Social production function theory asserts that people produce their own well-being by trying to optimize achievement of universal human goals (Ormel et al, 1997).*

- Address the client by name. Let the client know who is approaching and orient the client to the surroundings. *These interventions help the client with loss of ego boundaries to identify boundaries between himself or herself and the environment (Haber et al, 1992).*

- Provide communication, clear rules and aims, and safety procedures. **Nursing Research:** *One study demonstrated that with these interventions the use of seclusion for aggressive client behavior was substantially reduced (Mistral et al, 2002).*

- Have the client describe his or her perceptions of the environment as concretely as possible. *These descriptions provide feedback that confirms the client's existence.*

- Give the client permission to share his or her experiences. The client has always lived in secrecy and is not sure how much it is safe to reveal or who believes that the client's illness is an actual illness. **Clinical Research:** *An average of 6.8 years elapses between the time clients are first assessed and the time they receive an accurate diagnosis (Frye, 1990).*

- Use touch only after a thorough assessment and as appropriate. *Touch, which conveys caring, is an appropriate way of communicating unless it makes the person touched feel uncomfortable (Wells-Federman et al, 1995).* **Nursing Research:** *Some clients may touch people to identify separateness from others; other clients experience fusion with others when they touch (Haber et al, 1992).*

▲ Have all team members approach the client in a consistent manner. *Consistency promotes trust, which is necessary to establish a therapeutic relationship that helps the client develop interpersonal relationships.*

- Provide time for one-on-one interactions to establish a therapeutic relationship. **Nursing Research:** *Nursing presence, one-on-one interaction, connecting with the client's experience, going beyond the scientific data, and knowing what will work and when to act all support the nurse-client relationship and affirm the respective selves of nurse and client. As a result, the client grows in awareness of his or her own being (Doona, Chase, and Haggerty, 1999).*

- Encourage the client to verbalize feelings about self and body image. Have the client

• = **Independent;** ▲ = **Collaborative**

make a list of strengths. **Clinical Research:** *These verbalizations help the client recognize the self; listing strengths promotes self-exploration. In one study 48 women in a psychiatric outpatient clinic completed a survey whose results indicated a correlation between border-line personality and body weight/body image issues that were not necessarily a result of larger size (Sansone, Wiederman, and Monteith, 2001).*

- Hold the client responsible for age-appropriate behavior. Involve the client in the planning of self-care. *Involving clients in care gives them a sense of control and helps clients gain ego strength (Preston, 1994).*
- Give positive feedback when appropriate self-control is used. **Clinical Research:** *When given positive feedback, the boys in one study were able to relax their defensive posture and offer more realistic self-assessment (Diener and Milich, 1997).*
- ▲ Encourage participation in group therapy for building relationship skills and getting feedback from others with regard to behavior. **Clinical Research:** *Findings suggest that social skills training resulted in greater improvement in certain measures of social adjust-ment than supportive group therapy (Marder et al, 1996).* **Nursing Research:** *An adap-tive narcissistic client's need to depend on other people to feel whole suggests that group therapy could be a powerful tool for treating those who suffer profound wounds to self-esteem (Kurek-Ovshinsky, 1991).*
- Encourage the client to use a daily diary to set achievable and realistic goals and to monitor successes. *Journal writing has been found to improve physical and mental health measurably (Wells-Federman et al, 1995).*

Geriatric

- ▲ Monitor for signs of depression, grief, and withdrawal and make an appropriate refer-ral. *The disturbed personal identity may mask underlying depression.*
- Address the client by his or her full name preceded by the proper title (Mr., Mrs., Ms., Miss); use a nickname or first name only if suggested by the client, and do not use terms of endearment (e.g., "honey"). **Nursing Research:** *Research findings emphasize the importance of relationship-oriented experiences as part of assessment and interven-tion strategies for individuals with depression (Hagerty and Williams, 1999).*
- Practice reality orientation principles; ask specifically how the client feels about events that are happening. **Evidence-Based Research:** *Reality orientation therapy has ben-efits for both the cognition and behavior of dementia sufferers (Spector et al, 2000).*
- Ask the client about important past experiences. **Nursing Research:** *Factors that influ-ence self-efficacy beliefs are personal expectations, personality, role models, verbal encour-agement, progress, past experiences, spirituality, physical sensations, individualized care, social supports, and goals (Resnick, 2002).*
- ▲ If the client's symptoms are associated with a stroke, refer the client for longer rehabil-itation that includes physical programs addressing psychological as well as neuromus-cular issues. **Clinical Research:** *Clients who have had a stroke find the body unreliable, and the body appears separate from the self. These feelings may last a year or longer (Ellis-Hill, Payne, and Ward, 2000).*

Multicultural

- Assess for the influence of cultural beliefs, norms, and values on the family's percep-tions of infant/child behavior. **Nursing Research:** *What the family considers normal infant/child behavior may be based on cultural perceptions (Cochran, 1998; Doswell and Erlen, 1998; Guarnaccia, 1998; Leininger and McFarland, 2002).*

- **= Independent; ▲ = Collaborative**

- Use a neutral, indirect style when addressing areas in which improvement is needed (such as a need for verbal or oral stimulation) when working with Native American clients. **Nursing Research:** *Using indirect statements such as "Other mothers have tried . . . " or "I had a client who tried 'X' and it seemed to work very well" help to avoid resentment on the part of the parent (Seiderman et al, 1996).*
- Acknowledge and praise parenting strengths noted. **Nursing Research:** *This practice will increase trust and foster a working relationship with the parent (Seiderman et al, 1996).*
- Use therapeutic communication techniques that emphasize acceptance, offer the self, validate the client's concerns, and convey respect when discussing infant/child behavior. **Nursing Research:** *Validation is a therapeutic communication technique that lets the client know that the nurse has heard and understood what was said, and it promotes the nurse-client relationship (Heineken, 1998). Studies show that even when language is not a barrier, some ethnic clients may be reluctant to discuss their beliefs and practices because of fear of criticism or ridicule (Evans and Cunningham, 1996).*

Home care
- The interventions described previously may be adapted for home care use.
- Assess the client's immediate support system and family for relationship patterns and content of communication. *Knowledge of relationship dynamics in the client's environment assists the nurse in individualizing care.*
- Encourage the family to provide support and feedback regarding the client's identity and ego boundaries. *The family is a socially significant cultural group that generates behavior, defines roles, and promotes values.*
- ▲ If the client is involved in counseling or self-help groups, monitor and encourage attendance. Help the client identify the value of group participation after each group encounter. *Discussion of group participation identifies group feedback and support, and reinforces support for change.*
- ▲ If the client is taking prescribed psychotropic medications, assess for understanding of possible side effects and the reasons for taking medication. Teach as necessary.
- ▲ Assess medications for effectiveness and side effects and monitor for compliance. *Clients with poor ego strength may have difficulty adhering to a medication regimen.*
- ▲ If the client is homebound, refer for psychiatric home health care services for client reassurance and implementation of a therapeutic regimen. **Clinical Nursing:** *Psychiatric home care nurses can address issues relating to the client's identity, reality testing, and reaction to identity disturbance. Behavioral interventions in the home can help the client to participate more effectively in the treatment plan (Patusky, Rodning, and Martinez-Kratz, 1996).*

Client/Family Teaching
- Teach stress reduction and relaxation techniques. *These techniques can be used when the client becomes anxious about the loss of self.*
- ▲ Refer to community resources or other self-help groups appropriate for the client's underlying problem (e.g., Adult Children of Alcoholics, parent effectiveness group). **Nursing Research:** *Group therapy provides an arena in which clients can experience the interdependent mode of adaptation without assaults to self-esteem (Kurek-Ovshinsky, 1991).*

• = **Independent;** ▲ = **Collaborative**

▲ Refer to appropriate treatment as soon as signs of depression are noted. **Clinical Research:** *Effective acute-phase depression treatment reduced somatic distress and improved self-rated overall health (Simon et al, 1998). Results of a study using clinical significance methodology and encompassing 4761 clients undergoing standard psychotherapy in the United States revealed that between 15 and 19 treatment sessions were required for a 50% recovery rate (Hansen et al, 2003).*

• Be a role model for family members: talk to, not around, the client; give choices to the client when family members may be listening; always address the client by name; and do not interrupt when the client is attempting to communicate. **Nursing Research:** *Validation is a therapeutic communication technique that lets the client know that the nurse has heard and understood what was said, and it promotes the nurse-client relationship (Heineken, 1998).*

evolve WEBSITES FOR EDUCATION

See the EVOLVE website for World Wide Web resources for client education.

REFERENCES

Bowman ES, Coons PM: The differential diagnosis of epilepsy, pseudoseizures, dissociative identity disorder, and dissociative disorder not otherwise specified, *Bull Menninger Clin* 64(2):164, 2000.

Carpenito LJ: *Nursing diagnosis: application to clinical practice,* ed 5, Philadelphia, 1993, Lippincott.

Cochran M: Tears have no color, *Am J Nurs* 98(6):53, 1998.

Diener MB, Milich R: Effects of positive feedback on the social interactions of boys with attention deficit hyperactivity disorder: a test of the self-protective hypothesis, *J Clin Child Psychol* 26(3):256, 1997.

Doona M, Chase S, Haggerty L: Nursing presence: as real as Milky Way bar, *J Holist Nurs* 17(1):54, 1999.

Doswell W, Erlen J: Multicultural issues and ethical concerns in the delivery of nursing care interventions, *Nurs Clin North Am* 33(2):353, 1998.

Ellis-Hill CS, Payne S, Ward C: Self-body split: issues of identity in physical recovery following a stroke, *Disabil Rehabil* 22(16):725, 2000.

Evans CA, Cunningham BA: Caring for the ethnic elder, *Geriatr Nurs* 17(3):105, 1996.

Fetkewicz J, Sharma V, Merskey H: A note on suicidal deterioration with recovered memory treatment, *J Affect Disord* 58(2):155, 2000.

Frye B: Art and multiple personality disorder: an expressive framework for occupational therapy, *Am J Occup Ther* 44:1013, 1990.

Guarnaccia P: Multicultural experiences of family caregiving: a study of African American, European American, and Hispanic American families, *New Direct Ment Health Serv* 77:45, 1998.

Haber J et al: *Psychiatric nursing,* ed 4, St Louis, 1992, Mosby.

Hagerty BM, Williams RA: The effects of sense of belonging, social support, conflict, and loneliness on depression, *Nurs Res* 48(4):215, 1999.

Hansen NB, Lambert MJ: An evaluation of the dose-response relationship in naturalistic treatment settings using survival analysis, *Ment Health Serv Res* 5(1):1, 2003.

Harvey M: Managing agitation in critically ill patients, *Am J Crit Care* 5:7, 1996.

Heineken J: Patient silence is not necessarily client satisfaction: communication in home care nursing, *Home Healthc Nurse* 16(2):115, 1998.

Kurek-Ovshinsky C: Group psychotherapy in an acute inpatient setting: techniques that nourish self-esteem, *Issues Ment Health Nurs* 12:81, 1991.

Leininger MM, McFarland MR: *Transcultural nursing: concepts, theories, research and practices,* ed 3, New York, 2002, McGraw-Hill.

Marder SR et al: Two-year outcome of social skills training and group psychotherapy for outpatients with schizophrenia, *Am J Psychiatry* 153(12):1585, 1996.

Middleton W, Butler J: Dissociative identity disorder: an Australian series, *Aust N Z J Psychiatry* 32(6):794, 1998.

• = **Independent;** ▲ = **Collaborative**

Mistral W et al: Using therapeutic community principles to improve the functioning of a high care psychiatric ward in the UK, *Int J Ment Health Nurs* 11(1):10, 2002.

Ormel J et al: Quality of life and social production functions: a framework for understanding health effects, *Soc Sci Med* 45(7):1051, 1997.

Patusky KL, Rodning C, Martinez-Kratz M: Clinical lessons in psychiatric home care: a case study approach, *J Home Health Case Manag* 9:18, 1996.

Preston K: Rehabilitation nursing: a client-centered philosophy, *Am J Nurs* 94:66, 1994.

Resnick B: Geriatric rehabilitation: the influence of efficacy beliefs and motivation, *Rehabil Nurs* 27(4):152, 2002.

Sansone RA, Wiederman MW, Monteith D: Obesity, borderline personality symptomatology, and body image among women in a psychiatric outpatient setting, *Int J Eat Disord* 29(1):76, 2001.

Seiderman RY et al: Assessing American Indian families, *MCN Am J Matern Child Nurs* 21(6):274, 1996.

Simon G et al: Impact of improved depression treatment in primary care on daily functioning and disability, *Psychol Med* 28(3):693, 1998.

Spector A et al: Reality orientation for dementia (Cochrane Review), *Cochrane Database Syst Rev* 4(CD001119), 2000.

Wells-Federman C et al: The mind-body connection: the psychophysiology of many traditional nursing interventions, *Clin Nurse Spec* 9:59, 1995.

Functional urinary Incontinence

Mikel Gray

NANDA Definition

Impairment or loss of continence due to functional deficits, including altered mobility, dexterity, or cognition, or environmental barriers

Defining Characteristics

The relationship between functional limitations and urinary incontinence remains controversial (Hunskaar et al, 1999). While functional impairment clearly exacerbates the severity of urinary incontinence, the underlying factors that contribute to these functional limitations themselves contribute to abnormal lower urinary tract function and impaired continence.

Related Factors (r/t)

Cognitive disorders (delirium, dementia, severe or profound retardation); neuromuscular limitations impairing mobility or dexterity; environmental barriers to toileting

NOC Outcomes (Nursing Outcomes Classification)

Suggested NOC Outcomes

Urinary Continence; Urinary Elimination

Example NOC Outcome with Indicators

Urinary Continence as evidenced by the following indicators: Recognizes urge to void/Responds in timely manner to urge/Voids in appropriate receptacle/Underclothing remains dry during day/Underclothing or bedding remains dry during night (Rate each indicator of **Urinary Continence:** 1 = never demonstrated, 2 = rarely demonstrated, 3 = sometimes demonstrated, 4 = often demonstrated, 5 = consistently demonstrated [see Section I].)

• = Independent; ▲ = Collaborative

Client Outcomes

Client Will (Specify Time Frame):
- Eliminate or reduce incontinent episodes
- Eliminate or overcome environmental barriers to toileting
- Use adaptive equipment to reduce or eliminate incontinence related to impaired mobility or dexterity
- Use portable urinary collection devices or urine containment devices when access to the toilet is not feasible

NIC Interventions (Nursing Interventions Classification)

Suggested NIC Interventions
Urinary Habit Training; Urinary Incontinence Care

> **Example NIC Activities—Urinary Habit Training**
>
> Keep continence specification record for 3 days to establish voiding pattern; Establish interval for toileting of preferably not less than 2 hours

Nursing Interventions and Rationales
- Perform a history taking and physical assessment focusing on bothersome lower urinary tract symptoms, cognitive status, functional status (particularly physical mobility and dexterity), frequency and severity of leakage episodes, and alleviating and aggravating factors. *The history provides clues to the causes, the severity of the condition, and its management (Reuben et al, 1999; Vickerman, 2002).* **Nursing Research:** *Results of physical assessment, functional evaluation (mobility toileting skills, physical examination), and evaluation of cognitive status (Folstein Mini–Mental Status Examination) and psychological status (Geriatric Depression Scale) for a group of 90 homebound elders participating in a clinical trial revealed that functional impairments are associated with frequent and severe incontinence. Although these problems were perceived as particularly bothersome (despite multiple comorbid health issues) elders in this group remained optimistic about potential benefits of treatment (Folstein et al, 1975; McDowell et al, 1996).*
- ▲ Consult with the client and family, the client's physician, and other health care professionals concerning treatment of incontinence in the elderly client undergoing detailed geriatric evaluation. **Nursing Research:** *Geriatric assessment units are designed to evaluate and assist clients and their families to deal with multiple problems experienced by geriatric clients, including urinary incontinence. In a study of 128 older adults recruited into a randomized clinical trial of behavioral treatment for urinary incontinence, although treatment was recommended for two-thirds, nearly one third received no incontinence treatment recommendation. The recommendation for no treatment was based on a complex assessment of the client's physical health, comorbid conditions, and cognitive and psychological status (Silverman et al, 1997).*
- Complete a bladder log of diurnal and nocturnal urine elimination patterns, and patterns of urinary leakage. *A bladder log provides a more objective indication of urine elimination patterns than the history (Resnick et al, 1994) and a baseline against which the results of management can be evaluated.*
- ▲ Assess the client for potentially reversible or modifiable causes of acute/transient urinary incontinence (e.g., urinary tract infection; atrophic urethritis; constipation or

• = **Independent;** ▲ = **Collaborative**

impaction; use of sedatives or narcotics interfering with the ability to reach the toilet in a timely fashion, antidepressants or psychotropic medications interfering with efficient detrusor contractions, parasympatholytics, or alpha-adrenergic antagonists; polyuria caused by uncontrolled diabetes mellitus or insipidus). *Transient or acute incontinence may be relieved or eliminated by treating the underlying cause (Reilly, 2002).*

- Assess the client in an acute care or rehabilitation facility for risk factors for functional incontinence. **Nursing Research:** *Risk factors for urinary incontinence among elderly women admitted to an acute care facility include confusion, use of a wheelchair or assistive device for walking, and dependence on others for ambulation prior to admission (Palmer et al, 2002).*
- Assess the client for coexisting or premorbid urinary incontinence. *Research involving clients recovering from a stroke indicates that a history of premorbid urinary incontinence predicts a higher risk for persistent urinary leakage and poorer functional outcomes at 6 and 12 months (Jawad, Ward, and Jones, 1999; Thommessen, Bautz-Holter, and Laake, 1999).*
- Assess the home, acute care, or long-term care environment for accessibility to toileting facilities, paying particular attention to the following:
  - Distance of the toilet from the bed, chair, and living quarters
  - Characteristics of the bed, including presence of side rails and distance of the bed from the floor
  - Characteristics of the pathway to the toilet, including barriers such as stairs, loose rugs on the floor, and inadequate lighting
  - Characteristics of the bathroom, including patterns of use, lighting, height of the toilet from the floor, presence of handrails to assist transfers to the toilet, and breadth of the door and its accessibility for a wheelchair, walker, or other assistive device

  Functional continence requires access to a toilet; environmental barriers blocking this access can produce functional incontinence (Wells, 1992).
- Assess the client for mobility, including the ability to rise from chair and bed, transfer to the toilet, and ambulate, and the need for physical assistive devices such as a cane, walker, or wheelchair. *Functional continence requires the ability to gain access to a toilet facility, either independently or with the assistance of devices to increase mobility (Jirovec and Wells, 1990; Wells, 1992).*
- ▲ Assess the client for dexterity, including the ability to manipulate buttons, hooks, snaps, Velcro, and zippers as needed to remove clothing. Consult a physical or occupational therapist to promote optimal toilet access as indicated. *Functional continence requires the ability to remove clothing to urinate (Maloney and Cafiero, 1999; Wells, 1992).*
- Evaluate cognitive status with a Neecham Confusion Scale (Neelan et al, 1992) in cases of acute cognitive change or with a Folstein Mini-Mental State Examination (Folstein et al, 1975) or other tool as indicated. *Functional continence requires sufficient mental acuity to respond to sensory input from a filling urinary bladder by locating the toilet, moving to it, and emptying the bladder (Maloney and Cafiero, 1999; McDowell et al, 1996).*
- Remove environmental barriers to toileting in the acute care, long-term care, or home setting. Assist the client in removing loose rugs from the floor and improving lighting in hallways and bathrooms. *Functional continence requires ready access to a urinal (Wells, 1992).*
- Provide an appropriate, safe urinary receptacle such as a three-in-one commode, female or male hand-held urinal, no-spill urinal, or containment device when toilet-

- = **Independent**; ▲ = **Collaborative**

ing access is limited by immobility or environmental barriers. *These receptacles provide access to a substitute toilet and enhance the potential for functional continence (Rabin, 1998; Wells, 1992).*

▲ Help the client with limited mobility to obtain evaluation by a physical therapist and to obtain assistive devices as indicated; assist the client in selecting shoes with a nonskid sole to maximize traction when arising from a chair and transferring to the toilet. *A physical therapist is an important member of the interdisciplinary team needed to manage urinary incontinence in the client with functional impairments (Maloney and Cafiero, 1999).*

• Assist the client in altering the wardrobe to maximize toileting access. Select loose-fitting clothing with stretch waistbands rather than buttoned or zippered waist; minimize buttons, snaps, and multilayered clothing; and substitute Velcro or other easily loosened systems for buttons, hooks, and zippers in existing clothing.

• Begin a prompted voiding program or patterned urge response toileting program for the elderly client in the home or a long-term care facility who has functional incontinence and dementia:
  ■ Determine the frequency of current urination using an alarm system or check-and-change device.
  ■ Record urinary elimination and incontinent patterns in a bladder log to use as a baseline for assessment and evaluation of treatment efficacy.
  ■ Begin a prompted toileting program based on the results of this program; toileting frequency may vary from every 1.5 to 2 hours to every 4 hours.
  ■ Praise the client when toileting occurs with prompting.
  ■ Refrain from any socialization when incontinent episodes occur; change the client and make her or him comfortable.

  Nursing Research: *Prompted voiding or patterned urge response toileting has been shown to markedly reduce or eliminate functional incontinence in selected clients in long-term care facilities and in the community setting (Colling et al, 1992; Eustice, Roe, and Patterson, 2000).*

Geriatric
• Institute aggressive continence management programs for the cognitively intact, community-dwelling client in consultation with the client and family. *Uncontrolled incontinence can lead to institutionalization of an elderly person who prefers to remain in a home care setting (O'Donnell et al, 1992).*

• Monitor the elderly client in a long-term care facility, acute care facility, or home for dehydration. *Dehydration can exacerbate urine loss, produce acute confusion, and increase the risk of morbidity and morality, particularly in the frail elderly client (Colling, Owen, and McCreedy, 1994).*

Home care
• The interventions described previously may be adapted for home care use.

• Assess current strategies used to reduce urinary incontinence, including limitation of fluid intake, restriction of bladder irritants, prompted or scheduled toileting, and use of containment devices. *Many elderly clients and care providers use a variety of self-management techniques to control urinary incontinence, such as fluid limitation, avoidance of social contacts, and use of absorptive materials, that may or may not be effective for reducing urinary leakage or beneficial to general health (Johnson, 2000).*

• = Independent; ▲ = Collaborative

- Encourage a mind-set and program of self-care management. **Nursing Research:** *Addressing self-care activities through exercise, diet, fluid intake, and use of protective devices helps the client to exercise control over incontinence (Leenerts, Teel, and Pendleton, 2002).*
- Implement a bladder training program, including self-monitoring activities (reducing caffeine intake, adjusting amount and timing of fluid intake, decreasing long voiding intervals while awake, instituting dietary changes to promote bowel regularity), bladder training, and pelvic muscle exercise. **Nursing Research:** *In one study of women aged 55 years or older with involuntary urine loss associated with stress, urge, or mixed incontinence, clients responded to the aforementioned interventions with a 61% decrease in the severity of urinary incontinence at 2 years after intervention. Self-monitoring and bladder training accounted for most of the improvement (Dougherty et al, 2002).*
- For a memory-impaired elderly client, implement an individualized scheduled toileting program (on a schedule developed in consultation with the caregiver, approximately every 2 hours, with toileting reminders provided and existing patterns incorporated, such toileting before or after meals). **Nursing Research:** *Functional incontinence in memory-impaired elderly clients decreased significantly with the described intervention. The client must be able to cooperate for the intervention to be followed (Jirovec and Templin, 2001).*
- Teach the family the general principles of bladder health, including avoidance of bladder irritants, adequate fluid intake, and a routine schedule of toileting (refer to the care plan for **Impaired Urinary elimination**).
- Teach prompted voiding to the family and client for the client with mild to moderate dementia (refer to previous description) (Colling, 1996; McDowell et al, 1994).
- Teach the principles of perineal skin care, including routine cleansing following incontinent episodes, daily cleaning and drying of perineal skin, and the use of moisture barriers as indicated. *Routine cleansing and daily cleaning with appropriate products help maintain the integrity of perineal skin and prevent secondary cutaneous infections (Gray, Ratliff, and Donovan, 2002).*
- Advise the client about the advantages of using disposable or reusable insert pads, pad-pant systems, or replacement briefs specifically designed for urinary incontinence (or double urinary and fecal incontinence) as indicated. **Nursing Research:** *Many absorptive products used by community-dwelling elders are not designed to absorb urine, prevent odor, and protect the perineal skin (McClish et al, 1999). Disposable or reusable absorptive devices specifically designed to contain urine or double incontinence are more effective than household products, particularly in cases of moderate to severe incontinence (Gallo and Staskin, 1997; Shirran and Brazelli, 2000).*
- Assist the family with arranging care in a way that allows the client to participate in family or favorite activities without embarrassment. Elicit discussion of the client's concerns about the social or emotional burden of incontinence. **Nursing and Clinical Research:** *Careful planning can allow the dignity and integrity of family patterns to be retained. Urinary incontinence has a demonstrated influence on subjective well-being and quality of life, with depression, loneliness or sadness possible (Fultz and Herzog, 2001). Discussing emotional concerns helps the client to develop a sense of control over incontinence (Leenerts, Teel, and Pendleton, 2002).*
- ▲ Refer to occupational therapy for help in obtaining assistive devices and adapting the home for optimal toilet accessibility.
- ▲ Consider the use of an indwelling catheter for continuous drainage in the client who is both homebound and bed bound and is receiving palliative or end-of-life care (re-

• = **Independent;** ▲ = **Collaborative**

quires a physician's order). *An indwelling catheter may increase client comfort, ease care provider burden, and prevent urinary incontinence in bed-bound clients receiving end-of-life (palliative) care (Gray and Campbell, 2001).*

▲ When an indwelling catheter is in place, follow prescribed maintenance protocols for managing the catheter, drainage bag, perineal skin, and urethral meatus. Teach infection control measures adapted to the home care setting. *Proper care reduces the risk of catheter-associated urinary tract infection.* **Nursing Research:** *Multivariate analysis of data for a group of 106 home care clients demonstrated that frequent catheter changes increased the risk of a symptomatic urinary tract infection by approximately 12-fold compared with catheter changes every 4 weeks or less often (White and Ragland, 1995).*

• Assist the client in adapting to the catheter. Encourage discussion of the client's response to the catheter. **Nursing Research:** *Clients living with a catheter are keenly aware of its presence; adaptation is served by normalizing the experience. Instruction could include the fact that the client will be more aware of some sensations and sounds (e.g., urine sloshing in the bag, the weight of the bag, pressure or pain when urine flow has been altered). Rehearsing emptying of the bag when away from home will support resumption of activities. Discussion of the client's response will assist him or her in dealing with embarrassment or frustration (Wilde, 2002).*

Client/Family Teaching

• Work with the client, family, and their extended support systems to assist with needed changes in the environment and wardrobe, and other alterations required to maximize toileting access.

• Work with the client and family to establish a reasonable, manageable prompted voiding program using environmental and verbal cues to remind caregivers of voiding intervals, such as television programs, meals, and bedtime.

• Teach the family to use an alarm system for toileting or to carry out a check-and-change program and to maintain an accurate log of voiding and incontinence episodes.

evolve WEBSITES FOR EDUCATION

See the EVOLVE website for World Wide Web resources for client education.

REFERENCES

Colling JC: Noninvasive strategies to manage urinary incontinence among care-dependent persons, *J Wound Ostomy Continence Nurs* 23:302, 1996.

Colling JC, Owen TR, McCreedy MR: Urine volumes and voiding patterns among incontinent nursing home residents, *Geriatr Nurs* 15:188, 1994.

Colling JC et al: The effects of patterned urge response toileting (PURT) on urinary incontinence among nursing home residents, *J Am Geriatr Soc* 40:135, 1992.

Dougherty MC et al: A randomized trial of behavioral management for continence with older rural women, *Res Nurs Health* 25:3, 2002.

Eustice S, Roe B, Paterson J: Prompted voiding for the management of urinary incontinence in adults, *Cochrane Database System Rev* (CD002113), 2000.

Folstein MF, Folstein SE, McHugh PR: Mini-mental state: a practical method of grading the cognitive state of patients for the clinician, *J Psychiatr Res* 12(3):189, 1975.

Fultz NH, Herzog AR: Self-reported social and emotional impact of urinary incontinence, *J Am Geriatr Soc* 49: 892, 2001.

• = **Independent;** ▲ = **Collaborative**

Gallo M, Staskin DR: Patient satisfaction with a reusable undergarment for urinary incontinence, *J Wound Ostomy Continence Nurs* 24:226, 1997.

Gray M, Campbell F: Urinary tract disorders. In Ferrell B, Coyle N, editors: *Textbook of palliative nursing*, Oxford, UK, 2001, Oxford University Press.

Gray M, Ratliff C, Donovan A: Perineal skin care for the incontinent patient, *Adv Skin Wound Care* 15:170, 2002.

Hunskaar S et al: Epidemiology and natural history of urinary incontinence. In Abrams P, Khoury S, Wein A, editors. *Incontinence*, Plymouth, UK, 1998, Health Publication, Plymbridge Distributors.

Jawad SH, Ward AB, Jones P: Study of the relationship between premorbid urinary incontinence and stroke functional outcome, *Clin Rehabil* 13(5):447, 1999.

Jirovec MM, Templin T: Predicting success using individualized scheduled toileting for memory-impaired elders at home, *Res Nurs Health* 24:1, 2001.

Jirovec MM, Wells TJ: Urinary incontinence in nursing home residents with dementia: the mobility-cognition paradigm, *Appl Nurs Res* 3:112, 1990.

Johnson ST: From incontinence to confidence, *Am J Nurs* 100(2):69, 2000.

Leenerts MH, Teel CS, Pendleton MK: Building a model of self-care for health promotion in aging, *J Nurs Scholarsh* 34:355, 2002.

Maloney C, Cafiero M: Implementing an incontinence program in long-term care settings. A multidisciplinary approach, *J Gerontol Nurs* 25:47, 1999.

McClish DK et al: Use and costs of incontinence pads in female study volunteers, *J Wound Ostomy Continence Nurs* 26(4):207, 1999.

McDowell BJ et al: Effectiveness of behavioral therapy to treat incontinence in homebound older adults, *J Am Geriatr Soc* 15:303, 1994.

McDowell BJ et al: Characteristics of urinary incontinence in homebound older adults, *J Am Geriatr Soc* 44(8):963, 1996.

Neelan VJ et al: Use of the NEECHAM confusion scale to assess acute confusional states of hospitalized older patients. In Funk SG et al, editors: *Key aspects of elder care: managing falls, incontinence and cognitive impairment*, New York, 1992, Springer.

O'Donnell BF et al: Incontinence and troublesome behaviors predict institutionalization in dementia, *J Geriatr Psychiatry Neurol* 5:45, 1992.

Palmer MH et al: Risk factors for hospital acquired incontinence in elderly female hip fracture patients, *J Gerontol A Biol Sci Med Sci* 57(10):M672, 2002.

Rabin JM: Clinical use of the FemAssist device in female urinary incontinence, *J Med Syst* 22:257, 1998.

Reilly N: Assessment and management of acute or transient urinary incontinence. In Doughty D, editor: *Urinary and fecal incontinence: nursing management*, ed 2, St Louis, 2002, Mosby.

Resnick NM et al: Short term variability of self-report of incontinence in older persons, *J Am Geriatr Soc* 42:202, 1994.

Reuben DB: A randomized clinical trial of outpatient comprehensive geriatric assessment coupled with an intervention to increase adherence to recommendations, *J Am Geriatr Soc* 47(3):269, 1999.

Shirran E, Brazelli M: Absorbent products for the containment of urinary and/or fecal incontinence, *Cochrane Database Syst Rev* (CD0011406), 2000.

Silverman M et al: To treat or not to treat: issues in decisions not to treat older persons with cognitive impairment, depression, and incontinence, *J Am Geriatr Soc* 45(9):1094, 1997.

Thommessen B, Bautz-Holter E, Laake K: Predictors of outcome of rehabilitation of elderly stroke patients in a geriatric ward, *Clin Rehabil* 13(2):123, 1999.

Vickerman J: Thorough assessment of functional incontinence, *Nurs Times* 98(28):58, 2002.

Wells TJ: Managing incontinence through managing the environment, *Urol Nurs* 12:48, 1992.

White MC, Ragland KE: Urinary catheter related infections among home care patients, *J Wound Ostomy Continence Nurs* 22:286, 1995.

Wilde MH: Urine flowing: a phenomenological study of living with a urinary catheter, *Res Nurs Health* 25:14, 2002.

• = **Independent;** ▲ = **Collaborative**

Reflex urinary Incontinence

Mikel Gray

NANDA Definition

Involuntary loss of urine at somewhat predictable intervals when a specific bladder volume is reached (NANDA, 2003)

Involuntary loss of urine caused by a defect in the spinal cord between the nerve roots at or below the first cervical segment and those above the second sacral segment. Urine elimination occurs at unpredictable intervals; micturition may be elicited by tactile stimuli, including stroking of inner thigh or perineum (Gray, 2003).

Defining Characteristics

Absent or diminished sensation or urge to void; incomplete emptying caused by dyssynergia of striated sphincter mechanism, which produces functional outlet obstruction of bladder; may be associated with sweating and acute elevation in blood pressure and pulse rate in clients with spinal cord injury (see the care plan for **Autonomic dysreflexia**)

Related Factors (r/t)

Paralyzing spinal disorder affecting spinal segments C1 to S2

NOC Outcomes (Nursing Outcomes Classification)

Suggested NOC Outcomes

Urinary Continence; Urinary Elimination

> **Example NOC Outcome with Indicators**
>
> **Urinary Continence** as evidenced by the following indicators: Absence of urinary leakage between catheterizations or containment of micturition by condom catheter and drainage bag/Absence of urinary tract infection (absence of leukocytes and absence of bacterial growth or <100,000 colony-forming units per milliliter)/ Underclothing dry during day/Underclothing or bedding dry during night (Rate each indicator of **Urinary Continence:** 1 = never demonstrated, 2 = rarely demonstrated, 3 = sometimes demonstrated, 4 = often demonstrated, 5 = consistently demonstrated [see Section I].)

Client Outcomes

Client Will (Specify Time Frame):

- Follow prescribed schedule for bladder evacuation
- Demonstrate successful use of triggering techniques to stimulate voiding
- Have intact perineal skin
- Remain clear of symptomatic urinary tract infection
- Demonstrate how to apply containment device or insert indwelling catheter or be able to provide caregiver with instructions for performing these procedures
- Demonstrate awareness of risk of autonomic dysreflexia, its prevention and management

• = Independent; ▲ = Collaborative

| **NIC** | Interventions (Nursing Interventions Classification) |

Suggested NIC Interventions

Urinary Catheterization: Intermittent; Urinary Elimination Management; Urinary Incontinence Care

---

Example NIC Activities—Urinary Elimination Management

Monitor urinary elimination including frequency, consistency, odor, volume, and color as appropriate; Teach client signs and symptoms of urinary tract infection

---

Nursing Interventions and Rationales

- Assess the client's neurological status, including the type of neurological disorder, the functional level of neurological impairment, its completeness (effect on motor and sensory function), and the ability to perform bladder management tasks, including intermittent catheterization, application of a condom catheter, etc. *In clients with a single, well-circumscribed neurological lesion, knowledge of the level of the lesion strongly correlates with bladder function. In contrast, this correlation is weak in clients with multilevel cord trauma due to secondary bleeding or swelling (Weld, Graney, and Dmochowski, 2000).* Knowledge of functional impairments related to a spinal cord injury (including upper extremity function) is essential because it determines the client's ability to manage the bladder by self-catheterization (Gray, 2000).

- Perform a focused assessment of the urinary system, including perineal skin integrity. *Urinary and fecal incontinence associated with neurogenic bladder and bowel dysfunction in the client with a paralyzing disorder predisposes the perineal skin to irritant dermatitis and secondary infection, particularly when a urine containment device such as an adult containment brief or condom catheter is used (Gray, Ratliff, and Donovan, 2002).*

- Complete a bladder log to determine the pattern of urine elimination, incontinence episodes, and current bladder management program. *The bladder log provides an objective record of urine elimination that confirms the accuracy of the historical report, and a baseline for assessment and evaluation of treatment efficacy (Gray, 2000).*

- ▲ Consult with the physician concerning current bladder function and the potential of the bladder to produce upper urinary tract distress (hydronephrosis, vesicoureteral reflux, febrile urinary tract infection, or compromised renal function). **Nursing Research:** *Both nursing and medical research demonstrate that reflex incontinence is typically accompanied by detrusor striated sphincter dyssynergia, which increases the risk of upper urinary tract distress (Gray et al, 1991; Killorin et al, 1992; Weld et al, 2000).*

- ▲ Determine a bladder management program in consultation with the client, family, and rehabilitation team. **Nursing Research:** *The bladder management program profoundly affects the client and significant others; it is determined by holistic assessment that addresses the potential of the bladder to create upper urinary tract distress, the potential for incontinence and related complications, client and family preference, and the perceived impact of the bladder management program on the client's lifestyle (Anson and Gray, 1993; Gray, Rayome, and Anson 1995).*

- ▲ In consultation with the rehabilitation team, counsel the client and family concerning the merits and potential risks associated with each possible bladder management program, including spontaneous voiding, intermittent self-catheterization, reflex voiding with condom catheter containment, and indwelling catheterization. *All bladder*

- = Independent; ▲ = Collaborative

management programs carry some risk of urinary incontinence or serious urinary system com-plications (Wyndaele et al, 2001). **Nursing Research:** *Spontaneous voiding and inter-mittent catheterization carry greater risk of urine loss than condom catheter containment or indwelling catheter, but these latter strategies carry higher risk for serious urinary system complications, including upper urinary tract distress, when evaluated over a period of years (Anson and Gray, 1993; Gray, Rayome, and Anson, 1995).*

- Teach the client with reflex incontinence to consume an adequate amount of fluids on a daily basis (approximately 30 ml/kg of body weight). *Dehydration exacerbates urine loss and increases the risk of related complications, including constipation and urinary tract infection (Gray and Krissovich, in press).*

- Teach the client with reflex urinary incontinence that is managed by spontaneous voiding to self-administer an alpha-adrenergic blocking medication as directed and to recognize and manage potential side effects. *Clients who spontaneously urinate may take an alpha-adrenergic blocking drug to reduce urethral resistance during voiding (Linsenmeyer, Horton, and Benevento, 2002).*

▲ Begin intermittent catheterization using a modified clean or sterile technique based on facility policies. **Nursing Research:** *Modified clean intermittent catheterization may be used in an inpatient setting with appropriate staff and client education.*

▲ Teach intermittent catheterization as the client approaches discharge as directed. In-struct the client and at least one family member, spouse, or partner in the performance of catheterization using clean technique. Teach the client with quadriplegia how to instruct others to perform this procedure. **Nursing Research:** *Both nursing and medical research demonstrates that intermittent catheterization is a safe and effective bladder man-agement strategy for persons with reflex urinary incontinence. Inclusion of a family mem-ber, spouse, or significant other is particularly helpful for the client with limited upper extremity dexterity and reflex urinary incontinence (Anson and Gray, 1993; Chai et al, 1995; Gray, Rayome, and Anson, 1995; Shekelle et al, 1999).*

▲ Teach the client managed by intermittent catheterization to self-administer antispas-modic (parasympatholytic) medications as directed, and to recognize and manage potential side effects. *Persons who manage reflex incontinence by intermittent catheteriza-tion frequently require antispasmodic medications to manage the neurogenic overactive de-trusor contractions that produce urine loss (Pannek et al, 2000).*

▲ Consult with the physician and occupational therapist concerning the use of a neuro-prosthesis or other device designed to improve hand use for the quadriplegic client with partial hand function. *Use of a neuroprosthetic device designed to improve hand func-tion increases clients' independence when performing multiple functions, including bladder management. The high initial costs associated with these devices may be offset by reduc-tions in costs related to partially dependent bladder management over a period of approxi-mately 5 years (Creasey et al, 2000).*

▲ For a male client with reflex incontinence who cannot manage the condition effec-tively with spontaneous voiding, does not choose to perform intermittent catheteriza-tion, or cannot perform catheterization, teach the client and his family to obtain, select, and apply a condom catheter with drainage bag. Assist them in choosing a product that adheres to the penile shaft without allowing seepage of urine onto sur-rounding skin or clothing, contains a material and adhesive that does not produce hy-persensitivity reactions on the skin, and includes a leg bag that is easily concealed under the clothing and does not cause irritation to the skin of the thigh. *Multiple com-ponents of the condom catheter affect the product's ability to contain urinary leakage, pro-*

- = **Independent;** ▲ = **Collaborative**

tect underlying skin, and preserve the client's dignity (Joseph et al, 1998; Watson, 1989; Watson and Kuhn, 1990).

- Teach the client who uses a condom catheter to remove the condom device, inspect the skin, cleanse the penis thoroughly, and reapply a new catheter every day. *The risk of urinary tract infection increases if a condom catheter is worn for longer than 24 hours (Hirsh, Fainstein, and Musher, 1979).*
- Teach the client whose incontinence is managed by a condom catheter to routinely inspect the skin with each catheter change for evidence of lesions caused by pressure from the containment device or by exposure to urine. *Skin breakdown is a common complication associated with routine use of the condom catheter (Anson and Gray, 1993).*
- Teach the client managed by intermittent or indwelling catheter to recognize signs of significant urinary tract infection and to seek care promptly when these signs occur. The signs of significant infection are the following:
  - Discomfort over the bladder or during urination
  - Acute onset of urinary incontinence
  - Fever
  - Markedly increased spasticity of muscles below the level of the spinal lesion
  - Malaise, lethargy
  - Hematuria
  - Autonomic dysreflexia (hyperreflexia) (Siroky, 2002)

  Intermittent catheterization is typically associated with asymptomatic bacteriuria, and the indwelling catheter is routinely associated with asymptomatic colonization. Antibiotic treatment of asymptomatic bacteriuria has not proven helpful (Morton et al, 2002; Murphy and Lampert, 2003), but prompt management of significant infection is necessary to prevent urosepsis or related complications (Siroky, 2002).

Geriatric
- ▲ If difficulties are encountered in client teaching, refer the elderly client to a nurse who specializes in care of the aging client with urinary incontinence.

Home care
- The interventions described previously may be adapted for home care use.
- ▲ Teach the client what the complications of reflex incontinence are and when to report changes to a physician or primary nurse. *Early detection allows for rapid diagnosis and treatment before irreversible damage to the renal parenchyma occurs (Burns, Rivas, and Ditunno, 2001).*
- ▲ If the client is taught intermittent self-catheterization, arrange for contingency care in the event that the client is unable to perform self-catheterization. *Although self-catheterization has proved to be an effective and safe bladder management strategy, acute illness or surgery may render the client unable to perform self-catheterization and temporarily reliant on others to carry out this critical task (Joseph et al, 1998).*
- Assess and instruct the client and family in care of the catheter and supplies in the home. *Proper care of supplies reduces the risk of infection (Joseph et al, 1998).*
- Encourage a mind-set and program of self-care management. **Nursing Research:** *Addressing self-care activities through exercise, diet, fluid intake, and protective devices helps the client to exercise control over incontinence (Leenerts, Teel, and Pendleton, 2002).*
- Implement a bladder training program, including self-monitoring activities (reducing caffeine intake, adjusting the amount and timing of fluid intake, decreasing long

• = **Independent;** ▲ = **Collaborative**

voiding intervals while awake, making dietary changes to promote bowel regularity), bladder training, and pelvic muscle exercise. **Nursing Research:** *In one study of women aged 55 years or older with involuntary urine loss associated with stress, urge, or mixed incontinence, clients responded to the aforementioned interventions with a 61% decrease in the severity of urinary incontinence at 2 years after intervention. Self-monitoring and bladder training accounted for most of the improvement (Dougherty et al, 2002).*

- Assist the family with arranging care in a way that allows the client to participate in family or favorite activities without embarrassment. Elicit discussion of the client's concerns about the social or emotional burden of incontinence. **Nursing and Clinical Research:** *Careful planning can help the client retain dignity and maintain the integrity of family patterns. Urinary incontinence has a demonstrated influence on subjective well-being and quality of life, with depression, loneliness or sadness possible (Fultz and Herzog, 2001). Discussing emotional concerns helps the client to develop a sense of control over incontinence (Leenerts, Teel, and Pendleton, 2002).*

▲ If medications are ordered, instruct the family or caregivers and the client in medication administration, use, and side effects. *Adherence to a medication regimen increases its chances of success and decreases the risk of losing the regimen as an option for care when other alternatives are unacceptable.*

Client/Family Teaching

- Teach the client with a spinal injury the signs of autonomic dysreflexia, its relationship to bladder fullness, and management of the condition. (Refer to the care plan for **Autonomic dysreflexia.**)
- Teach the client and several significant others the techniques of intermittent catheterization, indwelling catheter care and removal, or condom catheter management as appropriate.
- Teach the client and family techniques to clean catheters used for intermittent catheterization, including washing with soap and water and allowing to air dry, and using microwave cleaning techniques.

𝗲𝘃𝗼𝗹𝘃𝗲 WEBSITES FOR EDUCATION

See the EVOLVE website for World Wide Web resources for client education.

REFERENCES

Anson C, Gray ML: Secondary complications after spinal cord injury, *Urol Nurs* 13:107, 1993.

Burns AS, Rivas DA, Ditunno JF: The management of neurogenic bladder and sexual dysfunction after spinal cord injury, *Spine* 26(24 suppl):S129, 2001.

Chai T et al: Compliance and complications of clean intermittent catheterization in the spinal cord injured patient, *Paraplegia* 33:161, 1995.

Creasey GH et al: Reduction of costs of disability using neuroprostheses, *Assist Technol* 12(1):67, 2000.

Dougherty MC et al: A randomized trial of behavioral management for continence with older rural women, *Res Nurs Health* 25:3, 2002.

Fultz NH, Herzog AR: Self-reported social and emotional impact of urinary incontinence, *J Am Geriatr Soc* 49:892, 2001.

Gray M: Reflex urinary incontinence. In: Doughty DB, editor: *Urinary and fecal incontinence: nursing management,* ed 2, St Louis, 2000, Mosby.

Gray M, Krissovich M: Evidence based report card: does fluid intake influence the risk for urinary incontinence, urinary tract infection and bladder cancer? *J Wound Ostomy Continence Nurs,* in press.

- = **Independent;** ▲ = **Collaborative**

Gray M, Ratliff C, Donovan A: Perineal skin care for the incontinent patient, *Adv Skin Wound Care* 15:170, 2002.

Gray M, Rayome RG, Anson C: Incontinence and clean intermittent catheterization following spinal cord injury, *Clin Nurs Res* 4:6, 1995.

Gray ML et al: Urethral pressure gradient in the prediction of upper urinary tract distress following spinal cord injury, *J Am Paraplegia Soc* 14:105, 1991.

Hirsh DD, Fainstein V, Musher DM: Do condom catheter collecting systems cause urinary tract infection? *JAMA* 242:340, 1979.

Joseph AC et al: Nursing clinical practice guideline: neurogenic bladder management, *SCI Nurs* 15(2):21, 1998.

Killorin WK et al: Evaluative urodynamics and bladder management in the prediction of upper urinary infection in male spinal cord injury, *Paraplegia* 30:437, 1992.

Leenerts MH, Teel CS, Pendleton MK: Building a model of self-care for health promotion in aging, *J Nurs Scholarsh* 34:355, 2002.

Linsenmeyer TA, Horton J, Benevento J: Impact of alpha$_1$-blockers in men with spinal cord injury and upper tract stasis, *J Spinal Cord Med* 25(2):124, 2002.

Morton SC et al: Antimicrobial prophylaxis for urinary tract infection in persons with spinal cord dysfunction, *Arch Phys Med Rehabil* 83(1):129, 2002.

Murphy DP, Lampert V: Current implications of drug resistance in spinal cord injury, *Am J Phys Med Rehabil* 82(1):72, 2003.

NANDA: *Nursing diagnoses: definitions & classification 2003-2004,* Philadelphia, 2003, The Association.

Pannek J et al: Combined intravesical and oral oxybutynin chloride in adult patients with spinal cord injury, *Urology* 55(3):358, 2000.

Shekelle PG et al: Systematic review of risk factors for urinary tract infection in adults with spinal cord dysfunction, *J Spinal Cord Med* 22(4):258, 1999.

Siroky MB: Pathogenesis of bacteriuria and infection in the spinal cord injured patient, *Am J Med* 113(suppl 1A):67S, 2002.

Watson R: A nursing trial of urinary sheath systems on male hospitalized patients, *J Adv Nurs* 14:467, 1989.

Watson R, Kuhn M: The influence of component parts on the performance of urinary sheath systems, *J Adv Nurs* 15:417, 1990.

Weld KJ, Graney MJ, Dmochowski RR: Clinical significance of detrusor sphincter dyssynergia in patients with post traumatic spinal cord injury, *Urology* 56:565, 2000.

Weld KJ et al. Influences on renal function in chronic spinal cord injured patients, *J Urol* 164(5):1490, 2000.

Wyndaele JJ, Madersbacher H, Kovindha A: Conservative treatment of the neuropathic bladder in spinal cord injured patients, *Spinal Cord* 39(6):294, 2001.

Stress urinary Incontinence

Mikel Gray

NANDA Definition

State in which the individual experiences urine loss of less than 50 ml accompanied by increased intra-abdominal pressure

NOTE: The value of less than 50 ml for the volume of urine loss may be exceeded by women and men with severe stress incontinence caused by intrinsic sphincter deficiency. This is sometimes classified as "total incontinence." In this book, however, "total incontinence" will be used to refer exclusively to incontinence due to extraurethral causes, and all forms of stress incontinence are reviewed under this diagnosis, regardless of severity.

Defining Characteristics

Observed urine loss with physical exertion (sign of stress incontinence); reported loss of urine associated with physical exertion or activity (symptom of stress incontinence); urine loss associated with increased abdominal pressure (urodynamic stress urinary incontinence) (Abrams et al, 2002)

- • = Independent; ▲ = Collaborative

Related Factors (r/t)

Urethral hypermobility/pelvic organ prolapse (familial predisposition, multiple vaginal deliveries, delivery of infant large for gestational age, forceps-assisted or breech delivery, obesity, changes in estrogen levels at climacteric, extensive abdominopelvic or pelvic surgery)

Intrinsic sphincter deficiency (multiple urethral suspensions in women, radical prostatectomy in men, uncommon complication of transurethral prostatectomy or cryosurgery of prostate, spinal lesion affecting sacral segments 2 to 4 or cauda equina, pelvic fracture)

NOC   Outcomes (Nursing Outcomes Classification)

Suggested NOC Outcomes
Urinary Continence; Urinary Elimination

> **Example NOC Outcome with Indicators**
>
> **Urinary Continence** as evidenced by the following indicators: Experiences no urine loss with physical activity or exertion, coughing, sneezing, or other maneuvers that precipitously raise abdominal pressure/Voids in appropriate receptacle/Able to move to toilet after strong desire to urinate is perceived/Underclothing remains dry during day/Underclothing or bedding remains dry during night (Rate each indicator of **Urinary Continence:** 1 = never demonstrated, 2 = rarely demonstrated, 3 = sometimes demonstrated, 4 = often demonstrated, 5 = consistently demonstrated [see Section I].)

Client Outcomes

Client Will (Specify Time Frame):
- Report relief from stress incontinence or report decrease in the incidence or severity of incontinence episodes
- Experience reduction in grams of urine loss measured objectively by a pad test
- Identify containment devices that assist in management of stress incontinence

NIC   Interventions (Nursing Interventions Classification)

Suggested NIC Intervention
Pelvic Muscle Exercise; Urinary Incontinence Care

> **Example NIC Activities—Urinary Incontinence Care**
>
> Explain etiology of problem and rationale for actions; Modify clothing and environment to provide easy access to toilet

Nursing Interventions and Rationales

- Take a focused history addressing duration of urinary leakage and related lower urinary tract symptoms, including daytime voiding frequency, urgency, frequency of nocturia, frequency of urinary leakage, and factors provoking urine loss. *A careful description of bothersome lower urinary tract symptoms helps identify the cause of urine loss and optimal treatment options (Addison, 1999).* **Nursing Research:** *A historical report of urine loss with physical exertion correlates well with objective findings of stress urinary incontinence on physical examination or urodynamic testing. In contrast, the symptom of urge incon-*

• = Independent; ▲ = Collaborative

tinence, when reported as an isolated finding, is a poor predictor of consistent urge inconti-nence. Querying clients about the symptom of urge incontinence, in combination with daytime voiding frequency and nocturia, greatly improves the predictive power of a nursing history in the evaluation of urinary incontinence.

- Perform a focused physical assessment, including perineal skin assessment, evaluation of the vaginal mucosa, reproduction of the sign of stress incontinence, and observation of urethral hypermobility and related pelvic descent (prolapse). *Urinary incontinence, particularly when combined with fecal incontinence or use of larger containment devices such as adult containment briefs, increases the risk for irritant dermatitis and secondary monilial or bacterial infection (Gray, Ratliff, and Donovan, 2002).* **Nursing Research:** *Reproduction of the sign of stress urinary incontinence using provocative maneuvers during physical examination (such as asking the client to cough or perform Valsalva's maneuver) provides clues as to the cause of urine loss, its association with pelvic organ prolapse and bladder base descent, and the severity of incontinence (Miller et al, 1998).*

- Determine the client's current use of containment devices; evaluate the devices for their ability to adequately contain urine loss, protect clothing, and control odor. Assist the client in identifying containment devices specifically designed to contain urinary leakage. **Nursing Research:** *Clients, particularly women, tend to select feminine hygiene pads for urine containment. These devices, designed to contain menstrual flow, are not well suited to address urine loss (McClish et al, 1999).*

- ▲ With the client and in close consultation with the physician, review treatment options, including behavioral management; drug therapy; use of a pessary, vaginal device, or urethral insert; and surgery. Outline their potential benefits, efficacy, and side effects. *Multiple treatments have been used to manage stress incontinence; behavioral management options should be offered initially (Burns, 2000).*

- ▲ Assess the client's pelvic muscle strength using pressure manometry, a digital evaluation technique, or urine stop test. **Nursing Research:** *A baseline of pelvic muscle strength is needed for initial assessment and for evaluation of treatment efficacy. Digital vaginal examination, a urine stream interruption test, or measurement of pelvic floor muscle contraction strength by a fluid-filled balloon are valid and reliable techniques for assessing pelvic floor muscle strength and contractile function (Brink et al, 1992; Sampselle and DeLancey, 1992; Worth, Dougherty, and McKey, 1986).*

- Begin a pelvic floor muscle rehabilitation program. *Pelvic floor muscle rehabilitation is effective in the treatment of stress and mixed urinary incontinence (Bo, Talseth, and Holme, 1999; Hay-Smith et al, 2001).*

- Teach the client undergoing pelvic muscle rehabilitation to identify, contract, and relax the pelvic floor muscles without contracting distant muscle groups (such as the abdominal muscles) using biofeedback techniques. *Pelvic muscle rehabilitation is enhanced by the use of biofeedback (Berghmann et al, 1996; Bump et al, 1991).*

- Incorporate principles of physiotherapy into a pelvic muscle training program using the following strategies:
  - Start a graded exercise program beginning with 5 to 10 repetitions and advancing gradually to 35 to 50 repetitions every day or every other day.
  - Continue exercise sessions over a period of 3 to 6 months.
  - Integrate muscle training into activities of daily living.
  - Assess progress every 2 weeks during the first month and every 4 to 6 weeks thereafter.

- = **Independent;** ▲ = **Collaborative**

Nursing Research: *Pelvic muscle rehabilitation alleviates or cures stress incontinence using a combination of techniques, including biofeedback and strength training. Application of principles of physiotherapy maximizes the value of pelvic muscle rehabilitation (Brink et al, 1992; Dougherty et al, 1991; Dougherty et al, 1992; Johnson, 2001; Nygaard et al, 1996).*

- Teach the female client to reeducate the pelvic muscles using weighted vaginal cones.
Nursing Research: *Weighted vaginal cones help women increase pelvic floor muscle tone and function and alleviate stress urinary incontinence (Laycock et al, 2001). A systematic review of existing research suggests that the efficacy of weighted cones may be comparable to that achieved by pelvic muscle rehabilitation, but more comparative studies are needed before a definitive conclusion can be reached.*

▲ Begin transvaginal or transrectal electrical stimulation therapy in selected persons with stress incontinence in consultation with the client and physician. *Electrical stimulation alleviates stress incontinence in selected clients, probably by strengthening the pelvic muscles and possibly via a biofeedback effect (Sand et al, 1995).*

- Teach the principles of bladder training to women with stress urinary incontinence.
  - Assist the client in completing a voiding diary over a period of a minimum of 3 days or up to 7 days.
  - Review the results with the client, determining typical voiding frequency and establishing goals for voiding frequency.
  - Using baseline voiding frequency, as determined by the diary, teach the client to urinate by the clock when awake, typically every 30 to 120 minutes.
  - Encourage adherence to the program with timing devices and verbal encouragement and support, and address individual reasons for schedule interruption.
  - Gradually increase the time between urinations to the negotiated goal. Time intervals between voiding are typically increased in increments of 15 to 30 minutes for clients with a baseline frequency of less than every 60 minutes and increments of 25 to 30 minutes for clients with a baseline frequency of more than every 60 minutes.

Nursing Research: *Bladder training reduces the frequency and severity of urinary leakage in women with stress incontinence, urge incontinence, and mixed incontinence. Research suggests that the results of bladder training in ambulatory, community-dwelling women is comparable to that achieved through pelvic floor muscle rehabilitation (Elser et al, 1999; Wyman et al, 1998).*

▲ Teach the client to self-administer alpha-adrenergic medications, imipramine, and topical or oral estrogens as directed. *Pharmacotherapeutic agents alleviate or temporarily cure stress incontinence in selected women (Andersson, 2000; Radley et al, 2000).*

▲ Refer the female client who wishes to employ a pessary, vaginal device, or urethral insert to manage stress incontinence to a nurse specialist or gynecologist with expertise in the placement and maintenance of these devices. *Pessaries, vaginal devices, and urethral inserts alleviate or correct stress incontinence; however, they may cause serious complications unless inserted correctly and monitored closely (Frazer et al, 2000).*

- Discuss potentially reversible or controllable risk factors with the client with stress incontinence and assist the client to formulate a strategy to alleviate or eliminate these conditions. *Although research supports a strong familial predisposition to stress incontinence among women, other risk factors associated with the condition, including obesity and chronic coughing from smoking, are reversible (Mushkat, Bukovsky, and Langer, 1996; Skoner, Thompson, and Caron, 1994).*

• = Independent; ▲ = Collaborative

▲ Provide information about support resources such as the Simon Foundation for Continence or the National Foundation for Continence.

▲ Refer the client with persistent stress incontinence to a continence service, physician, or nurse who specializes in the management of this condition. **Nursing Research:** *Complex stress incontinence can be successfully managed by a multidisciplinary approach (McDowell et al, 1996).*

Geriatric

• Evaluate the elderly client's functional and cognitive status to determine the impact of functional limitations on the frequency and severity of urine loss and on plans for management.

Home care

• The interventions described previously may be adapted for home care use.

• Elicit discussion of the client's concerns about the social or emotional burden of stress incontinence. **Nursing and Clinical Research:** *Urinary incontinence has a demonstrated influence on subjective well-being and quality of life, with depression, loneliness, or sadness possible (Fultz and Herzog, 2001). Discussing emotional concerns helps the client to develop a sense of control over incontinence (Leenerts, Teel, and Pendleton, 2002).*

• Encourage a mind-set and program of self-care management. **Nursing Research:** *Addressing self-care activities through exercise, diet, fluid intake, and protective devices helps the client to exercise control over incontinence (Leenerts, Teel, and Pendleton, 2002).*

• Implement a bladder training program, including self-monitoring activities (reducing caffeine intake, adjusting amount and timing of fluid intake, decreasing long voiding intervals while awake, making dietary changes to promote bowel regularity), bladder training, and pelvic muscle exercise. **Nursing Research:** *In one study of women aged 55 years or older with involuntary urine loss associated with stress, urge, or mixed incontinence, clients responded to the aforementioned interventions with a 61% decrease in the severity of urinary incontinence at 2 years after intervention. Self-monitoring and bladder training accounted for most of the improvement (Dougherty et al, 2002).*

▲ Consider the use of an indwelling catheter for continuous drainage in the client with severe stress urinary incontinence who is homebound, bed-bound, and receiving palliative or end-of-life care (requires a physician's order). *An indwelling catheter may increase client comfort, ease caregiver burden, and prevent urinary incontinence in bed-bound clients receiving end-of-life care.*

▲ When an indwelling catheter is in place, follow the prescribed maintenance protocols for managing the catheter, drainage bag, and perineal skin and urethral meatus. Teach infection control measures adapted to the home care setting. *Proper care reduces the risk of catheter-associated urinary tract infection.*

• Assist the client in adapting to the catheter. Encourage discussion of the client's response to the catheter. **Nursing Research:** *Clients living with a catheter are keenly aware of its presence; adaptation is served by normalizing the experience. Instruction could include the fact that the client will be more aware of some sensations and sounds (e.g., urine sloshing in the bag, the weight of the bag, pressure or pain when urine flow has been altered). Rehearsing emptying of the bag when away from home will support resumption of activities. Discussion of the client's response will help him or her to deal with embarrassment or frustration (Wilde, 2002).*

• = **Independent;** ▲ = **Collaborative**

- Begin a program of pelvic muscle rehabilitation in the homebound elderly client who is motivated to adhere to the program and has adequate cognitive function to understand and follow instructions. **Nursing Research:** *Homebound elders are capable of completing a program of pelvic muscle rehabilitation and achieving clinically relevant relief from stress and urge urinary incontinence.*

Client/Family Teaching

- Teach the client to perform pelvic muscle exercise using an audiotape or videotape if indicated.
- Teach the client the importance of avoiding dehydration and instruct the client to consume fluid at the rate of 30 ml/kg of body weight daily.
- Teach the client the importance of avoiding constipation by a combination of adequate fluid intake, adequate intake of dietary fiber, and exercise.
- Teach the client to apply and remove support devices such as a bladder neck support prosthesis.
- Teach the client to select and apply urine containment devices.

evolve WEBSITES FOR EDUCATION

See the EVOLVE website for World Wide Web resources for client education.

REFERENCES

Abrams PL et al: The standardization of terminology of lower urinary tract function: report from the Standardization Sub-committee of the International Continence Society, *Am J Obstet Gynecol* 187(1):116, 2002.

Addison R: Assessment of stress incontinence, *Nurs Times* 95(45 suppl 1-2):10, 1999.

Andersson KE: Drug therapy for urinary incontinence, *Best Pract Res Clin Obstet Gynecol* 14(2):291, 2000.

Berghmann LCM et al: Efficacy of biofeedback when included with pelvic muscle exercise treatment for stress incontinence, *Neurourol Urodyn* 15:37, 1996.

Bo K, Talseth T, Holme I: Single blind, randomized controlled trial of pelvic floor exercises, electrical stimulation, vaginal cones, and no treatment of genuine stress incontinence in women, *BMJ* 318:487, 1999.

Brink CA et al: Pelvic muscle exercise for elderly incontinence women. In Funk SG et al, editors: *Key aspects of elder care: managing falls, incontinence and cognitive impairment,* New York, 1992, Springer.

Bump RC et al: Assessment of Kegel pelvic muscle exercise performance after brief verbal instruction, *Am J Obstet Gynecol* 165(2):322, 1991.

Burns PA: Stress incontinence. In Doughty DB: *Urinary and fecal incontinence: nursing management,* ed 2, St Louis, 2000, Mosby.

Dougherty MC et al: Graded exercise: effect of pressures developed by the pelvic muscles. In Funk SG et al, editors: *Key aspects of elder care: managing falls, incontinence and cognitive impairment,* New York, 1992, Springer.

Dougherty MC et al: A randomized trial of behavioral management for continence with older rural women, *Res Nurs Health* 25:3, 2002.

Dougherty MC et al: Variations in intravaginal pressure measurements, *Nurs Res* 40:282, 1991.

Elser DM et al: The effect of bladder training, pelvic floor muscle training, or combination training on urodynamic parameters in women with urinary incontinence. Continence Program for Women Research Group, *Neurourol Urodyn* 18(5):427, 1999.

Frazer M et al: Mechanical devices for urinary incontinence in women, *Cochrane Database System Rev* Issue 4, 2000.

Fultz NH, Herzog AR: Self-reported social and emotional impact of urinary incontinence, *J Am Geriatr Soc* 49: 892, 2001.

Gray M, Ratliff C, Donovan A: Perineal skin care for the incontinent patient, *Adv Skin Wound Care* 15:170, 2002.

- = **Independent;** ▲ = **Collaborative**

Hay-Smith EJC et al: Pelvic floor muscle training for urinary incontinence in women, *Cochrane Database Syst Rev* 1:CD001407, 2001.

Johnson VY: How the principles of exercise physiology influence pelvic floor muscle training, *J Wound Ostomy Continence Nurs* 28(3):150, 2001.

Laycock J et al: Pelvic floor reeducation for stress incontinence: comparing three methods, *Br J Community Nurs* 6(5):230, 2001.

Leenerts MH, Teel CS, Pendleton MK: Building a model of self-care for health promotion in aging, *J Nurs Scholarsh* 34:355, 2002.

McClish DK et al: Use and costs of incontinence pads in female study volunteers, *J Wound Ostomy Continence Nurs* 26(4):207, 1999.

McDowell BJ et al: An interdisciplinary approach to the assessment and behavioral treatment of urinary incontinence in geriatric outpatients, *Kango Kenkyu* 29(5):425, 1996.

Miller JM, Ashton-Miller JA, Delancey JO: Quantification of cough-related urine loss using the paper towel test, *Obstet Gynecol* 91(5 pt 1):705, 1998.

Mushkat Y, Bukovsky I, Langer R: Female urinary stress incontinence—does it have familial prevalence? *Am J Obstet Gynecol* 174:617, 1996.

Nygaard IE et al: Efficacy of pelvic floor muscle exercise in women with stress, urge and mixed urinary incontinence, *Am J Obstet Gynecol* 174:120, 1996.

Radley SC et al: Alpha adrenergic drugs for urinary incontinence in women, *Cochrane Database System Rev* Issue 4, 2000.

Sampselle CM, DeLancey JOL: The urine stream interruption test and pelvic muscle function, *Nurs Res* 41:73, 1992.

Sand PK et al: Pelvic floor electrical stimulation in the treatment of genuine stress incontinence: a multicenter placebo controlled trial, *Am J Obstet Gynecol* 173:72, 1995.

Skoner MM, Thompson WD, Caron VA: Factors associated with risk of stress urinary incontinence in women, *Nurs Res* 43:301, 1994.

Wilde MH: Urine flowing: a phenomenological study of living with a urinary catheter, *Res Nurs Health* 25:14, 2002.

Worth AM, Dougherty MC, McKey PL: Development and testing of the circumvaginal muscle (CVM) rating scale, *Nurs Res* 35:166, 1986.

Wyman JF et al: Comparative efficacy of behavioral interventions in the management of female urinary incontinence. Continence Program for Women Research Group, *Am J Obstet Gynecol* 179(4):999, 1998.

Total urinary Incontinence

Mikel Gray

NANDA Definition

State in which the individual experiences continuous and unpredictable loss of urine
NOTE: In this book, the diagnosis **Total urinary Incontinence** will be used to refer to continuous urine loss due to an extraurethral cause, and the diagnosis **Stress urinary Incontinence** will be used to refer to leakage caused by urethral sphincter incompetence, regardless of severity.

Defining Characteristics

Continuous urine flow varying from dribbling incontinence superimposed on an otherwise identifiable pattern of voiding to severe urine loss without identifiable micturition episodes

Related Factors (r/t)

Ectopia (ectopic ureter opens into vaginal vault or cutaneously; bladder ectopia with exstrophy/epispadias complex)

• = Independent; ▲ = Collaborative

Fistula (opening from bladder or urethra to vagina or skin that bypasses urethral sphincter mechanism, allowing continuous urine loss)

| NOC | Outcomes (Nursing Outcomes Classification) |

Suggested NOC Outcomes

Tissue Integrity: Skin and Mucous Membranes; Urinary Continence; Urinary Elimination

> ### Example NOC Outcome with Indicators
>
> **Tissue Integrity: Skin and Mucous Membranes** as evidenced by the following indicators: Tissue lesion free/Skin intact (Rate each indicator of **Tissue Integrity: Skin and Mucous Membranes:** 1 = extremely compromised, 2 = substantially compromised, 3 = moderately compromised, 4 = mildly compromised, 5 = not compromised [see Section I].)

Client Outcomes

Client Will (Specify Time Frame):
- Experience urine loss that is adequately contained, with clothing remaining unsoiled and odor controlled
- Maintain intact perineal skin
- Maintain dignity, hide urine containment device in clothing, and minimize bulk and noise related to device

| NIC | Interventions (Nursing Interventions Classification) |

Suggested NIC Intervention

Urinary Incontinence Care

> ### Example NIC Activities—Urinary Incontinence Care
>
> Provide protective garments as needed; Cleanse genital skin at regular intervals

Nursing Interventions and Rationales

- Obtain a history of the duration and severity of urine loss, prior management, and aggravating or alleviating features. *Urinary incontinence from an extraurethral source (fistula or ectopia) is often confused with other forms of incontinence. Total incontinence should be suspected whenever the client reports continuous urine loss irrespective of physical exertion or associated urgency (Flores-Carreras et al, 2001).*
- Perform a focused physical assessment, including inspection of the perineal skin, examination of the vaginal vault, reproduction of the sign of stress incontinence (refer to the care plan for **Stress urinary Incontinence**), and testing of bulbocavernosus reflex and perineal sensations. *The physical examination will provide evidence supporting the diagnosis of extraurethral or another type of incontinence (stress, urge, or reflex) and provide the basis for further evaluation and/or treatment (Gray and Haas, 2000).*
- ▲ Consult a physician concerning the results of colposcopy, cystourethroscopy, intravenous urogram, cystogram, Pyridium pad test, or pelvic examination. *Evaluation of the location and characteristics of a urinary fistula or ectopic ureter requires direct visualiza-*

• = Independent; ▲ = Collaborative

tion or identification based on an imaging study of the urinary system (Flores-Carreras et al, 2001).

- Assist the client in selecting and applying a urine containment device(s). Review types of containment products with the client, including advantages and potential complications associated with each type of product. *Urine containment products include a variety of absorptive pads, incontinence briefs, underpads for bedding, absorptive inserts that fit into specially designed undergarments, and condom catheters. Careful selection of an absorptive product and education concerning its use maximizes its effectiveness in controlling urine loss in a particular individual (Dunn et al, 2002; Shirran and Brazelli, 2000).*

- Evaluate disposable vs. reusable products for urine containment, considering the setting (home care vs. acute care vs. long-term care), preferences of the client and caregiver(s), and immediate vs. long-term costs. *The economic and related impact of routine use of urine containment devices is significant, regardless of the setting. Economic factors as well as client and caregiver preferences affect the success and ultimate cost of a reusable vs. disposable urine containment device (Dunn et al, 2002; Shirran and Brazelli, 2000).* **Nursing Research:** *A study comparing a single reusable device with the "usual" containment device of a group of 175 community-dwelling subjects, which was most often a disposable pad, revealed that reusable garments provide comfort and perceived protection from visible urine loss equivalent to those of disposable pads (Gallo and Staskin, 1997).*

- Cleanse the perineal skin regularly using a cleanser capable of removing irritants (including urine, stool, and materials). Select a product with a slightly acidic pH close to that of normal skin, with a water base and surfactant designed to remove irritants from the skin with minimal physical force. Avoid vigorous scrubbing with water, soap and a washcloth. *Traditional soaps tend to be alkaline, interfering with the natural acid mantle of the integument and increasing its susceptibility to irritant dermatitis and secondary infection. Brisk scrubbing may exacerbate skin erosion and further increase the risk of irritation and infection (Gray, Ratliff, and Donovan, 2002).*

- Apply a skin moisturizer following cleansing. *Moisturizers contain humectants such as glycerin, methyl glucose esters, lanolin, and mineral oil that augment oils manufactured by the integument and create a moisture barrier protecting the skin from overhydration or dehydration (Gray, Ratliff, and Donovan, 2002).*

- Apply a moisture barrier containing zinc oxide to clients with severe and constant urine loss, and those with double urinary and fecal incontinence. *Although moisturizing creams containing humectants usually afford an adequate moisture barrier, clients with very severe incontinence and those with double fecal and urinary incontinence (particularly when the stool is liquified) often require a product with more vigorous moisture barrier qualities. Products containing zinc oxide can be applied to protect very compromised perineal skin exposed to highly irritating fecal effluent or constant, high-volume urinary leakage (Gray, Ratliff, and Donovan, 2002).*

- When cleansing a client with a moisture barrier containing zinc oxide, avoid vigorous scrubbing or use of a traditional washcloth to remove the paste. Instead, cleanse fecal materials away from the skin, leaving a clean layer of zinc oxide paste when cleansing after a single episode or gently removing the paste with mineral oil. *Pastes containing zinc oxide are difficult to remove, and it is not necessary to completely remove the product every time the perineal skin is cleansed. When deep cleansing and inspection of the underlying skin are indicated, mineral oil can be used to remove the paste without the need for brisk scrubbing.*

• = **Independent;** ▲ = **Collaborative**

▲ Consult the physician concerning use of an antifungal powder or ointment when perineal dermatitis is complicated by monilial infection. Teach the client to use the product sparingly when applying to affected areas. *Antifungal powders or ointments provide effective relief from monilial rash; however, application of excessive amounts of the product retains moisture and diminishes its effectiveness (Evans and Gray, 2003; Gray, Ratliff, and Donovan, 2002).*

▲ Consult the physician concerning placement of an indwelling catheter when severe urine loss is complicated by urinary retention, when careful fluid monitoring is indicated, when perineal dryness is required to promote healing of a stage 3 or 4 pressure ulcer, during periods of critical illness, or in the terminally ill client when use of absorbent products produces pain or distress. *Although not routinely indicated, the indwelling catheter provides an effective, transient management technique for carefully selected clients (Treatment of Pressure Ulcers Guideline Panel, 1994; Urinary Incontinence Guideline Panel, 1996).*

▲ Refer the client with "intractable" or extraurethral incontinence to a continence service or specialist for further evaluation and management of urine loss. *The successful management of complex, severe urinary incontinence requires specialized evaluation and treatment from a health care provider with special expertise.*

Geriatric

• Provide privacy and support when changing incontinent devices in elderly clients. *Elderly, hospitalized clients frequently express feelings of shame, guilt, and dependency when undergoing urinary containment device changes (Biggerson et al, 1993).*

• Avoid brisk scrubbing and use of a washcloth when cleansing the skin of an aging client. *Brisk washing with a washcloth tends to strip superficial layers of skin, which potentially exacerbates erosion or damage to subcutaneous connective tissues (Gray, Ratliff, and Donovan, 2002).*

• Employ meticulous infection control procedures when using an indwelling catheter.

Home care

• The interventions described previously may be adapted for home care use.

• Encourage a mind-set and program of self-care management. **Nursing Research:** *Addressing self-care activities through exercise, diet, fluid intake, and protective devices helps the client to exercise control over incontinence (Leenerts, Teel, and Pendleton, 2002).*

• Implement a bladder training program, including self-monitoring activities (reducing caffeine intake, adjusting amount and timing of fluid intake, decreasing long voiding intervals while awake, making dietary changes to promote bowel regularity), bladder training, and pelvic muscle exercise as appropriate. **Nursing Research:** *In one study of women aged 55 years or older with involuntary urine loss associated with stress, urge, or mixed incontinence, clients responded to the aforementioned interventions with a 61% decrease in the severity of urinary incontinence at 2 years after intervention. Self-monitoring and bladder training accounted for most of the improvement (Dougherty et al, 2002).*

• Assist the family with arranging care in a way that allows the client to participate in family or favorite activities without embarrassment. Elicit discussion of the client's concerns about the social or emotional burden of incontinence. **Nursing and Clinical Research:** *Careful planning can help the client retain dignity and maintain the integrity of family patterns. Urinary incontinence has a demonstrated influence on subjective*

• = Independent; ▲ = Collaborative

well-being and quality of life, with depression, loneliness, or sadness possible (Fultz and Herzog, 2001). Discussing emotional concerns helps the client to develop a sense of control over incontinence (Leenerts, Teel, and Pendleton, 2002).

▲ Consider the use of an indwelling catheter for continuous drainage in the client with severe urinary incontinence who is homebound, bed-bound, and receiving palliative or end-of-life care (requires a physician's order). *An indwelling catheter may increase client comfort, ease caregiver burden, and prevent urinary incontinence in bed-bound clients receiving end-of-life care.*

▲ When an indwelling catheter is in place, follow the prescribed maintenance protocols for managing the catheter, drainage bag, and perineal skin and urethral meatus. Teach infection control measures adapted to the home care setting. *Proper care reduces the risk of catheter-associated urinary tract infection.*

• Assist the client in adapting to the catheter. Encourage discussion of the client's response to the catheter. **Nursing Research:** *Clients living with a catheter are keenly aware of its presence; adaptation is served by normalizing the experience. Instruction could include the fact that the client will be more aware of some sensations and sounds (e.g., urine sloshing in the bag, the weight of the bag, pressure or pain when urine flow has been altered). Rehearsing emptying of the bag when away from home will support resumption of activities. Discussion of the client's response will help him or her to deal with embarrassment or frustration (Wilde, 2002).*

Client/Family Teaching

• Teach the family to obtain, apply, and dispose of or clean and reuse urine containment devices.
• Teach the family a routine perineal skin care regimen, including daily or every other day hygiene and cleansing with containment product changes.
• Teach the client and family to recognize and manage perineal dermatitis, ammonia contact dermatitis, and monilial rash.
• Teach the client to maintain adequate fluid intake (30 ml/kg of body weight per day).
• Teach the client and family to recognize and manage urinary tract infection.

evolve WEBSITES FOR EDUCATION

See the EVOLVE website for World Wide Web resources for client education.

REFERENCES

Biggerson AB et al: Elderly women's feelings about being incontinent, using napkins and being helped by nurses to change napkins, *J Clin Nurs* 2:165, 1993.

Dougherty MC et al: A randomized trial of behavioral management for continence with older rural women, *Res Nurs Health* 25(1):3, 2002.

Dunn S et al: Systematic review of the effectiveness of urinary continence products, *J Wound Ostomy Continence Nurs* 29(3):129, 2002.

Evans EC, Gray M: What interventions are effective for the prevention and treatment of cutaneous candidiasis? *J Wound Ostomy Continence Nurs* 30(1):11, 2003.

Flores-Carreras O et al: Fistulas of the urinary tract in obstetric surgery, *Int Urogynecol J Pelvic Floor Dysfunct* 12:203, 2001.

Fultz NH, Herzog AR: Self-reported social and emotional impact of urinary incontinence, *J Am Geriatr Soc* 49: 892, 2001.

• = **Independent**; ▲ = **Collaborative**

Gallo M, Staskin DR: Patient satisfaction with a reusable undergarment for urinary incontinence, *J Wound Ostomy Continence Nurs* 24(4):226, 1997.

Gray M, Haas J: Assessment of the patient with urinary incontinence. In Doughty DB, editor: *Urinary and fecal incontinence: nursing management,* St Louis, 2000, Mosby.

Gray M, Ratliff C, Donovan A: Perineal skin care for the incontinent patient, *Adv Skin Wound Care* 15:170, 2002.

Leenerts MH, Teel CS, Pendleton MK: Building a model of self-care for health promotion in aging, *J Nurs Scholarsh* 34:355, 2002.

Shirran E, Brazelli M: Absorbent products for the containment of urinary and/or fecal incontinence, *Cochrane Database System Rev* (CD0011406), 2000.

Treatment of Pressure Ulcers Guideline Panel: *Treatment of pressure ulcer: clinical practice guideline,* Rockville, Md, 1994, Agency for Health Care Policy and Research.

Urinary Incontinence Guideline Panel: *Urinary incontinence in adults: clinical practice guideline,* ed 2, Rockville, Md, 1996, Agency for Health Care Policy and Research.

Wilde MH: Urine flowing: a phenomenological study of living with a urinary catheter, *Res Nurs Health* 25:14, 2002.

Urge urinary Incontinence

Mikel Gray

NANDA   Definition

State in which the individual experiences involuntary passage of urine occurring with precipitous desire to urinate. Urge incontinence is usually defined within the context of overactive bladder syndrome. The overactive bladder is characterized by bothersome urgency, with or without urge incontinence, and accompanied by frequent daytime voiding and nocturia.

Defining Characteristics

Diurnal urinary frequency (voiding more than once every 2 hours while awake); urgency (subjective report of precipitous or immediate need to urinate when urgency is perceived); nocturia (awakening more than once per night to urinate for persons younger than 65 years of age and more than twice per night for persons older than 65 years of age); symptom of urge incontinence (urine loss associated with desire to urinate); enuresis (involuntary passage of urine while asleep)

Related Factors

- Neurological disorders (brain disorders, including cerebrovascular accident, brain tumor, normal pressure hydrocephalus, traumatic brain injury)
- Inflammation of bladder (calculi; tumor, including transitional cell carcinoma and carcinoma in situ; inflammatory lesions of the bladder; urinary tract infection)
- Bladder outlet obstruction (see **Urinary retention**)
- Stress urinary incontinence (mixed urinary incontinence; these conditions often coexist but relationship between them remains unclear)
- Idiopathic causes (implicated factors include depression, sleep apnea/hypoxia)

NOC   Outcomes (Nursing Outcomes Classification)

Suggested NOC Outcomes

Tissue Integrity: Skin and Mucous Membranes; Urinary Continence; Urinary Elimination

- • = Independent; ▲ = Collaborative

Client Outcomes

Client Will (Specify Time Frame):

- Report relief from urge urinary incontinence or a decrease in the incidence or severity of incontinent episodes
- Identify containment devices that assist in the management of urge urinary incontinence

NIC   Interventions (Nursing Interventions Classification)

Suggested NIC Interventions
Urinary Habit Training; Urinary Incontinence Care

Nursing Interventions and Rationales

- Take a nursing history focusing on duration of urinary incontinence, diurnal frequency, nocturia, severity of symptoms, and alleviating and aggravating factors. *A focused history helps determine the cause of urinary incontinence and guides its subsequent management.* **Nursing Research:** *Querying the client about the isolated symptom of urge incontinence shows a poor correlation with a diagnosis of detrusor overactivity incontinence. However, the agreement between urodynamic testing and the clinical diagnosis obtained by the history rises sharply when the client reports three symptoms: diurnal frequency, urge-related urine loss, and nocturia (Gray et al, 2001).*
- ▲ Complete a urinalysis, examining for the presence of nitrites, leukocytes, glucose, or hemoglobin (red blood cells). *The presence of nitrites and leukocytes raises a suspicion of urinary tract infection, the presence of glucosuria raises the risk of undiagnosed or poorly controlled diabetes mellitus, and the presence of red blood cells in the absence of signs of infection raises a suspicion of a bladder tumor. Each condition may produce acute urinary incontinence requiring treatment of the underlying cause (Fourcroy, 2001).*
- Complete a bladder log, including frequency of diurnal micturition and nocturia, patterns of incontinence, symptoms of accompanying urine loss, and the type and volume of fluids consumed. *The bladder log provides a more objective record of diurnal urinary frequency, nocturia, and patterns of urgency and urge incontinence than does the history (Resnick et al, 1994). Recording fluid consumption allows an evaluation of the volume of fluid consumed over a 24-hour period and the intake of bladder irritants.*

• = Independent; ▲ = Collaborative

▲ Review all medications the client is receiving, paying particular attention to sedatives, narcotics, diuretics, antidepressants, psychotropic drugs, and cholinergics. Consult the physician about altering or eliminating these medications if they are suspected of affecting incontinence. *The side effects of multiple medications may produce or exacerbate urge incontinence (Fourcroy, 2001).*

• Assess the client for urinary retention (see the care plan for **Urinary retention**). *Urinary retention associated with bladder outlet obstruction may be a contributing cause of urge incontinence (Zorn et al, 1999). Urinary retention associated with poor detrusor contraction strength has been described in frail elderly clients (Resnick and Yalla, 1987). Regardless of its cause, retention significantly affects the management of this condition (Gray, 2000).*

• Assess the client for functional limitations (environmental barriers, limited mobility or dexterity, impaired cognitive function (see the care plan for **Functional urinary Incontinence**). *Functional limitations affect the severity and management of urge urinary incontinence (Ouslander, 2002).*

▲ Consult the physician concerning diabetic management and pharmacotherapy for urinary tract infection when indicated. *In specific cases, urgency and an increased risk of urge incontinence may be related to urinary tract infection (Molander et al, 2000) or polyuria from undiagnosed or poorly managed diabetes mellitus (Samsioe et al, 1999).*

▲ Assess for signs and symptoms of atrophic vaginal changes in the perimenopausal or postmenopausal woman, including vaginal dryness, tenderness to touch, mucosal dryness, friability, and discomfort with gentle palpation. Specifically query the woman with atrophic vaginitis concerning irritative lower urinary tract symptoms (diurnal frequency, nocturia of more than two episodes per night, urgency, dysuria). Refer the woman with atrophic vaginal changes and bothersome lower urinary tract symptoms to a gynecologist, urologist, or women's health nurse-practitioner for further evaluation and management. *The relationship between atrophic vaginitis and urge incontinence risk remains unclear. However, several studies have observed a relationship between systemic estrogen replacement and urinary incontinence (Brown et al, 1999; Molander et al, 2000). Nevertheless, the nature of this relationship remains unknown, and additional evidence suggests that local hormone replacement therapy may reduce irritative lower urinary tract symptoms and the risk of urinary tract infection (Eriksen, 1999).*

• Establish bladder training (also called habit training or bladder retraining program) based on data gathered from the bladder log, physical assessment, and functional assessment. **Nursing Research:** *A randomized clinical trial encompassing 204 women revealed that bladder training was effective for urge and mixed urinary incontinence, and the magnitude of improvement is comparable to that achieved by women undergoing pelvic muscle rehabilitation or combination therapy (Elser et al, 1999).*

• Review with the client the types of beverages consumed, focusing on the intake of bladder irritants, including caffeine and alcohol. *A growing body of evidence supports limitation of caffeine as an effective means of reducing voiding frequency (Gray, 2001). Although epidemiological studies have failed to establish a statistically significant relationship between alcohol consumption and urinary incontinence risk (Bortolotti et al, 2000), alcohol is known to act as a diuretic and sedative, and clinical observations support its potential to transiently increase the risk of urine loss when consumed in significant quantities.*

• Review with the client the volume of fluids consumed and gradually adjust the fluid intake to meet the recommended daily allowance of 30 ml/kg of body weight

• = **Independent;** ▲ = **Collaborative**

(National Academy of Sciences, 1980). *Dehydration is postulated to exacerbate the symptoms of urgency (Pearson, 1992, 1993), and excessive fluid intake increases voided volume and urinary frequency (Fitzgerald and Brubaker, 2003). Increasing fluid intake in women with urinary incontinence may reduce the risk of urinary tract infection without increasing the frequency or severity of urine loss (Dougherty et al, 2002).*

- Instruct in techniques of urge suppression. Teach the client to identify, isolate, contract, and relax the pelvic floor muscles. When a strong or precipitous urge to urinate is perceived, teach the client to avoid running to the toilet. Instead, she or he should perform repeated, rapid pelvic muscle contractions until the urge is relieved. Relief is followed by micturition within 5 to 15 minutes, using nonhurried movements when locating a toilet and voiding. **Clinical Research:** *Randomized controlled trials comparing urge suppression techniques to pharmacotherapy or bladder training have shown it to be an effective method for reducing urge urinary incontinence episodes (Burgio and Engel, 2002).*

- ▲ Begin transvaginal or transrectal electrical stimulation using a low-frequency current (5 to 20 Hz) in consultation with the physician. *Electrical stimulation is an effective treatment for urge incontinence; in one randomized clinical trial it was found to completely eliminate symptoms of urge incontinence in 49% of a group of 121 subjects (Moore, Gray, and Rayome, 1995).*

- ▲ Teach the client to self-administer antimuscarinic (anticholinergic) drugs as directed. Teach dosage and administration of the medication and the importance of combining pharmacotherapy with scheduled voiding, adequate fluid intake, restriction of bladder irritants, and urge suppression techniques. *Antimuscarinic drugs increase bladder capacity, reduce the frequency of incontinence episodes, and diminish voiding frequency. However, they do not cure bladder dysfunction or reduce the time between perception of a strong urge and onset of an overactive detrusor contraction. The efficacy of pharmacotherapy for urge incontinence and overactive bladder dysfunction is enhanced when combined with behavioral interventions (Burgio, 2002; Burgio, Locher, and Goode, 2000).*

- ▲ Assist the client in selecting, obtaining, and applying a containment device for urine loss as indicated (see the care plan for **Total urinary Incontinence**).

- ▲ Provide the client with information about incontinence support groups such as the National Association for Continence and the Simon Foundation for Continence. *Self-help groups provide social support and a forum for sharing strategies for the management of all types of urinary incontinence (Irwin, 2000).*

Geriatric

- Assess the functional and cognitive status of the elderly client with urge incontinence. *Functional limitations affect the severity and management of urge urinary incontinence (Ouslander, 2002).*

- Plan care in long-term or acute care facilities based on knowledge of the elderly client's established voiding patterns, paying particular attention to patterns of nocturia.

- ▲ Carefully monitor the elderly client for potential adverse effects of antispasmodic medications, including a severely dry mouth interfering with the use of dentures, eating, or speaking, or confusion, nightmares, constipation, mydriasis, or heat intolerance. *Elderly persons are particularly susceptible to adverse effects associated with antispasmodic medications (Ghoneim and Hassouna, 1997).*

• = Independent; ▲ = Collaborative

Home care

- The interventions described previously may be adapted for home care use.
- Teach the importance of avoiding dehydration or excessive fluid consumption and the paradoxical relationship between dehydration and symptoms of urgency.
- Teach the family and client to identify and correct environmental barriers to toileting within the home.
- Encourage a mind-set and program of self-care management. **Nursing Research:** *Addressing self-care activities through exercise, diet, fluid intake, and protective devices helps the client to exercise control over incontinence (Leenerts, Teel, and Pendleton, 2002).*
- Implement a bladder training program as appropriate, including self-monitoring activities (reducing caffeine intake, adjusting amount and timing of fluid intake, decreasing long voiding intervals while awake, making dietary changes to promote bowel regularity), bladder training, and pelvic muscle exercise. **Nursing Research:** *In one study of women aged 55 years or older with involuntary urine loss associated with stress, urge, or mixed incontinence, clients responded to the aforementioned interventions with a 61% decrease in the severity of urinary incontinence at 2 years after intervention. Self-monitoring and bladder training accounted for most of the improvement (Dougherty et al, 2002).*
- Help the client and family to identify and correct environmental barriers to toileting within the home.

Client/Family Teaching

- Teach the client and family to recognize foods and beverages that are likely to irritate the bladder.
- Teach the family and client to recognize and manage side effects of antispasmodic medications used to treat urge incontinence.
- Help the client and family to recognize and manage side effect of anticholinergic medications used to manage irritative lower urinary tract symptoms.

REFERENCES

Bortolotti A et al: Prevalence and risk factors for urinary incontinence in Italy, *Eur Urol* 37(1):30, 2000.

Brown JS et al: Prevalence of urinary incontinence and associated risk factors in postmenopausal women, *Obstet Gynecol* 94:66, 1999.

Burgio KL: Influence of behavior modification on overactive bladder, *Urology* 60(5 suppl 1):72, 2002.

Burgio KL, Locher JL, Goode PS: Combined behavioral and drug therapy for urge incontinence in older women, *J Am Geriatr Soc* 48(4):370, 2000.

Dougherty MC et al: A randomized trial of behavioral management for continence with older rural women, *Res Nurs Health* 25(1):3, 2002.

Elser DM et al: The effect of bladder training, pelvic floor muscle training, or combination training on urodynamic parameters in women with urinary incontinence. Continence Program for Women Research Group, *Neurourol Urodyn* 18(5):427, 1999.

Eriksen B: A randomized, open, parallel group study on the preventive effect of an estradiol-releasing vaginal ring (Estring) on recurrent urinary tract infections in postmenopausal women, *Am J Obstet Gynecol* 180:1072, 1999.

Fitzgerald MP, Brubaker L: Variability of 24-hour voiding diary variables among asymptomatic women, *J Urol* 169(1):207, 2003.

Fourcroy JL: Overactive bladder: a practical overview of diagnosis and treatment, *Adv Nurse Practit* 9(3):59, 2001.

Ghoneim GM, Hassouna M: Alternatives for the pharmacologic management of urge and stress urinary incontinence in the elderly, *J Wound Ostomy Continence Nurs* 24:311, 1997.

Gray M: Urinary retention: management in the acute care setting, Part 2, *Am J Nurs* 100:36, 2000.

Gray M: Caffeine and urinary incontinence, *J Wound Ostomy Continence Nurs* 28:66, 2001.

- **= Independent;** ▲ **= Collaborative**

Gray M et al: A model for predicting motor urge urinary incontinence, *Nurs Res* 50:116, 2001.

Irwin B: User support groups in continence care, *Nurs Times* 96(31 suppl):24, 2000.

Leenerts MH, Teel CS, Pendleton MK: Building a model of self-care for health promotion in aging, *J Nurs Scholarsh* 34:355, 2002.

Molander U et al: A longitudinal cohort study of elderly women with urinary tract infection, *Maturitas* 34:127, 2000.

Moore KN, Gray ML, Rayome RG: Electric stimulation and urinary incontinence: research and alternatives, *Urol Nurs* 15: 94, 1995.

National Academy of Sciences, Food and Nutrition Board: *Recommended daily allowances,* ed 9, Washington, DC, 1980, The Academy.

Ouslander JG: Geriatric considerations in the diagnosis and management of overactive bladder, *Urology* 60(5 suppl 1):50, 2002.

Pearson BD: Urine control by elders: noninvasive strategies. In Funk SG et al: *Key aspects of elder care: managing falls, incontinence and cognitive impairment,* New York, 1992, Springer.

Pearson BD: Liquidate a myth: reducing liquids is not advisable for elderly with urine control problems, *Urol Nurs* 13:86, 1993.

Resnick NM, Yalla SV: Detrusor hyperactivity with impaired contractile function. An unrecognized but common cause of incontinence in elderly patients, *JAMA* 257:3076, 1987.

Resnick NM et al. Short term variability of self report of incontinence in older persons, *J Am Geriatr Soc* 42:202, 1994.

Samsioe G et al: Urogenital symptoms in women aged 50-59 years, *Gynecol Endocrinol* 13:113, 1999.

Zorn BH et al: Urinary incontinence and depression, *J Urol* 162:82, 1999.

Risk for urge urinary Incontinence

Mikel Gray

NANDA Definition

At risk for involuntary loss of urine associated with a sudden, strong sensation or urinary urgency

Risk Factors

Effects of medications, caffeine, alcohol; detrusor hyperreflexia from cystitis, urethritis, tumors, renal calculi, central nervous system disorders above the pontine micturition center; detrusor muscle instability with impaired contractility; involuntary sphincter relaxation; ineffective toileting habits; small bladder capacity

NOC Outcomes (Nursing Outcomes Classification)

Suggested NOC Outcomes

Tissue Integrity: Skin and Mucous Membranes; Urinary Continence; Urinary Elimination

---

Example NOC Outcome with Indicators

Urinary Continence as evidenced by the following indicators: Responds in timely manner to urge/Voids in appropriate receptacle/Has adequate time to reach toilet between urge and evacuation of urine/Underclothing remains dry during day/Underclothing or bedding remains dry during night (Rate each indicator of **Urinary Continence:** 1 = never demonstrated, 2 = rarely demonstrated, 3 = sometimes demonstrated, 4 = often demonstrated, 5 = consistently demonstrated [see Section I].)

• = Independent; ▲ = Collaborative

Client Outcomes

Client Will (Specify Time Frame):

- Report relief from urge urinary incontinence or a decrease in the incidence or severity of incontinent episodes
- Identify containment devices that assist in the management of urge urinary incontinence

NIC   Interventions (Nursing Interventions Classification)

Suggested NIC Interventions

Urinary Habit Training; Urinary Incontinence Care

Example NIC Activities—Urinary Habit Training

Keep continence specification record for 3 days to establish voiding pattern; Establish interval for toileting of preferably not less than 2 hours

---

Nursing Interventions and Rationales

- Take a nursing history focusing on the following lower urinary tract symptoms: daytime voiding frequency, nocturia, presence of bothersome urgency (precipitous desire to urinate that interferes with activities of daily living), and presence of urine loss. *Bothersome lower urinary tract symptoms are strongly correlated with urge incontinence in adult women (Alling-Moller, Lose, and Jorgensen, 2000).* **Nursing Research:** *Diurnal voiding frequency (voiding every 2 hours or less often), nocturia (arising to void more than once each night for younger clients and more than twice each night for adults older than 65 years of age), and bothersome urgency are associated with urge incontinence (Gray et al, 2001).*

- Query the client about specific risk factors for urge urinary incontinence, such as childhood enuresis, depression, prostate enlargement with bladder outlet obstruction, and neurological disorders, including stroke or parkinsonism. *Bladder outlet obstruction and neurological disorders affecting modulatory areas in the brain are strongly associated with detrusor overactivity, bothersome lower urinary tract symptoms, and an increased risk for urge incontinence (Mostwin, 2002). Childhood enuresis may be a risk factor for overactive bladder symptoms in adults (Kuh, Cardozo, and Hardy, 1999; Malmsten et al, 1997).*

- Assess the client's functional status, focusing on mobility, dexterity, and cognitive status. *The risk of urinary incontinence rises with increased impairment of mobility; clients who are bedridden are at greatest risk, followed by clients who are confined to a wheelchair, those relying on a walker, and those walking with minimal assistance (Aggazzotti et al, 2000). Cognitive impairment, particularly when accompanied by disoriented perception of time, is associated with an increased risk of urge urinary incontinence in the aging client (Griffiths et al, 2002).*

- ▲ Complete a urinalysis, focusing on the presence of nitrites, leukocytes, glucose, or hemoglobin (red blood cells). *The presence of nitrites and leukocytes raises a suspicion of urinary tract infection, the presence of glucosuria raises a risk of undiagnosed or poorly controlled diabetes mellitus, and the presence of red blood cells in the absence of signs of infection raises a suspicion of a bladder tumor. Each condition increases the risk of urgency symptoms and urge incontinence (Fourcroy, 2001).*

• = Independent; ▲ = Collaborative

- Complete a bladder log, including frequency of diurnal micturition and nocturia, and the type and volume of fluids consumed. *The bladder log provides a more objective record of diurnal urinary frequency, nocturia, and patterns of urgency than the history (Resnick et al, 1994). Recording fluid consumption allows an evaluation of the volume of fluid consumed over a 24-hour period and the intake of bladder irritants.*
- Review with the client the types of beverages consumed, focusing on the intake of bladder irritants, including caffeine and alcohol. Advise the client to reduce or eliminate intake of these substances to determine their effect on voiding frequency and symptoms of urgency. *A growing body of evidence supports limitation of caffeine as an effective means of reducing voiding frequency (Gray, 2001). Although epidemiological studies have failed to establish a statistically significant relationship between alcohol consumption and urinary incontinence risk (Bortolotti et al, 2000), alcohol is known to act as a diuretic and sedative, and clinical observations support its potential to transiently increase the risk of urine loss when consumed in significant quantities.*
- Additional bladder irritants, including aspartame, carbonated drinks, decaffeinated coffee or tea, citrus juices, highly spiced foods, chocolates, and vinegar-containing foods, may be eliminated from the diet and added back singly to determine their impact on bothersome lower urinary tract symptoms and urgency. *Evidence is limited in support of the role of these substances as potential bladder irritants in clients at risk of urge urinary incontinence, but they do play a more significant role for those with interstitial cystitis (Bade, Peeters, and Mensink, 1997; Interstital Cystitis Association, 1999).*
- Review with the client the volume of fluids consumed and gradually adjust the fluid intake to meet the recommended daily allowance of approximately 30 ml/kg of body weight in the ambulatory adult (National Academy of Sciences, 1980). *Dehydration is postulated to exacerbate symptoms of urgency (Pearson, 1992, 1993), and excessive fluid intake increases voided volume and urinary frequency. Consumption of fluids within the recommended daily allowance may reduce the risk of urinary tract infection without increasing the frequency or severity of urine loss (Dougherty, 1999).*
- ▲ Review all medications the client is receiving, paying particular attention to sedatives, narcotics, diuretics, antidepressants, psychotropic drugs, and cholinergics. Consult the physician about altering or eliminating these medications if they are suspected of affecting incontinence. *The side effects of multiple medications may produce or exacerbate urge incontinence (Fourcroy, 2001).*
- ▲ Consult the physician concerning diabetic management and pharmacotherapy for urinary tract infection when indicated. *In specific cases, urgency and an increased risk of urge incontinence may be related to urinary tract infection (Molander et al, 2000) or polyuria from undiagnosed or poorly managed diabetes mellitus (Samsioe et al, 1999).*
- ▲ Assess for signs and symptoms of atrophic vaginal changes in the perimenopausal or postmenopausal woman, including vaginal dryness, tenderness to touch, dryness of mucosa on touch with friability, and discomfort with gentle palpation. Specifically query the client with atrophic vaginitis concerning irritative lower urinary tract symptoms (diurnal frequency, nocturia of more than two episodes per night, urgency, dysuria). Refer the client with atrophic vaginal changes and bothersome lower urinary tract symptoms to a gynecologist, urologist, or women's health nurse-practitioner for further evaluation and management. *The relationship between atrophic vaginitis and urge incontinence risk remains unclear. However, several studies have found that systemic estrogen replacement slightly increases the frequency of urinary incontinence episodes (Brown et al, 1999; Molander et al, 2000). Nevertheless, the nature of this relationship remains unknown,*

- = **Independent**; ▲ = **Collaborative**

and additional evidence suggests that local hormone replacement therapy may reduce irritative lower urinary tract symptoms and the risk of urinary tract infection (Eriksen, 1999).

- Instruct in techniques of urge suppression. Teach the client to identify, isolate, contract, and relax the pelvic floor muscles. When a strong or precipitous urge to urinate is perceived, teach the client to avoid running to the toilet. Instead, she or he should perform repeated, rapid pelvic muscle contractions until the urge is relieved. Relief is followed by micturition within 5 to 15 minutes, using nonhurried movements when locating a toilet and voiding. *Urge suppression techniques reduce the risk of urine loss when a precipitous urge to urinate is experienced (Burgio et al, 1998; Wyman et al, 1998).*
- ▲ Provide the client with information about incontinence support groups such as the National Association for Continence and the Simon Foundation for Continence. *Self-help groups provide social support and a forum for sharing strategies for management of all types of urinary incontinence (Irwin, 2000).*

Geriatric

- Assess the functional and cognitive status of an elderly client with irritative lower urinary tract symptoms or urge incontinence.
- ▲ Advise a male client with bothersome lower urinary tract symptoms to see his physician or nurse-practitioner, since these symptoms may be related to prostate enlargement.
- ▲ Carefully monitor the elderly client for potential adverse effects of anticholinergic medications, including severe dry mouth interfering with the use of dentures, eating, or speaking, or the occurrence of confusion, nightmares, constipation, mydriasis, or heat intolerance. *Elderly persons are particularly susceptible to adverse effects associated with anticholinergic medications.*

Home care

- The interventions described previously may be adapted for home care use.
- Encourage a mind-set and program of self-care management. **Nursing Research:** *Addressing self-care activities through exercise, diet, fluid intake, and protective devices helps the client take control of incontinence (Leenerts, Teel, and Pendleton, 2002).*
- Implement a bladder training program, including self-monitoring activities (reducing caffeine intake, adjusting amount and timing of fluid intake, decreasing long voiding intervals while awake, making dietary changes to promote bowel regularity), bladder training, and pelvic muscle exercise. **Nursing Research:** *In one study of women aged 55 years or older with involuntary urine loss associated with stress, urge, or mixed incontinence, clients responded to the aforementioned interventions with a 61% decrease in the severity of urinary incontinence at 2 years after intervention. Self-monitoring and bladder training accounted for most of the improvement (Dougherty et al, 2002).*
- Teach the client and family to recognize foods and beverages that are likely to irritate the bladder.
- Teach the importance of avoiding dehydration or excessive fluid consumption and the paradoxical relationship between dehydration and symptoms of urgency.
- ▲ Teach the family and client to recognize and manage side effects of anticholinergic medications used to treat irritative lower urinary tract symptoms.
- Teach the family and client to identify and correct environmental barriers to toileting within the home.

- • = **Independent;** ▲ = **Collaborative**

- Assist the family with arranging care in a way that allows the client to participate in family or favorite activities without embarrassment. Elicit discussion of the client's concerns about the social or emotional burden of incontinence. **Nursing and Clinical Research:** *Careful planning can help the client retain dignity and maintain the integrity of family patterns. Urinary incontinence has a demonstrated influence on subjective well-being and quality of life, with depression, loneliness, or sadness possible (Fultz and Herzog, 2001). Discussing emotional concerns helps the client to develop a sense of control over incontinence (Leenerts, Teel, and Pendleton, 2002).*

Client/Family Teaching

- Teach the client and family to recognize foods and beverages that are likely to irritate the bladder.
- Teach the importance of avoiding dehydration or excessive fluid consumption and the paradoxical relationship between dehydration and symptoms of urgency.

evolve WEBSITES FOR EDUCATION

See the EVOLVE website for World Wide Web resources for client education.

REFERENCES

Aggazzotti G et al: Prevalence of urinary incontinence among institutionalized patients: a cross-sectional epidemiologic study in a midsized city in northern Italy, *Urology* 56(2):245, 2000.

Alling-Moller LA, Lose G, Jorgensen T: Risk factors for lower urinary tract symptoms in women 40 to 60 years of age, *Obstet Gynecol* 96:466, 2000.

Bade JJ, Peeters JM, Mensink HJ: Is the diet of patients with interstitial cystitis related to their disease? *Eur Urol* 32:179, 1997.

Brown JS et al: Prevalence of urinary incontinence and associated risk factors in postmenopausal women, *Obstet Gynecol* 94:66, 1999.

Burgio KL et al: Behavioral vs. drug treatment for urge urinary incontinence in older women: a randomized controlled trial, *JAMA* 280:1995, 1998.

Dougherty MC: *Establishing goals and lifestyle management,* WOCN Continence Conference, Austin, Tex, Feb 1999.

Dougherty MC et al: A randomized trial of behavioral management for continence with older rural women, *Res Nurs Health* 25(1):3, 2002.

Eriksen B: A randomized, open, parallel group study on the preventive effect of an estradiol-releasing vaginal ring (Estring) on recurrent urinary tract infections in postmenopausal women, *Am J Obstet Gynecol* 180:1072, 1999.

Fourcroy JL: Overactive bladder: a practical overview of diagnosis and treatment, *Adv Nurse Practit* 9(3):59, 2001.

Fultz NH, Herzog AR: Self-reported social and emotional impact of urinary incontinence, *J Am Geriatr Soc* 49:892, 2001.

Gray M: Caffeine and urinary incontinence, *J Wound Ostomy Continence Nurs* 28:66, 2001.

Gray M et al: A model for predicting motor urge urinary incontinence, *Nurs Res* 50:116, 2001.

Griffiths D et al: Urge incontinence and impaired detrusor contractility in the elderly, *Neurourol Urodyn* 21(2):126, 2002.

Interstitial Cystitis Association: *Interstitial cystitis and diet,* Rockville, Md, 1999, The Association.

Irwin B: User support groups in continence care, *Nurs Times* 96(31 suppl):24, 2000.

Kuh D, Cardozo L, Hardy R: Urinary incontinence in middle aged women: childhood enuresis and other lifetime risk factors in a British prospective cohort, *J Epidemiol Community Health* 53(8):453, 1999.

Leenerts MH, Teel CS, Pendleton MK: Building a model of self-care for health promotion in aging, *J Nurs Scholarsh* 34:355, 2002.

Malmsten UG et al: Urinary incontinence and lower urinary tract symptoms: an epidemiological study of men aged 45 to 99 years, *J Urol* 158(5):1733, 1997.

- **= Independent; ▲ = Collaborative**

Molander U et al: A longitudinal cohort study of elderly women with urinary tract infection, *Maturitas* 34:127, 2000.

Mostwin JL: Pathophysiology: the varieties of bladder overactivity, *Urology* 60(5 suppl 1):22, 2002.

National Academy of Sciences, Food and Nutrition Board: *Recommended daily allowances*, ed 9, Washington, DC, 1980, The Academy.

Pearson BD: Urine control by elders: noninvasive strategies. In Funk SG et al: *Key aspects of elder care: managing falls, incontinence and cognitive impairment*, New York, 1992, Springer.

Pearson BD: Liquidate a myth: reducing liquids is not advisable for elderly with urine control problems, *Urol Nurs* 13:86, 1993.

Resnick NM et al: Short term variability of self report of incontinence in older persons, *J Am Geriatr Soc* 42:202, 1994.

Samsioe G et al: Urogenital symptoms in women aged 50-59 years, *Gynecol Endocrinol* 13:113, 1999.

Wyman JF et al: Comparative efficacy of behavioral interventions in the management of female urinary incontinence. Continence Program for Women Research Group, *Am J Obstet Gynecol* 179:999, 1998.

Disorganized Infant behavior

T. Heather Herdman and Mary A. Fuerst-DeWys

NANDA Definition

Disintegrated physiological and neurobehavioral responses to the environment

Defining Characteristics

Regulatory problems; inability to inhibit startle; irritability

State-organization system

Active awake (fussy, worried gaze); diffuse/unclear sleep, state-oscillation; quiet-awake (staring, gaze aversion); irritable or panicky crying

Attention-interaction system

Abnormal response to sensory stimuli (e.g., difficult to soothe, inability to sustain alert status)

Motor system

Increased, decreased, or limp tone; finger splay, fisting, or hands to face; hyperextension of arms and legs; tremors, startles, twitches; jittery, jerky, uncoordinated movement; altered primitive reflexes

Physiological

Bradycardia, tachycardia, or dysrhythmias; pale, cyanotic, mottled, or flushed color; "time-out signals" (e.g., gaze, grasp, hiccough, cough, sneeze, sigh, slack jaw, open mouth, tongue thrust); oximeter reading: desaturation; feeding intolerances (aspiration or emesis)

Related Factors (r/t)

Prenatal

Congenital or genetic disorders; teratogenic exposure

• = Independent; ▲ = Collaborative

Postnatal
Malnutrition; oral/motor problems; pain; feeding intolerance; invasive/painful proce-dures; prematurity

Individual
Illness; immature neurological system, gestational age; postconceptual age

Environmental
Physical environment inappropriateness; sensory inappropriateness; sensory overstimula-tion; sensory deprivation

Caregiver
Cue misreading; cue-deficient knowledge; environmental stimulation contribution

| NOC | Outcomes (Nursing Outcomes Classification) |

Suggested NOC Outcomes
Child Development: 2 Months, 4 Months, 6 Months; Growth; Neurological Status; Newborn Adaptation; Nutritional Status: Food and Fluid Intake; Preterm Infant Organi-zation; Sleep; Thermoregulation: Newborn; Vital Signs

---

Example NOC Outcome with Indicators

Preterm Infant Organization as evidenced by the following indictors: O_2 saturation greater than 85%/Skin color/Feeding tolerance/Muscle tone relaxed/Smooth synchronous movement/Posture flexed/Hands brought to mouth/Appropriate time-out signals/Self-consolability/Deep sleep/Quiet-alert/active alert (Rate each indicator of **Preterm Infant Organization**: 1 = extreme deviation, 2 = substantial deviation, 3 = moderate deviation, 4 = mild deviation, 5 = no deviation [see Section I].)

Client Outcomes

Client Will (Specify Time Frame):

Infant/child
- Have stable vital signs
- Display smooth and synchronous body movements
- Display smooth transitions between sleep and wake states
- Demonstrate self-consoling behaviors
- Demonstrate ability to tolerate feedings
- Display stable color

Parents/significant other
- Recognize infant/child behaviors as a unique way of communicating needs and goals
- Recognize infant behavior used to communicate stress, avoidance and approach, and regulation
- Recognize and support infant's/child's drive and behaviors used to self-regulate
- Demonstrate ways of being more responsive to infant/child cues and needs
- Recognize the way their interactions affect the infant's/child's responses and that al-

• = **Independent**; ▲ = **Collaborative**

lowing the infant/child to take lead in the interaction fosters adaptive communication patterns

- Structure and modify the environment in response to infant/child behaviors
- Identify appropriate positioning and handling techniques to enhance comfort and normal development and prevent abnormalities

NIC   Interventions (Nursing Interventions Classification)

Suggested NIC Interventions

Developmental Care; Parent Education: Infant; Positioning; Sleep Enhancement

---

Example NIC Activities—Developmental Care

Teach parents to recognize infant states and cues; Point out infant's self-regulatory activities (e.g., hand-to-mouth, sucking, use of visual or auditory stimulus)

Nursing Interventions and Rationales

- Identify infant's/child's level of neurobehavioral organization as a unique way of communicating. *The infant's principal method of communicating goals, needs, and limits for stress and stability is by behavior; therefore, the infant's own behaviors provide a guide for individualizing care and interactions and promoting development (Als, 1982).*
- Recognize behavior used to communicate stress, avoid, approach, and regulate. *The ability to read and interpret infant/child behavior provides a framework for responding to an infant/child in a way that communicates both the infant's/child's importance and that he or she is able to affect his or her environment (Als, 1982; Blackburn and Vandenberg, 1991).*
- Identify and support the infant's/child's self-regulatory coping behaviors used for mastery of the environment. *A continuous interaction takes place between the infant and the environment; behaviors such as hand-to-mouth or hand-to-face, hand grasping, foot and leg bracing, sucking on fingers or fists, auditory and visual fixation, and postural changes are used to maintain or regain a balanced adaptation between the self and the environment. Supporting infant behaviors enhances the coregulatory fit between the infant and the environment (Als, 1986).*
- Cluster caregiving whenever possible to allow for longer periods of uninterrupted sleep. *Introduce one intervention at a time and observe infant responses. Take care to prevent overstimulation during clustering care (D'Apolito, 1991).*
- Correlate the evidence of stress or disorganization to internal factors (e.g., pain, hunger, discomfort) or external factors (e.g., lights, noise, handling). *Noise is one of the common stresses in hospital ICUs, resulting in sensory overload with the potential for alteration in development (Elander and Hellstrom, 1995; DePaul and Chambers, 1995). Infant colic characterized by increased irritability, diminished ability to be soothed, and excessive restlessness reflects immature sleep–wake regulation (an internal factor) (Keefe et al, 1996). Intrauterine cocaine exposure can result in disorganized behavior patterns of infants (DeWys and McComish-Fry, 1992).*
- Structure and modify care and environment. *A developmental care approach designed to reduce environmental and procedural stress and facilitate motor and sleep–wake organization results in improved behavioral organization during the preterm period (Als, 1998; Als et al, 1994; Becker et al, 1991; Buehler et al, 1995; D'Apolito, 1991; Newman, 1986). Patterns of sound, light, and caregiving tasks should minimize stress, conserve energy, and pro-*

- = Independent; ▲ = Collaborative

tect the developing neonate from inappropriate environmental stimuli (Blackburn and Vandenberg, 1991; D'Apolito, 1991).

- Facilitate the use of developmentally supportive positioning and handling. *Developmentally correct positioning (e.g., supporting/positioning in flexion or with containment, consoling infant, offering something to grasp) can be used to decrease stress, conserve energy, and enhance sleep and normal development of the preterm infant (Aita and Snider, 2003; D'Apolito, 1991; McGrath and Conliffe-Torres, 1996; Sweeney and Guitierrez, 2002).* **Nursing and Clinical Research:** *Some research has indicated that use of a prone position improves quality of sleep and decreases stress for ventilated preterm infants (Chang et al, 2002). However, recent research indicates that the development of posture and mobility in newborns requires an optimal balance between active and passive muscle tone. Although prone position is physiologically more beneficial for the preterm infant, prone position can lead to short- and long-term postural and associated developmental problems (Monterosso, Kristjanson, and Cole, 2002).*
- Consider the use of infant massage if appropriate. *Infant massage has been found to decrease stress levels, increase weight gain and improve motor function in preterm infants (Mainous, 2002).*
- Support parents' competence in appraising their infant's behavior and responses. *Parents must be supported and welcomed as active collaborators in their infant's care (Lawhon, 2002).*
- Facilitate Kangaroo Care/skin-to-skin contact to promote infant's adaptability to external environment. **Nursing and Clinical Research:** *Parents have been found to be more sensitive, to show more positive affect, touch and adaptation to infant cues when participating in skin-to-skin (Kangaroo) care (Feldman et al, 2002). Kangaroo Care provides an environment that supports autonomic stability and fosters improvement in basic physiological functions (Ludington-Hoe and Swinth, 1996). Infants have been found to benefit with cardiorespiratory stabilization, improved oxygenation, thermoregulation, increased weight gain, earlier feeding, easier breastfeeding, less crying, and decreased length of stay (Chwo et al, 2002; Ludington-Hoe et al, 1999). Kangaroo Care reduces the amount of time spent in active sleep and increases time spent in quiet, regular sleep (Ludington, 1990). Skin-to-skin care has been found to increase a favorable perception of the infant by the caregiver, and result in parents who feel more competent in caring for their infant (Tessier et al, 1998).*
- Identify techniques to assist development of state modulation and organization. *Providing care and stimulation contingent on the state of the infant is critical to state organization (Fajardo et al, 1990).*
- Identify and support infant's/child's attention capabilities. *In organized attentive states, infants are able to focus attention and interact with their environments purposefully (Burns et al, 1994).*
- Enhance normal developmental patterns through appropriate sensorimotor stimulation. *Healthy 33- to 34-week postconceptual age infants who received 15 minutes of auditory, visual, tactile, and vestibular stimulation each day were found to be better than others at state modulation. Their ability to maintain quiet-alertness enhances parent-infant interactions and feedings (White-Traut et al, 1996). Enhancing normal experiences through appropriate sensory stimulation, handling, and social interactions appropriate to an infant's developmental level can minimize secondary problems (Anderson and Auster-Liebhaber, 1984).*

• = **Independent;** ▲ = **Collaborative**

Multicultural

- Assess for the influence of cultural beliefs, norms, and values on the family's perceptions of infant/child behavior. **Nursing Research:** *What the family considers normal infant/child behavior may be based on cultural perceptions (Cochran, 1998; Doswell and Erlen, 1998; Guarnaccia, 1998; Leininger and McFarland, 2002).*
- Use a neutral, indirect style when addressing areas where improvement is needed (such as a need for verbal or oral stimulation) when working with Native American clients. **Nursing Research:** *Using indirect statements such as "Other mothers have tried . . ." or "I had a client who tried 'X' and it seemed to work very well" will assist in avoiding resentment from the parent (Seiderman et al, 1996).*
- Acknowledge and praise parenting strengths noted. **Nursing Research:** *This will increase trust and foster a working relationship with the parent (Seiderman et al, 1996).*
- Use therapeutic communication techniques that emphasize acceptance, offer the self, validate the client's concerns, and convey respect when discussing the infant/child behavior. **Nursing Research:** *Validation is therapeutic communication technique that lets the client know that the nurse has heard and understands what was said, and it promotes the nurse-client relationship (Heineken, 1998). Studies show that even when language is not a barrier, some ethnic clients may be reluctant to discuss their beliefs and practices because of fear of criticism or ridicule (Evans and Cunningham, 1996).*

Family Teaching

- Assist families/support systems in recognizing and responding to infant's unique behavioral cues. *Demonstrating and modeling appropriate interactional skills is an integral component of family education and will improve family-infant interaction (McGrath and Conliffe-Torres, 1996). Assisting parents with recognizing infant states and state modulation and self-consoling strategies provides caregivers with greater sense of competence (Nursing Child Assessment Satellite Training, 1994).*
- Give anticipatory guidance to parents about what infant/child behaviors are possible in given situations.
- Model calming interventions to provide parents with tools for positive interactions with their infant/child (Karl, 1999).
- Nurture parents so that they in turn can nurture their infant/child. *Establish a nurturing environment in which parents can interact with their infant/child (Goulet et al, 1998).*

Home care

- Above interventions may be adapted for home care use.
- Assist families in structuring home environment *Patterns of sound, light, and caregiving tasks should minimize stress, conserve energy, and protect the developing neonate from inappropriate environmental stimuli (Blackburn and Vandenberg, 1991; D'Apolito, 1991).*
- Encourage families to teach friends/visitors to recognize and respond to infant's unique behavioral cues. *It is important for families to feel comfortable obtaining support from their regular support systems; therefore, supportive persons need to be taught how to interact in the environment in a way that supports both the family and the infant. The ability to read and interpret infant behavior provides a framework for responding to infants in a way that communicates both the infant's/child's importance and the message that he or she is able to affect his or her environment (Als, 1982; Blackburn and Vandenberg, 1991).*

• = Independent; ▲ = Collaborative

REFERENCES

Aita M, Snider L: The art of developmental care in the NICU: a concept analysis, *J Adv Nurs* 41(3):223, 2003.

Als H: Toward a synactive theory of development: promise for the assessment and support of infant individuality, *Infant Ment Health* J 3:229, 1982.

Als H: A synactive model of neonatal behavioral organization: framework for the assessment and support of the neurobehavioral development of the premature infant and his parents in the environment of the neonatal intensive care unit, *Phys Occup Ther Pediatr* 6:3, 1986.

Als H: Developmental care in the newborn intensive care unit, *Curr Opin Pediatr* 10:138, 1998.

Als H et al: Individualized developmental care for the very low-birth-weight preterm infant: Medical and neurofunctional effects, *JAMA* 272 (11): 853, 1994.

Anderson J, Auster-Liebhaber J: Developmental therapy in the neonatal intensive care unit, *Phys Occup Ther Pediatr* 4:89, 1984.

Becker PT et al: Outcomes of developmentally supportive nursing care for very low birth weight infants, *Nurs Res* 40:150, 1991.

Blackburn S, Vandenberg K: Assessment and management of neonatal development. In Kenner C et al, editors: *Comprehensive neonatal nursing: a physiologic approach*, Toronto, 1991, WB Saunders.

Buehler D et al: Effectiveness of individualized developmental care for low-risk preterm infants: Behavioral and electrophysiologic evidence, *Pediatrics* 96(5):923, 1995.

Burns M et al: Infant stimulation: modification of an intervention based on physiologic and behavioral cues, *J Obstet Gynecol Neonatal Nurs* 23:581, 1994.

Chang Y, Anderson G, Lin C: Effects of prone and supine positions on sleep state and stress responses in mechanically ventilated preterm infants during the first postnatal week, *J Adv Nurs* 40(2):161, 2002.

Chwo M et al: A randomized controlled trial of early kangaroo care for preterm infants: Effects on temperature, weight, behavior, and acuity, *J Nurs Res* 10(2):129, 2002.

Cochran M: Tears have no color, *Am J Nurs* 98(6):53, 1998.

D'Apolito K: What is an organized infant? *Neonatal Netw* 10(1):23, 1991.

DePaul D, Chambers SE: Environmental noise in the neonatal intensive care unit: implications for nursing practice, *J Perinatal Neonatal Nurs* 8:71, 1995.

DeWys M, McComish-Fry J: *Infants states and cues: facilitating effective parent-infant interactions*. In *Caring for infants: a resource manual for caring for infant trainers*, East Lansing, Mich, 1992, Michigan State University Board of Trustees.

Doswell W, Erlen J: Multicultural issues and ethical concerns in the delivery of revising care interventions, *Nurs Clin North Am* 33(2):353, 1998.

Elander G, Hellstrom G: Reduction of noise levels in intensive care units for infants: evaluation of an intervention program, *Heart Lung* 24:376, 1995.

Evans CA, Cunningham BA: Caring for the ethnic elder, *Geriatr Nurs* 17(3):105, 1996.

Fajardo B et al: Effect of nursery environment on state regulation in very-low-birth-weight premature infants, *Infant Behav Dev* 13:287, 1990.

Feldman R et al: Comparison of skin-to-skin (kangaroo) and traditional care: Parenting outcomes and preterm infant behavior, *Pediatrics* 110(1):16, 2002.

Goulet C et al: A concept analysis of parent-infant attachment, *J Adv Nurs* 28(5):1071, 1998.

Guarnaccia, P: Multicultural experiences of family caregiving: a study of African American, European American, and Hispanic American families, *New Direct Ment Health Serv* 77:45, 1998.

Heineken J: Patient silence is not necessarily client satisfaction: communication in home care nursing, *Home Healthc Nurse* 16(2):115, 1998.

Karl D: The interactive newborn bath: using infant neurobehavior to connect parents and newborns, *MCN Am J Matern Child Nurse* 24(6):280, 1999.

Keefe M et al: A longitudinal comparison of irritable and nonirritable infants, *Nurs Res* 45:4, 1996.

Lawhon G: Facilitation of parenting the premature infant within the newborn intensive care unit, *J Perinat Neonatal Nurs* 16(1):71, 2002.

• = Independent; ▲ = Collaborative

Leininger MM, McFarland MR: *Transcultural nursing: concepts, theories, research and practices,* ed 3, New York, 2002, McGraw-Hill.

Ludington SM: Energy conservation during skin-to-skin contact between preterm infants and their mothers, *Heart Lung* 19(5 pt 1):445, 1990.

Ludington-Hoe SM, Swinth JY: Developmental aspects of kangaroo care, *J Obstet Gynecol Neonatal Nurs* 25(8): 691, 1996.

Ludington-Hoe SM et al: Birth-related fatigue in 34-36–week preterm neonates: rapid recovery with very early Kangaroo (skin-to-skin) care, *J Obstet Gynecol Neonatal Nurs* 28(1):94, 1999.

Mainous R: Infant massage as a component of developmental care: past, present, and future, *Holist Nurs Pract* 16(5):1, 2002.

McGrath J, Conliffe-Torres S: Integrating family-centered developmental assessment and intervention into routine care in the neonatal intensive care unit, *Nurs Clin North Am* 31(2):367, 1996.

Monterosso L, Kristjanson L, Cole J: Neuromotor development and the physiologic effects of positioning in very low birth weight infants, *J Obstet Gynecol Neonatal Nurs* 31(2):128, 2002.

Newman L: Social and sensory environment of low birth weight infants in a special care nursery, *J Nerv Ment Dis* 169:448, 1986.

Nursing Child Assessment Satellite Training: *NCAST caregiver/parent-child interaction feeding manual,* Seattle, 1994, University of Washington School of Nursing.

Seiderman RY et al: Assessing American Indian families, *MCN Am J Matern Child Nurs* 21(6):274, 1996.

Sweeney J, Gutierrez T: Musculoskeletal implications of preterm infant positioning in the NICU, *J Perinatal Neonatal Nurs* 16(1):58, 2002.

Tessier R et al: Kangaroo mother care and the bonding hypothesis, *Pediatrics* 102(2):e17, 1998.

White-Traut R: Environmental factors and alternative therapies in nursing, *Voice* 4(9):1, 1996.

White-Traut R et al: Patterns of physiological and behavioral response of intermediate care preterm infants to intervention, *Pediatr Nurs* 19:625, 1993.

Risk for disorganized Infant behavior

T. Heather Herdman and Mary A. Fuerst-DeWys

NANDA Definition

Risk for alteration in integrating and modulation of the physiological and neurobehavioral systems of functioning (i.e., autonomic, motor, state, organizational, self-regulatory, and attentional-interactional systems)

Risk Factors

Pain; invasive/painful procedures; lack of containment/boundaries; oral/motor problems; prematurity; environmental overstimulation

NOC Outcomes, Client Outcomes, NIC Interventions, Nursing Interventions and Rationales, Family Teaching, Websites for Education

• See care plan for **Disorganized Infant behavior.**

Readiness for enhanced organized Infant behavior

T. Heather Herdman and Mary A. Fuerst-DeWys

NANDA Definition

A pattern of modulation of the physiological and behavioral systems of functioning (i.e., autonomic, motor, state-organizational, self-regulatory, and attentional-interactional

• = Independent; ▲ = Collaborative

systems) in an infant that is satisfactory but that can be improved, resulting in higher levels of integration in response to environmental stimuli

Defining Characteristics

Definite sleep-wake states; use of some self-regulatory behaviors; response to visual/auditory stimuli; stable physiological measures

Related Factors (r/t)

Pain; prematurity

NOC   Outcomes (Nursing Outcomes Classification)

Suggested NOC Outcomes

Child Development: 2 Months, 4 Months, 6 Months; Growth; Neurological Status; Newborn Adaptation; Nutritional Status: Food and Fluid Intake; Preterm Infant Organization; Sleep; Thermoregulation: Newborn; Vital Signs

---

Example NOC Outcome with Indicators

Preterm Infant Organization as evidenced by the following indictors: O_2 saturation greater than 85%/Skin color/Feeding tolerance/Muscle tone relaxed/Smooth synchronous movement/Posture flexed/Hands brought to mouth/Appropriate time-out signals/Self-consolability/Deep sleep/Quiet-alert/Active-alert (Rate each indicator of **Preterm Infant Organization**: 1 = extreme deviation, 2 = substantial deviation, 3 = moderate deviation, 4 = mild deviation, 5 = no deviation [see Section I].)

Client Outcomes

Client Will (Specify Time Frame):

Infant/child

- Have stable vital signs
- Display smooth and synchronous body movements
- Display smooth transitions between sleep and wake states
- Demonstrate self-consoling behaviors
- Demonstrate ability to tolerate feedings
- Display stable color

Parents/significant other

- Recognize infant/child behaviors as a unique way of communicating needs and goals
- Recognize infant behavior used to communicate stress, avoidance and approach, and regulation
- Recognize and support infant's/child's drive and behaviors used to self-regulate
- Demonstrate ways of being more responsive to infant/child cues and needs
- Recognize the way interactions affect the infant's/child's responses and that allowing the infant/child to take lead in the interaction fosters adaptive communication patterns
- Structure and modify the environment in response to infant/child behaviors
- Identify appropriate positioning and handling techniques to enhance comfort and normal development and prevent abnormalities

• = **Independent;** ▲ = **Collaborative**

| **NIC** | Interventions (Nursing Interventions Classification) |

Suggested NIC Interventions

Developmental Care; Environmental Management; Kangaroo Care; Newborn Monitoring; Nonnutritive Sucking; Positioning; Sleep Enhancement

---

Example NIC Activities—Developmental Care

Provide water mattress and sheepskin as appropriate; Use smallest diaper to avoid hip abduction

---

Nursing Interventions and Rationales

- Identify infant's/child's level of neurobehavioral organization as a unique way of communicating. *The infant's principal method of communicating goals, needs, and limits for stress and stability is by behavior; therefore, the infant's own behaviors provide a guide for individualizing care and interactions and promoting development (Als, 1982).*
- Recognize behavior used to communicate stress, avoid and approach, and regulate. *The ability to read and interpret infant behavior provides a framework for responding to infants in a way that communicates both the infant's/child's importance and that he or she is able to affect his or her environment (Als, 1982; Blackburn and Vandenberg, 1991).*
- Identify and support the infant's/child's self-regulatory coping behaviors used for mastery of the environment. *A continuous interaction takes place between the infant and the environment; behaviors such as hand-to-mouth or hand-to-face, hand grasping, foot and leg bracing, sucking on fingers or fists, auditory and visual fixation, and postural changes are used to maintain or regain a balanced adaptation between the self and the environment. Supporting infant behaviors enhances the coregulatory fit between the infant and the environment (Als, 1986).*
- Cluster caregiving whenever possible to allow for longer periods of uninterrupted sleep. *Introduce one intervention at a time and observe infant responses. Take care to prevent overstimulation during clustering care (D'Apolito, 1991).*
- Correlate the evidence of stress or disorganization to internal factors (e.g., pain, hunger, discomfort) or external factors (e.g., lights, noise, handling). Increase stimulation toward the most mature systems (tactile and vestibular) while decreasing stimulation of the least mature systems (auditory and visual). *Noise is one of the common stresses in hospital ICUs, resulting in sensory overload with the potential for alteration in development (DePaul and Chambers, 1995; Elander and Hellstrom, 1995). Infant colic characterized by increased irritability, diminished ability to be soothed, and excessive restlessness reflects immature sleep-wake regulation (an internal factor) (Keefe et al, 1996). Intrauterine cocaine exposure can result in disorganized behavior patterns of infants (DeWys and McComish-Fry, 1992).*
- Structure and modify care and environment. *A developmental care approach designed to reduce environmental and procedural stress and facilitate motor and sleep-wake organization results in improved behavioral organization during the preterm period (Als, 1998; Als et al, 1994; Becker et al, 1991; Buehler et al, 1995; D'Apolito, 1991; Newman, 1986). Patterns of sound, light, and caregiving tasks should minimize stress, conserve energy, and protect the developing neonate from inappropriate environmental stimuli (Blackburn and Vandenberg, 1991; D'Apolito, 1991).*
- Facilitate the use of developmentally supportive positioning and handling. *Developmentally correct positioning (e.g., supporting/positioning in flexion or with contain-*

• = **Independent;** ▲ = **Collaborative**

ment, consoling infant, offering something to grasp) can be used to decrease stress, conserve energy, and enhance sleep and normal development of the preterm infant (Aita and Snider, 2003; D'Apolito, 1991; McGrath and Conliffe-Torres, 1996; Sweeney and Guitierrez, 2002). **Nursing and Clinical Research:** *Some research has indicated that use of a prone position improves quality of sleep and decreases stress for ventilated preterm infants (Chang et al, 2002). However, recent research indicates that the development of posture and mobility in newborns requires an optimal balance between active and passive muscle tone. Although prone position is physiologically more beneficial for the preterm infant, prone position can lead to short- and long-term postural and associated developmental problems (Monterosso, Kristjanson, and Cole, 2002).*

- Consider the use of infant massage if appropriate. *Infant massage has been found to decrease stress levels, increase weight gain, and improve motor function in preterm infants (Mainous, 2002).*
- Facilitate Kangaroo Care/skin-to-skin contact to promote infant's adaptability to external environment. **Nursing and Clinical Research:** *Kangaroo Care provides an environment that supports autonomic stability and fosters improvement in basic physiological functions (Ludington-Hoe and Swinth, 1996). Parents have been found to be more sensitive, to show more positive affect, touch and adaptation to infant cues when participating in skin-to-skin care (Feldman et al, 2002). Infants have been found to benefit with cardiorespiratory stabilization, improved oxygenation, thermoregulation, increased weight gain, earlier feeding, easier breastfeeding, less crying, and decreased length of stay (Chwo et al, 2002; Ludington-Hoe et al, 1999). Kangaroo Care reduces the amount of time spent in active sleep and increases time spent in quiet, regular sleep (Ludington, 1990). Skin-to-skin care has been found to increase a favorable perception of the infant by the caregiver, and result in parents who feel more competent in caring for their infant (Tessier et al, 1998).*
- Identify techniques to assist development of state modulation and organization. *Providing care and stimulation contingent on the state of the infant is critical to state organization (Fajardo et al, 1990).*
- Identify and support infant's/child's attention capabilities. *In organized attentive states, infants are able to focus attention and interact with their environments purposefully (Burns et al, 1994).*
- Enhance normal developmental patterns through appropriate sensorimotor stimulation. *Healthy 33- to 34-week postconceptual age infants who received 15 minutes of auditory, visual, tactile, and vestibular stimulation each day were found to be better than others at state modulation. Their ability to maintain quiet-alertness enhances parent-infant interactions and feedings (White-Traut et al, 1996). Enhancing normal experiences through appropriate sensory stimulation, handling, and social interactions appropriate to an infant's developmental level can minimize secondary problems (Anderson and Auster-Liebhaber, 1984).*

Multicultural

- Assess for the influence of cultural beliefs, norms, and values on the parent's/caregiver's perceptions of infant/child behavior. **Nursing Research:** *What the parent/caregiver considers normal infant/child behavior may be based on cultural perceptions (Cochran, 1998; Doswell and Erlen, 1998; Leininger and McFarland, 2002).*
- Use a neutral, indirect style when addressing areas where improvement is needed (such as a need for verbal or oral stimulation) when working with Native American clients. **Nursing Research:** *Using indirect statements such as "Other mothers have tried . . ." or*

- = Independent; ▲ = Collaborative

"I had a client who tried 'X' and it seemed to work very well" will assist in avoiding resentment from the parent (Seiderman et al, 1996).

- Acknowledge and praise parenting strengths and ability to respond to infant/child. **Nursing Research:** *This will increase trust and foster a working relationship with the parent (Seiderman et al, 1996).*
- Use therapeutic communication techniques that emphasize acceptance, offer the self, validate the client's concerns, and convey respect when discussing the infant/child behavior. **Nursing Research:** *Validation is therapeutic communication technique that lets the client know that the nurse has heard and understands what was said, and it promotes the nurse-client relationship (Heineken, 1998). Studies show that even when language is not a barrier, some ethnic clients may be reluctant to discuss their beliefs and practices because of the fear of criticism or ridicule (Evans and Cunningham, 1996).*

Family Teaching

- Assist families/support systems in recognizing and responding to infant's unique behavioral cues. *Demonstrating and modeling appropriate interactional skills is an integral component of family education and will improve family-infant interaction (McGrath and Conliffe-Torres, 1996). Assisting parents in recognizing infant states and state modulation and self-consoling strategies provides caregivers with a greater sense of competence (Nursing Child Assessment Satellite Training, 1994).*
- Support parents' competence in appraising their infant's behavior and responses. *Parents must be supported and welcomed as active collaborators in their infant's care (Lawhon, 2002).*
- Give anticipatory guidance to parents about what infant/child behaviors are possible in given situations. *Model calming interventions to provide parents with tools for positive interactions with their infant/child (Karl, 1999).*

Home care

- Assist families in structuring home environment. *Patterns of sound, light, and caregiving tasks should minimize stress, conserve energy, and protect the developing neonate from inappropriate environmental stimuli (Blackburn and Vandenberg, 1991; D'Apolito, 1991).*
- Encourage families to teach friends/visitors to recognize and respond to infant's unique behavioral cues. *It is important for families to feel comfortable obtaining support from their regular support systems; therefore, supportive people need to be taught how to interact in the environment in a way that supports both the family and the infant. The ability to read and interpret infant behavior provides a framework for responding to infants in a way that communicates both the infant's/child's importance and the message that he or she is able to affect his or her environment (Als, 1982; Blackburn and Vandenberg, 1991).*

evolve WEBSITES FOR EDUCATION

See the EVOLVE website for World Wide Web resources for client education.

REFERENCES

Aita M, Snider L: The art of developmental care in the NICU: a concept analysis, *J Adv Nurs* 41(3):223, 2003.
Als H: Toward a synactive theory of development: promise for the assessment and support of infant individuality, *Infant Ment Health* J 3:229, 1982.

- = Independent; ▲ = Collaborative

Als H: A synactive model of neonatal behavioral organization: framework for the assessment and support of the neurobehavioral development of the premature infant and his parents in the environment of the neonatal intensive care unit, *Phys Occup Ther Pediatr* 6:3, 1986.

Als H: Developmental care in the newborn intensive care unit, *Curr Opin Pediatr* 10:138, 1998.

Als H et al: Individualized developmental care for the very low-birth-weight preterm infant: Medical and neurofunctional effects, *JAMA* 272 (11): 853, 1994.

Anderson J, Auster-Liebhaber J: Developmental therapy in the neonatal intensive care unit, *Phys Occup Ther Pediatr* 4:89, 1984.

Becker PT et al: Outcomes of developmentally supportive nursing care for very low birth weight infants, *Nurs Res* 40:150, 1991.

Blackburn S, Vandenberg K: Assessment and management of neonatal development. In Kenner C et al, editors: *Comprehensive neonatal nursing: a physiologic approach,* Toronto, 1991, WB Saunders.

Buehler D et al: Effectiveness of individualized developmental care for low-risk preterm infants: Behavioral and electrophysiologic evidence, *Pediatrics* 96(5):923, 1995.

Burns M et al: Infant stimulation: modification of an intervention based on physiologic and behavioral cues, *J Obstet Gynecol Neonatal Nurs* 23:581, 1994.

Chang Y, Anderson G, Lin C: Effects of prone and supine positions on sleep state and stress responses in mechanically ventilated preterm infants during the first postnatal week, *J Adv Nurs* 40(2):161, 2002.

Chwo M et al: A randomized controlled trial of early kangaroo care for preterm infants: Effects on temperature, weight, behavior, and acuity, *J Nurs Res* 10(2):129, 2002.

Cochran M: Tears have no color, *Am J Nurs* 98(6):53, 1998.

D'Apolito K: What is an organized infant? *Neonatal Netw* 10(1):23, 1991.

DePaul D, Chambers SE: Environmental noise in the neonatal intensive care unit: implications for nursing practice, *J Perinat Neonatal Nurs* 8:71, 1995.

DeWys M, McComish-Fry J: *Infants states and cues: facilitating effective parent-infant interactions.* In *Caring for infants: a resource manual for caring for infant trainers,* East Lansing, Mich, 1992, Michigan State University Board of Trustees.

Doswell W, Erlen J: Multicultural issues and ethical concerns in the delivery of revising care interventions, *Nurs Clin North Am* 33(2):353, 1998.

Elander G, Hellstrom G: Reduction of noise levels in intensive care units for infants: evaluation of an intervention program, *Heart Lung* 24:376, 1995.

Evans CA, Cunningham BA: Caring for the ethnic elder, *Geriatr Nurs* 17(3):105, 1996.

Fajardo B et al: Effect of nursery environment on state regulation in very-low-birth-weight premature infants, *Infant Behav Dev* 13:287, 1990.

Feldman R et al: Comparison of skin-to-skin (kangaroo) and traditional care: Parenting outcomes and preterm infant behavior, *Pediatrics* 110(1):16, 2002.

Heineken J: Patient silence is not necessarily client satisfaction: communication in home care nursing, *Home Healthc Nurse* 16(2):115, 1998.

Karl D: The interactive newborn bath: using infant neurobehavior to connect parents and newborns, *MCN Am J Matern Child Nurse* 24(6):280, 1999.

Keefe M et al: A longitudinal comparison of irritable and nonirritable infants, *Nurs Res* 45:4, 1996.

Lawhon G: Facilitation of parenting the premature infant within the newborn intensive care unit, *J Perinat Neonatal Nurs* 16(1):71, 2002.

Leininger MM, McFarland MR: *Transcultural nursing: concepts, theories, research and practices,* ed 3, New York, 2002, McGraw-Hill.

Ludington SM: Energy conservation during skin-to-skin contact between preterm infants and their mothers, *Heart Lung* 19(5 pt 1):445, 1990.

Ludington-Hoe SM, Swinth JY: Developmental aspects of kangaroo care, *J Obstet Gynecol Neonatal Nurs* 25(8): 691, 1996.

Ludington-Hoe SM et al: Birth-related fatigue in 34-36–week preterm neonates: rapid recovery with very early Kangaroo (skin-to-skin) care, *J Obstet Gynecol Neonatal Nurs* 28(1):94, 1999.

Mainous R: Infant massage as a component of developmental care: past, present, and future, *Holist Nurs Pract* 16(5):1, 2002.

McGrath J, Conliffe-Torres S: Integrating family-centered developmental assessment and intervention into routine care in the neonatal intensive care unit, *Nurs Clin North Am* 31(2):367, 1996.

Monterosso L, Kristjanson L, Cole J: Neuromotor development and the physiologic effects of positioning in very low birth weight infants, *J Obstet Gynecol Neonatal Nurs* 31(2):128, 2002.

• = **Independent;** ▲ = **Collaborative**

Newman L: Social and sensory environment of low birth weight infants in a special care nursery, *J Nerv Ment Dis* 169:448, 1986.

Nursing Child Assessment Satellite Training: *NCAST caregiver/parent-child interaction feeding manual,* Seattle, 1994, University of Washington School of Nursing.

Seiderman RY et al: Assessing American Indian families, *MCN Am J Matern Child Nurs* 21(6):274, 1996.

Sweeney J, Gutierrez T: Musculoskeletal implications of preterm infant positioning in the NICU, *J Perinatal Neonatal Nurs* 16(1):58, 2002.

Tessier R et al: Kangaroo mother care and the bonding hypothesis, *Pediatrics* 102(2):e17, 1998.

White-Traut R: Environmental factors and alternative therapies in nursing, *Voice* 4(9):1, 1996.

White-Traut R et al: Patterns of physiological and behavioral response of intermediate care preterm infants to intervention, *Pediatr Nurs* 19:625, 1993.

Ineffective Infant feeding pattern

T. Heather Herdman, Vicki E. McClurg, and Virginia R. Wall

NANDA Definition

Impaired ability to suck or coordinate the suck-swallow response

Defining Characteristics

Inability to coordinate sucking, swallowing, and breathing; inability to initiate or sustain an effective suck

Related Factors (r/t)

Prolonged NPO; anatomic abnormality; neurological impairment/delay; oral hypersensitivity; prematurity

NOC Outcomes (Nursing Outcomes Classification)

Suggested NOC Outcomes

Breastfeeding Establishment: Infant, Maternal; Breastfeeding: Maintenance; Growth; Hydration; Knowledge: Breastfeeding; Neurological Status: Central Motor Control, Cranial Sensory/Motor Function; Nutritional Status: Food and Fluid Intake

---

Example NOC Outcome with Indicators

Breastfeeding Establishment: Infant as evidenced by the following indicators: Proper alignment and latch on/Proper areolar grasp/Proper areolar compression/Correct suck and tongue placement/Swallowing a minimum of 5 to 10 minutes per breast/Minimum eight feedings per day/Six or more urinations per day/Age appropriate weight gain (Rate each indicator of **Breastfeeding Establishment: Infant:** 1 = not adequate, 2 = slightly adequate, 3 = moderately adequate, 4 = substantially adequate, 5 = totally adequate [see Section I].)

• = Independent; ▲ = Collaborative

Client Outcomes

Client Will (Specify Time Frame):

Infant
- Receive adequate nourishment, without compromising autonomic stability
- Progress to a normal feeding pattern

Family
- Learn successful techniques for feeding the infant

NIC   Interventions (Nursing Interventions Classification)

Suggested NIC Interventions
Aspiration Precautions; Bottle Feeding; Breastfeeding Assistance; Enteral Tube Feeding; Fluid Monitoring; Kangaroo Care; Lactation Counseling; Nonnutritive Sucking; Swallowing Therapy; Teaching: Infant Safety; Tube Care: Umbilical Line

> **Example NIC Activities—Bottle Feeding**
>
> Place nipple on top of tongue; Increase infant alertness by loosening clothing, rubbing hands/feet or talking to infant

Nursing Interventions and Rationales

- Assess infant's oral reflexes (i.e., root, gag, suck, and swallow). *These reflexes are necessary for successful oral feedings. Feeding by nipple or breast should be encouraged to aid in the growth and maturity of the gastrointestinal tract and for comfort and oral gratification (Lau et al, 2000).*
- Determine infant's ability to coordinate suck, swallow, and breathing reflexes. *As infants develop they become more able to coordinate breathing with sucking and swallowing (Medoff-Cooper et al, 2000; Shiao, 1997).*
- ▲ Collaborate with other health care providers (e.g., physician, neonatal nutritionist, physical and occupational therapists, lactation specialists) to develop a feeding plan. *Various health care providers contribute expertise to the care of an infant with special needs (Baker and Rasmussen, 1997; Caretto et al, 2000).*
- ▲ Implement gavage feedings (or another alternative feeding method), using breast milk whenever possible, before infant's readiness for feedings by mouth. *Even after a preterm infant develops the ability to suck and swallow, the infant may require too much energy to do so and gavage feedings may be necessary. Serious illness can interfere with a neonate's ability to suck, and calorie and nutrient needs are increased by the stress of illness (Lucas et al, 1997; Medoff-Cooper et al, 2000).*
- Provide opportunities for nonnutritive sucking during gavage feedings (or other alternative feeding methods) and for 5 minutes before initiating oral feedings. **Nursing Research:** *Sucking helps calm infants, thus raising the oxygen level; may aid digestion and increase average daily weight gain; and may prepare infants for earlier nipple feedings and discharge (Pickler et al, 1996; Shiao, 1997).*
- Evaluate the feeding environment and minimize sensory stimuli. *Noxious stimuli must be kept to a minimum to decrease physiological stress on at-risk infants. The neonatal intensive care unit environment can interfere with normal development of the infant and*

• = Independent; ▲ = Collaborative

breastfeeding success; therefore, this environment must be modified to enhance attachment and normal development (Baker and Rasmussen, 1997; Brown and Heermann, 1997).

- Position preterm infant in a flexed feeding posture that is similar to the posture used for a full-term infant. **Nursing Research:** *The "total sucking pattern" of the full-term newborn combines strong physiological flexion and high rib cage position to provide support for the tongue and jaw, which is essential for effective nippling (Brandon, Holditch-Davis, and Beylea, 1999; Brown and Heermann, 1997).*

- Attempt to nipple feed baby only when infant is in a quiet-alert state. *The infant must be able to find and grasp the nipple effectively and then be ready and eager to suck. The quiet-alert state was found to be optimal for feeding preterm infants (Brandt, Andrews, and Kvale, 1998; McCain, 1997; Medoff-Cooper et al, 2000).*

- Allow appropriate time for nipple feeding to ensure infant's safety without exceeding calorie expenditure. **Nursing Research:** *Nipple feeding can lead to nutritional deficits because of the increased metabolic demands placed on the at-risk infant by thermoregulation, work of respiration and feeding, and decreased ability to absorb nutrients (Hill, Kurkowski, and Garcia, 2000; Shaio, 1997).*

- Monitor infant's physiological condition during feeding. *Cardiorespiratory stability is necessary for nipple feedings (Shaio, 1997).*

- Determine infant's active feeding behaviors without prodding. **Nursing and Clinical Research:** *Infants must be alert and eager to eat (rooting, latching on, and sucking readily) to ensure a successful feeding. Prodding compromises the infant's safety, interrupts learning, and may give an inaccurate picture of ability to take in adequate nutrients in preparation for discharge (Brandt, Andrews, and Kvale, 1998; Hill, Kurkowski, and Garcia, 2000; Shaio, 1997).*

- Assess parent-infant attachment. *Insecure attachment relationships may intensify feeding problems and may lead to more severe malnutrition (Chatoor et al, 1998).*

- Assess infant's ability to take in enough calories to sustain temperature and growth. Use electronic scale to estimate intake during breastfeeding sessions. Use nipple shield to increase milk intake during breastfeeding as needed. *Calories are needed to sustain basal metabolic rate, activity, digestive and metabolic processes, and growth.* **Clinical and Nursing Research:** *Electronic scales are the only accurate way to estimate breast milk intake. Nipple shield use increases milk intake without decreasing total duration of breastfeeding for preterm infants (Meier et al, 1996, 2000; Shaio, 1997).*

- Encourage family to participate in the feeding process. *Nurses can promote the psychosocial development of the at-risk infant and family by encouraging the caregiving ability of the parents (Moran et al, 1999).*

▲ Refer to a neonatal nutritionist, physical or occupational therapist, or lactation specialist as needed. *Collaborative practice with others who are specially trained to meet the needs of this vulnerable population will help ensure feeding and parenting success (Baker and Rasmussen, 1997; Caretto et al, 2000).*

Family Teaching

- Provide anticipatory guidance for infant's expected feeding course. *Knowing what to anticipate helps the family feel involved and enhances attachment (Huckabay, 1999; Jaeger, Lawson, and Filteau, 1997; Caretto et al, 2000).*

- Teach parents infant feeding methods. *Parents should be involved in the feeding process as soon as possible to enhance attachment through positive feedback about their ability to nurture a child (Bruschweiler, 1998; Huckabay, 1999).*

- **• = Independent; ▲ = Collaborative**

- Teach parents how to recognize infant cues. *Parents' understanding of infant's cues may increase their involvement in caring for the infant by improving their perception of the infant's abilities (Brandt, Andrews, and Kvale, 1998; Medoff-Cooper et al, 2000).*
- Provide anticipatory guidance for the infant's discharge. *Parents need assistance in assuming responsibility for infant care as the day of discharge approaches (Baker and Rasmussen, 1997; Davis et al, 1996; Elliott and Reimer, 1998).*

evolve WEBSITES FOR EDUCATION

See the EVOLVE website for World Wide Web resources for client education.

REFERENCES

Baker BJ, Rasmussen TW: Organizing and documenting lactation support of NICU families, *J Obstet Gynecol Neonatal Nurs* 26:515, 1997.

Brandon DH, Holditch-Davis D, Beylea M: Nursing care and the development of sleeping and waking behaviors in preterm infants, *Res Nurs Health* 22(3):217, 1999.

Brandt KA, Andrews CM, Kvale J: Mother-infant interaction and breast-feeding outcome 6 weeks after birth, *J Obstet Gynecol Neonatal Nurs* 27:169, 1998.

Brown LD, Heermann JA: The effect of developmental care on preterm infant outcome, *Appl Nurs Res* 10(4): 190, 1997.

Bruschweiler SN: Early emotional care for mothers and infants, *Pediatrics* 102(5 suppl E):1278, 1998.

Caretto V et al: Current parent education on infant feeding in the neonatal intensive care unit: the role of the occupational therapist, *Am J Occup Ther* 54(1):59, 2000.

Chatoor I et al: Attachment and feeding problems: A reexamination of nonorganic failure to thrive and attachment insecurity, *J Am Acad Child Adolesc Psychiatry* 37(11):1217, 1998.

Davis DW, Logsdon MC, Birkmer JC: Types of support expected and received by mothers after their infants' discharge from the NICU, *Issues Compr Pediatr Nurs* 19(4):263, 1996.

Elliott S, Reimer C: Postdischarge telephone follow-up program for breastfeeding preterm infants discharged from a special care nursery, *Neonatal Netw* 17(6):41, 1998.

Hill AS, Kurkowski TB, Garcia J: Oral support measures used in feeding the preterm infant, *Nurs Res* 49(1):2, 2000.

Huckabay LM: The effect on bonding behavior of giving a mother her premature baby's picture, *Sch Inq Nurs Pract* 13(4):349, 1999.

Jaeger MC, Lawson M, Filteau S: The impact of prematurity and neonatal illness on the decision to breast-feed, *J Adv Nurs* 25(4):729, 1997.

Lau C et al: Characterization of the developmental stages of sucking in preterm infants during bottle feeding, *Acta Paediatr* 89(7):846, 2000.

Lucas A et al: Breastfeeding and catch-up growth in infants born small for gestational age, *Acta Paediatr* 86:564, 1997.

McCain GC: Behavioral state activity during nipple feedings for preterm infants, *Neonatal Netw* 16(5):43, 1997.

Medoff-Cooper B, McGrath JM, Bilker W: Nutritive sucking and neurobehavioral development in preterm infants from 34 weeks PCA to term, *MCN Am J Matern Child Nurs* 25(2):64, 2000.

Meier PP et al: Estimating milk intake of hospitalized preterm infants who breastfeed, *J Hum Lact* 12(1):21, 1996.

Meier PP et al: Nipple shields for preterm infants: effect on milk transfer and duration of breastfeeding, *J Hum Lact* 16(2):106, 2000.

Moran M et al: Maternal kangaroo (skin-to-skin) care in the NICU beginning 4 hours postbirth, *MCN Am J Matern Child Nurs* 24(2):74, 1999.

Pickler RH et al: Effects of nonnutritive sucking on behavioral organization and feeding performance in preterm infants, *Nurs Res* 45(3):132, 1996.

Shiao SY: Comparison of continuous versus intermittent sucking in very-low-birth-weight infants, *J Obstet Gynecol Neonatal Nurs* 26:313, 1997.

• = **Independent;** ▲ = **Collaborative**

Risk for Infection

Gail B. Ladwig

NANDA Definition

At increased risk for being invaded by pathogenic organisms

Risk Factors

Invasive procedures; insufficient knowledge regarding avoidance of exposure to pathogens; trauma; tissue destruction and increased environmental exposure; rupture of amniotic membranes; pharmaceutical agents (e.g., immunosuppressants); malnutrition; increased environmental exposure to pathogens; immunosuppression; inadequate acquired immunity; inadequate secondary defenses (e.g., decreased hemoglobin, leukopenia, suppressed inflammatory response); inadequate primary defenses (e.g., broken skin, traumatized tissue, decrease in ciliary action, stasis of body fluids, change in pH secretions, altered peristalsis); chronic disease

Related Factors (r/t)

See Risk Factors

NOC   Outcomes (Nursing Outcomes Classification)

Suggested NOC Outcomes

Immune Status; Knowledge: Infection Control; Risk Control; Risk Detection

---

Example NOC Outcome with Indicators

Immune Status as evidenced by the following indicators: Recurrent infections not present/Skin and mucosa integrity/GI, Respiratory, GU/Weight and body temperature IER (Rate each indicator of **Immune Status:** 1 = extremely compromised, 2 = substantially compromised, 3 = moderately compromised, 4 = mildly compromised, 5 = not compromised [see Section I].)

GI, Gastrointestinal; *GU*, genitourinary; *IER*, in expected range.

Client Outcomes

Client Will (Specify Time Frame):
- Remain free from symptoms of infection
- State symptoms of infection of which to be aware
- Demonstrate appropriate care of infection-prone site
- Maintain white blood cell (WBC) count and differential within normal limits
- Demonstrate appropriate hygienic measures such as hand washing, oral care, and perineal care

NIC   Interventions (Nursing Interventions Classification)

Suggested NIC Interventions

Immunization/Vaccination Administration; Infection Control; Infection Protection

• = Independent; ▲ = Collaborative

> **Example NIC Activities—Infection Control**
>
> Wash hands before and after each patient care activity; Ensure aseptic handling of all intravenous lines; Ensure appropriate wound care technique

Nursing Interventions and Rationales

▲ Observe and report signs of infection such as redness, warmth, discharge, and increased body temperature. **Clinical Research:** *Prospective surveillance study for nosocomial infection on hematology-oncology units should include fever of unknown origin as the single most common and clinically important entity (Engelhart et al, 2002).*

▲ Assess temperature of neutropenic clients every 4 hours; report a single temperature of greater than 38.5° C or three temperatures of greater than 38° C in 24 hours. *Neutropenic clients do not produce an adequate inflammatory response; therefore, fever is usually the first and often the only sign of infection (Wujcik, 1993).*

• Oral or tympanic thermometers may be used to assess temperature in adults and infants. **Nursing Research:** *There was no significant difference between average tympanic and average oral temperatures in this study. The use of tympanic thermometers in addition to oral thermometers in obtaining temperatures is supported (Gilbert, Barton, and Counsell, 2002).* **Nursing Research:** *Tympanic membrane temperature recordings in healthy preterm neonates are safe, accurate, easy, and comfortable for the baby and appropriate with this client group provided staff are trained in the technique (Bailey and Rose, 2001)*

• Use oral thermometers for critically ill adults. **Nursing Research:** *Oral thermometry is recommended as the best practice method for temperature evaluation in critical care patients when measurement of core temperature via a pulmonary artery catheter is not possible (Giuliano, 2000).*

▲ Note and report laboratory values (e.g., WBC count and differential, serum protein, serum albumin, and cultures). **Clinical Research:** *The WBC count and the automated absolute neutrophil count are better diagnostic tests for adults and most children (Cornbleet, 2002). Laboratory values are correlated with the client's history and physical examination to provide a global view of the client's immune function and nutritional status and to develop an appropriate plan of care for the diagnosis (Lehmann, 1991).*

• Remove the granulocytopenic client from areas exposed to construction dust so that the client will not inhale fungal spores. Remove all plants and flowers from the client's room. Aspergillus, *an organism that can cause fungal pneumonia, is commonly found in soil, water, and decomposing vegetation. This fungus can enter the hospital through an unfiltered air system, in dust stirred up during construction, or in food or ornamental plants (Calianno, 1999).*

• Assess skin for color, moisture, texture, and turgor (elasticity). Keep accurate, ongoing documentation of changes. Preventive skin assessment protocol, including documentation, assists in the prevention of skin breakdown. *Intact skin is nature's first line of defense against microorganisms entering the body (Kovach, 1995).*

• Carefully wash and pat dry skin, including skinfold areas. Use hydration and moisturization on all at-risk surfaces. *Maintaining supple, moist skin is the best method of keeping skin intact. Dry skin can lead to inflammation, excoriations, and possible infection episodes (Kovach, 1995) (see care plan for* **Risk for impaired Skin integrity**).

• **= Independent; ▲ = Collaborative**

- Encourage a balanced diet, emphasizing proteins, fatty acids, and vitamins listed below. **Clinical Research:** *Nutrients that have been demonstrated to be required for the immune system to function efficiently include essential amino acids, the essential fatty acid linoleic acid, vitamin A, folic acid, vitamin B_6, vitamin B_{12}, vitamin C, vitamin E, Zn, Cu, Fe, and Se. Practically all forms of immunity may be affected by deficiencies in one or more of these nutrients (Calder and Kew, 2002).*
- Monitor weight loss, leaving 25% or more of food uneaten at most meals. **Nursing Research:** *This study demonstrated the above criteria as significant predictors of protein calorie malnutrition (Crogan et al, 2002).*
- Use strategies to prevent nosocomial pneumonia (NP): assess lung sounds, sputum, and redness or drainage around stoma sites; use sterile water rather than tap water for mouth care of immunosuppressed clients; provide a clean manual resuscitation bag for each client; use sterile technique when suctioning; suction secretions above tracheal tube before suctioning; drain accumulated condensation in ventilator tubing into a fluid trap or other collection device before repositioning the client; assess patency and placement of nasogastric tubes; elevate the client's head to 30 degrees or higher to prevent gastric reflux of organisms in the lung; institute feeding as soon as possible; assess for signs of feeding intolerance—no bowel sounds, abdominal distension, increased residual, emesis. **Clinical Research:** *Hospital-acquired pneumonia is the second most common nosocomial infection but has the highest mortality (30%) and morbidity rates. The strategies listed are used to prevent NP (Tasota et al, 1998). Once treatment for pneumonia has begun, it must continue for 48 to 72 hours, the minimum time to evaluate a clinical response (Ruiz et al, 2000).* **Nursing Research:** *NP is well documented as the second most common nosocomial infection. It is now more common in surgical patients than surgical-site or wound infection (Brooks, 2001).*
- Encourage fluid intake. *Fluid intake helps thin secretions and replace fluid lost during fever (Calianno, 1999).*
- Use appropriate "hand hygiene" (i.e., hand washing or use of alcohol-based hand rubs). *Improved adherence to hand hygiene has been shown to terminate outbreaks in health care facilities, to reduce transmission of antimicrobial resistant organisms (e.g., methicillin-resistant* Staphylococcus aureus*) and reduce overall infection rates (US Department of Health and Human Services, Centers for Disease Control and Prevention [CDC], 2002). Research has shown that health professionals, including nurses, do not decontaminate hands as often as they should (Gould, 2002).*
- When using an alcohol-based hand rub, apply product to palm of one hand and rub hands together, covering all surfaces of hands and fingers, until hands are dry. Note that the volume needed to reduce the number of bacteria on hands varies by product. **Clinical Research:** *By introducing the use of hand rubbing with an alcoholic solution, there was significant improved hand-cleansing compliance (Girou and Oppein, 2001).* **Clinical Research:** *Alcohols exert the strongest and fastest activity against a wide spectrum of bacteria and fungi (but not bacterial spores) as well as enveloped (but less so against nonenveloped) viruses, being little influenced by interfering substances. They are of low toxicity and offer acceptable skin tolerability when made up with suitable emollients. The mode of their application is simple and three to four times more economical of time than wash procedures, features that help to increase the compliance with the rules of hand hygiene (Rotter, 2001).*
- Follow Standard Precautions and wear gloves during any contact with blood, mucous membranes, nonintact skin, or any body substance except sweat. Use goggles, gloves,

• = Independent; ▲ = Collaborative

and gowns when appropriate. *The first and most important tier of the new CDC guidelines is Standard Precautions. Because client examination and medical history cannot reliably identify every client with blood-borne pathogens, Standard Precautions apply to all clients. You must assume all clients are carrying blood-borne pathogens such as human immunodeficiency virus (HIV) or hepatitis B or C virus (HBV or HCV). Standard Precautions exceed Universal Precautions. Transmission of blood-borne pathogens takes place via parenteral, mucous membrane, or nonintact skin exposure to blood and other body substances. You must take precautions whenever contact is likely with blood, mucous membranes, nonintact skin, or any body substance except sweat (CDC, 2002).* **Clinical Research:** *This study indicates that when risk for infection is high, powder-free gloves should be considered because powder may promote wound infection (Dave, Wilcox, and Kellett, 1999).*

- Follow Transmission-Based Precautions for airborne-, droplet-, and contact-transmitted microorganisms:
  - **Airborne:** Isolate the client in a room with monitored negative air pressure, with the room door closed, and the client remaining in the room. Always wear appropriate respiratory protection when you enter the room. For tuberculosis, you should wear an approved particulate respirator mask. Limit the movement and transport of the client from the room to essential purposes only. If at all possible, have the client wear a surgical mask during transport.
  - **Droplet:** Keep the client in a private room, if possible. If not possible, maintain a spatial separation of 3 feet from other beds or visitors. The door may remain open. You should wear a mask when you must come within 3 feet of the client. Some hospitals may choose to implement a mask requirement for droplet precautions for anyone entering the room. Limit transport to essential purposes and have the client wear a mask if possible.
  - **Transmission:** Place the client in a private room if possible or with someone who has an active infection from the same microorganism. Wear clean, nonsterile gloves when entering the room. When providing care, change gloves after contact with any infective material such as wound drainage. Remove the gloves and wash your hands before leaving the room and take care not to touch any potentially infectious items or surfaces on the way out. Wear a gown if you anticipate your clothing may have substantial contact with the client or other potentially infectious items. Remove the gown before leaving the room. Limit transport of the client to essential purposes and take care that the client does not contact other environmental surfaces along the way. Dedicate the use of noncritical client care equipment to a single client. If use of common equipment is unavoidable, adequately clean and disinfect equipment before use with other clients.

  Standard Precautions are based on the likely routes of transmission of pathogens. The second tier of the new CDC guidelines is Transmission-Based Precautions. This replaces many old categories of isolation precautions and disease-specific precautions with three simpler sets of precautions. These three sets of precautions are designed to prevent airborne transmission, droplet transmission, and contact transmission (CDC, 2002).
- Sterile technique must be used when inserting urinary catheters. Catheters must be cared for at least every shift. **Clinical Research:** *The genitourinary (GU) tract is the most common site of nosocomial infections in the acute care setting. Catheterization and instrumentation of the urinary tract are implicated as precipitating factors in approximately 80% of cases (Tasota et al, 1998).*

• = Independent; ▲ = Collaborative

- Use careful technique when changing and emptying urinary catheter bags; avoid cross-contamination. *Clients are most at risk for cross-infection during bag changing and emptying (Crow et al, 1993; Roe, 1993).*
▲ Use alternatives to indwelling catheters whenever possible (external catheters, incontinence pads, bladder control techniques). **Clinical Research:** *The GU tract is the most common site of nosocomial infections in the acute care setting. Catheterization and instrumentation of the urinary tract are implicated as precipitating factors in approximately 80% of cases (Tasota et al, 1998).*
- Provide well-designed site care for all peripheral, central venous, and arterial catheters: standardize insertion technique; select catheters with as few lumens as necessary; avoid use of femoral catheters in clients with fecal or urinary incontinence; use aseptic technique for insertion and care; stabilize cannula and tubing; maintain a sterile occlusive dressing (change every 72 hours per hospital policy); label insertion sites and all tubing with date and time of insertion, inspect every 8 hours for signs of infection, record and report; replace peripheral catheters per hospital policy (usually every 48 to 72 hours); when fever of unknown origin develops, obtain culture. **Clinical Research:** *More than 40% of bloodstream infections in ICUs are associated with short-term use of central venous catheters. Strict aseptic technique should be maintained. The risk of infection associated with use of triple-lumen catheters is as much as three times greater than the risk associated with single-lumen catheters. Clients with unexplained fever and signs of localized infection most likely have a catheter-related infection. The catheter should be removed and samples obtained for microbial culture (Tasota et al, 1998).* **Nursing Research:** *Care in selection of site and catheter is important. The shortest catheter and smallest size should be used when possible. Accommodate the need to replace catheters before they occlude (Schmid, 2000).*
- Use careful sterile technique wherever there is a loss of skin integrity. **Evidence-Based Practice:** *Extensive literature search revealed that sterile gloves should be used gloves for postoperative wound dressing changes (St Clair and Larrabee, 2002).*
- Ensure the client's appropriate hygienic care with hand washing; bathing; and hair, nail, and perineal care performed by either the nurse or the client. *Hygienic care is important to prevent infection in at-risk clients (Wujcik, 1993).*
▲ Recommend responsible use of antibiotics; use antibiotics sparingly. *Widespread use of certain antibiotics, particularly third-generation cephalosporins, has been shown to foster development of generalized beta-lactam resistance in previously susceptible bacterial populations. Reduction in the use of these agents (as well as imipenem and vancomycin) and concomitant increases in the use of extended-spectrum penicillins and combination therapy with aminoglycosides have been shown to restore bacterial susceptibility (Yates, 1999).*
Evidence-Based Research: *The reduction of endometritis by two thirds to three quarters and a decrease in wound infections justifies a policy of recommending prophylactic antibiotics to women undergoing elective or nonelective cesarean section (Smaill and Hofmeyr, 2002).*
Evidence-Based Research: *Antibiotic prophylaxis is effective in the prevention of postoperative complications in appendectomized patients, whether the administration is given preoperatively, peroperatively, and postoperatively, and could be considered for routine in emergency appendectomies (Andersen et al, 2001).*

Geriatric
- Recognize that geriatric clients may be seriously infected but have less obvious symptoms. The immune system declines with aging. *The elderly may present with atypical manifestations of infections (Madhaven, 1994).*

- = **Independent;** ▲ = **Collaborative**

- Suspect pneumonia when the client has symptoms of fatigue or confusion. *The only early indicators of pneumonia in an elderly client may be confusion and fatigue. An elderly client with pneumonia may not have such classic signs and symptoms as fever, cough, or an increased WBC count, or lung consolidation may be masked by chronic pulmonary disease. Clients older than 65 years are five times more likely than those in any other age group to die of a bacterial NP (Calianno, 1999).*
- Most clients develop NP by either aspirating contaminated substances or inhaling airborne particles. Refer to care plan for **Risk for Aspiration.**
▲ Foot care other than simple toenail cutting should be performed by a podiatrist.
▲ Observe and report if the client has a low-grade temperature or new onset of confusion. *The elderly can have infections with low-grade fevers. Be suspicious of any temperature rise or sudden confusion—these symptoms may be the only signs of infection (Madhaven, 1994).* **Evidence-Based Research:** *Residents of long-term care facilities who are suspected of having an infection and have one temperature reading of greater than 100° F (37.8° C), more than two readings of greater than 99° F (37.2° C), or an increase of 2° F (1.1° C) over baseline should be reported immediately to the on-site nurse, and appropriate testing should be done to determine site of infection (Bentley et al, 2002).*
- During the peak of the influenza epidemic, limit visits by relatives and friends. *Hospital- and nursing home–acquired influenza A virus infection leads to high mortality in the elderly (Madhaven, 1994).*
▲ Recommend that the geriatric client receive an annual influenza immunization and one-time pneumococcal vaccine. **Clinical Research:** *Immunization against influenza is an effective intervention that reduces serologically confirmed cases by between 60% and 70% (Hull et al, 2002). Among the many infections to which the aged are susceptible, pneumonia and influenza combined are responsible for the greatest mortality (Madhaven, 1994). Oseltamivir prophylaxis was very effective in protecting nursing home residents from influenza-like illnesses and in halting an outbreak of influenza B. A comparable nursing home in this study that did not use this treatment had double the number of cases (Parker, Loewen, and Skowronski, 2001).*
▲ Recognize that chronically ill geriatric clients, particularly those with depression, have an increased susceptibility to infection; practice meticulous care of all invasive sites. *Depression has been noted as a risk factor for lethal infectious disease in disabled older adults, with reduced reactivity in humoral and cellular immunity (Shinkawa et al, 2002).*
▲ Recognize that older adults are at risk for HIV/AIDS; institute Universal Precautions and appropriate instruction for all age groups. *Approximately 10% of AIDS cases occur in adults over age 50. Manifestations include* Pneumocystis carinii *pneumonia, herpes zoster, tuberculosis, cytomegalovirus, oral thrush,* Mycobacterium avium (M. intracellulare) *complex, and HIV dementia. Older women with HIV (compared with those without) are at higher risk for vaginal yeast infections, cervical dysplasia and carcinoma, condyloma, and pelvic inflammatory disease (Wooten-Bielski, 1999). Older adults are less likely to use a condom or to participate in routine HIV testing. Survival rates of elders with HIV are lower compared with younger patients (Chiao, Ries, and Sande, 1999) of all invasive sites.*

Home care

- Some of the above interventions may be adapted for home care use.
▲ Review standards for surveillance of infections in home care. *The Association for Professionals in Infection Control and Epidemiology has provided definitions for home care infec-*

• = Independent; ▲ = Collaborative

tion surveillance. While the current material is a draft, it is in use and will be revised periodically (Anonymous, 2001).

- • Assess home environment for general cleanliness, storage of food items, and appropriate waste disposal. Instruct as necessary in proper disposal and use of disinfecting agents. *Presence of waste and inappropriate storage of food items can contribute to the presence of pathogens.*
- ▲ Assess home care environment for appropriate disposal of used dressing materials. *Used dressing materials may contain or be a primary medium for growth of pathogens.*
- ▲ Role-model all preventive behaviors in care of the client (e.g., Universal Precautions). Do not visit the client when you are ill. *Demonstration is a more effective teaching strategy than verbalization.*
- ▲ Maintain the cleanliness of all irrigation and cleansing solutions. Change solutions when cleanliness has not been maintained—do not wait to finish bottle. *Solutions exposed to contaminants provide a medium for growth of pathogens.*
- ▲ Assess and teach clients about current medications and therapies that promote susceptibility to infection: corticosteroids, immunosuppressants, chemotherapeutic agents, and radiation therapy. *Knowledge of risk factors promotes vigilance in assessment, prompt reporting, and early treatment.*
- ▲ Assess the client for knowledge of infections that have been drug resistant.
- ▲ Instruct the client to complete any course of prophylactic antibiotic therapy unless experiencing adverse side effects. *Prophylactic antibiotic therapy decreases the risk of infection.*
- ▲ Monitor for the occurrence of infectious exacerbation of chronic obstructive pulmonary disease (COPD); refer to physician for treatment. *Nontypable* Haemophilus influenzae, Streptococcus pneumoniae, *and* Moraxella *can cause exacerbation of COPD (Sheikh and Sethi, 2001).*
- ▲ Refer for nutritional evaluation; implement dietary changes to support recovery and address antibiotic side effects. *Overgrowth of* Clostridium difficile *can cause abdominal pain, fever, and diarrhea. Inclusion of probiotics in the diet can counteract antibiotic-associated diarrhea (Vogelzang, 2001).*

Client/Family Teaching

- ▲ Teach the client risk factors contributing to surgical wound infection, smoking, and higher body mass index. **Evidence-Based Research:** *These are some of the factors associated with risk of surgical wound infection (Reilly, 2002).*
- ▲ Teach the client and family the symptoms of infection that should be promptly reported to a primary medical caregiver (e.g., redness; warmth; swelling; tenderness or pain; new onset of drainage or change in drainage from wound; increase in body temperature). **Clinical Research:** *Two thirds of wound infections occur after discharge (Reid et al, 2002).*
- ▲ Teach signs of hepatitis B virus (HBV)/AIDS symptoms: malaise, abdominal pain, vomiting or diarrhea, enlarged glands, rash; tuberculosis symptoms: cough, night sweats, dyspnea, changes in sputum, changes in breath sounds; insulin-dependent diabetes mellitus (IDDM) symptoms: sores or wounds that do not heal). *A high prevalence of HBV/AIDS, an increasing incidence of tuberculosis, and the general risk of diabetes are related to increased rate of infection.*
- ▲ Encourage high-risk persons, including health care workers, to have influenza vaccinations. *Vaccinations help to prevent viral NP (Calianno, 1999).*
- • Assess whether the client and family know how to read a thermometer; provide in-

• = **Independent;** ▲ = **Collaborative**

structions if necessary. Chemical dot thermometers are easy to use and decrease risk of infection. Clients need to know that the instructions should be followed carefully and that electronic thermometers may be the best choice for accuracy. *Single-use clinical thermometers provide a safe alternative to the traditional mercury in glass thermometers for routine temperature taking (MacQueen, 2001).*

- Instruct the client and family about the need for good nutrition (especially protein) and proper rest to prevent infection. *Optimal nutritional status contributes to health maintenance and the prevention of infection. The function of healthy cells is maintained by the provision of adequate nutrition (Felblinger, 2003).*
- If the client has AIDS, discuss the continued need to practice safe sex, avoid nonsterile needle use, and maintain a healthy lifestyle to prevent infection.
- ▲ Refer the client and family to social services and community resources to obtain support in maintaining a lifestyle that increases immune function (e.g., adequate nutrition and rest, freedom from excessive stress).

evolve WEBSITES FOR EDUCATION

See the EVOLVE website for World Wide Web resources for client education.

REFERENCES

Anonymous: Draft definitions of surveillance of infection in home healthcare, *Home Healthc Nurse* 19:439, 2001.

Bentley DW et al: Practice guidelines for evaluation of fever and infection in long-term care facilities, *Clin Infect Dis* 31(3):640, 2000, available on-line at http://www.guideline.gov/FRAMESETS/guideline_fs.asp?view=brief_summaryandguideline=1890andsynthesis_filename=andurl=andhidden=trueandsSearch_string, accessed March 16, 2003.

Brooks JA: Postoperative nosocomial pneumonia: nurse-sensitive interventions, *AACN Clin Issues* 12(2):305, 2001.

Calder PC, Kew S: The immune system: a target for functional foods? *Br J Nutr* 88(suppl 2):S165, 2002.

Calianno C: *Nosocomial pneumonia*, Springnet, Springhouse, available on-line at www.springnet.com/ce/ce965a.htm, accessed March 29, 1999.

CDC Hospital Infection Control Practices Advisory Committee: *Recommendations for isolation precautions in hospitals*, revised 11/09/2002, retrieved on March 16, 2003, from www http://www.cdc.gov/ncidod/hip/isolat/isopart2.htm.

Chiao EY, Ries KM, Sande MA: AIDS and the elderly, *Clin Infect Disease* 28:740, 1999.

Cornbleet PJ: Clinical utility of the band count, *Clin Lab Med* 22(1):101, 2002.

Crogan NL, Corbett CF, Short RA: The minimum data set: predicting malnutrition in newly admitted nursing home residents, *Clin Nurs Res* 11(3):341, 2002.

Crow R et al: *A study of patients with an indwelling urethral catheter and related nursing practice*, Guildford, Surrey, UK, 1996, Nursing Practice Unit, University of Surrey.

Dave J, Wilcox MH, Kellett M: Glove powder: implications for infection control, *J Hosp Infect* 42(4):283, 1999.

Engelhart S et al: Surveillance for nosocomial infections and fever of unknown origin among adult hematology-oncology patients, *Infect Control Hosp Epidemiol* 23(5):244, 2002.

Felblinger DM: Malnutrition, infection, and sepsis in acute and chronic illness, *Crit Care Nurs Clin North Am* 15(1):71, 2003.

Gilbert M, Barton AJ, Counsell CM: Comparison of oral and tympanic temperatures in adult surgical patients, *Appl Nurs Res* 15(1):42, 2002.

Girou E, Oppein F: Handwashing compliance in a French university hospital: new perspective with the introduction of hand-rubbing with a waterless alcohol-based solution, *J Hosp Infect* 48(Suppl A):S55, 2001.

Giuliano KK et al: Temperature measurement in critically ill adults: a comparison of tympanic and oral methods, *Am J Crit Care* 9(4):254, 2000.

Gould D: Hand decontamination, *Nurs Times* 98(46):48, 2002.

Hull S et al: Boosting uptake of influenza immunisation: a randomised controlled trial of telephone appointing in general practice, *Br J Gen Pract* 52(482):710, 2002.

- • = Independent; ▲ = Collaborative

Kovach T: The barrier defense: skin hydration as infection control, *J Pract Nurs* 45:13, 1995.

Lehmann S: Immune function and nutrition: the clinical role of the intravenous nurse, *J Intraven Nurs* 14:406, 1991.

Madhaven T: Infections in the elderly: current concepts in management, *Compr Ther* 20:465, 1994.

Parker R, Loewen N, Skowronski D: Experience with oseltamivir in the control of a nursing home influenza B outbreak, *Can Commun Dis Rep* 27(5):37, 2001.

Reid R et al: Postdischarge clean wound infections: incidence underestimated and risk factors overemphasized, *Aust N Z J Surg* 72(5):339, 2002.

Reilly J: Evidence-based surgical wound care on surgical wound infection, *Br J Nurs* 11(16 suppl):S4, 2002.

Roe B: Catheter-associated urinary tract infection: a review, *J Clin Nurs* 2:197, 1993.

Rotter ML: Arguments for alcoholic hand disinfection, *J Hosp Infect* 48(suppl A):S4, 2001.

Ruiz M et al: Diagnosis of pneumonia and monitoring of infection eradication, *Drugs* 60(6):1289, 2000.

Schmid MW: Risks and complications of peripherally and centrally inserted intravenous catheters, *Crit Care Nurs Clin North Am* 12(2):165, 2000.

Sheikh S, Sethi S: Management of infectious exacerbation of COPD, *Home Health Care Consult* 8(5):21, 2001.

Shinkawa M et al: Depression and immunoreactivity in disabled older adults, *J Am Geriatr Soc* 50:198, 2002.

St Clair K, Larrabee JH: Clean versus sterile gloves: which to use for postoperative dressing changes? *Outcomes Manag* 6(1):17, 2002.

Tasota F et al: Protecting ICU patients from nosocomial infections, *Crit Care Nurse* 18(1):54, 1998.

US Department of Health and Human Services, Centers for Disease Control and Prevention: *Hand hygiene guidelines fact sheet*, 2002, available on-line at http://www.cdc.gov/od/oc/media/pressrel/fs021025.=htm accessed Feb 12, 2003.

Vogelzang JL: Nutrition in home care. Nonfunctional gut? Try a probiotic food, *Home Healthc Nurse* 19:467, 2001.

Wujcik D: Infection control in oncology patients, *Nurs Clin North Am* 28:639, 1993.

Yates RR: New intervention strategies for reducing antibiotic resistance, *Chest* 115(suppl):24S, 1999.

Risk for Injury

Betty J. Ackley

NANDA   Definition

At risk of injury as a result of the interaction of environmental conditions interacting with the individual's adaptive and defensive resources

NOTE: This nursing diagnosis overlaps with other diagnoses such as **Risk for Falls, Risk for Trauma, Risk for Poisoning, Risk for Suffocation, Risk for Aspiration,** and if the client is at risk of bleeding, **Ineffective Protection.** See care plans for these diagnoses if appropriate.

Risk Factors

External

Mode of transport or transportation; people or provider (e.g., nosocomial agents; staffing patterns; cognitive, affective, and psychomotor factors); physical (e.g., design, structure, and arrangement of community, building, and/or equipment); nutrients (e.g., vitamins, food types); biological (e.g., immunization level of community, microorganism); chemical (e.g., pollutants, poisons, drugs, pharmaceutical agents, alcohol, caffeine, nicotine, preservatives, cosmetics, dyes)

Internal

Psychological (affective orientation); malnutrition; abnormal blood profile (e.g., leukocytosis/leukopenia; altered clotting factors; thrombocytopenia; sickle cell; thalassemia;

• = Independent; ▲ = Collaborative

decreased hemoglobin; immune-autoimmune dysfunction; biochemical, regulatory function (e.g., sensory dysfunction, integrative dysfunction, effector dysfunction, tissue hypoxia); developmental age (physiological, psychosocial); physical (e.g., broken skin, altered mobility)

Related Factors (r/t)

See Risk Factors.

NOC   Outcomes (Nursing Outcomes Classification)

Suggested NOC Outcomes

Fall Prevention Behavior; Fetal Status: Intrapartum; Immune Status; Maternal Status: Intrapartum; Parenting: Psychosocial Safety; Personal Safety Behavior; Risk Control; Safe Home Environment

> ### Example NOC Outcome with Indicators
>
> **Risk Control** as evidenced by the following indicators: Monitors environmental risk factors/Develops effective risk control strategies/Follows selected risk control strategies (Rate each indicator of **Risk Control**: 1 = never demonstrated, 2 = rarely demonstrated, 3 = sometimes demonstrated, 4 = often demonstrated, 5 = consistently demonstrated [see Section I].)

Client Outcomes

Client Will (Specify Time Frame):

- Remain free of injuries
- Explain methods to prevent injury

NIC   Interventions (Nursing Interventions Classification)

Suggested NIC Interventions

Behavior Modification; Health Education; Patient Contracting; Self-Modification Assistance

> ### Example NIC Activities—Health Education
>
> Identify internal or external factors that may enhance or reduce motivation for healthy behavior; Determine current health knowledge and lifestyle behaviors of individual, family, or target group

Nursing Interventions and Rationales

Prevent iatrogenic harm to the client by following these guidelines for giving care:
- ▲ Use at least two methods to identify the client before administering medications or blood products, such as the client's name and birth date.
- ▲ Prior to beginning any invasive or surgical procedure, have a final verification to confirm the correct client, the correct procedure, and the correct site for the procedure using active or passive communication techniques.
- • When taking verbal or telephone orders, always require a verification back of the complete order by the person taking the orders.

• = **Independent;** ▲ = **Collaborative**

- Standardize use of abbreviations and eliminate abbreviations that are prone to cause errors.
▲ Take high alert medications off the nursing unit, such as potassium chloride.
▲ Use only intravenous pumps that prevent free flow of intravenous solution when the tubing is taken out of the pump.
- Improve the effectiveness of alarm systems in the clinical area. *These are practical tips on improving client safety in a hospital or health care facility (Joint Commission Resources, 2003).*
- Thoroughly orient the client to environment. Place call light within reach and show how to call for assistance; answer call light promptly.
▲ Avoid use of restraints if at all possible. Obtain a physician's order if restraints are necessary. *If the elderly are restrained and fall, they can sustain severe injuries, including strangulation, asphyxiation, or head injury from leading with their heads to get out of the bed (DiMaio, Dana, and Bix, 1986; Evans and Strumpf, 1990). Restraint-free extended care facilities were shown to have fewer residents with activities of daily living (ADLs) deficiencies and fewer residents with bowel or bladder incontinence than facilities that use restraints (Castle and Fogel, 1998).* **Nursing and Clinical Research:** *A study demonstrated that there was no increase in falls or injuries in a group of clients that were not restrained, versus a similar group that was restrained in a nursing home (Capezuti et al, 1999). Restrained elderly clients often experience an increased number of falls, possibly as a result of muscle deconditioning or loss of coordination (Tinetti, Liu, and Ginter, 1992).*
- In place of restraints, use the following:
  ■ Alarm systems with ankle or wrist bracelets
  ■ Bed or wheelchair alarms
  ■ Increased observation of the client
  ■ Locked doors to unit
  ■ Bed with wheels removed to keep bed low (NOTE: may not conform to fire regulations)
  These are alternatives to restraints that can be helpful for preventing falls (Commodore, 1995; Wilson, 1998).
- For an agitated client, consider providing individualized music of the client's choice. **Nursing Research:** *One study demonstrated that hospitalized clients who previously were in restraints demonstrated more positive behaviors when listening to individualized music than did clients who were out of restraints but were not exposed to music (Janelli, Kanski, and Wu, 2002). Calming music was shown to be effective in decreasing agitation in persons with dementia (Remington, 2002).*
- If the client is extremely agitated, consider using a special safety bed that surrounds the client. If the client has a traumatic brain injury, use the Emory cubicle bed. *Special beds can be an effective alternative to restraints and can help keep the client safe during periods of agitation (Williams et al, 1990).*
- If the client has a new onset of confusion (delirium), provide reality orientation when interacting with him or her. Have family bring in familiar items, clocks, and watches from home to maintain orientation. If the client has chronic confusion with dementia, use validation therapy that reinforces feelings but does not confront reality. *Reality orientation can help prevent or decrease the confusion that increases risk of injury when the patient becomes agitated. Validation therapy is more effective for clients with dementia (Fine and Rouse-Bane, 1995).* (See Interventions for **Acute Confusion** if delirium or **Chronic Confusion** if dementia.)

- **= Independent; ▲ = Collaborative**

- Ask family to stay with the client to prevent the client from accidentally falling or pulling out tubes. *Remove all possible hazards in environment such as razors, medications, and matches.*
- Place an injury-prone client in a room that is near the nurses' station. *Such placement allows more frequent observation of the client.*
- Help clients sit in a stable chair with armrests. Avoid use of wheelchairs and geri-chairs except for transportation as needed. *Clients are likely to fall when left in a wheelchair or geri-chair because they may stand up without locking the wheels or removing the footrests. Wheelchairs do not increase mobility; people just sit in them the majority of the time (Lipson and, Braun, 1993; Simmons et al, 1995).*
- To ensure propulsion with legs or arms and ability to reach the floor, ensure that the chair or wheelchair fits the build, abilities, and needs of the client, eliminating footrests and minimizing problems with shearing. *The seating system should fit the needs of the client so that the client can move the wheels, stand up from the chair without falling, and not be harmed by the chair or wheelchair. Footrests can cause skin tears and bruising, as well as postural alignment and sitting posture problems (Lipson and Braun, 1993).*
- Avoid use of wheelchairs as much as possible because they can serve as a restraint device. Most people in wheelchairs do not move. **Clinical Research:** *Wheelchairs can be effective restraints. In one study, only 4% of residents in wheelchairs were observed to propel them independently and only 45% could propel them, even with cues and prompts. This study found that no residents could unlock the wheelchairs without help, wheelchairs were not fitted to residents, and residents were not trained in propulsion (Simmons et al, 1995).*
- ▲ Refer to physical therapy for strengthening exercises and gait training to increase mobility.
- ▲ Refer to occupational therapy for assistance with helping clients perform ADLs. *Gait training in physical therapy has been shown to effectively prevent falls (Galinda-Ciocon, Ciocon, and Galinda, 1995; Wilson, 1998).*
- ▲ For the agitated psychotic client, use nonphysical forms of behavior management, such as verbal intervention or show of force. If medication is required, use oral medications if at all possible. *Nonphysical behavior management is first-line strategy when dealing with the psychotic client; oral medications can be just as effective as intramuscular injections when used for agitation if the client will swallow them and avoid possible injury from intramuscular injections (Murphy, 2002).*

Pediatric

- Teach parents the need for close supervision of all young children playing near water. If child has epilepsy, recommend showers instead of tub baths, and no unsupervised swimming is ever allowed. *Most drowning accidents involving children are preventable if basic safety measures are taken (Bolte, 2000).*
- Teach parents and children the need to maintain safety for the exercising child, including wearing helmets when biking, using breakaway bases for baseball, and having the needed conditioning for the activity. **Clinical Research:** *Wearing helmets while bicycling was shown to reduce the rate of head injury by 85% (Thompson, Rivara, and Thompson, 1989). Use of breakaway bases was shown to reduce the number of injuries in baseball and softball by 96% (Janda, Bir, and Kedroske, 2001).*
- Teach both parents and children the need for gun safety. *There are a number of programs available to teach gun safety, including Eddie the Eagle Gun Safe Program, Straight*

• = **Independent;** ▲ = **Collaborative**

Talk about Risks (STAR), Steps to prevent Firearm Injury in the Home, and the Emergency Nurses Association Gun Safety Program (Howard, 2001).

Geriatric

- Encourage the client to wear glasses and hearing aids and to use walking aids when ambulating. *If the client experiences dizziness because of orthostatic hypotension when getting up, teach methods to decrease dizziness, such as rising slowly, remaining seated several minutes before standing, flexing feet upward several times while sitting, sitting down immediately if feeling dizzy, and trying to have someone present when standing. The elderly develop decreased baroreceptor sensitivity and decreased ability of compensatory mechanisms to maintain blood pressure when standing up, resulting in postural hypotension (Aaronson, Carlon-Wolfe, and Schoener, 1991; Matteson, McConnell, and Linton, 1997).*

Multicultural

- Acknowledge racial/ethnic differences at the onset of care. **Nursing Research:** *Acknowledgment of race/ethnicity issues will enhance communication, establish rapport, and promote treatment outcomes (D'Avanzo et al, 2001; Ludwick and Silva, 2000; Vontress and Epp, 1997).*
- Assess for the influence of cultural beliefs, norms, and values on the client's perceptions of risk for injury. **Nursing Research:** *What the client considers risky behavior may be based on cultural perceptions (Cochran, 1998; Doswell and Erlen, 1998; Leininger and McFarland, 2002).*
- Assess whether exposure to community violence is contributing to risk for injury. **Nursing Research:** *Exposure to community violence has been associated with increases in aggressive behavior and depression (Gorman-Smith and Tolan, 1998). Minority students, especially African American and Hispanic students in lower grades, may participate in and may more often be victims of school violence (Hill and Drolet, 1999).*
- Use culturally relevant injury prevention programs whenever possible. **Nursing Research:** *The Make It Safe program is a bilingual, culturally sensitive educational presentation for Hispanic families that focuses on living and working safely in a rural environment (National Rural Health Association, 1998).*
- Validate the client's feelings and concerns related to environmental risks. **Nursing Research:** *Validation is therapeutic communication technique that lets the client know that the nurse has heard and understands what was said, and it promotes the nurse-client relationship (Heineken, 1998).*

Home care

- Some of the above interventions may be adapted for home care use.
- Assess home environment for threats to safety: clutter, inappropriate storage of chemicals, slippery floors, scatter rugs, unsafe stairs and stairwells, blocked entries, dim lighting, extension cords across pathways, unsafe electrical or gas connections, unsafe heating devices, unsafe oxygen placement, high beds without rails, excessively hot water, pets, and pet excrement. *Clients suffering from impaired mobility, impaired visual acuity, and neurological dysfunction, including dementia and other cognitive functional deficits, are at risk for injury from common hazards.*
- ▲ Instruct the client and family or caregivers in correcting identified hazards. Refer to occupational therapy services for assistance if needed. Notify landlord or code enforcement office of any structural building hazards.

- **= Independent; ▲ = Collaborative**

▲ Refer to physical therapy services for the client and family education in safe transfers and ambulation and for strengthening exercises for ambulation and transfers.

• Avoid extreme hot and cold around clients at risk for injury (e.g., heating pads, hot water for baths/showers). Clients with decreased cognition or sensory deficits cannot discriminate extremes in temperature.

▲ Monitor blood glucose patterns for indicators of need for client instruction or referral to physician for treatment changes. *Pattern management of glucose levels is essential to client care (Linekin, 2002). Intensive management of blood glucose is possible, using multiple daily injections or continuous subcutaneous insulin pumps, with reduction of diabetes complications by up to 60%. Continuous glucose sensor monitoring is also available (Unger, 2001). Tools for diabetes education for the visually impaired are available (Camporeale, 2001), as well as "talking" glucometers.*

▲ Provide a signaling device for clients who wander or are at risk for falls. If the client lives alone, provide a Lifeline or similar call device. *Orienting a vulnerable client to a safety net relieves anxiety of the client and caregiver and allows for rapid response to a crisis situation.*

▲ Provide medical identification bracelet for clients at risk for injury from dementia, seizures, or other medical disorders.

Client/Family Teaching

• Teach how to safely ambulate at home, including using safety measures such as handrails in bathroom.

• If the client has visual impairment, teach the client and caregiver to label with bright colors such as yellow or red significant places in environment that must be easily located (e.g., stair edges, stove controls, light switches). **Clinical Research:** *Color cues can improve the legibility of the environment and increase the ability to target objects quickly (Cooper, 1999).*

• Teach the client to avoid excessive noise at work or at home, wearing hearing protection when necessary. Any noise that hurts the ears or is above 90 decibels is excessive. *Hearing loss from excessive noise is common and preventable (Lusk, 2002).*

• Teach clients winter safety information:
  ▪ Burn only untreated wood for heat.
  ▪ Keep portable space heaters at least 3 feet from anything that can burn.
  ▪ Install smoke alarms and carbon monoxide alarm near bedrooms.
  ▪ Check the chimney and flue each year.
  ▪ Avoid sitting in an idling car in winter when snow can obstruct the exhaust pipe.
  ▪ Follow safety guidelines for use of snow blowers.
  Winter presents many safety challenges both indoors and outdoors. These safety tips can help increase safety (National Center for Injury Prevention and Control, 2000).

evolve WEBSITES FOR EDUCATION

See the EVOLVE website for World Wide Web resources for client education.

REFERENCES

Aaronson L, Carlon-Wolfe W, Schoener S: Pressures that fall on rising, *Geriatr Nurs* 12:67, 1991.
Bolte R: Drowning: a preventable cause of death, *Patient Care* 34(7):129, 2000.

• = **Independent;** ▲ = **Collaborative**

Camporeale J: Client challenge. Teaching an insulin-dependent blind patient about self-care, *Home Healthc Nurse* 19:247, 2001.

Capezuti E et al: Outcomes of nighttime physical restrain removal for severely impaired nursing home residents, *Am J Alzheimer's Dis* 14(3):157, 1999.

Castle NG, Fogel B: Characteristics of nursing homes that are restraint free, *Gerontologist* 38(2):181, 1998.

Cochran M: Tears have no color, *Am J Nurs* 98(6):53, 1998.

Commodore DI: Falls in the elderly population: a look at incidence, risks, healthcare costs, and preventive strategies, *Rehabil Nurs* 20:84, 1995.

Cooper BA: The utility of functional colour cues: seniors' views, *Scand J Caring Sci* 13(3):186, 1999.

D'Avanzo CE et al: Developing culturally informed strategies for substance-related interventions. In Naegle MA, D'Avanzo CE, editors: *Addictions and substance abuse: strategies for advanced practice nursing*, St Louis, 2001, Mosby.

DiMaio V, Dana S, Bix R: Death caused by restraint vests, *JAMA* 255:905, 1986.

Doswell W, Erlen J: Multicultural issues and ethical concerns in the delivery of revising care interventions, *Nurs Clin North Am* 33(2):353, 1998.

Evans L, Strumpf N: Myths about elder restraint, *Image J Nurs Sch* 22:124, 1990.

Fine JI, Rouse-Bane S: Using validating techniques to improve communication with cognitively impaired older adults, *J Gerontol Nurs* 21:39, 1995.

Galinda-Ciocon DJ, Ciocon JO, Galinda DJ: Gait training and falls in the elderly, *J Gerontol Nurs* 21:11, 1995.

Gorman-Smith D, Tolan P: The role of exposure to community violence and developmental problems among inner city youth, *Dev Psychopathol* 10(1):101, 1998.

Howard PK: An overview of a few well-known national children's gun safety programs and ENA's newly developed program, *J Emerg Nurs* 27(5):485, 2001.

Joint Commission Resources: *Special Report! 2003 JCAHO national patient safety goals: practical strategies and helpful solutions for meeting these goals,* available on-line at http://www.jcrinc.com/subscribers/patientsafety.asp?durki+3746, accessed April 10, 2003.

Heineken J: Patient silence is not necessarily client satisfaction: communication in home care nursing, *Home Healthc Nurse* 16(2):115, 1998.

Hill SC, Drolet JC: School related violence among high school students in the United States 1993-1995, *J Sch Health* 69(7):264, 1999.

Janda DH, Bir C, Kedroske B: A comparison of standard versus breakaway bases: an analysis of a preventative intervention for softball and baseball foot and ankle injuries, *Foot Ankle Int* 22:810, 2001.

Janelli LM, Kanski GW, Wu YB. Individualized music—a different approach to the restraint issue, *Rehabil Nurs* 27(6):221, 2002.

Leininger MM, McFarland MR: *Transcultural nursing: concepts, theories, research and practices,* ed 3, New York, 2002, McGraw-Hill.

Linekin PL: Diabetes pattern management, *Home Healthc Nurse* 20:168, 2002.

Lipson J, Braun S: *Toward a restraint-free environment: reducing the use of physical and chemical restraint in long-term care and acute settings,* Baltimore, 1993, Health Professions Press.

Ludwick R, Silva M: Nursing around the world: cultural values and ethical conflicts, *Online J Issues Nurs,* available on-line at http://www.nursingworld.org/ojin/ethcol/ethics_4.htm.

Lusk SL: Preventing noise-induced hearing loss, *Nurs Clin North Am* 37(2):257, 2002.

Matteson MA, McConnell ES, Linton AD: *Gerontological nursing,* ed 2, Philadelphia, 1997, WB Saunders.

Murphy MC: The agitated psychotic patient: guidelines to ensure staff and patient safety, *J Am Psychiatr Nurses Assoc* 8(4 suppl):S2, 2002.

National Center for Injury Prevention and Control: Winter safety, *Int J Trauma Nurs* 6(4):138, 2000.

National Rural Health Association: Make it safe: an injury prevention program for Hispanic farm workers and families at work and play, *Int Electronic J Health Ed* 1(4):219, 1998.

Remington R: Calming music and hand massage with agitated elderly, *Nurs Res* 51(5):317, 2002.

Simmons S et al: Wheelchairs as mobility restraints: predictors of wheelchair activity in nonambulatory nursing home residents, *J Am Geriatr Soc* 43:384, 1995.

Thompson RS, Rivara FP, Thompson DC: A case-control study of the effectiveness of bicycle safety helmets, *N Engl J Med* 320:1361, 1989.

Tinetti ME, Liu W-L, Ginter SF: Mechanical restraint use and fall-related injuries among residents of skilled nursing facilities, *Ann Intern Med* 116:369, 1992.

Unger J: Intensive management of type I diabetes, *Home Health Care Consult* 8(6):7, 2001.

Vontress CE, Epp LR: Historical hostility in the African American client: implications for counseling, *J Multicult Counseling Dev* 25:170, 1997.

• = **Independent**; ▲ = **Collaborative**

Williams LM, Morton GA, Patrick CH: The Emory cubicle bed: an alternative to restraints for agitated traumatically brain injured clients, *Rehabil Nurs* 15:30, 1990.
Wilson EB: Preventing patient falls, *AACN Clin Issues* 9(1):100, 1998.

Risk for perioperative positioning Injury

Terri Foster

NANDA Definition

At risk for injury as a result of the environmental conditions found in the perioperative setting

Risk Factors

Disorientation; edema; emaciation; immobilization; muscle weakness; obesity; sensory/perceptual disturbances resulting from anesthesia (NANDA). High pressure for short periods of time and low pressure for extended periods of time are risk factors for tissue injury (AORN, 2002).

NOTE: The following systems are most frequently affected by surgical positioning: neurological, musculoskeletal, integumentary, respiratory, and cardiovascular. Risk factors contributing to the incidence of injury related to surgical positioning include but are not limited to the client's age; height; weight; nutritional status; skin condition; the presence of preexisting conditions such as diabetes, vascular, and/or respiratory disease; immunocompromise; impaired nerve function; physical mobility limitations such as arthritis, limited range of motion (ROM), implants/prosthesis, or malignancy; effects of anesthesia; staff's knowledge of the equipment; required position for the procedure; and the duration of the procedure (AORN, 2002). As a result of these factors, there is the potential for impaired tissue perfusion, impaired skin integrity, or neuromuscular or joint injury related to surgical positioning. The anesthetized client is at increased risk of injury due to positioning because anesthesia prevents the body's defense mechanism from warning the client of exaggerated stretching, twisting, or compression of his or her body (Powers, 2002).

Complications of surgical positioning

Complications of positioning include, but are not limited to, mechanical restriction of the rib cage, vasodilatation, hyper/hypotension, decreased cardiac output, inhibition of normal compensatory mechanisms, redistribution and congestion of the blood supply, and nerve and muscle trauma due to stretching and compression (AORN, 2002). **Nursing Research:** Several studies have shown that procedures lasting more than 2½ to 3 hours significantly increase the risk for pressure ulcer formation (AORN, 2002). Occlusion, causing restriction or blockage of blood flow, has been shown to occur when external pressure exceeds the normal capillary interface pressure of 23 to 32 mm Hg (AORN, 2002).

Transient physiological reactions to surgical positioning include skin redness and/or bruising, lumbar backache, stiffness in the limbs and neck, numbness, and generalized muscle aches that usually resolve within 24 to 48 hours without treatment. Lumbar back pain, previously considered a transient physiological reaction to positioning, may be an indication of rhabdomyolysis (Anema, 2000).

• = Independent; ▲ = Collaborative

More serious complications of surgical positioning include pressure ulcers, peripheral nerve injury, deep venous thrombosis, joint dislocation, compartment syndrome (impairment of microcirculation in soft tissue), rhabdomyolysis, and joint injury.

NOC   Outcomes (Nursing Outcomes Classification)

Suggested NOC Outcomes
Circulation Status; Neurological Status; Risk Control; Tissue Integrity: Skin and Mucous Membranes; Tissue Perfusion: Peripheral

> ### Example NOC Outcome with Indicators
>
> **Tissue Perfusion: Peripheral** as evidenced by the following indicators: Peripheral edema not present/ Localized extremity pain not present/Skin intact/Muscle function intact/Sensation level normal/Distal peripheral pulses strong (Rate each indicator of **Tissue Perfusion: Peripheral:** I = extremely compromised, 2 = substantially compromised, 3 = moderately compromised, 4 = mildly compromised, 5 = not compromised [see Section I].)

Client Outcomes

Client Will (Specify Time Frame):
- Be free of injury related to positioning during the surgical procedure
- Demonstrate unchanged or improved physical mobility from preoperative status
- Demonstrate unchanged or improved cardiovascular status from preoperative status
- Demonstrate unchanged or improved peripheral sensory integrity from preoperative status
- Maintain sense of privacy and dignity

NIC   Interventions (Nursing Interventions Classification)

Suggested NIC Interventions
Positioning: Intraoperative; Pressure Ulcer Prevention; Risk Identification; Skin Surveillance

> ### Example NIC Activities—Positioning: Intraoperative
>
> Use an adequate number of personnel to transfer the client; Maintain the client's proper body alignment

Nursing Interventions and Rationales

General interventions for any surgical patient
- Proper positioning requires knowledge of not only the equipment, but also anatomy and the application of physiological principles (Fortunato, 2002). **Nursing Research:** *Hypoxia, to some extent, is always present in the horizontal position (Fortunato, 2000). Tidal volume is reduced by as much as one third simply by lying down; therefore, it is necessary that no constriction occur around the client's neck or chest (Fortunato, 2000).*
- A preoperative assessment, which includes a determination of the client's ROM/ mobility, is necessary to determine the need for positioning aids and should be completed prior to the surgical procedure. *A proper preoperative assessment of the client is necessary to ensure appropriate positioning needs (AORN, 2002; Fortunato, 2000).*

• = Independent; ▲ = Collaborative

- Clients with limited mobility/ROM should be asked to position themselves under the nurse's guidance before induction of anesthesia so that the client can verify that a position of comfort has been obtained. **Nursing Research:** *Having the awake client assist in positioning is helpful for assessing range of comfort when the skeleton is distorted and for evaluating alternate positioning that will allow for maximum surgical site exposure (Martin, 2000).*
- Appropriate numbers of personnel should be present to assist in positioning the client. **Nursing Research:** *Two people should assist an awake client to transfer from a cart/bed to the OR table—one person on the stretcher side to assist the client onto the OR table and a second person on the far side of the OR table to prevent the client from falling off the table (Fortunato, 2000). A minimum of four persons are necessary when transferring/positioning an unconscious, obese, or weak client (Fortunato, 2000).*
- Monitor pressure being applied to the client intraoperatively by staff, equipment, and/or instruments. *Staff leaning on the client, or equipment and/or instruments resting on the client can cause redness and bruising and lead to pressure ulcers. Feet and protuberant parts should be protected from overbed tables, mayo stands, and frames. An adequate clearance of 2 to 3 inches should be maintained (Fortunato, 2000). During pelvic procedures, femoral nerve injuries, caused by retractors, have been observed (Fortunato, 2000). During hip surgery, sciatic nerve injuries can occur due to tissue retraction or manipulation (Fortunato, 2000). Head straps that are too tight or vigorous manual elevation of the mandible for airway maintenance can cause facial nerve injury (Fortunato, 2000).* **Nursing Research:** *A client undergoing cervical surgery sustained injury to her ulnar nerve due to pressure on the arm by a retractor bar, from the Thompson-Farley retractor system, during the procedure. As a result, continuous monitoring of somatosensory evoked potentials (SSEPs) is suggested with use of this retractor (Baumann, 2000).*
- Keep linens on the OR table free of wrinkles. *Folds and creases in linen can cause pressure indentations in the skin (Fortunato, 2000).*
- Maintain equipment in good working order and use according to manufacturer's instructions: Verify that the equipment is clean, operating properly, free of sharp edges, able to maintain normal capillary interface pressure, and nonallergenic to the client (AORN, 2002; Fortunato, 2000). Equipment that is working properly leads to client safety and aids in improved exposure of the surgical site (AORN, 2001). **Nursing Research:** *Many beds have a weight limit for safe use; therefore, it is necessary to check the equipment to ensure that it will tolerate the client's weight (Fortunato, 2000).*
- Reassess the client after positioning and during the procedure for maintenance of proper alignment and skin integrity. **Nursing Research:** *Changes in position can expose or injure body parts (e.g., shearing, friction, compression) that were protected previously (AORN, 2002). Once the client has been positioned, lifting him or her slightly for a moment may allow skin to realign with the skeleton (Meeker et al, 1999).*
- Do not allow extremities to extend beyond/off the OR. *Many beds have an extension that can be added to accommodate tall clients (Fortunato, 2000).*
- Avoid contact with metal when positioning the client.
- Avoid hyperextension of joints. **Nursing Research:** *Extension of the head for long periods of time can result in a stiff neck, which causes more pain then the incision site (Fortunato, 2000). Hyperextension of joints can cause permanent injury to extremities (Fortunato, 2000).*
- Any movement/positioning of the client should be done slowly. *Slow movement allows the body time to adjust to circulatory and respiratory changes and allows the abdominal*

- = **Independent;** ▲ = **Collaborative**

contents to reposition. It also allows the staff to have better control of the client's body (Fortunato, 2000).

- The OR table, cart, or bed should be locked and the mattress stabilized before transfer/positioning of the client (Fortunato, 2000). *An unlocked OR table, cart, or bed could lead to the client's sustaining a fall injury.*
- Use a full-length silicone gel pad to prevent pressure injuries. *Foam pads are ineffective in reducing capillary interface pressure due to their quick compression beneath heavy body areas (AORN, 2002). Pillows, blankets, and molded foam devices may only produce minimal pressure reduction (AORN, 2002). Towels and sheet rolls may contribute to friction injuries and they do not reduce pressure (AORN, 2002). Use of gel pads on the OR bed decreases pressure by redistributing the overall pressure across a larger surface area (AORN, 2002). The client's body weight is unevenly distributed when lying on the operating table (Fortunato, 2000).* **Nursing Research:** *Hoshowsky and Schramm (1998) have shown that the operating table surface affects the client's risk for pressure sore development.*
- Prevent pooling of preparative solutions, blood, irrigation, urine, and feces. *Prior to initiating the skin prep, absorbent pads should be placed to collect any preoperative solutions that run off the area being prepped. Clean up as necessary. Pooling in areas of high pressure can increase the chances for the development of a more severe pressure sore (Meeker et al, 1999).*
- Ensure privacy and dignity for the client during positioning, by reducing unnecessary exposure (AORN, 2002).
- The client should be kept warm during positioning to prevent hypothermia, which can lead to increased potential for infection and slower wound healing.
- Lift rather than pull or slide the client when positioning. *Sliding and pulling increase the incidence of skin injury (dermal abrasion or soft tissue injury) from shearing and friction (Fortunato, 2000). Pressure and/or shearing cause decreased circulation.* **Nursing Research:** *Use of a simple snow sled (the roll-up thin, flexible plastic type) to reposition the client up and down on the table can reduce shear or friction (Carris and Franczek, 1999).*
- Position the client's legs parallel and uncrossed. *Crossing of the client's ankles and legs creates occlusive pressure on blood vessels and nerves that can lead to pressure necrosis (Fortunato, 2000).*
- Maintain alignment of head with cervical, thoracic, and lumbar spine. *Misalignment, flexion, and twisting may cause muscle and nerve damage, as well as airway interference. Proper alignment of the head and spine prevents neuromuscular strain (Meeker et al, 1999).*
- Body supports and restraint straps (safety belt) should be loose and secured over waist or mid-thigh at least 2 inches above knees, avoiding bony prominences by placing a blanket between the strap and the client. *Adequate arterial circulation must be maintained to avoid changes in blood pressure, tissue perfusion (oxygenation), venous return, and thrombus formation. Occlusion and pressure on peripheral blood vessels should be avoided (Fortunato, 2000). The extremities and body should always be well supported so that prolonged pressure or stretching of peripheral nerves, which could result in sensory and/or motor loss, is avoided (Fortunato, 2000). Use of the safety belt during procedures performed in the lithotomy position can cause compression of abdominal structures and therefore should be used only when the client's legs are in the down position (Fortunato, 2000).*

Supine position (dorsal recumbent)
- Pad all bony prominences and positioning devices. *The occiput, scapulae, thoracic vertebrae, olecranon processes, sacrum/coccyx, calcanea, and knees are all pressure points (AORN,*

- = Independent; ▲ = Collaborative

2002). When weight is concentrated over bony prominences, pressure ulcers and deep tissue injury can occur (Fortunato, 2000). **Nursing Research:** *Skin overlying bony prominences supporting the weight of body parts can become relatively avascular with prolonged compression (Martin, 2000).*

- Support lumbar and popliteal areas. *Small pillows can be placed under the head, lumbar spine, and popliteal areas to relieve spine pressure. When placing a pillow under the client's knees, place it proximal to the popliteal space and examine the safety strap to make sure it is not too tight.* **Nursing Research:** *The popliteal artery, common peroneal nerve, and tibial nerve could be compressed between the pillow and the safety strap, causing nerve damage, impaired circulation, or thrombosis (Meeker and Rothrock, 1999).*
- Use a pillow, padded footboard, or donut under the heels. **Nursing Research:** *A support or footboard prevents prolonged plantar flexion and foot drop (Fortunato, 2000).*
- Arms positioned on armboards, should be in the palms down position, with the armboards at less than a 90-degree angle (some sources recommend less than 60 degrees) to the body and the armboard pads should be level with the OR table pad. **Nursing Research:** *Injury to the brachial plexus nerve, ulnar nerve, and axillary artery can occur when arms are placed at an angle greater then 90 degrees to the body (AORN, 2002; Fortunato, 2000). Arms placed in the palms up position prevent ulnar nerve pressure and abnormal shoulder rotation (Fortunato, 2000). Positioning the arm in this manner decreases pressure on the postcondylar groove of the humerus (American Society of Anesthesiologists Task Force, 2000). Hyperabduction of the arm can cause the brachial plexus to be stretched and compressed between the clavicle and the first rib. This pressure/compression increases when the client's head is turned toward the opposite shoulder/arm. Another complication of hyperabduction of the arm is thrombosis. The palms-up position increases stretching of the brachial plexus (Meeker et al, 1999).*
- Arms positioned at the sides of the body should have the palms against the sides of the body and fingers extended along the length of the body. The sheet flaps should be brought down over the arms and tucked under the client's sides. **Nursing Research:** *Lift sheets tucked under the side of the mattress can impair circulation or cause nerve torsion due to the combined weight of the mattress and the client's torso pressing on the arms (Fortunato, 2000).*
- When placing a pregnant client in the supine position, place a small roll under her right flank. **Nursing Research:** *In the supine position, there is increased pressure to the inferior vena cava from the abdominal contents and the fetus, which can decrease the return of blood to the heart (Meeker et al, 1999).*

Prone position (modification: kneeling, jackknife, or Kraske position)

- Provide an adequate number of personnel to accomplish "logroll" turning of the anesthetized client. **Nursing Research:** *At least four persons are necessary to "logroll" a client in order to maintain proper body alignment (Fortunato, 2000).*
- Place chest rolls from the acromioclavicular joint to the iliac crests. *Chest rolls allow for chest movement and decrease abdominal pressure (AORN, 2002).* **Nursing Research:** *Chest rolls allow for lung expansion and respirations by lifting the chest off the OR table, and raising the body weight off of the abdomen and thorax. This allows the weight of the abdomen to fall away from the diaphragm and keep pressure off the vena cava and aorta (Fortunato, 2000)* NOTE: *Some surgeons prefer to use a laminectomy frame, but the same rationale applies.*
- Male genitalia and female breasts should be checked and positioned to eliminate pres-

• = **Independent;** ▲ = **Collaborative**

sure. Male genitalia should be allowed to hang loosely and without pressure. **Nursing Research:** *Moving the female breasts laterally will reduce pressure on them (Fortunato, 2000).*

- Care must be taken when positioning obese clients in the Kraske position. *Dangling skin folds can drop down into table crevasses. If they come in contact with metal, a grounding burn could occur during cautery use. When the table is repositioned horizontally, the skin folds could become trapped, incised, or even amputated (Martin, 2000).*
- Place a bolster or pillow under the pelvis. **Nursing Research:** *Support of the pelvis decreases abdominal pressure on the inferior vena cava and male genitalia (Meeker et al, 1999).*
- Place padding under the knees to prevent undo pressure on the patellas.
- Rotate the client's arms from the side, to a "swimming" position to rest on armboards that are extended forward from the OR table.
- Shoulders should be kept in a neutral position with the elbows bent at 90 degrees and the hands resting alongside the head (Goettler et al, 2002). **Nursing Research:** *The most common neurological injury due to positioning in the operating room is brachial plexus injury. Conditions that appear to cause brachial plexus injuries are abduction of the arms with external rotation and posterior shoulder displacement (Goettler, 2002).*
- Place the head, turned to one side, on a padded headrest, maintain cervical alignment, and protect the client's ears and eyes. Pad the head and eyeballs to avoid pressure from the operating table. *A padded headrest provides airway access (AORN, 2001).* **Nursing Research:** *A reported incident of unilateral blindness occurred in a client after prolonged compression of the eyeball during cervical spine surgery. As a result, it is suggested that Halo traction on a Mayfield support might be helpful to avoid continuous contact of the face with the operating table (Manfredini et al, 2000).*
- Clients placed in the Kraske position should be observed for respiratory and circulatory changes. *In the Kraske position, the client has restricted diaphragm movement and increased blood volume in the lungs and feet because of venous pooling, which can lead to a decrease in mean arterial blood pressure, decreased ventilation, and decreased cardiac output (Meeker et al, 1999).*

Lateral position (lateral chest or kidney)
- Provide adequate personnel to properly position the client.
- Use a lift sheet to facilitate the turn. Lift sheets prevent skin injury resulting from shearing.
- Place a support under the head. *A pillow or support keeps the head properly aligned with the cervical spine and thoracic vertebrae and lessens stretching of the brachial plexus (Meeker et al, 1999).*
- Flex the bottom leg at the hip and knee. *Flexing the bottom leg helps to stabilize the client (Meeker et al, 1999).*
- Place beanbags, sandbags, or bolsters against the back and abdomen. *Additional positioning devices provide support and maintain body alignment (Meeker et al, 1999).*
- Pad the lateral aspect of the bottom knee.
- Place a pillow between the client's legs lengthwise so that the pillow also supports the foot. *Pressing the bony prominences of one extremity against the other may cause injury to the peroneal and tibial nerves (Meeker et al, 1999).*

• = Independent; ▲ = Collaborative

- Pad the lower shoulder and bring it forward slightly; the lower arm is extended on a padded armboard. *Bringing the shoulder forward relieves pressure on the brachial plexus and improves chest expansion (Meeker et al, 1999).*
- Place the upper arm on a padded raised armboard or over the lower arm with padding between the two arms. *Raising the upper arm elevates the scapula and widens the intercostal spaces, which provides access to the upper thoracic cavity (Meeker et al, 1999).*
- Place an axillary roll at the apex of the scapula in the axillary space of the dependent arm.
- When using positioning straps or tape to hold the client in the lateral position, place a towel or blanket between the client's skin and the strap/tape. **Nursing Research:** *Compression of the skin beneath the tape/strap can cause injury and should be avoided (Fortunato, 2000).*

NOTE: Some surgeons prefer the use of wide adhesive tape to secure the hips, arms, and legs. This practice would be contraindicated in clients with tape allergies or in the frail elderly with fragile skin. Some surgeons prefer to use a device known as the Montreal Positioning Device. When using this device, special care must be taken to pad the posts extremely well to prevent pressure injuries.

Lithotomy position

- Before placing the client in the lithotomy position, the stirrups should be checked to ensure that they are fastened securely in the sockets attached to the OR bed. *If the stirrups are not fastened securely and slip, the client could sustain a dislocated hip, muscle or nerve injury, or a fracture (Meeker et al, 1999).*
- Position the client's arms loosely secured across the abdomen, extended on padded armboards, or at the client's sides. *Extreme care must be taken when positioning the client's arms at the sides in this position because the hand and fingers could get crushed or pinched in the OR table when raising and lowering the lower third of the table for the procedure (Meeker et al, 1999).*

NOTE: Some surgeons prefer to have the left arm positioned at the client's side when they are doing a procedure such as a D and C with diagnostic laparoscopy. In this case, it is suggested that the arm is well padded and that, in the absence of a tape allergy, foam tape be used to tape the hands and fingers to the client's thigh. Extreme care must be taken to ensure that the hands and fingers have not come loose before raising and lowering the lower third of the OR table.

- Pad the sacral area and provide a small lumbar roll. The client's buttocks should be even with the table edge once the lower portion of the OR table has been lowered. *A lumbar roll helps maintain normal lumbar concavity (AORN, 2001; Meeker et al, 1999).* **Nursing Research:** *When the buttocks extend beyond the edge of the table it causes strain on the lumbosacral muscles and ligaments, due to the client's body weight resting on the sacrum (Fortunato, 2000). The greatest amount of force is placed on the lower back muscles when the client is in the lithotomy position (Anema et al, 2000).*
- Stirrups should be positioned at equal height and adjusted according to the length of the client's legs and at the level of the client's upper thighs. *Positioning stirrups at equal height helps to prevent knee and hip injury (AORN, 2002).*
- Place the client's legs in the stirrups simultaneously, using one hand to hold the foot and the other to hold the calf at the knee. **Nursing Research:** *Raising the legs slowly*

and simultaneously reduces lumbar and sacral pressure and vascular congestion (AORN, 2002; Fortunato, 2000).

- Lower the client's legs simultaneously and slowly, extending the legs fully. **Nursing Research:** *Lowering the legs slowly and simultaneously decreases lumbar and sacral pressure, and vascular congestion (AORN, 2002).*
- Minimize the height of the legs. *The height of the lower legs should be only slightly above the level of the left atria. Perfusion is decreased when the legs are elevated (Lampert et al, 1997).* **Nursing Research:** *Huge thighs can compress the outer abdomen and force abdominal contents midline, causing increased pressure on the diaphragm (Martin, 2000).*
- Avoid hyperabduction and excessive external rotation of the hip joint. *Acute flexion of the thigh increases intra-abdominal pressure against the diaphragm, thus decreasing tidal volume (Meeker et al, 1999). Excess flexion of the hip and knee can cause venous obstruction (Anema et al, 2000). Excess flexion of the hip can stretch the sciatic nerve (Meeker et al, 1999). Femoral, sciatic, and obturator nerves, along with the abductor muscles of the hip joint, are stretched when the legs are hyperabducted (Meeker et al, 1999).* **Nursing Research:** *To prevent wide abduction of the thighs when removing legs from the stirrups, the legs should be fully extended and then brought together (Fortunato, 2000). Overflexion of the hip can lead to injury to the sciatic nerve because of overstretching. In a study involving 1170 clients placed in the lithotomy position, nerve injury occurred in 12 and the study showed that the age of the client, the type of operation, length of the operation (over 180 minutes), and improper positioning by staff all contributed to those who sustained injury (Gumus et al, 2002).*
- Select lithotomy leg holders with optimal body alignment and weight bearing in mind (e.g., combination knee-crutch-and-boot). **Nursing Research:** *Product selection and evaluation should be based on identified needs and should promote client safety (AORN, 2001). Boot stirrups distribute weight evenly and allow controlled and limited abduction (Meeker et al, 1999).*
- Pad all bony prominences and surfaces that may contact the leg support system. *When using candy cane stirrups, the ankle strap presses on the distal sural and plantar nerves, which could cause neuropathies of the foot (Meeker et al, 1999). Knee crutch stirrups can put pressure on the posterior tibial, sural, and common peroneal nerves (Meeker et al, 1999). Well-padded stirrups can still create some pressure on the back of the knees and lower extremities and could jeopardize the popliteal vessels and nerves (Fortunato, 2000).* **Nursing Research:** *Research has shown that intramuscular pressures in the leg are increased, especially in the anterior and lateral compartments, with the leg in this position (Meyer et al, 2000).*
- NOTE: The hemilithotomy position (one leg in the lithotomy position) is often used when operating to repair a fractured hip or femur. *Studies have shown that the uninjured leg in the lithotomy holder can develop compartment syndrome because of elevated intramuscular pressures, decreased perfusion, and the length of the procedure. Therefore, it has been suggested that the uninjured leg be supported at the heel rather than at the calf (Meyer et al, 2000).*
- Arms should be positioned on armboards or loosely cradled over the lower abdomen and secured with the blanket. **Nursing Research:** *Arms should not rest on the chest due to possible impedance of respirations (Fortunato, 2000).*
- Assess the need for sequential compression stockings. *Sequential stockings aid in the prevention of thrombi/emboli.* **Nursing Research:** *Sequential compression stockings seem to closely resemble normal physiological conditions and could possibly decrease the risk of com-*

- = Independent; ▲ = Collaborative

partment syndrome (Anema et al, 2000). The lithotomy position is known to decrease venous blood flow and predispose clients to venous thrombus in the lower extremities (Canterbury, 1992). Deep vein thrombosis and pulmonary embolus are the most common complications of radical retropubic prostatectomy procedures, which are done in the lithotomy position (Michaels, Lish, and Mohler, 1998).

- Monitor the length of time the client remains in the lithotomy position. **Nursing Research:** *The potential for complications is directly proportional to the length of time a client is in the lithotomy position (Anema et al, 2000). During a study of 991 clients who underwent surgery in the lithotomy position, it was found that increased duration in the lithotomy position was associated with increased risk of lower extremity neuropathy. These clients had no previous neuropathies and were well padded, thus leading to this conclusion. The study also found that the frequency of neuropathy increased markedly after 2 hours in the lithotomy position (Warner et al, 2000). A study involving 153 women undergoing gynecological procedures in the lithotomy position showed that 41% had pain in their lower extremities, unrelated to incisional site pain, postoperatively and women who were in the position longer than 60 minutes had significantly more pain than those who were in the position for under 60 minutes (Powers, 2002).*
- NOTE: If assessment reveals conditions that place the client at increased risk for injury in this position, attempting this position while the client is awake and can report any discomfort may help prevent positioning complications.
- To decrease the length of time the client is in the lithotomy position, evaluate the procedure to determine if any portion can be done in the supine position. **Nursing Research:** *During urethral reconstruction, research has shown that the risk of positioning injury is directly proportional to the length of time the client is in the high lithotomy position, with procedures that take less than 5 hours having minimal risk (Anema et al, 2000). To decrease the length of time the client is in the lithotomy position, the authors perform the penile flap dissection, during urethral reconstruction procedures, with the client in the supine position (Anema et al, 2000).*

Trendelenburg/reverse Trendelenburg position

- Either of these positions (Trendelenburg or reverse Trendelenburg) may have adverse effects on both the circulatory system (i.e., increased blood pressure and intracranial pressure) and the respiratory system (i.e., diaphragm movement is impeded), which in most circumstances are monitored and controlled by anesthesia personnel.
- Modifications of both positions may be suggested and implemented by the nurse in collaboration with the surgeon and anesthesiologist.
- Padded shoulder braces may be used in the Trendelenburg position. They should be placed at an equal distance from the head of the table, and a ½-inch space allowed between the brace and the shoulder.
- The braces are placed over the acromion process and not over muscles and soft tissues near the neck (Fortunato, 2000). **Nursing Research:** *Allowing space between the shoulders and the braces prevents pressure from the braces to the shoulders (Fortunato, 2000).*
- Knees should be positioned at the break in the operating table. **Nursing Research:** *Positioning the knees at the break in the operating table prevent pressure on the peroneal nerves and leg veins (Fortunato, 2000).*
- Length of time in this position should be as short as possible. **Nursing Research:** *Lung volume is decreased, and the heart is compressed due to pressure of organs against the diaphragm in this position (Fortunato, 2000). It is recommended that specialized stirrups*

• = **Independent;** ▲ = **Collaborative**

that use a 30- to 45-degree angle be used for lengthy procedures as opposed to those with a 90-degree angle (Canterberry, 1992).

evolve **WEBSITES FOR EDUCATION**

See the EVOLVE website for World Wide Web resources for client education.

REFERENCES

American Society of Anesthesiologists Task Force on Prevention of Perioperative Peripheral Neuropathies: Practice advisory for the prevention of perioperative peripheral neuropathies, *Anesthesiology* 92(4):1168, 2000.

Anema JG et al: Complications related to the high lithotomy position during urethral reconstruction, *J Urol* 164:360, 2000.

AORN: *AORN standards and recommended practices for perioperative nursing,* Denver, 2001, The Association of PeriOperative Registered Nurses.

Baumann S, Welch W, Bloom M: Intraoperative SSEP detection of ulnar nerve compression or ischemia in an obese patient: a unique complication associated with a specialized spinal retraction system, *Arch Phys Med Rehabil* 81(1):130, 2000.

Canterbury TDW, Wheeler WE, Scott-Conner CEH: Effects of the lithotomy position on arterial blood flow in the lower extremities, *W V Med J* 88(3):100, 1992.

Carris J, Franczek T: Patient positioning: snow fun in the OR, Todays Surg Nurs 21:47, 1999.

Fortunato N: *Berry and Kohn's operating room technique, positioning the patient,* ed 9, St Louis, 2000, Mosby.

Goettler CE, Pryor JP, Reilly PM: Brachial plexopathy after prone positioning, *Crit Care* 6:6, 2002.

Gumus E et al: Neurapraxic complications in operations performed in the lithotomy position, *World J Urol* 20(1):68, 2002.

Hoshowsky VM: Surgical positioning, *Orthop Nurs* 17(5):55, 1998.

Lampert R et al: Compartment syndrome: a complication of the lithotomy position, *Dutch J Urol* 4:103, 1997.

Manfredini M et al: Unilateral blindness as a complication of intraoperative positioning for cervical spinal surgery, *J Spinal Disord* 13:3, 2000.

Martin JT: Positioning aged patients, *Geriatr Anesth* 18:1, 2000.

Meeker M, Rothrock J: *Alexander's care of the patient in surgery,* ed 11, St Louis, 1999, Mosby.

Meyer S et al: *Intramuscular and blood pressure in legs positioned in the hemi-lithotomy position on a fracture table,* 46th Annual Meeting of Orthopedics Research Society, Orlando, Fla, March 12-15, 2000.

Michaels MJ, Lish MC, Mohler JL: Patient positioning for radical retropubic prostatectomy, *Urology* 51:5, 1998.

Powers H: Patient positioning outcomes for women undergoing gynaecological surgeries, *Can Operating Room Nurs J,* September 2002.

Warner MA et al: Lower extremity neuropathies associated with lithotomy positions, *Anesthesiology* 93:4, 2000.

Decreased Intracranial adaptive capacity

Pamela H. Mitchell

NANDA Definition

Intracranial fluid dynamic mechanisms that normally compensate for increases in intracranial volumes are compromised, resulting in repeated disproportionate increases in intracranial pressure (ICP) in response to a variety of noxious and non-noxious stimuli (Mitchell, 1993)

• = Independent; ▲ = Collaborative

Defining Characteristics

Repeated increases in ICP of greater than 10 mm Hg for more than 5 minutes following a variety of external stimuli; disproportionate increases in ICP following a single environmental or nursing maneuver stimulus; baseline ICP greater than 10 mm Hg; elevated P2 component of ICP waveform; wide-amplitude ICP waveform; volume-pressure response test variation (volume-pressure ratio of 2, pressure-volume index of less than 10) (Rauch et al, 1990; Mitchell, 1993; Mitchell et al, 1998)

Related Factors (r/t)

Decreased cerebral perfusion less than 50 to 60 mm Hg; sustained increase in ICP greater than 10 to 15 mm Hg; systemic hypotension with intracranial hypertension; brain injuries

NOC   Outcomes (Nursing Outcomes Classification)

Suggested NOC Outcomes

Neurological Status; Neurological Status: Consciousness

> ### Example NOC Outcome with Indicators
>
> **Neurological Status** as evidenced by the following indicators: Neurological function: consciousness/Intracranial pressure WNL/Vital signs WNL/Neurological function: central motor control/Neurological function: cranial sensory-motor function/Neurological function: spinal sensory-motor function (Rate each indicator of **Neurological Status:** 1 = extremely compromised, 2 = substantially compromised, 3 = moderately compromised, 4 = mildly compromised, 5 = not compromised [see Section I].)

WNL, Within normal limits.

Client Outcomes

Client Will (Specify Time Frame):
- Experience fewer than five episodes of disproportionate increases in ICP (DIICP) in 24 hours
- Have neurological status changes that are not triggered by episodes of DIICP
- Have CPP remains greater than 60 to 70 mm Hg in adults

NIC   Interventions (Nursing Interventions Classification)

Suggested NIC Interventions

Cerebral Edema Management; Cerebral Perfusion Promotion; Intracranial Pressure (ICP) Monitoring; Neurological Monitoring

> ### Example NIC Activities—Cerebral Edema Management
>
> Monitor for confusion, changes in mentation, complaints of dizziness, syncope; Allow ICP to return to baseline between nursing activities

Nursing Interventions and Rationales

- For episodes of DIICP, do the following:
  - Reverse stimulus if readily apparent.
  - Evaluate position of the client. Head should be in midline without neck flexion to

• = **Independent;** ▲ = **Collaborative**

prevent intracranial trapping of jugular venous outflow. **Nursing and Clinical Research:** *Positional changes of the head and neck are the most consistent triggers of sustained ICP elevations. Forward, lateral, and rotational neck flexion will result in increased ICP until the neck position is restored to a neutral position (Bader and Littlejohns, 1999; Simmons, 1997; Mavrocordatos, Bissonnette, and Ravussin, 2000; Williams and Coyne, 1993; Yordy and Hanigan, 1985-1986).*

- Return the client to original position if a position change has triggered DIICP. **Nursing Research:** *No particular body position triggers DIICP unless combined with neck flexion; however, some individuals respond to passive turning to lateral or three-quarter prone positions. Routine physical therapy also does not trigger problematic increases in ICP (Brimioulle et al, 1997; Lee, 1989; Mitchell and Ackerman, 1992). Prone positioning may trigger significant increases in ICP and should be individually evaluated if used to improve lung functioning (Beuret et al, 2002).*
- Stop suctioning if routine suctioning is triggering DIICP. Follow preventive protocol if future suctioning is indicated. **Nursing and Clinical Research:** *A standard series of three suctioning passes can result in stair-step elevation of ICP with each successive pass, even with full hyperoxygenation and hyperinflation before suctioning. Brief hyperventilation may be protective against these increases (Kerr et al, 1997). In well-sedated patients, endotracheal suctioning is not associated with cerebral ischemia even though ICP rises (Gemma et al, 2002; Kerr et al, 1998, 1999).*
- Have clients who can follow directions exhale through their mouth if they are doing a Valsalva's maneuver. **Nursing Research:** *If client's nonvolitional movements such as posturing and unconscious straining are causing a Valsalva's maneuver, sedation or paralytics with sedation may be indicated (Kerr et al, 1998; McClelland et al, 1995).*
- Reduce environmental noise and painful or unexpected touching of the client. **Nursing and Clinical Research:** *All these factors have been shown to be potent noxious stimuli in individual adults and preterm infants but may not trigger DIICP in the majority of clients (Mitchell and Habermann, 1999; Yordy and Hanigan, 1985-1986).*

• Elevate head of bed if the client maintains CPP. **Nursing and Clinical Research:** *Head elevation reduces the average ICP in groups of clients, but individuals may exhibit either no change or even increased ICP (Ropper et al, 1982; Winkelman, 2000). In addition, when cerebral autoregulation is impaired, even a small systemic blood pressure drop with head elevation may decrease the CPP to an unacceptable level (Chesnut, 1997a; March et al, 1990). Patients with large hemispheric stroke and subarachnoid hemorrhage may be particularly susceptible to reduced CPP and cerebral blood flow with head elevation (Schwarz et al, 2002; Wojner, El-Mitwalli, and Alexandrov, 2002). Optimal head position needs to be determined individually, depending on both ICP and CPP measurement (Simmons, 1997).*

▲ For DIICP, if baseline ICP rises above 15 mm Hg or CPP (mean arterial blood pressure minus mean ICP) is less than 70 mm Hg in adults for 5 minutes or more, do the following:

- Initiate protocols for lowering ICP according to a collaborative plan with attending physician if ICP remains elevated or CPP decreases outside parameters—usually ICP greater than 15 to 20 mm Hg or CPP less than 60 to 70 mm Hg for 10 or more minutes. **Clinical Research:** *The Brain Trauma Foundation guidelines have been compiled by the American Association of Neurological Surgeons from systematic reviews of the research literature. Therapeutic option is to manage CPP to maintain pressure greater than 70 mm Hg for adults, based on observations that such a pressure level*

• = Independent; ▲ = Collaborative

may be associated with better outcomes (Brain Trauma Foundation, 2000a). A small controlled study in clients with severe head injury demonstrated better control of both ICP and CPP variations with a standardized protocol consistent with the Severe Head Injury Guidelines (McKinley, Parmley, and Tonneson, 1999). The plan will vary by region and individual physician preference but is increasingly likely to include interventions consistent with Brain Trauma Foundation guidelines (Bulger et al, 2002; Huizenga et al, 2002).

- Cerebrospinal fluid (CSF) drainage via ventriculostomy intermittently to maintain a given ICP level. **Clinical Research:** *CSF drainage will manage CPP by reducing ICP at least temporarily. It does not change adaptive capacity (intracranial compliance) (Chesnut, 1995).*

▲ Addition of sedation (e.g., morphine, midazolam, propofol) and analgesia with or without paralysis (e.g., atracurium, pancuronium [Pavulon]) if body movements or fighting respirator continuously stimulate a CPP decrease. **Nursing and Clinical Research:** *The short-acting agents allow rapid reversal of both sedation and paralysis for short periods to provide periodic neurological examination (McClelland et al, 1995) and appear useful in reducing ICP/CPP variations during suctioning (Gemma et al, 2002; Kerr et al, 1998, 1999). However there is recent evidence that ICP/CPP overall values do not differ in those head-injured patients who receive sedation and paralysis compared with those who do not (Juul et al, 2000).*

▲ Bolus administration of osmotic diuretic or other hyperosmotic agent (e.g., mannitol, mannitol plus furosemide) may be followed with continuous administration if CPP is not maintained with bolus administration. Note that it is essential to keep serum osmolality less than 320 mOsm/L to prevent hyperosmolality-related seizures. *These agents primarily reduce vascular volume and not cerebral edema. The older practice of keeping clients volume depleted in an attempt to prevent cerebral edema is no longer advocated (Chesnut, 1995).* **Clinical Research:** *Although mannitol produces dramatic changes in individual cases, the research base for on-going management is limited. The most recent Cochrane Review of use of mannitol for traumatic brain injury found few well-conducted studies and concluded that mannitol appears to be more beneficial than pentobarbital in reducing mortality and that treatment directed by ICP monitoring is more beneficial than that directed by observed neurological signs (Schierhout and Roberts, 2002a).*

▲ Control hyperventilation, maintaining Pco_2 of 30 to 35 mm Hg unless ICP continues to be refractory, in which case Pco_2 may be briefly decreased below 30 mm Hg if ICP is responsive. **Clinical Research:** *Older standards of early hyperventilation of clients to levels as low as 25 mm Hg have been shown to have poorer outcomes than in similar clients not hyperventilated. Prophylactic use of hyperventilation may induce cerebral ischemia (Brain Trauma Foundation, 2000b). Although many clinicians continue to use extreme hyperventilation, major trauma centers recommend this only as a last resort in refractory intracranial hypertension (Chesnut, 1995). Adequate randomized controlled trials have not yet been done to definitely settle the question of benefit or harm from aggressive hyperventilation (Schierhout and Roberts, 2002b).*

▲ To prevent DIICP in clients at risk (clients with elevated P2 waveforms and ICP of less than 10 mm Hg; clients previously responsive to general stimuli), do the following:
  - Maintain 15- to 30-degree head elevation if CPP is maintained at greater than 70 mm Hg.

- = **Independent;** ▲ = **Collaborative**

- Maintain systemic blood pressure adequate to keep CPP greater than 70 mm Hg by body positioning and use of vasoactive protocols.
- Maintain adequate respiratory status; suction if needed but not prophylactically. *If suctioning is required, may use aerosolized lidocaine or sedation to reduce associated coughing (Kerr et al, 1997, 1998, 1999). Preoxygenate, hyperventilate only very briefly, and limit number of catheter passes to one or two (Kerr et al, 1997).*
- Use gentle touching and talking or family visitations. **Nursing Research:** *These activities rarely stimulate DIICP (Schinner et al, 1995). Family voices and gentle string may help stabilize ICP (Hepworth et al, 1994; Mitchell and Ackerman, 1992; Mitchell and Habermann, 1999; Treloar et al, 1991).*
- Use mechanical turning beds if manual repositioning is a stimulus to DIICP. **Nursing Research:** *These beds keep the head and neck in a neutral alignment and have been shown not to alter ICP overall (Tillett et al, 1993; Mitchell, 1993).*
- Avoid 90-degree hip flexion and use of the knee gatch of the bed. **Nursing Research:** *Hip flexion may trap venous blood in the intra-abdominal space, increasing abdominal and intrathoracic pressure, which in turn reduces venous outflow from the head (Vos, 1993).*
- Sequence nursing care to allow for recovery of baseline ICP between noxious activities, such as suctioning, and position changes that involve neck flexion. **Nursing Research:** *Several studies have shown stair-step increases in ICP when a stimulus to DIICP is repeated several times within a short time (Kerr et al, 1993; Mitchell and Ackerman, 1992).*
▲ With regard to general ICP monitoring:
- Monitor ICP and CPP continuously with alarm settings on. **Nursing and Clinical Research:** *Secondary brain injury can result from even brief periods of hypoxia and hypotension. Data from the Traumatic Coma Data Bank and international studies have documented that even in well-attended intensive care units, periods of more than 5 minutes of systemic hypotension (systolic blood pressure of <90 mm Hg) or intracranial hypertension occur in 70% to 90% of clients (Jones et al, 1994; Miller, 1993) and that even a single recording of a hypotensive episode is generally associated with a doubling of mortality in clinical studies (Brain Trauma Foundation, 2000c).*
- Notify physician if nursing interventions and collaborative protocols do not maintain a CPP of greater than 70 mm Hg and an ICP of less than 20 mm Hg for adults; values may be lower for infants.
- Monitor neurological status and CPP, including level of arousal, ability to follow commands, response to painful stimuli if arousal is decreased, and brainstem signs (pupil response, respiratory pattern, symmetry of motor response, and vital signs). Notify physician of signs of neurological deterioration regardless of levels of ICP and CPP. *Brain shift and herniation will be manifested by these changes in neurological status and may occur at any level of ICP. If the client is sedated and paralyzed to control ICP, pupillary changes or changes in response to painful stimuli may be the only available sign of deterioration (Mitchell and Ackerman, 1992; Ross et al, 1989).*

Home care

NOTE: Clients experiencing potentially rapid changes in ICP are not candidates for home care. However, clients experiencing potentially gradual changes in ICP (i.e., clients with developmental delays resulting from genetic dysfunction), or clients post ICP changes

• = Independent; ▲ = Collaborative

secondary to brain trauma, may be served by home care with the following considerations:

- Some of the above interventions may be adapted for home care use.
- Identify baseline neurological data before discharge from institutional care. *Baseline data will help both to identify changes in status and to create an individualized care plan.*
- Evaluate neurological functioning at regular intervals. *Neurological function improvements require long-term intervention.*
- Instruct the caregiver about client-specific changes that will indicate increased ICP *Examples include changes in speech articulation and eye coordination, decreased ability to focus, increased seizure activity, and decreased coping ability. The nurse is cautioned that changes will be specific to the disability of the client. Early reporting of status changes allows for early intervention in neurologically impaired clients.*
- Instruct the client/family in appropriate expectations of cognitive recovery following minor brain injury. **Nursing Research:** *During the first 24 hours following minor brain injury, clients are likely to experience distractibility, impulsivity, irritability, and impaired executive function. The results of a study suggested that cognitive demands on clients should be reduced for at least 48 hours following injury and for 30 days or longer for clients who lost consciousness (Brewer, Metzger, and Therrien, 2002).*
- For clients with a history of traumatic brain injury, assess for mood, thought process, or personality disturbances and refer for appropriate mental health follow-up. *A 30-year follow-up study of individuals who suffered a traumatic brain injury found a substantial risk for depressive episodes, delusional disorder, or personality disturbances (Koponen et al, 2002).*
- Institute case management of frail elderly to support continued independent living. *Neurological difficulties represent and can lead to increasing needs for assistance in using the health care system effectively. Case management combines nursing activities of the client and family assessment, planning and coordination of care among all health care providers, delivery of direct nursing care, and monitoring of care and outcomes. These activities are able to address continuity of care, mutual goal setting, behavior management, and prevention of worsening health problems (Guttman, 1999).*

evolve WEBSITES FOR EDUCATION

See the EVOLVE website for World Wide Web resources for client education.

REFERENCES

Bader M, Littlejohns L: Intracranial pressure monitoring. In Bulechek GM, McCloskey JC, editors: *Nursing interventions: effective nursing treatments*, Philadelphia, 1999, WB Saunders.

Beuret P et al: Prone position as prevention of lung injury in comatose patients: a prospective, randomized, controlled study, *Intensive Care Med* 28(5):564, 2002.

Brain Trauma Foundation, American Association of Neurological Surgeons, Joint Section on Neurotrauma and Critical Care: Guidelines for cerebral perfusion pressure, *J Neurotrauma* 17(6-7):507, 2000a.

Brain Trauma Foundation, American Association of Neurological Surgeons, Joint Section on Neurotrauma and Critical Care: Hyperventilation, *J Neurotrauma* 17(6-7):513, 2000b.

Brain Trauma Foundation, American Association of Neurological Surgeons, Joint Section on Neurotrauma and Critical Care: Hypotension, *J Neurotrauma* 17(6-7):591, 2000c.

• = **Independent;** ▲ = **Collaborative**

Brewer TL, Metzger BL, Therrien B: Trajectories of cognitive recovery following a minor brain injury, *Res Nurs Health* 25:269, 2002.

Brimioulle S et al: Effects of positioning and exercise on intracranial pressure in a neurosurgical intensive care unit, *Phys Ther* 77:1682, 1997.

Bulger EM et al: Management of severe head injury: institutional variations in care and effect on outcome, *Crit Care Med* 30(8):1870, 2002.

Chesnut RM: Avoidance of hypotension: condition sine qua non of successful severe head-injury management, *J Trauma* 42(5 suppl):s4, 1997.

Chesnut RM: Medical management of severe head injury: present and future, *New Horiz* 3:581, 1995.

Gemma M et al: Intracranial effects of endotracheal suctioning in the acute phase of head injury, *J Neurosurg Anesthesiol* 14(1):50, 2002.

Guttman R: Case management of the frail elderly in the community, *Clin Nurs Spec* 13(4):174, 1999.

Hepworth JT, Hendrickson SG, Lopez J: Time series analysis of physiological response during ICU visitation, *West J Nurs Res* 16:704, 1994.

Huizenga JE et al: Guidelines for the management of severe head injury: are emergency physicians following them? *Acad Emerg Med* 9(8):806, 2002.

Jones PA et al: Measuring the burden of secondary insults in head-injured patients during intensive care, *J Neurosurg Anesthesiol* 6:4, 1994.

Juul N et al: Neuromuscular blocking agents in neurointensive care, *Acta Neurochir Suppl* 76:467, 2000.

Kerr ME et al: Head-injured adults: recommendations for endotracheal suctioning, *J Neurosci Nurs* 25:86, 1993.

Kerr ME et al: Effect of short-duration hyperventilation during endotracheal suctioning in severe head-injured adults, *Nurs Res* 46:195, 1997.

Kerr ME et al: Effect of neuromuscular blockers and opiates on the cerebrovascular response to endotracheal suctioning in adults with severe head injuries, *Am J Crit Care* 7:205, 1998.

Kerr ME et al: Effect of endotracheal suctioning on cerebral oxygenation in traumatic brain-injured patients, *Crit Care Med* 27(12):2776, 1999.

Koponen S et al: Axis I and II psychiatric disorders after traumatic brain injury: a 30-year follow-up study, *Am J Psychiatry* 159:1315, 2002.

Lee S: Intracranial pressure changes during positioning of patients with severe head injury, *Heart Lung* 18:411, 1989.

March K et al: Effects of backrest position on ICP and CPP, *J Neurosci Nurs* 22:375, 1990.

Mavrocordatos P, Bissonnette B, Ravussin P: Effects of neck position and head elevation on intracranial pressure in anaesthetized neurosurgical patients: preliminary results, *J Neurosurg Anesthesiol* 12(1):10, 2000.

McClelland M et al: Continuous midazolam/atracurium infusions for the management of increased intracranial pressure, *J Neurosci Nurs* 27:96, 1995.

McKinley BA, Parmley CL, Tonneson AS: Standardized management of intracranial pressure: a preliminary clinical trial, *J Trauma* 46:271, 1999.

Miller JD: Head injury, *J Neurol Neurosurg Psychiatry* 56:440, 1993.

Mitchell PH, Ackerman LL: Secondary brain injury reduction. In Bulechek GM, McCloskey JC, editors: *Nursing interventions*, ed 2, Philadelphia, 1992, WB Saunders.

Mitchell PH, Habermann B: Rethinking physiological stability: touch and intracranial pressure, *Biol Res Nurs* 1(1):12, 1999.

Mitchell PH et al: Waveform predictors: adverse response to nursing care: ICPX A, *Acta Neurochir Suppl* 71:420, 1998.

Mitchell PH: Decreased adaptive capacity. In Kinney MR, Packa DR, Dunbar SB, editors: *AACN's clinical reference for critical care nursing*, ed 3, St Louis, 1993, Mosby.

Rauch ME, Mitchell PH, Tyler ML: Validation of risk factors for the nursing diagnosis of decreased intracranial adaptive capacity, *J Neurosci Nurs* 22:173, 1990.

Ropper AH, O'Rourke D, Kennedy SK: Head position, intracranial pressure, and compliance, *Neurology* 32:1288, 1982.

Ross DA et al: Brain shift, level of consciousness and restoration of consciousness in patients with acute intracranial hematoma, *J Neurosurg* 71:498, 1989.

Schierhout G, Roberts I. Hyperventilation therapy for acute traumatic brain injury, *Cochrane Database Syst Rev* (2) Cochrane Library, Issue 4, Oxford, 2002b, Update software.

Schierhout G, Roberts I. Mannitol for acute traumatic brain injury, *Cochrane Database Syst Rev* (2), Cochrane Library, Issue 4, Oxford, 2002a, Update Software.

Schinner KM et al: Effects of auditory stimuli on intracranial pressure and cerebral perfusion pressure in traumatic brain injury, *J Neurosci Nurs* 27:348, 1995.

• = Independent; ▲ = Collaborative

Schwarz S et al: Effects of body position on intracranial pressure and cerebral perfusion in patients with large hemispheric stroke, *Stroke* 33(2):497, 2002.

Simmons BJ: Management of intracranial hemodynamics in the adult: a research analysis of head positioning and recommendations for clinical practice and future research, *J Neurosci Nurs* 29:44, 1997.

Tillett JM et al: Effect of continuous rotational therapy on intracranial pressure in the severely brain-injured patient, *Crit Care Med* 21(7):1005, 1993.

Treloar DM et al: The effect of familiar and unfamiliar voice treatments on intracranial pressure in head-injured patients, *J Neurosci Nurs* 23(5):295, 1991.

Vos HR: Making headway with intracranial hypertension, *Am J Nurse* 93:28, 1993.

Williams A, Coyne SM: Effects of neck position on intracranial pressure, *Am J Crit Care* 2:68, 1993.

Winkelman C: Effect of backrest position on intracranial and cerebral perfusion pressures in traumatically brain-injured adults, *Am J Crit Care* 9(6):373, 2000.

Wojner AW, El-Mitwalli A, Alexandrov AV: Effect of head positioning on intracranial blood flow velocities in acute ischemic stroke: a pilot study, *Crit Care Nurs Q* 24(4):57, 2002.

Yordy M, Hanigan WC: Cerebral perfusion pressure in the high-risk premature infant, *Pediatr Neurosci* 12:226, 1985-1986.

Deficient Knowledge (specify)

Gail B. Ladwig

NANDA Definition

Absence or deficiency of cognitive information related to a specific topic

Defining Characteristics

Verbalization of the problem; inaccurate follow-through of instruction; inaccurate performance of test; inappropriate or exaggerated behaviors (e.g., hysterical, hostile, agitated, apathetic)

Related Factors (r/t)

Lack of exposure; lack of recall; information misinterpretation; cognitive limitation; lack of interest in learning; unfamiliarity with information resources

NOC Outcomes (Nursing Outcomes Classification)

Suggested NOC Outcomes

Knowledge: Diet, Disease Process, Energy Conservation, Health Behavior, Health Resources, Infection Control, Medication, Personal Safety, Prescribed Activity, Substance Use Control, Treatment Procedure(s), Treatment Regimen

Example NOC Outcome with Indicators

Knowledge: Health Behavior as evidenced by the following indicators: Description of healthy nutritional practices/Benefits of exercise/Safe use of prescription and nonprescription drugs (Rate each indicator of **Knowledge: Health Behavior:** 1 = no knowledge, 2 = limited knowledge, 3 = moderate knowledge, 4 = substantial knowledge, 5 = extensive knowledge [see Section I].)

• = Independent; ▲ = Collaborative

Client Outcomes

Client Will (Specify Time Frame):
- Explain disease state, recognize need for medications, and understand treatments
- Explain how to incorporate new health regimen into lifestyle
- State an ability to deal with health situation and remain in control of life
- Demonstrate how to perform procedure(s) satisfactorily
- List resources that can be used for more information or support after discharge

NIC   Interventions (Nursing Interventions Classification)

Suggested NIC Interventions

Teaching: Disease Process, Individual, Infant Safety

> **Example NIC Activities—Teaching: Disease Process**
>
> Discuss therapy/treatment options; Explain rationale for management/therapy/treatment recommendations

Nursing Interventions and Rationales

- Observe the client's ability and readiness to learn (e.g., mental acuity, ability to see or hear, no existing pain, emotional readiness, absence of language or cultural barriers) and previous knowledge. **Nursing Research:** *Education in self-care must take into account physical, sensory, mobility, sexual, and psychosocial changes related to age (Bohny, 1997).* **Nursing Research:** *The client brings to the learning situation a unique personality, established social interaction patterns, cultural norms and values, and environmental influences (Bohny, 1997).*
- Assess barriers to learning (e.g., perceived change in lifestyle, financial concerns, cultural patterns, lack of acceptance by peers or coworkers). **Nursing Research:** *The client brings to the learning situation a unique personality, established social interaction patterns, cultural norms and values, and environmental influences (Bohny, 1997).*
- Involve clients in writing specific outcomes for the teaching session, such as identifying what is most important to learn from their viewpoint and lifestyle. **Nursing Research:** *This study indicated that clients were willing to take responsibility for playing their part in trying to optimize the outcome of their surgery (Edwards, 2002).*
- When teaching, build on the client's literacy skills. **Clinical Research:** *In clients with low literacy skills, materials should be short and have culturally sensitive illustrations (Mayeaux et al, 1996). The National Adult Literacy Survey reported that 44 million Americans could not read or write well enough to meet the needs of everyday living and working (Quirk, 2000).*
- Present material that is most significant to the client first, such as how to give injections or change dressings; present additional material once the client's most pressing educational needs have been met. *Information building begins with explaining simple concepts and moves on to explanations of complex application situations.*
- Determine the client's understanding of common medical terminology, such as "empty stomach," "emesis," and "palpation." **Clinical Research:** *Clients are expected to read and understand labels on medicine containers, appointment slips, and informed consents, yet an estimated 40 million adults are functionally illiterate (Williams et al, 1995).*
- Evaluate the readability of the material in pamphlets or written instructions. **Nursing Research:** *Nonadherence of older adults to new medication regimens appears to be a func-*

• = **Independent; ▲ = Collaborative**

tion of decreased cognitive ability and comprehension of instruction, poor communication, and increased physical limitations (Hayes, 1998).

▲ Use visual aids such as diagrams, pictures, videotapes, audiotapes, and interactive Internet websites. **Nursing Research:** *Verbal reinforcement of personalized, written instructions appears to be the best-tested intervention. Computer-generated, personalized instructions improved adherence when compared with handwritten instructions (Hayes, 1998).* **Evidence-Based Research:** *Leaflets are a useful resource for information provision (Kubba, 2000).* **Nursing Research:** *An intervention of an educational video and written instructions designed to reduce prehospital delays in patients with chest pain showed a significant increase in the use of ambulances for the intervention group (p = 0.03) but not for the control group (Blank and Smithline, 2002).*

▲ Provide preadmission self-instruction materials to prepare the client for postoperative exercises. **Nursing Research:** *Providing clients with preadmission information about exercises has been shown to increase positive feelings and the ability to perform prescribed exercises (Rice et al, 1992).*

▲ Assess willingness of family to incorporate new information, immunizations, medical/dental care, and diet/behavior modifications in support of the client. **Nursing Research:** *Attention needs to be directed at family adjustment factors. For example, women recovering from alcohol abuse are at risk for relapse if their spouse continues to drink alcohol (Murphy, 1993).* **Nursing Research:** *Modification of eating patterns plus social and partnership support have had more success than modification alone (Keller et al, 1997).*

▲ Help the client identify community resources for continuing information and support. **Clinical Research:** *Community resources can offer financial and educational support. For example, role modeling and skill training have been used to monitor symptoms and solve asthma problems (Bartholomew et al, 2000).*

• Evaluate the client's learning through return demonstrations, verbalizations, or the application of skills to new situations. *Presenting information along with examples of how to apply the information has been found more successful than providing information alone in a home care setting (Duffy, 1997).*

Geriatric

• Adapt the teaching process for the physical constraints of the aging process (e.g., speak clearly, use a variety of audio-visual-psychomotor methods, provide examples, and allow time for the client to repeat and review). **Nursing Research:** *Adults are capable of learning at any age. Age modifies but does not inhibit learning (Dellasega et al, 1994). Older adults need practice to use new technology (Westerman and Davies, 2000).*

• Ensure that the client uses necessary reading aids (e.g., eyeglasses, magnifying lenses, large-print text) or hearing aids. *Visual and hearing deficits require amplification or clarification of sensory input.*

• Use printed material, videotapes, lists, diagrams, and Internet addresses that the client can refer to at another time. **Clinical Research:** *These methods provide a reference that can be used in a less stressful setting, decreasing barriers to learning. This study demonstrated the effectiveness of printed material and a Web-based format for education. The Web-based format demonstrated two additional benefits when compared with printed material: increased social support and decreased anxiety (Scherrer-Bannerman et al, 2000).*

• Repeat and reinforce information during several brief sessions. *Understanding past information is essential to acquiring new knowledge. Brief sessions focus attention on essential information.*

• = Independent; ▲ = Collaborative

- Discuss healthy lifestyle changes that promote wellness for the older adult. **Nursing Research:** *Greater efforts must be made both to improve preventive health care and enhance quality of life interventions of older people (Nolan, 2001).*
- Evaluate readability of the material. **Nursing Research:** *Nonadherence of older adults to new medication regimens appears to be a function of decreased cognitive ability, comprehension of instruction, poor communication, and increased physical limitations (Hayes, 1998).*
- ▲ Consider health education programs using television and newspapers. *There was a significant increase in stroke knowledge (52% more likely to know a risk factor and 35% know a symptom, p = 0.032) following this health education program as demonstrated through a telephone pretest and posttest (Becker et al, 2001).*

Multicultural

- Acknowledge racial/ethnic differences at the onset of care. **Nursing Research:** *Acknowledgement of racial/ethnicity issues will enhance communication, establish rapport, and promote treatment outcomes (D'Avanzo et al, 2001, Ludwick and Silva, 2000; Vontress and Epp, 1997).*
- Assess for the influence of cultural beliefs, norms, and values on the client's knowledge base. **Nursing Research:** *The client's knowledge base may be influenced by cultural perceptions (Cochran, 1998; Doswell and Erlen, 1998; Leininger and McFarland, 2002).*
- Use a neutral indirect style when addressing areas where improvement is needed when working with Native American clients. **Nursing Research:** *Using indirect statements such as "I had a client who tried 'X' and it seemed to work very well" will help avoid resentment from the client (Seiderman et al, 1996).*
- Validate the client's feelings and concerns related to previous learning experiences. **Nursing Research:** *Validation is therapeutic communication technique that lets the client know that the nurse has heard and understands what was said, and it promotes the nurse-client relationship (Heineken, 1998).*
- Approach individuals of color with respect, warmth, and professional courtesy. **Nursing Research:** *Instances of disrespect and lack of caring have special significance for individuals of color (D'Avanzo et al, 2001; Vontress and Epp, 1997).*
- Provide health care information to mothers and grandmothers in African American families **Nursing Research:** *Mothers and grandmothers are considered the gatekeepers of health care in the African American Community (Sterling and Peterson, 2003).*

Home care

NOTE: Because home care is an intermittent model of care having a goal of safety and optimal wellness of the client between visits, the importance of teaching (by the nurse) and learning (by the client) should not be understated. All of the previously mentioned interventions are applicable to the home setting.

- ▲ Select a space and time for teaching in which the client and/or caregiver can focus on information to be learned. *The home setting provides many distractions that may impair the ability of the client to learn.*
- ▲ Consider the complexity of material or behaviors to be learned. Adjust care plan and respective teaching and learning experiences accordingly to build client confidence in ability to learn (and change). *Confidence in ability to learn and change is part of readiness to learn.*
- Assess the client for low or absent literacy. Use illustrations for instruction that are as

• = **Independent;** ▲ = **Collaborative**

closely equivalent as possible to written instructions. *Clients who are illiterate may assert their understanding of written instructions as a face-saving response. Clients with low literacy skills may demonstrate limitations in their understanding of written instructions.*

- Assess the client/family learning needs and current level of knowledge. *Adult learners bring preexisting knowledge to a situation. Building on that knowledge is more effective than assuming total client/family ignorance. At the same time, inaccuracies in preexisting knowledge may need to be corrected.*

- Assess for specific areas of learning that have the potential for strong emotional responses by the client or family/caregiver. Allow time for expression of feelings and encourage acceptance of need for learning. *An individual's perception of barriers and benefits has consistently been most predictive of subsequent behavior. Clinicians should develop interventions that increase benefits and decrease barriers (Fenn, 1998).*

- Use visual aids and other available media that engage multiple senses to maximize learning. Leave visually-oriented/written materials in home. Have the client/family practice and return-demonstrate manual skills. *Clients/family learn in different ways. Engaging as many senses as possible increases learning. Availability of materials serves as a reminder of information. Practicing skills enhances memory of how to do them.*

- Document the client's and caregivers' responses to learning. Clear documentation supports continuity in the learning experience.

- Explore resources for teaching relative to specific illnesses. **Nursing Research:** *The Learning Needs Assessment Tool (LNET) has been developed to assess family/environment, current knowledge, and learning style of clients with congestive heart failure (Lile, Buhmann, and Roders, 1999).*

- Encourage self care management of illness. Refer to care plan for **Powerlessness. Nursing Research:** *Enhancing the client's perception of his or her ability to perform specific diabetes activities increased self-efficacy for diabetes management (Corbett, 1999).*

▲ Consider high tech options for delivery of home-based instruction. **Nursing Research:** *Televideo technology has been used effectively to improve self-management of diabetes (Bowles and Dansky, 2002). Interactive teleconferencing and on-site training for family caregivers positively influenced knowledge, self-perceived competence, and resourcefulness, with no significant difference between the program delivery types (Rosswurm et al, 2002).*

evolve WEBSITES FOR EDUCATION

See the EVOLVE website for World Wide Web resources for client education.

REFERENCES

Bartholomew LK et al: Watch, discover, think, and act: a model for patient education program development, *Patient Educ Couns* 39(2-3):269, 2000.

Becker K et al: Community-based education improves stroke knowledge, *Cerebrovasc Dis* 11(1):34, 2001.

Blank FS, Smithline HA: Evaluation of an educational video for cardiac patients, *Clin Nurs Res* 11(4):403, 2002.

Bohny B: A time for self-care: role of the home healthcare nurse, *Home Healthc Nurse* 15(4):281, 1997.

Bowles KH, Dansky KH: Teaching self-management of diabetes, *Home Healthc Nurse* 20(1):36, 2002.

Cochran M: Tears have no color, *Am J Nurs* 98(6):53, 1998.

Corbett CF: Research-based practice implications for patients with diabetes: part II: diabetes self-efficacy, *Home Healthc Nurse* 17:587, 1999.

D'Avanzo CE et al: Developing culturally informed strategies for substance-related interventions. In Naegle

• = Independent; ▲ = Collaborative

MA, D'Avanzo CE, editors: *Addictions and substance abuse: strategies for advanced practice nursing*, St Louis, 2002, Mosby.

Dellasega D et al: Nursing process: teaching elderly clients, *J Gerontol Nurs* 31:20, 1994.

Doswell W, Erlen J: Multicultural issues and ethical concerns in the delivery of revising care interventions, *Nurs Clin North Am* 33(2):353, 1998.

Duffy B: Using a creative teaching process with adult patients, *Home Healthc Nurse* 15(2):102, 1997.

Edwards C: A proposal that patients be considered honorary members of the healthcare team, *J Clin Nurs* 11(3): 340 2002.

Fenn M: Health promotion: theoretical perspectives and clinical applications, *Holist Nurs Pract* 12(2):1, 1998.

Hayes K: Randomized trial of geragogy-based medication instruction in the emergency department, *Nurs Res* 47(4):211, 1998.

Heineken J: Patient silence is not necessarily client satisfaction: communication in home care nursing, *Home Healthc Nurse* 16(2):115, 1998.

Keller C et al: Strategies for weight control success in adults, *Nurse Pract* 22(3):37, 1997.

Kubba H: An evidence-based patient information leaflet about otitis media with effusion, *Clin Perform Qual Health Care* 8(2):93, 2000.

Leininger MM, McFarland MR: *Transcultural nursing: concepts, theories, research and practices*, ed 3, New York, 2002, McGraw-Hill.

Lile JB, Buhmann J, Roders S: Development of a learning needs assessment tool for patients with congestive heart failure, *Home Healthc Manag Pract* 11(6):11, 1999.

Ludwick R, Silva M: Nursing around the world: cultural values and ethical conflicts, *Online J Issues Nurs*, available on-line at http://www.nursingworld.org/ojin/ethcol/ethics_4.htm.

Mayeaux EJ et al: Improving patient education for patients with low literacy skills, *Am Physician* 53(1):205, 1996.

Murphy SP: Coping strategies of abstainers from alcohol 3 years to post treatment, *Image J Nurs Sch* 25:32, 1993.

Nolan J: Improving the health of older people: what do we do? *Br J Nurs* 10(8):524, 2001.

Quirk PA: Screening for literacy and readability: implications for the advanced practice nurse, *Clin Nurse Spec* 14(1):26, 2000.

Rice VH et al: Preadmission self-instruction effects on preadmission and postoperative indicators in CABG patients partial replication and extension, *Res Nurs Health* 15:253, 1992.

Rosswurm MA, Larrabee JH, Zhang J: Training family caregivers of dependent elderly adults through on-site and telecommunications programs, *J Gerontol Nurs* 28(7):27, 2002.

Scherrer-Bannerman A et al: Web-based education and support for patients on the cardiac surgery waiting list, *J Telemed Telecare* 6 (Suppl 2):S72, 2000.

Seiderman RY et al: Assessing American Indian families, *MCN Am J Matern Child Nurs* 21(6):274, 1996.

Sterling YM, Peterson JW: Characteristics of African American women caregivers of children with asthma, *MCN Am J Matern Child Nurs* 28(1):32, 2003.

Vontress CE, Epp LR: Historical hostility in the African American client: implications for counseling, *J Multicult Counsel Devel* 25:170, 1997.

Westerman SJ, Davies DR; Acquisition and application of new technology skills: the influence of age, *Occup Med* 50(7):478, 2000.

Williams M et al: Inadequate functional health literacy among patients at two public hospitals, *JAMA* 274:1677, 1995.

Readiness for enhanced Knowledge of (specify)

Gail B. Ladwig

NANDA Definition

The presence or acquisition of cognitive information related to a specific topic is sufficient for meeting health-related goals and can be strengthened

• = Independent; ▲ = Collaborative

Defining Characteristics

Expresses an interest in learning; Explains knowledge of the topic; Behaviors congruent with expressed knowledge; Describes previous experiences pertaining to the topic

Related Factors (r/t)

To be developed

NOC   Outcomes (Nursing Outcomes Classification)

Suggested NOC Outcome

Knowledge: Health Promotion

> **Example NOC Outcome with Indicators**
>
> **Knowledge: Health Promotion** as evidenced by the following indicator: Description of health behaviors/health resources (Rate each indicator of **Knowledge: Health Promotion:** 1 = no knowledge, 2 = limited knowledge, 3 = moderate knowledge, 4 = substantial knowledge, 5 = extensive knowledge [see Section I].)

Client Outcomes

Client Will (Specify Time Frame):

- Demonstrate knowledge of new information
- Meet personal health-related goals
- Explain how to incorporate new health regimen into lifestyle
- List sources to obtain information

NIC   Interventions (Nursing Interventions Classification)

Suggested NIC Interventions

Health Education; Learning Readiness Enhancement

> **Example NIC Activities—Learning Readiness Enhancement**
>
> Prioritize identified learner needs based on client preference, skills of nurse, resources available, and likelihood of successful goal attainment

Nursing Interventions and Rationales

- Include clients as members of the health care team when providing education. **Nursing Research:** *This study indicated that clients were willing to take responsibility for playing their part in trying to optimize the outcome of their surgery. Reconceptualization of clients as honorary members of the health care team may facilitate the development of a framework within which the potential contribution of clients to their own care could be valued and supported more effectively (Edwards, 2002).* **Nursing Research:** *Couples who had received a diagnosis of prostrate cancer in this study found that by engaging in the challenge of gathering a volume of facts and a variety of details, they felt could make informed decisions and regain a sense of control through the engagement in decision-making related to treatment, surgeon, and hospital (Maliski, Heilemann, and McCorkle, 2002).*
- Use open-ended questions and encourage two-way communication. **Nursing Re-**

• = Independent; ▲ = Collaborative

search: *Intervention strategies that use interpersonal communication, including the opportunity for mothers to ask questions, were most preferred. Strategies that involve one-way messages to mothers were least preferred (Gaffney and Altieri, 2001).*

- Provide appropriate individualized health education when clients visit health care providers. **Nursing Research:** *The low rate of lifestyle advice reported in this study by clients implies that more preventive advice should be provided in primary care settings. More effective health promotion should be planned according to the needs of the practice population (Duaso and Cheung, 2002).* **Clinical Research:** *Having a regular doctor was found to have a greater impact than having a regular site on discretional preventive services, such as blood pressure and cholesterol level checkups (Xu and Tom, 2002).*

- Ensure that clients receive appropriate health-oriented education during rehabilitation hospitalization. *The client rehabilitation setting provides an opportunity for a "teachable moment" to introduce the idea of smoking cessation to the active smoker or to encourage continued smoking cessation and relapse prevention to those clients who have not smoked since their admission to the acute care hospital (Guilmette et al, 2001).*

- When developing written information, assess and provide information that is important to clients. **Nursing Research:** *This randomized study of information compiled from focus group input led to major change in providing information and produced a leaflet that was clearer, more attractive, and more informative and that proved more satisfactory to clients (Chumbley et al, 2002).* **Nursing Qualitative Descriptive Research Study:** *During child psychiatric hospitalization, parents in this study identified needing informational, emotional, and instrumental support (Scharer, 2002).*

- Carefully develop written materials to ensure that the client's literacy levels, including English as a second language, are addressed. *Functional illiteracy contributes to negative long-term health consequences for clients who must understand and adhere to complex health care instructions and therefore is of primary importance to community health nurses. This problem is compounded when English is the client's second language (Horner, Surratt, and Juliusson, 2000).* **Nursing Research:** *Patients need and want comprehensible, written information (Semple and McGowan, 2002).*

- Assist clients to find access to the Internet, libraries, and schools to find health information. **Clinical Research:** *Access, demographics, and, in particular, motivational factors all influence clients' interest in the Internet as a health resource (Mead et al, 2003).*

- Assist clients with questions about health information to find quality sites on the Internet. **Evidence-Based Research:** *More popular sites according to Google rank were more likely than less popular ones to contain information on ongoing clinical trials, results of trials, and opportunities for psychosocial adjustment. These characteristics were also associated with higher number of links as reported by Google and AltaVista. More popular sites by number of linking sites were also more likely to provide updates on breast cancer research, information on legislation and advocacy, and a message board service (Meric et al, 2002).* **Nursing Research:** *Health care providers have important roles in helping their clients as well as the public locate, assess, and interpret health information (Houston and Ehrenberger, 2001).*

- ▲ Provide a previsit questionnaire to facilitate individualized proactive planning before the visit to health care provider. **Nursing Research:** *More than 75% of all women in this study wanted information to help them make decisions on breast cancer prevention options, benefits, and risks. The satisfaction survey (n = 61) revealed that most women's needs were met. A previsit questionnaire facilitates individualized proactive planning before the visit (Stacey, DeGrasse, and Johnston, 2002).*

- • = **Independent;** ▲ = **Collaborative**

▲ Provide appropriate health care information and screening for clients with physical disabilities. **Nursing Research:** *In this study of 170 women between 21 and 65 years of age with physical disabilities, most (96%) had not had routine preventive gynecological cancer screening services in the past 5 years or information and treatment for complications (fatigue, spasticity, deconditioning, joint pain, depression), which are preventable. Preventive health care services should be provided to clients with disabilities (Coyle and Santiago, 2002). The Americans with Disabilities Act requires that diabetes educators provide reasonable accommodations to people with disabilities in response to their particular individual needs (Position Statement, 2002).*

▲ Prior to the initiation of a mood stabilizer, the potential benefits, risks, and adverse effects should be communicated to the patient. Provide information on potential severe and life-threatening adverse cutaneous drug reactions (ACDRs) to all clients on mood-stabilizing agents such as carbamazepine, lithium carbonate, valproic acid, topiramate, lamotrigine, gabapentin, and oxcarbazepine. Patients should be advised to seek medical attention if they suspect a drug-induced skin reaction. *Of all the psychotropic medications currently available, the mood-stabilizing agents have the highest incidence of severe and life-threatening ACDRs. An exanthematous eruption in a patient treated with a mood-stabilizing agent should be viewed as possibly being the initial symptom of a severe and life-threatening ACDR, such as a hypersensitivity reaction, Stevens-Johnson syndrome, or toxic epidermal necrolysis (Warnock and Morris, 2003).*

▲ Refer to nurse practitioners for client education. Use the HOPE model (health-oriented patient education) instead of the DOPE model (disease-oriented health education). *The economics of prevention supports reimbursement of nurse practitioners for client education (Glanville, 2000).*

Refer to care plan for **Deficient Knowledge.**

Geriatric

▲ Consider using an interactive multimedia computer software program to disburse education. **Nursing Research:** *Users of PEP (Personal Education Program) designed for the learning styles and psychomotor skills of older adults had greater knowledge of potential interactions of prescription medications with OTC drugs and alcohol than controls. Participants indicated a high degree of satisfaction with the PEP and reported their intent to make specific changes in self-medication behaviors (Neafsey et al, 2001).* **Clinical Research:** *A total of 42 patients aged 51 to 92 years tested an interactive program on heart failure. They thought it was a better way of receiving information than reading a booklet or watching a video (Stromberg, Ahlen, and Fridlund, 2002).*

Multicultural

Refer to **Deficient Knowledge** care plan.

• Provide health care information to mothers and grandmothers in African American families. **Nursing Research:** *Mothers and grandmothers are considered the gatekeepers of health care in the African American Community (Sterling and Peterson, 2003).*

Home care

NOTE: Because home care is an intermittent model of care having a goal of safety and optimal wellness of the client between visits, the importance of teaching (by the nurse) and learning (by the client) should not be understated. All of the previously mentioned interventions are applicable to the home setting.

• = **Independent;** ▲ = **Collaborative**

▲ Consider high-tech options for delivery of home-based instruction. **Nursing Research:** *Televideo technology has been used effectively to improve self-management of diabetes (Bowles and Dansky, 2002). Interactive teleconferencing and on-site training for family caregivers positively influenced knowledge, self-perceived competence, and resourcefulness, with no significant difference between the program delivery types (Rosswurm and Larrabee, Zhang, 2002).*

evolve WEBSITES FOR EDUCATION

See the EVOLVE website for World Wide Web resources for client education.

REFERENCES

Bowles KH, Dansky KH: Teaching self-management of diabetes, *Home Healthc Nurse* 20(1):36, 2002.

Chumbley GM, Hall GM, Salmon P: Patient-controlled analgesia: what information does the patient want? *J Adv Nurs* 39(5):459, 2002.

Coyle CP, Santiago MC: Healthcare utilization among women with physical disabilities, *Medscape Womens Health* 7(4):2, 2002.

Duaso MJ, Cheung P: Health promotion and lifestyle advice in a general practice: what do patients think? *J Adv Nurs* 39(5):472, 2002.

Edwards C: A proposal that patients be considered honorary members of the healthcare team, *J Clin Nurs* 11(3):340, 2002.

Gaffney KF, Altieri LB: Mothers' ranking of clinical intervention strategies used to promote infant health, *Pediatr Nurs* 27(5):510, 2001.

Glanville IK: Moving towards health-oriented patient education (HOPE), *Holist Nurs Pract* 14(2):57, 2000.

Guilmette TJ et al: Promoting smoking cessation in the rehabilitation setting, *Am J Phys Med Rehabil* 80(8):560, 2001.

Horner SD, Surratt D, Juliusson S: Improving readability of patient education materials, *J Community Health Nurs* 17(1):15, 2000.

Houston TK, Ehrenberger HE: The potential of consumer health informatics, *Semin Oncol Nurs* 17(1):41, 2001.

Maliski SL, Heilemann MV, McCorkle R: From "death sentence" to "good cancer": couples' transformation of a prostate cancer diagnosis, *Nurs Res* 51(6):391, 2002.

Mead N et al: What predicts patients' interest in the Internet as a health resource in primary care in England, *J Health Serv Res Policy* 8(1):33, 2003.

Meric F et al: Breast cancer on the world wide web: cross sectional survey of quality of information and popularity of websites, *BMJ* 324(7337):577, 2002.

Neafsey PJ et al: Delivering health information about self-medication to older adults: use of touchscreen-equipped notebook computers, *J Gerontol Nurs* 27(11):19, 2001.

Position Statement: Diabetes education for people with disabilities, *Diabetes Educ* 28(6):916, 2002.

Rosswurm MA, Larrabee JH, Zhang J: Training family caregivers of dependent elderly adults through on-site and telecommunications programs, *J Gerontol Nurs* 28(7):27, 2002.

Scharer K: What parents of mentally ill children need and want from mental health professionals, *Issues Ment Health Nurs* 23(6):617, 2002.

Semple CJ, McGowan B: Need for appropriate written information for patients, with particular reference to head and neck cancer, *J Clin Nurs* 11(5):585, 2002.

Stacey D, DeGrasse C, Johnston L: Addressing the support needs of women at high risk for breast cancer: evidence-based care by advanced practice nurses, *Oncol Nurs Forum* 29(6):E77, 2002.

Sterling YM, Peterson JW: Characteristics of African American women caregivers of children with asthma, *MCN Am J Matern Child Nurs* 28(1):32, 2003.

Stromberg A, Ahlen H, Fridlund B: Interactive education on CD-ROM: a new tool in the education of heart failure patients, *Patient Educ Couns* 46(1):75, 2002.

Taylor KL et al: Improving knowledge of the prostrate cancer-screening dilemma among African American men: an academic-community partnership in Washington, DC, *Public Health Rep* 116(6):590, 2001.

• = **Independent;** ▲ = **Collaborative**

Warnock JK, Morris DW: Adverse cutaneous reactions to mood stabilizers, *Am J Clin Dermatol* 4(1):21, 2003.

Xu KT: Access to care: usual source of care in preventive service use: a regular doctor versus a regular site, *Health Serv Res* 37(6):1509, 2002.

Risk for Loneliness

Gail B. Ladwig

NANDA Definition

At risk for experiencing vague dysphoria

Risk Factors

Affectional deprivation; social isolation; cathectic deprivation; physical isolation

Related Factors (r/t)

See Risk Factors

NOC Outcomes (Nursing Outcomes Classification)

Suggested NOC Outcomes

Loneliness Severity; Social Interaction Skills; Social Involvement; Social Support

---
Example NOC Outcome with Indicators

Loneliness Severity: as evidenced by the following indicator: Expression of social isolation (Rate each indicator of **Loneliness Severity:** 1 = none, 2 = slight, 3 = moderate, 4 = substantial, 5 = severe [see Section I].)

Client Outcomes

Client Will (Specify Time Frame):

- Maintain one or more meaningful relationship (growth enhancing versus codependent or abusive in nature)—relationships allowing self-disclosure—and demonstrate a balance between emotional dependence and independence
- Participate in ongoing positive and relevant social activities and interactions that are personally meaningful
- Demonstrate positive use of time alone when socialization is not possible

NIC Interventions (Nursing Interventions Classification)

Suggested NIC Interventions

Family Integrity Promotion; Socialization Enhancement; Visitation Facilitation

---
Example NIC Activities—Socialization Enhancement

Encourage involvement in already established relationships; Use role-playing to practice improved communication skills and techniques

---

• = Independent; ▲ = Collaborative

Nursing Interventions and Rationales

- Use active listening skills. Establish therapeutic relationship and spend time with the client. **Nursing Research:** *In this study, being truly present was listed as one behavior that demonstrated caring (Yonge and Molzahn, 2002).* **Nursing Research:** *This study demonstrated the importance of presence and caring communication (Sundin et al, 2002).*
- Assess the client's perception of loneliness (Is the person alone by choice, or do others impose the aloneness?). **Nursing Research:** *Among persons with severe mental illness, more than half identify problems with loneliness and social isolation (Perese et al, 2003).* See care plan for **Social isolation.**
- Assist the client with identifying loneliness as a feeling and the causes related to loneliness. **Nursing Research:** *Loneliness was the number one fear identified. Chi square analysis showed that the homeless who did not stay in shelters were significantly longer-term residents (p < 0.0001) of the community and reported fear of loneliness significantly more frequently (Reichenbach et al, 1998).*
- Assess the client's ability and/or inability to meet physical, psychosocial, spiritual, and financial needs and how unmet needs further challenge the ability to be socially integrated (e.g., loss of job leading to inability to afford usual and familiar social interaction, fatigue; lack of energy necessary for social interaction and personal engagement; impaired skin integument and its relationship to real and/or perceived social isolation). NOTE: See care plan for **Disturbed Body image** if loneliness is associated with impaired skin integument. **Clinical Research:** *Existential loneliness is an issue that arises for women with HIV and needs to be given equal consideration alongside other forms of loneliness (Mayers and Svartberg, 2001).* **Nursing Research:** *Patients' perception of general health, symptoms, and social support influences outcome (Lindsay et al, 2001).*
- Use active listening skills including assessment and clarification of the client's verbal and nonverbal responses and interactions. *Using therapeutic observation and listening skills helps to accurately assess and validate this diagnosis. Clients are often unable to identify the problems or factors that directly contribute to their sense of isolation (O'Brien and Pheiffer, 1993).*
- Evaluate the client's desire for social interaction in relation to actual social interaction. **Clinical Research:** *The lonelier the student, the more dishonest, the more negative, and the less revealing was the quality of the self-disclosure in their ICQ ("I seek you") chat interaction (Leung, 2002).*
- Assess the client's interpersonal skills and address deficits and behaviors that are blocking communication.
- Encourage the client to be involved in meaningful social relationships that are characteristic of both giving and receiving support. **Nursing Research:** *It is important to recognize that the positive relevance of social relationships is related to the content and quality of relationships (Gulick, 1994).*
- Encourage social support for patients with visual impairments. **Clinical Research:** *Results of a large, nationwide study, conducted in 1994 through 1999 at the University of Amsterdam, on the meaning of personal networks and social support for Dutch adolescents with visual impairments indicate that social support, especially the support of peers, is important to adolescents with visual impairments (Kef, 2002).*
- Explore ways to increase the client's support system and participation in groups and organizations. **Nursing Research:** *Encouragement by nurses is important in helping clients with mental illness to become part of support groups (Perese et al, 2003).* **Clinical Research:** *Satisfaction with support networks was a potent predictor of self-esteem, emo-*

• = Independent; ▲ = Collaborative

tional health, and loneliness in female survivors of violence and abuse (Fry and Barker, 2002). Peer support is helpful for clients in the mental health system (Lynch, 2000).

- Encourage the client to develop closeness in at least one relationship. **Nursing Research:** *Dependence and independence should be balanced in healthy relationships. Previous research has indicated that the development of a balanced level of emotional dependence and the ability to self-disclose are important factors in reducing the risk for loneliness (Mahon and Yarcheski, 1992).*

Adolescents

- Assess the client's social support system. **Nursing Research:** *Use a social support tool or validated assessment tool if possible (e.g., UCLA Loneliness Scale for adolescents [Mahon et al, 1995]).* (See References for assessment tool.)
- Evaluate the depth and level of character traits, shyness, and self-esteem, particularly of younger and middle adolescent clients.
- Evaluate the family stability of younger and middle adolescent clients and advocate and encourage healthy, growth-producing relationships with family and support systems. **Clinical Research:** *This study showed a fear of intimacy and loneliness among adolescents who were taught during childhood not to trust strangers (Terrell, Terrell, and Von Drashek, 2000).*
- For older adolescents, encourage close relationships with peers and involvement with groups and organizations. **Nursing Research:** *Younger adolescents are at a higher risk for loneliness if they are shy or have low self-esteem. Younger adolescents rely more on parental relationships. An expanded set of relationships becomes increasingly important in alleviating loneliness as adolescents mature (Mahon and Yarcheski, 1992).*
- Consider use of pets to cope with loneliness. **Nursing Research:** *In this study of homeless youths, participants identified pets as companions that provide unconditional love and decrease feelings of loneliness (Rew, 2000).* **Nursing Research:** *Equine-facilitated psychotherapy, while not a new idea, is a little-known experiential intervention that offers the opportunity to achieve healing (Vidrine et al, 2002).*

Geriatric

- Assess caregivers for Alzheimer clients for depression related to loneliness. **Nursing Research:** *Loneliness was significantly related to depression in this secondary analysis of data from a sample of 242 husbands, wives, and daughters providing care for Alzheimer's disease family members (Beeson et al, 2000).*
- ▲ Identify community support systems specific to elderly populations. **Clinical Research:** *Aging is often accompanied by significant losses of family members and other social support systems, which may lead to loneliness and depression. A study of residents of a nursing facility showed that social relationships with other residents were a strong predictor of decreased depression and loneliness (Fessman and Lester, 2000).*
- Consider a retirement village. **Clinical Research:** *In this study of 323 residents in 25 retirement villages, participants reported that isolation and loneliness decreased when clients relocated to a retirement village (Buys, 2001).*
- Encourage support by friends and family when the decision to stop driving must be made. **Nursing Research:** *In this study, increased loneliness and isolation affected the older driver, although an enhanced sense of responsibility was evident among friends and family. Findings suggest that the support offered by friends and family played a significant role in the decision to stop driving (Johnson, 1998).*

- **= Independent; ▲ = Collaborative**

- Assess the client's adaptive sensory functions or any other health deviations that may limit or decrease his or her ability to interact with others. **Clinical Research:** *Greater loneliness was found to be associated with an increased probability of having a coronary condition, as were low levels of both emotional support and companionship (Sorkin et al, 2002).*
- ▲ Assess the client's potential or actual hearing loss or hearing impairment and make appropriate referrals if a problem is identified. *Because of the nature of this sensory deprivation, communication barriers are increased and human intimacy and self-esteem are negatively affected (Chen, 1994).* **Clinical Research:** *In addition, it is important to note that hearing impairments often go unnoticed and may not be obvious as are more visibly recognized handicaps (Chen, 1994).* **Clinical Research:** *This study demonstrated declines in speech understanding in noise and central auditory processing are common, in the growing population of older women (Garstecki and Erler, 2001).*
- Encourage physical activity such as aerobics or stretching and toning in a group. **Clinical Research:** *These activities decreased loneliness in former sedentary adults (n = 174, median age = 65.5 years) (McAuley et al, 2000).*
- Provide reading materials for clients who are able to read. *Older people who enjoyed reading for pleasure were rarely lonely (Rane-Szotak and Herth, 1994).*

Multicultural
- Acknowledge racial/ethnic differences at the onset of care. *Acknowledgment of racial/ethnicity issues will enhance communication, establish rapport, and promote treatment outcomes (D'Avanzo et al, 2001).*
- Assess for the influence of cultural beliefs, norms, and values on the client's perception of social activity and relationships. *What the client considers normal social interaction may be based on cultural perceptions (Leininger, 1996).*
- Approach individuals of color with respect, warmth, and professional courtesy. *Instances of disrespect and lack of caring have special significance for individuals of color and may impede efforts to increase social outlets (D'Avanzo et al, 2001).*
- Assess the use of personal space needs, communication styles, acceptable body language, eye contact, perception of touch, and use of paraverbals when communicating with the client. *Nurses need to consider these when interpreting verbal and nonverbal messages (Siantz, 1991). Native Americans may consider avoidance of direct eye contact as a sign of respect and asking questions to be rude and intrusive (Seiderman et al, 1996).*
- Use a family-centered approach when working with Latino, Asian American, African American, and Native American clients. *Latinos may perceive family as source of support, solver of problems, and a source of pride. Asian Americans may regard the family as the primary decision maker and influence on individual family members (D'Avanzo et al, 2001).*
- Promote a sense of ethnic attachment. *Older Korean clients with strong ethnic attachments had lower levels of loneliness than those without strong attachments (Kim, 1999).*
- Validate the client's feelings regarding isolation and loneliness. *Validation lets the client know that the nurse has heard and understands what was said, and it promotes the nurse-client relationship (Giger and Davidhizar, 1995; Stuart and Laraia, 2001).*

Home care
- Above interventions may be adapted for home care use.
- ▲ Assess for depression with lonely elderly client and make appropriate referrals. **Nurs-**

• = Independent; ▲ = Collaborative

ing **Research:** *Findings have related loneliness in older adults to mental health problems especially depression (McInnis and White, 2001).*

▲ If the client is experiencing somatic complaints, evaluate client complaints to ensure physical needs are being met, and then identify relationship between somatic complaints and loneliness. **Nursing Research:** *Three factors have been found to increase levels of loneliness among elderly individuals residing in a nursing home: lack of intimate relationships, increased dependency, and loss. Nurses in long-term care facilities are in a position to directly intervene with elderly resident (Hicks, 2000).*

▲ Help the client to identify periods when loneliness is greatest (e.g., certain times of day, anniversaries of past special events). With the client's permission, refer for services of visiting volunteers. *The only agenda of visiting volunteers is to meet the social needs of the client. Long-term friendships sometimes develop from volunteer experiences.*

• To keep older people independent, interventions to prevent loneliness should be explored. Consider using art as an intervention. *Study shows that extreme loneliness predicts admission to the nursing home (PSL Consulting Group, 1999).* **Nursing Research:** *The findings of a qualitative study, conducted between 1997 and 2000, to investigate the plausibility of integrating masterworks of art with care of the chronically ill elderly demonstrate that masterworks of art can generate energy exchange between the elderly and caregivers, providing a plausible catalyst for meaningful interventions that transcend age and practice settings (Hodges, Keeley, and Grier, 2001).*

• Identify alternatives to eating alone. *Clients are often susceptible to loneliness at mealtimes. Loneliness may contribute to nutritional deficiencies or excesses.*

• Identify alternatives to being alone (e.g., telephone contact). **Nursing Research:** *This research demonstrated social support can be provided to low-income pregnant women who may have little or no social support and feel alienated in a clinical setting by telephone (Bullock, Browning, and Geden, 2002).*

• Consider using computers and the Internet to alleviate or reduce loneliness and social isolation. **Nursing Research:** *This descriptive qualitative study used a Web page questionnaire and chat room interviews with online participants aged 65 years and older who were living alone. Seven of the 10 participants used the computer to combat loneliness (Clark, 2002). In this study, Internet use was found to decrease loneliness and depression significantly, while perceived social support and self-esteem increased significantly (Shaw and Gant, 2002). This randomized controlled trial assessed the psychosocial impact of providing Internet access to older adults over a 5-month period. Among Internet users (n = 29) in the intervention group, there were trends toward less loneliness and less depression (White et al, 2002).*

• Support religious beliefs. *Belief in a supreme being provides a feeling of ever-present help and prevents loneliness. If clients have regrets about their life, they may be separated from their usual source of religious comfort.*

• Discuss the meaning of death and fears associated with dying alone. Explore the possibility of significant others being with the client at the time of death. *In later stages of life, individuals give significant thought to death and the meaning of their life. If they perceive their life as undesirable, they may fear death.*

Client/Family Teaching

• Encourage positive use of solitude to prevent loneliness (e.g., reading, listening to music, enjoying nature and art). *A positive use of solitude plays a strong role in preventing or alleviating loneliness. The mentioned activities are flow activities—self-directed, inde-*

• = **Independent;** ▲ = **Collaborative**

pendent activities that enhance well-being and decrease feelings of loneliness (Rane-Szotak and Herth, 1994).

- Include the family in all client-teaching activities, and give them accurate information regarding the illness severity. **Nursing Research:** *In this study of residents and family members in the first year in long-term care listening to residents and family members, nurses can improve life for residents and dignify them as individuals (Iwasiw et al, 2003).*
- Give family members something to do such as holding a hand, applying lotion, or assisting with feeding. **Clinical Research:** *Perceived family support was predictive of reduced loneliness in this study of HIV-positive women (Serovich et al, 2001).*
- Encourage family members to express caring by telling the client where they will be and sending messages when they cannot be present. *If people could spare a smile or a word for others who might be perceived as lonely, even if in doing so they selfishly think "There but for the grace of God go I," such a small gesture might just make the day of a lonely person a little less of an ordeal (Killeen, 1998). Everyone is lonely to some degree, no matter how much they pretend they are not: it is part of the human condition. Loneliness is such an innate part of the human psyche that it cannot be solved like a puzzle; it can only be alleviated and made less painful. This can only be achieved by increasing humankind's awareness of this distressing condition that everyone has to endure in some way, shape, or form, sometime during their lives, about which there is nothing to be embarrassed (Killeen, 1998).*

evolve WEBSITES FOR EDUCATION

See the EVOLVE website for World Wide Web resources for client education.

REFERENCES

Beeson R et al: Loneliness and depression in caregivers of persons with Alzheimer's disease or related disorders, *Issues Ment Health Nurs* 21(8):779, 2000.

Bullock LF, Browning C, Geden E: Telephone social support for low-income pregnant women, *J Obstet Gynecol Neonatal Nurs* 31(6):658, 2002.

Buys LR: Life in a retirement village: implications for contact with community and village friends, *Gerontology* 47(1):55, 2001.

Chen H: Hearing in the elderly, relation of healing loss, loneliness, and self-esteem, *J Gerontol Nurs* 20:22, 1994.

Clark DJ: Older adults living through and with their computers, *Comput Inform Nurs* 20(3):117, 2002.

D'Avanzo CE et al: Developing culturally informed strategies for substance-related interventions. In Naegle MA, D'Avanzo CE, editors: *Addictions and substance abuse: strategies for advanced practice nursing*, St Louis, 2001, Mosby.

Fessman N, Lester D: Loneliness and depression among elderly nursing home patients, *Int J Aging Hum Dev* 51(2):137, 2000.

Fry PS, Barker LA: Quality of relationships and structural properties of social support networks of female survivors of abuse, *Genet Soc Gen Psychol Monogr* 128(2):139, 2002.

Garstecki DC, Erler SF: Personal and social conditions potentially influencing women's hearing loss management, *Am J Audiol* 10:2, 2001.

Giger JN, Davidhizar RE: *Transcultural nursing*, ed 2, St Louis, 1995, Mosby.

Gulick E: Social support among persons with multiple sclerosis, *Res Nurs Health* 17:195, 1994.

Hicks TJ Jr: What is your life like now? Loneliness and elderly individuals residing in nursing homes, *J Gerontol Nurs* 26(8):15, 2000.

Hodges HF, Keeley AC, Grier EC: Masterworks of art and chronic illness experiences in the elderly, *J Adv Nurs* 36(3), 2001.

• = Independent; ▲ = Collaborative

Iwasiw C et al: Resident and family perspectives. The first year in a long-term care facility, *J Gerontol Nurs* 29(1):45-54, 2003.

Johnson J: Older rural adults and the decision to stop driving: the influence of family and friends, *J Community Health Nurs* 15(4):205, 1998.

Kef S: Psychosocial adjustment and the meaning of social support for visually impaired adolescents, *J Visual Impairment Blindness* 96(1):22, 2002.

Killeen C: Loneliness: an epidemic in modern society, *J Adv Nurs* 28(4):762, 1998.

Kim O: Mediation effect of social support between ethnic attachment and loneliness in older Korean immigrants, *Res Nurs Health* 22(2):169, 1999.

Leininger MM: *Transcultural nursing: theories, research and practices*, ed 2, Hilliard, Ohio, 1996, McGraw-Hill.

Leung L: Loneliness, self-disclosure, and ICQ ("I seek you") use, *Cyberpsychol Behav* 5(3):241, 2002.

Lindsay GM et al: The influence of general health status and social support on symptomatic outcome following coronary artery bypass grafting, *Heart* 85(1):80, 2001.

Lynch K: The long road back, *J Clin Psychol* 56(11):1427, 2000.

Mahon NE, Yarcheski A: Alternate explanations of loneliness in adolescents: a replication and extension study, *Nurs Res* 41:151, 1992.

Mahon NE, Yarcheski T, Yarcheski A: Validation of the revised UCLA loneliness scale for adolescents, *Res Nurs Health* 18:263, 1995.

Mayers AM; Svartberg M: Existential loneliness: a review of the concept, its psychosocial precipitants and psychotherapeutic implications for HIV-infected women, *Br J Med Psychol* 74(Pt 4):539, 2001.

McAuley E et al: Social relations, physical activity, and well-being in older adults, *Prev Med* 31(5):608, 2000.

McInnis GJ, White JH: A phenomenological exploration of loneliness in the older adult, *Arch Psychiatr Nurs* 15(3):128, 2001.

O'Brien ME, Pheiffer W: Physical and psychosocial nursing care for patients with HIV infection, *Nurs Clin North Am* 28:303, 1993.

Perese EF; Getty C; Wooldridge P: Psychosocial club members' characteristics and their readiness to participate in a support group, *Issues Ment Health Nurs* 24(2):153, 2003.

PSL Consulting Group: Loneliness may foreshadow nursing home admission, doctor's guide, retrieved on March 31, 1999, from the World Wide Web. Website: www.pslgroup.com/dg/56afe.htm.

Rane-Szotak D, Herth K: A new perspective on loneliness in later life, *Issues Ment Health Nurs* 16:583, 1994.

Reichenbach E, McNamee M, Seibel L: The community health nursing implications of the self-reported health status of a local homeless population, *Public Health Nurs* 15(6):398, 1998.

Rew L: Friends and pets as companions: strategies for coping with loneliness among homeless youth, *J Child Adolesc Psychiatr Nurs* 13(3):125, 2000.

Seiderman RY et al: Assessing American Indian families, *MCN Am J Matern Child Nurs* 21(6):274, 1996.

Serovich JM et al: The role of family and friend social support in reducing emotional distress among HIV-positive women, *AIDS Care* 13(3):335, 2001.

Shaw LH, Gant LM: In defense of the internet: the relationship between Internet communication and depression, loneliness, self-esteem, and perceived social support, *Cyberpsychol Behav* 5(2):157, 2002.

Siantz ML: How can we be more aware of culturally specific body language and use this awareness therapeutically? *J Psychosocial Nurs Ment Health Serv* 29(11):38, 1991.

Sorkin D; Rook KS; Lu JL: Loneliness, lack of emotional support, lack of companionship, and the likelihood of having a heart condition in an elderly sample, *Ann Behav Med* 24(4):290, 2002.

Stuart GW, Laraia MT: Therapeutic nurse-patient relationship. In Stuart GW, Laraia MT, editors: *Principles and practice of psychiatric nursing*, St Louis, 2001, Mosby.

Sundin K, Jansson L, Norberg A: Understanding between care providers and patients with stroke and aphasia: a phenomenological hermeneutic inquiry, *Nursing Inquiry* 9(2):93, 2002.

Terrell F, Terrell IS, Von Drashek SR: Loneliness and fear of intimacy among adolescents who were taught not to trust strangers during childhood, *Adolescence* 35(140):611, 2000.

Vidrine M et al: Equine-facilitated group psychotherapy: applications for therapeutic vaulting, *Issues Ment Health Nurs* 23(6):587, 2002.

White H et al: A randomized controlled trial of the psychosocial impact of providing Internet training and access to older adults, *Aging Ment Health* 6(3):213, 2002.

Yonge O, Molzahn A: Exceptional nontraditional caring practices of nurses, *Scand J Caring Sci* 16(4):399, 2002.

• = **Independent;** ▲ = **Collaborative**

Impaired Memory

Betty J. Ackley

NANDA **Definition**

Inability to remember or recall bits of information or behavioral skills; impaired memory may be attributed to pathophysiological or situational causes that are either temporary or permanent

Defining Characteristics

Inability to recall factual information; inability to recall recent or past events; inability to learn or retain new skills or information; inability to determine whether a behavior was performed; observed or reported experiences of forgetting; inability to perform a previously learned skill; forgets to perform a behavior at a scheduled time

Related Factors (r/t)

Fluid and electrolyte imbalance; neurological disturbances; excessive environmental disturbances; anemia; acute or chronic hypoxia; decreased cardiac output

NOC **Outcomes (Nursing Outcomes Classification)**

Suggested NOC Outcomes

Cognitive Orientation; Memory; Neurological Status: Consciousness

> **Example NOC Outcome with Indicators**
>
> **Memory** as evidenced by the following indicators: Recalls immediate information accurately/Recalls recent information accurately/Recalls remote information accurately (Rate each indicator of **Memory:** 1 = never demonstrated, 2 = rarely demonstrated, 3 = sometimes demonstrated, 4 = often demonstrated, 5 = consistently demonstrated [see Section I].)

Client Outcomes

Client Will (Specify Time Frame):

- Demonstrate use of techniques to help with memory loss
- State has improved memory

NIC **Interventions (Nursing Interventions Classification)**

Suggested NIC Intervention

Memory Training

> **Example NIC Activities—Memory Training**
>
> Stimulate memory by repeating patient's last expressed thought, as appropriate; Provide opportunity to use memory for recent events, such as questioning patient about a recent outing

• = Independent; ▲ = Collaborative

Nursing Interventions and Rationales

- Assess neurological function; use an assessment tool such as the metamemory in adulthood (MIA) questionnaire or the Mini-Mental State Examination (MMSE). *The MIA is reliable and nonthreatening and has been validated to be effective (McDougall and Balyer, 1998). The MMSE can help determine whether the client has memory loss only or also has delirium or dementia and needs to be referred for further treatment (Breitner and Welsh, 1995).*

- ▲ Determine whether onset of memory loss is gradual or sudden. If memory loss is sudden, refer the client to a physician for evaluation. *Acute onset of memory loss may be associated with neurological disease, medication effect, electrolyte disturbances, hypoxia, hypothyroidism, mental illness, or many other physiological factors (Breitner and Welsh, 1995; Elliott, 2000).*

- Determine amount and pattern of alcohol intake. *Alcohol intake has been associated with blackouts; clients may function but not remember their actions. Long-term alcohol use causes Korsakoff's syndrome with associated memory loss (Vinson, 1989). Heavy alcohol use by adolescents can impair brain function, including memory (Brown et al, 2000).*

- ▲ Note the client's current medications and intake of any mind-altering substances such as benzodiazepines, ecstasy, marijuana, cocaine, or glucocorticoids. *Benzodiazepines can produce memory loss for events that occur after taking the medication; information is not stored in long-term memory (Fluck et al, 1998; Mejo, 1992). Cocaine abuse has been shown to decrease memory (Butler and Frank, 2000). The ingestion of ecstasy has been associated with impaired memory, both short term and possibly long term (Gowing et al, 2002; Morgan et al, 2002).* **Clinical Research:** *Glucocorticoid therapy can cause a mild decrease in memory function that is usually reversible once a person is off the medications (Wolkowitz et al, 1997). Clients receiving long-term prednisone performed significantly worse on memory tasks than matched control subjects (Keenan, 1996). Both infrequent and long-term use of marijuana is associated with impaired memory function (Curran et al, 2002; Solowij et al, 2002).*

- Note the client's current level of stress. Ask if there has been a recent traumatic event. *Post-traumatic stress and anxiety-inducing general life factors can cause memory problems (Mejo, 1992). Elevated cortisol levels associated with stress have been shown to impair memory (Greendale et al, 2000; Lupien et al, 1994, 1997).*

- ▲ If stress is associated with memory loss, refer to a stress reduction clinic. If not available, suggest that the client meditate, receive massages, or take whatever actions necessary to relieve the stress. *Nonpharmacological therapy for treatment of stress syndromes is preferable and less likely to aggravate memory loss than commonly used antianxiety medications (Mejo, 1992).*

- Determine the client's sleep patterns. If insufficient, refer to care plan for **Disturbed Sleep pattern. Clinical Research:** *Studies demonstrate that memory consolidation is enhanced by sleep (Gais et al, 2002; Peigneux et al, 2001).*

- ▲ Determine the client's blood sugar levels. If they are elevated, refer to physician for treatment and encourage healthy diet and exercise to improve memory. *Elevated blood sugar levels were associated with a small hippocampus and impaired memory (Convit, 2003).*

- ▲ If signs of depression such as weight loss, insomnia, or sad affect are evident, refer the client for psychotherapy. *Depression is commonly associated with memory loss (Mejo, 1992). Depression can result in source memory errors, in which case the client is not sure if he or she did something or just thought about doing it (Elias, 2001).*

- Encourage the client to develop an aerobic exercise program. **Clinical Research:**

• = **Independent;** ▲ = **Collaborative**

A study demonstrated that aerobic exercise improved memory and executive function in depressed middle-aged and older adults (Khatri et al, 2001).

▲ Perform a nutritional assessment. If nutritional status is marginal, confer with a dietitian and primary care practitioner to evaluate whether the client needs supplementation with foods or vitamins. Teach the client the need to eat a healthy diet with adequate intake of whole grains, fruits, and vegetables to decrease cerebrovascular infarcts. *Moderate, long-term deficiencies of nutrients may lead to loss of memory. This condition may be preventable or diminished through diet (Cataldo, DeBruyne, and Whitney, 1999). Adequate levels of vitamin E may help protect memory (Miller, 2000).* **Clinical Research:** *A large study demonstrated that people who ate mostly fruits and vegetables per day (9 or 10 servings) had decreased incidence of ischemic strokes (Joshipura et al, 1999). A study demonstrated that dementia and cognitive decline were positively associated with silent brain infarcts (Vermeer et al, 2003).*

▲ Question the client about cholesterol level. If it is high, refer to physician or dietitian for help in lowering. Encourage the client to eat a healthy diet, avoiding saturated fats and *trans*-fatty acids. **Clinical Research:** *One study demonstrated that individuals who were prescribed statin medications that lowered cholesterol had a substantially lowered risk of developing dementia (Jick et al, 2000). A study demonstrated that high intake of saturated or* trans-*fatty acids may increase the risk of Alzheimer's disease (Morris et al, 2003).*

• Encourage the client to use a calendar for appointments, keep reminder lists, place a string around finger or rubber band around wrist as reminders, or enlist someone else to remind him or her of important events. *Using reminders can serve as cues for memory-impaired clients.*

• Help the client set up a medication box that reminds the client to take medication at needed times; assist the client with refilling the box at intervals if necessary. *Medication boxes are effective because clients will know whether medication has been taken when corresponding compartments are empty.*

• If safety is an issue with certain activities (e.g., the client forgets to turn off stove after use or forgets emergency telephone numbers), suggest alternatives such as using a microwave or whistling teakettle for heating water and programming emergency numbers in telephone so that they are readily available. *These measures can increase client safety (Agostinelli et al, 1994).*

▲ Refer the client to a memory clinic (if available), a neuropsychologist, or an occupational therapist. *Memory clinics can help the client learn ways to improve memory. Clinics may be more effective if work is done in groups because of increased support, reinforcement, and motivation (McDougall, 1999). Neuropsychologists have expertise in working with the memory impaired, as do many occupational therapists (Robinson, 1992).*

• Suggest clients use cues, including alarm watches, electronic organizers, calendars, lists, or pocket computers, to trigger certain actions at designated times. *Cues can help remind clients of certain actions (Wilson and Moffat, 1992); these external cognitive strategies can be effective (McDougall, 1999).*

• For clients with memory impairments associated with dementia, see care plan for **Chronic Confusion.**

Geriatric

• Assess for signs of depression. *Depression is the most important affective variable for memory loss in the older adult (Byers, 1993; McDougall, 1999).* **Clinical Research:**

• = **Independent;** ▲ = **Collaborative**

Cognitive impairment is not an inevitable consequence of aging, even in very old age (Snowdon, 1997).

▲ Evaluate all medications that the client is taking to determine whether they are caus-ing the memory loss. *Many medications can cause memory loss in the elderly, including an-ticholinergics, H2-receptor antagonists, beta-blockers, digitalis, benzodiazepines, barbiturates, and even mild opiates (DeMaagd, 1995; Sjogren et al, 2000).*

• Recommend that elderly clients maintain a positive attitude and active involvement with the world around them and that they maintain good nutrition. **Clinical Research:** *Findings from the Nun Study demonstrated that it is possible to maintain good cognitive function until extreme old age if elderly persons maintain active involvement with their en-vironment and are able to avoid having vascular disease with infarction of brain tissue. Cog-nitive impairment is not an inevitable consequence of aging and disease (Snowdon, 1997).*

• Encourage the elderly to believe in themselves and to work to improve their memory. **Clinical Research:** *Elderly clients may be able to improve their memory function up to 50% if they use appropriate strategies and invest the energy and time (Keen, 1998). New re-search has shown that there is formation of new neurons in the brain, a process called neuro-genesis, throughout the lifespan, and stimulation of the brain is necessary for this forma-tion (Eriksson et al, 1998).*

▲ Refer the client to a memory class that focuses on helping older adults learn memory strategies. **Nursing and Clinical Research:** *Research has demonstrated that classes that focus on memory strategies can improve memory (McDougall, 2002; McDougall and Bayler, 1998). In memory impairment associated with strokes, there is insufficient evidence to de-termine if memory training is effective (Majid, Lincoln, and Weyman, 2002).*

• Help family develop a memory aid booklet or wallet that contains pictures and labels from the client's life, or develop a video movie that includes familiar pictures with nar-ration (Cohen, 2002). *Using memory aids helps clients with dementia make more factual statements and stay on topic and decreases the number of confused, erroneous, and repeti-tive statements made (Bourgeois, 1992).* **Clinical Research:** *Use of the memory book may also help decrease the number of depressive statements by the client (Bourgeois et al, 2001).*

• Help family label items such as the bathroom or sock drawer to increase recall. *A sup-portive environment that includes orientation can help increase the client's awareness (Green and Gildemeister, 1994).*

Multicultural

• Assess for the influence of cultural beliefs, norms, and values on the family or caregiv-er's understanding of impaired memory. If black male dealing with memory loss, en-courage him to believe in his abilities. **Nursing Research:** *What the family considers normal and abnormal health behavior may be based on cultural perceptions (Cochran, 1998; Doswell and Erlen, 1998; Leininger and McFarland, 2002). Nursing research demon-strated that there was no significant differences in the memories of black versus white men, but the black men had higher anxiety about memory function, used fewer memory strate-gies, and had a higher incidence of depression (McDougall and Holston, 2003).*

• Use bias-free instruments when assessing memory in the culturally diverse client. **Nursing Research:** *Use of the MMSE without modification for ethnic bias resulted in younger Hispanics being categorized as more severely impaired than others (Mulgrew et al, 1999).*

• Inform the client's family or caregiver of meaning of and reasons for common behav-ior observed in the client with impaired memory. *An understanding of impaired*

• = **Independent;** ▲ = **Collaborative**

memory behavior will enable the client family/caregiver to provide the client with a safe environment.

- Validate family members' feelings regarding the impact of the client's behavior on family lifestyle. **Nursing Research:** *Validation is therapeutic communication technique that lets the client know that the nurse has heard and understands what was said, and it promotes the nurse-client relationship (Heineken, 1998).*

Home care

- Above interventions may be adapted for home care use.
- Arrange cues for medication taking that are focused around daily events (e.g., meals and bedtimes). **Nursing Research:** *Older adults report the use of internal memory strategies to compensate for age-related memory loss; specifically they prefer event-based prescription medication instructions (Branin, 2001).*
- Assess the client's need for outside assistance with recall of treatment, medications, and willingness/ability of family to provide needed support. *During initial phase of home care, increased frequency of visits may be necessary to compensate for the client's inability to recall treatment, medications. Counting of medications may be needed to determine if the client is following medication regimen. Telephone calls from family/friends may help to remind the client of treatment schedule.*
- Identify a checking-in support system (e.g., Lifeline or significant others). *Checking in ensures the client's safety.*
- Keep furniture placement and household patterns consistent. *Change increases risk of impaired memory and decreased functioning.*
- ▲ In the presence of a medical disorder, institute case management of frail elderly to support continued independent living. *Memory difficulties often represent and can lead to increasing needs for assistance in using the health care system effectively. Case management combines nursing activities of the client and family assessment, planning and coordination of care among all health care providers, delivery of direct nursing care, and monitoring of care and outcomes. These activities are able to address continuity of care, mutual goal setting, behavior management, and prevention of worsening health problems (Guttman, 1999).*

Client/Family Teaching

- When teaching the client, determine what the client knows about memory techniques and then build on that knowledge. *New material is organized in terms of what knowledge already exists, and efficient teaching should attempt to take advantage of what is already known in order to graft on new material (Wilson and Moffat, 1992).*
- When teaching a skill to the client, set up a series of practice attempts. Begin with simple tasks so that the client can be positively reinforced and progress to more difficult concepts. *Distributed practice with correct recall attempts can be a very effective teaching strategy. Widely distribute practice over time if possible (Wilson and Moffat, 1992).*
- Teach clients to use memory techniques such as repeating information they want to remember, making mental associations to remember information, and placing items in strategic places so that they will not be forgotten. *These methods increase recall of information the client thinks is important. The internal methods of increasing memory can be effective, especially if used along with external methods such as calendars, lists, and other methods (McDougall, 1999).*

● = **Independent;** ▲ = **Collaborative**

WEBSITES FOR EDUCATION

See the EVOLVE website for World Wide Web resources for client education.

REFERENCES

Agostinelli B et al: Targeted interventions: use of the Mini-Mental State Exam, *J Gerontol Nurs* 20:15, 1994.

Bourgeois MS: *Conversing with memory impaired individuals using memory aids: a memory aid workbook,* Gaylord, Mich, 1992, Northern Speech Services.

Bourgeois MS et al: Memory aids as an augmentative and alternative communication strategy for nursing home residents with dementia, *AAC Augment Altern Commun* 17(3):196, 2001.

Branin JJ: The role of memory strategies in medication adherence among the elderly, *Home Health Care Serv Q* 20(2):1, 2001.

Breitner JC, Welsh KA: Diagnosis and management of memory loss and cognitive disorders among elderly persons, *Psychiatr Serv* 46:29, 1995.

Brown et al: Neurocognitive functioning of adolescents: effects of protracted alcohol use, *Alcohol Clin Exp Res* 24(2):164, 2000.

Butler LF, Frank EM: Neurolinguistic function and cocaine abuse, *J Med Speech Lang Pathol* 8(3):199, 2000.

Byers PH: Older adults' metamemory: coping, depression, and self-efficacy, *Appl Nurs Res* 6:28, 1993.

Cataldo CB, DeBruyne LK, Whitney EN: *Nutrition and diet therapy: principles and practice,* ed 5, Belmont, Calif, 1999, Wadsworth.

Cochran M: Tears have no color, *Am J Nurs* 98(6):53, 1998.

Cohen GD: Creative interventions for Alzheimer's disease: familiar activities, videos can help patients copy with memory loss, *Geriatrics* 57(3):62, 2002.

Convit A et al: Reduced glucose tolerance is associated with poor memory performance and hippocampal atrophy among normal elderly, *Proc Natl Acad Sci U S A* 100(4):2019, 2003.

Curran HV et al: Cognitive and subjective dose-response effects of acute oral Delta(9)-tetrahydrocannabinol in infrequent cannabis users, *Psychopharmacology* 164(1):61, 2002.

DeMaagd G: High-risk drugs in the elderly population, *Geriatr Nurs* 16:198, 1995.

Doswell W, Erlen J: Multicultural issues and ethical concerns in the delivery of revising care interventions, *Nurs Clin North Am* 33(2):353, 1998.

Elias J: Why caregiver depression and self-care abilities should be part of the PPS case mix methodology, *Home Healthc Nurse* 19(1):23, 2001.

Elliott B: Case report. Diagnosing and treating hypothyroidism, *Nurs Pract* 25(3):92, 2000.

Eriksson PS et al: Neurogenesis in the adult human hippocampus, *Nat Med* 4(11):1313, 1998.

Fluck E et al: Does the sedation resulting from sleep deprivation and lorazepam cause similar cognitive deficits? *Pharmacol Biochem Behav* 59(4):909, 1998.

Gais S et al: Learning-dependent increases in sleep spindle density, *J Neurosci* 22(15):6830, 2002.

Gowing LR et al: The health effects of ecstasy: a literature review, *Drug Alcohol Rev* 21(1):53, 2002.

Green PM, Gildemeister JE: Memory aging research and memory support in the elderly, *J Neurosci Nurs* 26: 241, 1994.

Greendale GA et al: Higher basal cortisol predicts verbal memory loss in postmenopausal women: Rancho Bernardo Study, *J Am Geriatr Soc* 48(12):1655, 2000.

Guttman R: Case management of the frail elderly in the community, *Clin Nurs Spec* 13(4):174, 1999.

Heineken J: Patient silence is not necessarily client satisfaction: communication in home care nursing, *Home Healthc Nurse* 16(2):115, 1998.

Jick H et al: Statins and risk of dementia, *Lancet* 356(9242):1627, 2000.

Joshipura KJ et al: Fruit and vegetable intake in relation to ischemic stroke, *JAMA* 6(282):1233, 1999.

Keen C: Elderly should ignore stereotypes about memory loss, 1998. Website: www.napa.ufl.edu/98news/eldermem.htm

Keenan PA: Chronic prednisone use causes memory loss, *Neurology* 47:1396, 1996.

Khatri P et al: Effects of exercise training on cognitive functioning among depressed older men and women, *J Aging Phys Activity* 9(1):43, 2001.

Leininger MM, McFarland MR: *Transcultural nursing: concepts, theories, research and practices,* ed 3, New York, 2002, McGraw-Hill.

Lupien SJ et al: Basal cortisol levels and cognitive deficits in human aging, *J Neurosci* (5 Pt 1):2893, 1994.

• = **Independent;** ▲ = **Collaborative**

Lupien SJ et al: Stress-induced declarative memory impairment in healthy elderly subjects: relationship to cortisol reactivity, *J Clin Endocrinol Metab* 82(7):2070-2075, 1997.

Majid MJ, Lincoln NB, Weyman N: Cognitive rehabilitation for memory deficits following stroke, *Cochrane Database Syst Rev* (CD002293), 2002.

McDougall GJ: Cognitive interventions among older adults, *Annu Rev Nurs Res* 17:219, 1999.

McDougall GJ. Memory improvement in octogenarians, *Appl Nurs Res* 15(1):2, 2002.

McDougall GJ, Balyer J: Decreasing mental frailty in at-risk elders, *Geriatr Nurs* 19(4):220, 1998.

McDougall GJ, Holston EC. Black and white men at risk for memory impairment, *Nurs Res* 52(1):42, 2003.

Mejo SL: Anterograde amnesia linked to benzodiazepines, *Nurse Pract* 17:44, 1992.

Miller JW: Vitamin E and memory: is it vascular protection? *Nutr Rev* 58(4):109-111, 2000.

Morgan MJ et al: Ectasy: are the psychological problems associated with its use reversed by prolonged abstinence? *Psychopharmacology* 159(3), 294-303, 2002.

Mulgrew CL et al: Cognitive functioning and impairment among rural elderly Hispanics and non-Hispanic whites as assessed by the Mini-Mental State Exam, *J Gerontol B Psychol Sci Soc Sci* 54B(4):223, 1999.

Peigneux P et al: Sleeping brain, learning brain. The role of sleep for memory systems, *Neuroreport* 12(18):A111, 2001.

Robinson S: Occupational therapy in a memory clinic, *Br J Occup Ther* 55:394, 1992.

Schwartz RH et al: Short-term memory impairment in cannabis-dependent adolescents, *Am J Dis Child* 143(8): 1214, 1989.

Sjogren P, Thomsen AB, Olsen AK: Impaired neuropsychological performance in chronic nonmalignant pain patients receiving long-term oral opioid therapy, *J Pain Symptom Manage* 19(2):100, 2000.

Snowdon DA: Aging and Alzheimer's disease: lessons from the Nun Study, *Gerontologist* 37(2):150, 1997.

Solowij N et al: Cognitive functioning of long-term heavy cannabis users seeking treatment, *JAMA* 287(9):1123, 2002.

Vermeer SE et al: Silent brain infarcts and the risk of dementia and cognitive decline, *N Engl J Med* 348:1215, 2003.

Wilson BA, Moffat N: *Clinical management of memory problems,* San Diego, 1992, Singular.

Wolkowitz OM et al: Glucocorticoid medication, memory and steroid psychosis in medical illness, *Ann NY Acad Sci* 823:81, 1997.

Impaired bed Mobility

Brenda Emick-Herring

NANDA Definition

Limitation of independent movement from one bed position to another

Defining Characteristics

Impaired ability to turn from side to side; impaired ability to move from supine to sitting or sitting to supine; impaired ability to "scoot" or reposition self in bed; impaired ability to move from supine to prone or prone to supine; impaired ability to move from supine to long sitting or long sitting to supine

Related Factors (r/t)

Intolerance to activity; decreased strength and endurance; pain or discomfort; perceptual or cognitive impairment; neuromuscular impairment; musculoskeletal impairment; depression; severe anxiety

Suggested functional level classifications include the following:
0—Completely independent
1—Requires use of equipment or device
2—Requires help from another person

• = Independent; ▲ = Collaborative

3—Requires help from another person and equipment device
4—Dependent (does not participate in activity)

NOC Outcomes (Nursing Outcomes Classification)

Suggested NOC Outcomes
Mobility; Self-Care: Activities of Daily Living (ADL)

> **Example NOC Outcome with Indicators**
>
> **Mobility** as evidenced by the following indicator: Self-initiated movement of the following joints: fingers/thumb/wrist/elbow/shoulder/ankle/knee/hip (Rate each indicator of **Mobility:** 1 = no motion, 2 = limited motion, 3 = moderate motion, 4 = substantial motion, 5 = full motion [see Section I].)

Client Outcomes

Client Will (Specify Time Frame):
- Demonstrate optimal independence in positioning, exercising, and performing functional activities in bed
- Demonstrate ability to direct others on how to do bed positioning, exercising, and functional activities

NIC Interventions (Nursing Interventions Classification)

Suggested NIC Intervention
Bed Rest Care

> **Example NIC Activities—Bed Rest Care**
>
> Position in proper alignment; Teach bed exercises as appropriate

Nursing Interventions and Rationales

- Perform accurate physical assessment to determine the client's risk for ICP, respiratory abnormalities, aspiration, pressure ulcer formation, muscle tone abnormalities, and pain levels. *These conditions warrant certain bed positions to prevent complications (Feldman et al, 1992; Mitchell et al, 1981; Palmer and Wyness, 1988; Panel for the Prediction and Prevention of Pressure Ulcers in Adults, 1992).*
- Use critical thinking and priority setting to decide the most therapeutic bed positions and frequency of turns based on the client's history, risk profile, and preventative needs. *Positioning for one condition may negatively affect another. For example, elevation of head of bed is therapeutic for persons with increased ICP, tube feedings, and difficulty breathing but is contraindicated in persons with intravascular volume deficit, cervical traction, abnormal tone, reflexive posturing, and high risk for pressure ulcers (Arbour, 1998; Feldman et al, 1992; Metzler and Harr, 1996).* **Nursing Research:** *The commonly recommended 2-hour schedule for turning clients to prevent pressure ulcers was not disproved in a literature review; however, nursing judgment should be used to lengthen or shorten turn intervals based on individual client risk (Buss et al, 2002).*

• = Independent; ▲ = Collaborative

- If the client has increased intracranial pressure, refer to care plan for **Decreased Intracranial adaptive capacity.**
- If the client is dysphagic, assist to sit upright during and after feedings or ingestion of pills. Refer to care plan for **Impaired Swallowing.** *Sitting upright helps prevent aspiration of food, liquids, and pills in clients with dysphasia (Glenn-Molali, 2002).*
- Position the client in an upright position at intervals as tolerated by condition. If possible, elevate head of bed incrementally. If vital signs, pulse pattern and oxygen saturation levels are stable, dangle the client or move the client from bed to a "stretcher chair"—a stretcher that turns into a chair—to get out of bed and into a more vertical position. *Being vertical reduces the work of the heart, changes intravascular pressure, and stimulates the neural reflexes. It improves lung ventilation and aeration at the base of the lungs, improves diaphragmatic movement, enhances symmetrical body alignment and awareness of the surroundings, and reduces abnormal posturing in the severely brain injured (Metzler and Harr, 1996; Palmer and Wyness, 1988).* **Clinical Research:** *A review of studies on the effects of bed rest demonstrated that generally there are few indications for bed rest and that bed rest may delay recovery or cause harm to the client (Allen, Glasziou, and Del Mar, 1999).*
- Maintain the head of the bed at the lowest degree of elevation consistent with medical conditions and other restrictions to prevent pressure ulcer formation. *Sacral shearing risk is high when the head of the bed is elevated past 30 degrees. Skin may stick to linens if clients slide down, causing skin to pull away from underlying tissue and potentially stretch or tear arteries, thereby reducing local blood flow (Panel for the Prediction of Pressure Ulcers in Adults, 1992). A 30-degree laterally inclined position puts less pressure on tissue than the 90-degree side lying position (Defloor, 2000; Hoeman, 2002).*
- Position the bed flat at intervals, unless contraindicated for a medical reason. *This helps maintain body alignment, which is a means of normalizing tone; prevents trunk and pelvic shortening in clients with hemiparesis; helps prevent forward head flexion in the elderly and those with Parkinson's disease or stroke; is the start position for most bed mobility tasks; and is the position of most clients' beds at home (Kumagai, 1998; Wilson, 1988).*
- Prevent complications of immobility. *The inability to be upright disturbs many body systems (Metzler and Harr, 1996; Murphy, 1997; Olson, 1967).*
- Assess risk for pressure ulcer development and place the client on static surface (foam, air, water, gel, overlay or air or water mattress) or dynamic surface (low air-loss overlay, dynamic flotation mattress) to reduce pressure. These are appropriate to prevent ulcer or for the client with stage I or II pressure ulcers. Consistently assess for "bottoming out" of overlays (body sinks into mattress so that the recommended 1 inch between the mattress/overlay and the client is absent). *Pressure-reducing devices such as these help prevent pressure ulcers caused by prolonged periods of lying in bed (Gutierrez, 2002; Johnson and Nolde-Lopez, 2002).*
- ▲ Place the client with stage II or III pressure ulcers on pressure-relieving surface (low-air-loss therapy, air fluidized or high-air-loss therapy, or kinetic or lateral rotation therapy). Consult enterostomal therapy nurse to help determine therapeutic surface for complex clients (Gutierrez, 2002; Johnson and Nolde-Lopez, 2002).
- Encourage the client to take deep breaths, cough, reposition self and drink adequate fluids at intervals. *This prevents atelectasis and possible pneumonia.*
- Ensure that the client receives adequate fiber and fluid, and recognize that he or she may need a stool softener or bulking agent to prevent constipation. Refer to care

• = **Independent;** ▲ = **Collaborative**

plan for **Constipation.** *Immobility leads to constipation; however, increased fiber, fluids, activity and medications can help prevent constipation (Folden, 2002; Wong and Kadakia, 1999).*

▲ Recognize the client at risk for deep vein thrombosis (DVT) and pulmonary emboli (PE) and implement prophylactic measures such as antiembolic stockings, Ace wrap, and sequential compression device to legs, encourage joint ROM, and movement of legs and fluid intake. Administer anticoagulant medications. Refer to care plan for **Ineffective Tissue perfusion.** *Immobility, history of abdominal or orthopedic surgery, trauma to blood vessel walls, previous DVT, and smoking; older age, obesity, and hypercoagulability are risk factors for DVT and PE (Epley, 2000).* **Nursing Research:** *Authors of a quantitative study concluded that changing the subcutaneous needle after withdrawing heparin from a vial did not reduce the size of ecchymoses at the injection site of study subjects (Klingman, 2000).*

• Encourage fluid intake of 2000 to 3000 ml/day as tolerated by medical condition. *Increased fluids help flush mobilized calcium and bacteria from the body to prevent kidney stones and urinary infection (Maas and Specht, 2001; McCourt, 1993).*

▲ Take scrupulous care of indwelling Foley catheter if present, and detect and report signs of urinary tract infection as early as possible. *Loss of weight bearing on bones and presence of an indwelling catheter can lead to increased urinary calculi and infection (McConnell, 1984; Murphy, 1997; Rubin, 1988).*

• Use the following interventions during bed mobility activities:
  ■ Place positioning devices such as pillows or foam wedges between bony prominences.
  ■ Use lifting or lateral transferring devices such as a trapeze, bed linen, mechanical lateral transfer aid, ceiling mounted lift, friction-reducing device or transfer chairs, and bed scales to move (rather than drag) dependent or obese individuals (Baptiste et al, 2002).
  ■ Use special equipment to reposition and move the bariatric (very obese) client, such as large bed, air mattress overlay with rotation function, and overhead trapeze. A stirrup and pulley attached to an overhead traction system can be used for the client to place one leg in to raise it during peri-care, etc. Only logroll and tilt a dependent bariatric client (avoid full side-lying position) until familiar with his or her ability to help and control turns in bed. *The air mattress overlay reduces skin shear and frictional burn plus decreases resistance for staff to overcome when moving a client up or over in bed. If the client would start to slide out of bed in the side-lying position, it is very difficult for staff to stop the motion (Dionne, 2002).*

  These interventions protect against external mechanical forces (e.g., pressure, friction, and shear). Note, however, that use of a trapeze may be contraindicated in persons with cardiac disease and stroke because of their isotonic effect. Trapeze use is discouraged with persons with hemiplegia because movement and gripping with the sound arm elicits an "associated reaction" of abnormal tone and flexion in the hemiplegic side (Bobath, 1978; Hoeman, 2002; Panel for the Prediction and Prevention of Pressure Ulcers in Adults, 1992).

• Avoid positioning persons directly on the trochanter bone when in side-lying position.
• Apply elbow pads if the client uses elbows to prop self up or to scoot self up in bed or if in coma or if arms are restrained. Apply nocturnal elbow splint to promote extension if a confirmed ulnar nerve palsy or if there is pain at the elbow and paresthesia in ulnar side of the 4th and 5th fingers. *Prolonged compression or repetitive flexion pro-*

• = **Independent;** ▲ = **Collaborative**

ducing pressure on the ulnar nerve can lead to neuropathy and nerve damage. The above strategies prevent pressure and compression of the nerve (Congress of Neurological Surgeons, 2002). Use of an enclosure bed for agitated and confused clients may reduce the risk of wrist and chest restraints.

- Allow and encourage client bed mobility, repositioning, and self-care activities to prevent contractures and disuse syndromes. Encourage extremity elevation, mild exercise, and compression such as an Isotoner glove to counteract lymphedema in the upper extremity. *Chronic spasticity, immobility, and muscle atrophy related to connective tissue changes contribute to contractures (Finocchiaro and Herzfeld, 1998). Bed mobility promotes lymph fluid accumulation thus venous insufficiency, which impedes movement, in the upper extremities of persons with dense hemiplegia (Borgman and Passarella, 1991). Leg and foot contractures may elicit discomfort in sitting or lying positions and may interfere with positioning options during sexual activity (Pires, 1984).*

- Explain the importance of exhaling when pulling self up in bed or rolling, or during any other activity that may precipitate breath holding or straining. *This prevents the Valsalva maneuver and increased intra-abdominal and intrathoracic pressure, which elevate blood pressure and impair myocardial and cerebral perfusion (Rodriguez, 1998).*

- ▲ Assess pain level and administer adequate analgesics before bed repositioning, mobility, or self-care activities. Develop a specific preventative analgesic schedule with clients if chronic pain is experienced. *Nurses must be willing to accept clients' definition and self-rating of pain and believe their need for analgesics (McCaffery and Pasero, 1999).*

- Assist clients to splint an incision, wound, or other painful abdominal area with a pillow as they change positions, cough, or perform functional activities.

- ▲ Administer oral antispasmodic medications as prescribed to help control muscle spasms that interfere with movement. *Spasticity is a primary cause of contractures and is painful. Therapeutic level is one that prevents spasms but does not produce muscle weakness (Finocchiaro and Herzfeld, 1998).*

- ▲ Apply ice as ordered by physician to sites after nerve and motor point blocks in children and adults and assess for side effects of pain, sensory deficits, or vascular problems. *Nerve blocks with phenol or* Botulinum toxin *type A is used locally via an injection to prevent contractures and reduce spasticity (in single areas such as the ankle/foot, or knee, or fingers) that interferes with hygiene, ROM, positioning, standing, gait, prevention of skin breakdown, and comfort (Gormley, 1999; Gracies et al, 1997).*

- ▲ Recognize that intractable chronic spasticity and pain can interrupt function, bed/chair positioning, hygiene, and quality of life. If conservative treatment fails, some pediatric and adult clients can benefit from continuous intrathecal baclofen infusion (CITB) via an implanted pump in the spinal canal. **Nursing Research:** *Follow-up with 18 clients receiving CITB treatment over 9 months to 12 years indicated the majority had a significant decrease in tone and nursing care and increased function (Rawicki, 1999).* **Clinical Research:** *Spasticity decreased in 25 subjects as measured by the Ashworth score, but quality of life scores did not reflect a change over 1 year. Subjects answers to two open-ended questions, however, suggest quality of life changed positively (Gianino et al, 1998).*

- ▲ Refer clients to a dietitian, or provide dietary information to promote normal body weight. *Excessive weight places extra work and stress on body parts during bed mobility activities and may prevent tolerance to prone positioning.*

- = Independent; ▲ = Collaborative

Exercising

- Perform passive ROM at least twice a day to those body parts that clients cannot actively range or move spontaneously. Support body parts above and below the joint being ranged (e.g., hold the forearm and hand while ranging the wrist). *Passive ROM maintains joint and muscle movement and prevents contracture. Muscles get stronger only by working, so progress clients to active ROM, self-movement, and functional activities as soon as possible. Adequate support of the joint allows for true range of movement and detection of ease or resistance to movement (Hoeman, 2002).*
- Range hemiplegic client's affected upper extremity with the shoulder in slight external rotation. *Spasticity often pulls hemiplegic shoulders into retraction, which prevents normal gliding movement. External rotation prevents soft tissue from becoming pinched between the head of the humerus and the acromion; thus, it reduces shoulder pain (Borgman and Passarella, 1991).*
- Perform ROM slowly and rhythmically. Do not range beyond the point of pain in those with sensation; range only to the point of resistance in those with poor sensation and mental awareness. *Fast, jerky ROM may create discomfort, thereby increasing abnormal tone. Slow, rhythmical movements may relax and lengthen tight (spastic) muscles so they can be ranged further. Slow joint movement with gentle stretch may also potentiate muscle relaxation.* NOTE: *This is not the case for those with rigidity, as in Parkinson's disease (Palmer and Wyness, 1988).*
- ▲ Reinforce clients' self-initiated practice of exercise programs, developed by physical or occupational therapists. Exercises may include muscle setting, active strengthening, contraction of muscles against resistance, and weight lifting as appropriate. *Clients will need to initiate exercise programs at home; allowing them to do so early on encourages self-responsibility and ownership. Active exercise and weight lifting helps maintain muscle tone and strength. Isometric (muscle setting) exercises shorten muscle fibers without actually moving limbs or joints. Progressive resistive exercises cause muscles to work against gentle force and gravity, which stimulates muscle lengthening (Hoeman, 2002, Finocchiaro and Herzfeld, 1998).*
- Assess and intervene for misalignment, asymmetry, abnormal tone (flaccidity and spasticity), synergistic flexor or extensor patterns, abnormal posture, inability to shift weight, poor coordination, reduced sensation, and excessive effort while moving in bed. *Therapeutic bed positioning and moving can counteract such problems; enhance sensation; and restore more normal tone, posture, and functioning (Bobath, 1978; Gee and Passarella, 1985; Johnston and Olson, 1980; Kumagai, 1998; Ossman and Campbell, 1990; Palmer and Wyness, 1988).*
- Use manual guidance and verbal cueing during bed positioning and mobility to facilitate more normal alignment, tone, posture, and movement. Wait for clients to respond and do as much of the activity as they can. *Clients need the opportunity to feel more normal tone, posture, and movements so they do not relearn abnormal patterns (Bobath, 1978; Gee and Passarella, 1985; Ossman and Campbell, 1990; Passarella and Lewis, 1987).*

Positioning

- Use the following measures for persons with neurological problems, especially hemiplegia, and persons with joint pain, inflammation, orthopedic problems, and the elderly. NOTE: Refer to the article by Ossman and Campbell (1990) for detailed sketches and instructions on positioning hemiplegics and to the article by Kumagai (1998) on positioning paralyzed clients.

- **• = Independent; ▲ = Collaborative**

- Position head and neck in neutral alignment. *Head, neck, and trunk alignment influences muscle tone in the extremities; therefore, positioning should begin proximally and proceed distally to normalize tone (Bobath, 1978).*
- Use a flat pillow when clients are supine if head/neck flexion occurs. Place a small towel or pillow behind the head and/or between the shoulder blades if extension occurs. *This prevents flexor or extensor tone and contractures of the head and neck (Bobath, 1978; Palmer and Wyness, 1988).*
- Place a sandbag under the pillow on one or both sides of the head when a client is supine, and one or two pillows under the head in the side-lying position to prevent lateral head flexion. *Lateral head flexion, extension, or rotation may occlude the internal jugular vein, preventing cerebral ventricular outflow and thus contributing to high ICP (Palmer and Wyness, 1988).*
- Change the position of clients' shoulders and arms frequently. Abduct the shoulders of persons with high paraplegia or quadriplegia horizontally (to 90 degrees) twice a day. The shoulders of hemiplegics should not be positioned out past 90 degrees. *Positioning paralyzed clients' arms in the horizontal plane provides full range of motion (Pires, 1989). Too much abduction may be contraindicated in hemiplegia because of spasticity around the scapula. Normal gliding movements are thus impaired so soft tissue can become pinched and painful (Borgman and Passarella, 1991).*
- Position elbows so they are extended or only slightly flexed with the wrist and fingers in extension (except for clients with increased ICP). *Extension counteracts flexor patterns (Bobath, 1978). However, arm extension increases cerebral ventricular fluid pressure in clients with acute head injury, thus worsening their increased ICP (Mitchell et al, 1981).*
- Apply resting forearm, wrist, and hand splints as ordered. On a routine schedule, check underlying skin for evidence of pressure and poor circulation. Strictly adhere to on/off orders. *Splints are used to maintain hands and wrists in neutral position or to immobilize inflamed joints as a means of controlling pain. The efficacy of splinting to inhibit spasticity is questionable.*
- Use hard cones in hands as ordered to help prevent contractures. Soft hand rolls should not be used for persons with spastic hands. **Nursing research:** *Soft rolls may elicit flexor patterns in the wrists and hands. Instead, a hard cone is suggested because it may inhibit the long flexors of the hand (Jamieson and Dayhoff, 1980).*
- Prevent external and internal rotation of the hips unless clients have a hip fracture, or have had a surgical hip pinning or replacement. *Neutral alignment of the hip and leg is obtained by placing a thin pillow or folded pad under the weak pelvic girdle, hip, and upper thigh. A pillow or folded pad should not be positioned under the knee. Persons with hip pinning and the like need legs in abduction to stabilize the new prosthesis in the joint; therefore, an abductor splint or pillows are used (Hoeman, 2002).*
- Position the leg and knees so that the toes point toward the ceiling; apply resting leg splints, boots, or high top tennis shoes. Assess underlying skin as mentioned. *These strategies help prevent foot and ankle plantar flexion by promoting neutral ankle alignment. Footboards are undesirable for persons with spasticity because pressure on the ball of the foot stimulates plantar flexion (Bobath, 1978; Hoeman, 2002; Palmer and Wyness, 1988).*
- Assist clients to lie prone or semiprone as part of the routine turn schedule (may be contraindicated in those with cardiopulmonary disturbances or increased intracranial pressure). *The prone-lying position promotes drainage and mobilization of re-*

• = Independent; ▲ = Collaborative

spiratory secretions from dependent lobes of the lung to improve lung aeration, thus oxygenation. It also enhances hip and trunk extension and is therapeutic for persons with lower extremity amputations, paraplegia, quadriplegia, and brain injury (Palmer and Wyness, 1988; Kumagai, 1998).

- Position hemiplegics on both the unaffected and affected sides. Position the affected shoulder well forward, moving it from the shoulder, not the arm. *Weight bearing relaxes tone in the hemiplegic side; protraction of the shoulder reduces its tone and prevents lying on the humerus. Moving the affected shoulder versus the arm prevents shoulder pain (Bobath, 1978; Borgman and Passarella, 1991).*
- Put a flat pad between the ribs and hip if trunk shortening occurs as hemiplegics lie on their affected side. *This helps elongate the trunk into neutral alignment (Bobath, 1978).*
- Use assistive devices (e.g., hydraulic or mechanical lift, friction reducer, or commercial repositioner) for severely dependent patients who need to be turned or moved up in bed. Do not use manual lifting such as the two-person under-axilla techniques. **Nursing Research:** *Manual lifting often causes overexertion back stress and injuries to staff and may be uncomfortable to clients (Owen, Welden, and Kane, 1999).*

Bed mobility—rolling

- Recognize components of normal movement with bed mobility activities (e.g., rolling, bridging, scooting, long sitting, and sitting upright). Most movements start with the client supine, flat in bed. *Normal movements are bilateral, segmental, well-timed, and effortless. They involve set positions, segmental action, weight bearing and shifting, trunk centering, and stabilization against gravity (Borgman and Passarella, 1991; Gee and Passarella, 1985; Kumagai, 1998).*
- Assist the client into the set position for rolling. For hemiplegics, this includes:
  - Moving the shoulder and arm on the side to which the client will turn outward with palm facing up
  - Flexing the knees with the feet flat on the bed
- For persons with bilateral paralysis, this includes:
  - Crossing the outside leg over the other leg or manually flexing the outside leg
  - Stretching the arms out in front of the chest with the handles clasped together if possible

  Set positions are those normal postures assumed to prepare the body for purposeful movements. Set positions and bilateral activity are often lost with neurological insult. Relearning these in bed prepares clients for bilateral activity as mobilization progresses to sitting, transfers, and standing (Gee and Passarella, 1985; Kumagai, 1998).
- Instruct and guide the client to roll over segmentally. Start the roll by lifting and turning the head in the direction of the turn, then moving the shoulders/arms/trunk, as the hips and knees follow. Be prepared to assist the affected shoulder and leg of hemiplegics. *This follows normal segmental patterns for rolling (Bobath, 1978; Ossman and Campbell, 1990; Kumagai, 1998).*

NOTE: For guidelines on how to assist the person with paraplegia or quadriplegia with rolling, refer to Kumagai (1998). For safety, always logroll a client with known or suspected spinal cord injury.

• = **Independent;** ▲ = **Collaborative**

Bed mobility—bridging

- Help the client to use bridging to move laterally or up in bed, or during functional activities such as using the bedpan, pulling up pants, or straightening bed linens. *Bridging is a bilateral activity that prepares the legs and feet for weight bearing while the hips are extended (Gee and Passarella, 1985).*
- Reinforce the set position for bridging (e.g., the knees flexed and the feet flat on the bed close to the buttocks). Assistance may be needed to keep the legs from externally rotating. *The hips can be lifted off the bed when the knees are flexed; the closer the feet are to the buttocks, the higher the hips can be lifted (Gee and Passarella, 1985). Lower extremity pain, limited range of motion, fractures, and so forth may limit knee flexion.*
- Help the client rest his or her arms and hands alongside the trunk. *Help lift or guide the pelvis as indicated. It may be difficult for persons with hemiplegia, obesity, or pain to extend their hips (Gee and Passarella, 1985).*

Bed mobility—scooting laterally

- Communicate which direction the client is to move.
- Help the client to bridge as described previously. Remind the client to place both feet flat on the bed and close to the buttocks.
- Support the client's pelvis to the extent needed as he or she moves over toward the side of the bed. *The lower body is moved first in lateral scooting.*
- Lower the client's pelvis down supine to the same starting position. Instruct the client to lift head and shoulders forward off the bed, then assist to move upper trunk over to the side of the bed. If the client has hemiplegia, support the affected shoulder from the scapula. The upper body and head move after the lower body does.
- Repeat above movements until the client is on the desired side of the bed.

Bed mobility—scooting up

- Assist the client to bridge, then move pelvis and buttocks up toward the head of the bed.
- Guide the client's buttocks back to the same starting position.
- Ask the client to tuck the chin and lift head and shoulders off the bed, then lay back down, straightening the trunk. *This elongates the trunk and moves the client up in bed bit by bit.*
- To move their shoulders up in bed, persons with hemiplegia can clasp hands together, outstretch them above the chest, then actively lower them toward the knees. Or, they can move the affected shoulder blade forward with the sound hand, lift their upper body and head forward, then lay back down. *Both methods help protract the affected shoulder forward to move and elongate the trunk while shifting upward. They also promote bilateral activity and sensory stimulation to the hemiplegic arm (Gee and Passarella, 1985; Ossman and Campbell, 1990).*
- Remind the client to move feet up toward buttocks each time before moving the lower body. Client should repeatedly raise the lower then the upper body and head until he or she is far enough up in bed.

Bed mobility—side-lying to sitting upright

- Assess whether the client is over to one side of the bed far enough; if not, help the client to move over. *This will reduce the risk of sliding off the edge of the bed while sitting up.*

- • = Independent; ▲ = Collaborative

- Plan the bed and furniture arrangement so that persons with hemiplegia can sit up using their affected side. *Weight bearing on the affected side is a means of increasing tone and promotes bilateral activity and sensory stimulation (Bobath, 1978).*
- Assist or cue the client into side-lying position (on their affected side if hemiplegic).
- Instruct the client to lower legs slowly over the edge of the bed with knees flexed and close to chest. If the client has recently had back or neck surgery or back pain, legs should instead be lowered slowly off the bed at the same time he or she pushes up with arms, keeping spine straight. *Hanging legs over the edge of the bed reduces the amount of weight to be shifted and managed while sitting up. However, in cases of back surgery or pain, legs are moved in unison with the body because the weight of freely hanging legs would aggravate back pain.*
- Ask the client to lift his or her head off the bed.
- Ensure that the bottom shoulder of hemiplegics is positioned forward before sitting up. If not, move it forward from the shoulder blade (not by pulling on the distal arm). *This allows the elbow to take weight as the body moves upright (Bobath, 1978; Ossman and Campbell, 1990).*
- Instruct the client to bear weight on the bottom arm and elbow while at the same time pushing against the mattress with the palm of other hand to sit up. Alternatively, instead of pushing up onto the elbow, the client is guided forward diagonally while pushing with the palm of his or her hand to sit himself or herself up (Kumagai, 1998).
- Help the client sit up by placing one of your hands under the bottom shoulder blade to keep it well forward and pushing down on the opposite iliac crest with your other hand. Shift the client's weight; do not lift it. Encourage the client to initiate and complete as much of the pushing and weight shifting as possible. *Protraction of the shoulder helps prevent abnormal tone and pain during movement. The shoulder and pelvis are key points of control for guiding the client's movements (Gee and Passarella, 1985; Ossman and Campbell, 1990). The nurse's weight shifts from the front foot (the one near the head of the bed) to the back foot using leverage, not strength (Gee and Passarella, 1985).*
- Assist clients to achieve a stable sitting posture with weight on both legs and buttocks. Hips and knees should flex to 90 degrees. If possible, feet should be flat on the floor. *Weight needs to shift so it is centered and distributed onto both sides of the body in a bilateral manner (Bobath, 1978).*

Bed mobility—long sitting

- Assess the client's ability for 100-degree straight leg raises; if this ability is absent, avoid long sitting position. Straight leg raise function indicates hamstring tone. *If hamstring muscles are too tight and long sitting is attempted, back extensor muscles will be overstretched and person will lose passive stability of the trunk (Kumagai, 1998).*
- Cue the client to start from the set position (flat and supine in bed).
- Instruct the client to grasp the side rails of the bed and pull himself or herself up to a sitting position. If hand function is poor, teach the client to raise head and trunk up by pushing against the mattress with flexed forearms until sitting upright. The legs remain in extension as the client sits up in bed.
- Assist quadriplegics and high paraplegics with the wrist extension method in the following manner:
  - Remind the client to wedge hands under hips and tuck chin.
  - Stand to the side and face the client.

• = Independent; ▲ = Collaborative

- Support the client from the scapula when raising trunk off the bed as he or she comes up onto elbows.
- Support the trunk and scapulas from behind as the client shifts weight side to side.
- Move behind the client to avoid getting in his or her way as the client unweights one arm and throws the other straightened arm back into an extended, locked position.
- Kneel on the bed behind the client to support upper trunk as weight is shifted onto the locked arm.
- Repeat the sequence for the remaining arm.
- Help the client with hand and arm positioning if necessary.
- Support the client's trunk (still kneeling from behind) as he or she shifts back and forth to bring extended arms closer to the body so that the client can support self sitting erect.

  Physical and occupational therapists teach the wrist extension method to persons with high-level quadriplegia or paraplegia; nurses may have to reinforce principles and assist the client as he or she practices outside of therapy (Kumagai, 1998).

NOTE: Refer to Kumagai (1998) for further information and sketches on how to assist quadriplegic or paraplegic clients with rolling to the semiprone and upright sitting position.

Geriatric

- Develop appropriate strategies for positioning and bed mobility based on the client's multiple chronic and disabling conditions. *The number of comorbid conditions in the elderly is high (Hoeman, 2002).*
- Assess the family caregivers' strength, health history, and cognitive status to predict ability and risk for helping clients with positioning and bed mobility tasks. Help family explore and develop other options if helping clients would place them at too high a risk. *Caregivers of elderly clients are often themselves frail elderly persons with chronic health problems. They would be at high risk for injury when helping clients with bed mobility, exercise, and ROM activities (McAnaw, 2001).*
- Prevent failure by assessing the client's stamina and energy level during exercising and bed mobility activities; give assistance or rest breaks as needed. *Elderly clients may have less energy reserves and may fatigue easily because of respiratory and circulatory impairments (McAnaw, 2001).*
- Spread out bed activities, exercise programs, and ADLs rather than clumping them together. *Anticipate that day-to-day abilities may fluctuate based on factors such as chronic disease, pain, restful sleep, constipation, nutritional intake, and mood.*
- Incorporate memory aids and strategies (e.g., written schedules, directions, sketches, or notes), timers, audiotaped instructions, etc, so that clients with cognitive decline can function independently.

Home care

- Some of the above interventions may be adapted for home care use.
- ▲ Begin discharge planning as soon as possible with case manager or social worker to assess need for home support systems, assistive devices, and community or home health services.
- ▲ Encourage use of the client's regular bed in the home unless contraindicated for specific medical reasons. *Emotionally, persons may benefit from sleeping in their own bed,*

• = Independent; ▲ = Collaborative

with their partner. Note that most of the bed activities described above did not require side rails or head elevation. Foam wedges or blocks can add elevation if necessary.

- Place indented or grooved-out areas in wood pieces under each leg of the bed and set bed against the walls in a corner of the room. *Such actions may prevent injury from bed movements because regular beds do not have brakes.*

- Suggest rearranging furniture at home to make it accessible to meet sleeping, toileting, and living needs. *Converting an existing room on a main level into a suite for living and sleeping purposes and decorating it so it is cozy yet functional may be emotionally soothing and prevent an institutional look (Yearns, 1995).*

- Discuss the psychological and physical benefits of allowing clients to be as self-sufficient as possible in bed mobility and repositioning, even though it may be time consuming. *Caregivers may try to help or save time by "doing for" their loved one. Discussion about prevention of helplessness, complications of disuse, and promoting self-esteem may change the caregiver's approach.*

- Prepare family members for potential regression in self-care during transition from hospital to home environment. *Relocation anxiety may interfere with independence. Confidence building, coaching, written instructions, sketches, instructional videotapes of proper techniques, and referrals may be needed (Theuerkauf, 1996).*

- ▲ Offer emotional support and suggest community resources and social supports to help with adjustment issues. *The home environment may trigger the reality of loss and change experienced with impaired physical mobility (Hoeman, 1996).*

- ▲ Consider referral for durable medical equipment as appropriate to the client's difficulty: bed frame or trapeze to assist the client with movement in bed.

- ▲ In the presence of a medical disorder, institute case management of frail elderly to support continued independent living. *Impaired mobility can lead to increasing needs for assistance in using the health care system effectively. Case management combines nursing activities of the client and family assessment, planning and coordination of care among all health care providers, delivery of direct nursing care, and monitoring of care and outcomes. These activities are able to address continuity of care, mutual goal setting, behavior management, and prevention of worsening health problems (Guttman, 1999).*

- See the Home Care Interventions section of the care plan for **Impaired physical Mobility.**

Client/Family Teaching

- Use various sensory modalities to teach the client, family, and caregivers correct techniques for ROM, exercising, repositioning, and bed mobility activities.
  - Give information visually (demonstrations, sketches, instructional videos, written instructions).
  - Give tactile stimulation (manual guidance, hand-on-hand technique, return demonstrations, note taking).
  - Give auditory information (verbal instructions, instructional audiotapes, verbal repeating of instructions, self-talk during motor activity, reading aloud written instructions).

    Developmentally, motor activities are first learned by trial and error, then by feeling normal movement, and last by repeated practice. Providing various sensory stimulation helps motor learning and memory retention (Bobath, 1978).

- Schedule time with family and caregivers for client education and practice sessions in addition to sharing information informally. Suggest that family members come

• = Independent; ▲ = Collaborative

prepared with their questions and wearing appropriate clothing and shoes for practice. *Practice—repetition promotes learning and retention.*

- Teach caregivers proper body mechanics and use of assistive devices (if applicable) while assisting clients with bed mobility activities. *This prevents injury and discomfort.*

evolve WEBSITES FOR EDUCATION

See the EVOLVE website for World Wide Web resources for client education.

REFERENCES

Allen C, Glasziou P, Del Mar C: Bed rest: a potentially harmful treatment needing more careful evaluation, *Lancet* 354(9186):1229, 1999.

Arbour R: Aggressive management of intracranial dynamics, *Crit Care Nurs* 18(3):30, 1998.

Bobath B: *Adult hemiplegia: evaluation and treatment,* London, 1978, William Heinemann Medical Books.

Borgman MF, Passarella PM: Nursing care of the stroke patient using Bobath principles: an approach to altered movement, *Nurs Clin North Am* 26(4):1019, 1991.

Buss IC, Halfens RJG, Abu-Saad HH: The most effective time interval for repositioning subjects at risk of pressure sore development: a literature review, *Rehabil Nurs* 27(2):59, 2002.

Congress of Neurological Surgeons: Medical student curriculum in neurosurgery. http://www.neurosurgery.org/cns/meetings/curriculum/d1.html.2002.

Defloor T: The effect of position and mattress on interface pressure, *Appl Nurs Res* 13(1):2, 2000.

Dionne M: 10 tips for safe mobility in the bariatric population, *Rehabil Manag* 15(8):28, 2002.

Epley D: Pulmonary emboli risk reduction, *J Vasc Nurs* XVIII(2):61, 2000.

Feldman Z et al: Effect of head elevation on intracranial pressure, cerebral perfusion pressure, and cerebral blood flow in head-injured patients, *J Neurosurg* 76(2):207, 1992.

Finocchiaro D, Herzfeld S: Neurological deficits associated with spinal cord injury. In Chin PA, Finocchiaro D, Rosebrough A: *Rehabilitation nursing practice,* New York, 1998, McGraw-Hill.

Folden S: Practice guidelines for the management of constipation in adults, *Rehabil Nurs* 27(5):169, 2002.

Gee ZL, Passarella PM: *Nursing care of the stroke patient: therapeutic approach,* Pittsburgh, 1985, AREN.

Gianino JM et al: Quality of life: effect of reduced spasticity from intrathecal baclofen, *J Neurosci Nurs* 30(1):47, 1998.

Glenn-Molali NH: Nourishment and swallowing. In Hoeman SP editor, *Rehabilitation nursing: process, application, and outcomes,* ed 3, St Louis, 2002, Mosby, pp. 322-346.

Gormley MH: Management of spasticity in children: part 1: chemical denervation, *J Head Trauma Rehabil* 14(1):97, 1999.

Gracies JM et al: Traditional pharmacological treatments for spasticity, part I: local treatments, *Muscle Nerve Suppl* 6:S61, 1997.

Gutierrez A: Pressure lessons, *Rehabil Manag* 15(9):44, 2002.

Guttman R: Case management of the frail elderly in the community, *Clin Nurs Spec* 13(4):174, 1999.

Hoeman SP: Coping with chronic, disabling, or developmental disorders. In Hoeman SP: *Rehabilitation nursing: process and application,* ed 2, St Louis, 1996, Mosby.

Hoeman SP: Movement, functional mobility, and activities of daily living. In Hoeman SP: *Rehabilitation nursing: process, application, and outcomes,* ed 3, St. Louis, 2002, Mosby.

Jamieson S, Dayhoff NE: A hard hand-positioning device to decrease wrist and finger hypertonicity: a sensorimotor approach for the patient with nonprogressive brain damage, *Nurs Res* 29:285, 1980.

Johnson KMM, Nolde-Lopez G: Skin integrity. In Hoeman SP, editor: *Rehabilitation nursing: process, application, and outcomes,* ed 3, St Louis, 2002, Mosby.

Johnston K, Olson E: Application of Bobath principles for nursing care of the hemiplegic patient, *Assoc Rehab Nurs J* 5:8, 1980.

Klingman L: Effects of changing needles prior to administering heparin subcutaneously, *Heart Lung* 29(1):70, 2000.

Kumagai KAS: Physical management of the neurologically involved client: techniques for bed mobility and transfers. In Chin PA, Finocchiaro D, Rosebrough A, editors: *Rehabilitation nursing practice,* New York, 1998, McGraw-Hill.

- **= Independent; ▲ = Collaborative**

- If geriatric client is scheduled for an elective surgery that will result in admission into ICU and immobility, or recovery from a knee replacement, initiate a prehabilitation program that includes a warm-up, aerobic strength, flexibility, and functional task work. **Nursing and Clinical Research:** *By increasing the functional capacity of the individual prior to the stressor of inactivity, the predictable declines in physical activity can be prevented or alleviated (Topp et al, 2002). In a study clients who performed strength activities preoperatively walked significantly greater distances postoperatively after total hip replacement (Whitney and Parkman, 2002).*

▲ Evaluate the client for signs of depression (flat affect, insomnia, anorexia, frequent somatic complaints) or cognitive impairment (use Mini-Mental State Exam [MMSE]). Refer for treatment or counseling as needed. **Nursing Research:** *Multiple studies have demonstrated that depression and decreased cognition in the elderly correlate with decreased levels of functional ability (Resnick, 1998).*

- Watch for orthostatic hypotension when mobilizing elderly clients. If relevant, have the client flex and extend feet several times after sitting up, then stand up slowly with someone watching. *Orthostatic hypotension as a result of cardiovascular system changes, chronic diseases, and medication effects is common in the elderly (Matteson et al, 1997).*

- Be very careful when getting a mostly immobile client up. Be sure to lock the bed and wheelchair and have sufficient personnel to protect the client from falls. *Elderly clients most commonly sustain the most serious injuries when they fall.* **Clinical Research:** *The most important preventative measure to reduce the risk of injurious falls for nonambulatory residents involves increasing safety measures while transferring, including careful locking of equipment such as wheelchairs and beds before moves (Thapa et al, 1996).*

- Help clients assume the prone position three times per week for 20 minutes each time. If clients are unable to do so, help them turn partially over and assume the position gradually. *The prone position helps prevent hip deformities that can interfere with balance and walking. This position may be contraindicated in some clients, such as morbidly obese clients, respiratory or cardiac clients who cannot lie flat, and neurological clients.*

- Do not routinely assist with transfers or bathing activities unless necessary. *The nursing staff may contribute to impaired mobility by helping too much. Encourage client independence (Mobily, Kelley, 1991).*

- Use gestures and nonverbal cues when helping clients move if they are anxious or have difficulty understanding and following verbal instructions. *Nonverbal gestures are part of a universal language that can be understood when the client is having difficulty with communication.*

- Recognize that wheelchairs are not a good mobility device and often serve as a mobility restraint. **Clinical Research:** *Wheelchairs can be very effective restraints. In one study, only 4% of residents in wheelchairs were observed to propel them independently; only 45% could propel them, even with cues and prompts; no residents could unlock them without help; the wheelchairs were not fitted to residents; and residents were not trained in propulsion (Simmons et al, 1995).*

- Ensure that chairs fit clients. Chair seat should be 3 inches above the height of the knee. Provide a raised toilet seat if needed. *Raising the height of a chair can dramatically improve the ability of many older clients to stand up. Low, deep, soft seats with armrests that are far apart reduce a person's ability to get up and down without help.*

- If the client is mainly immobile, provide opportunities for socialization and sensory stimulation (e.g., television and visits). See **Deficient Diversional activity.** *Immobility and a lack of social support and sensory input may result in confusion or depression in the*

• = **Independent;** ▲ = **Collaborative**

elderly (Mobily, Kelley, 1991). See interventions for **Acute Confusion** or **Hopelessness** as appropriate.

Home care

- Above interventions may be adapted for home care use.
- ▲ Begin discharge planning as soon as possible with case manager or social worker to assess need for home support systems, assistive devices, and community or home health services.
- ▲ Assess home environment for factors that create barriers to physical mobility. Refer to occupational therapy services if needed to assist the client in restructuring home and daily living patterns.
- ▲ Refer to home health aide services to support the client and family through changing levels of mobility. Reinforce need to promote independence in mobility as tolerated. *Providing unnecessary assistance with transfers and bathing activities may promote dependence and a loss of mobility (Mobily and Kelley, 1991).*
- ▲ Refer to physical therapy for gait training, strengthening, and balance training. *Physical therapists can provide direct interventions as well as assess need for assistive devices (e.g., cane, walker).*
- Assess skin condition at every visit. Establish a skin care program that enhances circulation and maximizes position changes. *Impaired mobility decreases circulation to dependent areas. Decreased circulation and shearing place the client at risk for skin breakdown.*
- Once the client is able to walk independently, and needs an exercise program, suggest the client enter an exercise program with a friend. **Nursing Research:** *Findings from a study of exercise behavior found that friends have the strongest influence to keep on an exercise program, more than family members or experts (Resnick, Orwig, and Magaziner, 2002).*
- Provide support to the client and family/caregivers during long-term impaired mobility. *Long-term impaired mobility may necessitate role changes within the family and precipitate caregiver stress (see care plan for* **Caregiver role strain**).
- ▲ Institute case management of frail elderly to support continued independent living. *Impaired mobility can lead to increasing needs for assistance in using the health care system effectively. Case management combines nursing activities of the client and family assessment, planning and coordination of care among all health care providers, delivery of direct nursing care, and monitoring of care and outcomes. These activities are able to address continuity of care, mutual goal setting, behavior management, and prevention of worsening health problems (Guttman, 1999).*

Client/Family Teaching

- Teach the client to get out of bed slowly when transferring from the bed to the chair.
- Teach the client relaxation techniques to use during activity.
- Teach the client to use assistive devices such as a cane, a walker, or crutches to increase mobility.
- Teach family members and caregivers to work with clients during self-care activities such as eating, bathing, grooming, dressing, and transferring rather than having the client be a passive recipient of care. *Maintaining as much independence as possible helps maintain mobility skills (Lipson and Braun, 1993).*
- Work with the client using the Transtheoretical Model of behavior change and determine if the client is in the precontemplation, contemplation, preparation, action, or

• = **Independent;** ▲ = **Collaborative**

maintenance state of behavior change about exercise. Provide appropriate strategies to support change to exercising based on determined state of change. **Nursing Research:** *The Transtheoretical Model of behavior change can be very useful for nurses to utilize to increase exercise behavior utilizing-stage appropriate interventions (Burbank, Reibe, and Padula, 2002). Use of the Transtheoretical Model of behavior change plus theory of self-efficacy suggests that both of these theories are helpful to increase exercise in the older adult (Resnick and Nigg, 2003).*

- Develop a series of contracts with mutually agreed on goals of increased activity. Include measurable landmarks of progress, consequences for meeting or not meeting goals, and evaluation dates. Sign the contracts with the client. **Nursing Research:** *Using a series of evolving contracts to modify behavior toward increasing activity helps the client learn skills to change behavior (Boehm, 1989; Steckel, 1974).*

evolve WEBSITES FOR EDUCATION

See the EVOLVE website for World Wide Web resources for client education.

REFERENCES

Allen C, Glasziou P, Del Mar C: Bed rest: a potentially harmful treatment needing more careful evaluation, *Lancet* 354(9186):1229, 1999.

Boehm S: Patient contracting, *Annu Rev Nurs Res* 7, 1989.

Burbank PM, Reibe D, Padula CA: Exercise and older adults: changing behavior with the transtheoretical model. *Orthop Nurs* 21:4, 2002.

Fried KM, Fried GW: Immobility. In Derstine JB, Hargrove SD: *Comprehensive rehabilitation nursing*, Philadelphia, 2001, WB Saunders.

Guttman R: Case management of the frail elderly in the community, *Clin Nurs Spec* 13(4):174, 1999.

Halfmann PL, Keller C, Allison M: Pragmatic assessment of physical activity, *Nurse Pract Forum* 8(4):160, 1997.

Hirvensalo M, Rantanen T, Heikkinen E: Mobility difficulties and physical activity as predictors of mortality and loss of independence in the community-living older population, *J Am Geriatr Soc* 48(5):493, 2000.

Koroknay VJ et al: Maintaining ambulation in the frail nursing home resident: a nursing administered walking program, *J Gerontol Nurs* 21:18, 1995.

Lipson J, Braun S: *Toward a restraint-free environment: reducing the use of physical and chemical restraint in long term care and acute settings,* Baltimore, 1993, Health Professions Press.

Matteson MA, McConnell ES, Linton AD: *Gerontological nursing,* Philadelphia, 1997, WB Saunders.

Mills EM: The effect of low-intensity aerobic exercise on muscle strength, flexibility, and balance among sedentary elderly persons, *Nurs Res* 43:207, 1994.

Mobily PR, Kelley LS: Iatrogenesis in the elderly: factors of immobility, *J Gerontol Nurs* 17:5, 1991.

Pedretti LW: *Occupational therapy: practice skills for physical dysfunction,* ed 4, St Louis, 1996, Mosby.

Resnick B: Predictors of functional ability in geriatric rehabilitation patients, *Rehabil Nurs* 23(1):21, 1998.

Resnick B: Testing the effect of the WALC intervention on exercise adherence in older adults, *J Gerontol Nurs,* 28(6), 2002.

Resnick B, Daly MP: Predictors of functional ability in geriatric rehabilitation patients, *Rehabil Nurs* 23(1):21, 1998.

Resnick B, Nigg C: Testing a theoretical model of exercise behavior for older adults, *Nurs Res* 52(2):80, 2003.

Resnick B, Orwig D, Magaziner J: The effect of social support on exercise behavior in older adults, *Clin Nurs Res* 11(1):52, 2002.

Resnick B, Zimmerman S, Orwig D: Model testing for reliability and validity of the outcome expectations for exercise scale, *Nurs Res* 50:5, 2001.

Simmons S et al: Wheelchairs as mobility restraints: predictors of wheelchair activity in nonambulatory nursing home residents, *J Am Geriatr Soc* 43:384, 1995.

Steckel SB: The use of positive reinforcement in order to increase patient compliance, *AANNT J* 1:1:1974.

• = **Independent;** ▲ = **Collaborative**

Tempkin T, Tempkin A, Goodman H: Geriatric rehabilitation, *Nurs Pract Forum* 8(2):59, 1997.

Thapa P et al: Injurious falls in nonambulatory nursing home residents: a comparative study of circumstances, incidence, and risk factors, *J Am Geriatr Soc* 44:273, 1996.

Topp R et al: The effect of bed rest and potential of prehabilitation on patients in the intensive care unit. *AACN Clin Issues* 13:2, 2002.

Vincent KR et al: Improved cardiorespiratory endurance following 6 months of resistance exercise in elderly men and women, *Arch Intern Med* 162:673, 2002.

Whitney JA, Parkman S: Preoperative physical activity, anesthesia, and analgesia: effects on early postoperative walking after total hip replacement, *Appl Nurs Res* 15:1, 2002.

Impaired wheelchair Mobility

Brenda Emick-Herring

NANDA Definition

Limitation of independent movement within the environment using a device equipped with wheels

Defining Characteristics

Impaired ability to operate a manual or power wheelchair on even or uneven surface; impaired ability to operate manual or power wheelchair on an incline or decline; impaired ability to operate wheelchair on curbs

Related Factors (r/t)

Intolerance to activity; decreased strength and endurance; pain or discomfort; perceptual or cognitive impairment; neuromuscular impairment; musculoskeletal impairment; depression; severe anxiety; amputation

Suggested functional level classifications include the following:

0—Completely independent

1—Requires use of equipment or device

2—Requires help from another person for assistance, supervision, or teaching

3—Requires help from another person and equipment or device

4—Dependent—does not participate in activity

NOC Outcomes (Nursing Outcomes Classification)

Suggested NOC Outcome

Ambulation: Wheelchair

Example NOC Outcome

Ambulation: Wheelchair as evidenced by the following indicators: Propels wheelchair safely/Transfers to and from wheelchair/Maneuvers curbs, doorways, ramps (Rate each indicator of **Ambulation: Wheelchair:** 1 = dependent—does not participate, 2 = requires assistive person and device, 3 = requires assistive person, 4 = independent with assistive device, 5 = completely independent [see Section I].)

• = Independent; ▲ = Collaborative

Client Outcomes

Client Will (Specify Time Frame):
- Demonstrate optimal independence in operating and moving a wheelchair or other device equipped with wheels
- Demonstrate the ability to direct others in operating and moving a wheelchair or other device equipped with wheels
- Demonstrate therapeutic positioning, pressure relief, and safety principles while operating and moving wheelchair or other device equipped with wheels

NIC   Interventions (Nursing Interventions Classification)

Suggested NIC Interventions
Exercise Therapy: Muscle Control; Positioning: Wheelchair

> **Example NIC Activities—Positioning: Wheelchair**
>
> Select the appropriate wheelchair for the patient; Monitor for patient's inability to maintain correct posture in wheelchair

Nursing Interventions and Rationales

- Assist or remind the client to don appropriate equipment (e.g., braces, corsets, shells, splints, orthoses, immobilizers, and abdominal binders) in bed before wheelchair mobility; loosen or remove equipment after the client returns to bed. *Provide stabilization and alignment of body parts; the abdominal binder helps prevent postural hypotension, supports abdominal contents, and increases vital capacity in persons with high spinal cord injury. For hemodynamic stability, the binder must be put on and taken off while the client is in bed.*

- ▲ Obtain referrals for physical therapy, occupational therapy, or a wheelchair seating clinic to ensure that the wheelchair and seating system fits the build, abilities, postural support needs, and pressure ulcer prevention of the client. The seating system should allow the client to propel the chair, safely and ably use the hands to complete ADLs/self-care/job/recreational activities, reach the foot rests and floor with the feet, stand up from the chair without falling, and not be harmed by the wheelchair legs and foot rests (Cooper et al, 2000; Minkel, 2001). *Wheelchair seating and cushion systems are the basis of postural support for clients. Poor posture (slouching, side leaning, and sliding down) can cause deformities, discomfort, high skin pressure, overuse of physical restraints, and trunk compression, which affects arousal, respiratory, circulatory, digestive, urinary, swallowing and speech functioning. Proper cushions lessen shock impact and repetitive vibration, both of which lead to fatigue, pain, and improper body mechanics over time. An individualized chair and seating system promotes independence, stability, balance, comfort, and prevention of medical complications. The sacrum and ischial tuberosities are at risk for pressure ulcer formation; therefore relief techniques, use of cushions/cutouts/supports that distribute mass to lower peak pressures, strict continence management, and adequate nutrition and hydration are key preventative strategies. Never use doughnut-type cushions (Cooper et al, 2000; Paleg 2002; Saur, 1999).* **Nursing Research:** *Healthy subjects were found to have maximum pressure at the buttock-seat interface during chair sitting on a pressure reducing cushion when they slid down or slouched in a chair. The least upright pressure was when the chair was tilted back and the legs (not heels) rested on a stool. Sitting up*

• = **Independent**; ▲ = **Collaborative**

but not reclined produced less pressure with the feet resting on the floor versus on a stool. The four cushions tested had varying pressure-reducing abilities (Defloor and Grypdonck, 1999). When the wheelchairs of two subjects with quadriplegia were tilted to 45 degrees or more, or reclined to at least 150 degrees, pressure at their ischial tuberosities decreased significantly (Pellow, 1999).

- For the client with loss of sensory and motor functioning, emphasize importance of weight shifts every 15 minutes. Reinforce side leans (leaning toward opposite side of chair), forward leans (leaning forward as arms lie alongside thighs; a safety belt is advised) and if balance and trunk control are present, push-ups (placing hands on the armrests and pushing to lift buttocks off the seat), and rear tilts (wheelchair is tilted backward by another person from 45 to 65 degrees). Client may also sit with the back of the wheelchair reclined (150 degrees) with legs on leg/foot rests to lower tissue pressure. *Weight shifts, push-ups, and reclined positioning should be used by clients for intermittent pressure relief to prevent pressure ulcers related to capillary occlusion from great force on a small bony area (McCourt, 1993; Minkel, 2000; Panel for the Prediction and Prevention of Pressure Ulcers in Adults, 1992).*

- Deliberately and frequently assess posture and help the client to position self in wheelchair in good alignment so that hips, knees, and ankles are close to 90-degree flexion and hips and pelvis are fully back in the chair. **Clinical Research:** *Nurses working with acute stroke patients only spent 6% of their time deliberately repositioning clients with poor posture and asymmetry. Nurses did indirectly change and improve these clients' posture while helping them with tasks such as getting ready to eat or take medications and so forth (Dowswell et al, 2000).*

- Consistently instruct the client to unlock wheelchair brakes, place feet securely on foot rests, and fasten safety restraints and seat belts (across the top of the thighs) before propelling chair. *Practicing and sequencing will help habituate steps of the safety plan. Securing feet on foot plates helps prevent foot injuries. Soft waist restraints may be needed to remind clients not to get up alone. Wheelchair seat belts help stabilize and hold the pelvis in place and should be strapped over thighs, not the abdomen (Rader et al, 1999).*

- Remove leg and foot rests from wheelchairs of the client who can actively move the wheelchair short distances by himself or herself by lifting the legs while propelling it, or by taking steps while sitting. *Foot rests can cause skin tears and bruising, as well as postural alignment problems. There is less pressure on sacral and buttock tissue sitting upright with feet on the floor than with feet on foot rests (Rader et al, 1999).*

- Implement precautionary measures, including leather gloves and use of friction-coated projection hand rims, to propel a manual wheelchair. *Persons without finger flexor function use palm action against the projection rims to propel a wheelchair. They are at risk for sores and calluses on the hands. Friction-coated projection rims are less invasive and slippery than aluminum hand rims.*

- Verbally reinforce and demonstrate placement of hand(s) on manual wheelchair rim(s) and propel wheelchair by (1) pushing forward on both wheel rims to go straight ahead, (2) pushing the right rim to turn left and vice versa, and (3) pulling backward on both wheels to back up (Wilson and Kerr, 1988).

- Guide or instruct the client with unilateral leg and arm functioning to propel the wheelchair by: (1) raising that foot plate and putting foot flat on the floor, (2) getting a lower wheelchair if whole foot doesn't reach the floor, (3) placing sound hand on the rim, (4) pushing as described above with the sound hand, and (5) "walking" the chair forward by extending the knee, then putting the heel then the entire foot on the

• = **Independent**; ▲ = **Collaborative**

tively affected role and occupational performance, responsibilities, interests, independence, self-esteem, and ability to adapt to ADLs (Buning, Angelo, and Schmeler, 2001).

▲ Prevent pain and overuse injury including carpal tunnel syndrome, ulna neuropathy, bilateral thumb and index finger hyperesthesia by activity modification, prescriptive exercises, ROM, strengthening, conditioning, and gentle stretching of the upper extremities, doing lateral weight shifts or forward leaning for pressure relief versus doing push-ups, and transferring between even height surfaces (Nyland et al, 2000). **Clinical Research:** *Individual forward adjustment of the axle position on manual wheelchairs, combined with personal fitting of the client to the wheelchair, improves the propulsion biomechanics and likely lessens the risk of upper extremity nerve injury (Boninger et al, 2000). Persons with tetraplegia had more frequent and intense shoulder pain than those with paraplegia. Both groups had elbow and hand pain. The functional tasks that created the greatest pain in both groups included pushing the wheelchair up an incline and wheeling longer than 10 minutes. Pain was also intense while sleeping for these clients (Curtis et al, 1999).*

Geriatric

- Alternate wheelchair mobility with rest periods when resting pulse rate, respiratory patterns, and blood pressure reading suggest compromised activity tolerance. *Chronic illness, debilitation and inactivity contribute to increased resting heart rate and blood pressure, and to decreased maximal oxygen uptake, vital capacity and strength in the elderly (Radwanski, 2002).*

- Avoid using restraints on elderly or confused clients, or those with deformities or spinal curvatures who are at risk for falling because they slide down in a wheelchair or try to reposition self. *Standard wheelchair seats and backs often sag; whereas a more solid seat and backrest, or a backrest with tension adjustable upholstery or segmented back supports, will provide more postural stability and comfort (Defloor and Grypdonck, 1999; Minkel, 2002; Rader et al, 1999). Elderly clients' lumbar spines tend to flatten, and hip flexion is often less than 90 degrees. A wheelchair with a reclining back offers support at the appropriate angle and may be more comfortable (Sussman and Bates-Jensen, 1998); however, compared with standard wheelchairs, reclining wheelchairs are heavier and harder to propel and may limit independence. Hamstring muscles may tighten and shorten behind the knees, preventing feet from reaching foot rests or the floor. Elderly clients may move to get comfortable or do a task, which may inadvertently result in poor posture and sliding down in the chair. Nurses may unnecessarily restrain such clients (Rader et al, 1999).* **Clinical Research:** *A gel- and air-filled wheelchair cushion provided pressure relief (low interface pressure readings) over the ischial tuberosities and sacrum of two persons with tetraplegia whereas a foam cushion did not; tilting their wheelchairs to 45 degrees and reclining them to 150 degrees also reduced pressure readings over the ischial tuberosities (Pellow, 1999).*

- Ensure proper lower extremity positioning when the client is sitting up. Do not use elevating leg rests as a means to prevent sliding down in the wheelchair. Custom foot rests may be needed. Place both feet either on foot rests or on the floor when wheelchair is stationary. *Tight hamstrings (posterior knee muscles) and a posterior pelvic tilt are common in the elderly. Tight hamstrings pull the client's pelvis toward the front of the chair. Special leg/foot rests may be needed to accommodate the short hamstrings. When the feet are not on an equal level, the tight hamstrings and posterior tilt are accentuated and may create further discomfort and malalignment (Gee and Passarella, 1985; Rader et al, 1999).*

• = **Independent;** ▲ = **Collaborative**

▲ Assess for side effects of medications and potential need for dosage readjustments related to increasing physical activity. *Antidepressants and benzodiazepines can cause postural hypotension and dizziness; antihypertensive and cardiac medications often create hypotension, dizziness, and may alter cardiac output; and diuretics cause postural hypotension (Halm, 2001; Skidmore-Roth, 2001).*

• Allow the client to move at his or her own speed. Avoid rushing. *The elderly normally move more slowly than younger people because of diminished ROM and strength, stiff joints, cardiopulmonary compromise, and discomfort.*

Home care

• Assess the client and obtain complete history with reference to reasons for impairment. *Complete understanding of the client problem promotes accurate determination of client needs and individualizes care.*

• Assess home environment for all barriers to wheelchair access. *If the client resides alone, assess support system for emergency and contingency care (e.g., Lifeline). Impaired mobility may pose a life threat during a crisis (e.g., falls, fire).*

• Assess for skin breakdown. Establish a skin care program to enhance circulation and decrease risk of skin breakdown. *Impaired mobility decreases circulation to dependent areas, placing the client at risk for skin breakdown.*

• Teach advantages, disadvantages, and long-term care involved with various cushions to reduce buttock and sacral pressure during chair sitting. *Air cushions can be changed to optimize flotation and are lightweight but they need reinflation. As flotation increases, a lightweight client's sense of stability may decrease. Gel cushions are durable, however, may be hot, heavy, and create a moist environment. The gel must be pushed back in place to provide pressure relief. Foam cushions are light and inexpensive but they change properties and break down, so may need to be replaced (Paleg 2002).* **Clinical Research:** *Manual wheelchair users identified seating discomfort and back pain as significant problems. Individual seating interventions focused on support for spinal and pelvic posture, pressure distribution, and wheelchair functionality. The majority of subjects experienced pain relief with ergonomic seating interventions (Samuelsson et al, 2001).*

▲ Supply home health aide services as appropriate for assistance with ADLs and skin care. *Mobility impairments may serve as a barrier to self-care.*

▲ Provide support to clients with long-term impairments and their caregivers. Refer to medical social services or mental health/support group services as necessary. *Long-term impairment may necessitate role changes and create anger and frustration. Counseling and support groups provide validation of feelings and alternative methods of problem solving.*

▲ Ensure that the client has information on advocacy, options for disability access, and related issues (e.g., education, personnel, and equipment availability) under the Americans with Disabilities Act. *Information creates the potential for independence (Minor and Minor, 1999).*

• Assess and help develop a plan for client accessibility to key spaces and functions (e.g., toileting upright, sleeping, bathing, and preparing and eating meals). *The ability to perform these activities is critical for staying in one's own home (Yearns and Huntoon, 1997).*

• Rearrange room functions, furniture, and cupboards so that toileting, sleeping, bathing, and preparing and eating meals can take place on one level of the home.

▲ Request a physical therapy referral to teach the client how to build endurance and propel wheelchair on carpet, over doorway thresholds, and on other irregular surfaces,

• = Independent; ▲ = Collaborative

plus how to get back into wheelchair if he or she falls (or intentionally moves) onto the floor.

- Remind clients and family to remove as many wheelchair parts as possible when lifting the chair into the car. Check that armrests or other parts of chair or device are fastened securely before picking them or the chair up. Check temperature of wheelchair or wheeled device in case the surface is excessively hot or cold. *Prevention is important. Removing parts reduces the weight that needs to be lifted, locking parts into place prevents dropping them, and checking temperature of chair and parts prevents skin from being burned or chilled from inadvertent exposure (Younker Rehabilitation Center, 1990).*

- Ensure that indoor traffic patterns are wide enough for a wheelchair or wheeled device to get around in. *Having adequate space prevents damage to skin (especially on knuckles of hands), wheelchair, walls, woodwork, and furniture (Yearns and Huntoon, 1997).*

- Familiarize yourself with literature on universal design concepts to make simple and economic changes such as replacing door hardware with fold-back hinges or doorway encasement removal if doorways are too narrow and removing or replacing doorway thresholds if existing ones are too high. *A branch of the universal design literature deals with ways to modify existing homes (and appliances) to make them more accessible.*

- Explain that a 5-foot turning space is necessary to maneuver a wheelchair in key areas of the home (bathroom, kitchen), doorways need to be 32 to 36 inches wide, ramps or paths ascending to an entrance should slope 1 inch per foot, and one outside entrance should have space enough to open the door and accommodate the wheelchair or wheeled device (Yearns and Huntoon, 1997).

▲ Investigate and share community resources and written information for locating wheelchair parts and services to repair and preventatively tune up devices if the client is not able to do it himself or herself (an annual tune-up is wise).

Client/Family Teaching

- Suggest that the client test-drive wheelchairs and try out cushions and postural supports before purchasing them. *Equipment is very expensive, and different makes and models have different advantages and disadvantages (Minkel, 2000).*

- Instruct and have the client return demonstrate reinflation of pneumatic tires; encourage the client to monitor tire pressure every 2 to 3 weeks. *Low tire pressure impacts the repetitive strain to the shoulder and wrist that occurs with manual wheelchair use.* **Clinical Research:** *Tire pressure that is at or below 50% of what the manufacturer recommends increases wheeling/rolling resistance and energy expenditure (Sawatzky et al, 2002).*

▲ Teach or secure social services referral to educate clients on financial coverage/ regulations of third-party payers and HCFA for durable medical equipment. Realize that light and ultralight wheelchairs may be easier to propel and may be more comfortable and adjustable than heavier models. They initially are expensive, but over time they cost less to operate than heavier chairs. *It is important to recognize the advantages, cost, and durability of different wheelchair models before deciding on a purchase (Cooper et al, 2000).*

- Supervise and reinforce the client's and family's correct performance of pressure relief techniques (which should be performed every 15 minutes). *Pressure relief techniques prevent prolonged pressure to the ischial tuberosities and sacrum during chair sitting (McCourt, 1993; Minkel, 2000).*

- Teach the client to prevent carpal tunnel syndrome and ulnar neuropathy by not putting pressure on the elbows. Client should redistribute pressure along the entire fore-

• = **Independent;** ▲ = **Collaborative**

arm, especially when doing weight shifts and pressure relief techniques. Rest, splints (especially nocturnal), elbow pads, assistance with transfers, and temporary use of an electric wheelchair may help treat upper extremity tendonitis. *Persons who are dependent on manual wheelchairs overwork their arms during transfers, repositioning, ADLs, and when propelling the chair. They are at risk for numerous painful syndromes (Minkel 2000; Congress of Neurological Surgeons 2002).* **Clinical Research:** *Persons with tetraplegia and paraplegia had chronic shoulder pain; the prevalence was higher in those with tetraplegia. Pushing wheelchairs up inclines, wheeling for more than 10 minutes, and sleeping caused pain in both subject groups; tetraplegics had more pain with pushing wheelchairs up ramps and inclines, donning pullover shirts, and driving (Curtis et al, 1999).*

- Teach the client the importance of using seatbelts or chair tie-downs when riding in motor vehicles. If unable to use seat belts or tie-down systems, clients in wheelchairs should be transported in large, heavy vehicles. *Clients need protection for abrupt vehicle maneuvers. They should be restrained with a seatbelt system and/or with a wheelchair tie-down for greater safety. If neither is available, they are more safely transported in large, heavy vehicles (Shaw, 2000).*

evolve WEBSITES FOR EDUCATION

See the EVOLVE website for World Wide Web resources for client education.

REFERENCES

Boninger ML et al: Manual wheelchair pushrim biomechanics and axle position, *Arch Phys Med Rehabil* 81:608, 2000.

Buning ME, Angelo JA, Schmeler MR: Occupational performance and the transition to powered mobility: a pilot study, *Am J Occup Ther* 55(3): 339, 2001.

Cooper RA et al: Long-term rehab: advanced seating systems, parts I and II, *Rehabil Manag* 13(2-3):58, 2000.

Congress of Neurological Surgeons: Medical student curriculum in neurosurgery: diagnosis and management of peripheral nerve injury and entrapment. http://www.neurosurgery.org/cns/meetings/curriculum/dl.html.

Curtis KA et al: Shoulder pain in wheelchair users with tetraplegia and paraplegia, *Arch Phys Med Rehabil* 80: 453, 1999.

Defloor T, Grypdonck MH: Sitting posture and prevention of pressure ulcers, Appl *Nurs Res* 12(3):136, 1999.

Dowswell G, Dowswell T, Young J: Adjusting stroke patients' poor position: an observational study, *J Adv Nurs* 32(2):286, 2000.

Gee ZL, Passarella PM: Nursing care of the stroke patient: therapeutic approach, Pittsburgh, 1985, America Rehabilitation Educational Network.

Halm M: Altered tissue perfusion. In Maas ML et al, editors: *Nursing care of older adults: diagnoses, outcomes, and interventions,* St Louis, 2001, Mosby.

McCourt A: *The specialty practice of rehabilitation nursing: a core curriculum,* ed 3, Skokie, Ill, 1993, Rehabilitation Nursing Foundation.

Minkel JL: Seating and mobility considerations for people with spinal cord injury, *Phys Ther* 80(7):701, 2000.

Minkel JL: Sitting outside of the box, *Rehabil Manag* 14(8):50, 2001.

Minor MAD, Minor SD: *Patient care skills,* ed 4, Stamford, Conn, 1999, Appleton and Lange.

Nyland J et al: Preserving transfer independence among individuals with spinal cord injury, *Spinal Cord* 38:649, 2000.

Paleg G: The prevention struggle, *Rehabil Manag* 15(8):40, 2002.

Panel for the Prediction and Prevention of Pressure Ulcers in Adults: Pressure ulcers in adults: prediction and prevention, Clinical Practice Guideline No. 3, AHCPR publication No. 92-0047, Rockville, Md, 1992, U.S. Department of Health and Human Services, Public Health Service.

• = **Independent;** ▲ = **Collaborative**

Pellow TR: A comparison of interface pressure readings to wheelchair cushions and positioning: a pilot study, *Can J Occup Ther* 66(3):140, 1999.

Pierce LL: Barriers to access: frustrations of people who use a wheelchair for full-time mobility, *Rehabil Nurs* 23(3):120, 1998.

Rader J, Jones D, Miller LL: Individualized wheelchair seating: reducing restraints and improving comfort and function, *Top Geriatr Rehabil* 15(2):34, 1999.

Radwanski MB: Gerontological rehabilitation nursing. In Hoeman SP, editor: *Rehabilitation nursing: process, application, and outcomes*, ed 3, St Louis, 2002, Mosby.

Samuelsson K et al: Wheelchair seating intervention. Results from a client-centered approach, *Disabil Rehabil* 23(15):677, 2001.

Saur T: Long-term rehab: seating and positioning in the newly injured, *Rehabil Manag* 12(6):70, 1999.

Sawatzky BJ, Denison I, Kim W: Rolling, rolling, rolling, *Rehabil Manag* 15(6):36, 2002.

Shaw G: Wheelchair rider risk in motor vehicles: a technical note, *J Rehabil Res Dev* 37(1):89, 2000.

Skidmore-Roth L: *Mosby's nursing drug reference,* St Louis, 2001, Mosby.

Sussman C, Bates-Jensen BM, editors: *Wound care: a collaborative practice manual for physical therapists and nurses,* Gaithersburg, Md, 1998, Aspen.

Wilson G, Kerr VL: Wheelchairs: selection, uses, adaptation, and maintenance. In Sine RD et al, editors: *Basic rehabilitation techniques: a self-instructional guide,* ed 3, Gaithersburg, Md, 1988, Aspen.

Yearns MH, Huntoon R: *A home for all ages: convenient, comfortable, and attractive,* Handout for 47th Annual Conference of the National Council on the Aging, HDFS-H-294, March 1997.

Younker Rehabilitation Center: *Wheelchair mobility class: do's and don'ts,* Physical Therapy Patient Teaching Sheet, No. 105, 1990 (Available from Younker Rehabilitation Center, Iowa Health System, 1200 Pleasant, Des Moines, IA 50309.)

Nausea

Betty J. Ackley and Gail B. Ladwig

NANDA Definition

An unpleasant wave-like sensation in the back of the throat, epigastrium, or throughout the abdomen that may or may not lead to vomiting

Defining Characteristics

Usually precedes vomiting, but may be experienced after vomiting or when vomiting does not occur; accompanied by pallor, cold and clammy skin, increased salivation, tachycardia, gastric stasis, and diarrhea; accompanied by swallowing movements affected by skeletal muscles; reports "nausea" or "sick to stomach"

Related Factors (r/t)

Treatment related

Gastric irritation: pharmaceuticals (e.g., aspirin, nonsteroidal anti-inflammatory drugs, steroids, antibiotics), alcohol, iron, and blood, gastric distention: delayed gastric emptying caused by pharmacological interventions (e.g., narcotics administration, anesthesia agents), pharmaceuticals (e.g., analgesics, antiviral for HIV, aspirin, opioids, chemotherapeutic agents), toxins (e.g., radiotherapy)

Biophysical

Biochemical disorders (e.g., uremia, diabetic ketoacidosis, pregnancy), cardiac pain, cancer of stomach or intra-abdominal tumors (e.g., pelvic or colorectal cancers), esophageal or pancreatic disease, gastric distention due to delayed gastric emptying, pyloric intestinal obstruction, genitourinary and biliary distention, upper bowel stasis, external

• = Independent; ▲ = Collaborative

compression of the stomach (liver, spleen, or other organ enlargement that slows the stomach functioning (squashed stomach syndrome), excess food intake, gastric irritation due to pharyngeal and/or peritoneal inflammation, liver or splenetic capsule stretch, local tumors (e.g., acoustic neuroma, primary or secondary brain tumors, bone metastases at base of skull), motion sickness, Menière's disease, or labyrinthitis

Physical factors
Examples included increased intracranial pressure, meningitis, and toxins (e.g., tumor-produced peptides, abnormal metabolites due to cancer)

Situational
Psychological factors (e.g., pain, fear, anxiety, noxious odors, taste, unpleasant visual stimulation)

NOC   Outcomes (Nursing Outcomes Classification)

Suggested NOC Outcomes
Comfort Level; Hydration; Nutritional Status: Food and Fluid Intake, Nutrient Intake

> **Example NOC Outcome with Indicators**
>
> **Comfort Level** as evidenced by the following indicators: Reported satisfaction with symptom control/ Reported physical well-being (Rate each indicator of **Comfort Level:** 1 = none, 2 = limited, 3 = moderate, 4 = substantial, 5 = extensive [see Section I].)

Client Outcomes

Client Will (Specify Time Frame):
- State relief of nausea
- Explain methods they can use to decrease nausea and vomiting (N&V)

NIC   Interventions (Nursing Interventions Classification)

Suggested NIC Interventions
Distraction; Medication Administration; Progressive Muscle Relaxation; Simple Guided Imagery; Therapeutic Touch

> **Example NIC Activities—Distraction**
>
> Encourage the client to choose the distraction technique(s) desired, such as music, engaging in conversation or telling a detailed account of event or story, guided imagery, or humor; Advise the client to practice the distraction technique before it is needed, if possible

Nursing Interventions and Rationales
- Determine cause of N&V (e.g., medication effects, viral illness, food poisoning, extreme anxiety, pregnancy). **Nursing Research:** *Nurses are in a position to identify clients at highest risk for developing anticipatory nausea and to implement strategies to prevent/ minimize it (Eckert, 2001).*
- Keep a clean emesis basin and tissues within the client's reach.

- = **Independent;** ▲ = **Collaborative**

- Provide oral care after the client vomits. *Oral care helps remove the taste and smell of vomitus, thus reducing the stimulus for further vomiting.*
- Stay with the client to give support, place hand on shoulder, and hold the emesis basin. *Human support can be helpful and comforting to an uncomfortable client (Morse, Bottorf, and Hutchinson, 1994).*
- Provide distraction from sensation of nausea using soft music, television, and videos per the client preference. *Distraction can help direct attention away from the sensation of nausea. Music therapy has been shown to decrease N&V (Ezzone et al, 1998).*
- Maintain a quiet, well-ventilated environment. *Odors from a kitchen or bathroom can trigger nausea (Pervan, 1990; Quinton, 1998).*
- Avoid sudden movement of the client; allow the client to lie still. *Movement can trigger further N&V.*
- After vomiting is controlled and nausea abates, begin feeding the client small amounts of clear fluids such as clear soda or preferably ginger ale, and then crackers; progress to a soft diet. *Ginger root (found in some ginger ales) has been shown to be more effective than a placebo for treatment of postoperative N&V (Hawthorn, 1995; Thompson, 1999).*
- Remove cover of food tray before bringing it into the client's room. *The sudden, concentrated food odors that come when the cover is removed in front of the client can trigger nausea (Hawthorn, 1995, Quinton, 1998).*
- ▲ Refer HIV-positive clients for management of antiretroviral-related nausea. **Nursing Research:** *A prospective time series design was used to assess the rate, severity, and distress of nausea in a cohort of 75 HIV-positive patients who were beginning or changing a combination of two or more antiretroviral medications. Nausea associated with combination antiretroviral therapy was quite common and may adversely affect medication adherence (Reynolds and Neidig, 2002).*

Nausea in pregnancy

- Recommend that the woman eat dry crackers or dry toast in bed before arising and then get up slowly. Also advise to chew gum or suck hard candies, eat small frequent meals, avoid foods with offensive odors, and avoid preparing food or shopping when nauseated. *These are traditional strategies for alleviating nausea (Whitney et al, 2001).*
- Recommend that she sit down when experiencing nausea. **Clinical Research:** *Women undergoing gynecological surgery presenting with orthostatic dysregulation and arterial hypotension in their history exhibit an increased risk of PONV (Pusch et al, 2002).*
- Determine if the woman is receiving adequate rest. *Fatigue predisposes to morning sickness (Rhodes et al, 1995).*
- ▲ Discuss with the client the possibility of using transcutaneous electrical stimulation in the form of Relief Band Device (Woodside Biomedical) to help relieve nausea. **Evidence-Based Research:** *The results of a systematic review of the studies showed that the results of using P6 acupressure are generally positive (Jewell and Young, 2002).*
- ▲ Consider the use of continuous acupressure at P6 applied by Sea-Bands with acupressure buttons to both wrists or P6 acupressure. **Nursing and Clinical Research:** *In this convenience sample of English-speaking, healthy pregnant women in their first trimester who had at least one episode of nausea, vomiting, or both before their prenatal clinic/office visit, Sea-Bands with acupressure buttons were demonstrated to be a noninvasive, inexpensive, safe, and effective treatment for the N&V of pregnancy (Steele et al, 2001).*

• = **Independent;** ▲ = **Collaborative**

Evidence-Based Research: *P6 acupressure reduced the frequency of nausea in early pregnancy (Jewell and Young, 2002).*
▲ Refer for acupuncture. Clinical Research: *Acupuncture is an effective treatment for women who experience nausea and dry retching in early pregnancy (Smith, Crowther, and Beilby, 2002).*
▲ Refer for antiemetic medication, vitamin B_6 (pyridoxine). Evidence-Based Research: *Pyridoxine appears to be more effective in reducing the severity of nausea in pregnancy, but there is very little information on fetal effects (Jewell and Young, 2002).*

Nausea following surgery

• Consider use of a recliner chair postoperatively if not contraindicated. Nursing Research and Clinical Study: *A randomized study was conducted to evaluate two methods of recovery positioning and to examine factors that affect home readiness (e.g., voiding, intake) for postsurgical laparoscopy patients. Subjects in the experimental group recovered in a "recliner-chair," which was adjustable by the patient for comfort. Patients in the recliner-chair group had fewer adverse symptoms such as nausea, severe pain, and delayed voiding (Agodoa et al, 2002).*
▲ Alleviate postoperative pain using ordered analgesic agents (refer to care plan for Acute Pain). *The pain sensation is known to be a factor in the development of postoperative N&V (Thompson, 1999).*
▲ If nausea is associated with the use of opioids, consult with primary care practitioner for possible use of alternative pain medication and consider the possible use of olanzapine as an antiemetic for advanced cancer patients. *Opioids can cause nausea in the postoperative client (Thompson, 1999).* Clinical Research: *This open-label pilot study suggest an antiemetic effect of olanzapine, an atypical antipsychotic, in patients with advanced cancer requiring opioid analgesics for pain (Passik et al, 2002).*
▲ Refer for possible use of isopropyl alcohol (IPA) inhalation for treatment of postoperative N&V for patients who have general anesthesia for a surgical procedure. Nursing Research: *The results of this show IPA to be effective for postoperative N&V and that there was no significant difference between the standard treatment protocol or antiemetics and treatment with IPA. Treatment with IPA was significantly more cost effective than standard drug treatment (Merritt, Okyere, and Jasinski, 2002).*
• Ensure that the nauseated client is not hypotensive. Check blood pressure and note signs of postural hypotension. *Postural hypotension can be caused by deficient fluid volume following surgery and can result in nausea (Thompson, 1999).*
▲ Consult with primary care practitioner for use of nonpharmacological techniques such as acupuncture, electroacupuncture, acupoint stimulation, transcutaneous electrical nerve stimulation, or acupressure as an adjunct for controlling postoperative N&V. Give the treatment soon after surgery. Clinical Research: *Nonpharmacological techniques demonstrated that they were equivalent to commonly used antiemetic drugs in preventing vomiting following surgery, especially within 6 hours of surgery in adults. These techniques were not of benefit in children (Lee and Done, 1999). Acupressure with sea bands can be taught to clients, is harmless, and may provide relief from postoperative N&V (Mann, 1999).*
▲ Teach the use of acupressure on two acupressure points on the wrist. Nursing and Clinical Research: *This study confirmed the effectiveness of acupressure in preventing postoperative N&V (Ming et al, 2002).*

• = Independent; ▲ = Collaborative

- Use relaxation and distraction techniques for nausea: encourage the client to take slow, deep breaths. *Deep breaths can serve as a distraction technique and can help rid the body of the anesthetic agent (Thompson, 1999).* **Nursing Research:** *Eight Chinese breast cancer patients receiving doxorubicin and cyclophosphamide demonstrated that progressive muscle relaxation treatment is an effective adjuvant method to decrease N&V in chemotherapy recipients (Molassiotis, 2000).*

Nausea following chemotherapy

▲ Use antiemetics and nursing interventions of increased access to support and increased information. **Nursing Research:** *In comparative antiemetic trials of 162 women with ovarian cancer receiving cisplatin-based chemotherapy, the group receiving antiemetics and the nursing intervention above reported less nausea (Borjeson et al, 2002).*

▲ Consult with physician regarding need for antiemetic medications. *N&V is among the most distressing side effects of chemotherapy (Bender et al, 2002). There are antiemetic drugs that can be very effective for clients with nausea from chemotherapy (Glicket et al, 1998; Goebel, 1996). Recognize that opioids used to treat pain may also result in nausea, but generally it is short in duration (Aparasu, 1999).*

▲ Consult with primary care provider on the use of transcutaneous electrical nerve stimulation as an adjunct for controlling chemotherapy-induced N&V. *Antiemetic medications may stop vomiting, but not nausea (Roscoe et al, 2000). Transcutaneous electric nerve stimulation, using the ReliefBand, was shown to be an effective adjunct to medications for controlling nausea in gynecological oncology clients (Pearl et al, 1999).*

▲ Help the client learn how to use acupressure for nausea, applying pressure bilaterally at P6 and ST36 acupressure points on the back of the wrist and by the knee. *Finger acupressure may be effective to relieve chemotherapy-induced nausea (Dibble et al, 2000).*

- Offer the nauseated client a 10-minute foot massage. **Nursing Research:** *Foot massage was shown to be an effective way to decrease nausea, pain, and anxiety in a group of oncology clients (Grealish, Lomasney, and Whiteman, 2000).*

▲ For clients who continue to experience nausea after antiemetic drugs or other treatments, consult with the primary care practitioner regarding the possibility of using acupuncture or transcutaneous nerve stimulation wristband. to control N&V. *Acupuncture has been shown to effectively control chemotherapy-induced N&V in adults (Acupuncture, 2000; Kaplan, LaRiccia, and Pian-Smith, 1999). Nerve stimulation for this patient receiving methotrexate demonstrated it as a valid alternative to other first-line antiemetic therapies (Wilson, 2002).*

Geriatrics

▲ Administer antiemetic drugs carefully; watch for side effects. *Elderly clients have increased risk of side effects, such as extrapyramidal effects or sedation, from antiemetic drugs (Johnson et al, 1997).*

Home care

- Above interventions may be adapted for home care use.
- Assist the client and family with identifying and avoiding irritants in the home setting that exacerbates nausea (e.g., strong odors from food, plants, perfume, and room deodorizers).

• = **Independent;** ▲ = **Collaborative**

Client/Family Teaching

- Teach the client techniques to use when uncomfortable, including relaxation techniques, guided imagery, hypnosis, and music therapy (Jablonski, 1993; Pervan, 1993; Rhodes et al, 1995). *Guided imagery has been shown to effectively decrease nausea associated with chemotherapy (Troesch, 1993). Behavioral interventions for nausea such as hypnosis, progressive muscle relaxation training, systematic desensitization, biofeedback, and distractions have also been shown to be effective (Dodd, 1993). Music therapy has been shown to be helpful for decreasing N&V in clients receiving high-dose chemotherapy (Ezzone et al, 1998).*

evolve WEBSITES FOR EDUCATION

See the EVOLVE website for World Wide Web resources for client education.

REFERENCES

Acupuncture: National Institutes of Health consensus development conference statement, *Dermatol Nurs* 12(2): 126, 2000.

Agodoa SE, Holder MA, Fowler SM: Effects of recliner-chair versus traditional hospital bed on postsurgical diagnostic laparoscopic recovery time, *J Perianesth Nurs* 17(5):318, 2002.

Aparasu R et al: Opioid-induced emesis among hospitalized nonsurgical patients: effect on pain and quality of life, *J Pain Sympt Manag* 8(4):280, 1999.

Bender CM et al: Chemotherapy-induced nausea and vomiting, *Clin J Oncol Nurs* 6(2):94, 2002.

Borjeson S et al: Treatment of nausea and emesis during cancer chemotherapy. Discrepancies between antiemetic effect and well-being, *J Pain Sympt Manag* 24(3):345, 2002.

Dibble SL et al: Acupressure for nausea: results of a pilot study, *Oncol Nurs Forum* 27(1):41, 2000.

Dodd MJ: Side effects of cancer chemotherapy, *Annu Rev Nurs Res* 11:77, 1993.

Eckert RM: Understanding anticipatory nausea, *Oncol Nurs Forum* 28(10):1553, 2001.

Ezzone S et al: Music as an adjunct to antiemetic therapy, *Oncol Nurs Forum* 25(9):1551, 1998.

Glick JH, Griffith RS, Mortimer JE: Cancer treatment, chemotherapy: helping the patient cope, *Patient Care* 32(1):49, 1998.

Goebel C: Prevention and control of nausea and vomiting for patients with cancer, *Home Healthc Nurse* 14:15, 1996.

Grealish L, Lomasney A, Whiteman B: Foot massage: a nursing intervention to modify the distressing symptoms of pain and nausea in patients hospitalized with cancer, *Cancer Nurs* 23(3):237, 2000.

Hawthorn J: *Understanding and management of nausea and vomiting,* Oxford, 1995, Blackwell Science.

Jablonski RS: Nausea: the forgotten symptom, *Holist Nurs Pract* 7:64, 1993.

Jewell D, Young G: Interventions for nausea and vomiting in early pregnancy, *Cochrane Database Syst Rev* (2): CD000145, 2002.

Johnson MH, Moroney CE, Gay CF: Relieving nausea and vomiting in patients with cancer: a treatment algorithm, *Oncol Nurs Forum* 24(1):51, 1997.

Kaplan G, LaRiccia PJ, Pian-Smith M: Acupuncture: another therapeutic choice? *Patient Care* 33(11):149, 1999.

Lee A, Done ML: The use of nonpharmacologic techniques to prevent postoperative nausea and vomiting: a meta-analysis, *Anesth Analg* 88(6):1362 1999.

Mann E: Using acupuncture and acupressure to treat postoperative emesis, *Prof Nurs* 14(10):691, 1999.

Merritt BA, Okyere CP, Jasinski DM: Isopropyl alcohol inhalation: alternative treatment of postoperative nausea and vomiting, *Nurs Res* 51(2):125, 2002.

Ming JL et al: The efficacy of acupressure to prevent nausea and vomiting in post-operative patients, *J Adv Nurs* 39(4):343, 2002.

Molassiotis A: A pilot study of the use of progressive muscle relaxation training in the management of post-chemotherapy nausea and vomiting, *Eur J Cancer Care (Engl)* 9(4):230, 2000.

Morse JM, Bottorff JL, Hutchinson S: The phenomenology of comfort, *J Adv Nurs* 20:189, 1994.

• = **Independent**; ▲ = **Collaborative**

Passik SD et al: A pilot exploration of the antiemetic activity of olanzapine for the relief of nausea in patients with advanced cancer and pain, *J Pain Sympt Manag* 23(6):526, 2002.

Pearl ML et al: Transcutaneous electrical nerve stimulation as an adjunct for controlling chemotherapy-induced nausea and vomiting in gynecologic oncology patients, *Cancer Nurs* 22(4):307, 1999.

Pervan V: Practical aspects of dealing with cancer therapy–induced nausea and vomiting, *Semin Oncol Nurs* 6:3, 1990.

Pervan V: Understanding anti-emetics, *Nurs Times* 89(10):36, 1993.

Pusch F et al: Preoperative orthostatic dysfunction is associated with an increased incidence of postoperative nausea and vomiting, *Anesthesiology* 96(6):1381, 2002.

Quinton D: Anticipatory nausea and vomiting in chemotherapy, *Prof Nurse* 13(10):663, 1998.

Reynolds NR, Neidig JL: Characteristics of nausea reported by HIV-infected patients initiating combination antiretroviral regimens, *Clin Nurs Res* 11(1):71, 2002.

Rhodes VA, Johnson MH, McDaniel RW: Nausea, vomiting, and retching: the management of the symptom experience, *Semin Oncol Nurs* 11:256, 1995.

Roscoe J et al: Nausea and vomiting remain a significant clinical problem: trends over time in controlling chemotherapy-induced nausea and vomiting in 1413 patients treated in community clinical practices, *J Pain Sympt Manag* 20(2):113, 2000.

Smith C, Crowther C, Beilby J: Acupuncture to treat nausea and vomiting in early pregnancy: a randomized controlled trial, *Birth* 29(1):1, 2002.

Steele NM et al: Effect of acupressure by Sea-Bands on nausea and vomiting of pregnancy, *J Obstet Gynecol Neonatal Nurs* 30(1):61, 2001.

Thompson HJ: The management of post-operative nausea and vomiting, *J Adv Nurs* 29(5):1130, 1999.

Troesch LM et al: The influence of guided imagery on chemotherapy-related nausea and vomiting, *Oncol Nurs Forum* 20:1179, 1993.

Whitney EN et al: *Nutrition for health and health care,* ed 2, Belmont, Calif, 2001, Wadsworth.

Wilson JK et al: Use of transcutaneous nerve stimulation wristband to treat methotrexate-induced nausea, *J Cutan Med Surg* 6(6):551, 2002.

Unilateral Neglect

Betty J. Ackley and Leslie Kalbach

NANDA Definition

Lack of awareness and attention to one side of the body

Defining Characteristics

Consistent inattention to stimuli on an affected side; does not look toward affected side; inadequate positioning and/or safety precautions with regard to the affected side; inadequate self-care; leaves food on plate on the affected side

Related Factors (r/t)

Effects of disturbed perceptual abilities (e.g., hemianopsia [one-sided blindness], neurological illnesses, trauma)

NOTE: Because the right hemisphere is dominant in directing attention, unilateral neglect is more common if neurological pathology occurs in the right hemisphere of the brain, which results in left-sided neglect (Katz et al, 2000). Also, unilateral neglect frequently occurs with damage to the right parietal lobe, the right frontal lobe, the thalamus, and basal ganglia (Pierce and Buxbaum, 2002).

• = Independent; ▲ = Collaborative

| **NOC** | Outcomes (Nursing Outcomes Classification) |

Suggested NOC Outcomes
Body Image; Body Positioning: Self-Initiated; Self-Care: Activities of Daily Living (ADL)

> **Example NOC Outcome with Indicators**
>
> **Body Image** as evidenced by the following indicators: Willingness to touch affected body part/Adjustment to changes in body function/Willingness to use strategies to enhance appearance and function (Rate each indicator of **Body Image**: 1 = never positive, 2 = rarely positive, 3 = sometimes positive, 4 = often positive, 5 = consistently positive [see Section I].)

Client Outcomes

Client Will (Specify Time Frame):
- Demonstrate techniques that can be used to minimize unilateral neglect
- Care for both sides of the body appropriately and keep affected side free from harm

| **NIC** | Interventions (Nursing Interventions Classification) |

Suggested NIC Intervention
Unilateral Neglect Management

> **Example NIC Activities—Unilateral Neglect Management**
>
> Provide realistic feedback about patient's perceptual deficit; Touch unaffected shoulder when initiating conversation

Nursing Interventions and Rationales

- Monitor the client for signs of unilateral neglect (e.g., not washing, shaving, or dressing one side of the body; sitting or lying inappropriately on affected arm or leg; failing to respond to stimuli on the contralateral side of lesion; eating food on only one side of plate; or failing to look to one side of the body). *Looking, listening, touching, and searching deficits occur on the affected side of the body and may or may not be associated with a loss of vision, sensation, or motion on the affected side (Herman, 1992; Kalbach, 1991).*
- If available, use the "star cancellation test" to evaluate presence of unilateral neglect. **Clinical Research:** *The star cancellation test consists of a series of big and little stars and words scattered on a page. When directed to cross out all the little stars, clients with unilateral neglect will miss stars on one side of the paper (Halligan et al, 1989; Taylor et al, 1994).*
- Use the Draw-A-Man test as a means of verifying the presence of unilateral neglect. **Clinical Research:** *The Draw-A-Man test is a valid and reliable method of determining clients who have unilateral neglect (Chen-Sea, 2000).*
- Provide a safe, well-lighted, and clutter-free environment. Place call light on unaffected side. Keep side rails up when the client is in bed. Cue the client to environmental hazards when mobile. *Cognitive impairment may accompany neglect; safety is of paramount importance.*

• = Independent; ▲ = Collaborative

- Nursing interventions for clients with unilateral neglect should be implemented in the following stages as the client progresses:
  Stage I: Focus attention mainly on nonneglected side.
  - Set up environment so that most activity is on unaffected side.
  - Keep the client's personal items within view and on unaffected side.
  - Position the client's bed so that activity is on unaffected side.
  The initial priority is client safety (Kalbach, 1991).
  Stage II: Help the client develop an awareness of neglected side.
  - Gradually focus the client's attention on affected side.
  - Gradually move personal items and activity to affected side.
  - Stand on the client's affected side when assisting with ambulation or ADLs.
  The goal now is for the client to develop an awareness of the neglected side (Kalbach, 1991).
  Stage III: Help the client develop ability to compensate for neglect.
  - Encourage the client to bathe and groom affected side first.
  - Focus touch and talking on affected side; use a positive approach (e.g., "Mary, turn your head to the left and you'll see your grandchildren" [Carnevali and Patrick, 1993]).
  - Use constant and positive reminders to keep the client scanning the entire environment.
  - Use bright yellow or red stickers on outer margins in reading or writing exercises. Have the client look for the sticker before reading or writing.
  - Help the client do ordinary tasks, compensating for their neglect situation.
  Use cues and anchors to promote attention to the neglected side and help the client develop compensatory mechanisms to deal with the neglect syndrome (Kalbach, 1991; Cooke, 1992; Riddoch and Humphreys, 1983). **Clinical Research:** *A study demonstrated that clients discovered and gradually compensated for their unilateral neglect during meaningful occupational or life situations (Tham, Borell, and Gustavsson, 2000).*
- ▲ Refer to a rehabilitation nurse specialist, a neuropsychologist, or an occupational therapist for continued help in dealing with unilateral neglect. *There are a number of different treatments for unilateral neglect, some of them effective, others with limited evidence of lasting improvement (Pierce and Buxbaum, 2002). Both the occupational therapist and the neuropsychologist can help to ameliorate symptoms of unilateral neglect (Freeman, 2001; Riddoch et al, 1995).* **Clinical Research:** *Research has shown that there is some evidence that cognitive rehabilitation for unilateral spatial neglect improves performance but its effect on disability is not clear. Further studies are needed (Bowen et al, 2002).*

Home care

- Many of the listed interventions may be adapted for use in the home care setting.

Client/Family Teaching

- Explain pathology and symptoms of unilateral neglect to both the client and family.
- Teach the client how to scan regularly to check the position of body parts and to regularly turn head from side to side for safety when ambulating, using a wheelchair, or doing other tasks. Recommend the client think of self like a horizon-illuminating lighthouse. **Clinical Research:** *The use of the visual image of being a lighthouse was shown to improve function in a neglect client when walking, using a wheelchair, or engaging in problem-solving activities (Niemeier, Cifu, and Kishore, 2001).*

- = Independent; ▲ = Collaborative

- Teach caregivers positive cueing (reminders to help the client remember to interact with entire environment).

evolve WEBSITES FOR EDUCATION

See the EVOLVE website for World Wide Web resources for client education.

REFERENCES

Bowen A, Lincoln NB, Dewey M: Cognitive rehabilitation for spatial neglect following stroke, *Cochrane Database Syst Rev* CD003586, 2002.

Carnevali DL, Patrick M: *Nursing management for the elderly,* ed 3, Philadelphia, 1993, Lippincott.

Cooke D: Remediation of unilateral neglect: what do we know? *Aust Occup Ther J* 39:19, 1992.

Freeman E: Unilateral spatial neglect: new treatment approaches with potential application to occupational therapy, *Am J Occup Ther* 55:401, 2001.

Halligan PW, Marshall JC, Wade DT: Visuospatial neglect: underlying factors and test sensitivity, *Lancet* 2(8668):908, 1989.

Herman EW: Spatial neglect: new issues and their implications for occupational therapy practice, *Am J Occup Ther* 46:207, 1992.

Kalbach LR: Unilateral neglect: mechanisms and nursing care, *J Neurosci Nurs* 23:125, 1991.

Katz N et al: Relationships of cognitive performance and daily function of clients following right hemisphere stroke: predictive and ecological validity of the LOTCA Battery, *Occup Ther J Res* 20(1):3, 2000.

Niemeier JP, Cifu DX, Kishore R: The lighthouse strategy: improving the functional status of patients with unilateral neglect after stroke and brain injury using a visual imagery intervention, *Top Stroke Rehabil* 8(2): 10, 2001.

Pierce SM, Buxbaum LJ: Treatments of unilateral neglect: a review, *Arch Phys Med Rehabil* 83:256, 2002.

Riddoch MF, Humphreys GW: The effect of cueing on unilateral neglect, *Neuropsychologist* 21:589, 1983.

Riddoch MF, Humphreys GW, Bateman A: Cognitive deficits following stroke, *Physiotherapy* 81:465, 1995.

Taylor D, Ashburn A, Ward CD: Asymmetrical trunk posture, unilateral neglect and motor performance following stroke, *Clin Rehabil* 8:48, 1994.

Tham K, Borell L, Gustavsson A: The discovery of disability: a phenomenological study of unilateral neglect, *Am J Occup Ther* 54(4):398, 2000.

Noncompliance

Betty J. Ackley and Gail B. Ladwig

NANDA Definition

Behavior of person and/or caregiver that fails to coincide with a health-promoting or therapeutic plan agreed on by the person (and/or family and/or community) and health care professional; in the presence of an agreed-on, health-promoting, or therapeutic plan, person's or caregiver's behavior is fully or partially nonadherent and may lead to clinically ineffective or partially ineffective outcomes

Defining Characteristics

Behavior indicative of failure to adhere (directly observed or verbalized by patient or significant others) (critical); objective tests (e.g., physiological measures, detection of markers); evidence of development of complications; evidence of exacerbation of symptoms; failure to keep appointments; failure to progress

• = Independent; ▲ = Collaborative

Related Factors (r/t)

Health care plan
Duration; significant others; cost; intensity; complexity

Individual factors
Personal and developmental abilities; health beliefs, cultural influences, spiritual values; individual's value system; knowledge and skill relevant to the regimen behavior; motivational forces

Health system
Satisfaction with care; credibility of provider; access and convenience of care; financial flexibility of plan; client-provider relationships; provider reimbursement of teaching and follow-up; provider continuity and regular follow-up; individual health coverage; communication and teaching skills of the provider

Network
Involvement of members in health plan; social value regarding plan; perceived beliefs of significant others

NOTE: The nursing diagnosis Noncompliance is judgmental and places blame on the client (Bakker, Kastermans, and Dassen, 1995; Ward-Collins, 1998). The author recommends use of the diagnosis Ineffective Therapeutic regimen management in place of the diagnosis **Noncompliance.** The diagnosis **Ineffective Therapeutic regimen management** has interventions that are developed by both the health care providers and the client. It is a more respectful and efficacious nursing diagnosis than **Noncompliance.**

NOC   Outcomes (Nursing Outcomes Classification)

Suggested NOC Outcomes
Adherence Behavior; Compliance Behavior; Pain Level; Symptom Control; Treatment Behavior: Illness or Injury

> **Example NOC Outcome with Indicators**
>
> **Adherence Behavior** as evidenced by the following indicators: Describes strategies to maximize health/ Describes strategies to eliminate unhealthy behavior/Provides rationale for adopting a regimen/Reports using strategies to eliminate unhealthy behavior (Rate each indicator of **Adherence Behavior:** 1 = never demonstrated, 2 = rarely demonstrated, 3 = sometimes demonstrated, 4 = often demonstrated, 5 = consistently demonstrated [see Section I].)

Client Outcomes

Client Will (Specify Time Frame):
- Describe consequence of continued noncompliance with treatment regimen
- State goals for health and the means by which to obtain them
- Communicate an understanding of disease and treatment
- List treatment regimens and expectations and agree to follow through
- List alternative ways to meet goals
- Describe the importance of family participation to help achieve goals

• = Independent; ▲ = Collaborative

| **NIC** | **Interventions (Nursing Interventions Classification)** |

Suggested NIC Interventions
Health System Guidance; Self-Modification Assistance

Example NIC Activities—Health System Guidance

Inform the client of appropriate community resources and contact persons; Inform the client how to access emergency services by telephone and vehicle, as appropriate

Nursing Interventions and Rationales

- Ask the client why he or she has not complied with the prescribed treatment. Have the client "tell his or her story." Listen nonjudgmentally. *Compliance assessment should begin with a nonthreatening discussion with the client (Kluckowski, 1992; London, 1998).* **Nursing Research:** *Nonadherence to antiretroviral (ARV) regimens has been associated with HIV drug resistance; 68% of respondents missed doses of ARV—54% because they forgot. Fifty-four percent stated that they did not report the nonadherence to their doctor. They were more likely to miss the lunchtime dosage (n = 49, p < 0.05) (Cummins et al, 2003).*
- Make the client an active partner in his or her own health care management. Recognize that the client has absolute control over whether he or she follows the health care regimen. Always treat the client with respect, and develop mutual outcomes for treatment. *If the client feels respected and is involved in decision making, compliance will increase. Many clients report that how they are treated by health professionals has a great impact on whether they follow advice (Lannon, 1997).*
- Observe for cause of noncompliance (see Related Factors). Recognize that noncompliance is very common. **Nursing Research:** *Adherence to treatment among persons with chronic disorders constitutes a significant problem; half of clients have difficulty following their regimen (Dunbar-Jacob et al, 2000).*
- Recognize that behavioral change comes slowly, and often in stages (Prochaska, 1994):
  - Precontemplation—change is not contemplated; unaware of problem or risk
  - Contemplation—aware that problem exists; no specific plans or commitment to change
  - Preparation—plan to take action within the next 30 days
  - Action—now taking action to improve health; often behavior not consistently carried out
  - Maintenance—consistently engages in healthful behavior for more than 6 months

  Individuals tend to cycle through the stages of change, often not in a linear progression, and may go through the cycle several times. The most important thing is unconditional acceptance of the person, understanding of the behavior, and subtle encouragement when asked. Make information available, but do not preach or force information on clients (Samuelson, 1998).
- If the client is in denial: provide information, communicate unconditional positive regard, avoid distancing yourself, and look for opportunities for authentic contact with your client, being present psychologically and physically. *The most important thing you can do for someone who appears to be in denial is to take the time to genuinely connect (Robinson, 1999).*

- = Independent; ▲ = Collaborative

- Determine the client's and family's knowledge of illness and treatment. Teach them about the illness and purpose of the treatment regimen if necessary. *Knowledge is power, and with it comes increased control; the more control clients have, the more likely they are to comply with the prescribed regimen (Kluckowski, 1992).*
- Observe whether locus of control is internal or external. Recognize that people with external locus of control are more likely to be noncompliant because they do not believe they can help themselves. They believe that it is a matter of luck or destiny that they are ill. *Clients with an internal locus of control are more compliant (Muscari, 1998; Warren, 1992).*
- ▲ Monitor the client for signs of depression that may cause noncompliance. Refer for treatment if appropriate. **Nursing Research:** *Depression can cause increased incidence of "source memory errors," resulting in the client being unable to remember if he or she did something or just thought about doing it, which can be very serious when it involves taking needed medications (Elias, 2001). Depression can also cause apathy, in which case the client does not care whether he or she takes needed actions for health.*
- Monitor the client's ability to follow directions, solve problems, concentrate, and read. **Clinical Research:** *A national survey found that almost half of the adult population has deficiencies in reading or computation skills. Literacy is defined as the basic ability to read and speak English, whereas functional health literacy is the ability to read, understand, and act on health information. Up to 48% of English-speaking patients do not have adequate functional health literacy (Andrus and Roth, 2002).* **Clinical Research:** *More than 90 million Americans have limited literacy skills. Almost 2 million U.S. residents cannot speak English, and millions more speak it poorly (Dreger and Tremback, 2001).*
- Avoid using threats, pressure, and inappropriate fear arousal to increase compliance. *These measures are unethical and generally ineffective. If clients are "browbeaten" and attempts are made to shame, induce guilt, or embarrass the client, the noncompliant client will only dig deeper in his or her resolve not to change (Samuelson, 1998).*
- Determine whether the client's support system helps or hinders therapy. Bring family members and significant others into the educational process as desired by the client. *A positive social support system is associated with increased compliance (Warren, 1992).* **Clinical Research:** *Schizophrenic clients who have little family support are more likely to be noncompliant than are those with family support, especially if there is a history of substance abuse and difficulty recognizing own symptoms (Olfson et al, 2000).*
- Develop therapeutic relationship based on active listening. *Good communication has been shown to increase compliance (Crane, Kirby, and Kooperman, 1996). Compliance is increased when the client feels that the health care provider is interested in and genuinely cares about the client (Warren, 1992).*
- Listen to the client's descriptions of abilities; encourage the client to use these abilities in self-care. When dealing with complex health care regimens, start the client with small behavioral changes (e.g., have chemotherapy client rinse mouth with a saliva substitute twice daily). When one step has been accomplished, add another step. *The client is often overwhelmed by what is expected and needs help with managing behavioral changes (Boehm, 1992).*
- Work with the client to develop cues that trigger-needed health care behaviors (e.g., checking blood sugar level before putting on makeup each morning), including weekends, holidays, and vacations. *Associating cues with desired behaviors increases the frequency of these behaviors. Compliance often decreases when the client no longer has a usual routine.*

- = Independent; ▲ = Collaborative

- Work with the client to develop an instruction and reminder sheet that fits medications and treatments into the client's lifestyle. *Visual reminders help increase compliance.*
- Observe the noncompliant client for possibility of secondary gain such as increased attention if the client continues to be ill and noncompliant. *Adolescent clients may use noncompliance as a passive form of manipulation to control their relationships with others to avoid school, work, or the legal system. Also, sometimes the illness has become part of the client's self-concept and identity and therefore meets needs (Muscari, 1998).*
- ▲ For a chronically ill client, develop a multidisciplinary team to provide care, including a nurse, physician, pharmacist, dietitian, and additional therapists as needed. Have team meetings to ensure continuity of care. *Multidisciplinary team care has been shown to increase compliance (Warren, 1992).*
- ▲ Consider allowing the client to take his or her own medications while in the hospital if appropriate. *Clients who learned to take medications successfully in the hospital were less likely to be readmitted in a group of mental health clients (DeProspero and Riffle, 1997).*
- Develop a mutually agreed-on written contract with the client regarding needed health care behaviors; give reinforcement as the client meets defined goals. *A client contract that helps the client analyze behaviors and choose behavioral strategies can be very effective in changing health care behaviors (Boehm, 1992; Simons, 1999).*
- ▲ Consult with primary care practitioner regarding the possibility of simplifying the health care regimen so that it more easily fits into the client's lifestyle (e.g., taking medications one time per day versus four times per day). *Complex regimens and inconvenient dose scheduling decrease compliance (Crane, Kirby, and Kooperman, 1996).*
- ▲ Refer for compliance therapy (motivational interviewing and cognitive behavioral therapy) for medication management for clients with schizophrenia **Nursing Research:** *Failure to keep up their antipsychotic medication is a major cause of relapse in people with psychosis. Compliance therapy is effective in enhancing concordance and reducing the risk of relapse (Gray, Robson, and Bressington, 2002).* **Nursing Research:** *Compliance therapy, based on cognitive-behavioral techniques, appears to be effective in enhancing compliance and preventing relapse in people with schizophrenia on antipsychotic medication (Gray, Wykes, and Gournay, 2002).*

Geriatric

- ▲ If the client has sensory and coordination deficits, use a medication organizer and have the home health nurse or family place the client's medications in daily compartments. *Careful labeling, self-administration of medicine programs, simplification of drug regimens, and the use of medication compliance devices can help to promote patient adherence in older patients (McGraw and Drennan, 2001).*
- Help the client feel like a partner in managing health care condition; use caring, encouragement, written goals, and a "power with" relationship with nurse. **Nursing Research:** *These methods have been shown to increase self-efficacy and empower both teenagers and elderly clients to manage their condition (Muscari, 1998; Resnick, 1996).*
- ▲ Ask clients if they can afford medications. Refer for financial help from social worker or case manager if needed. *The cost of therapeutic regimen may be a source of noncompliance, especially in the elderly (De Geest, 1998).*
- ▲ Monitor the client for signs of depression associated with noncompliance (e.g., refusing to eat or take medications). Refer the client for treatment of depression as needed. *Noncompliance in the elderly may be a form of indirect self-destructive behavior that is associated with depression and leads to suicide (Meisekothen, 1993).* **Nursing Re-**

- = Independent; ▲ = Collaborative

search: *One study demonstrated that depressed clients were three times more likely than non-depressed clients to be noncompliant (DiMatteo, Lepper, and Croghan, 2000).*

- Use repetition, verbal cues, and memory aids such as pictures, schedule, or reminder sheet when teaching the health care regimen. Use events such as meals, bedtime, etc, as reminders when to take medications. **Nursing Research:** *There may be age-related memory deficits that necessitate an increased use of measures that cue the client to perform needed health care behaviors (De Geest, 1998; Dunbar-Jacob et al, 2000). This research investigated the type of memory strategies used by older adults living independently in the community in adhering to their prescription medications. Older adults reported greater use of internal memory strategies and a preference for event-based over time-based prescription medication instructions (Branin, 2001).*
- Consider assistive medication technology: talking reminders, pill dispensers, etc. *Elderly clients are relying on technology to help them adhere to increasingly complex medication regimens (McGarry and Logue, 2002).*

Multicultural

- Assess for the influence of cultural beliefs, norms, and values on the client's ability to modify health behavior. **Nursing Research:** *What the client considers normal and abnormal health behavior may be based on cultural perceptions (Cochran, 1998; Doswell and Erlen, 1998; Leininger and McFarland, 2002).*
- Discuss with the client those aspects of their health behavior/lifestyle that will remain unchanged by their health status. **Nursing Research:** *Aspects of the client's life that are meaningful and valuable to him or her should be understood and preserved without change (Leininger and McFarland, 2002).*
- Negotiate with the client regarding the aspects of health behavior that will need to be modified. **Nursing Research:** *Give and take with the client will lead to culturally congruent care (Leininger and McFarland, 2002).*
- Assess the role of fatalism on the client's ability to modify health behavior. **Nursing Research:** *Fatalistic perspectives, which involve the belief that you cannot control your own fate, may influence health behaviors in some African American and Latino populations (Chen, 2001; Harmon et al, 1996; Phillips et al, 1999).*
- Validate the client's feelings regarding the impact of health status on current lifestyle. **Nursing Research:** *Validation is therapeutic communication technique that lets the client know that the nurse has heard and understands what was said, and it promotes the nurse-client relationship (Heineken, 1998).*

Home care

NOTE: Because the home care nurse enters the client's home as a guest, the ability of the nurse to establish a supportive, therapeutic relationship is especially important.

- Above interventions may be adapted for home care use.
- Before providing any care, review the Home Health Care Bill of Rights with the client, including the right to refuse treatment. *Identifying the rights of the client demonstrates respect of the health care system and its representatives for client wishes.*
  - If included in agency policies and procedures, also review patient responsibilities with the client (which is often part of a printed Bill of Rights). *Reviewing responsibilities helps the client define roles of mutual respect and partnership with the health care provider.*

• = Independent; ▲ = Collaborative

- When the client is noncompliant, redefine personal and health priorities (contract for services) with the client to determine alternative motivational strategies or health actions to meet health goals. *For clients to carry out desired health actions, they must perceive actions as beneficial to self and the cost of the health action as not being greater than the benefit (Rosenstock, 1974).*

- Institute self-care management to maximize client responsibility for own care. Refer to care plan for **Powerlessness.** *Client participation in care has been increased by using multiple components of self-regulation in interventions for asthma, anxiety, and smoking (Clark et al, 1992; Clark, Gong, and Kaciroti, 2001; Clark and Nothwehr, 1997; Clark and Starr-Schneidkraut, 1994).*

- Elicit and answer questions respectfully regarding illness and treatment, correcting any misconceptions and highlighting the importance of assisting the client to incorporate treatment plan into daily lifestyle. Do not use medical jargon in explanations. *Living situations that may interfere with adherence include inability to afford medications and lack of available transportation. Factors important to compliance with prescribed medications have been identified as the client's perceptions of his or her disease and treatment, physician's perceptions, manner assumed by physician, language used to communicate with the client, the client's living situation, regular medication review, and continuity of health care provision (Claesson et al, 1999).*

- Explore barriers to medical regimen adherence. Review medications and treatment regularly for needed modifications. Take complaints of side effects seriously and serve as the client advocate to address changes as indicated. *The presence of uncomfortable side effects frequently motivates clients to deviate from the medication regimen. A discussion of treatment regimen with coronary heart disease noted that physicians do not always adhere to guideline recommendations; adherence to guidelines and long term strategies would prompt use of the most effective agents with the lowest incidence of side effects, aiding client adherence (Erhardt, 1999). Older adults do not always take their antidepressant medications. They may not consider the medications helpful and may experience uncomfortable side effects. Their experience with the medications should be solicited (Prabhakaran and Butler, 2002).*

- ▲ If noncompliance compromises the client's health status, refer for psychiatric home health care services to assess the client's motivation and implement therapeutic regimen. *Psychiatric home care nurses can address issues relating to the client's nonadherence to treatment and inability to adjust to changes in health status. Behavioral interventions in the home can assist the client to participate more effectively in treatment plan (Patusky, Rodning, and Martinez-Kratz, 1996).*

- ▲ If noncompliant behavior continues and the client chooses not to cooperate with medical regimen, the home health care agency cannot continue to provide services. *Reimbursement guidelines and agency policies do not support the continued use of health care resources when the client makes an informed decision to not follow the prescribed regimen.*

- If care is to be terminated, identify all possible alternatives for the client, and assist with making an informed choice about future health actions. *Some regulatory guidelines require health care providers to give written notice of discontinuance of care using established time frames. Noncompliance and a plan for termination of care notwithstanding, it remains the goal and ethical responsibility of home health care providers to promote optimal wellness, independence, and safety.*

- Respect the wishes of terminally ill clients to refuse selected aspects of medical regimen. *With terminally ill clients, do not terminate care. Provide those aspects of care that the*

• = Independent; ▲ = Collaborative

client and family or caregivers will accept. The goal of hospice care is to provide comfort and dignity in the dying process.

Client/Family Teaching

▲ Teach clients about medication side effects (e.g., mental changes, sexual dysfunction) so that they understand them and feel comfortable discussing them. *Many medications can cause side effects such as changes in mental function and impotence, which can lead to noncompliance.*

• Teach clients to control their "self-talk" by giving themselves positive messages that will be used to promote desired behaviors, such as taking medications and controlling food intake. **Nursing Research:** *Self-talk has been shown to be a common motivating method for behavior changes (McSweeney, 1993).*

🔷 WEBSITES FOR EDUCATION

See the EVOLVE website for World Wide Web resources for client education.

REFERENCES

Andrus MR, Roth MT: Health literacy: a review, *Pharmacotherapy* 22(3):282, 2002.

Bakker RH, Kastermans MC, Dassen TW: An analysis of the nursing diagnosis in effective management of therapeutic regimen compared with noncompliance and Orem's self-care deficit theory of nursing, *Nurs Diagn* 6(4):161, 1995.

Boehm S: Patient contracting. In Bulechek GM, McCloskey JC, editors: *Nursing interventions: essential nursing treatments,* Philadelphia, 1992, WB Saunders.

Branin JJ: The role of memory strategies in medication adherence among the elderly, *Home Healthc Serv Q* 20(2):1, 2001.

Chen YC: Chinese values, health and nursing, *J Adv Nurs* 36(2):270, 2001.

Claesson S et al: Compliance with prescribed drugs: challenges for the elderly population, *Pharm World Sci* 21: 256, 1999.

Clark NM, Gong M, Kaciroti N: A model of self-regulation for control of chronic diseases, *Health Educ Behav* 28:769, 2001.

Clark NM, Nothwehr F: Self-management of asthma by adult patients, *Patient Educ Couns* 32:S5, 1997.

Clark NM, Starr-Schneidkraut NJ: Management of asthma by patients and families, *Am J Respir Crit Care Med* 149:S54, 1994.

Clark NM et al: Self-regulation of health behavior: the 'Take PRIDE' program, *Health Educ Q* 19:341, 1992.

Cochran M: Tears have no color, *Am J Nurs* 98(6):53, 1998.

Crane K, Kirby B, Kooperman D: Patient compliance for psychotropic medications, *J Psychosoc Nurs* 34(1):8, 1996.

Cummins D, Trotter G, Millar KH: Non-adherence to HIV antiretroviral medications: 'The drugs are working and I'm a continuing success story', *Aust J Adv Nurs* 20(2):15, 2003.

De Geest S: Compliance issues with the geriatric population, *Nurs Clin North Am* 33(3):467, 1998.

DeProspero T, Riffle WA: Improving patients' drug compliance, *Psychiatr Serv* 48(11):1468, 1997.

DiMatteo MR, Lepper HS, Croghan TW: Depression is a risk factor for noncompliance with medical treatment: meta-analysis of the effects of anxiety and depression on patient adherence, *J Psychosoc Nurs Ment Health Serv* 38(5):37, 2000.

Doswell W, Erlen J: Multicultural issues and ethical concerns in the delivery of revising care interventions, *Nurs Clin North Am* 33(2):353, 1998.

Dreger V, Tremback T: Optimize patient health by treating literacy and language barriers, *AORN J* 75(2):280, 287, 289; quiz 297, 303, 2002.

Dunbar-Jacob et al: Adherence in chronic disease, *Annu Rev Nurs Res* 18:48, 2000.

Elias JW: Why caregiver depression and self-care abilities should be part of the PPS case mix methodology, *Home Healthc Nurse* 19(1):23, 2001.

• **= Independent; ▲ = Collaborative**

Erhardt ER: The essence of effective treatment and compliance is simplicity, *Am J Hypertens* 12(10 Pt 2):105S, 1999.

Gray R, Robson D, Bressington D: Medication management for people with a diagnosis of schizophrenia, *Nurs Times* 98(47):38, 2002.

Gray R, Wykes T, Gournay K: From compliance to concordance: a review of the literature on interventions to enhance compliance with antipsychotic medication, *J Psychiatr Ment Health Nurs* 9(3):277, 2002.

Harmon MP, Castro FG, Coe K: Acculturation and cervical cancer: knowledge, beliefs, and behaviors of Hispanic women, *Women Health* 24(3):37, 1996.

Heineken J: Patient silence is not necessarily client satisfaction: communication in home care nursing, *Home Healthc Nurse* 16(2):115, 1998.

Kluckowski JC: Solving medication noncompliance in home care, *Caring* 11:34, 1992.

Lannon SL: Using a health promotion model to enhance medication compliance, *J Neurosci* 29(3):170, 1997.

Leininger MM, McFarland MR: *Transcultural nursing: concepts, theories, research and practices,* ed 3, New York, 2002, McGraw-Hill.

London F: Improving compliance: what you can do, *RN* 98(1):43, 1998.

McGarry Logue R: Self-medication and the elderly: how technology can help, *Am J Nurs* 102(7), 2002.

McGraw C, Drennan V: Self-administration of medicine and older people, *Nurs Stand* 15(18):33, 2001.

McSweeney JC: Making behavior changes after a myocardial infarction, *West J Nurs Res* 15(4):441, 1993.

Meisekothen LM: Noncompliance in the elderly: a pathway to suicide, *J Am Acad Nurs Pract* 5(2):67, 1993.

Muscari ME: Rebels with a cause, *Am J Nurs* 98(12):26, 1998.

Olfson M et al: Predicting medication noncompliance after hospital discharge among patients with schizophrenia, *Psychiatr Serv* 51(2):216, 2000.

Patusky KL, Rodning C, Martinez-Kratz M: Clinical lessons in psychiatric home care: a case study approach, *J Home Healthc Manag* 9:18, 1996.

Phillips JM, Cohen MZ, Moses G: Breast cancer screening and African American women: fear, fatalism, and silence, *Oncol Nurs Forum* 26(3):561, 1999.

Prabhakaran P, Butler R: What are older peoples' experiences of taking antidepressants? *J Affect Disord* 70:319, 2002.

Prochaska JO et al: *Changing for good: a revolutionary six stage program for overcoming bad habits and moving your life positively forward,* New York, Avon Books, 1994.

Resnick B: Motivation in geriatric rehabilitation, *Image* 28(1):41, 1996.

Robinson AW: Getting the heart of denial, *Am J Nurs* 99(5):38, 1999.

Rosenstock I: Health belief model and preventive behavior. In Becker M, editor: *The health belief model and personal health behavior,* Thorofare, NJ, 1974, CB Slack.

Samuelson M: Stages of change: from theory to practice, *Art Health Promotion* 2(5):1, 1998.

Simons MR: Patient contracting. In Bulechek GM, McCloskey JC, editors: *Nursing interventions: effective nursing treatments,* ed 3, Philadelphia, 1999, WB Saunders.

Ward-Collins D: Noncompliant: isn't there a better way to say it? *Am J Nurs* 98(5):27, 1998.

Warren JJ: Ethical concerns about noncompliance in the chronically ill patient, *Progr Cardiovasc Nurs* 7(4):10, 1992.

Readiness for enhanced Nutrition

Betty J. Ackley

NANDA   Definition

A pattern of nutrient intake that is sufficient for meeting metabolic needs and can be strengthened

Defining Characteristics

Expresses willingness to enhance nutrition; eats regularly; consumes adequate food and fluid; expresses knowledge of healthy food and fluid choices; follows an appropriate standard for intake (e.g., the food pyramid, US Dietary Guidelines or America Diabetic

• = **Independent;** ▲ = **Collaborative**

Association guidelines); safe preparation and storage for food and fluids; attitude toward eating and drinking is congruent with health goals

Related Factors (r/t)

Motivation to improve health through diet

NOC   Outcomes (Nursing Outcomes Classification)

Suggested NOC Outcomes

Nutritional Status; Nutritional Status: Food and Fluid Intake, Nutrient Intake; Weight Control

> #### Example NOC Outcome with Indicators
>
> **Nutritional Status** as evidenced by the following indicators: Food and fluid intake/Body mass index/Weight/Biochemical measures (Rate each indicator of **Nutritional Status:** 1 = extremely compromised, 2 = substantially compromised, 3 = moderately compromised, 4 = mildly compromised, 5 = not compromised [see Section I].)

Client Outcomes

Client Will (Specify Time Frame):

- Explain how to eat according to the US Dietary Guidelines
- Design dietary modifications to meet individual long-term goal of health, using principles of variety, balance, and moderation
- Weigh within normal range for height and age

NIC   Interventions (Nursing Interventions Classification)

Suggested NIC Interventions

Nutrition Management; Nutritional Counseling; Weight Reduction Assistance

> #### Example NIC Activities—Nutrition Management
>
> Determine the client's motivation for changing eating habits; Develop with the client a method to keep a daily record of intake

Nursing Interventions and Rationales

- Ask the client to keep a one day to three day food diary where everything eaten or drank is recorded. *Use of a Food Diary will be helpful for both the client and the nurse, to examine usual foods eaten and patterns of eating.* **Nursing Research:** *Self-monitoring helps the client assess adherence to self-determined performance criteria and progress toward desired goals. Self-monitoring serves an important role in the maintenance of internal standards of behavior (Fleury, 1991).*
- Determine the client's knowledge of a nutritious diet and need for supplements. *This information is useful for developing an individualized teaching plan based on the client's current state.*
- Determine the client's motivation to improve nutrition level, whether for appearance

• = Independent; ▲ = Collaborative

or health benefits. *Often a healthier body weight is only a 5% to 10% reduction from initial body weight (Nonas, 1998).*

- Recommend the client follow the U.S. Dietary Guidelines which can be found at this URL: http://www.health.gov/dietaryguidelines/dga2000/DIETGD.PDF. *The U.S. Dietary Guidelines are written by national experts and based on research in nutrition.*
- Help the client determine their body mass index (BMI). Use a chart or one of the formulas below:
  - Weight in kilograms divided by height (in meters) squared (kg/m^2)
  - Weight in pounds multiplied by 705, divided by height in inches, divided again by height in inches.

  A normal BMI is 20 to 25, 26 to 29 is overweight, and a BMI of greater than 30 is obese (Mokdad et al, 1998). If BMI is greater than 25, refer to **Imbalanced Nutrition: more than body requirements.**
- Review the client's current exercise level. With the client and primary health care provider, design a long-term exercise program. Encourage the client to adopt an exercise program that involves 45 minutes of exercise five times/week. *Exercise is important for increased energy expenditure, for maintenance of lean body mass, and as part of a total change in lifestyle, but a health risk appraisal should be performed on all previously sedentary individuals beginning a program of exercise (Lutz and Przytulski, 2001). Moderately intense physical activity for 30 to 45 minutes 5 to 7 days/week can expend the 1500 to 2000 calories/week that appear to be necessary to maintain weight loss. Cross-sectional and longitudinal studies illustrate that persons who increase their physical activity also increase their resting metabolic rate (Rippe and Hess, 1998).* **Clinical Research:** *Children receiving a 6-month classroom curriculum to reduce television, videotape, and video game use showed significant decreases in body mass index and triceps skinfolds compared with controls (Robinson, 1999).*
- Explain the value of the Food Pyramid to the client. With the client's input, evaluate the client's intake based on the Food Pyramid.
- Demonstrate the use of food labels to make healthful choices. Alert the client/family to focus on serving size, total fat, and simple carbohydrate. *The standardized food label in bold type simplifies the search for information. Fats and sugars contribute the least to a healthful diet and the most to excessive calorie intake. Generally clients should eat foods that are no more than 30% fat.*
- Recommend the client eat whole grains whenever possible, and explain how to find whole grains using the food label. **Clinical Research:** *Intake of whole grains (3 servings per day) has been shown to decrease the incidence of type 2 diabetes in men and women (McKeown et al, 2002; Meyer et al, 2000). It has also been shown to probably decrease heart disease (Liu et al, 1999).*
- Recommend the client eat five to nine fruits and vegetables per day, with a minimum of two servings of fruit and three servings of vegetables. Encourage them to eat a rainbow of fruits and vegetables because bright colors are associated with increased nutrients. *Both fruits and vegetables are excellent sources of vitamins and also phytochemicals that help protect from disease.* **Clinical Research:** *An epidemiological study demonstrated a decreased incidence of cardiovascular disease deaths and overall mortality with an increased intake of fruits and vegetables (Bazzano et al, 2002).*
- Recommend the client limit intake of saturated fats and *trans*-fatty acids; instead increase intake of vegetable oils such as canola oil, and olive oil. Limit fat intake to around 30% of total calories per day. *Intake of both saturated fat and* trans-*fatty acids*

• = **Independent;** ▲ = **Collaborative**

raise the low density lipoprotein level, which predisposes to atherosclerosis. Trans-*fatty acids also lower the high density lipoproteins, which are thought to be protective against heart disease (Cataldo, DeBruyne, and Whitney, 2003; Willett, 1994).*

- Recommend the client eat meatless meals at intervals and try alternative sources of protein including nuts (one handful), nut butters, and soy. Note: women with diagnosed cancer of the breast should generally avoid eating soy foods. **Clinical Research:** *Frequent nut consumption was associated with a reduced risk of coronary heart disease in a study of registered nurses (Hu et al, 1998). Consumption of nuts and peanut butter was shown to probably decrease the incidence of type 2 diabetes in women (Jiang et al, 2002) Nut consumption in a study done on physicians demonstrated that those whose diet included the most nuts had the lowest risk of dying from heart disease (Albert et al, 2002b). Eating soy as a substitute for animal products reduces the incidence of coronary artery disease by reducing blood lipids, oxidized LDL, homocysteine, and blood pressure (Jenkins et al, 2002).*

- Recommend that the client eat cold water fish such as salmon, tuna, or mackerel at least two times per week to ensure adequate intake of omega 3 fatty acids; if unwilling to eat fish suggest sources such as flaxseed, soy, or walnuts. Note: Fish oil capsules should be taken cautiously; some brands can be contaminated with mercury or pesticides. Intake of excessive omega 3 fatty acids can result in bleeding. **Clinical Research:** *Multiple studies have demonstrated that intake of omega 3 fatty acids by fish intake or fish oil capsules results in decreased incidence of sudden cardiac death (Albert et al, 2002a; Jones, 2002; Marchioli et al, 2002). In addition increasing intake of omega 3 fatty acids may be helpful in risk reduction for autoimmune disorders, some kinds of cancer, diabetes, and arthritis (Connor, 2000).*

- Encourage the client to decrease intake of sugars including intake of soft drinks, desserts, and candy. S*ugar predisposes to dental caries, and also is a source of calories that is empty of other nutrients (Cataldo, DeBruyne, and Whitney, 2003).*

- Recommend the client choose and prepare foods with less salt.

- If the client drinks alcohol, encourage to drink in moderation, no more than one drink per day for women, and two drinks per day for men.

- Advise the client to measure food periodically. Help the client learn usual portion sizes. *Measuring food alerts the client to normal portion sizes. Estimating amounts can be extremely inaccurate.*

- Evaluate the client's usual intake of fiber. *In general, high fiber foods take longer to eat and contain fewer calories than most other foods.* **Clinical Research:** *Dietary fiber was associated with lower body weight and waist–to–hip ratios and predicted weight gain more strongly than did fat consumption (Ludwig et al, 1999).*

Geriatric

- Assess changes in lifestyle and eating patterns. *Energy needs decrease an estimated 5% per decade after the age of 40 years but often eating patterns remain unchanged from youth (Lutz and Przytulski, 2001).*

- ▲ Recommend the client discuss the need for a low-dose balanced multiple vitamin and mineral supplement with physician. *It is generally recommended that anyone over 50 should take a multiple vitamin every day to ensure receives adequate amounts of vitamins and minerals.* **Clinical Research:** *Some studies have demonstrated increased immunity and decreased rate of infections in older people who take a vitamin supplement (Chandra, 1997; Johnson and Porter, 1997).*

- = Independent; ▲ = Collaborative

- Assess fluid intake. Recommend routine drinks of water whether thirsty or not. *The elderly are predisposed to deficient fluid volume because of decreased fluid in body, decreased thirst sensation, and decreased ability to concentrate urine (Bennett, 2000; Sheehy et al, 1999; Suhayda and Walton, 2002).*
- Observe for socioeconomic factors that influence food choices (e.g., funds, cooking facilities). *Even those on restricted budgets and with limited facilities can be assisted to choose food sources of a balanced diet.*
- Suggest a variety of seasonings. *The ability to taste sweet, bitter, sour, and salty declines in most, but not all, older persons (Morley, 1997).*

Multicultural
- Assess for dietary intake of essential nutrients. **Nursing Research:** *Studies have shown that black women have calcium intakes of less than 75% of the RDA (Zablah et al, 1999). Hispanics with type 2 diabetes also often have inadequate protein nutritional status (Castenada et al, 2000). Mexican American women have a higher prevalence of iron deficiency anemia than non-Hispanic white females (Frith-Terhune et al, 2000). Rural black men had low caloric intakes coupled with high fat intakes but nutrient deficiencies (Vitolins et al, 2000).*
- Assess for the influence of cultural beliefs, norms, and values on the client's nutritional knowledge. *What the client considers normal dietary practices may be based on cultural perceptions (Cochran, 1998; Doswell and Erlen, 1998; Leininger and McFarland, 2002).*
- Discuss with the client those aspects of their diet that will remain unchanged. *Aspects of the client's life that are meaningful and valuable to them should be understood and preserved without change (Leininger and McFarland, 2002).*
- Determine the motivational factors operating within the client at the present time. **Nursing Research:** *African American women were motivated to increase their physical activity by personal and familial histories of heart disease and related risk factors (Banks-Wallace, 2000).*
- Negotiate with the client regarding the aspects of his or her diet that will need to be modified. *Give and take with the client will lead to culturally congruent care (Leininger and McFarland, 2002).*
- Explore strategies that appeal to the client. **Nursing Research:** *Group interventions that include spiritual and community building may be especially effective for promoting physical activity among African American woman (Banks-Wallace, 2000). African American women tried more commercial diet products and ceased their weight loss efforts sooner than did Euro American women (Tyler, Allan, and Alcozer, 1997).*
- Validate the client's feelings regarding the impact of current lifestyle, finances, and transportation on ability to obtain nutritious food. **Nursing Research:** *Validation is therapeutic communication technique that lets the client know that the nurse has heard and understands what was said, and it promotes the nurse-client relationship (Heineken, 1998).*

Client/Family Teaching
- The majority of interventions above involve teaching.
- Work with the family members regarding information on how to improve nutritional status. *If the client and family select the nutritional plan, they are more likely to comply with it, particularly if the client does not do the marketing and cooking.*
- Teach the importance of exercise in a weight control program. *A physically conditioned person uses more fat for energy at rest and with exercise than a sedentary person does. The*

• = Independent; ▲ = Collaborative

majority of patients will benefit from establishing walking as a cornerstone of their physical activity program (Rippe, Crossley, and Ringer, 1998).

evolve WEBSITES FOR EDUCATION

See the EVOLVE website for World Wide Web resources for client education.

REFERENCES

Albert CM et al: Blood levels of long chain n-3 fatty acids and the risk of sudden death, *N Engl J Med* 346(15): 1113, 2002a.

Albert CM et al: Nut consumption and decreased risk of sudden cardiac death in the Physicians' Health Study, *Arch Intern Med* 162(2):1382, 2002b.

Banks-Wallace J: Staggering under the weight of responsibility: the impact of culture on physical activity among African American women, *Multicult Nurs Health* 6:24, 2000.

Bazzano LA et al: Fruit and vegetable intake and risk of cardiovascular disease in US adults: the first National Health and Nutrition Examination Survey epidemiologic follow-up study, *Am J Clin Nutr* 76:1, 2002.

Bennett JA: Dehydration: hazards and benefits, *Geriatr Nurs* 21(2):84, 2000.

Castenada C, Bermudez OI, Tucker KL: Protein nutritional status and functions are associated with type II diabetes in Hispanic elders, *Am J Clin Nutr* 72(1):89, 2000.

Cataldo CB, DeBruyne LK, Whitney EN: *Nutrition and diet therapy,* Belmont, Calif, 2003, Thomason Wadsworth.

Chandra RD: Graying of the immune system: can nutrient supplements improve immunity in the elderly? *JAMA* 277:1398, 1997.

Cochran M: Tears have no color, *Am J Nurs* 98(6):53, 1998.

Connor WE: Importance of n-3 fatty acids in health and disease, *Am J Clin Nutr* 71(1 suppl):171S, 2000.

Doswell W, Erlen J: Multicultural issues and ethical concerns in the delivery of revising care interventions, *Nurs Clin North Am* 33(2):353, 1998.

Fleury J: Empowering potential: a story of wellness motivation, *Nurs Res* 40:288, 1991.

Frith-Terhune AL et al: Iron deficiency anemia: higher prevalence in Mexican American than in non-Hispanic white females in the third National Health and Nutrition Examination Survey, 1988-1994, *Am J Clin Nutr* 72(4):963, 2000.

Heineken J: Patient silence is not necessarily client satisfaction: communication in home care nursing, *Home Healthc Nurse* 16(2):115, 1998.

Hu FB et al: Frequent nut consumption and risk of coronary heart disease in women: prospective cohort study, *BMJ* 317(7169):1341, 1998.

Jenkins DJ et al: Effects of high- and low-isoflavone soyfoods on blood lipids, oxidized LDL, homocysteine, and blood pressure in hyperlipidemic men and women, *Am J Clin Nutr* 76(2):365, 2002.

Jiang R et al: Nut and peanut butter consumption and risk of type 2 diabetes in women, *JAMA* 288(20):2554, 2002.

Johnson MA, Porter KH: Micronutrient supplementation and infection in institutionalized elders, *Nutr Rev* 55: 400, 1997.

Jones PJ: Effect of n-3 polyunsaturated fatty acids on risk reduction of sudden death, *Nutr Rev* 60:12, 2002.

Leininger MM, McFarland MR: *Transcultural nursing: concepts, theories, research and practices,* ed 3, New York, 2002, McGraw-Hill.

Liu S et al: Whole grain consumption and risk of coronary heart disease: results from the Nurses' Health Study, *Am J Clin Nutr* 70(3):412, 1999.

Ludwig DS et al: Dietary fiber, weight gain, and cardiovascular disease risk factors in young adults, *JAMA* 282: 1539, 1999.

Lutz CA, Przytulski KR: *Nutrition and diet therapy,* ed 3, Philadelphia, 2001, FA Davis.

Marchioli R et al: Early protection against sudden death by n-3 polyunsaturated fatty acids after myocardial infarction, *Circulation* 105(16):1987, 2002.

McKeown NM, Meigs JB, Liu S: Whole-grain intake is favorably associated with metabolic risk factors for type 2 diabetes and cardiovascular disease in the Framingham Offspring Study, *Am J Clin Nutr* 76:2, 2002.

• = Independent; ▲ = Collaborative

Meyer KA et al: Carbohydrates, dietary fiber, and incident type 2 diabetes in older women, *Am J Clin Nutr* 71(4):921, 2000.

Mokdad AH et al: The continuing epidemics of obesity and diabetes in the United States, *JAMA* 286:1195, 1998.

Morley JE: Anorexia of aging: physiologic and pathologic, *Am J Clin Nutr* 66:760, 1997.

Nonas CA: A model for chronic care of obesity through dietary treatment, *J Am Diet Assoc* 98(suppl 2):S16, 1998.

Rippe JM, Crossley S, Ringer R: Obesity as a chronic disease: modern medical and lifestyle management, *J Am Diet Assoc* 98(suppl 2):S9, 1998.

Rippe JM, Hess S: The role of physical activity in the prevention and management of obesity, *J Am Diet Assoc* 98(suppl 2):S31, 1998.

Robinson TN: Reducing children's television viewing to prevent obesity: a randomized controlled trial, *JAMA* 282:1561, 1999.

Sheehy CM, Perry PA, Cromwell SL: Dehydration: biological considerations, age-related changes, and risk factors in older adults, *Biol Res Nurs* 1(1):30, 1999.

Suhayda R, Walton JC: Preventing and managing dehydration, *Medsurg Nurs* 11(6):267, 2002.

Tyler DO, Allan JD, Alcozer FR: Weight loss methods used by African American and Euro American women, *Res Nurs Health*, 20:413, 1997.

Vitolins MZ et al: Ethnic and gender variation in the dietary intake of rural elders, *J Nutr Elderly* 19(3):15, 2000.

Willett WC: Diet and health: what should we eat? *Science* 264:532, 1994.

Zablah EM et al: Barriers to calcium intake in African American women, *J Hum Nutr* 12(2):123, 1999.

Imbalanced Nutrition: less than body requirements

Carroll A. Lutz

NANDA Definition

Intake of nutrients insufficient to meet metabolic needs

Defining Characteristics

Body weight less than 20% under ideal weight; pale conjunctival and mucous membranes; weakness of muscles required for swallowing or mastication; sore, inflamed buccal cavity; satiety immediately after ingesting food; reported or evidence of lack of food; reported inadequate food intake less than RDA (Recommended Dietary Allowance); reported altered taste sensation; perceived inability to ingest food; misconceptions; loss of weight with adequate food intake; aversion to eating; abdominal cramping; poor muscle tone; abdominal pain with or without pathology; lack of interest in food; capillary fragility; diarrhea and/or steatorrhea; excessive loss of hair; hyperactive bowel sounds; lack of information; misinformation

Related Factors (r/t)

Inability to ingest or digest food or absorb nutrients because of biological, psychological, or economic factors

NOC Outcomes (Nursing Outcomes Classification)

Suggested NOC Outcomes

Nutritional Status; Nutritional Status: Food and Fluid Intake, Nutrient Intake; Weight Control

• = Independent; ▲ = Collaborative

> ### Example NOC Outcome with Indicators
>
> **Nutritional Status** as evidenced by the following indicators: Food and fluid intake/Body mass index/ Weight/Biochemical measures (Rate each indicator of **Nutritional Status:** I = extremely compromised, 2 = substantially compromised, 3 = moderately compromised, 4 = mildly compromised, 5 = not compromised [see Section I].)

Client Outcomes

Client Will (Specify Time Frame):

- Progressively gain weight toward desired goal
- Weigh within normal range for height and age
- Recognize factors contributing to underweight
- Identify nutritional requirements
- Consume adequate nourishment
- Be free of signs of malnutrition

NIC   Interventions (Nursing Interventions Classification)

Suggested NIC Interventions

Eating Disorders Management; Electrolyte Management: Hypophosphatemia; Enteral Tube Feeding; Feeding; Nutrition Management; Nutrition Therapy; Nutritional Counseling; Nutritional Monitoring; Swallowing Therapy; Weight Gain Assistance; Weight Management

> ### Example NIC Activities—Nutrition Management
>
> Ascertain the client's food preferences; Provide the client with high-protein, high-calorie, nutritious finger foods and drinks that can be readily consumed, as appropriate

Nursing Interventions and Rationales

- Determine healthy body weight for age and height. Refer to dietitian for complete nutrition assessment if 10% under healthy body weight or if rapidly losing weight. Legal intervention may be necessary. *Early diagnosis and a holistic team treatment of eating disorders are desirable.* **Nursing Research:** *Of women who ran 15 to 30 miles per week, 20% to 25% had an increased risk of eating disorders (Estok and Rudy, 1996). In the developed world, protein-calorie malnutrition (PCM) most often accompanies a disease process. Surveys of hospitalized children in the United States revealed that 20% to 40% had PCM (Baker, 1997).* **Clinical Research:** *Over the short term, patients involuntarily committed for treatment of eating disorders progressed as well as those seeking treatment voluntarily (Watson et al, 2000).*
- Compare usual food intake with the U.S. Department of Agriculture Food Pyramid, noting slighted or omitted food groups. *Milk consumption has decreased among children while intake of fruit juices and carbonated beverages has increased.* **Clinical Research:** *A higher incidence of bone fractures in teenage girls has been associated with a greater consumption of carbonated beverages (Wyshak, 2000); possibly also related is the substitution of soda for milk. Omission of entire food groups increases risk of deficiencies.*

- = Independent; ▲ = Collaborative

- If the client is a vegetarian, evaluate vitamin B_{12} and iron intake. *Strict vegetarians may be at particular risk for vitamin B_{12} and iron deficiencies. Special care should be taken when implementing vegetarian diets for pregnant women, infants, children, and the elderly. A dietitian can usually furnish a balanced vegetarian diet (with adequate substitutes for omitted foods) for inpatients and can provide instruction for outpatients.*
- Assess the client's ability to obtain and use essential nutrients. **Clinical Research:** *Cases of vitamin D deficiency rickets have been reported among dark-skinned infants and toddlers who were exclusively breast fed and were not given supplemental vitamin D. The children resided in northern (Fitzpatrick et al, 2000), mid-south (Kreiter et al, 2000), and southern (Shah et al, 2000) states, indicating that the presence of natural sunlight does not eliminate the risk of disease.*
- Observe the client's ability to eat (time involved, motor skills, visual acuity, and ability to swallow various textures). *Clients in institutions are susceptible to protein-calorie malnutrition (PCM) or protein-energy malnutrition when they are unable to feed themselves.* **Clinical Research:** *Poor vision was associated with lower protein and energy (calorie) intakes in home care clients independent of other medical conditions (Payette et al, 1995).*

NOTE: If the client is unable to feed self, refer to Nursing Interventions and Rationales for **Feeding Self-care deficit.** If the client has difficulty swallowing, refer to Nursing Interventions and Rationales for **Impaired Swallowing.**

- If the client lacks endurance, schedule rest periods before meals and open packages and cut up food for the client. *Nursing assistance with activities of daily living (ADLs) will conserve the client's energy for activities that the client values. Clients who take longer than 1 hour to complete a meal may require assistance (Evans, 1992).*
- Evaluate the client's laboratory studies (serum albumin, serum total protein, serum ferritin, transferrin, hemoglobin, hematocrit, vitamins, and minerals). *An abnormal value in a single diagnostic study may have many possible causes, but serum albumin less than 3.2 g/dl was shown to be highly predictive of mortality in hospitals, and serum cholesterol of less than 156 mg/dl was the best predictor of mortality in nursing homes (Morley, 1997).*
- Maintain a high index of suspicion of malnutrition as a contributing factor in infections and vice versa. *Impaired immunity is a critical adjunct factor in malnutrition-associated infections in all age groups in all populations of the world (Chandra, 1997). Protein-energy malnutrition is associated with a significant impairment of cell-mediated immunity (Chandra, 2002). Infection may result in confusion, anorexia, and negative nitrogen balance, all of which contribute to protein-energy malnutrition (Kamel et al, 1998).*
- Be aware of clients at risk for refeeding syndrome: those with frank starvation, with anorexia nervosa, and those with chronic illness and malnutrition. *Refeeding syndrome, a potentially fatal condition, occurs in some malnourished clients when nutrients are given (orally, by tube feeding, or parenterally) in excess of the client's ability to metabolize them. Clients at risk of refeeding syndrome must be monitored carefully for electrolyte imbalances, congestive heart failure, and respiratory failure (Lutz and Przytulski, 2001).*
- Be alert for food-nutrient-drug interactions. *Individuals at greatest risk are those who are malnourished, consume alcohol, receive many drugs long-term for chronic diseases, or take medications with meals or through a feeding tube (Lutz, Przytulski, 2001). Clinical Research Case reports still appear in medical journals describing scurvy in persons with alcoholism (Garg, Draganescu, and Albornoz, 1998).*
- Assess for recent changes in physiological status that may interfere with nutrition. *The consequences of malnutrition can lead to a further decline in the patient's condition that then*

• = **Independent;** ▲ = **Collaborative**

becomes self-perpetuating if not recognized and treated. Extreme cases of malnutrition can lead to septicemia, organ failure, and death (Arrowsmith, 1997). **Clinical Research:** *Diarrhea in patients receiving warfarin has been suggested as possibly causing lower intake and/or malabsorption of vitamin K (Smith, Aljazairi, and Fuller, 1999). Oral supplements given to patients following elective gastrointestinal surgery produced significantly less weight loss and fewer complications than seen in control patients (Keele et al, 1997).*

- If the client is pregnant, ensure that she is receiving adequate amounts of folic acid by eating a balanced diet and taking prenatal vitamins as ordered. *All women of child-bearing potential are urged to consume 400 µg of synthetic folic acid from fortified foods or supplements in addition to food folate from a varied diet (National Academy of Sciences, 1998).*

- Observe the client's relationship to food. Attempt to separate physical from psychological causes for eating difficulty. *It may be difficult to tell if the problem is physical or psychological. Refusing to eat may be the only way the client can express some control, and it may also be a symptom of depression (Evans, 1992).*

- Provide companionship at mealtime to encourage nutritional intake. *Mealtime usually is a time for social interaction; often clients will eat more food if other people are present at mealtimes.* **Clinical Research:** *Compared to married subjects, mean weight loss and the prevalence of weight loss were significantly higher among widowed subjects who ate more solitary meals, more commercial meals per week, and fewer snacks and homemade meals (Shahar et al, 2001).*

- Consider six small nutrient-dense meals versus three larger meals daily to reduce the feeling of fullness. *Eating small, frequent meals reduces the sensation of fullness and decreases the stimulus to vomit (Love and Seaton, 1991).*

- Weigh the client weekly under same conditions.

- ▲ Monitor food intake; specify proportion of served food that is eaten (25%, 50%); consult with dietitian for actual calorie count.

- Monitor state of oral cavity (gums, tongue, mucosa, teeth). Provide good oral hygiene before and after meals. *Good oral hygiene enhances appetite; the condition of the oral mucosa is critical to the ability to eat. The oral mucosa must be moist, with adequate saliva production to facilitate and aid in the digestion of food.*

- If a client has anorexia and dry mouth from medication side effects, offer sips of fluids throughout the day. *Although artificial salivas are available, more often than not clients preferred water to the more expensive products (Ganley, 1995).*

- Determine relationship of eating and other events to onset of nausea, vomiting, diarrhea, or abdominal pain.

- Determine time of day when the client's appetite is the greatest. Offer highest calorie meal at that time. *Clients with liver disease often have their greatest appetite at breakfast time.*

- Offer small volumes of light liquids as an appetizer before meals. *Small volumes of liquids (less than 240 ml) stimulate the gastrointestinal tract, which enhances peristalsis and motility (Rogers-Seidel, 1991). Calories supplied by glucose (fruit juices) are less likely to interfere with appetite than those supplied by fat (Morley et al, 1998).*

- ▲ Administer antiemetics as ordered before meals. *Antiemetics are more effective when given before nausea occurs.*

- Prepare the client for meals. Clear unsightly supplies and excretions. Avoid invasive procedures before meals. *A pleasant environment helps promote intake.*

• = Independent; ▲ = Collaborative

- If food odors trigger nausea, remove food covers away from the client's bedside. *Trapped odors diffuse into air away from the client.*
- If vomiting is a problem, discourage consumption of favorite foods. *If favorite foods are consumed and then vomited, the client may later reject them.*
- Work with the client to develop a plan for increased activity. *Immobility leads to negative nitrogen balance that fosters anorexia.*
- If the client is anemic, offer foods rich in iron and vitamins B_{12}, C, and folic acid. *Heme iron in meat, fish, and poultry is absorbed more readily than nonheme iron in plants. Vitamin C increases the solubility of iron. Vitamin B_{12} and folic acid are necessary for erythropoiesis.*
- If the client is lactose intolerant (genetically or following diarrhea), suggest cheeses (natural or processed) with less lactose than fluid milk. Encourage the client to identify the extent of the intolerance. **Clinical Research:** *When lactose intake is limited to the equivalent of 240 ml of milk or less a day, symptoms are likely to be negligible and the use of lactose-digestive aids unnecessary (Suarez, Savaiano, and Levitt, 1995).*
- For the agitated client, offer finger foods (sandwiches, fresh fruit) and fluids. *If a client cannot be still, food can be consumed while pacing.*

Geriatric

- Assess for protein-energy malnutrition in elderly clients regardless of setting. *The majority of persons with weight loss in a nursing home either have protein-energy malnutrition or dehydration (Morley et al, 1998).* **Clinical Research:** *Twenty percent of hospitalized elderly veterans consumed less than 50% of their energy requirements and had higher rates of in-hospital and 90-day mortality (Sullivan et al, 1999). Protein-energy undernutrition at hospital discharge was a strong independent risk factor for mortality in outpatients followed for 4.5 years (Sullivan and Walls, 1998).* **Nursing Research:** *When followed for 6 months in a long-care hospital, 84% of patients had an intake below estimated energy expenditure and 30% had intakes below their estimated basal metabolic rates (Elmstahl et al, 1997).*
- Assess for factors contributing to a current acute illness. **Nursing Research:** *The strongest contributing factor to acute confusion in nursing home residents was inadequate fluid intake followed by dementia and a fall within 30 days (Mentes et al, 1999).* **Clinical Research:** *In one institution, only 26% of patients with femoral neck fractures had received a dietetic assessment despite low total lymphocyte counts in 71%, and only 6% were receiving medications for osteoporosis upon discharge (Miller et al, 2001).*
- Implement strategies to prevent recurrence of illness. **Clinical Research:** *Individuals with any amount of weight loss and no improvement in serum albumin levels during the first month following hospitalization for medical or surgical services were at a much higher risk of readmission than those who maintained or increased their discharge weight and repleted their serum albumin concentrations (Friedmann et al, 1997). Patients with osteoporotic hip fracture receiving protein supplements in addition to calcium and vitamin D had less bone loss and shorter stays on the rehabilitation units than controls who did not receive the protein supplements (Schurch et al, 1998).*
- Interpret laboratory findings cautiously. *Compromised kidney function makes reliance on urine samples for nutrient analyses less reliable in the elderly than in younger persons.* **Nursing Research:** *Because it is correlated to urine specific gravity and urine osmolality, observing urine color is a low-cost method of monitoring dehydration (Wakefield et al, 2002).*

- = Independent; ▲ = Collaborative

- Offer high protein supplements based on individual needs and capabilities. *Patients with decreased kidney function may not be able to excrete the waste products from protein metabolism.*
- Give the client a choice of supplements to increase personal control. If the client is unwilling to drink a glass of liquid supplement, offer 30 ml/hr in a medication cup. **Clinical Research:** *Alternatively, offer 3 ounces of supplement with each medication pass (Lewis, Boyle, 1998). Often the elderly will take medications when they will not take food. The supplement is then served as a medicine.*
- Offer liquid energy supplements. When given liquid preloads 60 minutes before the next meal, older persons consistently ate a greater total energy load (Morley, 1997). **Clinical Research:** *Elderly nursing home residents gained an average of 3.3 pounds in 60 days when consuming an average of 400 kilocalories per day of oral supplements (Lauque et al, 2000).* **Nursing Research:** *Inadequate kilocaloric intake has been correlated with increased mortality in the elderly (Elmstahl et al, 1997).*
- Unless medically contraindicated, permit self-selected seasonings and foods. *Older persons rate flavor as the most important determinant of their food choice but ability to taste declines in most but not all aging clients, most often affecting salt receptors and least often sweet receptors. Blindfolded older subjects have about one half the ability of younger subjects to recognize blended foods, which predominantly results from a decline in olfactory sense (Morley, 1997).* **Clinical Research:** *In hospitalized patients permitted their preferred food (ice cream) ad libitum, protein-energy malnutrition was reversed (Winograd and Brown, 1990).*
- Play relaxing dinner music during mealtime. **Nursing Research:** *On a nursing home ward for demented patients, the patients ate more calmly and spent more time with dinner when music was played (Ragneskog et al, 1996). Musical selections with a slow tempo, at or below the human heart rate, have usually been used to dampen environmental noises that might otherwise startle clients. Fewer incidents of agitated behaviors occurred during the weeks that music was played compared with weeks without music (Denney, 1997).*
- Assess components of bone health: calcium intake. *The adequate intake (AI) of calcium for adults aged 19 to 50 years is 1000 mg. For those greater than 50 years of age the amount is 1200 mg (National Academy of Sciences, 1998). Along with calcium, milk contains lactose that increases absorption of calcium and protein that the osteoblasts need to rebuild the bone matrix. In sum, milk is such an important source of calcium that it is virtually impossible to obtain adequate dietary calcium without milk or dairy products (Lutz and Przytulski, 2001).*
- Assess components of bone health: vitamin D status. *In the absence of adequate exposure to sunlight, the AI for vitamin D is set at 5 mg/day for persons 31 to 50 years of age, 10 mg for those 51 to 70 years of age, and 15 mg for persons greater than 70 years of age (National Academy of Sciences, 1998). An 80-year-old person requires almost twice as much time in the sun as a 20-year-old person would need to produce a given amount of vitamin D (Ryan, Eleazer, and Egbert, 1995).* **Clinical Research:** Postmenopausal community-living women who presented with hip fracture showed occult vitamin D deficiency (LeBoff et al, 1999).
- Assess components of bone health: regular exercise. **Clinical Research:** *In addition to increasing bone density, exercise also increases muscle mass and improves balance (Nelson et al, 1994).*
- Instruct in wise use of supplements. *The Modified Food Guide Pyramid for People Over 70 Years of Age specifies calcium, vitamin D, and vitamin B_{12} supplementation (Russell*

- = Independent; ▲ = Collaborative

floor and flexing the knee. NOTE: A hemi, one-arm drive wheelchair is recommended for persons with hemiplegia. *The sound foot propels the chair by repeating the process (Wilson and Kerr, 1988).*

- Suggest that the client back his or her wheelchair or wheeled device into an elevator, or if entering face first, instruct to turn chair around to face the elevator doors. *This allows the client to see the control panel, floor monitor display, and opening of doors. Client should exit by facing forward rather than backing out (Minor and Minor, 1999).*

- Reinforce concept of descending a curb backward ("popping a wheelie") if balance, trunk control, strength, and timing are adequate. Client needs to lean slightly forward and guide both wheels off curb at the same time. *Compared with a forward curb descent, a backward descent carries less risk of the client losing control and falling forward out of the wheelchair. If someone is helping the client, backing down the curb places less stress on the helper.*

- Reinforce principles of ascending curbs in a forward position by popping a wheelie or having an assistant tilt the chair back, placing the front wheels over the curb, and rolling the back wheels up. If surface is soft (muddy, sandy) go up curb backward via a wheelie. *The front casters will not roll on soft surfaces. A backward approach will require less energy and prevent getting stuck or injured from falling forward (Younker Rehabilitation Center, 1990).*

- During wheelies, hold the wheelchair until all four wheels are back on the ground and the client has balance and control of the wheelchair *Releasing your grip too soon may affect the client's balance and cause injury (Younker Rehabilitation Center, 1990).*

- When the client experiences unilateral neglect, agnosia, somatognosia, or proprioception deficits, cue the client and reinforce team intervention strategies for propelling the chair, entering doorways, and detecting and avoiding obstacles. *Too often nurses move the wheelchair or obstacle when clients run into doorways, furniture, etc, instead of cueing clients to detect and solve the problem. Scanning, self-talk, self-questioning about what could be wrong, and manual guiding are some cognitive strategies nurses should use.*

- Support clients and request referrals as needed to help clients cope and adjust to issues related to physical disability, loss of independence, and use of a wheelchair. *Clients may experience depression and anxiety with physical loss, especially with the inability to walk. Value systems of clients and nurses with regard to wheelchair use may vary greatly and create tension. Need for a wheelchair may symbolize weakness, disability, and loss of autonomy to clients, whereas it may symbolize increased independence and functioning to professionals (Minkel, 2000).* **Nursing Research:** *This phenomenological study found that full-time wheelchair users experience frustration with barriers and accessibility. Specifically there was frustration with independence issues, societal attitudes toward people with disability, lack of understanding by others, and lack of involvement of individuals with disability in decisions regarding development of accessible facilities (Pierce, 1998).*

▲ Nurses, therapists, or physicians may need to recommend and help the client transition from a manual to a powered wheelchair. The client may resist the idea of further dependency and need psychosocial support. *Shoulder/wrist pain and injury may result because of overuse from chronic weight bearing during transfers, performing push-ups to relieve sacral pressure, and from propelling a manual wheelchair. An electric wheelchair may be recommended to protect the integrity of the shoulder joints, reduce pain, reduce energy and time demands, and because of progression of physical illness or disability (Minkel, 2000).* **Clinical Research:** *Eight patients with progressive or static neuromuscular disability were interviewed 6 to 24 months after switching to a powered mobility device; the move posi-*

- • = **Independent;** ▲ = **Collaborative**

et al, 1999). **Clinical Research:** *Milk-alkali syndrome has occurred in women ingesting 4 to 12 g of calcium carbonate daily (Beall and Scofield, 1995). One should not exceed 2000 mg of calcium supplement per day, except at the advice of the health care provider, because excessive calcium could cause deficiencies of other minerals (Whiting et al, 1997).*

- Consider social factors that may interfere with nutrition (e.g., lack of transportation, inadequate income, lack of social support). *Nutritional deficiencies are seen in at least one third of the elderly in industrialized countries (Chandra, 1997). In most surveys, poverty was found to be the major social cause of food insecurity and weight loss, but friendship networks play an important role in maintaining adequate food intake (Morley, 1997).*

- Assess for psychological and mental factors that impact nutrition. Watch for signs of depression. **Clinical Research:** *Nutritional risk independently increased the likelihood of death in cognitively impaired older adults (Keller and Ostbye, 2000). In persons with depression, 90% of the elderly lose weight, compared with 60% of younger persons (Morley, 1997).*

- Consider the effects of medications on food intake. Appetite-stimulating drugs may have a role in some cases. *The side effects of drugs are a major cause of weight loss in older persons (Morley, 1997). Medications linked to protein-energy malnutrition in nursing home residents include digoxin, theophylline, nonsteroidal anti-inflammatory drugs, iron supplements, and psychoactive drugs (Kamel et al, 1998).* **Clinical Research:** *Compared with a placebo, megestrol acetate improved appetite and promoted weight gain in geriatric patients (Yeh et al, 2000).*

- ▲ Provide appropriate food textures for chewing ease. Insert dentures (if needed) before meals. Assess fit of dentures. Refer for dental consultation if needed. *The bony structure of jaws changes over time, requiring adjustment of dentures. The most common feeding difficulties among geriatric rehabilitation clients involved dentures (lack of or ill fitting) and oral infections (Keller, 1997).*

  NOTE: If the client is unable to feed self, refer to Nursing Interventions and Rationales for **Feeding Self-care deficit.**

Multicultural

- Assess for dietary intake of essential nutrients. **Clinical Research:** *Studies have shown that black women have calcium intakes of less than 75% of the RDA (Zablah et al, 1999). Hispanics with type 2 diabetes also often have inadequate protein nutritional status (Castaneda et al, 2000). Mexican American women have a higher prevalence of iron deficiency anemia than non-Hispanic white females (Frith-Terhune et al, 2000). Rural black men had low caloric intakes coupled with high fat intakes but nutrient deficiencies (Vitolins et al, 2000).*

- Assess for the influence of cultural beliefs, norms, and values on the client's nutritional knowledge. *What the client considers normal dietary practices may be based on cultural perceptions (Cochran, 1998; Doswell and Erlen, 1998; Leininger and McFarland, 2002).*

- Discuss with the client those aspects of their diet that will remain unchanged. *Aspects of the client's life that are meaningful and valuable to them should be understood and preserved without change (Leininger and McFarland, 2002).*

- Negotiate with the client regarding the aspects of his or her diet that will need to be modified. *Give and take with the client will lead to culturally congruent care (Leininger and McFarland, 2002).*

- Validate the client's feelings regarding the impact of current lifestyle, finances, and transportation on ability to obtain nutritious food. *Validation is a therapeutic commu-*

- • = **Independent;** ▲ = **Collaborative**

nication technique that lets the client know that the nurse has heard and understands what was said, and it promotes the nurse-client relationship (Heineken, 1998).

Home care

- Above interventions may be adapted for home care use.
- Monitor food intake. Instruct the client in intake of small frequent meals and liquid supplements (e.g., Ensure, Instant Breakfast). *Until definitive causes can be isolated for intervention, it is important for clients to maintain intake as much as possible. Reducing meal size and eating more frequently may help. Multiple causes of anorexia and weight loss in older adults have been suggested, from social isolation to gastrointestinal dysfunction. Altered neurochemistry has been implicated (Blanton et al, 1999).*
- ▲ Assess the client for depression. Refer for mental health services as indicated. *Decreased appetite with weight loss is part of the syndrome of depression. Return of appetite is unlikely unless the underlying depression is treated.*
- Recognize that older women may continue their younger preoccupation with weight and recurrent dieting, despite being at normal weight. Assess source of low weight or weight loss with this in mind. *Reports suggest that elderly women continue to be preoccupied with being thin. Increased awareness of eating habits and weight preoccupation in elderly women is recommended (Fallaz et al, 1999).*
- ▲ Monitor and effect total parenteral nutrition (TPN) as ordered by physician. TPN requires monitoring for potential complications and client/caregiver education (Gorski, 2001).
- ▲ In the presence of depression diagnosis, refer for psychiatric home health care services for client reassurance and implementation of therapeutic regimen. *Poor appetite and weight loss are symptoms of depression. Psychiatric home care nurses can address issues relating to assessment and treatment of the client's depression. Behavioral interventions in the home can assist the client to participate more effectively in a treatment plan (Patusky, Rodning, and Martinez-Kratz, 1996).*

Client/Family Teaching

- Help the client/family identify the area to change that will make the greatest contribution to improved nutrition. *Change is difficult. Multiple changes may be overwhelming.*
- Build on the strengths in the client's/family's food habits. Adapt changes to their current practices. *Accepting the client's/family's preferences shows respect for their culture.*
- Select appropriate teaching aids for the client's/family's background.
- Implement instructional follow-up to answer the client's/family's questions.
- ▲ Suggest community resources as suitable (food sources, counseling, Meals on Wheels, Senior Centers).
- Teach the client and family how to manage tube feedings or parenteral therapy at home.

ᴇᴠᴏʟᴠᴇ WEBSITES FOR EDUCATION

See the EVOLVE website for World Wide Web resources for client education.

• = Independent; ▲ = Collaborative

REFERENCES

Arrowsmith H: Malnutrition in hospital: detection and consequences, *Br J Nurs* 6:1131, 1997.

Baker SS: Protein-energy malnutrition in the hospitalized pediatric patient. In Walker WA, Watkins JB, editors: *Nutrition in pediatrics,* Hamilton, Ontario, 1997, BC Decker.

Beall D, Scofield R: Milk-alkali syndrome associated with calcium carbonate consumption, *Medicine* 74:89, 1995.

Castaneda C, Bermudez OI, Tucker KL: Protein nutritional status and functions are associated with type II diabetes in Hispanic elders, *Am J Clin Nutr* 72(1):89, 2000.

Chandra RK: Nutrition and the immune system: an introduction, *Am J Clin Nutr* 66:460S, 1997.

Chandra RK: Nutrition and the immune system from birth to old age, *Eur J Clin Nutr* 56 (suppl 3):S73, 2002.

Cochran M: Tears have no color, *Am J Nurs* 98(6):53, 1998.

Denney A: Quiet music: an intervention for mealtime agitation? *J Gerontol Nurs* 23:16, 1997.

Doswell W, Erlen J: Multicultural issues and ethical concerns in the delivery of revising care interventions, *Nurs Clin North Am* 33(2):353, 1998.

Elmstahl S et al: Malnutrition in geriatric patients: a neglected problem? *J Adv Nurs* 26:851, 1997.

Estok PJ, Rudy EB: The relationship between eating disorders and running in women, *Res Nurs Health* 19:377, 1996.

Evans NJ: Feeding. In Bulechek GM, McCloskey JC, editors: *Nursing interventions: essential nursing treatments,* ed 2, Philadelphia, 1992, WB Saunders.

Fitzpatrick S et al: Vitamin D-deficient rickets: a multifactorial disease, *Nutr Rev* 58:218, 2000.

Friedmann JM et al: Predicting early nonelective hospital readmission in nutritionally compromised older adults, *Am J Clin Nutr* 65:1714, 1997.

Frith-Terhune AL et al: Iron deficiency anemia: higher prevalence in Mexican American than in non-Hispanic white females in the third National Health and Nutrition Examination Survey, 1988-1994, *Am J Clin Nutr* 72(4):963, 2000.

Ganley BJ: Effective mouth care for head and neck radiation therapy patients, *Medsurg Nurs* 4:133, 1995.

Garg K, Draganescu JM, Albornoz MA: A rash imposition from a lifestyle omission, *Postgrad Med* 104:183, 1998.

Heineken J: Patient silence is not necessarily client satisfaction: communication in home care nursing, *Home Healthc Nurse* 16(2):115, 1998.

Kamel HK, Thomas DR, Morley JE: National deficiencies in long-term care: part II. Management of protein-energy malnutrition and dehydration, *Ann Long Term Care* 6:250, 1998.

Keele AM et al: Two phase randomised controlled clinical trial of postoperative oral dietary supplements in surgical patients, *Gut* 40:393, 1997.

Keller HH: Nutrition problems and their association with patient outcomes in a geriatric rehabilitation setting, *J Nutr Elderly* 17(2):1, 1997.

Keller HH, Ostbye T: Do nutrition indicators predict death in elderly Canadians with cognitive impairment? *Can J Public Health* 91:220, 2000.

Kreiter SR et al: Nutritional rickets in African American breast-fed infants, *J Pediatr* 137:153, 2000.

Lauque S et al: Protein-energy oral supplementation in malnourished nursing-home residents. A controlled trial, *Age Ageing* 29:51, 2000.

LeBoff MS et al: Occult vitamin D deficiency in postmenopausal US women with acute hip fracture, *JAMA* 281:1505, 1999.

Leininger MM, McFarland MR: *Transcultural nursing: concepts, theories, research and practices,* ed 3, New York, 2002, McGraw-Hill.

Lewis DA, Boyle KD: Nutritional supplement use during medication administration: selected case studies, *J Nutr Elderly* 17:53, 1998.

Love CC, Seaton H: Eating disorders: highlights of nursing assessment and therapeutics, *Nurs Clin North Am* 26:677, 1991.

Lutz CA, Przytulski KR: *Nutrition and diet therapy,* ed 3, Philadelphia, 2001, FA Davis.

Mentes J et al: Acute confusion indicators: risk factors and prevalence using MDS data, *Res Nurs Health* 22:95, 1999.

Miller M et al: Nutritional assessment and intervention in patients admitted with a femoral neck fracture: a chronicle of missed opportunities, *Aust J Nutr Diet* 58(2):86, 2001.

Morley JE: Anorexia of aging: physiologic and pathologic, *Am J Clin Nutr* 66:760, 1997.

Morley JE, Thomas DR, Kamel H: Nutritional deficiencies in long-term care: part I, *Ann Long Term Care* 6(5): 183, 1998.

• = **Independent;** ▲ = **Collaborative**

National Academy of Sciences: *Dietary reference intakes,* Washington, DC, 1998, National Academy Press.

Nelson ME et al: Effects of high-intensity strength training on multiple risk factors for osteoporotic fractures, *JAMA* 272(24):1909, 1994.

Patusky KL, Rodning C, Martinez-Kratz M: Clinical lessons in psychiatric home care: a case study approach, *J Home Healthc Manag* 9:18, 1996.

Payette H et al: Predictors of dietary intake in a functionally dependent elderly population in the community, *Am J Public Health* 85:677, 1995.

Ragneskog H et al: Dinner music for demented patients: analysis of video-recorded observations, *Clin Nurs Res* 5:262, 1996.

Rogers-Seidel FF, editor: *Geriatric nursing care plans,* St Louis, 1991, Mosby.

Russell RM, Rasmussen H, Lichtenstein AH: Modified food guide pyramid for people over 70 years of age, *J Nutr* 129:751, 1999.

Ryan C, Eleazer P, Egbert J: Vitamin D in the elderly, *Nutr Today* 30:228, 1995.

Schurch MA et al: Protein supplements increase serum insulin-like growth factor-1 levels and attenuate proximal femur bone loss in patients with recent hip fracture: a randomized, double-blind, placebo-controlled trial, *Ann Intern Med* 128:801, 1998.

Shah M et al: Nutritional rickets still afflict children in north Texas, *Tex Med* 96:64, 2000.

Shahar DR et al: The effect of widowhood on weight change, dietary intake, and eating behavior in the elderly population, *J Aging Health* 13:189, 2001.

Smith JK, Aljazairi A, Fuller SH: INR elevation associated with diarrhea in a patient receiving warfarin, *Ann Pharmacother* 33:301, 1999.

Suarez FL, Savaiano DA, Levitt MD: A comparison of symptoms after consumption of milk or lactose-hydrolyzed milk by people with self-reported severe lactose intolerance, *N Engl J Med* 333:1, 1995.

Sullivan DH, Sun S, Walls RC: Protein-energy undernutrition among elderly hospitalized patients: a prospective study, *JAMA* 281:2013, 1999.

Sullivan DH, Walls RC: Protein-energy undernutrition and the risk of mortality within six years of hospital discharge, *J Am Coll Nutr* 17:571, 1998.

Vitolins MZ et al: Ethnic and gender variation in the dietary intake of rural elders, *J Nutr Elderly* 19(3):15, 2000.

Wakefield B et al: Monitoring hydration status in elderly veterans, *West J Nurs Res* 24:132, 2002.

Watson T, Bowers WA, Andersen AE: Involuntary treatment of eating disorders, *Am J Psychiatry* 175:1806, 2000.

Whiting SJ, Wood R, Kim K: Calcium supplements, *J Am Acad Nurse Pract* 9:187, 1997.

Winograd CH, Brown EM: Aggressive oral refeeding in hospitalized patients, *Am J Clin Nutr* 52:967, 1990.

Wyshak G: Teenaged girls, carbonated beverage consumption, and bone fractures, *Arch Pediatr Adolesc Med* 154:610, 2000.

Yeh S et al: Improvement in quality-of-life measures and stimulation of weight gain after treatment with megesterol acetate oral suspension in geriatric cachexia: results of a double-blind, placebo-controlled study, *J Am Geriatr Soc* 48:485, 2000.

Zablah EM et al: Barriers to calcium intake in African American women, *J Hum Nutr* 12(2):123, 1999.

Imbalanced Nutrition: more than body requirements

Carroll A. Lutz

NANDA Definition

Intake of nutrients that exceeds metabolic needs

Defining Characteristics

Triceps skin fold of more than 25 mm in women; triceps skin fold of more than 15 mm in men; body weight more than 20% over ideal for height and frame; eating in response to external cues (e.g., time of day, social situation); eating in response to internal cues other than hunger (e.g., anxiety); reported or observed dysfunctional eating pat-

• = Independent; ▲ = Collaborative

tern pairing food with other activities; sedentary activity level; concentration of food intake at the end of the day

Related Factors (r/t)

Excessive intake in relation to metabolic need; deficient knowledge related to desirability of nutritional supplements

NOC   Outcomes (Nursing Outcomes Classification)

Suggested NOC Outcomes
Nutritional Status: Food and Fluid Intake, Nutrient Intake; Weight Control

> **Example NOC Outcome with Indicators**
>
> **Weight Control** as evidenced by the following indicators: Demonstrates progress toward target weight/ Balances exercise with caloric intake/Maintains recommended eating pattern/Controls preoccupation with food (Rate each indicator of **Weight Control:** 1 = never demonstrated, 2 = rarely demonstrated, 3 = sometimes demonstrated, 4 = often demonstrated, 5 = consistently demonstrated [see Section I].)

Client Outcomes

Client Will (Specify Time Frame):
- State pertinent factors contributing to weight gain
- Identify behaviors that remain under client's control
- Claim ownership for current eating patterns
- Design dietary modifications to meet individual long-term goal of weight control, using principles of variety, balance, and moderation
- Accomplish desired weight loss in a reasonable period (1 to 2 lb/wk)
- Incorporate appropriate activities requiring energy expenditure into daily life
- Use sound scientific sources to evaluate need for nutritional supplements

NIC   Interventions (Nursing Interventions Classification)

Suggested NIC Interventions
Eating Disorders Management; Nutrition Management; Nutritional Counseling; Weight Management; Weight Reduction Assistance

> **Example NIC Activities—Weight Management**
>
> Determine client's motivation for changing eating habits; Develop with client a method to keep daily record of intake

Nursing Interventions and Rationales

▲ Obtain a thorough history. Refer to a dietitian if the client has a medical condition. *The most appropriate clients for the nursing intervention of weight management are adults with no other major health problems requiring medical nutritional therapy.*

▲ Evaluate the client's physiological status in relation to weight control. Refer as appropriate. *Children have been included in weight management programs without sufficient consideration of their growth needs, which increases the risk of future health problems.*

• = Independent; ▲ = Collaborative

- Assess dietary intake through 24-hour recall or questions regarding the usual intake of food groups. *Information may not be completely accurate. Such assessment also permits an appraisal of the client's knowledge about diet.*
- Evaluate the client's usual intake of fiber. *In general, high-fiber foods take longer to eat and contain fewer calories than most other foods.* **Clinical Research:** *High dietary fiber intake was associated with lower body weight and waist-to-hip ratio and predicted weight loss more strongly than did level of fat consumption (Ludwig et al, 1999).*
- Determine the client's knowledge of a nutritious diet and need for supplements. *This information is useful for developing an individualized teaching plan based on the client's current state.*
- Calculate body mass index (BMI) using either of the following formulas.
  - Weight in kilograms divided by height (in meters) squared (kg/m^2)
  - Weight in pounds multiplied by 705, divided by height in inches, divided again by height in inches

  A normal BMI is 20 to 25; a BMI of 26 to 29 indicates overweight; and a BMI of more than 30 indicates obesity. A BMI of 40 is used by some programs as a criterion for surgical intervention.
- Compute the waist-to-hip ratio (WHR). *A WHR of over 0.85 in women and over 1.0 in men indicates increased risk of problems related to obesity (Lutz and Przytulski, 2001).* **Nursing Research:** A female peripheral fat pattern (gynecoid), predominant in most women, is associated with virtually no impairment of health (Allan, 1994).
- Determine the client's motivation to lose weight, whether for appearance or health benefits. *Often a healthier body weight is only a 5% to 10% reduction from the initial body weight (Nonas, 1998). Nondieting approaches focus on changing disturbed thoughts, emotions, and body image associated with obesity to help obese persons to accept themselves and resolve issues that may hinder long-term weight maintenance (Foreyt, Walker, and Poston, 1998). Overweight and obesity reduce immunity (Chandra, 2002).*
- Observe for situations that indicate a nutritional intake of more than body requirements. *Such observations help gain a clear picture of the client's dietary habits.* **Clinical Research:** *Post-trauma clients have been overfed due to lack of an interdisciplinary plan of care (Klein and Henry, 1999).*
- Suggest that the client keep a diary of food intake and the circumstances surrounding its consumption (methods of preparation, duration of meal, social situation, overall mood, activities accompanying consumption). **Nursing Research:** *Self-monitoring helps the client assess adherence to self-determined performance criteria and progress toward desired goals. Self-monitoring plays an important role in the maintenance of internal standards of behavior (Fleury, 1991).*
- Advise the client to measure food periodically. Help the client learn usual portion sizes. *Measuring food alerts the client to normal portion sizes. Estimation of amounts can be extremely inaccurate.*
- Review the client's current exercise level. With the client and primary health care provider, design a long-term exercise program. *Exercise is important for increased energy expenditure, for maintenance of lean body mass, and as part of a total change in lifestyle, but a health risk appraisal should be performed for all previously sedentary individuals before they begin an exercise program (Lutz and Przytulski, 2001). Loss of lean tissue is undesirable because muscle tissue is estimated to be as much as 70 times more metabolically active than fat tissue (Rippe and Hess, 1998). Women who consumed an energy-restricted diet in addition to performing aerobic and strength training exercise lost more weight than compari-*

• = **Independent;** ▲ = **Collaborative**

son study groups and slightly increased their lean muscle tissue *(Rippe and Hess, 1998).* **Clinical Research:** *Children receiving a 6-month classroom curriculum to reduce television, videotape, and video game use showed significant decreases in body mass index and triceps skin folds compared to controls (Robinson, 1999).*

- Establish a reasonable goal for the client's body weight and for weight loss (e.g., 1 to 2 lb/wk). **Clinical Research:** *Because subjects in one study achieved comparable weight loss on liquid formula diets of 420, 600, or 800 calories/day, choosing the higher-energy diets may minimize adverse side effects (Foster et al, 1992).*
- Determine the motivational factors operating in the client at the present time. **Nursing Research:** *African American women were motivated to increase their physical activity by personal and familial histories of heart disease and related risk factors (Banks-Wallace, 2000).*
- Explore strategies that appeal to the client. **Nursing Research:** *Group interventions that include spiritual practices and community building may be especially effective for promoting physical activity among African American women (Banks-Wallace, 2000). One study found that African American women tried more commercial diet products and ceased their weight loss efforts sooner than did Euro-American women (Tyler, Allan, and Alcozer, 1997).*
- Initiate a client contract that involves rewarding and reinforcing progressive goal attainment. *Client contracts can help clients learn to analyze their behavior and to choose effective behavioral strategies as well as provide a progress report to reinforce the behaviors.*
- Weigh the client twice a week under the same conditions. *It is important to most clients and contributes to their progress to have the tangible reward that the scale shows. Monitoring twice a week gives frequent feedback to encourage the client to continue with the program.*
- Instruct the client regarding adequate nutritional intake. A total plan permits occasional treats. *Because permanent lifestyle changes must occur for weight loss to be long lasting, eliminating all treats is unwise and not sustainable. Numerous studies have demonstrated that fewer than 5% of persons who lose weight through energy restriction alone are able to maintain this weight loss for 2 years or longer (Rippe and Hess, 1998). During energy restriction, a client should consume 72 to 80 g of high-biological-value protein per day to minimize the risk of ventricular arrhythmias (Nonas, 1998).*
- Familiarize the client with the following behavior modification techniques (Lutz and Przytulski, 2001):
  - Self-monitoring
  - Keeping a food and exercise diary
  - Graphing weight weekly
  - Controlling stimuli
  - Limiting food intake to one site in the home
  - Sitting down at the table to eat
  - Planning food intake for each day
  - Rearranging the schedule to avoid inappropriate eating
  - Saving or rescheduling everyday activities for times when one is hungry
  - Avoiding boredom; keeping a list of activities on the refrigerator
  - For a party, eating before arriving, sitting away from the snack foods, and substituting lower-calorie beverages for alcoholic ones
  - Deciding beforehand what to order in a restaurant
  - Slowing mealtime

- = **Independent**; ▲ = **Collaborative**

- Drinking a glass of water before each meal; taking sips of water between bites of food
- Swallowing food before putting more food on the utensil
- Trying to be the last one to finish eating
- Pausing for a minute during the meal and attempting to increase the number of pauses
- Rewarding oneself
- Charting one's progress
- Making an agreement with oneself or a significant other for a meaningful reward
- Not rewarding oneself with food
- Changing one's mind-set
- Viewing exercise as a means of controlling hunger
- Practicing relaxation techniques
- Imagining oneself ordering a side salad, diet dressing, low-fat milk, and a small hamburger at a fast-food restaurant
- Visualizing oneself enjoying a fresh apple in preference to apple pie

- Encourage the client to adopt an exercise program that involves 45 minutes of exercise five times a week. *Moderately intense physical activity for 30 to 45 minutes 5 to 7 days a week can expend the 1500 to 2000 calories/wk that appear to be necessary to maintain weight loss. Cross-sectional and longitudinal studies illustrate that persons who increase their physical activity also increase their resting metabolic rate (Rippe and Hess, 1998).* **Clinical Research:** *Diet plus exercise produced greater and better-sustained weight loss than either diet or exercise alone (Miller, 1997).*
- Assess for the use of nonprescription diet aids. *Herbal remedies are not subjected to the same scrutiny that the Food and Drug Administration devotes to prescription drugs and may be of varying strengths and/or have ingredients not listed on the label.* **Clinical Research:** *Ingestion of an herbal supplement containing ma-huang, the main plant source of ephedrine, for weight loss caused mania in a client with no history of psychiatric illness (Capwell, 1995).*
- Observe for overuse of particular nutrients. *Almost all nutrients given in quantities beyond a certain threshold will reduce immune responses (Chandra, 1997). Moreover, clients who are consuming excessive amounts of some nutrients may also be consuming less than adequate amounts of others.* **Clinical Research:** *Daily ingestion of 500 ml of tonic water containing 40 mg of quinine hydrochloride caused photosensitivity. Other conditions associated with tonic water consumption are disseminated intravascular coagulation, recurrent dermatitis, fixed drug eruption, and toxic epidermal necrolysis (Wagner et al, 1994).*
- Commit to the client for the long term. Follow up on a regular basis. *Lifestyle changes take time to accomplish. Reassurance may be needed frequently.* **Clinical Research:** *A telephone and mail follow-up resulted in better weight control in adolescents than did a single session of physician counseling (Saelens et al, 2002).*

Geriatric

- Assess changes in lifestyle and eating patterns. *Energy needs decrease an estimated 5% per decade after the age of 40 years, but often eating patterns remain unchanged from youth.*
- Assess fluid intake. Recommend routine drinks of water whether thirsty or not. *Thirst sensation becomes dulled in the elderly.*
- Observe for socioeconomic factors that influence food choices (e.g., inadequate funds

- = Independent; ▲ = Collaborative

or cooking facilities). *Even those on restricted budgets and with limited facilities can be helped to choose food sources for a balanced diet.*
- Suggest a variety of seasonings. *The ability to taste sweet, bitter, sour, and salty declines in most, but not all, older persons (Morley, 1997).*

Multicultural

- Assess for the influence of cultural beliefs, norms, and values on the client's nutritional knowledge and practices. *What the client considers normal dietary practices may be based on cultural perceptions (Cochran, 1998; Doswell and Erlen, 1998; Leininger and McFarland, 2002).*
- Assess for the influence of cultural beliefs, norms, and values on the client's ideal of acceptable body weight and body size. *Ideal body weight and size may be based on cultural perceptions (Leininger and McFarland, 2002).* **Clinical Research:** *African American women report more satisfaction with body size than other women (Miller et al, 2000). Overweight Hispanic women with high levels of binge eating and depression preferred a slim body ideal (Fitzgibbon et al, 1998).*
- Discuss with the client those aspects of his or her diet that will remain unchanged, and work with the client to adapt cultural core foods. *Aspects of the client's life that are meaningful and valuable to the client should be understood and preserved without change (Leininger and McFarland, 2002). Core foods are those foods that are universal, staple, important, and consistently used in the culture (Sanjur, 1995).* **Clinical Research:** *Dramatic weight loss was achieved in Hawaii using a culturally appropriate methodology (Shintani et al, 1991).*
- Negotiate with the client regarding the aspects of his or her diet that will need to be modified. *Give and take with the client will lead to culturally congruent care (Leininger and McFarland, 2002).*
- Validate the client's feelings regarding the impact of current lifestyle, finances, and transportation on the ability to obtain and prepare nutritious food. *Validation is a therapeutic communication technique that lets the client know that the nurse has heard and understood what was said, and it promotes the nurse-client relationship (Heineken, 1998).*

Client/Family Teaching

- Provide the client and family with information regarding the treatment plan options. *If the client and family select the treatment plan, they are more likely to comply with it, particularly if the client does not do the marketing and cooking.*
- Inform the client about the health risks associated with obesity for adults and children in the family. **Clinical Research:** *The risk of death from all causes, from cardiovascular disease, from cancer, and from other diseases increases throughout the range of moderate and severe overweight for both men and women in all age groups (Calle et al, 1999).*
- Treatment for childhood obesity should be started when weight gain exceeds established percentiles for age and gender (Nichols, 2002). *Guide the client toward changes that will have a major impact on health. Even modest weight loss contributes to diabetes and hypertension control.*
- Inform the client and family of the disadvantages of trying to lose weight by dieting alone. *Resting metabolic rate is decreased as much as 45% with extreme calorie restriction. The decrease persists after the diet period has ended, which leads to the "yo-yo effect." With a reduced-calorie diet alone, as much as 25% of the weight lost can be lean body mass rather than fat. Resting energy expenditure is positively related to lean body mass.*

- • = **Independent;** ▲ = **Collaborative**

- Teach the importance of exercise in a weight control program. *A physically conditioned person uses more fat for energy at rest and with exercise than a sedentary person does. The majority of clients will benefit from establishing walking as a cornerstone of their physical activity program (Rippe, Crossley, and Ringer, 1998).*
- Teach stress reduction techniques as alternatives to eating. *The client should have available a variety of healthy behaviors to substitute for unhealthy ones.*

evolve WEBSITES FOR EDUCATION

See the EVOLVE website for World Wide Web resources for client education.

REFERENCES

Allan JD: A biomedical and feminist perspective on women's experiences with weight management, *West J Nurs Res* 16:524, 1994.

Banks-Wallace J: Staggering under the weight of responsibility: the impact of culture on physical activity among African American women, *Multicult Nurs Health* 6:24, 2000.

Calle EE: Body-mass index and mortality in a prospective cohort of U.S. adults, *N Engl J Med* 34:1097, 1999.

Capwell R: Ephedrine-induced mania from an herbal diet supplement, *Am J Psychiatry* 152:647, 1995 (letter).

Chandra RK: Nutrition and the immune system: an introduction, *Am J Clin Nutr* 66:460S, 1997.

Chandra RK: Nutrition and the immune system from birth to old age, *Eur J Clin Nutr* 56(suppl 3):S73, 2002.

Cochran M: Tears have no color, *Am J Nurs* 98(6):53, 1998.

Doswell W, Erlen J: Multicultural issues and ethical concerns in the delivery of nursing care interventions, *Nurs Clin North Am* 33(2):353, 1998.

Fitzgibbon ML et al: Correlates of binge eating in Hispanic, black and white women, *Int J Eat Disord* 24(1):43, 1998.

Fleury J: Empowering potential: a theory of wellness motivation, *Nurs Res* 40:288, 1991.

Foreyt JP, Walker S, Poston II C: The role of the behavioral counselor in obesity treatment, *J Am Diet Assoc* 98(suppl 2):S27, 1998.

Foster GD et al: A controlled comparison of three very-low-calorie diets: effects on weight, body composition and symptoms, *Am J Clin Nutr* 55:811, 1992.

Heineken J: Patient silence is not necessarily client satisfaction: communication in home care nursing, *Home Healthc Nurse* 16(2):115, 1998.

Klein CJ, Henry SM: Acute nutrition interventions help identify indicators of quality in a trauma service, *Nutr Clin Pract* 14:85, 1999.

Leininger MM, McFarland MR: *Transcultural nursing: concepts, theories, research and practices,* ed 3, New York, 2002, McGraw-Hill.

Ludwig DS et al: Dietary fiber, weight gain, and cardiovascular disease risk factors in young adults, *JAMA* 282:1539, 1999.

Lutz CA, Przytulski KR: *Nutrition and diet therapy,* ed 3, Philadelphia, 2001, FA Davis.

Miller KJ et al: Comparisons of body image by race/ethnicity and gender in a university population, *Int J Eat Disord* 27(3):310, 2000.

Miller WC: A meta-analysis of the past 25 years of weight loss research using diet, exercise or diet plus exercise intervention, *Int J Obes Relat Metab Disord* 21:941, 1997.

Morley JE: Anorexia of aging: physiologic and pathologic, *Am J Clin Nutr* 66:760, 1997.

Nichols MR: Preventing pediatric obesity: assessment and management in the primary care setting, *J Am Acad Nurse Pract* 14:55, 2002.

Nonas CA: A model for chronic care of obesity through dietary treatment, *J Am Diet Assoc* 98(suppl 2):S16, 1998.

Rippe JM, Crossley S, Ringer R: Obesity as a chronic disease: modern medical and lifestyle management, *J Am Diet Assoc* 98(suppl 2):S9, 1998.

Rippe JM, Hess S: The role of physical activity in the prevention and management of obesity, *J Am Diet Assoc* 98(suppl 2):S31, 1998.

• = **Independent; ▲ = Collaborative**

Robinson TN: Reducing children's television viewing to prevent obesity: a randomized controlled trial, *JAMA* 282:1561, 1999.

Saelens BE et al: Behavior weight control for overweight adolescents initiated in primary care, *Obes Res* 10:22, 2002.

Sanjur D: *Hispanic foodways, nutrition, and health,* Needham Heights, Mass, 1995, Allyn and Bacon.

Shintani TT et al: Obesity and cardiovascular risk intervention through the ad libitum feeding of traditional Hawaiian diet, *Am J Clin Nutr* 53:1647S, 1991.

Tyler DO, Allan JD, Alcozer FR: Weight loss methods used by African American and Euro-American women, *Res Nurs Health* 20:413, 1997.

Wagner G et al: "I'll have mine with a twist of lemon": quinine photosensitivity from excessive intake of tonic water, *Br J Dermatol* 131:734, 1994 (letter).

Risk for imbalanced Nutrition: more than body requirements

Carroll A. Lutz

NANDA   Definition

At risk for intake of nutrients that exceeds metabolic needs

Risk Factors

Reported use of solid food as major food source before 5 months of age; concentration of food intake at end of day; reported or observed obesity in one or both parents; reported or observed higher baseline weight at beginning of each pregnancy; rapid transition across growth percentiles in infants or children; pairing of food with other activities; observed use of food as reward or comfort measure; eating in response to internal cues other than hunger (e.g., anxiety); eating in response to external cues (e.g., time of day, social situation); dysfunctional eating patterns

NOC   Outcomes (Nursing Outcomes Classification)

Suggested NOC Outcomes

Nutritional Status: Food and Fluid Intake, Nutrient Intake; Weight Control

> **Example NOC Outcome with Indicators**
>
> **Weight Control** as evidenced by the following indicators: Demonstrates progress toward target weight/Balances exercise with caloric intake/Maintains recommended eating pattern/Controls preoccupation with food (Rate each indicator of **Weight Control:** 1 = never demonstrated, 2 = rarely demonstrated, 3 = sometimes demonstrated, 4 = often demonstrated, 5 = consistently demonstrated [see Section I].)

Client Outcomes

Client Will (Specify Time Frame):
- Explain concept of a balanced diet
- Compare current eating pattern with recommended healthy one
- Design dietary modifications to meet individual long-term goal of weight control, using principles of variety, balance, and moderation
- Identify role of exercise in weight control
- Use sound scientific sources to evaluate need for nutritional supplements

• = **Independent; ▲ = Collaborative**

| **NIC** | **Interventions (Nursing Interventions Classification)** |

Suggested NIC Interventions

Nutrition Management; Nutritional Counseling; Weight Management

---

Example NIC Activities—Weight Management

Determine client's motivation for changing eating habits; Develop with client a method to keep daily record of intake

---

Nursing Interventions and Rationales

- Observe for the presence of risk factors (see Risk Factors). *Parents' obesity is the most important risk factor for childhood obesity.* **Clinical Research:** *Inheritance accounts for 25% to 40% of interindividual difference in adiposity (Maffeis, 2000).*
- Assess nutritional intake, including the use of supplements. *Clients may not volunteer information on supplements because they do not consider them pertinent; however, almost all nutrients given in quantities beyond a certain threshold will reduce immune responses (Chandra, 1997).*
- Determine the client's knowledge of nutrition. *Inform the client of the health risks associated with overconsumption of nutrients. Because fetal abnormalities have been related to vitamin A intake, women who are, or might become, pregnant should avoid consuming daily supplements containing more than 8000 IU of vitamin A and should consume liver and liver products only in moderation because they contain large amounts of vitamin A (Oakley and Erickson, 1995). The hazard is related to preformed vitamin A in animal products, not the provitamin A, carotene, in plants.* **Clinical Research:** *A client consuming more than ten times the recommended daily allowance (RDA) for vitamin A for 6 years developed fatal liver toxicity (Kowalski, 1994).*
- Assess the client's nutritional practices. **Clinical Research:** *Meal composition affects the metabolism of nutrients. Fat storage in children was eight times higher after a high-fat meal than after a low-fat meal (Maffeis et al, 2001).*
- Assess activity level and motivational factors. **Clinical Research:** *Television viewing, a promoter of inactivity and food intake, is a relevant risk factor for obesity in children. A low activity level is accompanied by a low fat oxidation rate in muscle, and a low fat oxidation rate is a risk factor for fat gain or fat regain after weight loss (Maffeis, 2000).* **Nursing Research:** *African American women were motivated to increase their activity by personal and familial histories of heart disease and related risk factors (Banks-Wallace, 2000).*
- Discuss the wise selection, use, and discontinuation of supplements. *If a client chooses to use calcium supplements, recommend those that have been tested and found free of lead.* **Clinical Research:** *Researchers have found lead in 38% (Ross, Szabo, and Tebbett, 2000) to 66% (Scelfo and Flegal, 2000) of calcium products tested.*
- Clients at risk for milk-alkali syndrome, such as those using thiazides and those with renal failure, should be monitored for hypercalcemia (Whiting, Wood, and Kim, 1997). **Clinical Research:** *Milk-alkali syndrome occurred in a man taking antacid tablets for epigastric pain (Vanpee et al, 2000).*
- Vitamin C rebound scurvy has occurred in clients who suddenly discontinued megadoses of vitamin C (ten times the RDA), because the body cannot adjust quickly enough and continues to absorb a meager proportion of the now-smaller dose (DePaola, Faine, and Palmer, 1999). **Clinical Research:** *Even without megadose*

• = Independent; ▲ = Collaborative

supplements, however, plasma levels of vitamin C fall to deficiency levels within 1 to 3 weeks of removal of vitamin-rich fruits and vegetables from the diet (Johnston, 1999).

- Establish a plan with the client, using techniques listed in the care plan for **Imbalanced Nutrition: more than body requirements.** *Intervening when the client is at risk allows relatively small changes in lifestyle to be effective. Lifestyle modification is one of the main predictors of success for weight management programs (Coulston, 1998).*

Geriatric

- Give the client credit for making enough wise choices to have lived to an advanced age. *Studies show that nutrition practices are related to health in certain ways. They are not predictive for individuals.*
- Encourage the use of varying suppliers of foodstuffs in the unlikely event of contamination.

Multicultural

- Assess for the influence of cultural beliefs, norms, and values on the client's nutritional knowledge and practices. *What the client considers normal dietary practices may be based on cultural perceptions (Cochran, 1998; Doswell and Erlen, 1998; Leininger and McFarland, 2002).* **Nursing Research:** *The perception that "big is healthy" drove the early introduction of solid food to infants among Puerto Rican Americans (Higgins, 2000).* **Clinical Research:** *African American grandmothers were the chief decision makers regarding the introduction of solid foods to infants of adolescent mothers (Bentley et al, 1999).*
- Assess for the influence of cultural beliefs, norms, and values on the client's ideal of acceptable body weight and body size. *Ideal body weight and size may be based on cultural perceptions (Leininger and McFarland, 2002).* **Clinical Research:** *African American women report more satisfaction than other women with body size (Miller et al, 2000). Overweight Hispanic women with high levels of binge eating and depression preferred a slim body ideal (Fitzgibbon et al, 1998).*
- Discuss with the client those aspects of the diet that will remain unchanged and work with the client to adapt cultural core foods. *Aspects of the client's life that are meaningful and valuable to the client should be understood and preserved without change (Leininger and McFarland, 2002). Core foods are those foods that are universal, staple, important, and consistently used in the culture (Sanjur, 1995).*
- Negotiate with the client regarding the aspects of his or her diet that will need to be modified. *Give and take with the client will lead to culturally congruent care (Leininger and McFarland, 2002).*
- Assess for the influence of the family on patterns of eating. *Women are the keepers and transmitters of culture in families. Female family members can play a dominant role in how infants and children are fed (Cesario, 2001; Pillitteri, 1999).*
- Validate the client's feelings regarding the impact of current lifestyle, finances, and transportation on his or her ability to obtain and prepare nutritious food. *Validation is a therapeutic communication technique that lets the client know that the nurse has heard and understood what was said, and it promotes the nurse-client relationship (Heineken, 1998).*

Client/Family Teaching

- Analyze the client's nutritional pattern and suggest lower-calorie substitutes for high-calorie dishes. *Ice milk contains 185 calories/cup, compared with 270 calories/cup for ice*

• = Independent; ▲ = Collaborative

cream. Low-calorie Italian dressing contains 5 calories/tbsp, compared with 80 calories/tbsp for regular Italian dressing.

- Demonstrate the use of food labels to make healthful choices. Alert the client and family to focus on serving size, total fat, and simple carbohydrates. *The standardized food label in bold type simplifies the search for information. Fats and sugars contribute the least to a healthful diet and the most to excessive caloric intake.*

evolve WEBSITES FOR EDUCATION

See the EVOLVE website for World Wide Web resources for client education.

REFERENCES

Banks-Wallace J: Staggering under the weight of responsibility: the impact of culture on physical activity among African American women, *Multicult Nurs Health* 6:24, 2000.

Bentley M et al: Infant feeding practices of low-income, African-American, adolescent mothers: an ecological, multigenerational perspective, *Soc Sci Med* 49(8):1085, 1999.

Cesario S: Care of the Native American woman: strategies for practice, education, and research, *J Gynecol Neonat Nurs* 30(1):13, 2001.

Chandra RK: Nutrition and the immune system: an introduction, *Am J Clin Nutr* 66:460S, 1997.

Cochran M: Tears have no color, *Am J Nurs* 98(6):53, 1998.

Coulston AM: Obesity as an epidemic: facing the challenge, *J Am Diet Assoc* 98(suppl 2):S6, 1998.

DePaola DP, Faine MP, Palmer CA: Nutrition in relation to dental medicine. In Shils ME et al, editors: *Modern nutrition in health and disease,* ed 9, Philadelphia, 1999, Lippincott Williams and Wilkins.

Doswell W, Erlen J: Multicultural issues and ethical concerns in the delivery of nursing care interventions, *Nurs Clin North Am* 33(2):353, 1998.

Fitzgibbon ML et al: Correlates of binge eating in Hispanic, black and white women, *Int J Eat Disord* 24(1):43, 1998.

Heineken J: Patient silence is not necessarily client satisfaction: communication in home care nursing, *Home Healthc Nurse* 16(2):115, 1998.

Higgins B: Puerto Rican cultural beliefs: influence on infant feeding practices in western New York, *J Transcult Nurs* 11(1):19, 2000.

Johnston CS: Biomarkers for establishing a tolerable upper intake level for vitamin C, *Nutr Rev* 57:71, 1999.

Kowalski T et al: Vitamin A hepatotoxicity: a cautionary note regarding 25,000 IU supplements, *Am J Med* 97: 523, 1994.

Leininger MM, McFarland MR: *Transcultural nursing: concepts, theories, research and practices,* ed 3, New York, 2002, McGraw-Hill.

Maffeis C: Aetiology of overweight and obesity in children and adolescents, *Eur J Pediatr* 159(suppl 1):S35, 2000.

Maffeis C et al: Meal-induced thermogenesis and obesity: is a fat meal a risk factor for fat gain in children? *J Clin Endocrinol Metab* 86:214, 2001.

Miller KJ et al: Comparisons of body image by race/ethnicity and gender in a university population, *Int J Eat Disord* 27(3):310, 2000.

Oakley GP, Erickson JD: Vitamin A and birth defects, *N Engl J Med* 333:1414, 1995.

Pillitteri A: Nutritional needs of the newborn. In Pillitteri A, editor: *Maternal and child health nursing: care of the childbearing and childrearing family,* Philadelphia, 1999, Lippincott.

Ross EA, Szabo NJ, Tebbett IR: Lead content of calcium supplements, *JAMA* 284:1425, 2000.

Sanjur D: *Hispanic foodways, nutrition, and health,* Needham Heights, Mass, 1995, Allyn and Bacon.

Scelfo GM, Flegal AR: Lead in calcium supplements, *Environ Health Perspect* 108:309, 2000.

Vanpee D et al: Ingestion of antacid tablets (Rennie) and acute confusion, *J Emerg Med* 19:169, 2000.

Whiting SJ, Wood R, Kim K: Calcium supplementation, *J Am Acad Nurse Pract* 9:187, 1997.

• = **Independent;** ▲ = **Collaborative**

Impaired Oral mucous membrane

Betty J. Ackley

NANDA Definition

Disruptions of lips and soft tissues of oral cavity

Defining Characteristics

Purulent drainage or exudates; gingival recession, pockets deeper than 4 mm; tonsils enlarged beyond what is developmentally appropriate; smooth, atrophic, sensitive tongue; geographic tongue; mucosal denudation; presence of pathogens; difficulty in speech; self-report of bad taste; gingival or mucosal pallor; oral pain/discomfort; xerostomia (dry mouth); vesicles, nodules, or papules; white patches/plaques, spongy patches, or white curdlike exudate; oral lesions or ulcers; halitosis; edema; hyperemia; desquamation; coated tongue; stomatitis; self-report of difficult eating or swallowing; self-report of diminished or absent taste; bleeding; macroplasia; gingival hyperplasia; fissures; cheilitis; red or bluish masses (e.g., hemangiomas)

Related Factors (r/t)

Chemotherapy; chemical exposure (e.g., alcohol, tobacco, acidic foods, regular use of inhalers); depression; immunosuppression; aging-related loss of connective, adipose, or bone tissue; barriers to professional care; cleft lip or palate; medication side effects; lack of or decreased salivation; chemical trauma (e.g., acidic foods, drugs, noxious agents, alcohol); pathological conditions—oral cavity (radiation to head or neck); nothing-by-mouth status for more than 24 hours; mouth breathing; malnutrition or vitamin deficiency; dehydration; infection; ineffective oral hygiene; mechanical factors (e.g., ill-fitting dentures, braces, tubes [endotracheal/nasogastric], surgery in oral cavity); decreased platelet count; immunocompromise; radiation therapy; barriers to oral self-care; diminished hormone levels (women); stress; loss of supportive structures

NOC   Outcomes (Nursing Outcomes Classification)

Suggested NOC Outcomes

Oral Hygiene; Tissue Integrity: Skin and Mucous Membranes

> **Example NOC Outcome with Indicators**
>
> **Oral Hygiene** as evidenced by the following indicators: Cleanliness of mouth/Moisture of oral mucosa and tongue/Healthy color of mucous membranes/Oral mucosa integrity (Rate each indicator of **Oral Hygiene:** 1 = extremely compromised, 2 = substantially compromised, 3 = moderately compromised, 4 = mildly compromised, 5 = not compromised [see Section I].)

Client Outcomes

Client Will (Specify Time Frame):

- Maintain intact, moist oral mucous membranes that are free of ulceration and debris
- Demonstrate measures to regain or maintain intact oral mucous membranes

• = Independent; ▲ = Collaborative

| **NIC** | **Interventions (Nursing Interventions Classification)** |

Suggested NIC Intervention
Oral Health Restoration

> **Example NIC Activities—Oral Health Restoration**
>
> Use soft toothbrush for removal of dental debris; Instruct client to avoid commercial mouthwashes

Nursing Interventions and Rationales

▲ Inspect the oral cavity at least once daily and note any discoloration, lesions, edema, bleeding, exudate, or dryness. Refer to a physician or specialist as appropriate. *Oral inspection can reveal signs of oral disease, symptoms of systemic disease, drug side effects, or trauma of the oral cavity (White, 2000).*

• Assess for mechanical agents such as ill-fitting dentures and chemical agents such as frequent exposure to tobacco that could cause or increase trauma to oral mucous membranes. *Irritative and causative agents for stomatitis should be eliminated (Rhodes, McDaniel, and Johnson, 1995).*

• Monitor the client's nutritional and fluid status to determine if it is adequate. Refer to the care plan for **Deficient Fluid volume** or **Imbalanced Nutrition: less than body requirements** if applicable. *Dehydration and malnutrition predispose clients to impaired oral mucous membranes.*

• Encourage fluid intake of up to 3000 ml/day if not contraindicated by the client's medical condition. *Fluids help increase moisture in the mouth, which protects the mucous membranes from damage and helps the healing process* (Rhodes, McDaniel, and Johnson, 1995; Roberts, 2000).

• Determine the client's mental status. If the client is unable to care for himself or herself, oral hygiene must be provided by nursing personnel. The nursing diagnosis **Bathing/Hygiene Self-care deficit** is then also applicable.

• Determine the client's usual method of oral care and address any concerns regarding oral hygiene. *Whenever possible, build on the client's existing knowledge base and current practices to develop an individualized plan of care.*

• If the client does not have a bleeding disorder and is able to swallow, encourage the client to brush the teeth with a soft pediatric-sized toothbrush using a fluoride-containing toothpaste after every meal. *The toothbrush is the most important tool for oral care. Brushing the teeth is the most effective method for reducing plaque and controlling periodontal disease (Brown and Yoder, 2002; Roberts, 2000).*

• If the client does not have a bleeding disorder, encourage the client to floss daily with approximately 18 inches of floss using a gentle rubbing up-and-down motion. *Floss is useful to remove plaque buildup between the teeth (Brown and Yoder, 2002).*

Chemotherapy/radiation

• Provide ice chips frequently to keep the mouth moist. **Clinical Research:** *There is some evidence that ice chips help prevent mucositis (Clarkson, Worthington, and Eden, 2002).*

▲ Provide an antifungal agent that is partially absorbed to prevent mucositis if physician so orders. **Clinical Research:** There is some evidence that a partially absorbed antifungal agent used prophylactically was more effective at preventing clinical signs of oral candidiasis than fully absorbed agents (Clarkson, Worthington, and Eden, 2002).

• = Independent; ▲ = Collaborative

- Use a mouth rinse of salt and soda every 1 to 2 hours for prevention and treatment of stomatitis. **Nursing Research:** *A study demonstrated that there was no difference in the rate of cessation of symptoms of stomatitis when three different mouthwashes were used: chlorhexidine, lidocaine, Benadryl and Maalox, and salt and soda (Dodd et al, 2000).*

▲ If the mouth is severely inflamed and it is painful to swallow, contact the physician for a topical anesthetic or analgesic order. Modification of oral intake (e.g., soft or liquid diet) may also be necessary to prevent friction trauma. The nursing diagnosis **Imbalanced Nutrition: less than body requirements** may apply.

- If the client's platelet count is lower than $50,000/mm^3$ or the client has a bleeding disorder, use a specially made toothbrush designed for sensitive or diseased tissue, or a toothette that is not soaked in glycerin or flavorings; if the client cannot tolerate a toothbrush or a toothettte, a piece of gauze wrapped around a finger can be used to remove plaque and debris (Brown and Yoder, 2002).

- Use tap water or normal saline to provide oral care; do not use commercial mouthwashes containing alcohol or hydrogen peroxide. Also, do not use lemon-glycerin swabs. *Alcohol dries the oral mucous membranes (Rogers, 2001).* **Nursing Research:** *Hydrogen peroxide can cause mucosal damage and is extremely foul-tasting to clients (Tombes and Gallucci, 1993). Use of lemon-glycerin swabs can result in decreased salivary amylase and oral moisture, as well as erosion of tooth enamel (Foss-Durant and McAffee 1997; Poland, 1987).*

- Use foam sticks to moisten the oral mucous membranes, clean out debris, and swab out the mouth of the edentulous client. Do not use to clean the teeth unless the platelet count is very low and the client is prone to bleeding gums. *Foam sticks are useful for cleansing the oral cavity of a client who is edentulous (Curzio and McCowan, 2000).* **Nursing Research:** *Foam sticks are not effective for removing plaque; the toothbrush is much more effective (DeWalt, 1975; Pearson and Hutton, 2002).*

- If the client's oral cavity is dry, keep the inside of the mouth moist with frequent sips of water and saltwater rinses (1/2 tsp salt in 8 oz of warm water) or artificial saliva. *Moisture promotes the cleansing effect of saliva and helps avert mucosal drying, which can result in erosions, fissures, or lesions (Rhodes, McDaniel, and Johnson, 1995). Sodium chloride rinses have been shown to be effective for the prevention and treatment of stomatitis (Feber, 1994).*

- Keep the lips well lubricated using petroleum jelly or a similar product (Yeager et al, 2000).

▲ For a client with stomatitis, increase the frequency of oral care to up to every hour while awake if necessary. *Increasing the frequency of oral care has been shown to be effective in decreasing stomatitis (Armstrong, 1994).*

- Provide scrupulous oral care to a critically ill client. *Cultures of the teeth of critically ill clients have yielded significant bacterial colonization, which can lead to nosocomial pneumonia (Scannapieco, Stewart, and Mylotte, 1992).*

▲ If whitish plaques are present in the mouth or on the tongue and can be rubbed off readily with gauze, leaving a red base that bleeds, suspect a fungal infection and contact the physician for follow-up. *Oral candidiasis (moniliasis) is extremely common secondary to antibiotic therapy, steroid therapy, HIV infection, diabetes, or treatment with immunosuppressive drugs, and should be treated with oral or systemic antifungal agents (Epstein and Chow, 1999; Fauci et al, 1998).*

- If the client is unable to swallow, keep suction nearby when providing oral care.

• = **Independent;** ▲ = **Collaborative**

- Refer to the care plan for **Impaired Dentition** if the client has problems with the teeth.

Geriatric

- Determine the functional ability of the client to provide his or her own oral care. If the client has problems with self-care function, ensure that oral care is provided. Refer to **Bathing/Hygiene Self-Care Deficit.** *Interventions must be directed toward both treatment of the functional loss and care of oral health (Avlund, Holm-Pedersen, and Schroll, 2001).*
- Carefully observe the oral cavity and lips for abnormal lesions such as white or red patches, masses, ulcerations with an indurated margin, or a raised granular lesion. *Malignant lesions are more common in elderly persons than in younger persons (especially if there is a history of smoking or alcohol use), and many elderly persons rarely visit a dentist (Aubertin, 1997).*
- Ensure that dentures are removed and scrubbed at least once daily, removed and rinsed thoroughly after every meal, and removed and kept in an appropriate solution at night. *This is an evidence-based protocol for denture care (Curzio and McCowan, 2000). Denture plaque containing* Candida *organisms can cause denture-induced stomatitis, which is more common in clients with unhealthy lifestyles and poor oral hygiene than in others (Nikawa, Hamada, and Yamamoto, 1998; Sakki et al, 1997).*
- If the client has xerostomia, evaluate medications to see if they could be the cause, provide synthetic saliva products to moisten the oral cavity, and offer frequent sips of water and sugarless gum or candy to provide lubrication. *Xerostomia is common in the elderly for many reasons, including medication use and aging. The goal is to keep the mouth moist to prevent stomatitis (Walton, Miller, and Tordecilla, 2001).*
- Provide appropriate oral care to the elderly, brushing the teeth after every meal. **Clinical Research:** *In one study the rate of pneumonia was decreased by providing oral care after every meal (Yoneyama et al, 2002).*

Home care

- The interventions described previously may be adapted for home care use.
- ▲ If dryness is a side effect of the client's medication(s), instruct the client in the use of artificial saliva. Monitor sodium intake in hypertensive clients (Humphrey, 1994). Use alternatives to sodium chloride rinses. *Frequent rinsing with sodium chloride places the client at risk for exacerbation of hypertension or heart failure.*
- Instruct the client to avoid alcohol-based or hydrogen peroxide–based commercial products for mouth care and to avoid other irritants to the oral cavity (e.g., tobacco, spicy foods). *Oral irritants can further damage the oral mucosa and increase the client's discomfort.*
- Instruct the client in ways to soothe the oral cavity (e.g., cool beverages, Popsicles, viscous lidocaine) (Jaffe and Skidmore-Roth, 1993).
- If the client often breathes by mouth, add humidity to the room unless contraindicated.
- ▲ If necessary, refer for home health aide services to support the family in oral care and observation of the oral cavity.

• = **Independent;** ▲ = **Collaborative**

Client/Family Teaching

- Teach the client how to inspect the oral cavity and monitor for signs and symptoms of infection or complications, and when to call the health care practitioner (Rogers, 2001).

evolve WEBSITES FOR EDUCATION

See the EVOLVE website for World Wide Web resources for client education.

REFERENCES

Armstrong TS: Stomatitis in the bone marrow transplant patient, *Cancer Nurs* 17(5):403, 1994.

Aubertin MA: Oral cancer screening in the elderly: the home healthcare nurse's role, *Home Healthc Nurse* 15(9): 594, 1997.

Avlund K, Holm-Pedersen P, Schroll M: Functional ability and oral health among older people: a longitudinal study from age 75 to 80, *J Am Geriatr Soc*, 49:7, 2001.

Brown CG, Yoder LH: Stomatitis: an overview, *Am J Nurs* 102(suppl 4):20, 2002.

Clarkson JE, Worthington HV, Eden OB: Interventions for preventing oral mucositis or oral candidiasis for patients with cancer receiving chemotherapy, *The Cochrane Library* (CD000978), 2002.

Curzio J, McCowan M: Getting research into practice: developing oral hygiene standards, *Br J Nurs* 9(7):434, 2000.

DeWalt EM: Effect of timed hygienic measures on oral mucosa in a group of elderly subjects, *Nurs Res* 24:104, 1975.

Dodd MJ et al: Randomized clinical trial of the effectiveness of three commonly used mouthwashes to treat chemotherapy-induced mucositis, *Oral Surg Oral Med Oral Pathol Oral Radiol Endod* 90:1, 2000.

Epstein JB, Chow AW: Oral complications associated with immunosuppression and cancer therapies, *Infect Dis Clin North Am* 13(4):901, 1999.

Fauci AS et al, editors: *Harrison's principles of internal medicine*, New York, 1998, McGraw-Hill.

Feber T: Mouth care for patients receiving oral irradiation, *Prof Nurse* 10(10):666, 1994.

Foss-Durant AM, McAffee A: A comparison of three oral care products commonly used in practice, *Clin Nurs Res* 6:1, 1997.

Humphrey C: *Home care nursing handbook,* ed 2, Gaithersburg, Md, 1994, Aspen.

Jaffe MS, Skidmore-Roth L: *Home health care nursing care plans,* ed 2, St Louis, 1993, Mosby.

Nikawa H, Hamada T, Yamamoto T: Denture plaque—past and recent concerns, *J Dent* 26(4):299, 1998.

Pearson LS, Hutton JL: A controlled trial to compare the ability of foam swabs and toothbrushes to remove dental plaque, *J Adv Nurs* 39:5, 2002.

Poland JM: Comparing Moi-Stir to lemon-glycerin swabs, *Am J Nurs* 87(4):422, 1987.

Rhodes VA, McDaniel RW, Johnson MH: Patient education: self care guide, *Semin Oncol Nurs* 11(4):298, 1995.

Roberts J: Developing an oral assessment and intervention tool for older people: 2, *Br J Nurs* 9(18):2033, 2000.

Rogers BB: Mucositis in the oncology patient, *Nurs Clin North Am* 36:4, 2001.

Sakki TK et al: The association of yeasts and denture stomatitis with behavioral and biologic factors, *Oral Surg Oral Med Oral Pathol Oral Radiol Endod* 84(6):624, 1997.

Scannapieco FA, Stewart EM, Mylotte JM: Colonization of dental plaque by respiratory pathogens in medical intensive care patients, *Crit Care Med* 20(6):740, 1992.

Tombes MB, Gallucci B: The effects of hydrogen peroxide rinses on the normal oral mucosa, *Nurs Res* 42(6): 332, 1993.

Walton JC, Miller J, Tordecilla L: Elder oral assessment and care, *MedSurg Nurs* 10:1, 2001.

White R: Nurse assessment of oral health: a review of practice and education, *Br J Nurs* 9(5):260, 2000.

Yeager KA et al: Implementation of an oral care standard for leukemia and transplantation patients, *Cancer Nurs* 23(1):40, 2000.

Yoneyama T et al: Oral care reduces pneumonia in older patients in nursing homes, *J Am Geriatr Soc* 50(3), 2002.

• = **Independent;** ▲ = **Collaborative**

Pain: Assessment Guide and Equianalgesic Chart

Margo McCaffery and Chris Pasero

ASSESSMENT: USE OF PAIN RATING SCALES

Nursing Assessment/Diagnosis of Pain Sensation

Ask the client about the current level of pain if at all possible. The client's self-report of pain is the single most reliable indicator of how much pain the client is experiencing. The rating given by the client is always what is recorded in the patient's record.

Basic Measures of Pain

The hierarchy of importance of basic measures of pain is as follows (Agency for Health Care Policy and Research: Quick reference on acute pain in childhood, Rockville, Md, 1992, The Agency; Schechter NL, Altman A, Weisman S, editors: Report of the Consensus Conference on the Management of Pain in Childhood Cancer, *Pediatrics* 86:813, 1990):
- Client's self-report
- Report of parent, family, or others close to client
- Behaviors (e.g., facial expressions, body movements, crying)
- Physiological measures, "neither sensitive nor specific as indicators of pain" (Agency for Health Policy and Research: *Quick ref. Acute pain in children,* Rockville, Md, 1992, The Agency, p 7)

Client/Family Teaching—Use of Pain Rating Scale

NOTE: When it is obvious that pain is severe (e.g., following trauma or major surgery), a pain rating scale need not be used initially. Give an analgesic and wait until the client is better able to cooperate.
- Explain the primary purposes of a pain rating scale. Show the client and family the scale. *This step allows quick, consistent communication between client and caregiver/nurse/physician. Emphasize that the client must volunteer information because the caregivers may not know when the client has pain. This step also helps establish a pain relief goal that is satisfactory to the client.*
- Explain the specific pain rating scale (e.g., 0 to 10; 0 = no pain and 10 = worst possible pain). When a numerical scale is used, verify that the client can count to the number used. If the client does not understand whatever scale is standard in that clinical setting, use another scale.
- Discuss the word *pain*. Explain that pain is discomfort that may occur anywhere in the body; may have various characteristics such as aching, hurting, pulling, tightness, burning, or pricking; and may be mild to severe. If the client prefers some other term such as *hurt*, use that word. *To verify that the client understands how the word* pain *(or other word preferred by client) is used, ask client to give two examples of pain he or she has now or has experienced.*
- Ask client to practice using the pain rating scale by rating the current pain or past painful experiences.
- Ask the client what pain rating would be acceptable or satisfactory while at rest and

• = Independent; ▲ = Collaborative

active. This helps set a realistic, initial goal. Zero pain is not always possible. Once the initial goal is achieved, the possibility of better pain relief can be considered. Emphasize to the client that satisfactory pain relief is a level of pain that is noticeable but not distressing and enables the client to sleep, eat, and perform other required or desired physical activities.

Wong-Baker FACES Pain Rating Scale

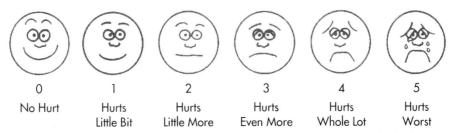

0	1	2	3	4	5
No Hurt	Hurts Little Bit	Hurts Little More	Hurts Even More	Hurts Whole Lot	Hurts Worst

From Wong DL, Hockenberry-Eaton M, Wilson D, Winkelstein ML: *Wong's essentials of pediatric nursing,* ed 6, St Louis, 2001, Mosby. Reprinted with permission.

Original instructions: Explain to the person that each face is for a person who feels happy because he has no pain (hurt) or sad because he has some or a lot of pain. **Face 0** is very happy because he doesn't hurt at all. **Face 1** hurts just a little bit. **Face 2** hurts a little more. **Face 3** hurts even more. **Face 4** hurts a whole lot. **Face 5** hurts as much as you can imagine, although you do not have to be crying to feel this bad. Ask the person to choose the face that best describes how he or she is feeling.

The rating scale is recommended for persons 3 years and older.

Brief word instructions: Point to each face using the words to describe the pain intensity. Ask the child to choose face that best describes his or her own pain and record the appropriate number.

SELECTED REFERENCES

For more complete information and additional references, see: Pasero C, Portenoy RK, McCaffery M: Opioid analgesics. In McCaffery M, Pasero C: *Pain clinical manual,* St Louis, 1999, Mosby.

American Pain Society (APS): *Principles of analgesic use in the treatment of acute and cancer pain,* ed 4, Glenview, Ill, 1999, The Society.

Lawlor P et al: Dose ratio between morphine and hydromorphone in patients with cancer pain: a retrospective study, *Pain* 72(1):79-85, 1997.

Mandfredi PL et al: Intravenous methadone for cancer pain unrelieved by morphine and hydromorphone: clinical observations, *Pain* 70:99, 1997.

Portenoy RK: Opioid analgesics. In Portenoy RK, Kanner RM, editors: *Pain management: theory and practice,* Philadelphia, 1996, FA Davis.

A GUIDE TO USING EQUIANALGESIC CHARTS

- Equianalgesic means approximately the same pain relief.
- The equianalgesic chart is a guideline. Doses and intervals between doses are titrated according to the individual's response.
- The equianalgesic chart is helpful when switching from one drug to another, or switching from one route of administration to another.
- Dosages in the equianalgesic chart for moderate to severe pain are not necessarily start-

• = **Independent; ▲ = Collaborative**

ing doses. The doses suggest a ratio for comparing the analgesia of one drug to another.

- For elderly patients, initially reduce the recommended adult opioid dose for moderate to severe pain by 25% to 50%.
- The longer the patient has been receiving opioids, the more conservative the starting doses of a **new** opioid.

Equianalgesic Chart: Approximate Equivalent Doses of Opioids for Moderate to Severe Pain

Analgesic	Parenteral (IM, SC, IV) Route*† (mg)	PO Route* (Mg)	Comments
MU Opioid Agonists			
Morphine	10	30	Standard for comparison. Multiple routes of administration. Available in immediate-release and controlled-release formulations. Active metabolic M6G can accumulate with repeated dosing in renal failure.
Codeine	130	200 NR	IM has unpredictable absorption and high side-effect profile; used PO for mild to moderate pain; usually compounded with nonopioid (e.g., Tylenol #3).
Fentanyl	100 µg/h parenterally and transdermally $\cong$ 4 mg/h morphine parenterally; 1 µg/h transdermally $\cong$ 2 mg/24 h morphine PO	—	Short half-life, but at a steady state, slow elimination from tissues can lead to a prolonged half-life (up to 12 h). Start opioid-naïve patients on no more than 25 µg/h transdermally. Transdermal fentanyl NR for acute pain management. Available by oral transmucosal route.
Hydrocodone (as in Vicodin, Lortab)		30? (MR)	Equianalgesic information lacking.
Hydromorphone (Dilaudid)	1.5	7.5	Useful alternative to morphine. No evidence that metabolites are clinically relevant; shorter duration than morphine. Available in high-potency parenteral formulation (10 mg/ml) useful for SC infusion; 3 mg rectal $\cong$ 650 mg aspirin PO. With repeated dosing (e.g., PCA), it is more likely that 2-3 mg parenteral hydromorphone = 10 mg parenteral morphine.

• = Independent; ▲ = Collaborative

Analgesic	Parenteral (IM, SC, IV) Route*† (mg)	PO Route* (Mg)	Comments
Levorphanol (Levo-Dromoran)	2	4	Longer acting than morphine when given repeatedly. Long half-life can lead to accumulation within 2-3 days of repeated dosing.
Meperidine	75	300 NR	No longer preferred as a first-line opioid for the management of acute or chronic pain due to potential toxicity from accumulation of metabolite, normeperidine. Normeperidine has 15-20 h half-life and is not reversed by naloxone. NR in elderly or patients with impaired renal function; NR by continuous IV infusion.
Methadone (Dolophine)	10	29	Longer acting than morphine when given repeatedly. Long half-life can lead to delayed toxicity from accumulation within 3-5 days. Start PO dosing on PRN schedule; in opioid-tolerant patients converted to methadone, start with 10-25% of equianalgesic dose.
Oxycodone	—	20	Used for moderate pain when combined with a nonopioid (e.g., Percocet, Tylox). Available as a single entity in immediate-release and controlled-release formulations (e.g., OxyContin); can be used like PO morphine for severe pain.
Oxymorphone (Numorphan)	1	10 rectal	Used for moderate to severe pain. No PO formulation
Agonist-Antagonist Opioids: Not recommended for severe, escalating pain. If used in combination with mu agonists, may reverse analgesia and precipitate withdrawal in opioid-dependent patients			
Buprenorphine (Buprenex)	0.4	—	Not readily reversed by naloxone; NR for laboring patients
Butorphanol (Stadol)	2	—	Available in nasal spray
Dezocine (Dalgan)	10	—	
Nalbuphine (Nubain)	10	—	
Pentazocine (Talwin)	60	180	

From McCaffery M, Pasero C: *Pain: clinical manual,* St Louis, 1999, Mosby.
FDA, Food and Drug Administration; *NR,* not recommended; ≅, roughly equal to.
*Duration of analgesia is dose-dependent; the higher the dose, usually the longer the duration.
†IV boluses may be used to produce analgesia that lasts approximately as long as IM or SC doses. However, of all routes of administration, IV produces the highest peak concentration of the drug, and the peak concentration is associated with the highest level of toxicity, e.g., sedation. To decrease the peak effect and lower the level of toxicity, IV boluses may be administered more slowly, e.g., 10 mg of morphine over a 15 minute period or smaller doses may be administered more often, e.g., 5 mg of morphine every 1-1.5 hours.

Acute Pain

Chris Pasero and Margo McCaffery

NANDA **Definition**

Pain is whatever the experiencing person says it is, existing whenever the person says it does (McCaffery, 1968); unpleasant sensory and emotional experience arising from actual or potential tissue damage or described in terms of such damage (International Association for the Study of Pain); sudden or slow onset of pain of any intensity from mild to severe with anticipated or predictable end (NANDA)

Defining Characteristics

Subjective

Pain is always subjective and cannot be proved or disproved. A client's report of pain is the most reliable indicator of pain (Acute Pain Management Guideline Panel, 1992). A client with cognitive ability who can speak or point should use a pain rating scale (e.g., 0 to 10) to identify the current level of pain intensity (self-report) and determine a comfort/function goal (McCaffery and Pasero, 1999). Establishment of a comfort/function goal involves helping the client to select a pain rating level that will allow the client to easily perform identified functional goals (e.g., a pain rating of 3 on a scale of 0 to 10 to cough, deep breathe, and ambulate).

Objective

Expressions of pain are extremely variable and cannot be used in lieu of self-report. Neither behavior nor vital signs can substitute for the client's self-report (McCaffery and Ferrell, 1991, 1992; McCaffery and Pasero, 1999). However, observable responses to pain may be helpful in assessing clients who cannot or will not use a self-report pain rating scale. Observable responses may be loss of appetite and inability to deep breathe, ambulate, sleep, or perform activities of daily living. Clients may show guarding, self-protective behavior, self-focusing or narrowed focus, distraction behavior ranging from crying to laughing, and muscle tension or rigidity. In sudden and severe pain, autonomic responses such as diaphoresis, blood pressure and pulse changes, pupillary dilation, or increases or decreases in respiratory rate and depth may be present.

Related Factors (r/t)

Actual or potential tissue damage (mechanical [e.g., incision or tumor growth], thermal [e.g., burn], or chemical [e.g., toxic substance])

NOC **Outcomes (Nursing Outcomes Classification)**

Suggested NOC Outcomes

Comfort Level; Pain Control; Pain: Disruptive Effects; Pain Level

• = Independent; ▲ = Collaborative

States/demonstrates achievement of the comfort/function goal. (Rate pain intensity: 0 = no pain, 1 to 3 = mild pain, 4 to 6 = moderate pain, 7 to 9 = severe pain, 10 = worst possible pain.) In cognitively impaired clients, demonstrates reduction in pain behaviors or improved function.

Client Outcomes

Client Will (Specify Time Frame):

- Use pain rating scale to identify current pain intensity and determine comfort/function goal (if client has cognitive abilities)
- Describe how unrelieved pain will be managed
- Report that pain management regimen relieves pain to satisfactory level with acceptable and manageable side effects
- Perform activities of recovery with reported acceptable level of pain (if pain is above comfort/function goal, take action that decreases pain or notify a member of health care team)
- If cognitively impaired, demonstrate a reduction in pain behaviors, have manageable and tolerable side effects, and perform recovery activities satisfactorily
- State ability to obtain sufficient amounts of rest and sleep
- Describe nonpharmacological method that can be used to help control pain

NIC   Interventions (Nursing Interventions Classification)

Suggested NIC Interventions

Analgesic Administration; Pain Management; Patient-Controlled Analgesia (PCA) Assistance

Example NIC Activities—Pain Management

Ensure that client receives attentive analgesic care; Perform comprehensive assessment of pain, including location, characteristics, onset and duration, frequency, quality, intensity or severity, and precipitating factors

Nursing Interventions and Rationales

- ▲ Determine whether the client is experiencing pain at the time of the initial interview. If so, intervene at that time to provide pain relief (McCaffery and Pasero, 1999). Assess and document the intensity, character, onset, duration, and aggravating and relieving factors of pain during the initial evaluation of the client. *The initial assessment and documentation provides direction for the pain treatment plan. A comprehensive pain assessment includes all characteristics of the pain that the client can provide. The client's report of the pain is considered the single most reliable datum (Acute Pain Management Guideline Panel, 1992; American Pain Society Quality of Care Committee, 1995; Joint Commission on Accreditation of Healthcare Organizations [JCAHO], 2000).*
- Ask the client to describe past experiences with pain and the effectiveness of methods used to manage pain, including experiences with side effects, typical coping responses, and the way the client expresses pain. **Nursing Research:** *A study involving 270 people with cancer pain revealed that those surveyed had a number of concerns (barriers) that affected their willingness to report pain and use analgesics (Ward et al, 1993). Many*

• = Independent; ▲ = Collaborative

harbored fears and misconceptions regarding the use of analgesics, management of side effects, and risk of addiction.

- Describe the adverse effects of unrelieved pain. **Nursing and Clinical Research:** *Numerous pathophysiological and psychological morbidity factors may be associated with pain. One study demonstrated that persistent unrelieved pain suppressed immune function, which can lead to infection and other complications (Page and Ben-Eliyahu, 1997). Analgesics, such as opioids and local anesthetics, have been shown to block immunosuppression (Page and Ben-Eliyahu, 1997). Another study showed that critically ill clients with severe pain had a significantly higher incidence of atelectasis than those with less pain (Puntillo and Weiss, 1994).*

- Tell the client to report the location, intensity (using a pain rating scale), and quality when experiencing pain. Assess and document the intensity of the pain and discomfort after any known pain-producing procedure, with each new report of pain, and at regular intervals. *Systematic ongoing assessment and documentation provide direction for the pain treatment plan; adjustments are based on the client's responses. The client's report of pain is the single most reliable indicator of pain (Acute Pain Management Guideline Panel, 1992; Jacox et al, 1994; JCAHO, 2000).*

- If the client is cognitively impaired and unable to report pain and use a pain rating scale, assess and document behaviors that might be indicative of pain (e.g., change in activity, loss of appetite, guarding, grimacing, moaning) (Herr, 2002). *The absence of behaviors thought to be indicative of pain does not necessarily mean that pain is absent (McCaffery and Pasero, 1999).* **Nursing Research:** *Certain behaviors have been shown to be indicative of pain and can be used to assess pain in clients who cannot use a self-report pain rating tool (e.g., in the cognitively impaired client). The clinician should be aware that pain expression is highly individual and what may be a pain behavior in one client may not be in another. Pain assessment must be individualized (Herr, 2002).*

- Assume that pain is present and treat accordingly in a client who has a pathological condition or who is undergoing a procedure thought to be painful. *Pain is associated with certain pathological conditions (e.g., fractures) and procedures (e.g., surgery). In the absence of the client's report of pain (e.g., anesthetized, critically ill, or cognitively impaired client), the clinician should assume pain is present and treat accordingly (McCaffery and Pasero, 1999).*

- Determine the client's current medication use. *To aid in planning pain treatment, obtain a medication history (Acute Pain Management Guideline Panel, 1992). Obtaining a complete history of medications the client is taking or has taken can help to prevent drug-drug interactions and toxicity problems that can occur when incompatible drugs are combined or when allergies are present. The history will also provide the clinician with an understanding of what medications have been tried and were or were not effective in treating the client's pain (Acute Pain Management Guideline Panel, 1992; McCaffery and Pasero, 1999).*

- ▲ Explore the need for both opioid (narcotic) and nonopioid analgesics. *Pharmacological interventions are the cornerstone of management of moderate to severe pain (Acute Pain Management Guideline Panel, 1992; McCaffery and Pasero, 1999). All analgesic options are considered. Unless contraindicated, all clients with acute pain should receive a nonopioid agent around the clock (ATC) (Acute Pain Management Guideline Panel, 1992). The analgesic regimen should include a nonopioid even if pain is severe enough to require the addition of an opioid (Jacox et al, 1994; McCaffery and Pasero, 1999). Combining analgesics can result in acceptable pain relief with lower dosages of each analgesic than would be*

• = Independent; ▲ = Collaborative

possible with one analgesic alone. Lower dosages can result in fewer or less severe side effects (McCaffery and Pasero, 1999).

▲ Obtain a prescription to administer a nonopioid (acetaminophen), a nonselective nonsteroidal anti-inflammatory drug (NSAID), or a selective NSAID (cyclo-oxygenase-2 [COX-2] inhibitor) ATC, unless contraindicated. *NSAIDs act mainly in the periphery to inhibit the initiation of pain impulses (Dahl and Kehlet, 1991). Unless contraindicated, all clients with acute pain should receive a nonopioid ATC (Acute Pain Management Guideline Panel, 1992). The analgesic regimen should include a nonopioid, even if pain is severe enough to require the addition of an opioid (Jacox et al, 1994; McCaffery and Pasero, 1999).*

▲ Obtain a prescription to administer an opioid analgesic if indicated, especially for severe pain. *Opioid analgesics are indicated for the treatment of moderate to severe pain (Jacox et al, 1994; McCaffery and Pasero, 1999).*

▲ Administer opioids orally or intravenously (IV), not intramuscularly (IM). Use a preventive approach to keep pain at or below an acceptable level. Provide PCA and intraspinal routes of administration when appropriate and available. *The least invasive route of administration capable of providing adequate pain control is recommended. The IM route is avoided because of unreliable absorption, pain, and inconvenience. The IV route is preferred for rapid control of severe pain. For ongoing pain, give analgesia ATC. For intermittent pain, prn dosing is appropriate (Jacox et al, 1994; McCaffery and Pasero, 1999).*

• Explain to the client the pain management approach that has been ordered, including therapies, medication administration, side effects, and complications. *One of the most important steps toward improved control of pain is a better client understanding of the nature of pain, its treatment, and the role the client needs to play in pain control (Jacox et al, 1994).*

• Discuss the client's fears of undertreated pain, overdose, and addiction. *Because of the many misconceptions regarding pain and its treatment, education about the ability to control pain effectively and correction of myths about the use of opioids should be included as part of the treatment plan (Jacox et al, 1994; McCaffery and Pasero, 1999). Addiction is extremely unlikely after clients use opioids for pain management (Acute Pain Management Guideline Panel, 1992).* **Nursing Research:** *A survey of 270 people with cancer pain revealed that many harbored fears and misconceptions regarding the use of analgesics, management of side effects, and risk of addiction (Ward et al, 1993).*

▲ When opioids are administered, assess pain intensity, sedation, and respiratory status at regular intervals. Assess sedation and respiratory status at least every 2 hours in opioid-naïve clients (those who have not been taking regular daily doses of opioids) during the first 24 hours of opioid therapy. Decrease the opioid dose if the client is excessively sedated. *Opioids may cause respiratory depression because they reduce the responsiveness of carbon dioxide chemoreceptors located in the respiratory centers of the brain. Because even more opioid is required to produce respiratory depression than is required to produce sedation, clients with clinically significant respiratory depression are usually also sedated. Respiratory depression can be prevented by assessing sedation and decreasing the opioid dose when the client is arousable but has difficulty staying awake (McCaffery and Pasero, 1999; Pasero and McCaffery, 1994).*

▲ Review the client's flow sheet and medication records to determine overall degree of pain relief, side effects, and analgesic requirements during the previous 24 hours. **Nursing Research:** *One study showed that systematic tracking of pain was an important factor in improving pain management (Faries et al, 1991).*

• = **Independent;** ▲ = **Collaborative**

▲ Administer supplemental opioid doses as needed to keep pain ratings at or below the comfort/function goal. *An order for prn supplementary opioid doses between regular doses is an essential backup (American Pain Society, 1999; McCaffery and Pasero, 1999).*

▲ Obtain prescriptions to increase or decrease opioid doses as needed; base prescriptions on the client's report of pain severity and response to the previous dose in terms of relief, side effects, and ability to perform the activities of recovery. Increase or decrease the dosage of opioid based on assessment of the client's response. *Clients' responses, and therefore their analgesic requirements, vary widely, so it is less important to focus on the amount given than on the response (McCaffery and Pasero, 1999; Pasero and McCaffery, 1994).*

▲ When the client is able to tolerate oral analgesics, obtain a prescription to change to the oral route; use an equianalgesic chart to determine initial dose. (See Appendix E for an equianalgesic chart.) *The oral route is preferred because it is the most convenient and cost effective (Jacox et al, 1994). Use of equianalgesic doses when switching from one opioid or route of administration to another will help to prevent loss of pain control from underdosing and side effects from overdosing (McCaffery and Pasero, 1999).*

• In addition to administering analgesics, support the client's use of nonpharmacological methods to help control pain, such as distraction, imagery, relaxation, massage, and application of heat and cold. *Cognitive-behavioral strategies can restore the client's sense of self-control, personal efficacy, and active participation in his or her own care (Jacox et al, 1994).*

• Teach and implement nonpharmacological interventions when pain is relatively well controlled with pharmacological interventions. *Nonpharmacological interventions should be used to supplement, not replace, pharmacological interventions (Acute Pain Management Guideline Panel, 1992).*

• Plan care activities around periods of greatest comfort whenever possible. *Pain diminishes the client's activity. Performing care actions at times when the client is rested and pain is well controlled will make it easier for the client to achieve recovery or rehabilitation milestones (Jacox et al, 1994; McCaffery and Pasero, 1999).*

▲ Ask the client to describe appetite, bowel elimination, and ability to rest and sleep. Administer medications and treatments to improve these functions. Obtain a prescription for a peristaltic stimulant to prevent opioid-induced constipation. *Because there is great individual variation in the development of opioid-induced side effects, these side effects should be monitored and, if their development is inevitable (e.g., constipation), prophylactically treated. Opioids cause constipation by decreasing bowel peristalsis (Jacox et al, 1994; McCaffery and Pasero, 1999).*

Geriatric

▲ Always take the elderly client's reports of pain seriously and ensure that the pain is relieved. *In spite of what many professionals and clients believe, pain is not an expected part of normal aging (American Geriatric Society Panel on Persistent Pain in Older Persons, 2002; McCaffery and Pasero, 1999).*

• When assessing pain, speak clearly, slowly, and loudly enough for the client to hear, and if the client uses a hearing aid, be sure it is in place; repeat information as needed. Be sure the client can see well enough to read the pain scale (use an enlarged scale) and written materials. *Elderly clients often have difficulty hearing and seeing. Comprehension is improved when instructions are given slowly and clearly and when the client can see visual aids (Herr, 2002).*

• = **Independent;** ▲ = **Collaborative**

- Handle the client's body gently. Allow the client to move at his or her own speed. *The elderly are particularly susceptible to injury during care activities. Caregivers must be patient and expect that the elderly will move more slowly than younger clients; they may also perform better and experience less pain during care activities when they are allowed to move themselves (McCaffery and Pasero, 1999).*

▲ Use acetaminophen and NSAIDs with low side-effect profiles, such as the selective COX-2 NSAIDs (COX-2 inhibitors), choline and magnesium salicylates (Trilisate), and diflunisal (Dolobid), and watch for side effects, such as gastrointestinal disturbances and bleeding problems. *Elderly people are at increased risk for gastric and renal toxicity from NSAIDs (Acute Pain Management Guideline Panel, 1992; American Geriatric Society Panel on Persistent Pain in Older Persons, 2002; Griffin et al, 1991).*

▲ Avoid or use with caution drugs with a long half-life, such as the NSAID piroxicam (Feldene), the opioids methadone (Dolophine) and levorphanol (Levo-Dromoran), and the benzodiazepine diazepam (Valium). *The higher prevalence of renal insufficiency in the elderly than in younger persons can result in toxicity from drug accumulation (Acute Pain Management Guideline Panel, 1992; American Geriatric Society Panel on Persistent Pain in Older Persons, 2002; American Pain Society, 1999; McCaffery and Pasero, 1999).*

▲ Use opioids with caution in the elderly client. *The elderly are more sensitive to the analgesic effects of opioid drugs because they experience a higher peak effect and a longer duration of pain relief. Reduce the initial recommended adult starting dosage of opioids by 25% to 50%, especially if the client is frail and debilitated, then increase the dosage if safe and necessary (Acute Pain Management Guideline Panel, 1992).*

▲ Avoid the use of opioids with toxic metabolites, such as meperidine (Demerol) and propoxyphene (Darvon, Darvocet), in elderly clients. *Meperidine's metabolite, normeperidine, can produce central nervous system (CNS) irritability, seizures, and even death; propoxyphene's metabolite, norpropoxyphene, can produce CNS toxicity. Both of these metabolites are eliminated by the kidneys, which makes meperidine and propoxyphene particularly poor choices for elderly clients, many of whom have at least some degree of renal insufficiency (Acute Pain Management Guideline Panel, 1992; McCaffery and Pasero, 1999).*

Multicultural

- Assess pain in a client from a different culture using a self-report 0 to 10 numerical pain rating scale or the Wong Baker Faces pain rating scale (see Appendix E). Have the scale translated into the client's native language if necessary. *Inadequate pain management is widespread, especially among minority groups, and a major reason is the failure to assess pain properly. The more cultural differences between the client and the nurse, the more difficult it is for the nurse to assess and treat pain. Self-report of pain is the single most reliable indicator of pain, regardless of culture (McCaffery, 1999; McCaffery and Pasero, 1999).*

▲ Administer analgesics on a preventive basis to keep pain ratings at or below an acceptable level. *Regardless of the client's cultural background, pain rated at higher than 3 on a 0 to 10 pain rating scale interferes significantly with daily function. Perceived quality of life appears to be comparable across cultures, with pain ratings of higher than 5 interfering markedly with a person's ability to enjoy life (McCaffery, 1999; McCaffery and Pasero, 1999).*

- = **Independent;** ▲ = **Collaborative**

- Assess for the influence of cultural beliefs, norms, and values on the client's perception and experience of pain. **Nursing Research:** *One study showed that the client's experience of pain may be influenced by cultural perceptions (Leininger, 1996).*
- Assess for the effect of fatalism on the client's beliefs regarding the current state of comfort. **Nursing Research:** Fatalistic perspectives, which involve the belief that one cannot control one's own fate, may influence health behaviors in some African American and Latino populations (Harmon, Castro, and Coe, 1996; Phillips, Cohen, and Moses, 1999).
- Incorporate safe and effective folk health care practices and beliefs into care whenever possible. *It is the responsibility of the caregiver to ensure that safe and effective pain management is provided. Although support of an individual's health care beliefs is recommended, when research does not support the safety or effectiveness of a method or when research does not exist, this should be explained fully to the client (McCaffery and Pasero, 1999).* **Nursing Research:** *Incorporating folk health care beliefs and practices into pain management care increased compliance with the treatment plan (Juarez, Ferrell, and Borneman, 1998).*
- Use a family-centered approach to care. **Nursing Research:** *Involving the family in pain management care increased compliance with the treatment regimen (Juarez, Ferrell, and Borneman, 1998).*
- Use culturally relevant pain scales (e.g., the Oucher Scale), if available, to assess pain in the client. **Nursing Research:** *Clients from minority cultures may express pain differently than clients from the majority culture. The Oucher Scale is available in African American and Hispanic versions and is used to assess pain in children (Beyer, Denyes, and Villarruel, 1992).*
- Ensure that directions for medication use are available in the client's language of choice and are understood by the client and caregiver. **Nursing Research:** *Use of bilingual instructions for medication administration increased compliance with the pain management plan (Juarez, Ferrell, and Borneman, 1998).*

Home care

- Develop the treatment plan with the client and caregivers. **Nursing Research:** *Compliance with the medical regimen for treating pain improves the likelihood of successful management (Humphrey, 1994).*
- ▲ Develop a full medication profile, including medications prescribed by all physicians and all over-the-counter medications. Assess for drug interactions. Instruct the client to refrain from mixing medications without physician approval. *Pain medications may significantly affect or be affected by other medications and may cause severe side effects. Some combinations of drugs are specifically contraindicated (Jacox et al, 1994).*
- Assess the client's and family's knowledge of side effects and safety precautions associated with pain medications (e.g., use caution in operating machinery when opioids are first taken or dosage has been increased significantly). *The cognitive effects of opioids usually subside within a week of initial dosing or dosage increases (McCaffery and Pasero, 1999). The use of long-term opioid treatment does not appear to affect neuropsychological performance.* **Clinical Research:** *Pain itself may reduce performance on neuropsychological tests more than oral opioid treatment (Sjogren et al, 2000).*
- If medication is administered using highly technological methods, assess the home for the necessary resources (e.g., electricity) and ensure that there will be responsible caregivers available to assist the client with administration. *Some routes of medication*

- = Independent; ▲ = Collaborative

administration require special conditions and procedures to be safe and accurate (McCaffery and Pasero, 1999).

▲ Assess the knowledge base of the client and family with regard to highly technological medication administration. Teach as necessary. Be sure the client knows when, how, and whom to contact if analgesia is unsatisfactory. *Appropriate instruction in the home increases the accuracy and safety of medication administration (McCaffery and Pasero, 1999).*

Client/Family Teaching

NOTE: To avoid the negative connotations associated with the words *drugs* and *narcotics*, use the term *pain medicine* when teaching clients.

• Provide written materials on pain control such as *Understanding Your Pain: Using a Pain Rating Scale* (McCaffery, Pasero, and Portenoy, 2001) (see pages 706-707 for instructions on the use of pain rating scales). *Written materials are provided in addition to verbal instructions so that the client will have a reference during treatment (McCaffery and Pasero, 1999).*

• Discuss the various discomforts encompassed by the word *pain* and ask the client to give examples of previously experienced pain. Explain the pain assessment process and the purpose of the pain rating scale. *It is often difficult for clients to understand the concept of pain and describe their pain experience. Using alternative words and providing a complete description of the assessment process, including the use of scales, will ensure that an accurate treatment plan is developed (McCaffery and Pasero, 1999).*

▲ Teach the client to use the pain rating scale to rate the intensity of past or current pain. Ask the client to set a comfort/function goal by selecting a pain level on the rating scale that makes it easy to perform recovery activities (e.g., turn, cough, deep breathe). If pain is above this level, the client should take action that decreases pain or notify a member of the health care team. (See pages 706-707 for information on teaching clients to use the pain rating scale.) *The use of comfort/function goals provides direction for the treatment plan. Changes are made according to the client's response and achievement of the goals of recovery or rehabilitation (McCaffery and Pasero, 1999).*

▲ Demonstrate medication administration and the use of supplies and equipment. If PCA is ordered, determine the client's ability to press the appropriate button. Remind the client and staff that the PCA button is for client use only. *Appropriate instruction increases the accuracy and safety of medication administration (McCaffery and Pasero, 1999).*

• Reinforce the importance of taking pain medications to keep pain under control. *Teaching clients to stay on top of their pain and prevent it from getting out of control will improve the ability to accomplish the goals of recovery (McCaffery and Pasero, 1999).*

• Reinforce that taking opioids for pain relief is not addiction and that addiction is very unlikely to occur. *The development of addiction when opioids are taken for pain relief is extremely rare (Acute Pain Management Guideline Panel, 1992; American Pain Society, 1999; Jacox et al, 1994).*

• Demonstrate the use of appropriate nonpharmacological approaches in addition to pharmacological approaches for helping to control pain, such as application of heat and/or cold, distraction techniques, relaxation breathing, visualization, rocking, stroking, music listening, and television watching. *Nonpharmacological interventions are used to complement, not replace, pharmacological interventions (Acute Pain Management Guideline Panel, 1992; McCaffery and Pasero, 1999).*

• = Independent; ▲ = Collaborative

ⓔⓥⓞⓛⓥⓔ WEBSITES FOR EDUCATION

See the EVOLVE website for World Wide Web resources for client education.

REFERENCES

Acute Pain Management Guideline Panel: *Acute pain management operative or medical procedures and trauma: clinical practice guideline,* Agency for Health Care Policy and Research Pub No. 92-0032, Rockville, Md, 1992, Public Health Service, US Department of Health and Human Services.

American Geriatric Society Panel on Persistent Pain in Older Persons: The management of persistent pain in older persons, *J Am Geriatr Soc* 50:S205, 2002.

American Pain Society: *Principles of analgesic use in the treatment of acute pain and cancer pain,* ed 4, Glenview, Ill, 1999, The Society.

American Pain Society Quality of Care Committee: Quality improvement guidelines for the treatment of acute pain and cancer pain, *JAMA* 274:1874, 1995.

Beyer J, Denyes M, Villarruel A: The creation, validation, and continuing development of the Oucher: a measure of pain intensity in children, *J Pediatr Nurs* 7(5):335, 1992.

Dahl JB, Kehlet H: Non-steroidal anti-inflammatory drugs: rationale for use in severe postoperative pain, *Br J Anaesth* 66:703, 1991.

Faries JE et al: Systematic pain records and their impact on pain control, *Cancer Nurs* 14:306, 1991.

Griffin MR et al: Nonsteroidal anti-inflammatory drug use and increased risk for peptic ulcer disease in elderly persons, *Ann Intern Med* 11(4):257, 1991.

Harmon MP, Castro FG, Coe K: Acculturation and cervical cancer: knowledge, beliefs, and behaviors of Hispanic women, *Women Health* 24(3):37, 1996.

Herr K: Pain assessment in cognitively impaired older adults, *Am J Nurs* 102(12):65, 2002.

Humphrey C: *Home care nursing handbook,* ed 2, Gaithersburg, Md, 1994, Aspen.

Jacox A et al: *Management of cancer pain,* Clinical Practice Guideline No. 9, Agency for Health Care Policy and Research Pub No. 94-0592, Rockville, Md, 1994, Public Health Service, US Department of Health and Human Services.

Joint Commission on Accreditation of Healthcare Organizations: *2000 Hospital accreditation standards,* Oakbrook, Ill, 2000, The Organization.

Juarez G, Ferrell BR, Borneman T: Influence of culture on cancer pain management in Hispanic clients, *Cancer Pract* 6(5):262, 1998.

Leininger MM: *Transcultural nursing: theories, research and practices,* ed 2, Hilliard, Ohio, 1996, McGraw-Hill.

McCaffery M: *Nursing practice theories related to cognition, bodily pain and man-environment interactions,* Los Angeles, 1968, University of California at Los Angeles Students' Store.

McCaffery M: Culturally sensitive pain assessment, *Am J Nurs* 99(8):18, 1999.

McCaffery M, Ferrell BR: How would you respond to these clients in pain? *Nursing* 21(6):34, 1991.

McCaffery M, Ferrell BR: How vital are vital signs? *Nursing* 22(1):42, 1992.

McCaffery M, Pasero C: *Pain: clinical manual,* St Louis, 1999, Mosby.

McCaffery M, Pasero C, Portenoy RK: *Understanding your pain: using a pain rating scale,* Chadds Ford, Pa, 2001, Endo Pharmaceuticals, Inc. Call 800-462-3636 to order.

Page GG, Ben-Eliyahu S: The immune-suppressive nature of pain, *Semin Oncol Nurs* 13(1):10, 1997.

Pasero C, McCaffery M: Avoiding opioid-induced respiratory depression, *Am J Nurs* 94:25, 1994.

Phillips JM, Cohen MZ, Moses G: Breast cancer screening and African American women: fear, fatalism, and silence, *Oncol Nurs Forum* 26(3):561, 1999.

Puntillo K, Weiss SJ: Pain: its mediators and associated morbidity in critically ill cardiovascular surgical clients, *Nurs Res* 43(3):1, 1994.

Sjogren P et al: Neuropsychological performance in cancer clients: the role of oral opioids, pain and performance status, *Pain* 86:237, 2000.

Stuart GW, Laraia MT: Therapeutic nurse-client relationship. In Stuart GW, Laraia MT, editors: *Principles and practice of psychiatric nursing,* St Louis, 2001, Mosby, p 30.

Ward S et al: Client-related barriers to management of cancer pain, *Pain* 52:319, 1993.

• = Independent; ▲ = Collaborative

Chronic Pain

Chris Pasero and Margo McCaffery

NANDA Definition

Pain is whatever the experiencing person says it is, existing whenever the person says it does (McCaffery, 1968); unpleasant sensory and emotional experience arising from actual or potential tissue damage or described in terms of such damage (International Association for the Study of Pain); sudden or slow onset of pain of any intensity from mild to severe, constant or recurring, without anticipated or predictable end (NANDA); state in which the individual experiences pain that persists for a period of time beyond the usual course of acute illness or a reasonable duration for the injury to heal, is associated with a chronic pathological process, or recurs at intervals for months or years (Bonica, 1990)

Defining Characteristics

Subjective

Pain is always subjective and cannot be proved or disproved. The client's report of pain is the most reliable indicator of pain (Acute Pain Management Guideline Panel, 1992). Clients with cognitive abilities who can speak or point should use a pain rating scale (e.g., 0 to 10) to identify their current level of pain intensity (self-report) and determine a comfort/function goal (McCaffery and Pasero, 1999). Establishment of a comfort/function goal involves assisting clients in selecting a pain rating that will allow them to easily perform identified functional goals, e.g., a pain rating of 3 on a scale of 0 to 10 to work or walk the dog.

Objective

Expressions of pain are extremely variable and cannot be used in lieu of self-report. Neither behavior nor vital signs can substitute for the client's self-report (McCaffery and Ferrell, 1991, 1992; McCaffery and Pasero, 1999). However, observable responses to pain may be helpful in pain assessment, especially in clients who cannot or will not use a self-report pain rating scale. Observable responses may be loss of appetite or the inability to ambulate, perform activities of daily living (ADLs), work, or sleep. Clients may show guarding, self-protective behavior, self-focusing or narrowed focus, distraction behavior ranging from crying to laughing, and muscle tension or rigidity. In sudden severe pain, autonomic responses such as diaphoresis, blood pressure and pulse changes, pupillary dilation, and increase or decrease in respiratory rate and depth may be present but are usually not seen with chronic pain that is relatively stable. Clients with chronic or persistent cancer or nonmalignant pain may experience threats to self-image, a perceived lack of options for coping, and worsening helplessness, anxiety, and depression. Chronic pain may affect almost every aspect of the client's daily life, including concentration, work, and relationships.

Related Factors (r/t)

Actual or potential tissue damage; tumor progression and related pathology; diagnostic and therapeutic procedures; central or peripheral nerve injury (neuropathic pain)

NOTE: The cause of chronic nonmalignant pain may not be known because pain study is a new science and an area encompassing diverse types of problems.

• = Independent; ▲ = Collaborative

| **NOC** | Outcomes (Nursing Outcomes Classification) |

Suggested NOC Outcomes

Comfort Level; Pain Control; Pain: Disruptive Effects; Pain Level

States/demonstrates achievement of the comfort/function goal. (Rate pain intensity: 0 = no pain, 1 to 3 = mild pain, 4 to 6 = moderate pain, 7 to 9 = severe pain, 10 = worst possible pain.) In cognitively impaired clients, demonstrates a reduction in pain behaviors or improved function.

Client Outcomes

Client Will (Specify Time Frame):

- Use pain rating scale to identify current level of pain intensity, determine comfort/function goal, and maintain a pain diary (if client has cognitive abilities)
- Describe total plan for pharmacological and nonpharmacological pain relief, including how to safely and effectively take medicines and integrate nondrug therapies
- Demonstrate ability to pace self, taking rest breaks before they are needed
- Function on acceptable ability level with minimal interference from pain and medication side effects (if pain is above comfort/function goal, take action that decreases pain or notify a member of health care team)
- If cognitively impaired, demonstrate a reduction in pain behaviors, have manageable and tolerable side effects, and perform ADLs satisfactorily

| **NIC** | Interventions (Nursing Interventions Classification) |

Suggested NIC Interventions

Analgesic Administration; Pain Management

Example NIC Activities—Pain Management

Ensure that client receives attentive analgesic care; Perform comprehensive assessment of pain, including location, characteristics, onset and duration, frequency, quality, intensity or severity, and precipitating factors

Nursing Interventions and Rationales

▲ Determine whether the client is experiencing pain at the time of the initial interview. If so, intervene at that time to provide pain relief. Assess and document the intensity, character, onset, duration, and aggravating and relieving factors of pain during the initial evaluation of the client. *The initial assessment and documentation provide direction for the pain treatment plan. A comprehensive pain assessment includes all characteristics of the pain that the client can provide. The client's report of the pain is considered the single most reliable datum (Acute Pain Management Guideline Panel, 1992; American Pain Society Quality of Care Committee, 1995; Joint Commission on Accreditation of Healthcare Organizations [JCAHO], 2000).*

• Ask the client to describe past and current experiences with pain and the effectiveness of the methods used to manage the pain, including experiences with side effects, typical coping responses, and the way the client expresses pain. **Nursing Research:** *A study of 270 people with cancer pain revealed that those surveyed had a number of con-*

• = Independent; ▲ = Collaborative

cerns (barriers) that affected their willingness to report pain and use analgesics (Ward et al, 1993). Many harbored fears and misconceptions regarding the use of analgesics, management of side effects, and risk of addiction.

- Describe the adverse effects of unrelieved pain. **Nursing and Clinical Research:** *Numerous pathophysiological and psychological morbidity factors may be associated with pain. One study demonstrated that persistent unrelieved pain suppressed immune function, which can lead to infection, increased tumor growth, and other complications (Page and Ben-Eliyahu, 1997). Analgesics such as opioids and local anesthetics have been shown to block immunosuppression (Page and Ben-Eliyahu, 1997).*

- Tell the client to report pain location, intensity, and quality when experiencing pain. Assess and document the intensity of pain and discomfort after any known pain-producing procedure, with each new report of pain, and at regular intervals. *Systematic ongoing assessment and documentation provide direction for the pain treatment plan; adjustments are based on the client's response. The client's report of pain is the single most reliable indicator of pain (Acute Pain Management Guideline Panel, 1992; Jacox et al, 1994; JCAHO, 2000).*

- Ask the client to maintain a diary of pain ratings, timing, precipitating events, medications, treatments, and steps that work best to relieve pain. **Nursing Research:** *One study showed that systematic tracking of pain was an important factor in improving pain management (Faries et al, 1991).*

- If the client is cognitively impaired and unable to report pain and use a pain rating scale, assess and document behaviors that might be indicative of pain (e.g., change in activity, loss of appetite, guarding, grimacing, moaning). *The absence of behaviors thought to be indicative of pain does not necessarily mean that pain is absent (Herr, 2002; McCaffery and Pasero, 1999).* **Nursing Research:** *Certain behaviors have been shown to be indicative of pain and can be used to assess pain in clients who cannot use a self-report pain rating tool (e.g., in the cognitively impaired client). The clinician should be aware that pain expression is highly individual, and what may be a pain behavior in one client may not be in another. Pain assessment must be individualized (Herr, 2002).*

- ▲ Assume that pain is present and treat accordingly in clients who have a pathological condition or are undergoing a procedure thought to be painful. *Pain is associated with certain pathological conditions (e.g., arthritis) and procedures (e.g., surgery). In the absence of the client's report of pain (e.g., in critically ill or cognitively impaired clients), the clinician should assume that pain is present and treat accordingly (McCaffery and Pasero, 1999).*

- ▲ Determine the client's current medication use. *To aid in planning pain treatment, obtain a medication history (Acute Pain Management Guideline Panel, 1992).* Obtaining a complete history of medications the client is taking or has taken can help to prevent drug-drug interactions and toxicity problems that can occur when incompatible drugs are combined or when allergies are present. The history will also provide the clinician with an understanding of what medications have been tried and were or were not effective in treating the client's pain (Acute Pain Management Guideline Panel, 1992; McCaffery and Pasero, 1999).

- ▲ Explore the need for medications from the three classes of analgesic: opioids (narcotics), nonopioids (acetaminophen, nonselective nonsteroidal anti-inflammatory drugs [NSAIDs], and selective NSAIDs [cyclo-oxygenase-2 or COX-2 inhibitors]), and adjuvant medications. For chronic neuropathic pain, consider adjuvant medications that are analgesic, such as anticonvulsants and antidepressants. *NSAIDs act mainly in the pe-*

- • = Independent; ▲ = Collaborative

riphery to inhibit the initiation of pain signals (Dahl and Kehlet, 1991). The analgesic regimen should include a nonopioid drug around the clock (ATC), even if pain is severe enough to require the addition of an opioid (American Pain Society, 1999, 2002). Some types of pain respond to nonopioid drugs alone. If the pain is not responding, however, consider increasing the dosage or adding an opioid. At any level of pain, analgesic adjuvants may be useful (American Pain Society, 1999, 2002). Analgesic combinations may enhance pain relief. Combining analgesics can result in acceptable pain relief with lower dosages of each analgesic than would be possible with one analgesic alone. Lower dosages can result in fewer or less severe side effects (McCaffery and Pasero, 1999).

▲ For persistent cancer pain, obtain a prescription to administer opioid analgesics. *When pain persists or increases, an opioid such as oxycodone should be added to the nonopioid (Jacox et al, 1994). If this is not effective, switch to morphine or other single-entity opioids (McCaffery and Pasero, 1999).*

▲ For persistent chronic nonmalignant pain, discuss the use of opioid analgesics with the health care team and obtain a prescription to administer if appropriate. *The use of opioid analgesics for chronic nonmalignant pain is both legal and clinically important. These agents should be used for clients with chronic nonmalignant pain (e.g., osteoarthritis, rheumatoid arthritis) when other medications and nonpharmacological interventions produce inadequate pain relief and the client's quality of life is affected by the pain (American Pain Society, 2002).*

▲ The oral route is preferred. If the client is receiving parenteral analgesia, use an equianalgesic chart to convert to an oral or other noninvasive route as smoothly as possible. (See Appendix E for an equianalgesic chart.) *The least invasive route of administration capable of providing adequate pain control is recommended. The oral route is the most preferred because it is the most convenient and cost effective. Avoid the intramuscular (IM) route because of unreliable absorption, pain, and inconvenience. Repeated IM injections can produce sterile abscesses (Jacox et al, 1994).*

▲ Establish ATC dosing and administer supplemental opioid doses as needed to keep pain ratings at or below the comfort/function goal. *An order for prn supplementary opioid doses between regular doses is an essential backup (American Pain Society, 1999).*

▲ Ask the client to describe appetite, bowel elimination, and ability to rest and sleep. Administer medications and treatments to improve these functions. Always obtain a prescription for a peristaltic stimulant to prevent opioid-induced constipation. *Because there is great individual variation in the development of opioid-induced side effects, they should be monitored and, if their development is inevitable (e.g., constipation), prophylactically treated. Opioids cause constipation by decreasing bowel peristalsis (Jacox et al, 1994; McCaffery and Pasero, 1999).*

• Explain to the client the pain management approach that has been ordered, including therapies, medication administration, side effects, and complications. *One of the most important steps toward improved control of pain is a better client understanding of the nature of pain, its treatment, and the role the client needs to play in pain control (Jacox et al, 1994).*

• Discuss the client's fears of undertreated pain, addiction, and overdose. *Because of the many misconceptions regarding pain and its treatment, education about the ability to control pain effectively and correction of myths about the use of opioids should be included as part of the treatment plan (Jacox et al, 1994; McCaffery and Pasero, 1999). Opioid tolerance and physical dependence are expected with long-term opioid treatment and should not be confused with addiction (Jacox et al, 1994). Addiction is extremely unlikely after clients use opioids*

• = **Independent;** ▲ = **Collaborative**

for pain relief (Acute Pain Management Guideline Panel, 1992; Jacox et al, 1994). **Nursing Research:** *A survey of 270 people with cancer pain revealed that many harbor fears and misconceptions regarding the use of analgesics, management of side effects, and risk of addiction (Ward et al, 1993).*

▲ Review the client's pain diary, flow sheet, and medication records to determine the overall degree of pain relief, side effects, and analgesic requirements for an appropriate period (e.g., 1 week). **Nursing Research:** *Systematic tracking of pain was found to be an important factor in improving pain management (Faries et al, 1991; JCAHO, 2000).*

▲ Obtain prescriptions to increase or decrease analgesic doses when indicated. Base prescriptions on the client's report of pain severity and the comfort/function goal and response to previous dose in terms of relief, side effects, and ability to perform ADLs and comply with the prescribed therapeutic regimen. *Analgesic dosages should be adjusted to achieve pain relief with manageable and tolerable adverse effects (Jacox et al, 1994; McCaffery and Pasero, 1999).*

▲ If opioid dose is increased, monitor sedation and respiratory status for a brief time. *Clients receiving long-term opioid therapy generally develop tolerance to the respiratory depressant effects of these agents (Jacox et al, 1994; McCaffery and Pasero, 1999).*

▲ In addition to the use of analgesics, support the client's use of nonpharmacological methods to help control pain, such as physical therapy, group therapy, distraction, imagery, relaxation, massage, and application of heat and cold. *Cognitive-behavioral strategies can restore the client's sense of self-control, personal efficacy, and active participation in his or her own care (Jacox et al, 1994).*

• Teach and implement nonpharmacological interventions when pain is relatively well controlled with pharmacological means. *Nonpharmacological interventions should be used to supplement, not replace, pharmacological interventions (Acute Pain Management Guideline Panel, 1992).*

• Encourage the client to plan activities around periods of greatest comfort whenever possible. *Pain diminishes activity. Clients will find it easier to perform their ADLs and enjoy social activities when they are rested and pain is under control (Jacox et al, 1994; McCaffery and Pasero, 1999).*

▲ Explore appropriate resources for management of pain on a long-term basis (e.g., hospice, pain care center). *Most clients with cancer or chronic nonmalignant pain are treated for pain in outpatient and home care settings. Plans should be made to ensure ongoing assessment of the pain and the effectiveness of treatments in these settings (Jacox et al, 1994).*

• If the client has progressive cancer pain, assist the client and family with handling issues related to death and dying. *Peer support groups and pastoral counseling may increase the client's and family's coping skills and provide needed support (Jacox et al, 1994).*

• Assist the client and family in minimizing the effects of pain on interpersonal relationships and daily activities such as work and recreation. **Nursing Research:** *Pain can reduce clients' options to exercise control, diminish psychological well-being, and make them feel helpless and vulnerable. Therefore, clinicians should encourage active client involvement in effective and practical methods to manage pain (Hitchcock, Ferrell, and McCaffery, 1994).*

Geriatric

▲ Always take an elderly client's reports of pain seriously and ensure that the pain is relieved. *In spite of what many professionals and clients believe, pain is not an expected part of*

• = **Independent;** ▲ = **Collaborative**

normal aging *(American Geriatric Society Panel on Persistent Pain in Older Persons, 2002; McCaffery and Pasero, 1999).*

- When assessing pain, speak clearly, slowly, and loudly enough for the client to hear, and if the client uses a hearing aid, be sure it is in place; repeat information as needed. Be sure the client can see well enough to read the pain scale (use an enlarged scale) and written materials. **Nursing Research:** *Elderly clients often have difficulty hearing and seeing. Comprehension is improved when instructions are given slowly and clearly and when clients can see visual aids (Herr, 2002).*

- Handle the client's body gently. Allow the client to move at his or her own speed. *The elderly are particularly susceptible to injury during care activities. Caregivers must be patient and expect that the elderly will move more slowly than younger clients; they may also perform better and experience less pain when they are allowed to move themselves (McCaffery and Pasero, 1999).*

- ▲ Use acetaminophen and NSAIDs with low side-effect profiles, such as the selective COX-2 NSAIDs (COX-2 inhibitors), choline and magnesium salicylates (Trilisate), and diflunisal (Dolobid), and watch for side effects, such as gastrointestinal disturbances and bleeding problems. *Elderly people are at increased risk for gastric and renal toxicity from NSAIDs (Acute Pain Management Guideline Panel, 1992; American Geriatric Society Panel on Persistent Pain in Older Persons, 2002; Griffin et al, 1991). Opioids ATC are preferable to long-term administration of nonselective NSAIDs in the elderly client because of an increased risk for NSAID adverse effects (American Geriatric Society Panel on Persistent Pain in Older Persons, 2002).*

- ▲ Avoid or use with caution drugs with a long half-life, such as the NSAID piroxicam (Feldene), the opioids methadone (Dolophine) and levorphanol (Levo-Dromoran), and the benzodiazepine diazepam (Valium). *The higher prevalence of renal insufficiency in the elderly than in younger persons can result in toxicity from drug accumulation (Acute Pain Management Guideline Panel, 1992; American Geriatric Society Panel on Persistent Pain in Older Persons, 2002; American Pain Society, 1999; McCaffery and Pasero, 1999).*

- ▲ Use opioids with caution in the elderly client. *The elderly are more sensitive to the analgesic effects of opioid drugs because they experience a higher peak effect and a longer duration of pain relief. Reduce the initial recommended adult starting opioid dosage by 25% to 50%, especially if the client is frail and debilitated; then increase the dosage if safe and necessary (Acute Pain Management Guideline Panel, 1992).*

- ▲ Avoid the use of opioids with toxic metabolites, such as meperidine (Demerol) and propoxyphene (Darvon, Darvocet), in elderly clients. *Meperidine's metabolite, normeperidine, can produce central nervous system (CNS) irritability, seizures, and even death; propoxyphene's metabolite, norpropoxyphene, can produce CNS toxicity. Both of these metabolites are eliminated by the kidneys, which makes meperidine and propoxyphene particularly poor choices for elderly clients, many of whom have at least some degree of renal insufficiency (Acute Pain Management Guideline Panel, 1992; McCaffery and Pasero, 1999).*

Multicultural

- Assess pain in a client from a different culture using a self-report 0 to 10 numerical pain rating scale or the Wong Baker Faces pain rating scale (see Appendix E). Have the scale translated into the client's native language if necessary. *Inadequate pain management is widespread, especially among minority groups, and a major reason is the failure*

- = Independent; ▲ = Collaborative

to assess pain properly. The more cultural differences between the client and the nurse, the more difficult it is for the nurse to assess and treat pain. Self-report of pain is the single most reliable indicator of pain, regardless of culture (McCaffery, 1999; McCaffery and Pasero, 1999).

▲ Administer analgesics on a preventive basis to keep pain ratings at or below an acceptable level. *Regardless of the client's cultural background, pain rated at higher than 3 on a 0 to 10 pain rating scale interferes significantly with daily function. Perceived quality of life appears to be comparable across cultures, with pain ratings of higher than 5 interfering markedly with a person's ability to enjoy life (McCaffery, 1999; McCaffery and Pasero, 1999).*

• Assess for the influence of cultural beliefs, norms, and values on the client's perception and experience of pain. **Nursing Research:** *One study showed that the client's experience of pain may be influenced by cultural perceptions (Leininger, 1996).*

• Assess for the effect of fatalism on the client's beliefs regarding the current state of comfort. **Nursing Research:** *Fatalistic perspectives, which involve the belief that one cannot control one's own fate, may influence health behaviors in some African American and Latino populations (Harmon, Castro, and Coe, 1996; Phillips, Cohen, and Moses, 1999).*

• Incorporate safe and effective folk health care practices and beliefs into care whenever possible. *It is the responsibility of the caregiver to ensure that safe and effective pain management is provided. Although support of an individual's health care beliefs is recommended, when research does not support the safety or effectiveness of a method or when research does not exist, this should be explained fully to the client (McCaffery and Pasero, 1999).* **Nursing Research:** *Incorporating folk health care beliefs and practices into pain management care increased compliance with the treatment plan (Juarez, Ferrell, and Borneman, 1998).*

• Use a family-centered approach to care. **Nursing Research:** *Involving the family in pain management care increased compliance with the treatment regimen (Juarez, Ferrell, Borneman, 1998).*

• Use culturally relevant pain scales (e.g., the Oucher Scale), if available, to assess pain in the client. **Nursing Research:** *Clients from minority cultures may express pain differently than clients from the majority culture. The Oucher Scale is available in African American and Hispanic versions and is used to assess pain in children (Beyer, Denyes, and Villarruel, 1992).*

• Ensure that directions for medication use are available in the client's language of choice and are understood by the client and caregiver. **Nursing Research:** *Use of bilingual instructions for medication administration increased compliance with the pain management plan (Juarez, Ferrell, and Borneman, 1998).*

Home care

• Develop the treatment plan with the client and caregivers. *Clients and caregivers will be more likely to follow the treatment plan when their input is considered (McCaffery and Pasero, 1999).* **Nursing Research:** *Compliance with the medical regimen for treating pain improves the likelihood of successful management (Humphrey, 1994).*

▲ Develop a full medication profile, including medications prescribed by all physicians and all over-the-counter medications. Assess for drug interactions. Instruct the client to refrain from mixing medications without physician approval. *Pain medications may significantly affect or be affected by other medications and may cause severe side effects. Some combinations of drugs are specifically contraindicated (Jacox et al, 1994).*

• = **Independent;** ▲ = **Collaborative**

- Assess the client's and family's knowledge of side effects and safety precautions associated with pain medications (e.g., use caution if operating machinery when opioids are first taken or dosage has been increased significantly). *The cognitive effects of opioids usually subside within a week of initial dosing or dose increases (McCaffery and Pasero, 1999). The use of long-term opioid treatment does not appear to affect neuropsychological performance.* **Clinical Research:** *Pain itself may reduce performance on neuropsychological tests more than oral opioid treatment (Sjogren et al, 2000).*
- ▲ Collaborate with the health care team (including the client and family) on an ongoing basis to determine an optimal pain control profile. Identify the most effective interventions and the medication administration routes most acceptable to the client and family. **Nursing Research:** *Success in pain control is partially dependent on the acceptability of the suggested intervention. Acceptability promotes compliance. Dosages vary among routes and will need to be adjusted accordingly to avoid breakthrough or transitional pain (Bohnet, 1995).*
- ▲ If medication is administered using highly technological methods, assess the home for necessary resources (e.g., electricity) and ensure that responsible caregivers will be available to assist the client with administration. *Some routes of medication administration require special conditions and procedures to be safe and accurate (McCaffery and Pasero, 1999).*
- ▲ Assess the knowledge base of the client and family for highly technological medication administration. Teach as necessary. Be sure the client knows when, how, and whom to contact if analgesia is unsatisfactory. *Appropriate instruction in the home increases the accuracy and safety of medication administration (McCaffery and Pasero, 1999).*
- Support the client and family in the use of opioid analgesics. *Well-intentioned friends and family may create added stress by expressing judgment or fears regarding the use of opioid analgesics (McCaffery and Pasero, 1999).*

Client/Family Teaching

NOTE: To avoid the negative connotations associated with the words *drugs* and *narcotics,* use the term *pain medicine* when teaching clients.
- Provide written materials on pain control such as *Understanding Your Pain: Using a Pain Rating Scale* (McCaffery, Pasero, and Portenoy, 2001) (see pages 706-707 for instructions on the use of a pain rating scale). *Written materials are provided in addition to verbal instructions so that the client will have a reference during treatment (McCaffery and Pasero, 1999).*
- Discuss the various discomforts encompassed by the word *pain* and ask the client to give examples of previously experienced pain. Explain the pain assessment process and the purpose of the pain rating scale. *It is often difficult for clients to understand the concept of pain and describe their pain experience. Using alternative words and providing a complete description of the assessment process, including the use of scales, will ensure that an accurate treatment plan is developed (McCaffery and Pasero, 1999). Teach clients to use the pain rating scale to rate the intensity of past or current pain.*
- ▲ Ask the client to set a comfort/function goal by selecting a pain level on the rating scale that makes it easy to perform recovery activities (e.g., turn, cough, deep breathe). If pain is above this level, the client should take action that decreases pain or notify a member of the health care team. (See pages 706-707 for information on teaching clients to use the pain rating scale.) *The use of comfort/function goals provides direction for*

• = Independent; ▲ = Collaborative

the treatment plan. Changes are made according to the client's response and achievement of the goals of recovery or rehabilitation (McCaffery and Pasero, 1999).

▲ Discuss the total plan for pharmacological and nonpharmacological treatment, including the medication plan for ATC administration and supplemental doses, the maintenance of a pain diary, and the use of supplies and equipment. *Appropriate instruction increases the accuracy and safety of medication administration (McCaffery and Pasero, 1999).*

• Reinforce the importance of taking pain medications to keep pain under control. *Teaching clients to stay on top of their pain and prevent it from getting out of control will improve their ability to perform ADLs and accomplish goals (McCaffery and Pasero, 1999).*

• Reinforce that taking opioids for pain relief is not addiction and that addiction is very unlikely to occur. *The development of addiction when opioids are taken for pain relief is extremely rare (Acute Pain Management Guideline Panel, 1992; American Pain Society, 1999; Jacox et al, 1994).*

• Explain to a client with chronic neuropathic pain the process of taking adjuvant analgesics (e.g., tricyclic antidepressants). *A low dose of adjuvant analgesic is used initially and the dose is increased gradually. Pain relief is delayed, and the adjuvant analgesics must be taken daily. Teaching clients that, although the medicine is an antidepressant, it is used for analgesia and not depression will increase understanding of the drug. Comparable teaching should take place when an anticonvulsant is prescribed for analgesia (McCaffery and Pasero, 1999).*

• Emphasize to the client the importance of pacing himself or herself and taking rest breaks before they are needed. *Clients will find they are able to perform their ADLs and achieve goals better when they are rested (McCaffery and Pasero, 1999).*

▲ Demonstrate the use of appropriate nonpharmacological approaches in addition to pharmacological approaches for helping to control pain (e.g., physical therapy, group therapy, distraction, imagery, and application of heat and cold).

• Teach and implement nonpharmacological interventions when pain is relatively well controlled with pharmacological means. *Nonpharmacological interventions are used to supplement, not replace, pharmacological interventions (Acute Pain Management Guideline Panel, 1992; McCaffery and Pasero, 1999).*

evolve WEBSITES FOR EDUCATION

See the EVOLVE website for World Wide Web resources for client education.

REFERENCES

Acute Pain Management Guideline Panel: *Acute pain management operative or medical procedures and trauma: clinical practice guideline,* Agency for Health Care Policy and Research Pub No. 92-0032, Rockville, Md, 1992, Public Health Service, US Department of Health and Human Services.

American Geriatric Society Panel on Persistent Pain in Older Persons: The management of persistent pain in older persons, *J Am Geriatr Soc* 50:S205, 2002.

American Pain Society: *Principles of analgesic use in the treatment of acute pain and cancer pain,* ed 4, Glenview, Ill, 1999, The Society.

American Pain Society: *Guideline for the management of pain in osteoarthritis, rheumatoid arthritis, and juvenile chronic arthritis,* Glenview, Ill, 2002, The Society.

American Pain Society Quality of Care Committee: Quality improvement guidelines for the treatment of acute pain and cancer pain, *JAMA* 274:1874, 1995.

• = Independent; ▲ = Collaborative

Beyer J, Denyes M, Villarruel A: The creation, validation, and continuing development of the Oucher: a measure of pain intensity in children, *J Pediatr Nurs* 7(5):335, 1992.

Bohnet N: Chronic pain management in the home care setting, *J Wound Ostomy Continence Nurs* 22:135, 1995.

Bonica JJ: Definitions and taxonomy of pain. In Bonica JJ, editor: *The management of pain*, Philadelphia, 1990, Lea and Febiger.

Dahl JB, Kehlet H: Non-steroidal anti-inflammatory drugs: rationale for use in severe postoperative pain, *Br J Anaesth* 66:703, 1991.

Faries JE et al: Systematic pain records and their impact on pain control, *Cancer Nurs* 14:306, 1991.

Griffin ME et al: Nonsteroidal anti-inflammatory drug use and increased risk for peptic ulcer disease in elderly persons, *Ann Intern Med* 11:257, 1991.

Harmon MP, Castro FG, Coe K: Acculturation and cervical cancer: knowledge, beliefs, and behaviors of Hispanic women, *Women Health* 24(3):37, 1996.

Herr K: Pain assessment in cognitively impaired older adults, *Am J Nurs* 102(12):65, 2002.

Hitchcock LS, Ferrell BR, McCaffery M: The experience of chronic nonmalignant pain, *J Pain Symptom Manage* 9:312, 1994.

Humphrey C: *Home care nursing handbook*, ed 2, Gaithersburg, Md, 1994, Aspen.

Jacox A et al: *Management of cancer pain*, Clinical Practice Guideline No. 9, Agency for Health Care Policy and Research Pub No. 94-0592, Rockville, Md, 1994, Public Health Service, US Department of Health and Human Services.

Joint Commission on Accreditation of Healthcare Organizations: *2000 Hospital accreditation standards*, Oakbrook, Ill, 2000, The Organization.

Juarez G, Ferrell B, Borneman T: Influence of culture on cancer pain management in Hispanic clients, *Cancer Pract* 6(5):262, 1998.

Leininger MM: *Transcultural nursing: theories, research and practices*, ed 2, Hilliard, Ohio, 1996, McGraw-Hill.

McCaffery M: *Nursing practice theories related to cognition, bodily pain, and man-environment interactions*, Los Angeles, 1968, University of California at Los Angeles Students' Store.

McCaffery M: Culturally sensitive pain assessment, *Am J Nurs* 99(8):18, 1999.

McCaffery M, Ferrell BR: How would you respond to these clients in pain? *Nursing* 21(6):34, 1991.

McCaffery M, Ferrell BR: How vital are vital signs? *Nursing* 22(1):42, 1992.

McCaffery M, Pasero C: *Pain: clinical manual*, St Louis, 1999, Mosby.

McCaffery M, Pasero C, Portenoy RK: *Understanding your pain: using a pain rating scale*, Chadds Ford, Pa, 2001, Endo Pharmaceuticals, Inc. Call 800-462-3636 to order.

Page GG, Ben-Eliyahu S: The immune-suppressive nature of pain, *Semin Oncol Nurs* 13(1):10, 1997.

Phillips JM, Cohen MZ, Moses G: Breast cancer screening and African American women: fear, fatalism, and silence, *Oncol Nurs Forum* 26(3):561, 1999.

Sjogren P et al: Neuropsychological performance in cancer clients: the role of oral opioids, pain and performance status, *Pain* 86:237, 2000.

Ward S et al: Client-related barriers to management of cancer pain, *Pain* 52:319, 1993.

Readiness for enhanced Parenting

Gail B. Ladwig

NANDA   Definition

Pattern of providing environment for children or other dependent person(s) that is sufficient to nurture growth and development and can be strengthened

Defining Characteristics

Expresses willingness to enhance parenting; children or other dependent person(s) express satisfaction with home environment; emotional and tacit support of children or dependent person(s) is evident; bonding or attachment is evident; physical and emotional needs of children or other dependent person(s) are met; realistic expectations of children or other dependent person(s) are exhibited

• = **Independent;** ▲ = **Collaborative**

| NOC | Outcomes (Nursing Outcomes Classification) |

Suggested NOC Outcomes

Child Development: 1 Month, 2 Months, 4 Months, 6 Months, 12 Months, Preschool, Middle Childhood, Adolescence; Growth; Health-Promoting Behavior; Health-Seeking Behavior; Immunization Behavior; Knowledge: Breastfeeding, Child Physical Safety, Diet, Health Behavior, Health Resources, Infection Control, Medication, Personal Safety; Leisure Participation; Nutritional Status; Parent-Infant Attachment; Parenting Performance; Parenting: Psychosocial Safety; Risk Control; Risk Detection; Role Performance; Safe Home Environment; Self-Esteem

Example NOC Outcome with Indicators

Parenting Performance as evidenced by the following indicators: Provides regular preventive and episodic health care/Stimulates cognitive and social development/Stimulates emotional and spiritual growth/Interacts positively with child/Demonstrates empathy toward child/Expresses satisfaction with parenting role/Demonstrates positive self-esteem (Rate each indicator of **Parenting Performance:** 1 = never demonstrated, 2 = rarely demonstrated, 3 = sometimes demonstrated, 4 = often demonstrated, 5 = consistently demonstrated [see Section I].)

Client Outcomes

Client/Family Will (Specify Time Frame):

- Affirm desire to improve parenting skills to further support growth and development of children
- Demonstrate loving relationship with children
- Provide a safe, nurturing environment
- Assess risks in home/environment and takes steps to prevent possibility of harm to children
- Meet physical, psychosocial, and spiritual needs or seek appropriate assistance

| NIC | Interventions (Nursing Interventions Classification) |

Suggested NIC Interventions

Anticipatory Guidance; Attachment Promotion; Developmental Enhancement: Adolescent, Child; Family Integrity Promotion: Childbearing Family; Infant Care; Newborn Care; Parent Education: Adolescent, Childrearing Family, Infant; Parenting Promotion; Teaching: Infant Stimulation

Example NIC Activities—Parenting Promotion

Assist parents to have realistic expectations appropriate to developmental and ability level of child; Assist parents with role transition and expectations of parenthood

Nursing Interventions and Rationales

- Use family-centered care and role modeling for holistic care of families. **Nursing Research:** *Specific techniques of role modeling and reflective practice are suggested as effec-*

• = Independent; ▲ = Collaborative

tive approaches to teach the family sensitive care in clinical settings in which families are part of the care environment (Tomlinson et al, 2002).

- Assess parents' feelings when dealing with a child who has a chronic illness. **Nursing Research:** *Knowing how parents feel about a child's asthma is the first step in helping them manage this common chronic disease (Clark and Chalmers, 2003).*

- Encourage positive parenting: respect for children, understanding of normal development, and use of creative and loving approaches to meet parenting challenges. **Nursing Research:** *Understanding normal development is a first step so that parents can distinguish common behaviors for a given stage of development from "problems." Central to positive parenting is developing approaches that can be used in place of anger, manipulation, punishment, and rewards (Ahmann, 2002).*

- Provide opportunities for mother-infant skin-to-skin contact (kangaroo care [KC]) for preterm infants. **Clinical Research:** *One study showed that the neurodevelopmental profile was more mature for infants receiving KC. Results underscore the role of early skin-to-skin contact in the maturation of the autonomic and circadian systems in preterm infants (Feldman and Eidelman, 2003).*

- Provide the parent with the opportunity to assist in the newborn's first bath, allowing a flexible bath time. **Nursing Research:** *A flexible bathing time is recommended depending on the characteristics and stability of the newborn and family desires. Axillary temperatures as measured at four different times did not differ significantly between infants bathed within 1 hour of birth and those bathed 4 to 6 hours after birth (Behring, Vezeau, and Fink, 2003).*

- When the person who is ill is the parent, use family-centered assessment skills to determine the impact of an adult's illness on the child and then guide the parent through those topics that are most likely to be of concern, including (a) the name of the illness, (b) the cause of the illness, (c) the potential contagion or spread of the illness, and (d) the ultimate impact of the illness on the life of the child. **Nursing Research:** *The pediatric nurse, by embracing core principles of openness and honesty and by providing concrete developmental information, can empower parents to support their own children (McCue and Bonn, 2003).*

▲ Have family members participate in client conferences that involve all members of the health care team. *Conferences allow for distribution of information, input by all members at one time, and a decrease in anxiety levels of family members.*

Multicultural

- Assess for the influence of cultural beliefs, norms, and values on the client's perception of parenting. **Nursing Research:** *What the client considers normal parenting may be based on cultural perceptions (Cochran; 1998; Doswell and Erlen, 1998; Leininger and McFarland, 2002).*

- Acknowledge racial/ethnic differences at the onset of care. *Acknowledgment of racial/ethnicity issues will enhance communication, establish rapport, and promote treatment outcomes (D'Avanzo et al, 2001).*

- Acknowledge that value conflicts from acculturation stresses may contribute to increased anxiety and significant conflict with children. **Nursing Research:** *Challenges to traditional beliefs and values are anxiety provoking. Less acculturated parents may experience conflict with their more acculturated children as the children demand greater independence and freedom (True, 1995).*

• = **Independent;** ▲ = **Collaborative**

- Acknowledge and praise parenting strengths noted. **Nursing Research:** *Such acknowledgment will increase trust and foster a working relationship with the parent (Seiderman et al, 1996).*
- Refer to the care plans for **Impaired Parenting, Risk for impaired Parenting,** and **Risk for impaired parent/infant/child Attachment** for additional interventions that could be used with slight modification.

Home care
The nursing interventions described previously should be used in the home environment with adaptations as necessary.
- ▲ Refer to a parenting program to facilitate learning of parenting skills. **Nursing Research:** *At the end of an 8-week parenting program, parents demonstrated statistically significant reduced levels of clinical anxiety and depression. Parents showed an increase in more positive ratings of personality states, such as not shouting at their children and being more calm and energetic, at the end of the program (Long et al, 2001).*

Client/Family Teaching
Refer to Client/Family Teaching for **Impaired Parenting** and **Risk for impaired Parenting** for suggestions that may be used with minor adaptations.
- Teach parents home safety: reduction of hot water temperature, proper poison storage, use of smoke alarms, installation of safety gates for stairs, and use of ipecac syrup. **Clinical Research:** *Counseling coupled with convenient access to reduced-cost products appears to be an effective strategy for promoting children's home safety (Gielen, McDonald, and Wilson, 2002).*
- Teach parents and young teens conflict resolution using a hypothetical conflict solution with and without a structured conflict resolution guide. **Nursing Research:** *Parents and young teens do not use a systematic method of solving disagreements, but with structured guidance, the parents and teens are able to resolve conflicts (Riesch et al, 2003).*
- ▲ Refer mothers of children with type 1 diabetes for community support in baby-sitting, child care, or respite. **Nursing Research:** *A study of mothers raising young children older than 4 years of age with type 1 diabetes highlights the importance of identifying family and/or community resources that could reduce some of the tremendous stress and burden of responsibility experienced after a child is diagnosed with diabetes (Sullivan-Bolyai et al, 2003).*
- Support empowerment of parents of children with asthma. **Nursing Research:** *Asthma is the most common chronic illness in children and has a significant impact on children and their families. Empowering parents by facilitating their sense of control resulted in increased knowledge and ability to make decisions regarding their child's care (McCarthy et al, 2002).*
- Teach families the importance of monitoring television viewing and limiting exposure to violence. **Nursing Research:** *Media violence can be hazardous to children's health, and studies point overwhelmingly to a causal connection between media violence and aggressive attitudes, values, and behaviors in some children. Nurses can teach children and parents about the effects of media violence and advise them on how to avoid exposure (Muscari, 2002).*

• = **Independent;** ▲ = **Collaborative**

evolve WEBSITES FOR EDUCATION

See the EVOLVE website for World Wide Web resources for client education.

REFERENCES

Ahmann E: Promoting positive parenting: an annotated bibliography, *Pediatr Nurs* 28(4):382, 2002.

Behring A, Vezeau TM, Fink R: Timing of the newborn first bath: a replication, *Neonatal Netw* 22(1):39, 2003.

Clark BA, Chalmers KL: Helping parents cope, *Can Nurse* 99(2):19, 2003.

Cochran M: Tears have no color, *Am J Nurs* 98(6):53, 1998.

D'Avanzo CE et al: Developing culturally informed strategies for substance-related interventions. In Naegle MA, D'Avanzo CE, editors: *Addictions and substance abuse: strategies for advanced practice nursing*, St Louis, 2001, Mosby.

Doswell W, Erlen J: Multicultural issues and ethical concerns in the delivery of nursing care interventions, *Nurs Clin North Am* 33(2):353, 1998.

Feldman R, Eidelman A: Skin-to-skin contact (kangaroo care) accelerates autonomic and neurobehavioural maturation in preterm infants, *Dev Med Child Neurol* 45(4):274, 2003.

Gielen AC, McDonald EM, Wilson ME: Effects of improved access to safety counseling, products, and home visits on parents' safety practices: results of a randomized trial, *Arch Pediatr Adolesc Med* 156(1):33, 2002.

Leininger MM, McFarland MR: *Transcultural nursing: concepts, theories, research and practices*, ed 3, New York, 2002, McGraw-Hill.

Long A et al: The effectiveness of parenting programmes facilitated by health visitors, *J Adv Nurs* 34(5):611, 2001.

McCarthy MJ et al: Empowering parents through asthma education, *Pediatr Nurs* 28(5):465, 2002.

McCue K, Bonn R: Helping children through an adult's serious illness, *Pediatr Nurs* 29(1):47, 2003.

Muscari M: Media violence: advice for parents, *Pediatr Nurs* 28(6):585, 2002.

Riesch SK et al: Conflict and conflict resolution: parent and young teen perceptions, *J Pediatr Health Care* 17(1): 22, 2003.

Seiderman RY et al: Assessing American Indian families, *MCN Am J Matern Child Nurs* 21(6):274, 1996.

Sullivan-Bolyai S et al: Constant vigilance: mothers' work parenting young children with type 1 diabetes, *J Pediatr Nurs* 18(1):21, 2003.

Tomlinson PS et al: Clinical innovation for promoting family care in paediatric intensive care: demonstration, role modelling and reflective practice, *J Adv Nurs* 38(2):161, 2002.

True RH: Mental health issues of Asian/Pacific island women. In Adams DL, editor: *Health issues for women of color: a cultural diversity perspective*, Thousand Oaks, Calif, 1995, Sage.

Impaired Parenting

T. Heather Herdman and Gail B. Ladwig

NANDA Definition

Inability of primary caretaker to create, maintain, or regain an environment that promotes optimum growth and development of the child

Defining Characteristics

Infant/child

Poor academic performance; frequent illness; running away; physical and psychological trauma or abuse; frequent accidents; lack of attachment; failure to thrive; behavioral disorders; poor social competence; lack of separation anxiety; poor cognitive development

• = Independent; ▲ = Collaborative

Parental

Inappropriate child care arrangements; rejection of or hostility toward child; statements of inability to meet child's needs; inflexibility in meeting needs of child or situation; poor or inappropriate caretaking skills; regular punitive behavior; inconsistent care; child abuse; inadequate child health maintenance; unsafe home environment; verbalization of inability to control child; negative statements about child; verbalization of role inadequacy or frustration; inappropriate visual, tactile, or auditory stimulation of child; abandonment; insecure attachment or lack of attachment to infant; inconsistent behavior management; child neglect; little cuddling; maternal-child interaction deficit; poor parent-child interaction

Related Factors (r/t)

Social

Lack of access to resources; social isolation; lack of resources; poor home environment; lack of family cohesiveness; inadequate child care arrangements; lack of transportation; unemployment or job problems; role strain or overload; marital conflict, declining satisfaction; lack of value of parenthood; change in family unit; low socioeconomic class; unplanned or unwanted pregnancy; presence of stress (e.g., financial or legal difficulties, recent crisis, cultural move); lack of or poor parental role model; single parenthood; lack of social support network; lack of involvement of father of child; history of being abusive; history of being abused; financial difficulties; maladaptive coping strategies; poverty; poor problem-solving skills; inability to put child's needs before own; low self-esteem; relocation; legal difficulties

Knowledge

Lack of knowledge about child health maintenance; lack of knowledge about parenting skills; unrealistic expectations for self, infant, partner; limited cognitive functioning; lack of knowledge about child development; inability to recognize and act on infant cues; low educational level or attainment; poor communication skills; lack of cognitive readiness for parenthood; preference for physical punishment

Physiological

Physical illness

Infant/child

Premature birth; illness; prolonged separation from parent; not desired gender; attention deficit hyperactivity disorder; difficult temperament; separation from parent at birth; lack of goodness of fit (temperament) with parental expectations; unplanned or unwanted child; handicapping condition or developmental delay; multiple births; altered perceptual abilities

Psychological

History of substance abuse or dependencies; disability; depression; difficult labor and/or delivery; young age, especially adolescence; history of mental illness; high number of or closely spaced pregnancies; sleep derivation or disruption; lack of or late prenatal care; separation from infant/child

• = Independent; ▲ = Collaborative

NOTE: It is important to reaffirm that adjustment to parenting in general is a normal maturational process that elicits nursing behaviors to prevent potential problems and to promote health.

NOC   Outcomes (Nursing Outcomes Classification)

Suggested NOC Outcomes

Abuse Cessation; Abuse Protection; Abuse Recovery: Emotional; Abusive Behavior Self-Restraint; Child Development: 2 Months, 4 Months, 6 Months, 2 Years, 3 Years, 4 Years, Preschool, Middle Childhood, Adolescence; Coping; Knowledge: Child Physical Safety; Neglect Recovery; Parent-Infant Attachment; Parenting Performance; Parenting: Psychosocial Safety; Role Performance; Safe Home Environment; Social Support

Example NOC Outcome with Indicators

Abuse Recovery: Emotional as evidenced by the following indicators: Demonstration of confidence/Demonstration of impulse control, self-advocacy/Expressions of feeling empowered/Demonstration of positive interpersonal relationships/Demonstration of provision of safety for child (Rate each indicator of **Abuse Recovery: Emotional:** 1 = none, 2 = limited, 3 = moderate, 4 = substantial, 5 = extensive [see Section I].)

Client Outcomes

Client Will (Specify Time Frame):
- Affirm desire to develop constructive parenting skills to support infant/child growth and development
- Initiate appropriate measures to develop a safe, nurturing environment
- Acquire and display attentive, supportive parenting behaviors
- Identify strategies to protect child from harm and/or neglect and initiate action when indicated

NIC   Interventions (Nursing Interventions Classification)

Suggested NIC Interventions

Abuse Protection Support: Child; Attachment Promotion; Caregiver Support; Developmental Enhancement: Adolescent, Child; Environmental Management: Attachment Process; Family Integrity Promotion; Family Support; Family Therapy; Infant Care; Parent Education: Adolescent, Childrearing Family, Infant

Example NIC Activities—Abuse Protection Support: Child

Identify whether adult at risk has close friends or family available to help with children when needed; Monitor for signs of neglect in high-risk families

Nursing Interventions and Rationales

- Use the Parenting Risk Scale to assess parenting. **Clinical Research:** *One study demonstrated that the Parenting Risk Scale is a reliable and valid measure for the systemic assessment of five key dimensions of parenting (Mrazek, Mrazek, and Klinnert, 1995).*

- = Independent; ▲ = Collaborative

- Examine the characteristics of parenting style and behaviors, including the following:
  - Emotional climate at home
  - Attribution of negative traits to the child
  - Failure to support the child's increases in autonomy
  - Type of interaction with the infant/child
  - Competition with the child for attention of spouse/significant other
  - Lack of knowledge/concern about health maintenance or behavioral problems
  - Other behaviors or concerns

  Clinical Research: *Children are at risk for neglect, abuse, and other negative psychosocial outcomes in families with dysfunctions (Mrazek, Mrazek, and Klinnert, 1995).*

▲ Institute abuse/neglect protection measures if there is evidence of an inability to cope with family stressors or crisis, signs of parental substance abuse are observed, or a significant level of social isolation is apparent. *The risk of abuse/neglect is higher in families with high levels of stress, substance abuse, or lack of social support systems (Devlin and Reynolds, 1994).* **Nursing Research:** *Maternal difficult life circumstances, psychiatric-mental health symptoms, educational level, maternal experience in the family of origin, and parenting stress explained 74% of the variance in maternal sensitivity and responsiveness of mothers with their toddlers in the laboratory setting (LeCuyer-Maus, 2003).*

▲ For a mother with a toddler, assess maternal depression, perceptions of difficult temperament in the toddler, and low maternal self-efficacy. Make appropriate referral. **Nursing Research:** *Self-efficacy is defined as one's judgment of how effectively one can execute a task or manage a situation that may contain novel, unpredictable, and stressful elements. A cyclic relationship among depression, perceived difficult temperament, and self-efficacy has been identified. Negative feelings about oneself and one's child are likely to negatively influence the parent-child relationship (Gross et al, 1994).*

- Appraise the parent's resources and the availability of social support systems. Determine the single mother's particular sources of support, especially the availability of her own mother and partner. Encourage the use of healthy, strong support systems. *Before adequate interventions and education can be initiated, the current support system and concerns must be understood. The mother's partner and her mother are often important sources of support (Zacharia, 1994).*

- Provide education to at-risk parents on behavioral management techniques such as looking ahead, giving good instructions, providing positive reinforcement, redirecting, planned ignoring, and instituting time-outs. **Clinical Research:** *These behavioral management techniques are effective approaches for dealing with ineffective parent-child interactions and improving family relationships (Nicholson et al, 2002).*

- Support parents' competence in appraising their infant's behavior and responses. **Nursing Research:** *Parents must be supported and welcomed as active collaborators in their infant's care (Lawhon, 2002).*

- Encourage skin-to-skin care by parents of preterm infants. **Clinical Research:** *Parents have been found to be more sensitive and to show more positive affect, touch, and adaptation to infant cues when participating in skin-to-skin (kangaroo) care (Feldman et al, 2002).*

- Model age-appropriate and cognitively appropriate caregiver skills by doing the following:
  - Communicating with the child at an appropriate cognitive level of development
  - Giving the child tasks and responsibilities appropriate to age or functional age/level
  - Instituting safety considerations such as the use of assistive equipment

- = **Independent;** ▲ = **Collaborative**

■ Encouraging the child to perform activities of daily living as appropriate
These activities illustrate parenting and childrearing skills and behaviors for parents and family (McCloskey and Bulechek, 1992).

▲ Provide programs for homeless mothers with severe mental illness who have lost physical custody of their children. **Nursing Research:** *One study suggests that programs for homeless mothers with severe mental illness can effect changes that promote family reunification. Changes in housing, psychosis, substance use, and therapeutic relationships predicated reunification (Hoffman and Rosenheck, 2001).*

▲ Provide a recovery program that includes instruction in parenting skills and child development for mothers who are addicted to cocaine. **Nursing Research:** *Women addicted to cocaine who are parenting children need strong encouragement from the health care system to begin a recovery program and also to gain parenting skills. Lack of parenting knowledge may be a major barrier for them (Coyer, 2003).*

Multicultural

• Assess for the influence of cultural beliefs, norms, and values on the client's perception of parenting. **Nursing Research:** *What the client considers normal parenting may be based on cultural perceptions (Cochran; 1998; Doswell and Erlen, 1998; Leininger and McFarland, 2002).*

• Acknowledge racial/ethnic differences at the onset of care. **Nursing Research:** *Acknowledgment of racial/ethnicity issues will enhance communication, establish rapport, and promote treatment outcomes (D'Avanzo et al, 2001; Ludwick and Silva, 2000; Vontress and Epp, 1997).*

• Approach individuals of color with respect, warmth, and professional courtesy. **Nursing Research:** *Instances of disrespect have special significance for individuals of color (D'Avanzo et al, 2001; Vontress and Epp, 1997).*

• Give a rationale when assessing African American individuals about sensitive issues. **Nursing Research:** *African Americans may expect white caregivers to hold negative and preconceived ideas about them. Giving a rationale for questions will help reduce this perception (D'Avanzo et al, 2001; Vontress and Epp, 1997).*

• Acknowledge that value conflicts from acculturation stresses may contribute to increased anxiety and significant conflict with children. **Nursing Research:** *Challenges to traditional beliefs and values are anxiety provoking. Less acculturated parents may experience conflict with their more acculturated children as the children demand greater independence and freedom (True, 1995).*

• Use a neutral, indirect style when addressing areas in which improvement is needed (such as a need for verbal stimulation) when working with Native American clients. **Nursing Research:** *Using indirect statements such as "Other mothers have tried . . ." or "I had a client who tried 'X' and it seemed to work very well" will help to avoid resentment from the parent (Seiderman et al, 1996).*

• Provide support for Chinese families caring for children with disabilities. **Nursing Research:** *The care of children with handicaps strains and violates the Chinese culturally expected order of parental obligations. The following themes emerged: disruptions to natural order, public opinions on what constitutes personhood and ordered bodies, and the establishment of moral reputations linked to shame and blame and the gendered division of parenting (Holroyd, 2003).*

• Acknowledge and praise parenting strengths noted. **Nursing Research:** *Such acknowl-*

• = **Independent;** ▲ = **Collaborative**

edgment will increase trust and foster a working relationship with the parent (Seiderman et al, 1996).

- Validate the client's feelings regarding parenting. **Nursing Research:** *Validation is a therapeutic communication technique that lets the client know that the nurse has heard and understood what was said, and it promotes the nurse-client relationship (Heineken, 1998).*
- Facilitate modeling and role playing to help the family improve parenting skills. **Nursing Research:** *It is helpful for the family and the client to practice parenting skills in a safe environment before trying them in real-life situations (Rivera-Andino and Lopez, 2000).*

Home care

- The interventions described previously may be adapted for home care use.
- ▲ Assess the single mother's history regarding childhood and partner abuse, and current status regarding depressive symptoms, abusive parenting attitudes (lack of empathy, favorable opinion of corporal punishment, parent-child role-reversal, inappropriate expectations). Refer for mental health services as indicated. **Nursing Research:** *In a study of low-income single mothers, findings indicated high levels of abuse, depressive symptoms, and abusive parenting attitudes, with little history of previous mental health treatment. Past history of partner and child abuse predicted higher daily stress leading to lower self-esteem. The presence of more depressive symptoms and daily stressors was associated with greater anger. Greater anger was associated with lower parental empathy. Partner abuse predicted higher levels of abusive parenting attitudes (Lutenbacher, 2002).*
- ▲ Implement behavioral parent training (BPT), including enhancement of skills in child-directed play, effective use of commands, use of discipline measures such as imposing time-outs and providing immediate and natural consequences, problem solving, and communication strategies. **Nursing Research:** *Initial work (Gross, Fogg, and Tucker, 1995) and follow-up at 1 year (Tucker et al, 1998) of a behavioral training program for parents showed improvements in maternal self-efficacy and stress reduction, and in the quality of maternal-infant interaction. A higher amount of BPT was associated with fewer maternal critical statements and negative physical behaviors.*

Client/Family Teaching

- Explain individual differences in children's temperaments and compare and contrast with the parents' expectations. Help parents determine and understand the implications of their child's temperament. **Nursing Research:** *Promoting parental understanding of temperament facilitates development of more realistic expectations (McClowry, 1992; Melvin, 1995).*
- Discuss sound disciplinary techniques, which include catching children being good, listening actively, conveying positive regard, ignoring minor transgressions, giving good directions, using praise, and imposing time-outs. *A variety of opinions exist about disciplinary methods. Proper discipline provides children with security, and clearly enforced rules help them learn self-control and social standards. Parenting classes can be beneficial when the parent has had little formal or informal preparation (Herman-Staab, 1994).*
- Encourage positive parenting: respect for children, understanding of normal development, and creative and loving approaches to meet parenting challenges. **Nursing Research:** *Understanding normal development is a first step so parents can distinguish common behaviors for a given stage of development from "problems." Central to positive parenting is developing approaches that can be used in place of anger, manipulation, punishment. and rewards (Ahmann, 2002).*

- • = Independent; ▲ = Collaborative

- Plan parental education directed toward the following age-related parental concerns:
  - Birth to 2 years—transition, sleep, aggression
  - 3 to 5 years—transition, parent-child relationship, sleep
  - 6 to 10 years—school, parent-child relationship, divorce
  - 11 to 18 years—parent-child relationship, divorce, school

  Parents with children of any age may seek basic information about a variety of concerns, which can be anticipated and addressed by providing ongoing information and support (Jones, Maestri, and McCoy, 1993).
- ▲ Initiate referrals to community agencies, parent education programs, stress management training, and social support groups. *The parent needs support to manage angry or inappropriate behaviors. Use of support systems and social services can provide an opportunity to decrease feelings of inadequacy (Baker, 1994; Campbell, 1992).*
- ▲ Provide information regarding available telephone counseling services. *Telephone counseling services can provide confidential advice and support to families who might not otherwise have access to help in dealing with behavioral problems and parenting concerns (Jones, Maestri, and McCoy, 1993).*
- Refer to the care plan for **Delayed Growth and development** for additional teaching interventions.

evolve WEBSITES FOR EDUCATION

See the EVOLVE website for World Wide Web resources for client education.

REFERENCES

Ahmann E: Promoting positive parenting: an annotated bibliography, *Pediatr Nurs* 28(4):382, 2002.
Baker NA: Avoid collisions with challenging families, *MCN Am J Matern Child Nurs* 19:97, 1994.
Campbell JM: Parenting classes: focus on discipline, *J Community Health Nurs* 9:197, 1992.
Cochran M: Tears have no color, *Am J Nurs* 98(6):53, 1998.
Coyer SM: Women in recovery discuss parenting while addicted to cocaine, *MCN Am J Matern Child Nurs* 28(1):45, 2003.
D'Avanzo CE et al: Developing culturally informed strategies for substance-related interventions. In Naegle MA, D'Avanzo CE, editors: *Addictions and substance abuse: strategies for advanced practice nursing,* St Louis, 2001, Mosby.
Devlin BK, Reynolds E: Child abuse: how to recognize it, how to intervene, *Am J Nurs* 94:26, 1994.
Doswell W, Erlen J: Multicultural issues and ethical concerns in the delivery of nursing care interventions, *Nurs Clin North Am* 33(2):353, 1998.
Feldman R et al: Comparison of skin-to-skin (kangaroo) and traditional care: parenting outcomes and preterm infant behavior, *Pediatrics* 110(1):16, 2002.
Gross D, Fogg L, Tucker S: The efficacy of parent training for promoting positive parent-toddler relationships, *Res Nurs Health* 18:489, 1995.
Gross D et al: A longitudinal model of maternal self-efficacy, depression, and difficult temperament during toddlerhood, *Res Nurs Health* 17:207, 1994.
Heineken J: Patient silence is not necessarily client satisfaction: communication in home care nursing, *Home Healthc Nurse* 16(2):115, 1998.
Herman-Staab B: Screening, management and appropriate referral for pediatric behavior problems, *Nurs Pract* 19:40, 1994.
Hoffman D, Rosenheck R: Homeless mothers with severe mental illnesses and their children: predictors of family reunification, *Psychiatr Rehabil J* 25(2):163, 2001.
Holroyd EE: Chinese cultural influences on parental caregiving obligations toward children with disabilities, *Qual Health Res* 13(1):4, 2003.

• = **Independent;** ▲ = **Collaborative**

Jones LC, Maestri BO, McCoy K: Why parents use the warm line, *MCN Am J Matern Child Nurs* 18:258, 1993.

Lawhon G: Facilitation of parenting the premature infant within the newborn intensive care unit, *J Perinat Neonatal Nurs* 16(1):71, 2002.

LeCuyer-Maus E: Stress and coping in high-risk mothers: difficult life circumstances, psychiatric-mental health symptoms, education, and experiences in their families of origin, *Public Health Nurs* 20(2):132, 2003.

Leininger MM, McFarland MR: *Transcultural nursing: concepts, theories, research and practices,* ed 3, New York, 2002, McGraw-Hill.

Ludwick R, Silva M: Nursing around the world: cultural values and ethical conflicts, *Online J Issues Nurs* August 14, 2000, available online at http://www.nursingworld.org/ojin/ethcol/ethics_4.htm, accessed June 19, 2003.

Lutenbacher M: Relationships between psychosocial factors and abusive parenting attitudes in low-income single mothers, *Nurs Res* 51:158, 2002.

McCloskey JC, Bulechek GM, editors: *Nursing interventions classification (NIC),* St Louis, 1992, Mosby.

McClowry SG: Temperament theory and research, *Image* 24:319, 1992.

Melvin N: Children's temperament: intervention for parents, *J Pediatr Nurs* 10:152, 1995.

Mrazek DA, Mrazek P, Klinnert M: Clinical assessment of parenting, *J Am Acad Child Adolesc Psychiatry* 34: 272, 1995.

Nicholson B et al: One family at a time: a prevention program for at-risk parents, *J Couns Dev* 80(3):362, 2002.

Rivera-Andino J, Lopez L: When culture complicates care, *RN* 63(7):47, 2000.

Seiderman RY et al: Assessing American Indian families, *MCN Am J Matern Child Nurs* 21(6):274, 1996.

True RH: Mental health issues of Asian/Pacific island women. In Adams DL, editor: *Health issues for women of color: a cultural diversity perspective,* Thousand Oaks, Calif, 1995, Sage.

Tucker S et al: The long-term efficacy of a behavioral parent training intervention for families with 2-year-olds, *Res Nurs Health* 21:199, 1998.

Vontress CE, Epp LR: Historical hostility in the African American client: Implications for counseling, *J Multicult Counseling Dev* 25:170, 1997.

Zacharia R: Perceived social support and social network of low-income mothers of infants and preschoolers: pre- and postparenting program, *J Community Health Nurs* 11:11, 1994.

Risk for impaired Parenting

T. Heather Herdman and Gail B. Ladwig

NANDA Definition

Risk for inability of primary caretaker to create, maintain, or regain an environment that promotes optimum growth and development of the child

Risk Factors

Social

Marital conflict, declining satisfaction; history of being abused; poor problem-solving skills; role strain/overload; social isolation; legal difficulties; lack of access to resources; lack of value of parenthood; relocation; poverty; poor home environment; lack of family cohesiveness; lack of or poor parental role model; lack of involvement of father of child; history of being abusive; financial difficulties; low self-esteem; lack of resources; unplanned or unwanted pregnancy; inadequate child care arrangements; maladaptive coping strategies; low socioeconomic class; lack of transportation; change in family unit; unemployment or job problems; single parenthood; lack of social support network; inability to put child's needs before own; stress

Knowledge

Low educational level or attainment; unrealistic expectations of child; lack of knowledge about parenting skills; poor communication skills; preference for physical punishment; in-

• = Independent; ▲ = Collaborative

ability to recognize and act on infant cues; low cognitive functioning; lack of knowledge about child health maintenance; lack of knowledge about child development; lack of cognitive readiness for parenthood

Physiological
Physical illness

Infant/child
Multiple births; handicapping condition or developmental delay; illness; altered perceptual abilities; lack of goodness of fit (temperament) with parental expectations; unplanned or unwanted child; premature birth; not desired gender; difficult temperament; attention deficit hyperactivity disorder; prolonged separation from parent; separation from parent at birth

Psychological
Separation from infant/child; large number of closely spaced children; disability; sleep deprivation or disruption; difficult labor and/or delivery; young age (especially adolescence); depression; history of mental illness; lack of or late prenatal care; history of substance abuse or dependence

NOTE: It is important to reaffirm that adjustment to parenting in general is a normal maturational process that elicits nursing behaviors to prevent potential problems and to promote health.

Related Factors (r/t)

Lack of available role models; ineffective role models; physical and psychosocial abuse by nurturing figure; lack of support from significant others; unmet social, emotional, or maturational needs of parenting figures; interruption in bonding process (e.g., maternal, paternal); unrealistic expectations for self, infant, or partner; perceived threat to own physical and emotional survival; mental or physical illness; presence of stressor (e.g., financial difficulties, legal issues, recent crisis, cultural move); lack of knowledge; limited cognitive functioning; lack of role identity; absent or inappropriate response of child to relationship; multiple pregnancies

NOC   Outcomes (Nursing Outcomes Classification)

Suggested NOC Outcomes
Abuse Recovery: Emotional, Physical, Sexual; Abusive Behavior Self-Restraint; Caregiver Emotional Health; Caregiver Stressors; Coping; Parent-Infant Attachment; Parenting Performance; Risk Control: Unintended Pregnancy; Social Interaction Skills

---

Example NOC Outcome with Indicators

Parenting Performance as evidenced by the following indicators: Provides for child's needs/Interacts positively with child/Has realistic expectations of parental role/Demonstrates a loving relationship with child/Expresses satisfaction with parental role (Rate each indicator of **Parenting Performance:** 1 = not adequate, 2 = slightly adequate, 3 = moderately adequate, 4 = substantially adequate, 5 = totally adequate [see Section I].)

• = Independent; ▲ = Collaborative

Client Outcomes

Client Will (Specify Time Frame):
- Successfully establish a nurturing parenting role
- Affirm desire to acquire and maintain constructive parenting skills to support infant/child growth and development
- Maintain appropriate measures to develop a safe, nurturing environment
- Display attentive, supportive parenting behaviors
- Have knowledge of strategies to protect child from harm and/or neglect

NIC   Interventions (Nursing Interventions Classification)

Suggested NIC Interventions

Abuse Protection Support: Child; Attachment Promotion; Caregiver Support; Developmental Enhancement: Adolescent, Child; Environmental Management: Attachment Process; Family Integrity Promotion; Family Support; Family Therapy; Infant Care; Kangaroo Care; Parent Education: Adolescent, Childrearing Family, Infant; Risk Identification: Childbearing Family; Role Enhancement

Example NIC Activities—Kangaroo Care

Determine and monitor parent's level of confidence in caring for infant; Encourage parent to initiate infant care

Nursing Interventions and Rationales

NOTE: Management of a risk diagnosis necessitates approaches using primary and secondary prevention. Primary prevention interventions include activities such as safety instruction and focus on forestalling the development of a disease or condition. Early detection through screening, monitoring, and surveillance is secondary prevention (Shortridge and Valanis, 1992).

- Conduct risk identification, noting the presence of a history of abuse, parental/family stressors, strength and adequacy of social support systems, established coping styles, and other related factors (see Related Factors). *Identification of a family at risk signals special teaching and referral needs (McCloskey and Bulechek, 1992).*
- Screen for maternal psychiatric-mental health symptoms and negative experiences in the mother's family of origin. **Nursing Research:** *Early detection can provide opportunities for intervention with these mothers (LeCuyer-Maus, 2003). One study partially explains the relationship between maternal abuse history and mental health status, and parenting attitudes. The findings underscore the need for health care providers to consider the mental health status and abuse histories of low-income single mothers (Lutenbacher, 2002).*
- Support parents' competence in appraising their infant's behavior and responses. **Nursing Research:** *Parents must be supported and welcomed as active collaborators in their infant's care (Lawhon, 2002).*
- Encourage skin-to-skin care by parents of preterm infants. **Clinical Research:** *Parents have been found to be more sensitive and to show more positive affect, touch, and adaptation to infant cues when participating in skin-to-skin (kangaroo) care (Feldman et al, 2002).*
- Provide education to at-risk parents on behavioral management techniques such as looking ahead, giving good instructions, providing positive reinforcement, redirecting, planned ignoring, and using time-outs. **Clinical Research:** *These behavioral manage-*

- **= Independent; ▲ = Collaborative**

ment techniques are effective approaches for dealing with ineffective parent-child interactions and improving family relationships (Nicholson et al, 2002).

- Monitor parent-infant interactions that may signal interrupted or inadequate attachment or other parenting issues. *Early detection can lead to early intervention, which can prevent or limit problems (McCloskey and Bulechek, 1992).*
- Refer to the care plan for **Impaired Parenting** for other interventions as appropriate to the situation.

Multicultural

- Assess for the influence of cultural beliefs, norms, and values on the client's perception of parenting. **Nursing Research:** *What the client considers normal parenting may be based on cultural perceptions (Cochran, 1998; Doswell and Erlen, 1998; Leininger and McFarland, 2002).*
- Acknowledge racial/ethnic differences at the onset of care. **Nursing Research:** *Acknowledgment of racial/ethnicity issues will enhance communication, establish rapport, and promote treatment outcomes (D'Avanzo et al, 2001; Ludwick and Silva, 2000; Vontress and Epp, 1997).*
- Approach individuals of color with respect, warmth, and professional courtesy. **Nursing Research:** *Instances of disrespect have special significance for individuals of color (D'Avanzo et al, 2001; Vontress and Epp, 1997).*
- Give a rationale when assessing African American individuals about sensitive issues. **Nursing Research:** *Many African Americans expect white caregivers to hold negative and preconceived ideas about them. Giving a rationale for questions will help reduce this perception (D'Avanzo et al, 2001; Vontress and Epp, 1997).*
- Acknowledge that value conflicts from acculturation stresses may contribute to increased anxiety and significant conflict with children. **Nursing Research:** *Challenges to traditional beliefs and values are anxiety provoking. Less acculturated parents may experience conflict with their more acculturated children as the children demand greater independence and freedom (True, 1995).*
- Use a neutral, indirect style when addressing areas in which improvement is needed (such as a need for verbal stimulation) when working with Native American clients. **Nursing Research:** *Using indirect statements such as "Other mothers have tried . . ." or "I had a client who tried 'X' and it seemed to work very well" will assist in avoiding resentment from the parent (Seiderman et al, 1996).*
- Acknowledge and praise parenting strengths noted. **Nursing Research:** *Such acknowledgment will increase trust and foster a working relationship with the parent (Seiderman et al, 1996).*
- Validate the client's feelings regarding parenting. **Nursing Research:** *Validation is a therapeutic communication technique that lets the client know that the nurse has heard and understood what was said, and it promotes the nurse-client relationship (Heineken, 1998).*
- Facilitate modeling and role playing to help the family improve parenting skills. **Nursing Research:** *It is helpful for the family and the client to practice parenting skills in a safe environment before trying them in real-life situations (Rivera-Andino and Lopez, 2000).*

Home care

- The interventions described previously may be adapted for home care use.

• = **Independent;** ▲ = **Collaborative**

Client/Family Teaching

▲ Initiate referrals to an appropriate community agency for early follow-up if an actual problem is identified.

• Refer to the care plan for **Impaired Parenting** for additional teaching interventions.

evolve WEBSITES FOR EDUCATION

See the EVOLVE website for World Wide Web resources for client education.

REFERENCES

Cochran M: Tears have no color, *Am J Nurs* 98(6):53, 1998.

D'Avanzo CE et al: Developing culturally informed strategies for substance-related interventions. In Naegle MA, D'Avanzo CE, editors: *Addictions and substance abuse: strategies for advanced practice nursing,* St Louis, 2001, Mosby.

Doswell W, Erlen J: Multicultural issues and ethical concerns in the delivery of nursing care interventions, *Nurs Clin North Am* 33(2):353, 1998.

Feldman R et al: Comparison of skin-to-skin (kangaroo) and traditional care: parenting outcomes and preterm infant behavior, *Pediatrics* 110(1):16, 2002.

Heineken J: Patient silence is not necessarily client satisfaction: communication in home care nursing, *Home Healthc Nurse* 16(2):115, 1998.

Lawhon G: Facilitation of parenting the premature infant within the newborn intensive care unit, *J Perinat Neonatal Nurs* 16(1):71, 2002.

LeCuyer-Maus E: Stress and coping in high-risk mothers: difficult life circumstances, psychiatric-mental health symptoms, education, and experiences in their families of origin, *Public Health Nurs* 20(2):132, 2003.

Leininger MM, McFarland MR: *Transcultural nursing: concepts, theories, research and practices,* ed 3, New York, 2002, McGraw-Hill.

Ludwick R, Silva M: Nursing around the world: cultural values and ethical conflicts, *Online J Issues Nurs* August 14, 2000, available online at http://www.nursingworld.org/ojin/ethcol/ethics_4.htm, accessed June 19, 2003.

Lutenbacher M: Relationships between psychosocial factors and abusive parenting attitudes in low-income single mothers, *Nurs Res* 51(3):158, 2002.

McCloskey JC, Bulechek GM, editors: *Nursing interventions classification (NIC),* St Louis, 1992, Mosby.

Nicholson B et al: One family at a time: a prevention program for at-risk parents, *J Couns Dev* 80(3):362, 2002.

Rivera-Andino J, Lopez L: When culture complicates care, *RN* 63(7):47, 2000.

Seiderman RY et al: Assessing American Indian families, *MCN Am J Matern Child Nurs* 21(6):274, 1996.

Shortridge L, Valanis B: The epidemiological model applied in community health nursing. In Stanhope M, Lancaster J, editors: *Community health nursing: process and practice for promoting health,* ed 3, St Louis, 1992, Mosby.

True RH: Mental health issues of Asian/Pacific island women. In Adams DL, editor: *Health issues for women of color: a cultural diversity perspective,* Thousand Oaks, Calif, 1995, Sage.

Vontress CE, Epp LR: Historical hostility in the African American client: implications for counseling, *J Multicult Counseling Dev* 25:170, 1997.

Risk for Peripheral neurovascular dysfunction

Betty J. Ackley

NANDA Definition

At risk for disruption in circulation, sensation, or motion of an extremity

• = **Independent; ▲ = Collaborative**

Risk Factors

Trauma; fractures; mechanical compression (e.g., tourniquet, cast, brace, dressing, restraints); orthopedic surgery; immobilization; burns; vascular obstruction

NOC   Outcomes (Nursing Outcomes Classification)

Suggested NOC Outcomes

Circulation Status; Joint Movement: Passive; Neurological Status: Spinal Sensory/Motor Function; Risk Detection; Tissue Perfusion: Peripheral

---

Example NOC Outcome with Indicators

Tissue Perfusion: Peripheral will be intact as evidenced by the following indicators: Distal peripheral pulses strong/Sensation level normal/Skin color normal/Muscle function intact/Skin intact/Peripheral edema not present/Localized extremity pain not present (Rate each indicator of **Tissue Perfusion: Peripheral:** 1 = extremely compromised, 2 = substantially compromised, 3 = moderately compromised, 4 = mildly compromised, 5 = not compromised [see Section I].)

Client Outcomes

Client Will (Specify Time Frame):

- Maintain circulation, sensation, and movement of an extremity within client's own normal limits
- Explain signs of neurovascular compromise and ways to prevent venous stasis

NIC   Interventions (Nursing Interventions Classification)

Suggested NIC Interventions

Exercise Therapy: Joint Mobility; Peripheral Sensation Management

---

Example NIC Activities—Peripheral Sensation Management

Monitor for paresthesia: numbness, tingling, hyperesthesia, and hypoesthesia; Monitor for thrombophlebitis and deep vein thrombosis (DVT)

Nursing Interventions and Rationales

- Perform neurovascular assessment every 1 to 4 hours or every 15 minutes as ordered. Use the six *P*s of assessment:
  - **Pain**—Assess severity (on a scale of 1 to 10), quality, radiation, and relief by medications. *Diffuse pain that is aggravated by passive movement and is unrelieved by medication can be an early symptom of compartment syndrome or a symptom of limb ischemia (Kasirajan and Ouriel, 2002; Walls, 2002).*
  - **Pulses**—Check the pulses distal to the injury. Check the uninjured side first to establish a baseline for a bilateral comparison. *An intact pulse generally indicates a good blood supply to the extremity (Dykes, 1993), although compartment syndrome may be present even if the pulse is intact (Gulli and Templeman, 1994; Walls, 2002).*
  - **Pallor/Poikilothermia**—Check color and temperature changes below the injury site. Check capillary refill. If pallor is present, record the level of coldness care-

• = Independent; ▲ = Collaborative

fully. *A cold, pale, or bluish extremity indicates arterial insufficiency or arterial damage, and a physician should be notified (Kasirajan and Ouriel, 2002). A reddened, warm extremity may indicate infection (Feldman, 1998). Normal capillary refill time is 3 seconds or less (Dykes, 1993).*

- **Paresthesia** (change in sensation)—Check by lightly touching the skin proximal and distal to the injury. Ask if the client has any unusual sensations such as hypersensitivity, tingling, prickling, decreased feeling, or numbness. *Changes in sensation are indicative of nerve compression and damage and can also indicate compartment syndrome (Kasirajan and Ouriel, 2002; Walls, 2002).*
- **Paralysis**—Ask the client to perform appropriate range-of-motion exercises in the unaffected and then the affected extremity. *Paralysis is a late and ominous symptom of compartment syndrome or limb ischemia (Kasirajan and Ouriel, 2002; Walls, 2002).*
- **Pressure**—Check by feeling the extremity; note new onset of firmness of the extremity. *With compartment syndrome, the affected area becomes taut and feels firm when touched (Walls, 2002).*

▲ Monitor the client for symptoms of compartment syndrome evidenced by decreased sensation, weakness, loss of movement, pain with passive movement, pain greater than expected, absence of pulse, and tension in the skin that surrounds the muscle compartment. These symptoms are not always present and can be difficult to assess. *Compartment syndrome is characterized by increased pressure within the muscle compartment, which compromises circulation, viability, and function of tissues (Tumbarello, 2000; Walls, 2002).*

• Monitor appropriate application and function of corrective device (e.g., cast, splint, traction) every 1 to 4 hours as needed. *An improperly applied device can cause nerve damage, circulatory impairment, or pressure ulcers.*

• Position the extremity in correct alignment with each position change; check every hour to ensure appropriate alignment.

▲ Get the client out of bed and mobilize the client as soon as possible, after consultation with the physician. *Immobility is a risk factor for deep vein thrombosis (DVT); early ambulation can help prevent clot formation (Launius and Graham, 1998).*

▲ Monitor for signs of DVT, especially in high-risk populations, including persons older than 40 years of age; persons with immobility or obesity; persons taking estrogen or oral contraceptives; persons with a history of trauma, surgery, or previous DVT; and persons with a cerebrovascular accident, varicose veins, malignancy, or cardiovascular disease. *There are identified risk factors that increase the incidence of DVT and have been validated using a DVT risk scale (Autar, 1996; Hyers, 1999).*

▲ Apply graduated compression stockings if ordered; measure carefully to ensure proper fit, removing at least daily to assess circulation and skin condition. **Nursing and Clinical Research:** *A meta-analysis of 11 studies encompassing 1752 subjects demonstrated that graduated compression stockings reduced the incidence of deep vein thrombosis in a high-risk orthopedic surgical population and that additional antithrombotic measures along with stocking use decreased the incidence even further (Joanna Briggs Institute, 2001). The use of graduated compression stockings, alone or in conjunction with other prevention modalities, prevents DVT in hospitalized clients (Amarigiri and Lees, 2000).*

▲ Watch for and report signs of DVT as evidenced by pain, deep tenderness, swelling in the calf and thigh, and redness in the involved extremity. Take serial leg measure-

• = Independent; ▲ = Collaborative

ments of the thigh and leg circumferences. In some clients a tender venous cord can be felt in the popliteal fossa. Do not rely on Homans' sign. *Thrombosis with clot formation is usually first detected as edema of the involved leg and then as pain. Leg measurement discrepancies greater than 2 cm warrant further investigation. Homans' sign is not reliable (Herzog, 1992). Unfortunately, symptoms of DVT will not be found on examination in 25% of clients with DVT (Eftychiou, 1996).*

▲ Help the client perform prescribed exercises every 4 hours as ordered.

• Provide a nutritious diet and adequate fluid replacement. *Good nutrition and sufficient fluids are needed to promote healing and prevent complications.*

Geriatric

• Use heat and cold therapies cautiously; elderly clients often have decreased sensation and circulation.

Home care

• Assess the knowledge base of the client and family following any institutional care. Teach about the disease process and care as necessary. *The length of time of institutional care and teaching may have been very short and insufficient for learning.*

• If risk is related to fractures and cast care, teach the family to complete a neurovascular assessment; it may be performed as often as every 4 hours but is more commonly done two to three times per day. *A risk requiring monitoring more often than every 4 hours for longer than 24 hours indicates a need for institutionally based care.*

• If the fracture is peripheral, position the limb for comfort and change position frequently, avoiding dependent positions for extended periods. *Changes in position enhance circulation.*

▲ Refer to physical therapy services as necessary to establish an exercise program and safety in transfers or mobility within limitations of physical status.

• Establish an emergency plan. *Having a predetermined plan will save valuable time in the event of emergency.*

Client/Family Teaching

• Teach the client and family to recognize signs of neurovascular dysfunction and to report signs immediately to the appropriate person.

• Emphasize proper nutrition to promote healing.

▲ If necessary, refer the client to a rehabilitation facility for instruction in proper use of assistive devices and measures to improve mobility without compromising neurovascular function.

🌐 WEBSITES FOR EDUCATION

See the EVOLVE website for World Wide Web resources for client education.

REFERENCES

Amarigiri SV, Lees TA: Elastic compression stockings for prevention of deep vein thrombosis, *Cochrane Database Syst Rev* 3:(CD001484), 2000.

Autar R: Nursing assessment of clients at risk of deep vein thrombosis (DVT): the Autar DVT scale, *J Adv Nurs* 23:763, 1996.

• = **Independent;** ▲ = **Collaborative**

Dykes PC: Minding the five P's of neurovascular assessment, *Am J Nurs* 93(6):38, 1993.

Eftychiou V: Clinical diagnosis and management of the patient with deep venous thromboembolism and acute pulmonary embolism, *Nurse Pract* 21:50, 1996.

Feldman CB: Caring for feet: patients and nurse practitioners working together, *Nurse Pract Forum* 9(2):87, 1998.

Gulli B, Templeman D: Compartment syndrome of the lower extremity, *Orthop Clin North Am* 25(4):677, 1994.

Herzog JA: Deep vein thrombosis in the rehabilitation client, *Rehabil Nurs* 17(4):196, 1992.

Hyers TM: Venous thromboembolism, *Am J Respir Crit Care Med* 159:1, 1999.

Joanna Briggs Institute: Best practice: graduated compression stockings for the prevention of post-operative venous thromboembolism, *Evidenced Based Practice Information Sheets for Health Professions* 5:2, 2001.

Kasirajan K, Ouriel K: Current options in the diagnosis and management of acute limb ischemia, *Prog Cardiovasc Nurs* 17:1, 2002.

Launius BK, Graham BD: Understanding and preventing deep vein thrombosis and pulmonary embolism, *AACN Clin Issues* 9(1):91, 1998.

Tumbarello C: Acute extremity compartment syndrome, *J Trauma Nurs* 7(2):30, 2000.

Walls M: Orthopedic trauma, *RN* 65:7, 2002.

Risk for Poisoning

Betty J. Ackley and Gail B. Ladwig

NANDA Definition

Accentuated risk of accidental exposure to, or ingestion of, drugs or dangerous products in doses sufficient to cause poisoning

Risk Factors

External

Unprotected contact with heavy metals or chemicals; storage of medicines in unlocked cabinets accessible to children or confused persons; presence of poisonous vegetation; presence of atmospheric pollutants, paint, lacquer, etc., in poorly ventilated areas or without effective protection; flaking, peeling paint or plaster in presence of young children; chemical contamination of food and water; availability of illicit drugs potentially contaminated by poisonous additives; presence of large supplies of drugs in home; placement or storage of dangerous products within reach of children or confused persons

Internal

Verbalization that occupational setting is without adequate safeguards; reduced vision; lack of safety or drug education; lack of proper precautions; insufficient finances; cognitive or emotional difficulties

Related Factors (r/t)

See Risk Factors.

NOC Outcomes (Nursing Outcomes Classification)

Suggested NOC Outcomes

Knowledge: Child Physical Safety, Medication, Personal Safety; Parenting Performance; Risk Control; Risk Control: Alcohol Use, Drug Use; Risk Detection; Safe Home Environment

• = Independent; ▲ = Collaborative

> ### Example NOC Outcome with Indicators
>
> **Risk Control** as evidenced by the following indicators: Monitors environmental risk factors/Develops effective risk control strategies (Rate each indicator of **Risk Control:** 1 = never demonstrated, 2 = rarely demonstrated, 3 = sometimes demonstrated, 4 = often demonstrated, 5 = consistently demonstrated [see Section I].)

Client Outcomes

Client Will (Specify Time Frame):

- Prevent inadvertent ingestion of or exposure to toxins or poisonous substances
- Explain and undertake appropriate safety measures to prevent ingestion of or exposure to toxins or poisonous substances

NIC   Interventions (Nursing Interventions Classification)

Suggested NIC Interventions

Environmental Management: Safety; First Aid; Health Education; Medication Management; Surveillance; Surveillance: Safety

> ### Example NIC Activities—Environmental Management: Safety
>
> Identify safety hazards in the environment (i.e., physical, biological, and chemical); Remove hazards from the environment when possible

Nursing Interventions and Rationales

- Identify risk factors for poisoning, noting special circumstances in which preventive or protective measures are indicated. *Identification of a family at risk signals the need for special teaching and referral (McCloskey and Bulechek, 1996).*
- ▲ Evaluate lead exposure risk and consult the health care provider regarding lead screening measures as indicated (public/ambulatory health). *Lead poisoning is one of the most common and preventable types of childhood poisoning today. Assessment of exposure risk and blood level testing are important preventive measures (Dennis, Staley, and Curtis, 2002).*
- ▲ Properly label medications, using large print for the visually impaired. Supply "Mr. Yuk" labels for families with children. *Implementing poisoning prevention program strategies benefits the client and family (Jones, 1993; Dart and Ramack, 2003).*
- ▲ Detect possible interactions and cumulative or other adverse effects among prescribed medications, self-administered over-the-counter products, culturally based home treatments, and foods. *Serious consequences may occur if interactions are not identified (Weitzel, 1992).*
- Prevent iatrogenic harm to client caused by receiving the wrong medication or dose by following these guidelines for giving care:
  - Use at least two methods to identify the client, such as client name and birth date, before administering medications or blood products.
  - When giving verbal or telephone orders, always require the person taking the orders to verify them by repeating them back.
  - Standardize use of abbreviations and eliminate abbreviations that are prone to cause errors.

- **• = Independent; ▲ = Collaborative**

- ■ Remove high-alert medications such as potassium chloride from the nursing unit.
- ■ Use only IV pumps that prevent free flow of IV solution when the tubing is taken out of the pump.

  These are practical tips on improving client safety in a hospital or health care facility (Joint Commission Resources, 2003).
- Complete an exposure history in the work environment if toxic exposure occurs (occupational concerns exist). Early exposure detection and treatment and prevention of sequelae are important in the work setting (Agency Toxic Substance and Disease Registry, 1995).

Home care

- The interventions described previously may be adapted for home care use.
- Provide the client and/or family with a poison control diagram to be kept on the refrigerator or a bulletin board. Ensure that the telephone number for local poison control information is readily available.
- Prepour medications for a client who is at risk of ingesting too much of a given medication because of mistakes in preparation. Delegate this task to the family or caregivers if possible. *Elderly clients who live alone are at greatest risk of poisoning.*
- Identify poisonous substances in the immediate surroundings of the home, such as a garage or barn, including paints and thinners, fertilizers, rodent and bug control substances, animal medications, gasoline, and oil. Label with the name, a poison warning sign, and a poison control center number. Lock out of the reach of children. *Dangerous poisonous substances can be found in areas other than the internal home setting. Curious children are at risk for ingestion when exploring.*
- Identify the risk of toxicity from environmental activities such as spraying trees or roadside shrubs. Contact local departments of agriculture or transportation to obtain material substance data sheets or to prevent the activity in desired areas. *Very young children, women who are of childbearing age or who are pregnant, and the elderly are at greatest risk.*
- Avoid carbon monoxide poisoning. Instruct the client and family in the importance of using a carbon monoxide detector in the home, having the chimney professionally cleaned each year, having the furnace professionally inspected each year, ensuring that all combustion equipment is properly vented, and installing a chimney screen and cap to prevent small animals from moving into the chimney. *Many deaths each year are attributed to carbon monoxide poisoning. Take these precautions to protect the child and family (Jordan, 2002).*

Client/Family Teaching

- Counsel the client and family members regarding medication safety:
  - ■ Avoid sharing prescriptions.
  - ■ Read and follow labeling instructions on all products; adjust dosage for age.
  - ■ Avoid excessive amounts and/or frequency of doses ("If a little does some good, a lot should do more").

    Each year, thousands of adverse drug-related events occur, including poisoning. Poisoning is a major cause of morbidity and mortality.
- Advise the family to post first aid charts and poison center instructions in an accessible location. Poison control center telephone numbers should be posted close to the telephone. A poison control center should always be called immediately before initiating any first aid measures. Advise family when calling the poison control center to:

• = Independent; ▲ = Collaborative

- Give as much information as possible, including your name, location, and telephone number, so that the poison control operator can call back in case you are disconnected or summon help if needed.
- Give the name of the potential poison ingested and, if possible, the amount and time of ingestion. If the bottle or package is available, give the trade name and ingredients if they are listed.
- Describe the state of the poisoning victim. Is the victim conscious? Are there any symptoms? What is the person's general appearance, skin color, respiration, breathing difficulties, mental status (alert, sleepy, unusual behavior)? Is the person vomiting? Having convulsions?

Rapid initiation of proper treatment reduces mortality and morbidity and decreases emergency department visits and inpatient admissions (Jones, 1993). Consultation with a poison control center is necessary to assess and treat poisoned clients (Larsen and Cummings, 1998; Tapley et al, 2003).

- Encourage the client and family to take first aid and other types of safety-related programs. *These programs raise participants' level of emergency preparation.*
- ▲ Initiate referrals to peer group interventions, peer counseling, and other types of substance abuse prevention/rehabilitation programs when substance abuse is identified as a risk factor. **Nursing Research:** *Clients with substance abuse problems are at risk for contact with tainted substances or for overdose. The peer pressure factor is extremely strong for adolescents; rehabilitation programs providing nonpunitive and skill-focused approaches are most effective (Anderson, 1996).*

Infant/child

- Provide guidance for parents/caregivers regarding age-related safety measures, including the following:
  - Store potentially harmful substances in the original containers with safety closures intact.
  - Avoid storage of medications or toxic substances in food containers.
  - Place poisonous house plants out of the reach of infants and children; preferably remove from the home.
  - Keep cleaning agents, disinfectants, and other hazardous materials out of sight and out of children's reach; preferably keep them locked up.
  - Do not take medications in front of children; children mimic parents' behaviors.
  - Do not suggest that medications such as aspirin and children's vitamins are candy.
  - If interrupted when using a harmful product, take it with you; children can get into it within seconds.
  - Use extreme caution with pesticides and gardening materials close to children's play areas.
  - Keep perfume and makeup out of reach of children.

Infants have a high level of hand-to-mouth behavior and will ingest anything. Young children may inadvertently ingest poisonous materials, particularly if those materials are thought to be food or beverage (Mitchell et al, 1995; Dart and Rumack, 2003).

- Teach the family to keep the home safe for children by keeping harmful cleaning products and all liquids containing hydrocarbons away from children and using child-resistant packaging as available. *Liquid products that contain more than 10% hydrocarbons (cosmetics such as hair oils, automotive chemicals, cleaning solvents, water repellents) are now required to be in child-resistant packaging. When these products enter the lungs inadvertently, they can cause chemical pneumonia and death in children (Barone, 2002).*

- Review the need to keep prescription and over-the-counter medications secure and out of the reach of children. For example, iron pills are the most common substance causing fatal poisoning in children (Rudolph et al, 2003). Lock the cupboard if a toddler is prone to climbing. *Once infants learn to crawl, they explore and are persistent. When children begin to walk, climb, and develop the concept of object and object permanence, they can reach most heights, open cupboards, and unscrew lids. Many toxic substances are not protected by the use of safety caps alone (Corbett, 1995; Kuhn, 1992; Liebelt and Shannon, 1993).*
- Advise families that syrup of ipecac is generally no longer recommended to be kept and used in the home. *Many poison control centers have reconsidered the former recommendation to keep syrup of ipecac in the home; it is not considered very effective and can delay or hamper administration of charcoal admixture that may be more effective (Rudolph et al, 2003). There is a high aspiration potential with these clients. Giving ipecac may delay the administration or reduce the effectiveness of activated charcoal, oral antidotes, and whole bowel irrigation (Krenzelok, McGuigan, and Lheur, 1997).*

Community

- Propane-fueled ice-resurfacing machines should not be used in indoor ice arenas. **Clinical Research:** *An outbreak of acute respiratory illness among adolescent ice hockey players was attributed to the high level of nitrogen dioxide that resulted from poor ventilation and malfunctioning of an ice-resurfacing machine (Rosenlund and Bluhm, 1999).*

Geriatric

- Caution the client and family to avoid storing medications with similar appearances close to one another (e.g., nitroglycerin ointment near toothpaste or denture creams). *Confusion and visual impairment can place the older person at risk of incorrectly identifying of the contents (Weitzel, 1992).*
- Place medications in a medication box that indicates when medications are to be taken. *Failing eyesight, the use of multiple drugs, and difficulty in remembering whether a medication was taken are among the causes of accidental poisoning in older persons (Tapley et al, 2003).*
- Remind the older client to store medications out of reach when young children come to visit. *Children are inquisitive and may ingest medicines in containers without safety caps.*

Multicultural

- Assess housing for pathways of lead poisoning. **Clinical Research:** *Minority individuals are more likely to reside in older and substandard housing. About 74% of privately owned, occupied housing units in the United States built before 1980 contain lead-based paint (Centers for Disease Control and Prevention, 2001).*

evolve WEBSITES FOR EDUCATION

See the EVOLVE website for World Wide Web resources for client education.

REFERENCES

Agency Toxic Substance and Disease Registry: Taking an exposure history, *Am Assoc Occup Health Nurs J* 43: 380, 1995.

Anderson NLR: Decisions about substance abuse among adolescents in juvenile detention, *Image J Nurs Sch* 28: 65, 1996.

Barone S: Child-resistant packaging, *Consumer Product Safety Review* 6(3):2002155337, 2002.

• = Independent; ▲ = Collaborative

Centers for Disease Control and Prevention: Sources and pathways of lead exposure. In *Preventing lead poisoning in young children,* Atlanta, 2001, The Center.

Corbett JV: Pharmacopeia: accidental poisoning with iron supplements, *MCN Am J Matern Child Nurs* 20:234, 1995.

Dart RC, Rumack BA: Poisoning. In Hay WW et al, editors: *Current pediatrics: diagnosis and treatment,* ed 16, New York, 2003, McGraw Hill.

Joint Commission Resources: *Special Report! 2003 JCAHO national patient safety goals: practical strategies and helpful solutions for meeting these goals,* available on-line at http://www.jcrinc.com/subscribers/patientsafety.asp?durki+3746, accessed April 10, 2003.

Jones NE: Childhood residential injuries, *MCN Am J Matern Child Nurs* 18:1168, 1993.

Jordan RA: Preventing CO poisoning: carbon monoxide, *Consumer Product Safety Review* 6(3):2002155338, 2002.

Kim DY, Staley F, Curtis G: Relation between housing age, housing value and childhood blood levels in children in Jefferson County, Ky, *Am J Public Health* 92(5):769, 2002.

Krenzelok E, McGuigan M, Lheur P: Position statement: ipecac syrup—American Academy of Clinical Toxicology; European Association of Poisons Centres and Clinical Toxicologists, *J Toxicol Clin Toxicol* 35(7):699, 1997.

Kuhn MM: Drug overdose: salicylates, *Crit Care Nurse* 12:16, 1992.

Larsen LC, Cummings D: Oral poisonings: guidelines for initial evaluation and treatment, *Am Fam Physician* 57(1):85, 1998.

Liebelt E, Shannon MW: Small doses, big problems: a selected review of highly toxic common medications, *Pediatr Emerg Care* 9:292, 1993.

McCloskey JC, Bulechek GM, editors: *Nursing interventions classification (NIC),* ed 2, St Louis, 1996, Mosby.

Mitchell A et al: Acute organophosphate pesticide poisoning in children, *MCN Am J Matern Child Nurs* 20:261, 1995.

Rosenlund M, Bluhm G: Health effects resulting from nitrogen dioxide exposure in an indoor ice arena, *Arch Environ Health* 54(1):2, 1999.

Rudolph CD et al: *Rudolph's pediatrics,* ed 21, New York, 2003, McGraw-Hill.

Tapley DF et al: Poisoning. *Columbia University College of P & S complete home medical guide 2003,* available on-line at http://www.cpmcnet.columbia.edu/texts/guide/hmg14_0020.html, accessed April 22, 2003.

Weitzel EA: Medication management. In McCloskey JC, Bulechek GM, editors: *Nursing interventions classification (NIC),* ed 2, St Louis, 1992, Mosby.

Post-trauma syndrome

Gail B. Ladwig and Michele Walters

NANDA Definition

Sustained maladaptive response to a traumatic, overwhelming event

Defining Characteristics

Avoidance; repression; difficulty in concentrating; grief; intrusive thoughts; neurosensory irritability; palpitations; enuresis (in children); anger and/or rage; intrusive dreams; nightmares; aggression; hypervigilance; exaggerated startle response; hopelessness; altered mood state; shame; panic attack; alienation; denial; horror; substance abuse; depression; anxiety; guilt; fear; gastric irritability; detachment; psychogenic amnesia; irritability; numbing; compulsive behavior; flashbacks; headaches

Related Factors (r/t)

Events outside range of usual human experience; physical and psychosocial abuse; tragic occurrence involving multiple deaths; epidemic; sudden destruction of one's home or community; confinement as prisoner of war or criminal victimization (torture); war; rape; natural and/or manmade disaster; serious accident; witnessing of mutilation, violent

• = Independent; ▲ = Collaborative

death, or other horror; serious threat or injury to self or loved ones; industrial or motor vehicle accident; military combat

| NOC | **Outcomes (Nursing Outcomes Classification)** |

Suggested NOC Outcomes

Abuse Cessation; Abuse Protection; Abuse Recovery: Emotional, Sexual; Coping; Impulse Self-Control; Self-Mutilation Restraint

> **Example NOC Outcome with Indicators**
>
> **Abuse Recovery: Emotional** as evidenced by the following indicator: Resolution of trauma-induced psychoneurotic behaviors, conduct disorders, and learning difficulties (Rate indicator of **Abuse Recovery: Emotional:** 1 = none, 2 = limited, 3 = moderate, 4 = substantial, 5 = extensive [see Section I].)

Client Outcomes

Client Will (Specify Time Frame):

- Return to pretrauma level of functioning as quickly as possible
- Acknowledge traumatic event and begin to work with the trauma by talking about the experience and expressing feelings of fear, anger, anxiety, guilt, and helplessness
- Identify support systems and available resources and be able to connect with them
- Return to and strengthen coping mechanisms used in previous traumatic event
- Acknowledge event and perceive it without distortions
- Assimilate event and move forward to set and pursue life goals

| NIC | **Interventions (Nursing Interventions Classification)** |

Suggested NIC Interventions

Counseling; Support System Enhancement

> **Example NIC Activities—Counseling**
>
> Encourage expression of feelings; Assist client in identifying strengths and reinforcing these

Nursing Interventions and Rationales

- Observe for a reaction to a traumatic event in all clients regardless of age. *Groups at risk are those who have a history of emotional problems, have experienced domestic violence, have lost a friend or family member by homicide, are homeless, have been sexually assaulted (especially those abused as children), and have previous involvement with a traumatic event. Give serious attention to childhood loss (Irwin, 1994). Post-traumatic stress disorder (PTSD) is the expected outcome of youths exposed to suicide, loss, and abuse (Brent, 1995).* **Clinical Research:** *In a survey of 5877 persons, 1703 reported experiencing a traumatic event, and combat was reported as the worst trauma. Men who have faced combat are more likely to have lifetime PTSD, delayed PTSD symptom onset, and unresolved symptoms and are more likely to be unemployed, fired, and divorced, and to be physically abusive spouses (Prigerson, Maciejewski, and Rosenheck, 2001).*
- Provide a safe and therapeutic environment that enables the client to regain control. **Clinical Research:** *Safety and empowerment are vital to recovery, as are treating the per-*

- = Independent; ▲ = Collaborative

son with dignity and sensitivity and being able to tolerate high emotional arousal. Intervention must strike a balance between protection of the client and confrontation about the reality of the event. A study showed that individuals found the confrontational aspects of intervention, such as viewing the body of a lost loved one and returning to the site of the traumatic event, to be helpful (Winje and Ulvik, 1995).

- Remain with the client and provide support during periods of overwhelming emotions. *Being able to withstand a client's strong emotions can be difficult for an unskilled nurse. The client may initially be in shock and appear dazed or confused.*
- Use touch with the client's permission (e.g., a hand on the shoulder, holding a hand). **Nursing Research:** *A meta-analysis of therapeutic touch indicated that therapeutic touch has a positive, medium effect on physiological and psychological variables (Peters, 1999).*
- For a client who is uncomfortable with physical touch, consider the use of therapeutic touch techniques. (See the care plan for **Disturbed Energy field.**) *Therapeutic touch, when provided by the nurse, can promote feelings of comfort, peace, calm, and security (Hayes and Cox, 1999).*
- Provide opportunities for emotional expression through activities.
- Avoid pressuring the client to express emotions if he or she is not ready to do so.
- Explore and enhance available support systems. **Clinical Research:** *Social supports clearly benefit the client. Social support was the most important factor in predicting adaptive coping among family members of the seriously mentally ill (Solomon and Draine, 1995). Support systems decrease isolation, encourage communication, and provide diversional activities. Nurses should help traumatized children by strengthening their social relationships and enhancing their ability to self-soothe and process information, which helps them cope with traumatic memories (Burgess, Hartman, and Clements, 1995).*
- Assist the client in regaining previous sleeping and eating habits. *Disrupted sleep is the most prevalent symptom following a traumatic event (Schwartz, Kettley, and Rizzo, 1992). Consider short-term drug treatment such as the use of a short-acting benzodiazepine for the first few days following a traumatic event. Imipramine, fluoxetine, clonidine, and carbamazepine have shown promise (Marshall and Kleine, 1995).*
- ▲ Consider the use of medication. **Evidence-Based Research:** *Medications can be effective for treating PTSD. The largest trials showing efficacy have been with selective serotonin reuptake inhibitors (Stein et al, 2000).*
- Help the client use positive cognitive restructuring to reestablish feelings of self-worth. **Clinical Research:** *In two studies of 159 and 138 motor vehicle accidents survivors, cognitive strategies to control intrusive negative thoughts played a major role in reducing post-traumatic stress in accident victims (Steil and Ehlers, 2000).* **Clinical Research:** *In one study, cognitive-behavioral interventions were shown to be more effective than other interventions for reducing occupational stress (van der Klink et al, 2001).*
- Provide the means for the client to express feelings through therapeutic drawing. *Expressive techniques such as therapeutic drawing can be used to facilitate the emotional work of coping with chronic trauma issues (Glaister and McGuinness, 1992).*
- Normalize symptoms; help the client to understand that his or her feelings and thoughts are a result of the trauma and do not indicate mental illness. *Many symptoms of a trauma response are mistaken for mental illness, when actually they are normal responses to an abnormal event (Forster, 1994).*
- Encourage the client to return to the normal routine as quickly as possible. *Nurses can help traumatized children and adolescents relearn flexible responses in order to begin processing traumatic memories.*

- • = **Independent;** ▲ = **Collaborative**

- Talk to and support a child after a traumatic event. *The International Critical Incident Stress Foundation (2001) suggests telling children the facts that are appropriate to their age group. Listen to what they have to say. Tell them how you feel. Provide reassurance of safety by touch and holding. Allow children to grieve and mourn and validate the normalcy of their reactions.*

Geriatric

- Use environmental assessment skills to identify elderly clients who are traumatized by disaster, loss, or both. *The elderly who live alone are at greatest risk. Early intervention can minimize the response.*
- Observe the client for concurrent losses that may affect coping skills. *As the elderly grow older, losses are multiplied and compounded.*
- Allow the client more time to establish trust and express anger, guilt, and shame about the trauma. Review past coping skills and give the client positive reinforcement for successfully dealing with other life crises. *Clients who have adjusted positively to aging and can put events into proper perspective may adjust to loss more positively.*
- Monitor the client for clinical signs of depression and anxiety; refer to a physician for medication if appropriate. *Depression in the elderly is underestimated in this country.*
- Instill hope. *The therapeutic technique of reminiscence can renew hope (Forbes, 1994). The energy generated by hope can help the elderly cope, overcome obstacles, and maintain normal functioning.*

Multicultural

- Assess for the influence of cultural beliefs, norms, and values on the client's ability to cope with a traumatic experience. **Nursing Research:** *What the client views as healthy coping may be based on cultural perceptions (Cochran, 1998; Doswell and Erlen, 1998; Leininger and McFarland, 2002).*
- Acknowledge racial/ethnic differences at the onset of care. **Nursing Research:** *Acknowledgment of race/ethnicity issues will enhance communication, establish rapport, and promote positive treatment outcomes (D'Avanzo et al, 2001, Ludwick and Silva, 2000; Vontress and Epp, 1997).*
- Use a family-centered approach when working with Latino, Asian, African American, and Native American clients. **Nursing Research:** *Latinos may perceive the family as a source of support, solver of problems, and source of pride. Asian Americans may regard the family as the primary decision maker and influence on individual family members (D'Avanzo et al, 2001).*
- When working with an Asian American client, provide opportunities by which the family can save face. **Nursing Research:** *Asian American families may avoid situations and discussion of issues that they perceive will bring shame on the family unit (D'Avanzo et al, 2001).*
- Validate the client's feelings regarding the trauma. **Nursing Research:** *Validation is a therapeutic communication technique that lets the client know that the nurse has heard and understood what was said, and it promotes the nurse-client relationship (Heineken, 1998).*

Home care

- Assess family support and the response to the client's coping mechanisms. Refer the family for medical social services or other counseling as necessary. *Persons who have not shared the client's traumatic experience may have unrealistic expectations about recovery and recovery time. Support may be denied if the client's response to the trauma does not stay within support system expectations.*

- **• = Independent; ▲ = Collaborative**

- Provide a stable routine of day-to-day activities consistent with pretrauma experience. Do not force a new routine on the client. *Resuming a pretrauma routine can be reassuring to the client and can help place the trauma in perspective. Imposing an undesired routine can further isolate the client.*
- ▲ If the client is receiving medications, assess the client's self-medicating ability. Assign a responsible person to administer medications if necessary. *Crisis creates a feeling of helplessness. Then the client may be unable to make the simplest decisions (Spradley, 1990).*
- ▲ Assess the impact of the trauma on significant others (e.g., a father may have to take over his partner's parenting responsibility after she has been raped and injured). Provide empathy and caring to significant others. Refer for additional services as necessary. *Traumatic events can pose a crisis for significant others as well as for the involved client.*

Client/Family Teaching

- Explain to the client and family what to expect the first few days after the traumatic event and in the future. *Knowing what to expect can minimize much of the anxiety that accompanies a traumatic response.*
- Teach positive coping skills and avoidance of negative coping skills. **Nursing Research:** *Taking a direct action to resolve the problem itself is associated with higher levels of coping efficacy, while wishful thinking coping is associated with lower levels of coping efficacy (Tsay, Tuls Halstead, and McCrone, 2001). Depressive coping is found to have a high correlation with PTSD (Schnyder et al, 2000).*
- Teach stress reduction methods such as deep breathing, visualization, meditation, and physical exercise. Encourage their use especially when intrusive thoughts or flashbacks occur. *After a traumatic event, it is tempting for clients to maladaptively cope with their overwhelming emotions, which can establish unhealthy patterns for the future.*
- Encourage other healthy living habits of proper diet, adequate sleep, regular exercise, family activities, and spiritual pursuits.
- ▲ Refer the client to peer support groups. *Peer support decreases the sense of social isolation, enhances knowledge, and increases coping skills (Solomon and Draine, 1995).*
- ▲ Refer the client who has been in an accident to counseling for PTSD. **Clinical Research:** *It is estimated that PTSD occurs in at least 25% of traffic accident victims who sustain physical injuries. This percentage is probably higher among clients with chronic whiplash complaints. A case report showed that improvement of PTSD symptoms can have a beneficial effect on coping with the chronic whiplash complaints (Jaspers, 1998).*
- ▲ Refer the client who has suffered traumatic brain injury (TBI) for counseling for PTSD. **Clinical Research:** *One study highlights the significant number of clients who experience an acute traumatic response after TBI and raises the possibility that those with acute stress disorder represent those for whom an early intervention may prevent long-term psychopathology (Harvey and Bryant, 1998).*
- Instruct the family in ways to be helpful to and supportive of the traumatized person. Emphasize the importance of listening and being there. Also emphasize that there are no magic phrases capable of easing the person's emotional suffering.
- Consider the use of complementary and alternative therapies. **Clinical Research:** *Suggest the use of humanistic treatments (complementary and alternative medicine) for clients who have catastrophic illness or injuries (Halstead, 2001).*

REFERENCES

Brent D: Risk factors for adolescent suicide and suicidal behavior, mental and substance abuse disorders, family environmental factors, and life stress, *Suicide Life Threat Behav* 25(suppl):52, 1995.

Burgess A, Hartman C, Clements P: Biology of memory and childhood trauma, *J Psychosoc Nurs Ment Health Serv* 33:16, 1995.

Cochran M: Tears have no color, *Am J Nurs* 98(6):53, 1998.

D'Avanzo CE et al: Developing culturally informed strategies for substance-related interventions. In Naegle MA, D'Avanzo CE, editors: *Addictions and substance abuse: strategies for advanced practice nursing,* St Louis, 2001, Mosby.

Doswell W, Erlen J: Multicultural issues and ethical concerns in the delivery of nursing care interventions, *Nurs Clin North Am* 33(2):353, 1998.

Forbes S: Hope: an essential human need in the elderly, *J Gerontol Nurs* 20:5, 1994.

Forster K: Traumatic stress reactions and the psychiatric emergency, *Psychiatr Ann* 24:603, 1994.

Glaister JA, McGuinness T: The art of therapeutic drawing: helping chronic trauma survivors, *J Psychosoc Nurs Ment Health Serv* 30(5):9, 1992.

Halstead LS: The John Stanley Coulter lecture: the power of compassion and caring in rehabilitation healing, *Arch Phys Med Rehabil* 82(2):149, 2001.

Harvey AG, Bryant R: Acute stress disorder after mild traumatic brain injury, *J Nerv Ment Dis* 186(6):333, 1998.

Hayes J, Cox C: The experience of therapeutic touch from a nursing perspective, *Br J Nurs* 8(18):1249, 1999.

Heineken J: Patient silence is not necessarily client satisfaction: communication in home care nursing, *Home Healthc Nurse* 16(2):115, 1998.

International Critical Incident Stress Foundation: *Children's reactions and needs after disaster,* 2001, available online at http://www.icisf.org/articles/Acrobat%20Documents/TerrorismIncident/Children_and_terroristattack.html, accessed Jan 13, 2003.

Irwin J: Proneness to dissociation and traumatic childhood, *J Nerv Ment Dis* 182:456, 1994.

Jaspers J: Whiplash and posttraumatic stress disorder, *Disabil Rehabil* 20(11):397, 1998.

Leininger MM, McFarland MR: *Transcultural nursing: concepts, theories, research and practices,* ed 3, New York, 2002, McGraw-Hill.

Ludwick R, Silva M: Nursing around the world: cultural values and ethical conflicts, *Online J Issues Nurs* August 14, 2000, available online at http://www.nursingworld.org/ojin/ethcol/ethics_4.htm, accessed June 19, 2003.

Marshall R, Kleine D: Pharmacotherapy in the treatment of posttraumatic stress disorder, *Psychiatr Ann* 25:588, 1995.

Peters R: The effectiveness of therapeutic touch: a meta-analytic review, *Nurs Sci Q* 12(1):52, 1999.

Prigerson HG, Maciejewski PK, Rosenheck RA: Combat trauma: trauma with highest risk of delayed onset and unresolved posttraumatic stress disorder symptoms, unemployment, and abuse among men, *J Nerv Ment Dis* 189(2):99, 2001.

Schnyder U, Morgeli H, Nigg C et al: Early psychological reactions to life-threatening injuries, *Crit Care Med* 28(1):86, 2000.

Schwartz J, Kettley J, Rizzo J: Predictors of vulnerability after trauma, unpublished manuscript, 1992.

Solomon P, Draine J: Adaptive coping among family members of persons with serious mental illness, *Psychiatr Serv* 46:1156, 1995.

Spradley B: *Community health nursing, concepts and practice,* ed 3, Glenview, Ill, 1990, Scott, Foresman/Little, Brown.

Steil R, Ehlers A: Dysfunctional meaning of posttraumatic intrusions in chronic PTSD, *Behav Res Ther* 38(6): 537, 2000.

Stein DJ et al: Pharmacotherapy for posttraumatic stress disorder (Cochrane Review), *Cochrane Database Syst Rev* 4(CD002795), 2000.

Tsay S-L, Tuls Halstead M, McCrone S: Predictors of coping efficacy, negative moods and post-traumatic stress syndrome following major trauma, *Int J Nurs Pract* 7:74, 2001.

van der Klink JJ et al: The benefits of interventions for work-related stress, *Am J Public Health* 91(2), 2001.

Vontress CE, Epp LR: Historical hostility in the African American client: implications for counseling, *J Multicult Counseling Dev* 25:170, 1997.

Winje D, Ulvik A: Confrontations with reality: crises intervention services for traumatized families after a school bus accident in Norway, *J Trauma Stress* 8(3):429, 1995.

Risk for Post-trauma syndrome

Gail B. Ladwig and Michele Walters

NANDA Definition

At risk for sustained maladaptive response to a traumatic, overwhelming event

Risk Factors

Exaggerated sense of responsibility; perception of event; survivor's role in the event; occupation (e.g., police, fire, rescue, corrections, emergency department, mental health worker); displacement from home; inadequate social support; nonsupportive environment; diminished ego strength; duration of event

NOC **Outcomes (Nursing Outcomes Classification)**

Suggested NOC Outcomes

Abuse Cessation; Abuse Protection; Abuse Recovery: Emotional; Aggression Self-Control; Anxiety Self-Control; Coping; Grief Resolution; Sleep

Example NOC Outcome with Indicators

Abuse Recovery: Emotional as evidenced by the following indicator: Resolution of trauma-induced psychoneurotic behaviors, conduct disorders, and learning difficulties (Rate indicator of **Abuse Recovery: Emotional:** 1 = none, 2 = limited, 3 = moderate, 4 = substantial, 5 = extensive [see Section I].)

Client Outcomes

Client Will (Specify Time Frame):

- Identify symptoms associated with post-traumatic stress disorder (PTSD) and seek help
- Identify the event in realistic, cognitive terms
- State that he or she is not to blame for the event

NIC **Interventions (Nursing Interventions Classification)**

Suggested NIC Interventions

Counseling; Support System Enhancement

Example NIC Activities—Counseling

Encourage expression of feelings; Assist client in identifying strengths and reinforcing these

Nursing Interventions and Rationales

- Assess for PTSD in a client who has chronic illness, anxiety, or personality disorder; was a witness to serious injury or death; or experienced sexual molestation. **Clinical Research:** *PTSD has emerged as the most common anxiety disorder in women. There are also high rates of PTSD in chronically ill and psychiatric clients (McFarlane, 2000; Stein et al, 2000; Yen et al, 2002).*
- Consider the use of the Stanford Acute Stress Reaction Questionnaire to evaluate anxiety and dissociation symptoms after traumatic events. *This test was developed to assess dissociative and anxiety symptoms that research suggests trauma victims experience after the traumatic event (Cardena et al, 2000).*
- Consider screening for PTSD in a client who is a high utilizer of medical care. **Clinical Research:** *Traumatized clients who are at risk for PTSD are found to be high utilizers of medical care (Stein et al, 2000).*
- Provide peer support to contact co-workers experiencing trauma to remind them that

• = **Independent;** ▲ = **Collaborative**

others in the organization are concerned about their welfare; provide an opportunity to discuss the traumatic incident and assess for the need for further post-trauma services. *The purpose of peer support in a post-trauma program is to ensure that each person involved in potentially traumatic incidents will receive the support and services necessary to make a successful recovery. Without the availability of peers, some individuals will certainly be overlooked. Peer supporters are not counselors. Their tasks include contacting co-workers to remind them that others in the organization are concerned about their welfare, providing the opportunity to discuss the incident, and assessing for the need for further post-trauma services (Post Trauma Resources, 1998).*

- Provide post-trauma debriefings. Effective post-trauma coping skills are taught, and each participant creates a plan for his or her recovery. During the debriefing, the facilitators assess participants to determine their needs for further services in the form of post-trauma counseling. For maximum effectiveness, the debriefing should occur within 2 to 5 days of the incident. *A debriefing is a specially designed group meeting that provides the opportunity to discuss the traumatic incident experiences and post-trauma consequences (Post Trauma Resources, 1998). The need for debriefing remains acute to accelerate recovery from traumatic events before harmful stress reactions have a chance to damage the performance, careers, health, and families of personnel responding to emergencies (Hayes, 1997).*
- Provide post-trauma counseling. Counseling sessions are extensions of debriefings and include continued discussion of the traumatic event and post-trauma consequences, and the further development of coping skills. *Immediate post-trauma responses cannot be prevented. Long-term problems can develop if post-trauma consequences are not managed. With immediate and effective responses to duty-related trauma, most of these long-term problems can be prevented (Post Trauma Resources, 1998).*
- Instruct the client to use the following critical incident stress management techniques:

Things to Try: Critical Incident Stress Debriefing (CISD)

- Within the first 24 to 48 hours, engaging in periods of appropriate physical exercise alternated with relaxation will alleviate some of the physical reactions.
- Structure your time—keep busy.
- You're normal and are having normal reactions—don't label yourself as crazy.
- Talk to people—talk is the most healing medicine.
- Be aware of numbing the pain with overuse of drugs or alcohol; you don't need to complicate the stress with a substance abuse problem.
- Reach out—people do care.
- Maintain as normal a schedule as possible.
- Spend time with others.
- Help your co-workers as much as possible by sharing feelings and checking out how they are doing.
- Give yourself permission to feel rotten and share your feelings with others.
- Keep a journal—write your way through those sleepless hours.
- Do things that feel good to you.
- Realize that those around you are under stress.
- Don't make any big life changes.
- Do make as many daily decisions as possible to give you a feeling of control over your life (i.e., if someone asks you what you want to eat, answer them even if you're not sure).
- Get plenty of rest.

- = **Independent**; ▲ = **Collaborative**

- Reoccurring thoughts, dreams, or flashbacks are normal—don't try to fight them; they'll decrease over time and become less painful.
- Eat well-balanced and regular meals (even if you don't feel like it).

The CISD process is specifically designed to prevent or mitigate the development of PTSD among emergency services professions. CISD represents an integrated "system" of interventions that is designed to prevent and/or alleviate the adverse psychological reactions that are so often experienced by those engaged in emergency services, public safety, and disaster response functions. CISD interventions are especially directed toward the mitigation of post-traumatic stress reactions (International Critical Incident Stress Foundation, 1999).

- Assess for a history of life-threatening illness such as cancer and provide appropriate counseling. *People with histories of cancer can now be considered to be at risk for PTSD. The physical and psychological impact of having a life-threatening disease, of undergoing cancer treatment, and of living with recurring threats to physical integrity and autonomy constitute traumatic experiences for many cancer clients (National Cancer Institute, 1999).*
- Children with cancer should continue to be assessed for PTSD into adulthood. **Nursing Research:** *In children surviving childhood cancer, PTSD symptoms may continue to emerge into young adulthood (Hobbie et al, 2000; Meeske et al, 2001).*
- Provide protection for a child who has witnessed violence or who has had traumatic injuries. Help the child to acknowledge the event and to express grief over the event. **Clinical Research:** *Children who witness violent events that threaten the family's integrity are at highest risk for development of PTSD (Silva et al, 2000). Prevention measures during the first stage focus on protection and advocacy, whereas second-stage interventions help the child acknowledge and tolerate the realities of the violent event (Rollins, 1997). One study supported the need for psychological evaluation and treatment for children who have had disfiguring traumatic injuries (Rusch et al, 2000).*
- Consider implementation of a school-based program for children to decrease PTSD after catastrophic events. **Nursing Research:** *The Catastrophic Stress Intervention was implemented following Hurricane Hugo to decrease mental stress by increasing the children's understanding of stress, enhancing their self-efficacy and social support, and thus decreasing the symptoms of PTSD (Hardin et al, 2002).*

Geriatric

- Carefully assess the elderly client's response to a traumatic event (e.g., a natural disaster) and use the critical incident stress techniques described previously to prevent symptoms associated with PTSD. *Older adults appeared to be especially vulnerable to PTSD. Nurses, who are aware of the effects of natural disasters, particularly flooding, may be better able to identify vulnerable populations and understand the health needs of other survivors (Keene, 1998).*

Multicultural

- Assess for the influence of cultural beliefs, norms, and values on the client's ability to cope with a traumatic experience. **Nursing Research:** *What the client views as healthy coping may be based on cultural perceptions (Cochran, 1998; Doswell and Erlen, 1998; Leininger and McFarland, 2002).*
- Acknowledge racial/ethnic differences at the onset of care. **Nursing Research:** *Acknowledgment of race/ethnicity issues will enhance communication, establish rapport, and promote positive treatment outcomes (D'Avanzo et al, 2001; Ludwick and Silva, 2000).*
- Assure the client of confidentiality. **Nursing Research:** *Many Indo-Chinese women will*

● = **Independent;** ▲ = **Collaborative**

not discuss traumatic events like rape if they think that other staff members, their families, their husbands, or their community may find out (Mollica and Lavelle, 1988).

- Validate the client's feelings regarding the trauma and allow the client to tell the trauma story. **Nursing Research:** *Validation is a therapeutic communication technique that lets the client know that the nurse has heard and understood what was said, and it promotes the nurse-client relationship (Heineken, 1998). Through the trauma story, the clinician can bridge the disrupted social connection that exists between the client, his or her family, and the community (Mollica and Lavelle, 1988).*

Home care

- ▲ Assess the client's ability to meet primary needs of shelter, nourishment, and safety. Refer to medical social services, state departments of human services, or other organizations as appropriate. *Clients in need of primary life requirements are unable to master a higher level of coping.*
- Identify other losses or stressors that may affect coping ability (e.g., role or relationship changes, deaths). *The presence of other stressors can compound the risk of post-trauma stress response and ineffective coping.*
- ▲ Assess the family's response to the client's risk. Refer the family to medical social services or mental health services or support groups as necessary. Provide nursing support. *Individuals in the client's support systems may not understand or be able to cope with the risk involved in selected occupations or the response to selected traumatic events in the client's experience. This is a barrier to the provision of immediate and ongoing support to the client.*
- ▲ If the client is on medication, assess its effectiveness and the client's compliance with the regimen. Identify who administers the medication. *Clients with diminished ego strength may have difficulty adhering to a medication regimen.*
- Assist the client in the home in identifying and establishing daily patterns that have meaning for the client. *Daily patterns provide the client and support system with structure, stability, and a point of reference for perspective development.*
- ▲ For a client who is displaced from the home, identify internal values that can be maintained while the client is displaced, such as respite, contact with specific persons, and honesty. *Maintaining internal values reinforces ego strength, supports dignity, and promotes hope. Caution: Hope should not be misconstrued to mean that a client displaced from the home can return home if this is not possible.*
- ▲ Encourage the client to verbalize feelings of risk and trauma to therapeutic staff or other supportive persons. Refer to medical social services or mental health/support group services as appropriate. *Expressing feelings validates client feelings, fears, and needs. Professional support systems may be a necessary substitute for inadequate personal support systems on a temporary basis.*
- ▲ Evaluate the client's response to a traumatic or critical event. If screening warrants, refer to a therapist for counseling/treatment. *Critical incident debriefing has become a controversial intervention. A review of psychological debriefing has concluded that little evidence exists to support its use. Early intervention recommendations are to assess the need for sustained treatment, provide psychological first aid, and provide education about trauma and information about treatment resources. Recommendations for secondary prevention of PTSD include education, anxiety management, cognitive restructuring, exposure, and relapse prevention (Litz et al, 2002).*
- See the care plan for **Post-trauma syndrome.**

• = **Independent;** ▲ = **Collaborative**

Client/Family Teaching

- Instruct the family and friends to use the following critical incident stress management techniques (International Critical Incident Stress Foundation, 1999):

  For Family Members and Friends:
  - Listen carefully.
  - Spend time with the traumatized person.
  - Offer your assistance and a listening ear, even if the person has not asked for help.
  - Help the person with everyday tasks like cleaning, cooking, caring for the family, and minding children.
  - Give the person some private time.
  - Don't take the individual's anger or other feelings personally.
  - Don't tell the person that he or she is "lucky it wasn't worse"; such statements do not console traumatized people. Instead, tell the person that you are sorry such an event has occurred and you want to understand and assist him or her.
- Teach the client and family to recognize symptoms of PTSD and to seek treatment when the client does the following (de Vries, Aiko, Kassam-Adams, 1999; McDermott and Cvitanovich, 2000):
  - Relives the traumatic event by thinking or dreaming about it frequently
  - Is unsettled or distressed in other areas of his or her life such as in school, at work, or in personal relationships
  - Avoids any situation that might cause him or her to relive the trauma
  - Demonstrates a certain amount of generalized emotional numbness
  - Shows a heightened sense of being on guard
- Instruct the parents to monitor a child who sustained minor injuries for symptoms of PTSD. **Clinical Research:** *The child's perception of threat and fear of death at the time of or immediately after the accident is significantly more related to development of the symptoms of PTSD than is the severity of the injuries sustained (de Vries, Aiko, Kassam-Adams, 1999; McDermott and Cvitanovich, 2000).*
- ▲ Refer a client with a history of substance abuse and PTSD for appropriate counseling. *One study suggested that women with PTSD and substance abuse can be helped when provided with a treatment designed for them (Najavits et al, 1998).*

🄴🄿🄾🄻🅅🄴 WEBSITES FOR EDUCATION

See the EVOLVE website for World Wide Web resources for client education.

REFERENCES

Cardena E et al: Psychometric properties of the Stanford Acute Stress Reaction Questionnaire (SASRQ): a valid and reliable measure of acute stress, *J Trauma Stress* 13(4):719, 2000.

Cochran M: Tears have no color, *Am J Nurs* 98(6):53, 1998.

D'Avanzo CE et al: Developing culturally informed strategies for substance-related interventions. In Naegle MA, D'Avanzo CE, editors: *Addictions and substance abuse: strategies for advanced practice nursing*, St Louis, 2001, Mosby.

de Vries C, Aiko PJ, Kassam-Adams N: Looking beyond the physical injury: posttraumatic stress disorder in children and parents after pediatric traffic injury, *Pediatrics* 104(6):1293, 1999.

Doswell W, Erlen J: Multicultural issues and ethical concerns in the delivery of nursing care interventions, *Nurs Clin North Am* 33(2):353, 1998.

• = Independent; ▲ = Collaborative

Hardin S et al: Effects of a long-term psychosocial nursing intervention on adolescents exposed to catastrophic stress, *Issues Ment Health Nurs* 23(6):537, 2002.

Hayes L: Jail suicide and the need for debriefing, *Crisis* 18(4):150, 1997.

Heineken J: Patient silence is not necessarily client satisfaction: communication in home care nursing, *Home Healthc Nurse* 16(2):115, 1998.

Hobbie WL et al: Symptoms of posttraumatic stress in young adult survivors of childhood cancer, *J Clin Oncol* 18(24):4060, 2000.

International Critical Incident Stress Foundation: *Critical incident stress information, signs and symptoms,* available online at http://www.icisf.org/CIS.html, accessed June 20, 2003.

Keene EP: Phenomenological study of the North Dakota flood experience and its impact on survivors' health, *Int J Trauma Nurs* 4(3):79, 1998.

Leininger MM, McFarland MR: *Transcultural nursing: concepts, theories, research and practices,* ed 3, New York, 2002, McGraw-Hill.

Litz BT et al: Early intervention for trauma: current status and future direction, *Clin Psychol Sci Pract* 9:112, 2002.

Ludwick R, Silva M: Nursing around the world: cultural values and ethical conflicts, *Online J Issues Nurs* August 14, 2000, available online at http://www.nursingworld.org/ojin/ethcol/ethics_4.htm, accessed June 19, 1993.

McDermott BM, Cvitanovich A: Posttraumatic stress disorder and emotional problems in children following motor vehicle accidents: an extended case series, *Aust N Z J Psychiatry* 34:446, 2000.

McFarlane AC: Traumatic stress in the 21st century, *Aust N Z J Psychiatry* 34(6):919, 2000.

Meeske KA et al: Posttraumatic stress, quality of life, and psychological distress in young adult survivors of childhood cancer, *Oncol Nurs Forum* 28(3):481, 2001.

Mollica RF, Lavelle J: Southeast Asian refugees. In Comas-Diaz L, Griffith EEH, editors: *Clinical guidelines in cross-cultural mental health,* New York, 1988, John Wiley and Sons.

Najavits LM et al: Seeking safety: outcome of a new cognitive-behavioral psychotherapy for women, *J Trauma Stress* 11(3):437, 1998.

National Cancer Institute: *Posttraumatic stress disorder,* available on-line at http://www.cancer.gov/cancerinfo/pdq/supportivecare/post-traumatic-stress/HealthProfessional, accessed June 20, 2003.

Post Trauma Resources: *Tools for an unsafe world, 2001,* available on-line at http://www.posttrauma.com/tools.htm, accessed June 20, 2003.

Rollins JA: Minimizing the impact of community violence on child witnesses, *Crit Care Nurs Clin North Am* 9(2):211, 1997.

Rusch MD et al: Psychological adjustment in children after traumatic disfiguring injuries: a 12-month follow-up, *Plast Reconstr Surg* 106(7):1451, 2000.

Silva RR et al: Stress and vulnerability to posttraumatic stress disorder in children and adolescents, *Am J Psychiatry* 157(8):1229, 2000.

Stein MB et al: Posttraumatic stress disorder in the primary care medical setting, *Gen Hosp Psychiatry* 22(4):261, 2000.

Yen S et al: Traumatic exposure and posttraumatic stress disorder in borderline schizotypal, avoidant, and obsessive-compulsive personality disorders: findings from the Collaborative Longitudinal Personality Disorders Study, *J Nerv Ment Dis* 190(8):510, 2002.

Powerlessness

Kathleen L. Patusky

NANDA Definition

Perception that one's own actions will not significantly affect an outcome; perceived lack of control over current situation or immediate happening

Defining Characteristics

Low

Expressions of uncertainty about fluctuating energy levels; passivity

• = Independent; ▲ = Collaborative

Moderate

Nonparticipation in care or decision making when opportunities are provided; resentment, anger, and guilt; reluctance to express true feelings; passivity; dependence on others that may result in irritability; fearing alienation from caregivers; expressions of dissatisfaction and frustration because of inability to perform previous tasks/activities; expression of doubt regarding role performance; failure to monitor progress; failure to defend self-care practices when challenged; inability to seek information regarding care

Severe

Verbal expressions of having no control over self-care, or influence over situation, or influence over outcome; apathy; depression regarding physical deterioration that occurs despite client's compliance with regimens

Related Factors (r/t)

Health care environment; interpersonal interactions; lifestyle of helplessness; illness-related regimen

NOC Outcomes (Nursing Outcomes Classification)

Suggested NOC Outcomes

Depression Self-Control; Health Beliefs; Health Beliefs: Perceived Ability to Perform, Perceived Control, Perceived Resources; Participation in Health Care Decisions

> ### Example NOC Outcome with Indicators
>
> **Health Beliefs: Perceived Control** as evidenced by the following indicators: Perceived responsibility for health decisions/Beliefs that own decisions and actions control health outcomes (Rate each indicator of **Health Beliefs: Perceived Control:** 1 = very weak belief, 2 = weak belief, 3 = moderately strong belief, 4 = strong belief, 5 = very strong belief [see Section I].)

Client Outcomes

Client Will (Specify Time Frame):

- State feelings of powerlessness and other feelings related to powerlessness (e.g., anger, sadness, hopelessness)
- Identify factors that are uncontrollable
- Participate in planning and implementing care; make decisions regarding care and treatment when possible
- Ask questions about care and treatment
- Verbalize hope for the future and sense of participation in planning and implementing care

NIC Interventions (Nursing Interventions Classification)

Suggested NIC Interventions

Cognitive Restructuring; Complex Relationship Building; Mutual Goal Setting; Self-Esteem Enhancement; Self-Responsibility Facilitation

• = Independent; ▲ = Collaborative

Example NIC Activities—Self-Responsibility Facilitation
Encourage independence but assist client when unable to perform; Assist client to identify areas in which client could readily assume more responsibility

Nursing Interventions and Rationales

NOTE: Prior to implementation of interventions in the face of client powerlessness, nurses should examine their own philosophies of care to ensure that control issues or lack of faith in client capabilities will not bias the ability to intervene sincerely and effectively.

- Observe for factors contributing to powerlessness (e.g., immobility, hospitalization, unfavorable prognosis, lack of support system, misinformation about situation, inflexible routine, chronic illness). *Powerlessness can be experienced by people suffering from acute or chronic illness, as well as by those attempting health promotion (Kubsch and Wichowski, 1997). Correctly identifying the actual or perceived problem is essential to providing appropriate support measures.* **Nursing Research:** *Complaints of powerlessness by people with chronic complaints, such as fatigue or low back pain, are often dismissed (Dzurec et al, 2002; Lane, 2000).*
- Assess for ineffective therapeutic regimen management or noncompliance. **Nursing Research:** *Ineffective adherence to the therapeutic regimen or noncompliance can be an assertion of the need for control (Gibson and Kenrick, 1998).*
- Assess the client's locus of control related to his or her health. **Nursing Research:** *An external locus of control can lead a client to believe that he or she has no power over a situation (Gibson and Kenrick, 1998).*
- Assess for signs/symptoms of hopelessness depression and pay particular attention to the availability of social support. Hopelessness depression is characterized by a negative cognitive style (i.e., a tendency to perceive negative events as stable and global). *When negative life events occur, depression based on hopelessness can result, especially when social support is low or absent (Johnson et al, 2001; Joiner et al, 2001). Lack of social support for men with HIV has been shown to increase hopelessness and thereby increase the risk for onset of depressive symptoms (Johnson et al, 2001).*
- Establish a therapeutic relationship with the client by spending one-on-one time with him or her, assigning the same caregiver, keeping commitments (e.g., saying, "I will be back to answer your questions in the next hour"), providing encouragement, and being empathetic. **Nursing Research:** *In mothers undergoing the loss of a newborn, empowerment was experienced when the mothers felt a sense of nearness, encouragement, and empathy. Powerlessness was experienced when there was a sense of distance, violation, or disconnection (Lundqvist, Nilstun, and Dykes, 2002).*
- Allow the client to express hope, which may range from "I hope my coffee will be hot" to "I hope I will die with my significant other here." Listen to the client's priorities and incorporate those priorities in the therapeutic regimen wherever possible. *Hope is a way of coping with a stressful situation and motivates the client to continue living. Motivation is necessary in the change process. Listening to priorities without addressing them leads to frustration for the client.*
- Allow the client to share feelings. Evaluate the influence those feelings could have on the client's decision making and actions. Help the client to focus on objective elements of his or her situation, rather than on the emotionally threatening aspects of the experience. The experience of feeling overwhelmed by a medical situation can increase

- = Independent; ▲ = Collaborative

feelings of powerlessness. **Nursing Research:** *Sharing feelings often leads to the realization that similar feelings are experienced by others, and this realization can lead to a feeling of solidarity and reduce powerlessness (de Schepper, Francke, and Abu-Saad, 1997). Emotional responses to illness influence client behavior, coping efforts, and motivation for change; focusing on emotional rather than objective features of a threatening situation can increase negative emotional responses (Johnson, 1999).*

- Encourage the client to participate in self-regulation and self-care management of the client's illness. Have the client assist in planning care whenever possible (e.g., determining what time to bathe, taking pain medication before uncomfortable procedures, expressing food and fluid preferences). Document specifics in the care plan. *Self-regulation is a component of self-care management in which the client learns to monitor his or her own symptoms, make judgments about the meaning and seriousness of the symptoms, select strategies to manage the illness, try out the strategies, and evaluate whether or not they were successful (Allen and Hagerty, 2003). Self-regulation and self-care management promote feelings of self-efficacy; confidence about managing chronic illness increases (Lorig et al, 2001). The more that clients participate in their own care, the less powerless they feel.* **Nursing Research:** *Clients' participation in their own care provides a sense of control (Gibson and Kenrick, 1998) and can increase their self-esteem and maintain their dignity (Kasten, 1998).*

- Encourage the client to share his or her beliefs, thoughts, and expectations about his or her illness. *Self-regulation theory assumes that clients use perceptions, interpretations, and expectations about the illness experience to regulate their responses and behaviors (Johnson, 1999).*

- Assist the client in specifying the health goals he or she would like to achieve, prioritizing those goals with regard to immediate concerns, and identifying actions that will achieve the goals. Offer feedback and education to ensure that goals and the expected time frame for meeting them are realistic. Goals may need to be small to be attainable (e.g., dangle legs at bedside for 2 days, then sit in chair 10 minutes for 2 days, then walk to window). *Self-regulation theory assumes that people develop a hierarchy of goals and that the discrepancy between what these goals are and what exists motivates action to reduce the discrepancy (Johnson, 1999). Goals must be realistic and achievable; otherwise, the inability to perceive progress will increase hopelessness and powerlessness.*

- Help the client identify factors not under his or her control. *Identifying factors within the client's control encourages the client to take some control of the situation. Acknowledging those factors not under the client's control provides the opportunity to address irritations and frustrations, while providing information crucial to insuring realistic goal setting.*

- Assist the client in identifying a repertoire of strategies to implement in managing his or her symptoms. **Nursing Research:** *Clients who have multiple strategies to choose from in addressing situations have more success in managing symptoms than clients who use only one behavior (Taylor, 1999).*

- Discuss with the client areas in which he or she feels the need to protect himself or herself or others, and the strategies used. Support appropriate protective measures while assisting the client in identifying more effective and stress-reducing measures. *The ability to protect the self is an important part of retaining a sense of power or control over one's life.* **Nursing Research:** *In a study of individuals living with a catastrophic illness or injury, participants felt the need to protect themselves from insensitive statements by others, including health care providers. A need to protect significant others was felt because of the additional physical and emotional burdens on caregivers. Protective strategies used*

• = Independent; ▲ = Collaborative

included hiding the extent of the problem, concealing distress, trying to do things themselves, and trading what assistance they could provide to friends in exchange for physical care. The strategies were directed at maintaining social support but were themselves stressful (Dewar, 2001).

- Recognize the client's need to experience a sense of reciprocity in dealing with others. Negotiate actions that the client can contribute to the caregiving partnership with both family and nurse; e.g., have the client prepare a cup of tea for the nurse during visits if the client is able. *A sense of control is promoted when the client feels he or she is able to exchange something of equitable value.* **Nursing Research:** *Ill or injured individuals made attempts to exchange what skills they could for physical care in attempts to gain a feeling of equity (Dewar, 2001). For older adults, a lack of reciprocity (equitable exchange) was associated with depression, although older adults receiving home care services seemed to have adjusted to the lack of reciprocity (Patusky, 2000).*

- Help the client to identify and persist with self-care strategies that are effective; extinguish strategies that are ineffective. *Evaluation of strategies used is an important part of self-care management.*

- Allow time for questions (15 to 20 minutes each shift); have the client write down questions; encourage the client to record a summary of answers received if desired or practicable, or provide written material that reinforces answers. *Encouraging the client to write down questions and answers emphasizes the importance of client input and nurses' willingness to attend to that input; facilitates memory of questions and answers when the client may be distracted by health or other concerns; and provides the client with material that can be reviewed to refresh memory of the answers and offer reassurance in the absence of the nurse.*

- Keep items the client uses and needs, such as a urinal, tissues, telephone, and television controls, within reach. *Well-being can be affected much more by choices related to activities of daily living (ADLs) like eating, sleeping, and grooming than by those related to larger, occasional events (Tolley, 1997). The client is able to participate in his or her own care if care devices are accessible. Participation in care provides a sense of control.*

- Give realistic and sincere praise for accomplishments. *Giving realistic praise assists the client in developing positive feelings and enhances self-concept (Meddaugh and Peterson, 1997).* **Nursing Research:** *Sincerity promotes a sense of connectedness with the nurse. Clients with chronic obstructive pulmonary disease reported that they value a sense of effectiveness and connectedness in their attempts to maintain personal integrity (Leidy and Haase, 1999).*

- Keep interactions with the client focused on the client, not on the family or physician. Actively listen to the client. *For a teen, this will support the developing ego. Directly focusing on the client also aids the client in practicing decision-making skills and increases the client's investment in adapting behavior (Hennessy-Harstad, 1999). It is important to convey the message that the client is unique and valued. Letting the client know that the schedule is tailored to meet his or her needs instead of tailored to the institution helps the client maintain a sense of self (Tolley, 1997). The client can expend a lot of energy holding in unacceptable or frightening feelings. Listening to the client and encouraging these feelings to be expressed allows the energy to be released and used in other ways (Clark, 1993).*

- Acknowledge subjective concerns or fears. *All feelings are personal and have meaning for the client.*

- Encourage the client to take control of as many ADLs as possible; keep the client informed of all care that will be given. *Clients are more amenable to therapy if they know*

• = **Independent;** ▲ = **Collaborative**

what to expect and can perform some tasks independently. **Nursing Research:** *Providing an opportunity for control is an important intervention for people experiencing powerlessness (Kasten, 1998).*

- Develop a contract with the client that states the client's and nurse's responsibilities and privileges. *Contracting can encourage the client to assume responsibility and increase motivation (Kubsch and Wichowski, 1997). A contract helps give a situation structure and clarifies what may or may not happen and who has responsibility for the client's care.*
- See the care plans for **Hopelessness** and **Spiritual distress**.

Geriatric

▲ Initiate focused assessment questioning and education regarding syndromes common in the elderly. **Nursing Research:** *Older adults may not recognize the need for treatment when they misjudge symptoms and may initiate ineffective self-care treatment or seek no treatment at all (Edwardson and Dean, 1999).*

- Explore feelings of powerlessness—the feeling that the client's behavior will not affect outcomes. *Powerlessness can be exhibited as apathy, depression, expressions of no control, nonparticipation, indecisiveness, and passivity (Meddaugh and Peterson, 1997).* **Nursing Research:** *Older adults who engaged in effective strategies to control their health problems experienced fewer depressive symptoms, particularly in the presence of acute physical symptoms (Wrosch, Schulz, and Heckhausen, 2002). Older adults who reported restricted activity due to arthritis and low levels of perceived control used more health services, had more physician visits, required more laboratory tests, and had longer hospital stays over a 1-year period than did study participants who expressed perceived high control (Chipperfield and Greenslade, 1999).*
- Explore personality resources and inner strengths that the client has used in the past. Incorporate these into the treatment plan. **Nursing Research:** *While resources and strengths cultivated by older adults over the years often go unrecognized, they contribute to the older adult's sense of coherence (perception that life is meaningful, comprehensible, and manageable) and have been shown to optimize quality of life in older women with chronic health problems (Nesbitt and Heidrich, 2000).*
- Establish therapeutic relationships by listening; participate with the client in generating choices and incorporate his or her statement of limitations. **Nursing Research:** *An individualized approach to health promotion, providing education that will support the individual client's needs, creates a partnership relationship that permits the nurse to enhance self-care practices of the older adult and thereby promote self-care ability and activity (Leenerts, Teel, and Pendleton, 2002; Resnick, 2001).*
- Emphasize client control in all possible ADLs. *A study of older adults in nursing homes demonstrated that exposing older hospitalized adults to uncontrollable, disempowering circumstances could lead to the development of dependence based on learned helplessness. The dependence could be alleviated by fostering an expectation of control over activities, which lead to the development of a sense of mastery (Faulkner, 2001).*
- Encourage the positive use of solitude—reading, listening to music, enjoying nature—to prevent loneliness. Encourage socialization with others when possible; advocate for the client regarding family visitation if relationships are viewed positively by the client. **Nursing Research:** *Loneliness, helplessness, and boredom can occur in older adults in nursing homes who lack companionship, have no opportunity to care for others, and find little variety in their lives (Slama and Bergman-Evans, 2000).*

▲ Monitor the use of alternative therapies but do not intervene unless the therapy inter-

• = Independent; ▲ = Collaborative

acts negatively with the existing therapeutic regimen. Ensure that all health care providers involved with the client are aware of the alternative therapies being used. *Older women in particular may use alternative therapies learned in their roles as mothers, midwives, and shamans. Familiarity with these alternatives to a patriarchal medical model can increase control over health and enhance prevention and self-care (Gaylord, 1999).*

Multicultural

- Assess for the influence of cultural beliefs, norms, and values on the client's feelings of powerlessness. The client's expressions of powerlessness may be based on cultural perceptions or expectations (Leininger, 1996). **Nursing Research:** *Older Chinese adults who had fallen reported powerlessness, fear, and care seeking. Powerlessness was expressed as lack of control, self-comforting, and lack of emotion. Falls were perceived as unpredictable and not preventable, which provoked fear that the older adult might become dependent and a care burden on others (Kong et al, 2002). Elderly Taiwanese men with heart trouble identified powerlessness as arising from lacking choice in living arrangements, having no control over discomfort, being unable to obtain care and companionship from families and friends, failing to get medical information about their disease and treatment options, or expecting deteriorating health and receiving no assistance (Shih et al, 2000).*
- Assess the effect of fatalism on the client's expression of powerlessness. *Fatalistic perspectives, which involve the belief that one cannot control one's own fate, may influence health behaviors in some African American, Latino, and Native American populations (Harmon, Castro, and Coe, 1996; Phillips, Cohen, and Moses, 1999; Ramirez et al, 2002).*
- Encourage spirituality as a source of support to decrease powerlessness. *African Americans and Latinos may identify spirituality, religiousness, prayer, and church-based approaches as coping resources (Bourjolly, 1998; Mapp and Hudson, 1997; Samuel-Hodge et al, 2000).*
- Validate the client's feelings regarding the impact of health status on current lifestyle. **Nursing Research:** *Validation lets the client know that the nurse has heard and understood what was said, and it promotes the nurse-client relationship (Heineken, 1998). In focus groups convened to determine the elements clients wanted to be addressed in diabetes education, powerlessness was reported as a concern of African American clients. Previous diabetes education programs had not addressed this element, but its inclusion in future programming was recommended (Blanchard et al, 1999).*
- For inner-city clients, help the client to redefine behaviors as ways of coping with a hostile environment and to reconnect with community supports. **Nursing Research:** *Powerlessness among inner-city African Americans can arise in reaction to inner-city environments, poverty, and racism. Strategies that involve redefining behavior and reconnecting to the community promote empowerment (Dancy et al, 2001).*

Home care

- ▲ Include an initial and ongoing assessment and evaluation of potential abuse and neglect. Photograph evidence of abuse or neglect when possible. *A common dynamic of abusive situations is powerlessness. Victims of abuse perceive themselves to be powerless to change the situation. Indeed, the abuser fosters this perception and may threaten violence or death if the victim attempts to leave. Chronic abuse and neglect of the elderly by the spouse or other family member is often hidden until home care personnel are actively involved.*

• = Independent; ▲ = Collaborative

▲ If neglect or abuse is suspected, identify an emergency plan that addresses the problem immediately, ensures client safety, and includes a report to the appropriate authorities. *Client safety is a nursing priority. An emergency plan should address either immediate removal to a safe environment or identification of appropriate steps to take in the event of abuse, and the securing of resources for anticipated action (e.g., telephone is accessible, bag is packed, alternative living arrangements are available). Reporting abuse is a legal requirement of health care workers.*

• Develop a therapeutic relationship in the home setting that respects the client's domain. **Nursing Research:** *Effective home care involves negotiation between the nurse and the client within the context of territoriality, shared perception of situations, an amicable working relationship, role synchronization, knowledge, and taboo topics. The process empowers and makes vulnerable both nurse and client (Spiers, 2002).*

• Develop a written contract with the client that designates what care will be given and who has responsibility for care elements. Focus should be on care that is controlled by the client. Enable the client to develop his or her own resources actively. *A written contract reassures the client that the designation of control of care will be honored.*

▲ Empower the client by encouraging the client to guide specifics of care such as wound care procedures and dressing and grooming details. Confirm the client's knowledge and document in the chart that the client is able to guide procedures. Document in the home and in the chart the preferred approach to procedures. Orient the family and caregivers to the client's role. *Accurate documentation of the client's knowledge and abilities supports teamwork with the health care team and avoids conflict.* **Nursing Research:** *Negotiation, reciprocity, shared decision making, creation of opportunities, and effective information and support are key elements of empowerment in the home. Empowerment is not a transfer of power from one person to another; it involves recognizing the power that each person has and assisting the client in identifying and using his or her own power (Houston and Cowley, 2002).*

▲ Identify the client's concerns and implement interventions to address the consequences of disability in clients with medical illness. **Clinical Research:** *In a study of cancer clients being cared for at home, primary factors influencing vulnerability to depression and suicide were identified as real or feared loss of autonomy and independence, concerns about being a burden on others, hopelessness about their condition, and fear of suffering (Filberti et al, 2001).*

• Enhance self-efficacy by creating an environment that supports physical activities; provide support in the form of encouragement, anticipatory guidance, sharing of how others perform, and realistic assessment of the client's abilities. **Nursing Research:** *Increasing self-efficacy in clients with heart failure can decrease symptomatology and improve quality of life (Borsody et al, 1999).*

• Respect the client's choices regarding desired assistance. Identify knowledge deficits and provide education to address them to ensure that the client's choice is accurately informed. **Nursing Research:** *The client may identify a problem but choose not to receive help at this time. Assessment is an opportunity to discuss health needs, not a condition for treatment (Houston and Cowley, 2002).*

• Assess the affective climate within the family and family support system. Instruct the family in appropriate expectations of the client and in the specifics of the client's illness. Encourage the family and client in efforts toward educating friends and coworkers regarding appropriate expectations for the client. Serve as the client's advocate. *Negative affective climate may interfere with the client's ability to adhere to the treat-*

• = Independent; ▲ = Collaborative

ment plan as well as with adjustment to health changes. **Clinical Research:** *Positive family affective climate and family support have been found to enhance social adjustment (Langfitt et al, 1999). Recognize that clients with an illness requiring extensive physical assistance may become caught in a dilemma: they may be dependent on others for assistance but that very dependence may hamper their ability to respond naturally within the relationship or to require that caregivers meet certain standards.* **Nursing Research:** *Clients suffering a catastrophic illness or injury felt distressed by family members' or friends' comments that indicated a lack of understanding of the illness experience (Dewar, 2001).*

▲ Refer for homemaker or psychiatric home health care services for respite, client reassurance, and implementation of a therapeutic regimen. *Responsibility for a person who perceives himself or herself to be powerless can promote high caregiver stress. Respite decreases caregiver stress. The presence of caring individuals is reassuring to both the client and caregivers, especially during periods of client anxiety or depression. For a client with powerlessness, especially if accompanied by depression, the interventions described earlier can be used, modified for the home setting.*

Client/Family Teaching

▲ Explain all relevant symptoms, procedures, treatments, and expected outcomes. *By increasing knowledge and adapting new behaviors, clients learn that they have some control over their health (Hennessy-Harstad, 1999). With knowledge comes power; the health care professional must ensure that clients have a sound knowledge base from which to make informed decisions (Meddaugh and Peterson, 1997). Clients are more amenable to therapy and better able to initiate appropriate self-care if they know what to expect.*

▲ Provide written instructions for treatments and procedures for which the client will be responsible. *A written record provides a concrete reference so that the client and family can clarify any verbal information that was given. People tend to forget half of what they hear within a few minutes, so it is important for nurses to supplement oral instructions with written material (Wong, 1992).*

▲ Continually assess the client for signs of inappropriate exercise of self-care. Confront such applications of self-care; instruct the client in the dangers that inappropriate care may present and in alternatives for care that would be more effective. *Although inappropriate self-care may represent an attempt to exercise personal power, clients who elect this action without sufficient knowledge of illness syndromes or treatment alternatives may deny themselves necessary and effective treatment.* **Nursing Research:** *Clients frequently attempt to implement treatment on their own (e.g., through the use of previous prescribed medications, home remedies, or over-the-counter medication) and may not be aware that they are misjudging a need for professional services or selecting less than optimal treatment options (Edwardson and Dean, 1999).*

• Teach stress reduction, relaxation, and imagery. Many cassette tapes are available on relaxation and meditation. Assist the client with relaxation based on the client's preference indicated in the initial assessment. *These techniques can restore power in the client by allowing the client to learn how to control the autonomic nervous system and other physiological mechanisms (Johnson, Dahlen, and Roberts, 1997). Relaxation techniques, desensitization, and guided imagery can help clients to cope, increase their control, and allay anxiety (Narsavage, 1997).*

• Teach cognitive-behavioral activities, such as active problem solving, reframing (reappraising the situation from a different perspective), or thought stopping (in response to a negative thought, picturing a large stop sign and replacing the image with a prear-

• = Independent; ▲ = Collaborative

ranged positive alternative). Teach the client to confront his or her own negative thought patterns (or cognitive distortions), such as catastrophizing (expecting the very worst), dichotomous thinking (perceiving events as belonging in only one of two opposite categories), or magnification (placing distorted emphasis on a single event). *Cognitive-behavioral activities address clients' assumptions, beliefs, and attitudes about their situations, fostering modification of these elements to be as realistic and optimistic as possible. Persons with negative cognitive styles tend to perceive situations as overwhelming, resistant to improvement, and all-encompassing. Through cognitive-behavioral interventions, clients become more aware of their cognitive choices in adopting and maintaining their belief systems, thereby exercising greater control over their own reactions (Hagerty and Patusky, 2003; Sinclair et al, 1998).*

- Help the client practice assertive communication techniques. **Nursing Research:** *Clients with conditions such as quadriplegia need to be assertive so that they can direct their care and be as independent as possible (Bach and McDaniel, 1993).*

- Role play (e.g., say, "Tell me what you are going to ask your doctor"). *Role playing is the most commonly used technique in assertiveness training. It deconditions the anxiety that arises from interpersonal encounters by allowing the client to practice how he or she might respond in a given situation. Anxiety levels tend to be higher in situations that are unfamiliar.*

- Identify the strengths of the caregiver and efforts to gain control of unpredictable situations. Help the caregiver to stay connected with a client who may be behaving differently than usual, to make life as routine as possible, to help the client set goals and sustain hope, and to allow the client space to experience progress. **Nursing Research:** *Identifying positive caregiver responses to the client's illness will assist the caregiver in tolerating his or her own feelings of powerlessness. Family members of persons with severe mental illness have found it helpful to work at staying connected to the person with mental illness, finding a role that they can feel comfortable with, and helping the relative move forward (Rose, 1998).*

- ▲ Refer the client to support groups, pastoral care, or social services. *There is an assignment of power in the imparting of advice (Bonhote, Romano-Egan, and Cornwell, 1999). These services help decrease levels of stress, increase levels of self-esteem, and reassure clients that they are not alone.*

ⓔⓥⓞⓛⓥⓔ WEBSITES FOR EDUCATION

See the EVOLVE website for World Wide Web resources for client education.

REFERENCES

Allen KS, Hagerty BM: Depression in primary care: empowering depressed patients to monitor their recurrent depression, in preparation, 2003.

Bach C, McDaniel R: Quality of life in quadriplegic adults: a focus group study, *Rehabil Nurs* 18:364, 1993.

Blanchard MA et al: Using a focus group to design a diabetes education program for an African American population, *Diabetes Educ* 25:917, 1999.

Bonhote K, Romano-Egan J, Cornwell C: Altruism and creative expressions in a long-term older adult psychotherapy group, *Issues Ment Health Nurs* 20(6):603, 1999.

Borsody JM et al: Using self-efficacy to increase physical activity in patients with heart failure, *Home Healthc Nurs* 17:113, 1999.

Bourjolly JN: Differences in religiousness among black and white women with breast cancer, *Soc Work Health Care* 28(1):21, 1998.

• = Independent; ▲ = Collaborative

Chipperfield JG, Greenslade L: Perceived control as a buffer in the use of health care services, *J Gerontol B Psychol Sci Soc Sci* 54B:146, 1999.

Clark S: Challenges in critical care nursing: helping patients and families cope, *Crit Care Nurs* 13(4 suppl):1, 1993.

Dancy et al: Empowerment: a view of two low-income African-American communities, *J Natl Black Nurses Assoc* 12(2):49, 2001.

de Schepper AM, Francke AL, Abu-Saad HH: Feelings of powerlessness in relation to pain: ascribed causes and reported strategies, *Cancer Nurs* 20(6):422, 1997.

Dewar A: Protecting strategies used by sufferers of catastrophic illness and injuries, *J Clin Nurs* 19:600, 2001.

Dzurec LC et al: Acknowledging unexplained fatigue of tired women, *J Nurs Scholarsh* 34:41, 2002.

Edwardson SR, Dean, KJ: Appropriateness of self-care responses to symptoms among elders: identifying pathways of influence, *Res Nurs Health* 22:329, 1999.

Faulkner M: The onset and alleviation of learned helplessness in older hospitalized people, *Aging Ment Health* 5:379, 2001.

Filberti A et al: Characteristics of terminal cancer patients who committed suicide during a home palliative care program, *J Pain Symptom Manage* 22:544, 2001.

Gaylord S: Alternative therapies and empowerment of older women, *J Women Aging* 11(2-3):29, 1999.

Gibson JM, Kenrick M: Pain and powerlessness: the experience of living with peripheral vascular disease, *J Adv Nurs* 27(4):737, 1998.

Hagerty B, Patusky K: Mood disorders: depression and mania. In Fortinash KM, Holoday-Worret PA, editors: *Psychiatric mental health nursing*, ed 3, St Louis, 2003, Mosby.

Harmon MP, Castro FG, Coe K: Acculturation and cervical cancer: knowledge, beliefs, and behaviors of Hispanic women, *Women Health* 24(3):37, 1996.

Heineken J: Patient silence is not necessarily client satisfaction: communication in home care nursing, *Home Healthc Nurse* 16(2):115, 1998.

Hennessy-Harstad EB: Empowering adolescents with asthma to take control through adaptation, *J Pediatr Health Care* 13:273, 1999.

Houston AM, Cowley S: An empowerment approach to needs assessment in health visiting practice, *J Clin Nurs* 11:640, 2002.

Johnson JE: Self-regulation theory and coping with physical illness, *Res Nurs Health* 22:435, 1999.

Johnson JG et al: Hopelessness as a mediator of the association between social support and depressive symptoms. Findings of a study of men with HIV, *J Consult Clin Psychol* 69:1056, 2001.

Johnson LH, Dahlen R, Roberts SL: Supporting hope in congestive heart failure patients, *Dimens Crit Care Nurs* 16(2):65, 1997.

Joiner TE et al: Hopelessness depression as a distinct dimension of depressive symptoms among clinical and non-clinical samples, *Behav Res Ther* 39:523, 2001.

Kasten AA: Case study: clinical opportunities and challenges related to diagnosis of and interventions for loss of control, *Nurs Diagn* 9(3):90, 1998.

Kong KS et al: Psychosocial consequences of falling: the perspective of older Hong Kong Chinese who had experienced recent falls, *J Adv Nurs* 37:234, 2002.

Kubsch S, Wichowski HC: Restoring power through nursing intervention, *Nurs Diagn* 8(1):7, 1997.

Lane P: Adults with chronic low back pain feel frustrated, unsupported, and powerless with healthcare, social, and legal systems, *Evid Based Nurs* 3(1):29, 2000.

Langfitt JT et al: Family interactions as targets for intervention to improve social adjustment after epilepsy surgery, *Epilepsia* 40(6):735, 1999.

Leenerts MH, Teel CS, Pendleton MK: Building a model of self-care for health promotion in aging, *J Nurs Scholarsh* 34:355, 2002.

Leidy NK, Haase JE: Functional status from the patient's perspective: the challenge of preserving personal integrity, *Res Nurs Health* 22:67, 1999.

Leininger MM: *Transcultural nursing: theories, research and practices*, ed 2, Hilliard, Ohio, 1996, McGraw-Hill.

Lorig K et al: Chronic disease self-management program: 2-year health status and health care utilization outcomes, *Med Care* 39:1217, 2001.

Lundqvist A, Nilstun T, Dykes A: Both empowered and powerless: mothers' experiences of professional care when their newborn dies, *Birth* 29(3):192, 2002.

Mapp I, Hudson R: Stress and coping among African American and Hispanic parents of deaf children, *Am Ann Deaf* 142(1):48, 1997.

Meddaugh D, Peterson B: Removing powerlessness from the nursing home, *Nurs Homes* 46(8):32, 1997.

• = **Independent;** ▲ = **Collaborative**

Narsavage GL: Promoting function in clients with chronic lung disease by increasing their perception of control, *Holist Nurs Pract* 12(1):17, 1997.

Nesbitt BJ, Heidrich SM: Sense of coherence and illness appraisal in older women's quality of life, *Res Nurs Health* 23:25, 2000.

Patusky KL: Event-generated dependence and its psychological sequelae in older adults, doctoral dissertation, Ann Arbor, Mich, 2000, University of Michigan.

Phillips JM, Cohen MZ, Moses G: Breast cancer screening and African American women: fear, fatalism, and silence, *Oncol Nurs Forum* 26(3):561, 1999.

Ramirez JR et al: Effects of fatalism and family communication on HIV/AIDS awareness variations in American and Anglo parents and children, *AIDS Educ Prev* 14(1):29, 2002.

Resnick B: Motivating older adults to engage in self-care, *Pat Care Nurs Pract* 4:13, 2001.

Rose LE: Gaining control: family members relate to persons with severe mental illness, *Res Nurs Health* 21:363, 1998.

Samuel-Hodge CD et al: Influences on day-to-day self-management of type 2 diabetes among African-American women: spirituality, the multi-caregiver role, and other social context factors, *Diabetes Care* 23(7): 928, 2000.

Shih S et al: The forgotten faces: the lonely journey of powerlessness experienced by elderly single Chinese men with heart disease in Taiwan, *Geriatr Nurs* 21:254, 2000.

Sinclair VG et al: Effects of a cognitive-behavioral intervention for women with rheumatoid arthritis, *Res Nurs Health* 21:315, 1998.

Slama CA, Bergman-Evans B: A troubling triangle: an exploration of loneliness, helplessness, and boredom of residents of a veterans home, *J Psychosoc Nurs Ment Health Serv* 38(12):36, 2000.

Spiers JA: The interpersonal contexts of negotiating care in home care nurse-patient interactions, *Qual Health Res* 12:1033, 2002.

Taylor D: Effectiveness of professional peer group treatment: symptom management for women with PMS, *Res Nurs Health* 22:496, 1999.

Tolley M: Power to the patient, *J Gerontol Nurs* 23(10):7, 1997.

Wong M: Self-care instructions: do patients understand educational materials? *Focus Crit Care* 19:47, 1992.

Wrosch C, Schulz R, Heckhausen J: Health stresses and depressive symptomatology in the elderly. The importance of health engagement control strategies, *Health Psychol* 21:340, 2002.

Risk for Powerlessness

Kathleen L. Patusky

NANDA Definition

At risk for perceived lack of control over a situation and/or one's ability to significantly affect an outcome

Related Factors (r/t)

Physiological

Chronic or acute illness (hospitalization, intubation, ventilator use, suctioning); acute injury or progressive debilitating disease process (e.g., multiple sclerosis); aging (e.g., decreased physical strength, decreased mobility); dying

Psychosocial

Lack of knowledge of illness or health care system; lifestyle of dependency with inadequate coping patterns; absence of integrality (e.g., essence of power); decreased self-esteem; low or unstable body image

• = Independent; ▲ = Collaborative

NOC   Outcomes (Nursing Outcomes Classification)

Suggested NOC Outcomes

Depression Self-Control; Health Beliefs; Health Beliefs: Perceived Ability to Perform, Perceived Control, Perceived Resources; Participation in Health Care Decisions

---

Example NOC Outcome with Indicators

Health Beliefs: Perceived Control as evidenced by the following indicators: Perceived responsibility for health decisions/Beliefs that own decisions and actions control health outcomes (Rate each indicator of **Health Beliefs: Perceived Control:** 1 = very weak belief, 2 = weak belief, 3 = moderately strong belief, 4 = strong belief, 5 = very strong belief [see Section I].)

Client Outcomes

Client Will (Specify Time Frame):

- State feelings of powerlessness and other feelings related to powerlessness (e.g., anger, sadness, hopelessness)
- Identify factors that are uncontrollable
- Participate in planning and implementing care; make decisions regarding care and treatment when possible
- Ask questions about care and treatment
- Verbalize hope for the future and sense of participation in planning and implementing care

NIC   Interventions (Nursing Interventions Classification)

Suggested NIC Interventions

Cognitive Restructuring; Complex Relationship Building; Mutual Goal Setting; Self-Esteem Enhancement; Self-Responsibility Facilitation

---

Example NIC Activities—Self-Responsibility Facilitation

Encourage independence but assist client when unable to perform; Assist client in identifying areas in which he or she could readily assume more responsibility

---

Nursing Interventions and Rationales, Client/Family Teaching

See the care plan for **Powerlessness.**

evolve WEBSITES FOR EDUCATION

See the EVOLVE website for World Wide Web resources for client education.

• = Independent; ▲ = Collaborative

Ineffective Protection

Betty J. Ackley and Gail B. Ladwig

NANDA   Definition

Decrease in ability to guard self from internal or external threats such as illness or injury

Defining Characteristics

Maladaptive stress response; neurosensory alteration; impaired healing; deficient immunity; altered clotting; dyspnea; insomnia; weakness; restlessness; pressure ulcers; perspiring; itching; immobility; chilling; fatigue; disorientation; cough; anorexia

Related Factors (r/t)

Abnormal blood profiles (e.g., leukopenia, thrombocytopenia, anemia, coagulation); extremes of age; inadequate nutrition; alcohol abuse; drug therapies (e.g., antineoplastic, corticosteroid, immune, anticoagulant, thrombolytic); treatments (e.g., surgery, radiation); diseases such as cancer and immune disorders

NOC   Outcomes (Nursing Outcomes Classification)

Suggested NOC Outcomes

Abuse Protection; Blood Coagulation; Endurance; Immune Status

---

Example NOC Outcome with Indicators

Immune Status as evidenced by the following indicators: Recurrent infections not present/Tumors not present/Gastrointestinal status IER/Respiratory status IER/Weight IER/Body temperature IER/Absolute WBC values WNL (Rate each indicator of **Immune Status:** 1 = extremely compromised, 2 = substantially compromised, 3 = moderately compromised, 4 = mildly compromised, 5 = not compromised [see Section I].)

IER, In expected range; *WBC,* white blood cell; *WNL,* within normal limits.

Client Outcomes

Client Will (Specify Time Frame):

- Remain free of infection
- Remain free of any evidence of new bleeding
- Explain precautions to take to prevent infection
- Explain precautions to take to prevent bleeding

NIC   Interventions (Nursing Interventions Classification)

Suggested NIC Interventions

Bleeding Precautions; Infection Control; Infection Protection

---

Example NIC Activities—Infection Control

Monitor for systemic and localized signs and symptoms of infection; Inspect skin and mucous membranes for redness, extreme warmth, or drainage

---

• = Independent; ▲ = Collaborative

Nursing Interventions and Rationales

- Take temperature, pulse, and blood pressure (e.g., q 1 to 4 hours). *Prospective surveillance study for nosocomial infection on hematology-oncology units should include fever of unknown origin as the single most common and clinically important entity (Engelhart et al, 2002). Changes in vital signs can indicate the onset of bleeding or infection.*
- ▲ Observe nutritional status (e.g., weight, serum protein and albumin levels, muscle mass, usual food intake). Work with the dietitian to improve nutritional status if needed. All clients diagnosed with HIV should have a dietary consult. *Early assessment of nutrition, good management of nutrition, and psychological support are essential for meeting the needs of the neutropenic client (Rust, Simpson, and Lister, 2000).* **Clinical Research:** *Nutrient status is an important factor contributing to immune competence: undernutrition impairs the immune system (Calder and Kew, 2002). Good nutrition is needed to maintain immune function and support formation of clotting elements. Most people who die of AIDS actually die of starvation. Malnutrition is almost universal among persons with AIDS because of malabsorption (Woznicki and D'Alessandro, 1997).*
- Observe the client's sleep pattern; if altered, see Nursing Interventions and Rationales for **Disturbed Sleep patterns.**
- Determine the amount of stress in the client's life. If stress is uncontrollable, see Nursing Interventions and Rationales for **Ineffective Coping.** *Uncontrolled stress depresses immune system function (Carter, 1993).*

Prevention of infection

- ▲ Monitor for and report any signs of infection (e.g., fever, chills, flushed skin, drainage, edema, redness, abnormal laboratory values, and pain) and notify the physician promptly. *The immune system is stimulated with the onset of infection, which results in classic signs of infection. In the neutropenic client, antibiotics must be given promptly because a delay increases morbidity and mortality (Quadri and Brown, 2000).* **Nursing Research:** *In many cases, changes in hematological parameters may be the initial sign of an occult infectious or inflammatory disorder (Szymanski, 2001).*
- Use appropriate "hand hygiene" (i.e., hand washing or use of alcohol-based hand rubs). *Improved adherence to hand hygiene has been shown to terminate outbreaks of infection in health care facilities, to reduce transmission of antimicrobial-resistant organisms (e.g., methicillin-resistant* Staphylococcus aureus) *and to reduce overall infection rates (US Department of Health and Human Services, 2002).*
- When using an alcohol-based hand rub, apply product to palm of one hand and rub hands together, covering all surfaces of hands and fingers, until hands are dry. Note that the volume needed to reduce the number of bacteria on hands varies by product. **Clinical Research:** *Introducing the use of hand rubbing with an alcoholic solution resulted in significantly improved hand-cleansing compliance (Girou and Oppein, 2001). Alcohols exert the strongest and fastest activity against a wide spectrum of bacteria and fungi (but not bacterial spores) as well as enveloped viruses (but less so against nonenveloped viruses) and are little influenced by interfering substances. They are of low toxicity and offer acceptable skin tolerability when formulated with suitable emollients. The mode of their application is simple and they are three to four times more economical of time than wash procedures, features that help to increase compliance with the rules of hand hygiene (Rotter, 2001).*
- Consider warming the client before elective surgery. **Evidence-Based Nursing Research:** *In clients undergoing elective hernia repair, varicose vein surgery, or breast surgery,*

• = Independent; ▲ = Collaborative

preoperative warming using a local device or a warm air blanket reduced the incidence of wound infection after surgery (Borbasi and Brougham, 2002).

▲ If the client's immune system is depressed, notify the physician of elevated temperature, even in the absence of other symptoms of infection. *Clients with depressed immune function are unable to mount the usual immune responses to the onset of infection; fever may be the only sign of infection. A neutropenic client with fever represents an absolute medical emergency (Burney, 2000; Quadri and Brown, 2000).*

• If white blood cell count is severely decreased (absolute neutrophil count of <1000/mm³), initiate the following precautions:
  ▪ Take vital signs every 4 hours.
  ▪ Complete a head-to-toe assessment twice daily, including inspection of oral mucosa, invasive sites, wounds, urine, and stool; monitor for onset of new complaints of pain.
  ▪ Avoid any invasive procedures, including catheterization, injections, or rectal or vaginal procedures.
  Infectious agents can invade when a treatment damages the skin or mucous membranes, which are natural barriers against infection (Flyge, 1993).

▲ Administer granulocyte growth factor therapy as ordered. *Myeloid growth factors for granulocytes are more useful for preventing than for treating neutropenic infections in cancer clients (Glaspy, 2000). Clinical trials suggest that granulocyte-macrophage colony-stimulating factor (sargramostim [Leukine], Immunex Corporation, Seattle, WA) has clinical benefits beyond enhancing neutrophil recovery, including shortening the duration of mucositis and diarrhea, stimulating dendritic cells, preventing infection, acting as an adjuvant vaccine agent, and facilitating antitumor activity (Buchsel et al, 2002).*

• Take meticulous care of all invasive sites; use chlorhexidine gluconate for cleansing. **Nursing Research:** *Use of chlorhexidine gluconate for vascular catheter site care reduced catheter-related bloodstream infections and catheter colonization more than use of povidone iodine (Chaiyakunapruk et al, 2003).*

• Provide frequent oral care. *The effects of chemotherapy or radiation leave the mouth inflamed; combined with immunosuppression, this can result in stomatitis. Good oral care can help prevent this complication (Dose, 1995).*

▲ Refer for prophylactic medication to prevent oral candidiasis. **Evidence-Based Research:** *There is strong evidence from randomized controlled trials that drugs absorbed or partially absorbed from the gastrointestinal (GI) tract prevent oral candidiasis in the client receiving treatment for cancer. There is also evidence that these drugs are significantly better at preventing oral candidiasis than drugs not absorbed from the GI tract (Worthington, Clarkson, and Eden, 2002).*

▲ Refer for appropriate prophylactic antifungal treatment and avoid pathogen exposure (through air filtration, regular hand hygiene, avoidance of plants and flowers). *Practical measures can be taken to avoid exposing the client to fungi (Maertens, Vrebos, and Boogaerts, 2001).* **Evidence-Based Research:** *Intravenous amphotericin B is the only antifungal agent for which there is evidence suggesting that its use might reduce mortality. It should therefore be preferred when prophylactic or empirical antifungal therapy is indicated in cancer clients with neutropenia (Gotzsche and Johansen, 2002).*

• Have the client wear a mask when leaving the room. **Clinical Research:** *To prevent nosocomial pulmonary aspergillosis during hospital construction, neutropenic clients with hematological malignancy were required to wear high-efficiency filtering masks when leaving their rooms. The rate of nosocomial aspergillosis decreased from 0.73 per 1000 hospital*

• = **Independent;** ▲ = **Collaborative**

client-days during fiscal years 1993 to 1996 to 0.24 per 1000 hospital client-days during fiscal years 1996 to 1999 (Raad et al, 2002).

- Limit and screen visitors to minimize exposure to contagion.
- Help the client bathe daily.
- Serve the client well-cooked food only; avoid all raw foods, including salads. Avoid serving processed meats, cheeses, yogurt, and beer or wine. Have the client drink sterile or boiled water only, and make ice cubes out of sterile water (Fenelon, 1998; Rust, Simpson, and Lister, 2000). *Data are lacking to confirm that consumption of neutropenic diets diminishes the rate of infection. Most centers use guidelines that recommend specific dietary restrictions during a period of immunosuppression (Rust, Simpson, and Lister, 2000; Smith and Besser, 2000).*
- Ensure that the client is well nourished. Provide food with protein and consider vitamin supplements. If appetite is suppressed, institute a dietary referral. Keep track of serum albumin levels as well as transferrin and prealbumin levels. **Clinical Research:** *It is essential that the nurse ensure adequate nutrition for the neutropenic client. If the client cannot eat and the GI system is temporarily damaged, it may be necessary for the client to receive total parenteral nutrition. Levels of the visceral proteins (albumin, transferrin, and prealbumin) are an indirect measure of nutritional status (Rust, Simpson, and Lister, 2000). Nutrients that have been demonstrated (in either animal or human studies) to be required for the immune system to function efficiently include essential amino acids, the essential fatty acid linoleic acid, vitamin A, folic acid, vitamin B_6, vitamin B_{12}, vitamin C, vitamin E, zinc, copper, iron, and selenium. Practically all forms of immunity may be affected by deficiencies in one or more of these nutrients (Calder and Kew, 2002).*
- Help the client to cough and practice deep breathing regularly. Maintain an appropriate activity level.
- Obtain a private room for the client. Take ordered precautions, including the use of a protective isolation or laminar airflow room, a Shinki bioclean room (SBCR), and/or high-energy particulate air (HEPA) filters if available and appropriate. Recognize that cotton cover gowns may not be effective in decreasing infection. *A private room is always necessary for neutropenic clients. There is no standardization of infection prevention practices nationwide for bone marrow transplant clients (Poe et al, 1994). A client with an absolute neutrophil count of less than $1000/mm^3$ is severely neutropenic, has an impaired immune function, and is extremely prone to infection. Precautions should be taken to limit exposure to pathogens (Wujcik, 1993).* **Nursing Research:** *A pilot study investigating the routine use of cotton cover gowns in the care of neutropenic clients found that the rates of infection were no different than when cover gowns were not used (Kenny and Lawson, 2000). Protective contact isolation with gowns, gloves, and hand washing is not superior to the use of gloves and hand washing alone in the prevention of airway colonization and nosocomial pneumonia in SICU clients and may in fact be detrimental (Koss et al, 2001).* **Clinical Research:** *In a retrospective cohort study, the use of HEPA filters provided protection for highly immunocompromised clients with hematological malignancies and demonstrated effectiveness in controlling outbreaks of infection due to air contamination with* Aspergillus conidia *(Hahn et al, 2002).* **Nursing Research:** *The SBCR is equal or superior to the laminar airflow room in preventing infection during neutropenia. Other advantages for the SBCR are a low level of noise (40 dB), easy control of temperature and humidity, and efficient removal of odor (Shinjo et al, 2002).*
- ▲ Watch for signs of sepsis, including change in mental status, fever, shaking, chills, and

• = **Independent;** ▲ = **Collaborative**

hypotension. If present, notify the physician promptly. *Change in mental status, fever, shaking, chills, and hypotension are indicators of sepsis (Flyge, 1993).*

Geriatric

- If not contraindicated, promote exercise to strengthen the immune system in the elderly. **Clinical Research:** *The results of a study of adults aged 62 years and older suggest that lifestyle factors, including exercise, may influence immune response to influenza immunization. The practice of regular, vigorous exercise was associated with enhanced immune response following influenza vaccination in older adults (Kohut et al, 2002).*
- Give elderly clients with imbalanced nutrition a nutritional supplement to enhance immune function. **Clinical Research:** *Nineteen subjects aged 65 years and older with a body mass index of 25 or less received either a complete liquid nutritional supplement containing energy, vitamins, and minerals, including enhanced levels of antioxidants, or a noncaloric placebo drink for 7 months. The study indicated that consumption of this complete liquid nutritional supplement may have a beneficial effect on antibody response to influenza vaccination in the elderly population (Wouters-Wesseling et al, 2002).*
- See the care plan for **Risk for Infection** for more interventions related to the prevention of infection.

Prevention of bleeding

- Monitor the client's risk for bleeding; evaluate results of clotting studies and platelet counts. *Laboratory studies give a good indication of the seriousness of the bleeding disorder.*
- Watch for hematuria, melena, hematemesis, hemoptysis, epistaxis, bleeding from mucosa, petechiae, and ecchymoses. *These types of bleeding can be detected in a bleeding disorder (Ellenberger, Hass, and Cundiff, 1993; Paschall, 1993).*
- ▲ Give medications orally or intravenously only; avoid giving them intramuscularly, subcutaneously, or rectally (Shuey, 1996). Apply pressure for a longer time than usual to invasive sites such as venipuncture or injection sites. *Additional pressure is needed to stop bleeding of invasive sites in clients with bleeding disorders.*
- Take vital signs frequently; watch for changes associated with fluid volume loss. *Excessive bleeding causes decreased blood pressure and increased pulse and respiratory rates.*
- Monitor menstrual flow if relevant; have the client use pads instead of tampons. *Menstruation can be excessive in clients with bleeding disorders. Use of tampons can increase trauma to the vagina.*
- Have the client use a moistened toothette instead of a toothbrush, or a very soft child's toothbrush. Have the client use alcohol-free dental products and avoid flossing. *These actions help prevent trauma to the oral mucosa, which could result in bleeding (Shuey, 1996).*
- Ask the client either not to shave or to use an electric razor only. *This helps to prevent any unnecessary trauma that could result in bleeding (Shuey, 1996).*
- To decrease risk of bleeding, avoid administering salicylates or nonsteroidal anti-inflammatory drugs (NSAIDs) if possible. *Salicylates and NSAIDs can cause GI bleeding; salicylates interfere with platelet function and can increase bleeding.*

Home care

- Some of the interventions described previously may be adapted for home care use.
- Consider institution of a nurse-administered mobile care unit for monitoring anticoagulant therapy. **Nursing Research:** *Establishment of anticoagulation therapy management (ATM) clinics led to improvements in quality of care, in terms of improved control*

● = Independent; ▲ = Collaborative

of international normalized ratio (INR) and reduced complications. From the year before to the year after implementation of an ATM program, the percentage of in-range INRs increased from 40.7% to 58.5%. The percentage in the modified target range also increased (50.0% to 62.9%) (Gill and Landis, 2002).

▲ For terminally ill clients, teach and institute all of the aforementioned noninvasive precautions that will maintain quality of life. Discuss with the client, family, and physician the consequences of contracting infection. Determine which precautions do not maintain quality of life and should not be used (e.g., physical assessment twice daily, multiple vital sign assessments). *Multiple assessments and other invasive procedures are recovery-based, cure-focused activities. The client and physician must agree on an approach to care for the client's remaining life.*

Client/Family Teaching
Depressed immune function

- Teach precautions to take to decrease the chance of infection (e.g., avoiding uncooked fruits or vegetables, using appropriate self-care, ensuring a safe environment).
- Teach the client and family how to take a temperature. Encourage the family to take the client's temperature between 3 PM and 7 PM at least once daily. *For most people, the difference between high and low values throughout the day is about 1.1° C (2.0° F) (36.1° to 37.2° C [97° to 99° F]) with the lowest value typically occurring in the early morning hours (2:00 AM to 5:00 AM) and the highest values commonly occurring in the evening (7:00 PM to 10:00 PM) (Round-the-Clock Systems, 2003).*
▲ Teach the client and family to notify the physician of elevated temperature, even in the absence of other symptoms of infection. *Clients with depressed immune function are unable to mount the usual immune response to the onset of infection; fever may be the only sign of infection present (Wujcik, 1993).*
- Teach the client to avoid crowds and contact with persons who have infections. *Teach the need for good nutrition, avoidance of stress, and adequate rest to maintain immune system function. Client education to increase nutrition, manage stress, and perform self-care can reduce the risk of neutropenic infection (Carter, 1993).*

Bleeding disorder

▲ Teach the client to wear a medical alert bracelet and notify all health care personnel of the bleeding disorder. *Emergency identification schemes such as medical alert bracelets use emblems that alert health care professionals to potential problems and can ensure appropriate and prompt treatment (Morton et al, 2002).*
- Teach the client and family the signs of bleeding, precautions to take to prevent bleeding, and action to take if bleeding begins. Caution the client to avoid taking over-the-counter medications without the permission of the physician. *Medications containing salicylates can increase bleeding.*
- Teach the client to wear loose-fitting clothes and avoid physical activity that might cause trauma.

evolve WEBSITES FOR EDUCATION

See the EVOLVE website for World Wide Web resources for client education.

• = Independent; ▲ = Collaborative

REFERENCES

Borbasi S, Brougham L: Warming patients before clean surgery reduced the incidence of postoperative wound infection, *Evid Based Nurs* 5(2):48, 2002.

Buchsel PC et al: Granulocyte macrophage colony-stimulating factor: current practice and novel approaches, *Clin J Oncol Nurs* 6(4):198, 2002.

Burney KY: Tips for timely management of febrile neutropenia, *Oncol Nurs Forum* 27(4):617, 2000.

Calder PC, Kew S: The immune system: a target for functional foods? *Br J Nutr* 88(suppl 2):S165, 2002.

Carter LW: Influences of nutrition and stress on people at risk for neutropenia: nursing implications, *Oncol Nurs Forum* 20(8):1241, 1993.

Chaiyakunapruk N et al: Chlorhexidine compared with povidone-iodine solution for vascular catheter-site care: a meta-analysis, *Ann Intern Med* 136:792, 2002.

Dose AM: The symptom experience of mucositis, stomatitis, and xerostomia, *Semin Oncol Nurs* 11:248, 1995.

Ellenberger BJ, Hass L, Cundiff L: Thrombotic thrombocytopenia purpura: nursing during the acute phase, *Dimens Crit Care Nurs* 12:58, 1993.

Engelhart S et al: Surveillance for nosocomial infections and fever of unknown origin among adult hematology-oncology patients, *Infect Control Hosp Epidemiol* 23(5):244, 2002.

Fenelon L: Strategies for prevention of infection in short-duration neutropenia, *Infect Control Hosp Epidemiol* 19(8):590, 1998.

Flyge HA: Meeting the challenge of neutropenia, *Nursing* 23(7):60, 1993.

Gill JM, Landis MK: Benefits of a mobile, point-of-care anticoagulation therapy management program, *Jt Comm J Qual Improv* 28(11):625, 2002.

Girou E, Oppein F: Handwashing compliance in a French university hospital: new perspective with the introduction of hand-rubbing with a waterless alcohol-based solution, *J Hosp Infect* 48(suppl A):S55, 2001.

Glaspy JA: Hematologic supportive care of the critically ill cancer patient, *Semin Oncol* 27(3):375, 2000.

Gotzsche PC, Johansen HK: Routine versus selective antifungal administration for control of fungal infections in patients with cancer, *Cochrane Database Syst Rev* (CD000026), 2002.

Hahn T et al: Efficacy of high-efficiency particulate air filtration in preventing aspergillosis in immunocompromised patients with hematologic malignancies, *Infect Control Hosp Epidemiol* 23(9):525, 2002.

Kenny H, Lawson E: The efficacy of cotton cover gowns in reducing infection in nursing neutropenic patients: an evidence-based study, *Int J Nurs Pract* 6(3):135, 2000.

Kohut ML et al: Exercise and psychosocial factors modulate immunity to influenza vaccine in elderly individuals, *J Gerontol A Biol Sci Med Sci* 57(9):M557, 2002.

Koss WG et al: Nosocomial pneumonia is not prevented by protective contact isolation in the surgical intensive care unit, *Am Surg* 67(12):1140, 2001.

Maertens J, Vrebos M, Boogaerts M: Assessing risk factors for systemic fungal infections, *Eur J Cancer Care (Engl)* 10(1):56, 2001.

Morton L et al: Importance of emergency identification schemes, *Emerg Med J* 19(6):584, 2002.

Paschall FE: Thrombotic thrombocytopenic purpura: the challenges of a complex disease process, *AACN Clin Issues* 4:655, 1993.

Poe SS et al: A national survey of infection prevention practices on bone marrow transplant units, *Oncol Nurs Forum* 21(10):1687, 1994.

Quadri TL, Brown AE: Infectious complications in the critically ill patient with cancer, *Semin Oncol* 27(3):335, 2000.

Raad I et al: Masking of neutropenic patients on transport from hospital rooms is associated with a decrease in nosocomial aspergillosis during construction, *Infect Control Hosp Epidemiol* 23(1):41, 2002.

Rotter ML: Arguments for alcoholic hand disinfection, *J Hosp Infect* 48(suppl A):S4, 2001.

Round-the-Clock Systems: *Circadian rhythms*, available online at http://www.matrices.com/Workplace/Learning/sw.circadian.html, accessed March 16, 2003.

Rust DM, Simpson JK, Lister J: Nutritional issues in patients with severe neutropenia, *Semin Oncol Nurs* 16(2):152, 2000.

Shinjo K et al: Efficacy of the Shinki bioclean room for preventing infection in neutropenic patients, *J Adv Nurs* 37(3):227, 2002.

Shuey KM: Platelet-associated bleeding disorders, *Semin Oncol Nurs* 12(1):15, 1996.

Smith LH, Besser SG: Dietary restrictions for patients with neutropenia: a survey of institutional practices, *Oncol Nurs Forum* 27(3):515, 2000.

Szymanski N: Infection and inflammation in dialysis patients: impact on laboratory parameters and anemia. Case study of the anemic patient, *Nephrol Nurse J* 28(3):337, 2001.

• = Independent; ▲ = Collaborative

US Department of Health and Human Services, Centers for Disease Control and Prevention, *Hand hygiene guidelines fact sheet*, 2002, available online at http://www.cdc.gov/od/oc/media/pressrel/fs021025.htm, accessed Feb 12, 2003.

Worthington HV, Clarkson JE, Eden OB: Interventions for preventing oral candidiasis for patients with cancer receiving treatment, *Cochrane Database Syst Rev* (CD003807), 2003.

Wouters-Wesseling W et al: Effect of a complete nutritional supplement on antibody response to influenza vaccine in elderly people, *J Gerontol A Biol Sci Med Sci* 57(9):M563, 2002.

Woznicki D, D'Alessandro G: Nutrition against AIDS, *Health Priorities* 9(2), 1997, available at http://www.acsh.org/publications/priorities/0902/nutrition.html, accessed June 20, 2003.

Wujcik D: Infection control in oncology patients, *Nurs Clin North Am* 28:639, 1993.

Rape-trauma syndrome

Linda Hutson

NANDA | Definition

Sustained maladaptive response to forced, violent sexual act (penetration may not actually occur) (Ohio Revised Code) against victim's will and consent

Defining Characteristics

Fear disorganization; change in relationships; confusion; physical trauma (e.g., bruising, tissue irritation; injuries identified by use of new technology); suicide attempt; denial; guilt; paranoia; humiliation; embarrassment; aggression; muscle tension and/or spasms; mood swings; dependence; powerlessness; nightmares and sleep disturbances; sexual dysfunction; desire for revenge; phobias; loss of self-esteem; inability to make decisions; dissociative disorders; self-blame; hyperalertness; vulnerability; substance abuse; depression; helplessness; anger; anxiety; agitation; shame; shock

Related Factors (r/t)

Rape; sexual assault; abuse

NOC | Outcomes (Nursing Outcomes Classification)

Suggested NOC Outcomes

Abuse Cessation; Abuse Protection; Abuse Recovery: Emotional, Sexual; Coping; Impulse Self-Control; Self-Mutilation Restraint

> **Example NOC Outcome with Indicators**
>
> **Abuse Recovery** as evidenced by the following indicators: Acknowledgment of right to disclose abusive situation/Expression of right to have been protected from abuse (Rate each indicator of **Abuse Recovery:** 1 = none, 2 = limited, 3 = moderate, 4 = substantial, 5 = extensive [see Section I].)

Client Outcomes

Client Will (Specify Time Frame):

- Share feelings, concerns, and fears
- Recognize that the rape or attempt was not client's own fault
- State that, no matter what the situation, no one has the right to assault another
- Describe medical/legal treatment procedures and reasons for treatment

• = Independent; ▲ = Collaborative

- Report absence of physical complications or pain
- Identify support people and be able to ask them for help in dealing with this trauma
- Function at same level as before crisis, including sexual functioning
- Recognize that it is normal for full recovery to take a minimum of 1 year

NIC   Interventions (Nursing Interventions Classification)

Suggested NIC Interventions
Counseling; Rape-Trauma Treatment

Example NIC Activities—Counseling

Explain rape protocol and obtain consent to proceed through protocol; Encourage expression of feelings

---

Nursing Interventions and Rationales

- Observe the client's responses, including anger, fear, self-blame, sleep pattern disturbances, and phobias.
- Monitor the client's verbal and nonverbal psychological state (e.g., crying, hand wringing, avoidance of interactions or eye contact with staff, silence and denial). **Clinical Research:** *The most depressed victims are those most concerned with being stigmatized and blamed for the crime (Frable, Blackstone, and Sherbaum, 1990).*
- ▲ Stay with (or have a trusted person stay with) the client initially. If a law enforcement interview is permitted, provide support by staying with the client, but only at the client's request. **Nursing Research:** *Allow the client to make the decision about whom the client wishes to have present during any interviews or examinations to allow a return of control to the client (Ledray, 1998a).*
- Explain the entire medical/legal examination to the client before beginning any procedures. Obtain written permission to perform the examination but explain to the client that at any time during the examination the client may withdraw consent. Discuss with the client the importance of participating in the entire examination and the importance of the collection of evidence. The examination will include several procedures that might be uncomfortable or painful and the client should know this in advance. Before moving on to each procedure, repeat the explanation and offer the client the right to skip any part of the examination in which the client feels unable to fully participate. Discuss the importance of performing a speculum examination rather than a pelvic examination. If it is the client's first examination, explain the instruments and let the client know when and where you will touch. Encourage the presence of either an advocate or a person the client trusts during any physical examination. Do this with the client's permission. Most often the examiner is busy collecting evidence and photographs and cannot offer the emotional support the client may need during this portion of the examination. **Nursing Research:** *This returns control to the client. Explain that a speculum examination will be performed for the purpose of identifying any injury and collecting evidence (Hutson, 2002).*
- Do not wait for the client to ask questions; explain everything you are doing, clarify why it must be done, and describe when and where you will touch. *Eye contact is very important because it helps the client feel worthy and alive (Ruckman, 1992).*
- ▲ Observe for signs of physical injury as you are asking the client to undress and collecting the client's clothing for evidence. Ask the client where it hurts without asking

• = **Independent;** ▲ = **Collaborative**

leading questions. Do not ask specific questions but allow the client to give you a history of the sexual assault in the client's own words. If further clarification is needed by the examiner, ask the client to point to areas that were injured or touched. Inform the client that photographs of any injuries are necessary for forensic evidence. Obtain specific written permission for photographs to be taken and released to law enforcement personnel. **Nursing Research:** *The aforementioned nonleading questions are recommended. Do not ask questions that could indicate to the defense attorney and the jury that the examiner was leading the client and may have influenced the client's report of the assault (Ledray, 1998b).*

▲ Instruct the client to return for additional photographs either to the medical facility or to law enforcement personnel if bruises become more pronounced in a few days. It is recommended that all medical treatment be completed at the initial encounter due to the difficulty in getting clients to return for follow-up medical care. **Nursing Research:** *Clients are reluctant to return for any medical evaluation and have a poor history of doing so (Dandino-Abbott, 1999). Sore areas can be visible using the new technology employed in these examinations (Sommers et al, 2001).*

• Documentation of a sexual assault examination is critical to evidentiary reports. It is important to document the client's exact description of the assault and then to collect evidence and photographs that validate the history the client reports. **Nursing Research:** *It is very important that the examiner not offer any subjective information on the documentation (Ledray, 1998a).*

• It is also very important for the examiner not to offer any opinions in the documentation about whether or not the assault occurred according to the physical findings. **Nursing Research:** *These opinions should be offered to the legal system only when they are requested for prosecution (Ledray, 1998b).*

▲ Document a one- or two-sentence summary of what happened. The chief complaint of the client reporting sexual assault should always be given as "reported sexual assault"; obtaining the details of the sequence of events is the police officer's job. **Nursing Research:** *The chief complaint of the client reporting sexual assault should always be listed as "reported sexual assault." Other terms, such as "alleged sexual assault," "rape," or "sexual assault," imply an opinion by the person taking the history (Hutson, 2002). It is important to remember that sexual assault clients are often very traumatized in the acute phase of the assault and may give several different histories of the event. They may remember certain aspects of the assault at different times. If the details given during the medical/legal examination differ from the details given to law enforcement personnel, the law enforcement agency will obtain the information needed to support or contradict the client's history of events (Ledray, 1998a). If some details that are not in the nurse's notes were told to the police, the defense attorney may attempt to make this look like a discrepancy in facts, which can cause reasonable doubt and result in an acquittal (Ledray, 1992).*

• Encourage the client to verbalize feelings. *Listening to clients helps them gain self-control by feeling acceptance from others (Ruckman, 1992).*

• Escort the client to the treatment room immediately to remove the client from the general population; do not question the client in the triage area, close curtains and door, and avoid other interruptions during contact with the client (e.g., telephone calls, absence from the room, outside stimuli such as radios). **Nursing and Clinical Research:** *It is preferable that the client have a dedicated caregiver such as a sexual assault nurse examiner (SANE) specially trained in sexual assault medical/forensic examinations so that interruptions can be avoided. This not only serves the client but allows for the accurate*

• = **Independent;** ▲ = **Collaborative**

collection and preservation of evidence (Ledray, 1999; McGregor, DuMont, and Myhr, 2002).

▲ Provide a sexual assault response team that includes a SANE, rape counseling advocate, and representative of law enforcement. **Nursing Research:** *This team maximizes care to the client. In many cases, the advocate will be the person to assist the client through the legal system up to and including accompaniment to the courtroom. The quality of care the client receives from "first responders" may determine the client's willingness to continue with long-term treatment (Ledray, 1998a). Evidence-based practice indicates that this model brings quality care to women (Selig, 2000). Comparing a baseline group of 130 sexual assault victims with 39 clients who were evaluated after the SANE approach was implemented indicated that the SANE approach increased clinical interaction and completeness of evaluation and information gathered (Derhammer et al, 2000).*

▲ The rape crisis center advocate should be part of the sexual assault response team (SART) and respond when the SANE responds. This person can encourage follow-up at the rape crisis center. *The advocate can talk with the client during the acute phase; the client does not need to make an immediate decision about whether the client would like the advocate called for follow-up. Because advocates are better trained and prepared to talk to clients of acute sexual assault, they are usually more successful in encouraging further follow-up than the medical/nursing staff.* **Clinical Research:** *Clients want control but may have difficulty making decisions during the initial visit to the emergency department. Involvement of social service agencies will help to guarantee a timely follow-up home visit (Jones, 1994).*

• Provide items for self-care after examination (e.g., for cleansing the vaginal and rectal area). **Nursing Research:** *Many facilities that provide care for sexual assault clients have "survivor packs" available for post-treatment care. These include items for personal hygiene, i.e., shampoo, soap, toothbrush, toothpaste, new underwear and outer clothing to replace those secured for evidential purposes, etc. (Hutson, 2002).*

▲ Most states provide sexual assault evidence collection kits that have been reviewed by the SART members to provide adequate evidence for analysis by the forensic laboratory. Explain to the client that all or some of the client's clothing may be kept for evidential purposes. Also explain that the client will receive replacement clothing or that the client can request that a friend or family member bring clothing from home to replace the clothing kept for evidence. Explain to the client that, if the clothing worn during the assault is still at the scene, the client should disclose this information to law enforcement officials so that law enforcement personnel can go to the scene and collect the evidence appropriately. **Nursing Research:** *If the client arrives at the medical facility with the evidentiary clothing already in a bag, explain to the client that you will notify law enforcement personnel to pick it up directly from the client (Hutson, 2002). No clothing or evidence should be placed in a plastic bag because of the potential for deterioration or destruction. SANEs are specifically trained in the appropriate procedure.*

• An alternative light source will be used for direct inspection of the body for the presence of body fluids. *This is part of the examination and should be explained by the SANE (Ledray, 1999; O'Brien, 1998).*

▲ Discuss the possibility of pregnancy and sexually transmitted diseases (STDs) and the treatments available. *Administering a urine pregnancy test is routine before giving medications to prevent pregnancy or treat STDs. Most clients prefer to prevent pregnancy rather than face the possibility of terminating it in the future. The risk of HIV exposure is a*

• = Independent; ▲ = Collaborative

- A culturally sensitive approach should be part of the training of all SARTs and members of the teams. *Compassion and familiarity in a care plan will allow all care providers to create a comfortable environment for the client (McCleary, 1994).*

Home care

- Some of the interventions described previously may be adapted for home care use.
- Interact with the client supportively and nonjudgmentally; this supports the client's self-worth. *Rape victims usually experience a loss of self-worth.*
- Assist the client with realistically assessing the home setting for safety and/or selecting a safe environment in which to live. *Rape clients may be unable to make a realistic assessment of home safety both immediately after the rape and during long-term recovery.*
- ▲ Ensure that the client has a support system in place for long-term support. Instruct the family that recovery may take a long time. Refer for medical social work services to assist in setting up a support system if necessary. Refer for counseling if necessary. *The long-term response to rape (up to 4 years) requires ongoing support for the client to reorganize and reintegrate.*
- ▲ Make sure that physical symptoms from the rape or other physical conditions are followed up. Follow-up should include a visit to the primary care physician or the local health department in 3 to 4 weeks for repeat pregnancy testing and STD testing. Explain to the client that additional medication may be necessary for the treatment of STDs or pregnancy (Ohio Chapter of the International Association of Forensic Nurses [IAFN], 2002). *Stress response to rape can precipitate reemergence of other physical conditions that may be ignored because of the rape.*
- ▲ If the client is homebound, refer for psychiatric home health care services for client reassurance and implementation of a therapeutic regimen. *Psychiatric home care nurses can address issues relating to the client's rape-trauma syndrome. Behavioral interventions in the home can help the client to participate more effectively in the treatment plan (Patusky, Rodning, and Martinez-Kratz, 1996).*

Client/Family Teaching

- ▲ Provide information on prophylactic antibiotic therapy, hepatitis B vaccination, and tetanus prophylaxis for nonimmunized clients with trauma. *Prophylactic treatment for STDs should be provided as part of the initial examination (Ohio Chapter of the IAFN, 2002).*
- Discharge instructions should be written out for the client. *Anxiety can hamper comprehension and retention of information; repeat instructions and provide them in a written form.*
- Give instructions to significant others. *Significant others need many of the same supportive and caring interventions as the client; suggest that they too might benefit from counseling.*
- ▲ Explain the purpose of the "morning-after pill." *The morning-after pill—norgestrel (Ovral)—often prevents pregnancy and is used only in emergencies. It must be taken within 72 hours (3 days) of sexual contact to be effective. It will not cause a miscarriage if the client is already pregnant, but it could harm the baby.*
- ▲ Explain the potential for common side effects related to treatment with norgestrel, such as breast swelling or nausea and vomiting. (Call the emergency department if the client vomits within 1 hour of taking the pill because the pill may need to be taken again.) (Discuss any issues about prophylactic medications at the follow-up visit in 3 to 4 weeks.) It may take 3 to 30 days for the menstrual period to start; if menstruation has not begun in 30 days, contact a physician.

- **• = Independent; ▲ = Collaborative**

▲ Explain the potential for severe side effects related to treatment with norgestrel, such as severe leg or chest pain, trouble breathing, coughing up of blood, severe headache or dizziness, and trouble seeing or talking.

- Advise the client to call or return if new problems develop. *Physical injuries may not be recognized because of the client's emotional numbness during the initial examination or because the client may have forgotten or not understood some of the instructions.*
- Teach relaxation techniques.
- Discuss practical lifestyle changes within the client's control to reduce the risk of future attacks. *A client's financial situation may limit some options, such as moving to another home. Provide other alternatives such as keeping doors locked, checking the car before getting in, not walking alone at night, keeping someone informed of whereabouts, asking someone to check if the client has not arrived at a destination within a reasonable amount of time, keeping lights on in an entryway, having keys in hand when approaching the car or house, and having a remote key entry car or garage.*

▲ Teach the client to use self-defense techniques to surprise an attacker and create an opportunity to run for help. Refer the client to a self-defense school.

- Teach the client appropriate outlets for anger. *Encourage the significant other to direct anger at the event and the attacker, not at the client.*
- Emphasize the vulnerability of the client and ensure that reactions are appropriate for the victim of sexual assault. *Females are at higher risk for depression than males, and the risk is significantly higher between the ages of 18 and 44 (Mackey et al, 1992).*

NOTE: Post-traumatic stress disorder (PTSD) has a high probability of being a psychological sequela to rape. Research demonstrated two effective treatments for improvement of PTSD in rape victims—prolonged exposure and stress inoculation training (Foa et al, 1991). Prolonged exposure involves reliving the rape experience by imagining it as vividly as possible, describing it aloud in the present tense, taping this description, and listening to the tape at least once daily. Stress inoculation training uses breathing exercises to diminish anxiety and instruction in coping skills, thought stopping, cognitive restructuring, self-dialogue, and role playing. Research suggests that a combination of both treatments may provide the optimal effect.

evolve WEBSITES FOR EDUCATION

See the EVOLVE website for World Wide Web resources for client education.

REFERENCES

Adams JA, Girardin B, Faugno D: Signs of genital trauma in adolescent rape victims examined acutely, *J Pediatr Adolesc Gynecol* 13(2):88, 2000.

Cochran M: Tears have no color, *Am J Nurs* 98(6):53, 1998.

Crowley SA: *Sexual assault: the medical-legal examination,* ed 1, Stamford, Conn, 1999, Appleton and Lange.

Dandino-Abbott D: Sexual assault: clinical issues. Birth of a sexual assault response team: the first year of the Lucas County/Toledo, Ohio SART program, *J Emerg Nurs* 25(4):333, 1999.

D'Avanzo CE et al: Developing culturally informed strategies for substance-related interventions. In Naegle MA, D'Avanzo CE, editors: *Addictions and substance abuse: strategies for advanced practice nursing,* St Louis, 2001, Mosby.

Delorey C, Wolf KA: Sexual violence and older women, *AWHONNS Clin Issues Perinat Womens Health Nurs* 4:173, 1993.

Derhammer F et al: Using a SANE interdisciplinary approach to care of sexual assault victims, *Jt Comm J Qual Improv* 26(8):488, 2000.

- = Independent; ▲ = Collaborative

Doswell W, Erlen J: Multicultural issues and ethical concerns in the delivery of nursing care interventions, *Nurs Clin North Am* 33(2):353, 1998.

Dunn SF, Gilchrist VJ: Sexual assault, *Prim Care* 20(2):359, 1993.

Foa EB et al: Treatment of posttraumatic stress disorder in rape victims: a comparison between cognitive-behavioral procedures and counseling, *J Consult Clin Psychol* 59(5):715, 1991.

Frable D, Blackstone T, Sherbaum C: Marginal and mindful: deviants in social interaction, *J Pers Soc Psychol* 59: 140, 1990.

Heineken J: Patient silence is not necessarily client satisfaction: communication in home care nursing, *Home Healthc Nurse* 16(2):115, 1998.

Hutson L: Development of sexual assault nurse examiner programs, *Nurs Clin North Am* 35:79, 2002.

Jones J: Elder abuse and neglect: responding to a national problem, *Ann Emerg Med* 23:845, 1994.

Laurent C: Male rape, *Nurs Times* 89(6):18, 1993.

Ledray L: The sexual assault nurse clinician: a 15-year experience in Minneapolis, *J Emerg Nurs* 18(3):217, 1992.

Ledray L: Sexual assault: clinical issues. SANE development and operation guide, *J Emerg Nurs* 24(2):197, 1998a.

Ledray L: Sexual assault: clinical issues. SANE expert and factual testimony, *J Emerg Nurs* 24(3):284, 1998b.

Ledray LE: Sexual assault: clinical issues, IAFN Sixth Annual Scientific Assembly highlights, *J Emerg Nurs* 25(1):63, 1999.

Leininger MM, McFarland MR: *Transcultural nursing: concepts, theories, research and practices,* ed 3, New York, 2002, McGraw-Hill.

Ludwick R, Silva M: Nursing around the world: cultural values and ethical conflicts, *Online J Issues Nurs,* August 14, 2000, available online at http://www.nursingworld.org/ojin/ethcol/ethics_4.htm, accessed June 19, 2003.

Mackey T et al: Factors associated with long-term depressive symptoms of sexual assault victims, *Arch Psychiatr Nurs* 6:10, 1992.

McCleary PH: Female genitalia mutilation and childbirth: a case report, *Birth* 21(4):221, 1994.

McGregor MJ, DuMont J, Myhr TL: Sexual assault forensic medical examination: is evidence related to successful prosecution? *Ann Emerg Med* 39:6, 2002.

Mollica RF, Lavelle J: Southeast Asian refugees. In Comas-Diaz L, Griffith EEH, editors: *Clinical guidelines in cross-cultural mental health,* New York, 1988, John Wiley and Sons.

O'Brien C: Light staining microscope: clinical experience in a Sexual Assault Nurse Examiner (SANE) program, *Emerg Nurs* 24(1):95, 1998.

Ohio Chapter of the International Association of Forensic Nurses, *The Ohio adolescent and adult sexual assault nurse examiner training manual,* Cleveland, Ohio, Summer 2002, Ohio Office of the Attorney General.

Patusky KL, Rodning C, Martinez-Kratz M: Clinical lessons in psychiatric home care: a case study approach, *J Home Health Case Manag* 9:18, 1996.

Ruckman LM: Rape: how to begin the healing, *Am J Nurs* 92:48, 1992.

Selig C: Sexual assault nurse examiner and sexual assault response team (SANE/SART) program, *Nurs Clin North Am* 35(2):311, 2000.

Sommers M et al: Injury patterns in women resulting from sexual assault, *Trauma, Violence, and Abuse* 2(3):240. 2001.

Tyra PA: Older women: victims of rape, *J Gerontol Nurs* 19(5):7, 1993.

Vontress CE, Epp LR: Historical hostility in the African American client: implications for counseling, *J Multicult Counseling Dev* 25:170, 1997.

Rape-trauma syndrome: compound reaction

Linda Hutson

NANDA   Definition

Forced violent sexual act (penetration may not actually occur) (Ohio Revised Code) against victim's will and consent resulting in a trauma syndrome that includes an acute phase of disorganization of victim's lifestyle and a long-term process or reorganization of lifestyle

- • = Independent; ▲ = Collaborative

Defining Characteristics

Change in lifestyle (e.g., changing residence, dealing with repetitive nightmares and phobias, seeking family support, seeking social network support in long-term phase); emotional reaction (e.g., anger, embarrassment, fear of physical violence and death, humiliation, desire for revenge, self-blame in acute phase); multiple physical symptoms (e.g., gastrointestinal irritability, genitourinary discomfort, muscle tension, sleep pattern disturbance in acute phase); reactivated symptoms of previous conditions (i.e., physical illness, psychiatric illness in acute phase); reliance on alcohol and/or drugs (acute phase)

Related Factors (r/t)

Rape; sexual assault; abuse

NOC   Outcomes (Nursing Outcomes Classification)

Suggested NOC Outcomes

Abuse Cessation; Abuse Protection; Abuse Recovery: Emotional, Sexual; Coping; Impulse Self-Control; Self-Mutilation Restraint

---

Example NOC Outcome with Indicators

Abuse Recovery: Emotional as evidenced by the following indicators: Acknowledgment of right to disclose abusive situation/Expression of right to have been protected from abuse (Rate each indicator of **Abuse Recovery: Emotional:** 1 = none, 2 = limited, 3 = moderate, 4 = substantial, 5 = extensive [see Section I].)

Client Outcomes

Client Will (Specify Time Frame):

- Share feelings, concerns, and fears
- Recognize that the rape or attempt was not client's own fault
- State that, no matter what the situation, no one has the right to assault another
- Describe medical/legal treatment procedures and reasons for treatment
- Report absence of physical complications or pain
- Identify support people and be able to ask them for help in dealing with this trauma
- Function at same level as before crisis, including sexual functioning
- Recognize that it is normal for full recovery to take a minimum of 1 year

NIC   Interventions (Nursing Interventions Classification)

Suggested NIC Interventions

Counseling; Rape-Trauma Treatment

Example NIC Activities—Counseling

Encourage expression of feelings; Help client to identify strengths and reinforce these

---

• = Independent; ▲ = Collaborative

Nursing Interventions and Rationales

- See the care plans for **Rape-trauma syndrome, Powerlessness, Ineffective Coping, Dysfunctional Grieving, Anxiety, Fear, Risk for self-directed Violence,** and **Sexual dysfunction.**

Geriatric

▲ A new subgroup of rape victims resides in nursing homes. Treatment is necessary. *Nursing home victims can suffer both compound and silent rape trauma (Burgess, Dowdell, and Prentky, 2000).*

Risk for compound reaction

See the care plan for **Rape-trauma syndrome.**

Multicultural

- Assess for the influence of cultural beliefs, norms, and values on the client's ability to cope with the trauma of the rape experience. **Nursing Research:** *What the client views as healthy coping may be based on cultural perceptions (Cochran, 1998; Doswell and Erlen, 1998; Leininger and McFarland, 2002).*
- Provide opportunities by which the family and individual can save face when working with Asian American clients. **Nursing Research:** *Asian American families may avoid situations and discussion of issues that they perceive will bring shame on the family unit (D'Avanzo et al, 2001).*
- Assure the client of confidentiality. **Nursing Research:** *Many Indo-Chinese women will not discuss rape if they think that other staff members, their families, their husbands, or their community may find out (Mollica and Lavelle, 1988).*
- Validate the client's feelings regarding the rape and allow the client to tell his or her rape story. **Nursing Research:** *Validation lets the client know that the nurse has heard and understood what was said, and it promotes the nurse-client relationship (Heineken, 1998). Through the trauma story, the clinician can bridge the disrupted social connection that exists between the client, family, and community (Mollica and Lavelle, 1988).*
- A culturally sensitive approach should be part of the training of all sexual assault response team teams and members of the teams. *Compassion and familiarity in a care plan will allow all care providers to provide a comfortable environment for the client (McCleary, 1994).*

Home care

▲ If the client has pursued psychiatric counseling, monitor and encourage attendance. *Reliving the rape experience and the accompanying feelings is painful. The client may need additional support to continue.*

▲ If the client is receiving medication, assess the client's knowledge of its purpose, side effects, and interactions with medications for other diagnoses. Monitor for effectiveness, side effects, and interactions. *Ongoing stress may leave the client overwhelmed and less able to cope with the impact of changing medical status.*

▲ Establish an emergency plan including use of hotlines. Contract with the client to use the emergency plan. Role play using the hotlines. *Having an emergency plan reassures the client and decreases the risk of suicide.*

- For other home care and hospice considerations, see the care plan for **Rape-trauma syndrome.**

- = Independent; ▲ = Collaborative

Client/Family Teaching

- Teach the client what reactions to expect during the acute and long-term phases: acute phase—anger, fear, self-blame, embarrassment, vengeful feelings, physical symptoms, muscle tension, sleeplessness, stomach upset, genitourinary discomfort; long-term phase—changes in lifestyle or residence, nightmares, phobias, seeking of family and social network support. *Of assessed rape victims, 16.5% were diagnosed with posttraumatic stress disorder an average of 17 years after the assault (Mackey et al, 1992).*
- ▲ Encourage psychiatric consultation if the client is suicidal, violent, or unable to continue activities of daily living. *Rape victims are four times more likely than the general population to attempt suicide, which is an 8.7% higher rate than that of nonrape victims (Mackey et al, 1992).*
- ▲ Discuss any of the client's current stress-relieving medications that may result in substance abuse. *The initial response to trauma is for the noradrenergic system to maintain the arousal state, increase vigilance, and be protective to prevent subsequent trauma. Following massive trauma, neurotransmitters are depleted at the synapse level, which is associated with long-term depression and numbing. This depletion also leaves clients with a different threshold of sensitivity to their medications, which increases vulnerability to subsequent stress (Mackey et al, 1992).*

evolve WEBSITES FOR EDUCATION

See the EVOLVE website for World Wide Web resources for client education.

REFERENCES

Burgess AW, Dowdell EB, Prentky RA: Sexual abuse of nursing home residents, *J Psychosoc Nurs Ment Health Serv* 38(6):10, 2000.

Cochran M: Tears have no color, *Am J Nurs* 98(6):53, 1998.

D'Avanzo CE et al: Developing culturally informed strategies for substance-related interventions. In Naegle MA, D'Avanzo CE, editors: *Addictions and substance abuse: strategies for advanced practice nursing,* St Louis, 2001, Mosby.

Doswell W, Erlen J: Multicultural issues and ethical concerns in the delivery of nursing care interventions, *Nurs Clin North Am* 33(2):353, 1998.

Heineken J: Patient silence is not necessarily client satisfaction: communication in home care nursing, *Home Healthc Nurse* 16(2):115, 1998.

Leininger MM, McFarland MR: *Transcultural nursing: concepts, theories, research and practices,* ed 3, New York, 2002, McGraw-Hill.

Mackey T et al: Factors associated with long-term depressive symptoms of sexual assault victims, *Arch Psychiatr Nurs* 6(1):10, 1992.

McCleary PH: Female genitalia mutilation and childbirth: a case report, *Birth* 21(4):221, 1994.

Mollica RF, Lavelle J: Southeast Asian refugees. In Comas-Diaz L, Griffith EEH, editors: *Clinical guidelines in cross-cultural mental health,* New York, 1988, John Wiley and Sons.

Rape-trauma syndrome: silent reaction

Linda Hutson

NANDA Definition

Forced violent sexual act (penetration may not actually occur) (Ohio Revised Code) against victim's will and consent resulting in a trauma syndrome that includes an acute

● = Independent; ▲ = Collaborative

phase of disorganization of victim's lifestyle and a long-term process of reorganization of lifestyle

Defining Characteristics

Increased anxiety during interview (e.g., blocking of associations, long periods of silence, minor stuttering, physical distress); sudden onset of phobic reactions; lack of verbalization about the rape; abrupt changes in relationships with males; increased nightmares; pronounced changes in sexual behavior

Related Factors (r/t)

Rape; sexual assault; abuse

NOC   Outcomes (Nursing Outcomes Classification)

Suggested NOC Outcomes
Abuse Cessation; Abuse Protection; Abuse Recovery: Emotional, Sexual; Coping; Impulse Self-Control; Self-Mutilation Restraint

> **Example NOC Outcome with Indicators**
>
> **Abuse Recovery: Emotional** as evidenced by the following indicators: Acknowledgment of right to disclose abusive situation/Expression of right to have been protected from abuse (Rate each indicator of **Abuse Recovery: Emotional:** 1 = none, 2 = limited, 3 = moderate, 4 = substantial, 5 = extensive [see Section I].)

Client Outcomes

Client Will (Specify Time Frame):
- Resume previous level of relationships with significant others
- State improvement in sleep and fewer nightmares
- Express feelings about and discusses the rape (Nondisclosure about a sexual assault may arise out of self-protection, but this defensive coping style acts as a pressure cooker and is associated with more intense depressive symptoms. Clients should be assured that disclosure of an incident of sexual assault to a care provider or advocate has guaranteed confidentiality and does necessitate notification of law enforcement [Mackey et al, 1992].)
- Return to usual pattern of sexual behavior (Women who are sexually active after the assault report lower levels of depression [Mackey et al, 1992]. However, being sexually active cannot be construed to mean that the client has adjusted to or resolved the sexual trauma.)
- Remain free of phobic reactions

See the care plan for **Rape-trauma syndrome.**

NIC   Interventions (Nursing Interventions Classification)

Suggested NIC Interventions
Counseling; Support System Enhancement

• = Independent; ▲ = Collaborative

> **Example NIC Activities—Counseling**
>
> Encourage expression of feelings; Help client to identify strengths and reinforce these

Nursing Interventions and Rationales

- See the care plans for **Rape-trauma syndrome, Powerlessness, Ineffective Coping, Dysfunctional Grieving, Anxiety, Fear, Risk for self-directed Violence, Sexual dysfunction,** and **Impaired verbal Communication.**
- Observe for disruptions in relationships with significant others. *Poorly adjusted clients may elicit nonsupportive behavior from others or perceive the actions of others in a negative way.*
- Monitor for signs of increased anxiety (e.g., silence, stuttering, physical distress, irritability, unexplained crying spells).
- Focus on the client's coping strengths.
- Observe for changes in sexual behavior. *More than 80% of sexually active victims reported some sexual dysfunction as a result of the assault (Mackey et al, 1992). Some victims engage in sexual intimacy to prove to themselves and their partners that they are normal or unaffected by the assault.*
- Identify phobic reactions to persons or objects in the environment (e.g., strangers, doorbells, groups of people, knives).
- Provide support by listening when the client is ready to talk. **Clinical Research:** *In one study, delayed disclosure of childhood rape was very common and long delays were typical. Close friends are the most common confidants (Smith et al, 2000).*
- Be nonjudgmental when feelings are expressed. Explain that anger is normal and needs to be verbalized. Reassure the client with phrases such as, "I'm sorry this happened to you."
- Remain with an anxious client even if the client is silent. Use gentle speech and actions; move slowly.
- Evaluate somatic complaints. *Women are at higher risk for depression than men (Mackey et al, 1992).*

Geriatric

- A new subgroup of rape victims resides in nursing homes. Treatment is necessary. **Nursing Research:** *Nursing home victims can suffer both compound and silent rape trauma (Burgess, Dowdell, and Prentky, 2000).*
- See the care plan for **Rape-trauma syndrome.**

Multicultural

- Assess for the influence of cultural beliefs, norms, and values on the client's ability to cope with the trauma of the rape experience. **Nursing Research:** *What the client views as healthy coping may be based on cultural perceptions (Cochran, 1998; Doswell and Erlen, 1998; Leininger and McFarland, 2002).*
- Provide opportunities by which the family and individual can save face when working with Asian American clients. **Nursing Research:** *Asian American families and individuals may avoid situations and discussion of issues that they perceive will bring shame on the family unit (D'Avanzo et al, 2001).*

- = Independent; ▲ = Collaborative

- Assure the client of confidentiality. **Nursing Research:** *Many Indo-Chinese women will not discuss rape if they think that other staff members, their families, their husbands, or their community may find out (Mollica and Lavelle, 1988).*
- Allow the client to tell his or her rape story without probing. **Nursing Research:** *Through the rape story, the clinician can bridge the disrupted social connection that exists between the client, family, and community (Mollica and Lavelle, 1988).*

Home care
- See the care plan for **Rape-trauma syndrome.**

Client/Family Teaching
- Reassure the client that he or she is not bad and is not at fault. Avoid questions beginning with "why." *"Why" questions may sound judgmental and feed into self-blame.*
- ▲ Refer the client to a sexual assault counselor. *Long-term counseling may be necessary.*
- ▲ Offer information about testing, treatment, and procedures related to pregnancy, hepatitis B, and sexually transmitted infection. Do not wait for the client to request information.
- See the care plan for **Rape-trauma syndrome.**

evolve WEBSITES FOR EDUCATION

See the EVOLVE website for World Wide Web resources for client education.

REFERENCES

Burgess AW, Dowdell EB, Prentky RA: Sexual abuse of nursing home residents, *J Psychosoc Nurs Ment Health Serv* 38(6):10, 2000.
Cochran M: Tears have no color, *Am J Nurs* 98(6):53, 1998.
D'Avanzo CE et al: Developing culturally informed strategies for substance-related interventions. In Naegle MA, D'Avanzo CE, editors: *Addictions and substance abuse: strategies for advanced practice nursing,* St Louis, 2001, Mosby.
Doswell W, Erlen J: Multicultural issues and ethical concerns in the delivery of nursing care interventions, *Nurs Clin North Am* 33(2):353, 1998.
Leininger MM, McFarland MR: *Transcultural nursing: concepts, theories, research and practices,* ed 3, New York, 2002, McGraw-Hill.
Mackey et al: Factors associated with long-term depressive symptoms of sexual assault victims, *Arch Psychiatr Nurs* 6:10, 1992.
Mollica RF, Lavelle J: Southeast Asian refugees. In Comas-Diaz L, Griffith EEH, editors: *Clinical guidelines in cross-cultural mental health,* New York, 1988, John Wiley and Sons.
Smith DW et al: Delay in disclosure of childhood rape: results from a national survey, *Child Abuse Negl* 24(2):273, 2000.

Relocation stress syndrome

Betty J. Ackley and Gail B. Ladwig

NANDA Definition

Physiological and/or psychosocial disturbances that result from transfer from one environment to another

- • = Independent; ▲ = Collaborative

NOTE: Recent research on the nursing diagnosis of relocation stress syndrome may indicate that the nursing diagnosis is not valid or may not be valid when applied to group moves of clients (Mallick and Whipple, 2000). More research is needed in this area to validate this nursing intervention.

Defining Characteristics

Temporary and/or permanent move; voluntary and/or involuntary move; aloneness, alienation, or loneliness; depression; anxiety (e.g., separation); sleep disturbance; withdrawal; anger; loss of identity, self-worth, or self-esteem; increased verbalization of needs, unwillingness to move or concern over relocation; increased physical symptoms/illness (e.g., gastrointestinal disturbance, weight change); dependency; insecurity; pessimism; frustration; worry; fear

Related Factors (r/t)

Unpredictability of experience/isolation from family/friends; passive coping; language barrier; decreased health status; impaired psychosocial health; past, concurrent, and recent losses; feeling of powerlessness; lack of adequate support system/group; lack of predeparture counseling

NOC   Outcomes (Nursing Outcomes Classification)

Suggested NOC Outcomes

Anxiety Self-Control; Child Adaptation to Hospitalization; Coping; Depression Level; Depression Self-Control; Loneliness Severity; Psychosocial Adjustment: Life Change; Quality of Life

> ### Example NOC Outcome with Indicators
>
> **Anxiety Self-Control** as evidenced by the following indicators: Seeks information to reduce anxiety/Plans coping strategies for stressful situations/Uses effective coping strategies/Uses relaxation techniques to reduce anxiety/Maintains social relationships/Reports adequate sleep/Reports absence of physical manifestations of anxiety (Rate each indicator of **Anxiety Self-Control:** 1 = never demonstrated, 2 = rarely demonstrated, 3 = sometimes demonstrated, 4 = often demonstrated, 5 = consistently demonstrated [see Section I].)

Client Outcomes

Client Will (Specify Time Frame):

- Recognize and know the name of at least one staff member
- Express concern about move when encouraged to do so during individual contacts
- Carry out activities of daily living (ADLs) in usual manner
- Maintain previous mental and physical health status (e.g., nutrition, elimination, sleep, social interaction)

NIC   Interventions (Nursing Interventions Classification)

Suggested NIC Interventions

Anxiety Reduction; Coping Enhancement; Discharge Planning; Hope Instillation; Self-Responsibility Facilitation

• = Independent; ▲ = Collaborative

> **Example NIC Activities—Anxiety Reduction**
>
> Stay with client to promote safety and reduce fear; Provide objects that symbolize safeness

Nursing Interventions and Rationales

- Obtain a history, including the reason for the move, the client's usual coping mechanisms, history of losses, and family support for the client. *A history helps determine the amount of support needed and appropriate interventions to decrease relocation stress (Manion and Rantz, 1995).*
- If the client is an adolescent, try to avoid a move in the middle of the school year, find a newcomers' club for the adolescent to join, and refer for counseling if needed. *An adolescent who is relocating can experience emotional, social, and cognitive dysfunctions. The interventions listed can be helpful (Puskar and Dvorsak, 1991).*
- Provide support for a child and family who must relocate to be near a transplant center. **Nursing Research:** *Recognizing the unique needs of parents who must relocate for a child's transplantation procedure supports the delivery of individualized nursing care and the effective allocation of program resources (Stubblefield and Murray, 2002).*
- Observe the following procedures if the client is being transferred to a nursing home or adult foster care:
  - Allow the client to have a choice of placement and arrange a preadmission visit if possible. Having some control over the event strengthens problem-solving and coping strategies (Nypaver, Titus, and Brugler, 1996; Oleson and Shadick, 1993) and may help reduce mortality (Thorson and Davis, 2000).
  - If the client cannot choose placement, arrange for a visit or telephone call by a member of the staff to welcome the client and show a videotape or at least provide pictures of the new care facility.
  - Have a familiar person accompany the client to the new facility. This lessens client and family anxiety, confusion, and dissatisfaction (Manion and Rantz, 1995).
  - Validate the caregiver's feelings of difficulty with putting a loved one in a different environment. This is a distressing experience, and caregivers feel responsible. Validating their feelings will help establish a trusting relationship (Dellasega and Mastrian, 1995).
- Identify previous routines for ADLs. Try to maintain as much continuity with the previous schedule as possible. *Continuity of routines has been shown to be a crucial factor in positively influencing adjustment to a new environment (Manion and Rantz, 1995).*
- Bring in familiar items from home (e.g., pictures, clocks, afghans).
- Establish the way the client would like to be addressed (Mr., Mrs., Miss, first name, nickname). *Calling clients by the desired name shows respect.*
- Thoroughly orient the client to the new environment and routines; repeat directions as needed. *The stress of the move may interfere with the client's ability to remember directions (Harkulich, 1992).*
- Spend one-on-one time with the client. Allow the client to express feelings and convey acceptance of them; emphasize that the client's feelings are real and individual and that it is acceptable to be sad or angry about moving. *Expressing feelings can help the client adjust to the situation.*

- = Independent; ▲ = Collaborative

- Assign the same staff members to the client; maintain consistency in the personnel the client interacts with. *Consistency hastens adjustment (Harkulich, 1992).*
- Ask the client to state one positive aspect of the new living situation each day. *Helping the client to focus on the positive aspects of the move can help change attitude and reframe the situation in a positive fashion.*
- Monitor the client's health status and provide appropriate interventions for problems with social interaction, nutrition, sleep, new onset of infection, or elimination problems. *Stress from the transfer can cause physiological and psychological disturbances (Barnhouse, Brugler, and Harkulich, 1992; Lander, Brazill, and Ladrigan, 1997).* **Clinical Research:** *Clients who moved showed lower natural killer cell immunity 1 month after moving than was shown by a control group of elderly who did not move (Lutgendorf et al, 1999).*
- If the client is being transferred within a facility, have staff members from the new unit visit the client before transfer.
- Once the client is transferred, have previous staff make occasional visits until the client is comfortable in the new surroundings. **Nursing Research:** *Participants in one study discussed a desire for normality and indicated that leaving the ICU staff was the most negative component of transfer (McKinney and Deeny, 2002).*
- Watch for coping problems (e.g., withdrawal, regression, or angry behavior) and intervene immediately. *Failure to cope in a timely manner may cause a permanent pattern of impaired adjustment (Oleson and Shadick, 1993).*
- Allow the client to grieve for the loss of the old situation; explain that it is normal to feel sadness over change and loss.
- Allow the client to participate in care as much as possible and make decisions when possible (e.g., placement of the bed, choice of roommate, bathing routines). Make an effort to accommodate the client. *Having choices helps prevent feelings of powerlessness that may lead to depression.*

Geriatric

- Monitor the need for transfer and transfer only when necessary. *Elderly clients often adapt poorly to transfer; they can lose normal functioning in areas such as self-care (Lander, Brazill, and Ladrigan, 1997), and relocation may even cause death (Rantz and Egan, 1987; Thorson and Davis, 2000).*
- Protect the client from injuries such as falls. *An increase in the number of accidents in frail elderly can occur with relocation (Lander, Brazill, and Ladrigan, 1997).*
- After the transfer, determine the client's mental status. Document and observe for any new onset of confusion. *Confusion can follow relocation because of the overwhelming stress and sensory overload.*
- Refer for music therapy. **Nursing Research:** *One case study indicated that music therapy may facilitate a resident's adjustment to life in a long-term-care facility (Kydd, 2001).*
- Use reality orientation if needed (e.g., "Today is . . .," "The date is . . .," "You are at . . . facility"). Repeat the information as needed and provide a clock or calendar. *Reality orientation can be helpful to prevent new onset of confusion (Manion and Rantz, 1995).*

Client/Family Teaching

- Teach family members about relocation stress syndrome. Encourage them to monitor for signs of the syndrome. *Acceptance of the new living situation begins within 6 to*

● = **Independent;** ▲ = **Collaborative**

8 weeks after institutionalization, and adjustment is usually complete within 3 to 6 months (Manion and Rantz, 1995).

- Help significant others learn how to support the client in the move by setting up a schedule of visits, arranging for holidays, bringing familiar items from home, and establishing a system for contact when the client needs support.

evolve WEBSITES FOR EDUCATION

See the EVOLVE website for World Wide Web resources for client education.

REFERENCES

Barnhouse AH, Brugler CJ, Harkulich JT: Relocation stress syndrome, *Nurs Diagn* 3(4):166, 1992.
Dellasega C, Mastrian K: The process and consequences of institutionalizing an elder, *West J Nurs Res* 17(2): 123, 1995.
Harkulich JT: Relocation stress. In Gettrust K, Brabeck PD, editors: *Nursing diagnosis in clinical practice: guides for care planning*, Albany, NY, 1992, Delmar.
Kydd P: Using music therapy to help a client with Alzheimer's disease adapt to long-term care, *Am J Alzheimers Dis Other Demen* 16(2):103, 2001.
Lander SM, Brazill AL, Ladrigan PM: Intrainstitutional relocation: effects on residents' behavior and psychosocial functioning, *J Gerontol Nurs* 23(4):35, 1997.
Lutgendorf SK et al: Sense of coherence moderates the relationship between life stress and natural killer cell activity in healthy older adults, *Psychol Aging* 14(4):552, 1999.
Mallick MJ, Whipple TW: Validity of the nursing diagnosis of relocation stress syndrome, *Nurs Res* 49(2):97, 2000.
Manion PD, Rantz MJ: Relocation stress syndrome: a comprehensive plan for long-term care admissions, *Geriatr Nurs* 16(3):108, 1995.
McKinney AA, Deeny P: Leaving the intensive care unit: a phenomenological study of the patients' experience, *Intensive Crit Care Nurs* 18(6):320, 2002.
Nypaver JM, Titus M, Brugler CJ: Patient transfer to rehabilitation: just another move? Relocation stress syndrome, *Rehabil Nurs* 21(2):94, 1996.
Oleson M, Shadick KM: Application of Moos' and Schaefer's model to nursing care of elderly persons relocating to a nursing home, *J Adv Nurs* 18:479, 1993.
Puskar KR, Dvorsak KG: Relocation stress in adolescents: helping teenagers cope with a moving dilemma, *Pediatr Nurs* 17(3):295, 1991.
Rantz M, Egan K: Reducing death from translocation syndrome, *Am J Nurs* 87(9):1351, 1987.
Stubblefield C, Murray RL: Waiting for lung transplantation: family experiences of relocation, *Pediatr Nurs* 28(5):501, 2002.
Thorson JA, Davis RE: Relocation of the institutionalized aged, *J Clin Psychol* 56(1):131, 2000.

Risk for Relocation stress syndrome

Betty J. Ackley and Gail B. Ladwig

NANDA Definition

At risk for physiological and/or psychosocial disturbances that result from transfer from one environment to another

Risk Factors

Moderate to high degree of environmental change (e.g., physical, ethnic, cultural); temporary and/or permanent move; voluntary and/or involuntary move; lack of adequate sup-

- = Independent; ▲ = Collaborative

port system/group; feelings of powerlessness; moderate mental competence (e.g., alert enough to experience changes); unpredictability of experiences; decreased psychosocial or physical health status; lack of predeparture counseling; passive coping; past, current, or recent losses

NOC Outcomes (Nursing Outcomes Classification)

Suggested NOC Outcomes

Anxiety Self-Control; Child Adaptation to Hospitalization; Coping; Loneliness Severity; Psychosocial Adjustment: Life Change; Quality of Life

---

Example NOC Outcome with Indicators

Anxiety Self-Control as evidenced by the following indicators: Seeks information to reduce anxiety/ Plans coping strategies for stressful situations/Uses effective coping strategies/Uses relaxation techniques to reduce anxiety/Maintains social relationships/Reports adequate sleep/Reports absence of physical manifestations of anxiety (Rate each indicator of **Anxiety Self-Control**: 1 = never demonstrated, 2 = rarely demonstrated, 3 = sometimes demonstrated, 4 = often demonstrated, 5 = consistently demonstrated [see Section I].)

Client Outcomes

Client Will (Specify Time Frame):

- Recognize and know name of at least one staff member
- Express concern about move when encouraged to do so during individual contacts
- Carry out activities of daily living in usual manner
- Maintain previous mental and physical health status (e.g., nutrition, elimination, sleep, social interaction)

NIC Interventions (Nursing Interventions Classification)

Suggested NIC Interventions

Anxiety Reduction; Coping Enhancement; Discharge Planning; Hope Instillation; Self-Responsibility Facilitation

---

Example NIC Activities—Anxiety Reduction

Stay with the client to promote safety and reduce fear; Provide objects that symbolize safeness

---

Nursing Interventions and Rationales and Client/Family Teaching

- Adequately prepare the client and family for transfer from the ICU. *Discharge from specialized care environments can actually be as traumatic as admission. This phenomenon has become known as transfer anxiety, relocation anxiety, or translocation anxiety when routines, environments, and/or invasive monitoring procedures are altered or ceased without prior knowledge, preparation, or adequate explanation (Coyle, 2001).*
- Assist caregivers with the use of respite care for family members, acknowledge the importance of the caregivers' role, and seek their assistance in planning the client's

• = Independent; ▲ = Collaborative

care. **Nursing Research:** *The research findings highlight the need for nurses and other formal caregivers to place themselves in a secondary and supporting caregiving role, to acknowledge the family caregivers as the primary caregivers, and to use family caregivers' in-depth and intimate knowledge of the needs of their relative to inform care within the institutional setting (Gilmour, 2002).*

- Relocation to more supportive housing is a potentially stressful life event for an older adult. Nurses have a critical role to play in helping the family identify the most appropriate housing alternative, assisting in planning the relocation, and helping older adults, especially ethnic elders, adjust to their new homes. *Relocation is particularly stressful for ethnic elders who may not understand the housing options available or may fear prejudicial treatment and exclusion in the various settings. Nurses need to take time to carefully assess the older adults' preferences and to provide information needed to help them make relocation decisions within the context of their existing support networks (Johnson and Tripp-Reimer, 2001).*

▲ Consider 24-hour in-home care as an alternative to nursing home placement. **Nursing Research:** *In one community, programs of home care services for the elderly were reorganized to provide around-the-clock in-home nursing and home help services 7 days a week (ACC). Evidence from the analysis indicated that ACC might contribute to less use of institutionalization as an alternative to home care, even though, in some instances, institutionalization is the only appropriate alternative (Murashima and Asahara, 2003).*

- Provide support for spouses who have placed a partner in a care home. Support a continued relationship with the partner. *One article indicates that the relationship between care home staff and families is often superficial and strained. There is a need for more proactive efforts to facilitate a partnership between care home staff and families (Sandberg, Lundh, and Nolan, 2001).*

- Refer to the care plan for **Relocation stress syndrome.**

evolve WEBSITES FOR EDUCATION

See the EVOLVE website for World Wide Web resources for client education.

REFERENCES

Coyle MA: Transfer anxiety: preparing to leave intensive care, *Intensive Crit Care Nurs* 17(3):138, 2001.

Gilmour JA: Dis/integrated care: family caregivers and in-hospital respite care, *J Adv Nurs* 39(6):546, 2002.

Johnson RA, Tripp-Reimer T: Relocation among ethnic elders. A review—part 2, *J Gerontol Nurs* 27(6):22, 2001.

Murashima S, Asahara K: The effectiveness of the around-the-clock in-home care system: did it prevent the institutionalization of frail elderly? *Public Health Nurs* 20(1):13, 2003.

Sandberg J, Lundh U, Nolan MR: Placing a spouse in a care home: the importance of keeping, *J Clin Nurs* 10(3):406, 2001.

• = **Independent;** ▲ = **Collaborative**

Ineffective Role performance

Gail B. Ladwig

NANDA Definition

Patterns of behavior and self-expression that do not match the environmental context, norms, and expectations

Defining Characteristics

Change in self-perception of role; role denial; inadequate external support for role enactment; inadequate adaptation to change or transition, system conflict; change in usual patterns of responsibility; discrimination; domestic violence; harassment uncertainty; altered role perceptions; role strain; inadequate self-management; role ambivalence; pessimistic attitude; inadequate motivation; inadequate confidence; inadequate role competency and skills; inadequate knowledge; inappropriate developmental expectations; role conflict; role confusion; powerlessness; inadequate coping; anxiety or depression; role overload; change in other's perception or role; role dissatisfaction; inadequate opportunities for role enactment

Related Factors (r/t)

Social

Inadequate or inappropriate linkage with the health care system; job schedule demands; young age; developmental level; lack of rewards; poverty; family conflict; inadequate support system; inadequate role socialization (e.g., role model, expectations responsibilities); low socioeconomic status; stress and conflict; domestic violence; lack of resources

Knowledge

Inadequate role preparation (e.g., role transition, skill, rehearsal, validation); lack of knowledge about role, role skills; role transition; lack of opportunity for role rehearsal; developmental transitions; unrealistic role expectations; education attainment level; lack of or inadequate role model

Physiological

Inadequate/inappropriate linkage with health care system; substance abuse; mental illness; body image alteration; physical illness; cognitive deficits; health alterations (e.g., physical health, body image, self-esteem, mental health, psychosocial health, cognitive, learning style, neurological health); depression; low self-esteem; pain; fatigue

NOTE: There is typology of roles: sociopersonal (friendship, family, marital, parenting, community), home management intimacy (sexuality, relationship building), leisure/exercise/recreation, self-management, socialization (developmental transitions), community contributor, and religious.

NOC Outcomes (Nursing Outcomes Classification)

Suggested NOC Outcomes

Coping; Psychosocial Adjustment: Life Change

• = Independent; ▲ = Collaborative

> **Example NOC Outcome with Indicators**
>
> **Coping** as evidenced by the following indicators: Identifies effective and ineffective coping patterns/Modifies lifestyle as needed (Rate each indicator of **Coping:** 1 = never demonstrated, 2 = rarely demonstrated, 3 = sometimes demonstrated, 4 = often demonstrated, 5 = consistently demonstrated [see Section I].)

Client Outcomes

Client Will (Specify Time Frame):
- Identify realistic perception of role
- State personal strengths
- Acknowledge problems contributing to inability to carry out usual role
- Accept physical limitations regarding role responsibility and consider ways to change lifestyle to accomplish goals associated with role performance
- Demonstrate knowledge of appropriate behaviors associated with new or changed role
- State knowledge of change in responsibility and new behaviors associated with new responsibility
- Verbalize acceptance of new responsibility

NIC   Interventions (Nursing Interventions Classification)

Suggested NIC Intervention
Role Enhancement

> **Example NIC Activities—Role Enhancement**
>
> Help the client to identify behaviors needed for new or changed roles; Help the client to identify positive strategies for managing role changes

Nursing Interventions and Rationales
- Observe the client's knowledge of behaviors associated with role. *Ability to perform perceived roles is easily hampered by illness. It is important to note whether or not the client feels capable of functioning in the usual role.*
- Allow the client to express feelings regarding the role change. **Nursing Research:** *In a study to determine how cancer affects men's role as a father this central theme—change in self-image as a man and as a parent—was generated. This theme consists of the subthemes gaining control, balancing emotions, subjective well-being, being open or not toward the family, and challenges in family life and to family well-being (Elmberger and Bolund, 2002).*
- Ask the client direct questions regarding new roles and how the health care system can help him or her continue in roles. **Nursing Research:** *This article suggests that best practice with regard to communication in palliative care could be achieved by using a sensitive assessment of how each client chooses to cope with his or her situation rather than a uniform approach to care (Dean, 2002).*
- Assist new parents to adjust to changes in workload associated with childbirth. **Clinical Research:** *Expectant parents in this study anticipated increase in workload after childbirth. Work increases were greater for women than men (Gjerdingen, 2000).*

- • = Independent; ▲ = Collaborative

- Reinforce the client's strengths, have the client identify past coping skills, and support the continued use of these skills. **Clinical Research:** *Behavioral change is facilitated by a personal sense of control. If people believe that they can take action to solve a problem instrumentally, they become more inclined to do so and feel more committed to this decision (Schwarzer and Fuchs, 1995).*
- Have the client make a list of strengths that are needed for the new role. Acknowledge which strengths the client has and which strengths need to be developed. Work with the client to set goals for desired role. *In setting valued goals, people adapt their world to self-generated needs and projects rather than adapting themselves to a given world (Nuttin, 1992).*
- Have the client list problems associated with the new role and identify ways of overcoming them (e.g., if pain is worse late in day, have the client complete necessary role tasks early in day). *There are many ways to accomplish tasks; help the client recognize this and make the appropriate accommodations.*
- Provide parents with coping skills when the role change is associated with a critically ill child. **Nursing Research:** *Results from mothers who received the Creating Opportunities for Parent Empowerment (COPE) program indicate the need to educate parents regarding their children's responses as they recover from critical illness and how they can assist their children in coping with the stressful experience (Melnyk et al, 1997).*
- Assist parents in coping with infants with colic, a condition common in infants. **Nursing Research:** *Even though nursing interventions do not cure infant colic, the amount of crying may be reduced and life made easier for the families if the parents are offered help in coping with the situation (Helseth et al, 2002).*
- Assist families with life beyond the hospital when living with the illness of a child. Teach family members to value the small things children do, connect with other families, locate community resources, and understand the short- and long-term needs of the child. *Family-focused activities can help families cope better with the hospital experience. To promote optimal healing, health care providers must recognize that a family's life goes on after the hospital stay. Many stresses make life difficult for families. Most families are resilient, but many can benefit from help with managing the transition from hospital to home (Worthington, 1995).*
- Support the client's religious practices. **Clinical Research:** *Religion plays a role in helping clients cope with illness and the outcomes of illness (Koenig, Larson, and Larson, 2001).*
- Identify ways to compensate for physical disabilities (e.g., have a ramp built to provide access to house, put household objects within the client's reach from wheelchair). *Helping clients to help themselves by modifying the environment enhances self-esteem and fosters a sense of power because they remain able to function in their role.*
- See care plans for **Readiness for enhanced family Coping, Impaired Home maintenance, Impaired Parenting, Risk for Loneliness, Readiness for enhanced community Coping,** and **Ineffective Sexuality patterns.**

Geriatric

▲ Support the client's religious beliefs and activities and provide appropriate spiritual support persons. **Clinical Research:** *The findings from this study suggest that religious coping is a common behavior that is inversely related to depression in hospitalized elderly men (Koenig et al, 1992).*
- Encourage the use of humor by family caregivers to describe their role reversal. **Clini-**

• = **Independent;** ▲ = **Collaborative**

cal Research: *This study suggested that humor is a useful communication tool for family caregivers that release nervous energy (Bethea et al, 2000).*

▲ Explore community needs after assessing the client's strengths. Suggest functional activities (e.g., being a foster grandparent or a mentor for small businesses). *If physical strength is declining, activities that require less physical prowess and more mental expertise are sometimes appropriate (Ringsven and Bond, 1991).*

▲ Refer to appropriate support groups for adjustment to role changes. **Nursing Research:** *Health care professionals should provide information on PD symptom management, identify appropriate resources to reduce caregiver burden, and use of support groups (Edwards et al, 2002).* **Nursing Research:** *Significant differences were found for distress levels and quality of life, with the mutual support group having greater improvements than the control group for dementia family caregivers (Fung and Chien, 2002).*

▲ Refer to home health agency for home visits when there is an infant who has excessive crying. **Nursing Research:** *Almost every aspect of family life was disrupted when there was an infant who cried excessively, resulting in strained relationships, feelings of guilt, and concerns about losing control. This study showed the benefit of a health visitor to support parents. This visitor needed to visit frequently, stay for a prolonged period; demonstrate engagement with the family and its difficulties, and impart specific messages with conviction and sincerity (Long and Johnson, 2001).*

▲ Refer to therapy to improve memory for patients with Alzheimer disease. **Clinical Research:** *The available evidence shows that alternative and innovative ways of memory rehabilitation for Alzheimer's patients can indeed be clinically effective or pragmatically useful with a great potential for use within the new culture of a more graded and proactive type of Alzheimer's disease care (De Vreese et al, 2001).*

Multicultural

• Assess for the influence of cultural beliefs, norms, values, and expectations on the individual's role. **Nursing Research:** *The individual's role may be based on cultural perceptions (Cochran, 1998; Doswell and Erlen, 1998; Leininger and McFarland, 2002).*

• Assess for conflicts between the caregiver's cultural role obligations and competing factors like employment. **Nursing Research:** *Conflicts between cultural expectations and competing factors can increase role stress (Jones, 1996).*

• Negotiate with the client regarding the aspects of their role that can be modified and still honor cultural beliefs. **Nursing Research:** *Give and take with the client will lead to culturally congruent care (Leininger and McFarland, 2002).*

• Encourage family to use support groups or other service programs to assist with role changes. **Nursing Research:** *Studies indicate that minority families of clients with dementia use few support programs even though these programs could have a positive impact on caregiver well-being (Cox, 1999).*

• Validate the individual's feelings regarding the impact of role changes on family and personal lifestyle. **Nursing Research:** *Validation lets the client know that the nurse has heard and understands what was said (Heineken, 1998).*

Home care

• Above interventions may be adapted for home care use.

• Determine the anticipated duration of role change. *Knowing the anticipated duration of role change helps the client and significant others determine the acceptability of role change, role conflict, and changes in communication patterns.*

• = **Independent;** ▲ = **Collaborative**

- Assess family's ability to physically or psychologically assume responsibilities of decrease or change in the client's role function. *The health, abilities, or other role expectations of caregivers or significant others may prohibit the assumption of responsibilities once held by the client.*
- ▲ Offer a referral to medical social services to assist with assessing the short- and long-term impacts of role change. *Social workers may assist clients with life care planning (Rice et al, 2000). Collaboration with specialists provides the client with greater resources for adaptation. Terminally ill clients may see the transition of role responsibilities as a task that must be completed before dying. Resolution of role transition will reassure the client, allow remaining energy to be focused elsewhere, and may give the client permission to die.*

Client/Family Teaching

- Teach significant others about health care changes to expect when the client returns home. **Nursing Research:** *All spouses, male and female, expressed uncertainty about their roles and what their partner could do after discharge (McSweeney, 1993).*
- ▲ Help the client identify resources for assistance in caring for a disabled or aging parent (e.g., adult day care). **Nursing Research:** *The wives of men with COPD in this phenomenological study were dissatisfied with their lack of recreation, as well as support from friends, families and health care providers (Bergs, 2002).*
- ▲ Refer to appropriate community agencies to learn skills for functioning in the new or changed role (e.g., vocational rehabilitation, parenting classes, hospice, respite care). *As one person changes, other family members need to alter their patterns of communication and behavior to maintain balance. Family members also need assistance with developing these new skills (Barry, 1994).*

evolve WEBSITES FOR EDUCATION

See the EVOLVE website for World Wide Web resources for client education.

REFERENCES

Barry P: *Mental health and mental illness,* ed 5, Philadelphia, 1994, Lippincott.
Bergs D: "The Hidden Client"—women caring for husbands with COPD: their experience of quality of life, *J Clin Nurs* 11(5):613, 2002.
Bethea LS, Travis SS, Pecchioni L: Family caregivers' use of humor in conveying information about caring for dependent older adults, *Health Commun* 12(4):361, 2000.
Cochran M: Tears have no color, *Am J Nurs* 98(6):53, 1998.
Cox C: Race and caregiving: patterns of service use by African American and white caregivers of persons with Alzheimer's, *J Gerontol Soc Work* 32(2):5, 1999.
De Vreese LP et al: Memory rehabilitation in Alzheimer's disease: a review of progress, *Int J Geriatr Psychiatry* 16(8):794, 2001.
Dean A: Talking to dying clients of their hopes and needs, *Nurs Times* 98(43):34, 2002.
Doswell W, Erlen J: Multicultural issues and ethical concerns in the delivery of revising care interventions, *Nurs Clin North Am* 33(2):353, 1998.
Edwards NE et al: Predictors of burden for caregivers of patients with Parkinson's disease, *J Neurosci Nurs* 34(4):184, 2002.
Elmberger E, Bolund C: Men with cancer. Changes in attempts to master the self-image as a man and as a parent, *Cancer Nurs* 25(6):477, 2002.
Fung WY, Chien WT: The effectiveness of a mutual support group for family caregivers of a relative with dementia, *Arch Psychiatr Nurs* 16(3):134, 2002.

• = **Independent;** ▲ = **Collaborative**

Gjerdingen D: Expectant parents' anticipated changes in workload after the birth of their first child, *J Fam Pract* 49(11):993, 2000.

Heineken J: Patient silence is not necessarily client satisfaction: communication in home care nursing, *Home Healthc Nurse* 16(2):115, 1998.

Helseth S et al: Help in times of crying: nurses' approach to parents with colicky infants, *J Adv Nurs* 40(3):267, 2002.

Jones PS: Asian American women caring for elderly parents, *J Fam Nurs* 2(1):56, 1996.

Koenig HG, Larson DB, Larson SS: Religion and coping with serious medical illness, *Ann Pharmacother* 35(3): 352, 2001.

Koenig H et al: Religious coping and depression among elderly, hospitalized medically ill men, *Am J Psychiatry* 149(12):1693, 1992.

Leininger MM, McFarland MR: *Transcultural nursing: concepts, theories, research and practices,* ed 3, New York, 2002, McGraw-Hill.

Long T, Johnson M: Living and coping with excessive infantile crying, *J Adv Nurs* 34(2):155, 2001.

McSweeney J: Making behavior changes after a myocardial infarction, *West J Nurs Res* 5:441, 1993.

Melnyk B et al: Helping mothers cope with a critically ill child: a pilot test of the COPE intervention, *Res Nurs Health* 20(1):3, 1997.

Nuttin J: Motivation, intention, and volition. In Fleury J, editor: The application of motivational theory to cardiovascular risk reduction, *Image J Nurs Sch* 24:229, 1992.

Rice J, Hicks PB, Wiehe V: Life care planning: a role for social workers, *Soc Work Health Care* 31(1):85, 2000.

Ringsven M, Bond D: *Gerontology and leadership skills for nurses,* Albany, NY, 1991, Delmar.

Schwarzer R, Fuchs R: Self-efficacy and health behaviors. In Conner M, Norman P, editors: *Predicting health behaviour: research and practice with social cognition models,* Buckingham, 1995, Open University Press.

Worthington R: Effective transitions for families: life beyond the hospital, *Pediatr Nurs* 21(1):86, 1995.

Bathing/hygiene Self-care deficit

Linda S. Williams

NANDA Definition

Impaired ability to perform or complete bathing/hygiene activities for oneself

Defining Characteristics

Inability to: wash body or body parts; obtain or get to water source; regulate temperature or flow of bath water; get bath supplies; dry body; get in and out of bathroom
Impaired physical mobility-functional level classification:
0—Completely independent
1—Requires use of equipment or device
2—Requires help from another person for assistance, supervision, or teaching
3—Requires help from another person and equipment or device
4—Dependent (does not participate in activity)

Related Factors (r/t)

Decreased or lack of motivation; weakness and tiredness; severe anxiety; inability to perceive body part or spatial relationship; perceptual or cognitive impairment; pain; neuromuscular impairment; musculoskeletal impairment; environmental barriers

NOC Outcomes (Nursing Outcomes Classification)

Suggested NOC Outcomes
Self-Care: Activities of Daily Living (ADL), Bathing, Hygiene

• = Independent; ▲ = Collaborative

> ### Example NOC Outcome with Indicators
>
> **Self-Care: Activities of Daily Living (ADLs)** as evidenced by the following indicators: Bathing/Hygiene (Rate each indicator of **Self-Care: Activities of Daily Living [ADL]:** 1 = severely compromised, 2 = substantially compromised, 3 = moderately compromised, 4 = mildly compromised, 5 = not compromised [see Section I].)

Client Outcomes

Client Will (Specify Time Frame):

- Remain free of body odor and maintain intact skin
- State satisfaction with ability to use adaptive devices to bathe
- Bathe with assistance of caregiver as needed without anxiety
- Explain and use methods to bathe safely and with minimal difficulty

NIC   Interventions (Nursing Interventions Classification)

Suggested NIC Interventions

Bathing; Self-Care Assistance: Bathing/Hygiene

> ### Example NIC Activities—Self-Care Assistance: Bathing/Hygiene
>
> Monitor the client's ability for independent self-care; Provide assistance until the client is fully able to assume self-care

Nursing Interventions and Rationales

- If in a typical bathing setting for the client, assess the client's ability to bathe self via direct observation using physical performance tests for ADLs. *Observation of bathing performed in an atypical bathing setting may result in false data for which use of a physical performance test compensates to provide more accurate ability data (Guralnik, 1994).*
- Ask the client for input on bathing habits and cultural bathing preferences. *Creating opportunities for guiding personal care honors long-standing routines, increases control, prevents learned helplessness, and preserves self-esteem (Miller, 1997). Cultural preferences are respected (Freeman, 1997).*
- Develop a bathing care plan based on the client's own history of bathing practices that addresses skin needs, self-care needs, client response to bathing and equipment needs. *Bathing is a healing rite and should not be routinely scheduled with a task focus. It should be a comforting experience for the client that enhances health (Rader et al, 1996).*
- Individualize bathing by identifying function of bath (e.g., odor or urine removal), frequency required to achieve function, and best bathing form (e.g., towel bathing, tub, or shower) to meet client preferences, preserve client dignity, make bathing a soothing experience, and reduce client aggression. *Individualized bathing produces a more positive bathing experience and preserves client dignity. Client aggression is increased with shower (especially) and tub bathing. Towel bathing increases privacy and eliminates need to move the client to central bathing area; therefore it is a more soothing experience than either showering or tub bathing (Hoeffer et al, 1997; Miller, 1997; Rader et al, 1996).*
- ▲ Request referrals for occupational and physical therapy. *Collaboration and correlation of*

• = **Independent;** ▲ = **Collaborative**

activities with interdisciplinary team members increases the client's mastery of self-care tasks (Schemm and Gitlin, 1998).

- Plan activities to prevent fatigue during bathing and seat the client with feet supported. *Energy conservation increases activity tolerance and promotes self-care.*
- Provide pain relief measures: ice packs, heat, analgesics 45 minutes before bathing if needed. *Pain relief promotes participation in self-care.*
- Consider environmental and human factors that may limit bathing ability, such as bending to get into tub, reaching required for bathing items, grasping force needed for faucets, and lifting of self. Adapt environment by placing items within easy reach, lowering faucets, and using a handheld shower. *Environmental factors affect task performance. Function can be improved based on engineering principles that adapt environmental factors to the meet the client's capabilities (Rogers et al, 1998).*
- Use any necessary adaptive bathing equipment (e.g., long-handled brushes, soap-on-a-rope, washcloth mitt, wall bars, tub bench, shower chair, commode chair without pan in shower). *Adaptive devices extend the client's reach, increase speed and safety, and decrease exertion. Identification of the client's likelihood using devices such as the long-handled brush allows for alternate device planning (Rogers et al, 2002).*
- Provide privacy: have only one caregiver providing bathing assistance, encourage a traffic-free bathing area, and post privacy signs. *The client perceives less privacy if more than one caregiver participates or if bathing takes place in a central bathing area in a high-traffic location that allows staff to enter freely during care (Miller, 1997).*
- Keep the client warmly covered. *Clients, especially elderly clients, who are prone to hypothermia may experience evaporative cooling during and after bathing, which produces an unpleasant cold sensation (Miller, 1997).*
- Allow the client to participate as able in bathing. Smile and provide praise for accomplishments in a relaxed manner. *The client's expenditure of energy provides the caregiver the opportunity to convey respect for a well-done task, which increases the client's self-esteem. Smiling and being relaxed are associated with a calm, functional client response (Maxfield et al, 1996).*
- Inspect skin condition during bathing. *Observation of skin allows detection of skin problems.*
- Use or encourage caregiver to use an unhurried, caring touch. *The basic human need of touch offers reassurance and comfort.*
- If the client is bathing alone, place assistance call light within reach. *A readily available signaling device promotes safety and provides reassurance for the client.*
- Nurture personal attributes such as humor, positive attitude, faith and hope and control of stress for clients with multiple sclerosis. **Nursing Research:** *For those with multiple sclerosis, personal attributes intervene between emotional distress and ADL functioning by decreasing a stress appraisal response (Gulick, 2001).* **Nursing Research:** *Continue rehabilitation efforts with poststroke client's long term to achieve optimal functioning. Client improvement may continue 6 months or longer post-stroke (Cavanagh et al, 2002).*

Geriatric

- Develop client muscle strength building plan to build the client's physiological capacity. **Nursing Research:** *Elders may have little reserve capacity but building physiological capacity may allow continued functioning during periods of illness or stress (Leidy and Haase, 1999).*

- = Independent; ▲ = Collaborative

- Include exercise and walking program in plan of care. *Exercise for flexibility, strengthening and a walking program in the hospital promotes ADLs, prevents injury, increases quality of life and may delay admission to a long-term care facility (Hart et al, 2002; Penninx, 2001).* **Nursing Research:** *Discuss in advance with client bathing schedule and identify specific bathing tasks the client will perform. Client's task performance may be affected by a loss of individual control due to frustration from not being able to anticipate timing of care events, an inability to predict if nurse or client would perform tasks and perception that nurse permission is necessary before performing a task (Brubaker, 1996).*
- Assess self-efficacy (The Self-Efficacy for Functional Activities scale); assess outcome expectations (Outcome Expectations for Functional Activities scale). Based on assessment promote motivation and self-efficacy for ADL functioning by: role modeling via videotape or partnering; verbal encouragement; individualize care using humor, kindness, joy and excitement with achievements; social supports; and decrease unpleasant sensations with the ADL function. *Assessment and interventions for self-efficacy strengthen client efficacy expectations and improve functional performance (Resnick, 2002).*
- Provide same type of bathrobe and bathing articles, such as scented dusting powder and bath oil, that the client used previously. *Use of sensory channels to stimulate memory may help foster understanding of bathing and self-care (Danner et al, 1993).*
- Assess for grieving resulting from loss of function. *Grief resulting from loss of function can inhibit relearning of self-care.*
- Arrange bathing environment to promote sensory comfort: reduce noise of voices and water and decrease glare from tiles, white walls, and artificial lights. *Noise discomfort can result from high-echo tiled walls, loud voices, and running water. Glare can cause visual discomfort, especially in clients with visual changes or cataracts (Miller, 1997).*
- When bathing a cognitively impaired client, have all bathing items ready for the client's needs before bathing begins. *Injury often occurs when cognitively impaired client is left alone to obtain forgotten items (Sloane et al, 1995).*
- Bathe elderly clients before bedtime to improve sleep. *An evening bath helps elderly clients sleep better (Kanda et al, 1999).*
- Bathe cognitively impaired clients before bedtime. *Bathing a cognitively impaired client in the evening helps improve symptoms of dementia (Deguchi et al, 1999).*
- Limit bathing to once or twice a week; provide a partial bath at other times. *Frequent bathing promotes skin dryness. Reducing frequency of bathing decreases aggressive behavior in cognitively impaired clients (Hoeffer et al, 1997).*
- Allow the client or caregiver adequate time to complete the bathing activity. *Significant aging increases the time required to complete a task; therefore, elderly individuals with a self-care deficit require more time to complete a task.*
- Use a nondetergent, no-rinse cleanser for bed-bathing rather than soap and water. **Nursing Research:** *Nondetergent, no-rinse cleanser bathing reduces skin tears and saves money for skin tear treatment costs, reduces bathing time and eliminates soap residue on the skin (Burch and Coggins, 2003).*
- Avoid soap or use only mild soap on genital and axillary areas; rinse well. *Soap can alter skin pH and thus skin defenses, and it may increase skin dryness that results from decreased oil and perspiration production in the elderly (Skewes, 1997).*
- Use tepid water: test water temperature before use with armometer. *Hot water promotes skin dryness and may burn a client with decreased sensation.*
- Use a gentle touch when bathing; avoid vigorous scrubbing motions. *Aging skin is thinner, more fragile, and less able to withstand mechanical friction than younger skin.*

- **= Independent; ▲ = Collaborative**

- Add hydrating bath oils to tub bath water 15 minutes after the client immerses in water. *Client's skin is coated with oil rather than being hydrated if bath oil is placed in water before the client's skin is moistened with water (Skewes, 1997).*

Home care

▲ Based on functional assessment and rehabilitation capacity, refer for home health aide services to assist with bathing and hygiene. *Support by home health aides preserves the energy of the client and provides respite for caregivers.*
- Turn down temperature of hot water heater. **Nursing Research:** *Prevent accidental scalding by reducing thermostat on water heater (Gerdner, 2002).*
- Show caregiver videotape of caregiver self-care activities (organizing day, talking when frustrated, self-time, and nonjudgmental person with whom to talk) followed by a discussion. **Nursing Research:** *Videotape intervention and discussion can model self-care activities and buffer caregiver stress (Clark and Lester, 2000).*
- Cue cognitively impaired clients in steps of hygiene. *Cognitively impaired clients can successfully participate in many activities with cueing, and participation in self-care can enhance their self-esteem.*
- Respect the preference of terminally ill clients to refuse or limit hygiene care. *Maintaining hygiene, even with assistance, may require excessive energy demands from terminally ill clients. Pain on touch or movement may be intractable and not resolved by medication.*
- If a terminally ill client requests hygiene care, make an extra effort to meet request and provide care when client and family will most benefit (e.g., before visitors, at bedtime, in the early morning). *When desired, improved hygiene greatly boosts the morale of terminally ill clients.*
- Maintain temperature of home at a comfortable level when providing hygiene care to terminally ill clients. *Terminally ill clients may have difficulty with thermoregulation, which will add to the energy demand or decrease comfort during hygiene care.*

Client/Family Teaching

- Teach the client and family how to use adaptive devices for bathing, and teach bathing techniques that promote safety (e.g., getting into tub before filling it with water, emptying water before getting out, using an antislip mat, wall-grab bars, tub bench). *Adaptive devices can provide independence, safety, and speed (Schemm and Gitlin, 1998).*
- Teach the client and family an individualized bathing routine that includes a schedule, privacy, skin inspection, soap or lubricant, and chill prevention. *Teaching methods to meet the client's needs increases client's satisfaction with the bathing experience.*

evolve WEBSITES FOR EDUCATION

See the EVOLVE website for World Wide Web resources for client education.

REFERENCES

Brubaker B: Self care in nursing home residents, *J Gerontol Nurs* 22(7):22, 1996.
Burch S, Coggins T: No rinse, one step bed bath: the effects on the occurrence of skin tears in a long-term care setting, *Ostomy/Wound Manag* 49(1):64, 2003.
Cavanagh S et al: Assessing cognitive function after stroke using the FIMTM instrument, *J Neurosci Nurs* 34(2): 99, 2002.

- = Independent; ▲ = Collaborative

Clark M, Lester J: The effect of video-based interventions on self-care, *West J Nurs Res* 22(8):895, 2000.

Danner C et al: Cognitively impaired elders: using research findings to improve nursing care, *J Gerontol Nurs* 19:5, 1993.

Deguchi A et al: Improving symptoms of senile dementia by a night time spa bathing, *Arch Gerontol Geriatr* 29(3):267, 1999.

Freeman E: International perspectives on bathing, *J Gerontol Nurs* 23(5):40, 1997.

Gerdner L et al: Impact of a psychoeducational intervention on caregiver response to behavioral problems, *Nurs Res* 51(6):363, 2002.

Gulick E: Emotional distress and activities of daily living functioning in persons with multiple sclerosis, *Nurs Res* 50(3):147, 2001.

Guralnik JM: A short physical performance battery assessing lower extremity function: association with self-reported disability and prediction of mortality and nursing home admission, *J Gerontol Med Sci* 49:M85, 1994.

Hart B et al: Promoting positive outcomes for elderly persons in the hospital: prevention and risk factor modification, *AACN Clin Issues* 13(1):22, 2002.

Hoeffer B et al: Reducing aggressive behavior during bathing cognitively impaired nursing home residents, *J Gerontol Nurs* 23(5):16, 1997.

Kanda K, Tochihara Y, Ohnaka T: Bathing before sleep in the young and in the elderly, *Eur J Appl Physiol* 80: 71, 1999.

Leidy N, Haase J: Functional status from the patient's perspective: the challenge of preserving personal integrity, *Res Nurs Health* 22:67, 1999.

Maxfield MC et al: Training staff to prevent aggressive behavior of cognitively impaired elderly patients during bathing and grooming, *J Gerontol Nurs* 22(1):37, 1996.

Miller M: Physically aggressive resident behavior during hygienic care, *J Gerontol Nurs* 23(5):24, 1997.

Penninx B et al: Physical exercise and the prevention of disability in activities of daily living in older persons with osteoarthritis, *Arch Intern Med* 161(19):2309, 2001.

Rader J, Hoeffer B, McKenzie D: Individualizing the bathing process, *J Gerontol Nurs* 22(3):32, 1996.

Resnick B: The impact of self-efficacy and outcome expectations on functional status in older adults, *Top Geriatr Rehabil* 17(4):1, 2002.

Rogers J, Holm M, Perkins L: Trajectory of assistive device usage and user and non-user characteristics: long-handled bath sponge, *Arthritis Rheum* 47(6):645, 2002.

Rogers WA et al: Functional limitations to daily living tasks in the aged: a focus group analysis, *Hum Factors* 40(1):111, 1998.

Schemm RL, Gitlin LN: How occupational therapists teach older patients to use bathing and dressing devices in rehabilitation, *Am J Occup Ther* 52(4):276, 1998.

Skewes S: Bathing: it's a tough job! *J Gerontol Nurs* 23(5):45, 1997.

Sloane P et al: Bathing the Alzheimer's patient in long-term care: results and recommendation from three studies, *Am J Alzheimers Dis* 10(4):3, 1995.

Dressing/grooming Self-care deficit

Linda S. Williams

NANDA Definition

Impaired ability to perform or complete dressing and grooming activities for self

Defining Characteristics

Impaired ability to put on or take off necessary items of clothing; impaired ability to fasten clothing; impaired ability to obtain or replace articles of clothing; inability to clothe upper body; inability to clothe lower body; inability to choose clothing; inability to use assistive devices; inability to use zippers; inability to remove clothes; inability to put on socks; inability to maintain appearance at a satisfactory level; inability to pick up clothing; inability to put on shoes

• = Independent; ▲ = Collaborative

Related Factors (r/t)

Decreased or lack of motivation; pain; severe anxiety; perceptual or cognitive impairment; weakness or tiredness; neuromuscular impairment; musculoskeletal impairment; discomfort; environmental barriers

NOTE: See suggested Functional Level Classification in care plan for **Impaired physical Mobility.**

NOC Outcomes (Nursing Outcomes Classification)

Suggested NOC Outcomes

Self-Care: Activities of Daily Living (ADL), Dressing, Hygiene

> **Example NOC Outcome with Indicators**
>
> **Self-Care: Activities of Daily Living (ADL)** as evidenced by the following indicators: Gets clothes from closet and puts on upper body, lower body/Shampoos, combs, brushes hair/Applies makeup (Rate each indicator of **Self-Care: Activities of Daily Living [ADL]:** 1 = severely compromised, 2 =substantially compromised, 3 = moderately compromised, 4 = mildly compromised, 5 = not compromised [see Section I].)

Client Outcomes

Client Will (Specify Time Frame):
- Dress and groom self to optimal potential
- Use adaptive devices to dress and groom
- Explain and use methods to enhance strengths during dressing and grooming
- Dress and groom with assistance of caregiver as needed

NIC Interventions (Nursing Interventions Classification)

Suggested NIC Interventions

Dressing; Hair Care; Self-Care Assistance: Dressing/Grooming

> **Example NIC Activities—Self-Care Assistance: Dressing/Grooming**
>
> Be available for assistance in dressing as necessary; Reinforce efforts to dress, groom self

Nursing Interventions and Rationales

- Observe the client's ability to dress and groom self through direct observation and from the client/caregiver report, noting specific deficits and their causes. *Use of both observation and report of function provides complementary assessment data for goal and intervention planning (Reuben et al, 1992).*
- Consider environmental and human factors that may limit dressing/grooming ability, such as reaching for clothes or grooming aids in closets or drawers. Help the client arrange clothing and grooming devices within easy reach. Installing turntables and closet rods or drawers between eye and hip level is helpful. *Environmental factors affect task performance. Function can be improved based on engineering principles that adapt environmental factors to meet the client's capabilities (Rogers et al, 1998).*
- Identify and include the client's strengths in dressing and grooming to individualize

• = Independent; ▲ = Collaborative

dressing process. *Incorporating the client's strengths into a dressing and grooming program increases self-care independence (Vogelpohl et al, 1996).*

- Ask the client for input on clothing choices and how to increase the ease of dressing. **Nursing Research:** *Client's task performance may be affected by a loss of individual control due to frustration from not being able to anticipate timing of care events, an inability to predict if nurse or client would perform tasks and perception that nurse permission is necessary before performing a task (Brubaker, 1996).*
▲ Request referrals for occupational and physical therapy. *Collaboration and correlation of activities with interdisciplinary team members increases the client's mastery of self-care tasks.*
▲ Provide medication for pain 45 minutes before dressing and grooming if needed. *Pain relief promotes participation in self-care.*
- Plan activities to prevent fatigue while dressing and grooming. *Energy conservation increases activity tolerance and promotes self-care.*
- Provide privacy and limit people/caregivers in room. **Nursing Research:** *Privacy conveys respect and increases dressing ability (Beck et al, 1997).*
- Select larger-sized clothing, clothing with elastic waistbands, wide sleeves and pant legs, dresses that open down the back for wheelchair-bound women; and Velcro fasteners or larger buttons. *Simplifying clothing facilitates dressing for those with impaired mobility.*
- Use adaptive dressing and grooming equipment as needed (e.g., long-handled brushes, grasping devices, Velcro closures, zipper pulls, button hooks, elastic shoelaces, large buttons, soap-on-a-rope, suction holders). *Adaptive devices increase speed and safety and decrease exertion.*
- Lay clothing out in the order that it will be put on by the client. Dress bottom half, then top half of body. **Nursing Research:** *Simplifying dressing tasks increases self-care ability (Beck et al, 1997).*
- Encourage the client to dress appropriately for time of day. Perform dressing and grooming activities in a consistent sequence each day. *An established routine of waking and dressing provides a sense of normalcy and increases motivation to perform self-care. Prolonged repetition promotes increased relearning of self-care tasks (Giles and Shore, 1989). Use verbal prompting to complete dressing task and provide positive reinforcement immediately for accomplished steps of task (Vogelpohl et al, 1996).*
- Encourage participation; guide the client's hand through task if necessary. **Nursing Research:** *Experiencing the normal process of a task through guided practice facilitates optimal relearning (Beck et al, 1997).*
- Nurture personal attributes such as humor, positive attitude, faith and hope and control of stress for clients with multiple sclerosis. **Nursing Research:** *For those with multiple sclerosis, personal attributes intervene between emotional distress and ADL functioning by decreasing a stress appraisal response (Gulick, 2001).*

Geriatric
- Assess for grieving resulting from loss of function. *Grief resulting from loss of function can inhibit relearning of self-care tasks.*
▲ Provide medication for pain if needed and plan activities to prevent fatigue before dressing/grooming. **Nursing Research:** *Level of functioning is increased for older adults with chronic medical conditions if pain and fatigue are controlled (Bennett et al, 2002).*
- Assess self-efficacy (The Self-Efficacy for Functional Activities scale); assess outcome

- **• = Independent; ▲ = Collaborative**

expectations (Outcome Expectations for Functional Activities scale). Based on assessment, promote motivation and self-efficacy for ADL functioning by: role modeling via videotape or partnering; verbal encouragement; individualize care using humor, kindness, joy and excitement with achievements; social supports; and decrease unpleasant sensations with the ADL function. *Assessment and interventions for self-efficacy strengthen client efficacy expectations and improve functional performance (Resnick, 2002).*

- Assess tasks the client can complete, noting areas of independence and difficulty to make adaptations. **Nursing Research:** *Some areas of a task can be performed independently but certain dressing tasks are reported as most difficult: tying shoelaces, fastening pants and buttoning shirts; difficult grooming tasks are applying toothpaste and hair combing at the top and back of the head (Johnson et al, 1992).*
- Allow the client or caregiver adequate time to complete dressing (e.g., do not insist that the client is dressed at an early hour). *Significant aging increases the time required to complete a task; elderly clients with a self-care deficit require more time than others to complete a task.*
- Telehomecare can be an effective way to assess and monitor ADL performance for older adults. **Nursing Research:** *Telehomecare improves patient education and self-management outcomes (Bowles and Dansky, 2002). Telehealth is a cost-effective opportunity for gerontological home nursing practice for frequent monitoring and reassurance (Wakefield et al, 2001).*

Home care

- Involve the client in planning of informal care and provide access to health professionals and financial support for the care. **Nursing Research:** *Clients receiving informal care including dressing assistance reported concerns showing a need to increase their involvement in planning services related to informal care (McCann and Evans, 2002).*
- ▲ Based on functional assessment and rehabilitation capacity, refer for home health aide services to assist with dressing and grooming. *Support by home health aides preserves the energy of the client and provides respite for caregivers.*
- Have caregiver view videotape showing caregiver self-care activities (organizing day, talking when frustrated, self-time and nonjudgmental person with whom to talk) followed by a discussion. **Nursing Research:** *Videotape intervention and discussion can model self-care activities and buffer caregiver stress (Clark and Lester, 2000).*
- Cue cognitively impaired clients in steps of dressing and grooming. *Cognitively impaired clients can participate successfully in many activities with cueing, and participation in self-care can enhance their self-esteem.*
- Respect the preference of the terminally ill client to refuse dressing and limit grooming. *Dressing and grooming, even with assistance, may require excessive energy demands from the terminally ill. Pain on touch or movement may be intractable and not resolved by medication.*
- If terminally ill clients request dressing and grooming, make an extra effort to meet the request and provide care when the client and family will most benefit (e.g., before visitors, in early morning). *When desired, dressing and grooming are a great boost to the morale of terminally ill clients and their families.*
- Maintain the temperature of the home at a comfortable level when dressing terminally ill client. *Terminally ill clients may have difficulty with thermoregulation, which will add to the energy demand or decrease comfort during hygiene activities.*

- **= Independent; ▲ = Collaborative**

Client/Family Teaching

- Teach the client to dress the affected side first, then the unaffected side. *Dressing the affected side first allows for easier manipulation of clothing.*
- Teach the simplest step in a task until mastered, and then proceed to more complicated steps. Give praise. **Nursing Research:** *Simplifying dressing and grooming tasks that consist of many small steps promotes mastery (Beck et al, 1997).*
- Teach the client how to use adaptive devices for dressing and grooming. *Adaptive devices can provide independence and safety and promote speed.*
- Teach the client and family to select clothes appropriate for the season, temperature, and weather. *Clients with altered sensation need to understand the factors that influence body temperature and the environment.*

evolve WEBSITES FOR EDUCATION

See the EVOLVE website for World Wide Web resources for client education.

REFERENCES

Beck C et al: Improving dressing behavior in cognitively impaired nursing home residents, *Nurs Res* 46(3):126, 1997.

Bennett J et al: The mediating effect of pain and fatigue on level of functioning in older adults, *Nurs Res* 51(4): 254, 2002.

Bowles K, Dansky K: Teaching self-management of diabetes via telehomecare, *Home Healthc Nurse* 20(1):36, 2002.

Brubaker B: Self care in nursing home residents, *J Gerontol Nurs* 22(7):22, 1996.

Clark M, Lester J: The effect of video-based interventions on self-care, *West J Nurs Res* 22(8):895, 2000.

Giles G, Shore M: A rapid method for teaching severely brain injured adults how to wash and dress, *Arch Phys Med Rehabil* 70:156, 1989.

Gulick E: Emotional distress and activities of daily living functioning in persons with multiple sclerosis, *Nurs Res* 50(3):147, 2001.

Johnson P et al: Applying nursing diagnosis and nursing process to activities of daily living and mobility, *Geriatric Nurs* 13:25, 1992.

McCann S, Evans D: Informal care: the views of people receiving care, *Health Soc Care Community* 10(4):221, 2002.

Resnick B: The impact of self-efficacy and outcome expectations on functional status in older adults, *Top Geriatr Rehabil* 17(4):1, 2002.

Reuben DB et al: The predictive validity of self-report and performance-based measures of function and health, *J Gerontol Med Sci* 47:M106, 1992.

Rogers WA et al: Functional limitations to daily living tasks in the aged: a focus group analysis, *Hum Factors* 40(1):111, 1998.

Vogelpohl TS et al: "I can do it!" dressing: promoting independence through individualized strategies, *J Gerontol Nurs* 22(3):39, 1996.

Wakefield B et al: Telehealth: an opportunity for gerontological nursing practice, *J Gerontol Nurs,* 27(1):10, 2001.

Feeding Self-care deficit

Linda S. Williams

NANDA Definition

Impaired ability to perform or complete feeding activities

- **• = Independent; ▲ = Collaborative**

Defining Characteristics

Inability to swallow food; inability to prepare food for ingestion; inability to handle utensils; inability to chew food; inability to use assistive device; inability to get food onto utensils; inability to open containers; inability to ingest food safely; inability to manipulate food in mouth; inability to bring food from a receptacle to the mouth; inability to complete a meal; inability to ingest food in a socially acceptable manner; inability to pick up cup or glass; inability to ingest sufficient food

Related Factors (r/t)

Weakness or tiredness; severe anxiety; neuromuscular impairment; pain; perceptual or cognitive impairment; discomfort; environmental barriers; decreased or lack of motivation; musculoskeletal impairment

NOTE: See suggested Functional Level Classification in the care plan **Impaired physical Mobility.**

NOC   Outcomes (Nursing Outcomes Classification)

Suggested NOC Outcomes

Self-Care: Activities of Daily Living (ADL), Eating

> **Example NOC Outcome with Indicators**
>
> **Self-Care: Activities of Daily Living (ADL)** as evidenced by the following indicators: Opens containers/Handles utensils/Completes a meal (Rate each indicator of **Self-Care: Activities of Daily Living [ADL]:** 1 = dependent (does not participate), 2 = requires assistive person and device, 3 = requires assistive person, 4 = independent with assistive device, 5 = completely independent [see Section I].)

Client Outcomes

Client Will (Specify Time Frame):

- Feed self
- State satisfaction with ability to use adaptive devices for feeding
- Provide assistance with feeding when necessary (caregiver)

NIC   Interventions (Nursing Interventions Classification)

Suggested NIC Interventions

Feeding; Self-Care Assistance: Feeding

> **Example NIC Activities—Self-Care Assistance: Feeding**
>
> Provide adaptive devices to facilitate the client's feeding self (e.g., long handles, handle with large circumference, or small strap on utensils) as needed; Provide frequent cueing and close supervision as appropriate

Nursing Interventions and Rationales

- Assess the client's ability to feed self. Test gag reflex bilaterally, and note specific deficits. *Functional assessment provides ADLs task analysis data for matching the client's ability to feed self with caregiver's level of assistance (Van Ort and Phillips, 1995).*
- Observe for cause of inability to feed self independently (see Related Factors). *Self-care*

• = Independent; ▲ = Collaborative

requires multisystem competence. Restorative program planning is specific to problems that interfere with self-care (Phaneuf, 1996).

- Ask the client for input on methods to facilitate eating and feeding (e.g., cultural foods, other food and fluid preferences), and provide four entrée choices, including ethnic choice. *When clients are given a choice, their food intake increases (Kayser-Jones, 1997).*
- ▲ Request referral for occupational and physical therapy; request a dietician. *Collaboration and correlation of activities with interdisciplinary team members increases the client's mastery of self-care tasks.*
- Ensure that the client has dentures, hearing aids, and glasses in place. *Adaptive devices increase opportunity for self-care.*
- Use any necessary adaptive feeding equipment (e.g., rocker knives, plate guards, suction mats, built-up handles on utensils, scoop dishes, large-handled cups). *Adaptive devices increase independence.*
- Seat the client at table using name card and place mat with meal in visual range next to role model who can eat, if applicable. *Familiar feeding patterns and cues increase self-feeding (Van Ort and Phillips, 1995).*
- Help the client into sitting position; ensure that the client's head is flexed slightly forward and shoulders are supported while eating and for 1 hour after a meal. *Gravity assists with swallowing, and aspiration is decreased when sitting upright.*
- Prepare meal items before the client begins eating. *Preparing items for the client conserves energy for hand-to-mouth activities.*
- Provide small portions of favorite foods, one entrée at a time, at proper serving temperature. *Food intake is increased when meal appeals to the client and is simplified (Kayser-Jones and Schell, 1997).*
- Provide consistency in caregiver and meal activities. *Assigning caregivers to clients rather than dining areas allows caregiver to learn the client's needs and promotes a positive attitude between caregiver and the client (Kennedy-Holzapfel et al, 1996).*
- Caregiver should sit beside the client (on the client's unaffected side) at eye level. *Sitting at eye level with the client increases eye contact and promotes a relaxed atmosphere that increases consumed food (Kennedy-Holzapfel et al, 1996).*
- Caregiver should sit at a half circle table if interacting with a group of clients and should remain with clients until meal is completed. *Environmental strategies that reduce interruptions and distractions increase food intake (Van Ort and Phillips, 1995).*
- Encourage participation; guide the client's hand through task if needed; provide cues and pantomime desired behaviors. *Experiencing the normal process of a task through guided practice facilitates optimal relearning (Tappen, 1994).*
- Allow the client to participate in feeding as able; provide verbal prompting; provide praise for all feeding attempts; increase tasks as able. *The client should be an active participant in feeding instead of a passive recipient of food (Osburn and Marshall, 1993).*
- Provide the client with a pleasant social meal environment. Keep the environment free of toileting devices and odors, avoid painful procedures before meals, remove lids from tray, and provide clean utensils for separate courses. *Attention to the aesthetics of feeding increases food intake (Kayser-Jones and Schell, 1997).*
- Do not mix different foods together when assisting the client with eating. *Mixing foods together decreases client dignity and reduces appeal of food, decreasing food intake (Kayser-Jones and Schell, 1997).*
- Play slow-tempo, quiet music during meals. *Agitated behaviors may communicate anxi-*

• = Independent; ▲ = Collaborative

ety from a noisy, overwhelming environment; quiet music can mask this, resulting in relaxed and smiling clients (Denney, 1997).

- Encourage the client to keep food on the unaffected side of mouth with a rocking motion to deposit the food, if applicable. *Keeping food away from the affected side of the mouth prevents pocketing of food (Donahue, 1990).*
- Be prepared to intervene if choking occurs; have suction equipment readily available and know the Heimlich maneuver. *Dysphagia increases the risk of choking (Donahue, 1990).*
- Provide oral hygiene after eating and check for pocketing of food. *Aspiration can occur from food left in the mouth.*
- ▲ Continue rehabilitation efforts with poststroke clients long term to achieve optimal functioning. **Nursing Research:** *Client improvement may continue 6 months or longer poststroke (Cavanagh et al, 2002).*

Geriatric

- Develop client muscle strength building plan to build the client's physiological capacity. **Nursing Research:** *Elders may have little reserve capacity but building physiological capacity may allow continued functioning during periods of illness or stress (Leidy and Haase, 1999).*
- Implement Hospital Elder Life Program, a model of care to prevent functional and cognitive decline of older persons during hospitalization. *The Hospital Elder Life Program successfully prevents cognitive and functional decline in at-risk older patients (Inouye et al, 2000).*
- ▲ Provide medication for pain before meals if needed and plan activities to prevent fatigue before meals. **Nursing Research:** *Level of functioning is increased for older adults with chronic medical conditions if pain and fatigue are controlled (Bennett et al, 2002).*
- Assess and maintain documentation about poststroke client's eating and nutrition (include weight) upon admission to long-term care. **Nursing Research:** *Poststroke clients may have multiple nutritional deficits that require early and ongoing assessment to enable appropriate care and promotion of health (Kumlien and Axelsson, 2002).*
- Serve meals "family-style" with food in serving bowls and an empty plate to be filled by patient. **Nursing Research:** *Institutional practices foster "excess disability," with eating often the first skill to go, family-style meal serving rather than prepared meal plates allows opportunity for food and portion size selection, self-serving, passing serving bowls, selecting seconds and social engagement. An added benefit is that less staff time is needed to prepare plates (Altus et al, 2002).*
- Obtain and value patient's view of agency's food selection and presentation. Present views to administration. **Nursing Research:** *Patient barriers to eating are the dislike of presented foods, feeling that the food is not appetizing and nonvaluing of patient's food reports from nursing assistants and the need for administration to value these reports (Crogan et al, 2001).*
- ▲ Ensure adequate staffing at meal times. **Nursing Research:** *Short staffing results in decreased time for feeding (Crogan et al, 2001).*
- Choose soft foods rather than liquids, or use dietary thickeners. *Choking occurs more easily with clear liquids than with solid or soft foods.*
- Assess for intolerance to food texture and, if found, reverse food texture pattern as tolerated, progressing finally to texture stage of thick liquids. *Dementia clients lose ability*

- **• = Independent; ▲ = Collaborative**

to tolerate texture-pattern reverses from regular to soft to mechanical soft with chopped meat to puree to thick liquids, and pocketing of food is seen, along with statements of choking and spitting of food (Boylston et al, 1995).

- Provide finger foods for clients with Alzheimer's disease and place in hands as needed to cue. *Finger foods attract patient attention and increase involvement in meal. They are easier to handle than utensils, and as a result, weight is maintained (Slotesz and Dayton, 1995). Finger foods can be nutritious and can allow independence and the choice of what and when to eat (Kennedy-Holzapfel et al, 1996).*
- Allow the client with dentures adequate time to chew. *Chewing with dentures takes four times longer to reach a certain level of mastication than chewing with natural teeth.*
- Provide emotionally neutral nonverbal cues to improve table-sitting behavior if patient rises from table early such as a firm hand on dominant shoulder indicating to resit. **Nursing Research:** *Wanderers often receive positive social engagement from staff when leaving the table early so emotionally neutral behavior extinguishing cues are useful to increase table sitting and food intake (Beattie and Algase, 2002).*

Home care

- ▲ Based on functional assessment and rehabilitation capacity, refer for home health aide services to assist with feeding. *Support by home health aides preserves the energy of the client and provides respite for caregivers.*
- Telehomecare can be an effective way to assess and monitor ADL performance for older adults. **Nursing Research:** *Telehomecare improves patient education and self-management outcomes (Bowles and Dansky, 2002). Telehealth is a cost-effective opportunity for gerontological home nursing practice for frequent monitoring and reassurance (Wakefield et al, 2001).*
- Cue cognitively impaired client when feeding. *Cognitively impaired clients can participate successfully in many activities with cueing. Participation in self-care can enhance the self-esteem of cognitively impaired clients.*
- Respect the preference of terminally ill clients to refuse nutrition or assistance with eating. Refer to care plans for **Imbalanced Nutrition: less than body requirements** and **Impaired Swallowing.**
- If terminally ill client requests nutrition, take special care to provide foods and assistive devices that protect the client from aspiration, minimize energy requirements, and meet the client's taste preferences. *Terminally ill clients have altered taste and other sensations, which impacts their willingness to eat or to invest time or energy in eating.*

Client/Family Teaching

- Teach the client how to use adaptive devices. *Adaptive devices increase independence.*
- Teach the client with hemianopsia to turn head so that the plate is in the line of vision. *Compensation for hemianopsia is done by turning head to place items in line of vision (Needham, 1993).*
- Teach visually impaired client to locate foods according to numbers on a clock. *Teach caregiver-feeding techniques that prevent choking (e.g., sitting beside the client on the unaffected side, feeding the client slowly, checking food temperature, providing fluid between bites, establishing a method to communicate readiness for next bite, limiting conversation while chewing).*

• = **Independent**; ▲ = **Collaborative**

evolve **WEBSITES FOR EDUCATION**

See the EVOLVE website for World Wide Web resources for client education.

REFERENCES

Altus D et al: Using family-style meals to increase participation and communication in persons with dementia, *J Gerontol Nurs* 28(9):47, 2002.

Beattie E, Algase D: Improving table-sitting behavior of wanderers, *J Gerontol Nurs* 28(10):6, 2002.

Bennett J et al: The mediating effect of pain and fatigue on level of functioning in older adults, *Nurs Res* 51(4): 254, 2002.

Bowles K, Dansky K: Teaching self-management of diabetes via telehomecare, *Home Healthc Nurse* 20(1):36, 2002.

Boylston E et al: Increase oral intake in dementia patients by altering food texture, *Am J Alzheimers Dis* 10(6): 37, 1995.

Cavanagh S et al: Assessing cognitive function after stroke using the FIMTM instrument, *J Neurosci Nurs* 34(2): 99, 2002.

Crogan N et al: Barriers to Nutrition Care for Nursing home residents, *J Gerontol Nurs* 27(12):25, 2001.

Denney A: Quiet music: an intervention for mealtime agitation, *J Gerontol Nurs* 23(7):16, 1997.

Donahue P: When it's hard to swallow: feeding techniques for dysphagia management, *J Gerontol Nurs* 16:6, 1990.

Inouye S et al: The Hospital elder life program: a model of care to prevent cognitive and functional decline in older hospitalized patients, *J Am Geriatr Soc* 48(12):1697, 2000.

Kayser-Jones J: Inadequate staffing at mealtime: implications for nursing and health policy, *J Gerontol Nurs* 23(8):4, 1997.

Kayser-Jones J, Schell E: The mealtime experience of a cognitively impaired elder: ineffective and effective strategies, *J Gerontol Nurs* 23(7):33, 1997.

Kennedy-Holzapfel S et al: Feeder position and food and fluid consumed by nursing home residents, *J Gerontol Nurs* 22(4):6, 1996.

Kumlien S, Axelsson K: Stroke patients in nursing homes: eating, feeding, nutrition and related care, *J Clin Nurs* 11(4):498, 2002.

Leidy N, Haase J: Functional status from the patient's perspective: the challenge of preserving personal integrity. *Res Nurs Health* 22:67, 1999.

Needham J: *Gerontological nursing: a restorative approach,* Albany, NY, 1993, Delmar.

Osburn C, Marshall M: Self-feeding performance in nursing home residents, *J Gerontol Nurs* 19:7, 1993.

Phaneuf C: Screening elders for nutritional deficits, *Am J Nurs* 96:58, 1996.

Slotesz KS, Dayton JH: The effects of menu modification to increase dietary intake and maintain the weight of Alzheimer's residents, *Am J Alzheimers Dis* 10(6):20, 1995.

Tappen R: The effect of skill training on functional abilities of nursing home residents with dementia, *Res Nurs Health* 17:159, 1994.

Van Ort S, Phillips L: Nursing interventions to promote functional feeding, *J Gerontol Nurs* 21:6, 1995.

Wakefield B et al: Telehealth: an opportunity for gerontological nursing practice, *J Gerontol Nurs* 27(1):10, 2001.

Toileting Self-care deficit

Linda S. Williams

NANDA Definition

Impaired ability to perform or complete own toileting activities

• = **Independent;** ▲ = **Collaborative**

Defining Characteristics

Inability to get to toilet or commode; inability to sit on or rise from toilet or commode; inability to manipulate clothing for toileting; inability to carry out proper toilet hygiene; inability to flush toilet or commode

Related Factors (r/t)

Environmental barriers; weakness or tiredness; decreased or lack of motivation; severe anxiety; impaired mobility status; impaired transfer ability; musculoskeletal impairment; neuromuscular impairment; pain; perceptual or cognitive impairment

NOTE: See suggested Functional Level Classification in care plan for **Impaired physical Mobility.**

NOC   Outcomes (Nursing Outcomes Classification)

Suggested NOC Outcomes

Self-Care: Activities of Daily Living (ADL), Toileting

Example NOC Outcome with Indicators

Self-Care: Activities of Daily Living (ADL) as evidenced by the following indicators: Recognizes and responds to a full bladder and urge to have a bowel movement/Gets to and from toilet (Rate each indicator of **Self-Care: Activities of Daily Living [ADL]:** I = severely compromised, 2 =substantially compromised, 3 = moderately compromised, 4 = mildly compromised, 5 = not compromised [see Section I].)

Client Outcomes

Client Will (Specify Time Frame):
- Remain free of incontinence and impaction with no urine or stool on skin
- State satisfaction with ability to use adaptive devices for toileting
- Explain and use methods to be safe and independent in toileting

NIC   Interventions (Nursing Interventions Classification)

Suggested NIC Interventions

Environmental Management; Self-Care Assistance: Toileting

Example NIC Activities—Self-Care Assistance: Toileting

Assist the client to toilet/commode/bedpan/fracture pan/urinal at specified intervals; Institute a toileting schedule as appropriate

---

Nursing Interventions and Rationales

- Observe cause of inability to toilet independently (see Related Factors). *Self-care requires multisystem competence. Restorative program planning is specific to problems that interfere with self-care.*
- Assess ability to toilet; note specific deficits. *Functional assessment provides analysis data for ADLs tasks for use in goal and intervention planning.*
- Ask the client for input on toileting methods and timing and how to better provide toileting activity assistance. **Nursing Research:** *Client's task performance may be affected*

• = Independent; ▲ = Collaborative

by a loss of individual control due to frustration from not being able to anticipate timing of care events, an inability to predict if nurse or client would perform tasks, and perception that nurse permission is necessary before performing a task (Brubaker, 1996).

- Assess the client's usual bowel and bladder toileting patterns and the terminology used for toileting. *Individuals develop a unique pattern of toileting over time for faster, normal elimination.*
- ▲ Request referral for occupational and physical therapy for help in working with the client to transfer from bed to commode. *Collaboration and correlation of activities with interdisciplinary team members increase the client's mastery of self-care tasks.*
- Use any necessary assistive toileting equipment (e.g., raised toilet seat, suction mats, spill-proof urinals, support rails next to toilet, toilet safety frames, Sanifems [allows a woman to void standing], fracture bedpans, long-handled toilet paper holders). *Adaptive devices promote independence and safety.*
- Provide privacy. *Privacy can prevent suppression of elimination resulting from embarrassment about noise and odor.*
- Develop toileting schedule using clocks, written schedules, or verbal prompting as cues for the client and provide assistance at scheduled times. *Toileting schedules convey continence is valued, and maintain continence (Hart et al, 2002).*
- Schedule toileting to occur when defecation urge is strongest or voiding is likely (e.g., in the morning, every 2 hours, after meals, at bedtime). Assist the client until self-care ability increases. *The defecation urge is strongest in the morning or within 1 hour after meals or warm beverages. Approximately 50 to 75 ml of urine is produced hourly, and the urge to void occurs when 200 ml has accumulated. Therefore a 2-hour schedule can reduce incontinence.*
- Allow the client to participate as able in toileting, and provide praise for accomplishments. Increase tasks as the client is able, and work with the client to aim toward independence in toileting. *Client's expenditure of energy provides caregiver the opportunity to convey respect for a well-done task, which increases self-esteem.*
- Obtain a bedside commode if necessary and adapt it for the client's needs; avoid bedpans if possible. If the client is acutely ill, provide bedpan at appropriate intervals. *A sitting position uses gravity and is more conducive to normal elimination than a lying position.*
- Make assistance call button readily available to the client and answer call light promptly. *To decrease incontinence, the client needs rapid access to toileting facilities.*
- Assess and remove physical barriers to toilet, such as cluttered walkways. *Environmental assessment identifies barriers that can increase incontinence episodes (Penn et al, 1996).*
- Keep toilet paper and hand-washing items within easy reach of the client. Provide prompt skin care and linen changes after incontinence episodes. *The presence of urine or stool on the skin leads to skin breakdown.*

Geriatric

- Develop client muscle strength building plan to build the client's physiological capacity. **Nursing Research:** *Elderly clients may have little reserve capacity but building physiological capacity may allow continued functioning during periods of illness or stress (Leidy and Haase, 1999).*
- Include exercise and walking program in plan of care. *Exercise for flexibility, strengthening and a walking program in the hospital promotes ADLs, prevents injury, increases quality of life, and may delay admission to a long-term care facility (Hart et al, 2002).*

- = **Independent;** ▲ = **Collaborative**

▲ Implement Hospital Elder Life Program, a model of care to prevent functional and cognitive decline of older persons during hospitalization. *The Hospital Elder Life Program successfully prevents cognitive and functional decline in at-risk older patients (Inouye et al, 2000).*

• Assess self-efficacy (The Self-Efficacy for Functional Activities scale); assess outcome expectations (Outcome Expectations for Functional Activities scale). Based on assessment, promote motivation and self-efficacy for ADL functioning by: role modeling via videotape or partnering; verbal encouragement; individualize care using humor, kindness, joy and excitement with achievements; social supports; and decrease unpleasant sensations with the ADL function. *Assessment and interventions for self-efficacy strengthen client efficacy expectations and improve functional performance (Resnick, 2002).*

• Monitor clients with dementia for behavioral toileting cues (e.g., pacing, restlessness, fidgeting) and assist with prompt toileting, or use an individualized scheduled toileting for memory impaired elderly. *Assisting clients promptly when toileting cues are observed can reduce toileting accidents and the resulting upsetting client reactions that occur (Hutchinson, 1996).* **Nursing Research:** *An individual toileting schedule helps prevent incontinence in moderately cognitively impaired elders (Jirovec and Templin, 2001).*

• Assess the client's mobility status and speed of movement. **Nursing Research:** *Elderly women with slower mobility have more incontinent episodes than others (Wyman and Eiswick, 1993).*

• Reassure the client that call light will be answered promptly. *The elderly cannot respond quickly to the urge to void because of limited functional ability and environmental barriers; they are also unable to delay voiding because of decreased muscle tone and neurological changes (Palmer, 1994).*

• Provide a small footstool in front of toilet or commode. *Intra-abdominal pressure is increased by elevating knees above the hips, which facilitates elimination in elderly persons with weak abdominal muscles.*

• Assess the client's functional ability to manipulate clothing for toileting. If necessary, modify clothing with Velcro fasteners and elastic waists. *Delays caused by having to manipulate zippers and buttons may cause functional incontinence (Penn et al, 1996).*

• Avoid use of indwelling or condom catheters if possible. *An indwelling urinary catheter is a source of infection and keeps the bladder empty, which reduces bladder capacity and decreases the opportunity for independent toileting.*

Home care

• Have caregiver view videotape showing caregiver self-care activities (organizing day, talking when frustrated, self-time, and nonjudgmental person with whom to talk) followed by a discussion. **Nursing Research:** *Videotape intervention and discussion can model self-care activities and buffer caregiver stress (Clark and Lester, 2000).*

▲ Based on functional assessment and rehabilitation capacity, refer for home health aide services to assist with toileting. *Support by home health aides preserves the energy of the client and provides respite for caregivers.*

• Cue cognitively impaired clients in steps of toileting. *Cognitively impaired persons can participate successfully in many activities with cueing, and participation in self-care can enhance their self-esteem.*

▲ Avoid the use of medications that place undue toileting stress on the client who is terminally ill.

▲ Provide pain medication for terminally ill clients 20 to 45 minutes before toileting in

• = Independent; ▲ = Collaborative

anticipation of possible pain (e.g., in coordination with a bowel stimulation program). See care plan for constipation. *Pain from touch or movement may be intractable and not resolved by medication, but medication may decrease the pain enough to allow limited movement and passing of stool.*

▲ Consider use of an indwelling catheter for terminally ill clients in too much pain to move when hygiene and skin integrity are difficult to maintain. *The goal of hospice care is to promote comfort and dignity in the dying process.*

Client/Family Teaching

- Teach the client and family how to toilet the client with adaptive and safety devices. *Adaptive devices can provide independence and safety and promote speed.*
- Have family install toilet seat of a contrasting color. **Nursing Research:** *Visualization of toilet is aided by installing toilet seat of a contrasting color (Gerdner, 2002).*
- Prepare the client for toileting needs by teaching the action of medications such as diuretics. *Medications that promote elimination require prompt responses to toileting needs.*
- Help the visually impaired client to develop a plan for locating bathrooms in new environments. *Clients with visual impairments may find locating bathrooms in unfamiliar settings difficult.*

evolve WEBSITES FOR EDUCATION

See the EVOLVE website for World Wide Web resources for client education.

REFERENCES

Brubaker B: Self care in nursing home residents, *J Gerontol Nurs* 22(7):22, 1996.

Clark M, Lester J: The effect of video-based interventions on self-care, *West J Nurs Res* 22(8):895, 2000.

Gerdner L et al: Impact of a psychoeducational intervention on caregiver response to behavioral problems, *Nurs Res* 51(6):363, 2002.

Hart B et al: Promoting positive outcomes for elderly persons in the hospital: prevention and risk factor modification, *AACN Clin Issues* 13(1):22, 2002.

Hutchinson S, Leger-Krall S, Wilson HS: Toileting: a biobehavioral challenge in Alzheimer's dementia care, *J Gerontol Nurs* 22(10):18, 1996.

Inouye S et al: The hospital elder life program: a model of care to prevent cognitive and functional decline in older hospitalized patients, *J Am Geriatr Soc* 48(12):1697, 2000.

Jirovec MM, Templin T: Predicting success using individualized scheduled toileting for memory-impaired elders at home, *Res Nurs Health* 24:1, 2001.

Leidy N, Haase J: Functional status from the patient's perspective: the challenge of preserving personal integrity. *Res Nurs Health* 22:67, 1999.

Palmer M: Level 1: basic assessment and management of urinary incontinence in nursing homes, *Nurs Pract Forum* 5:152, 1994.

Penn C et al: Assessment of urinary incontinence, *J Gerontol Nurs* 22:8, 1996.

Resnick B: The impact of self-efficacy and outcome expectations on functional status in older adults, *Top Geriatr Rehabil* 17(4):1, 2002.

Wyman J, Eiswick R: Influence of functional, urological, and environmental characteristics on urinary incontinence in community-dwelling older women, *Nurs Res* 42:270, 1993.

• = Independent; ▲ = Collaborative

Readiness for enhanced Self-concept

Gail B. Ladwig

NANDA   Definition

A pattern of perceptions or ideas about the self that is sufficient for well-being and can be strengthened

Defining Characteristics

Expresses willingness to enhance self-concept; Expresses satisfaction with thoughts about self, sense of worthiness, role performance, body image, and personal identity; Actions are congruent with expressed feelings and thoughts; Expresses confidence in abilities; Accepts strengths and limitations

Related Factors (r/t)

To be developed

NOC   Outcomes (Nursing Outcomes Classification)

Suggested NOC Outcome
Self-Esteem

> #### Example NOC Outcome with Indicators
>
> **Self-Esteem** as evidenced by the following indicators: Verbalizations of self-acceptance/Open communication/ Confidence level/Description of pride in self (Rate each indicator of **Self-Esteem**: 1 = never positive, 2 = rarely positive, 3 = sometimes positive, 4 = often positive, 5 = consistently positive [see Section I].)

Client Outcomes

Client Will (Specify Time Frame):
- State willingness to enhance self-concept
- State satisfaction with thoughts about self, sense of worthiness, role performance, body image, and personal identity
- Demonstrate actions that are congruent with expressed feelings and thoughts
- State confidence in abilities
- Accept strengths and limitations

NIC   Interventions (Nursing Interventions Classification)

Suggested NIC Intervention
Self-Esteem Enhancement

> #### Example NIC Activities—Self-Esteem Enhancement
>
> Encourage the client to identify strengths; Assist the client in setting realistic goals to achieve higher self-esteem

• = Independent; ▲ = Collaborative

Nursing Interventions and Rationales

- Assess and support activities that promote self-concept developmentally. **Clinical Research:** *Cohort sequential longitudinal design: This study evaluated domains of self-concept in school-aged children and adolescents that included academic competence, physical appearance, behavioral conduct, social acceptance, and sports competence (Cole et al, 2001).* **Clinical Research:** *High self-esteem is associated with high academic achievement, involvement in sport and physical activity, and development of effective coping, and peer pressure resistance skills (Gurney et al, 1987, in King, 2002).* **Nursing Research:** *Social support, self-esteem, and optimism were all positively related to positive health practices (McNicholas, 2002).*

- ▲ Consider the development of a Healthy Kids mentoring program that has four components: (1) relationship building, (2) self-esteem enhancement, (3) goal setting, and (4) academic assistance (tutoring). Mentors met with students twice each week for $1^{1}/_{2}$ hours each session on school grounds. During each meeting, mentors devoted time to each program component. **Clinical Research:** *Paired sample t-tests were conducted to assess The Healthy Kids Mentoring Program impact on mentored students' self-esteem and connectedness scores from pretest to posttest. Results indicated students' overall self-esteem, school connectedness, peer connectedness, and family connectedness were significantly higher at posttest than at pretest (King et al, 2002).*

- ▲ Assess and provide referrals to mental health professionals for clients with unresolved worries associated with terrorism. **Nursing Research:** *NAPNAP initiated a new national campaign entitled Keep Your Children/Yourself Safe and Secure (KySS). The first phase of this campaign was to conduct a national survey. Results of this survey indicated that interventions are urgently needed to assist children and teens in coping with the multitude of stressors related to growing up in today's society (Melnyk et al, 2002).*

- ▲ Provide an alternative school based program for pregnant and parenting teenagers. **Nursing Research:** *Analysis of the data revealed four major themes: nurture and positive regard, sisterhood and belonging, mentoring and sense of family, and proactive learning environment and academic pride. The girls who attended the program developed close relationships with their peers and teachers. Many of them experienced academic success for the first time and reported that pregnancy and impending motherhood motivated them to do better in school (Spear, 2002).*

- ▲ Support the client's choice of alternative therapies and provide information on appropriate therapies (e.g., using a certified massage therapist when massage is the treatment of choice). *Nurses need to instruct the client to report special considerations, such as the presence of neutropenia or thrombocytopenia.*

- ▲ Clients with cancer often use massage therapy as an adjunct treatment. *Safe and effective massage therapy to clients with cancer only is achieved when the client, health care providers, and LMT (licensed massage therapist) collaborate effectively (Gecsedi, 2002).*

- ▲ Support establishing a church-based community health promotion programs (CBHPPs) with the following key elements: partnerships, positive health values, availability of services, access to church facilities, community-focused interventions, health behavior change, and supportive social relationships. *CBHPPs have effectively promoted health behaviors within certain communities. To promote health and wellness in light of our diverse society and health needs, health promotion professionals and churches can be dynamic partners (Peterson, Atwood, and Yates, 2002).*

- ▲ For clients who have had breast surgery and need prosthesis provide the appropriate prosthesis before the client leaves the health care facility. *A diagnosis of breast cancer*

• = **Independent;** ▲ = **Collaborative**

carries enormous implications for the client in terms of physical and psychological health. For this reason, it is vital that nurses respond sensitively to these needs and assist women to cope with the changes in body image and have the appropriate knowledge to fit the soft breast prosthesis (Keeton and McAloon, 2002).

Multicultural
- Carefully assess each client and allow families to participate in providing care that is acceptable based on the client's cultural beliefs; silent presence, quiet prayers (Hasidic Jewish families), telling stories and singing songs in their native language. *Health services in a pluralistic society require interventional approaches that recognize the significance of culture in shaping a person's conception of self as well as mental health and illness (Carnevale, 1999).*
- Provide support for health promoting behaviors and self-concept for clients from diverse cultures. **Nursing Research:** *In this convenience sample regression analyses demonstrated that the internalization racial identity stage (beta = 0.12; p < 0.001) and self-esteem (beta = 0.50; p < 0.001) contributed to the variance in health-promoting lifestyles (Johnson, 2002).*
- Refer to care plans **Disturbed Body Image; Chronic low Self-esteem;** and **Readiness for enhanced Spiritual well-being.**

Home care
- Above interventions may be used in the home care setting.

evolve WEBSITES FOR EDUCATION

See the EVOLVE website for World Wide Web resources for client education.

REFERENCES

Carnevale FA: Toward a cultural conception of the self, *J Psychosoc Nurs Ment Health Serv* 37(8):26, 1999.
Cole DA et al: The development of multiple domains of child and adolescent self-concept: a cohort sequential longitudinal design, *Child Dev* 72(6):1723, 2001.
Gecsedi RA: Massage therapy for patients with cancer, *Clin J Oncol Nurs* 6(1):52, 2002.
Keeton S, McAloon L: The supply and fitting of a temporary breast prosthesis, *Nurs Stand* 16(41):43, 2002.
King K, Vidourek R, Davis B: Increasing self-esteem and school connectedness through a multidimensional mentoring program, *J School Health* 72(7):294, 2002.
McNicholas SL: Social support and positive health practices, *West J Nurs Res* 24(7):772, 2002.
Melnyk BM et al: Mental health worries, communication, and needs in the year of the U.S. terrorist attack: national KySS survey findings, *J Pediatr Health Care* 16(5):222, 2002.
Peterson J, Atwood JR, Yates B: Key elements for church-based health promotion programs: outcome-based literature review, *Public Health Nurs* 19(6):401, 2002.
Spear HJ: Reading, writing, and having babies: a nurturing alternative school program, *J School Nurs* 18(5):293, 2002.
Walter R, Davis K, Glass N: Discovery of self: exploring, interconnecting and integrating self (concept) and nursing, *Collegian* 6(2):12, 1999.

Chronic low Self-esteem

Judith R. Gentz

NANDA Definition

Long-standing negative self-evaluations/feelings about self or self-capabilities

Defining Characteristics

Rationalizes away/rejects positive feedback and exaggerates negative feedback about self (long-standing or chronic); self-negating verbalization (long-standing or chronic); hesitant to try new things/situations (long-standing or chronic); expressions of shame/guilt (long-standing or chronic); evaluates self as unable to deal with events (long-standing or chronic); lack of eye contact; nonassertive/passive; frequent lack of success in work or other life events; excessively seeks reassurance; overly conforming, dependent on others' opinions; indecisive

Related Factors (r/t)

To be developed

NOC   Outcomes (Nursing Outcomes Classification)

Suggested NOC Outcome

Self-Esteem

Example NOC Outcome with Indicators

Self-Esteem as evidenced by the following indicators: Verbalizations of acceptance of self and limitations/ Open communication (Rate each indicator of **Self-Esteem**: 1 = never positive, 2 = rarely positive, 3 = sometimes positive, 4 = often positive, 5 = consistently positive [see Section I].)

Client Outcomes

Client Will (Specify Time Frame):

- Demonstrate improved ability to interact with others (e.g., maintains eye contact, expresses feelings)
- Verbalize increased self-acceptance through use of positive self-statements
- Identify personal strengths
- Set small, achievable goals
- Attempt independent decision-making

NIC   Interventions (Nursing Interventions Classification)

Suggested NIC Intervention

Self-Esteem Enhancement

Example NIC Activities—Self-Esteem Enhancement

Encourage the client to identify strengths; Assist the client in setting realistic goals to achieve higher self-esteem

Nursing Interventions and Rationales

- Actively listen to and respect the client. **Nursing Research:** *Listening was identified as positive communication in the nurse-client relationship (Gilbert, 1998).*
- Assist the client with identifying and confronting problems of not valuing self or enduring abuse from others. *Tolerance of abusive or violent behavior may be developed over time (Norris, 1992).*
- Assess existing strengths and coping abilities, and provide opportunities for their ex-

• = **Independent;** ▲ = **Collaborative**

pression and recognition. **Nursing Research:** *Nursing home residents supported in completing ADLs by nursing staff had significantly higher self-esteem than residents who were overly assisted (Blair, 1999).*

• Reinforce the personal strengths and positive self-perceptions that the client identifies. **Nursing Research:** *Lower levels of depressive symptoms were associated with higher optimism scores in rural adolescents (Puskar et al, 1999).*

• Identify and limit the client's negative self-assessments. **Nursing Research:** *Negative thinking had a greater effect on depressive symptoms than self-esteem (Peden et al, 2000).*

• Encourage realistic and achievable goal setting, resources, and impediments to achievement. **Nursing Research:** *Clients infected with HIV who had higher self-esteem focused on resources and perceived fewer threats (Anderson, 2000).*

• Demonstrate and promote effective communication techniques; spend time with the client. **Nursing Research:** *This study demonstrated the importance of presence and caring communication (Sundin et al, 2002).*

• Encourage independent decision-making by reviewing options and their possible consequences with the client. Autonomy enhances self-esteem (Pierce and Hicks, 2001). **Nursing Research:** *Perceived autonomy and control in nursing home residents increased motivation and self-esteem (Blair, 1999).*

• Assist the client to challenge negative perceptions of self and performance. *Reduction in negative thinking is correlated with increase in self-esteem (Peden et al, 2000).*

• Use failure as an opportunity to provide valuable feedback. *Allows a client to change expectations of what would happen given the reality of what did happen (Pierce and Hicks, 2001).*

• Promote a positive environment and activities that enhance self-esteem. *Self-esteem is positively correlated with the ability to meet self-care requirements (Blair, 1999).*

• Assist the client with evaluating the impact of family and peer group on feelings of self-worth. *Strong negative societal messages may decrease self-esteem and increase depression (Peden et al, 2000).*

• Support socialization and communication skills. Teach conflict resolution skills. **Nursing Research:** *Socialization increases opportunities for support and validation from others. Conflict was found to have negative effects on psychological sense of belonging (Haggerty and Williams, 1999). Social support increases the client's ability to cope with problems (Beebe, 2002).*

• Help the client to identify a range of feelings in response to situations. *Shame is decreased when acceptance of all feelings occurs (Merritt, 1997).*

• Help the client to increase sense of belonging. **Nursing Research:** *A sense of belonging and socialization reduce vulnerability to depression and low self-esteem (Haggerty and Williams, 1999).*

Geriatric

• Support the client in identifying and adapting to functional changes. *Accurate evaluation allows the client to establish realistic expectations of self.*

• Use reminiscence therapy to identify patterns of strength and accomplishment. *Identifying strengths and accomplishments counteracts pervasive negativity.*

• Encourage participation in peer group activities. *Withdrawal and social isolation are detrimental to feelings of self-worth.*

• Encourage activities in which the client can support/help others. *Helping others increases self-esteem in older adults (Krause and Shaw, 2000).*

• = Independent; ▲ = Collaborative

Multicultural
- Assess for the influence of cultural beliefs, norms, and values on the client's sense of self-esteem. **Nursing Research:** *How the client values self may be based on cultural perceptions (Cochran, 1998; Doswell and Erlen, 1998; Leininger and McFarland, 2002).*
- Validate the client's feelings regarding ethnic or racial identity. **Nursing Research:** Validation lets the client know that the nurse has heard and understands what was said, and it promotes the nurse-client relationship (Heineken, 1998). Individuals with strong ethnic affiliation have higher levels of self-esteem than others (Phinney, 1995).

Home care
- Above interventions may be adapted for home care use.
- Assess the client's immediate support system/family for relationship patterns and content of communication. *Knowledge of client relationships helps the nurse to individualize care.*
- Encourage family to provide support and feedback regarding client value or worth. *The family is a socially significant cultural group that generates behavior, defines roles, and promotes values.*
- Encourage/assist the client to identify interest areas; ways of becoming involved with interest areas; ways of becoming involved with and helping others. *Clients with chronic low self-esteem tend to be self-focused in a negative way. Accomplishing objectives in interest areas (e.g., learning to read if illiterate), receiving positive feedback for those accomplishments, and focusing on something else aid in improving self-esteem.*
- Encourage the client to become involved in self-care management. *Low self-esteem generates a sense of powerlessness. Refer to care plan for* **Powerlessness.**
- ▲ Refer to medical social services to assist the family in pattern changes that could benefit the client. *The best nursing plan may be to access specialty services for the client and family.*
- ▲ If the client is involved in counseling or self-help groups, monitor and encourage attendance. Help the client identify value of group participation after each group encounter. *Discussion about group participation clarifies and reinforces group feedback and support.*
- ▲ If the client is taking prescribed psychotropic medications, assess for knowledge of medication side effects and reasons for taking medication. Teach as necessary. *Understanding the medical regimen supports compliance.*
- ▲ Assess medications for effectiveness and side effects and monitor the client for compliance. *Clients with poor ego strength may have difficulty adhering to a medication regimen. Clients who experience negative side effects are less likely than others to adhere to medication regimen.*

Client/Family Teaching
- ▲ Refer to community agencies for psychotherapeutic counseling.
- ▲ Refer to psychoeducational groups on stress reduction and coping skills.
- ▲ Refer to self-help support groups specific to needs.

𝗲𝘃𝗼𝗹𝘃𝗲 WEBSITES FOR EDUCATION

See the EVOLVE website for World Wide Web resources for client education.

• = Independent; ▲ = Collaborative

REFERENCES

Anderson E: Self-esteem and optimism in men and women infected with HIV, *Nurs Res* 49:5, 2000.

Beebe LH: Problems in community living identified by people with schizophrenia, *J Psychosoc Ment Health Nurs* 40:2, 2002.

Blair C: Effects of self-care ADL's on self-esteem of intact nursing home residents, *Issues Ment Health Nurs* 20: 559, 1999.

Cochran M: Tears have no color, *Am J Nurs* 98(6):53, 1998.

Doswell W, Erlen J: Multicultural issues and ethical concerns in the delivery of revising care interventions, *Nurs Clin North Am* 33(2):353, 1998.

Gilbert DA: Relational message themes in nurses' listening behavior during brief client-nurse interactions, *Scholarly Inquiry Nurs Pract* 12 (1), 1998.

Haggerty B, Williams R: The effects of sense of belonging, social support, conflict and loneliness on depression, *Nurs Res* 48:4, 1999.

Heineken J: Patient silence is not necessarily client satisfaction: Communication in home care nursing, *Home Healthc Nurse* 16(2):115, 1998.

Krause N, Shaw BA: Giving social support to others: socioeconomic status and self-esteem in late life, *J Gerontol B Psychol Sci Soc Sci* 55:11, 2000.

Leininger MM, McFarland MR: *Transcultural nursing: concepts, theories, research and practices,* ed 3, New York, 2002, McGraw-Hill.

Merritt P: Guilt and shame in recovering addicts: a personal account, *J Psychosoc Nurs Ment Health Serv* 35:7, 1997.

Norris J: Nursing interventions for self-esteem disturbance, *Nurs Diagn* 3:48, 1992.

Peden A et al: Negative thinking mediates the effects of self-esteem on depressive symptoms in college women, *Nurs Res* 49:4, 2000.

Phinney JS: Ethnic identity and self-esteem. In Padilla A, editor: *Hispanic psychology: critical issues in theory and research,* Thousand Oaks, Calif, 1995, Sage.

Pierce P, Hicks F: Client decision-making behavior: an emerging paradigm for nursing science, *Nurs Res* 50:5, 2001.

Puskar et al: Optimism and it's relationship to depression, coping, anger and life events in rural adolescents, *Issues Ment Health Nurs* 20:15, 1999.

Sundin K, Jansson L, Norberg A: Understanding between care providers and clients with stroke and aphasia: a phenomenological hermeneutic inquiry, *Nurs Inq* 9(2), 2002.

Situational low Self-esteem

Judith R. Gentz

NANDA Definition

Development of a negative perception of self-worth in response to a current situation (specify)

Defining Characteristics

Verbally reports current situational challenge to self-worth; self-negating verbalizations; indecisive, nonassertive behavior; evaluation of self as unable to deal with situations or events; expressions of helplessness and uselessness

Related Factors (r/t)

Developmental changes (specify); disturbed body image; functional impairment (specify); loss (specify); social role changes (specify); lack of recognition/rewards; behavior inconsistent with values; failures/rejections

• = Independent; ▲ = Collaborative

| NOC | Outcomes (Nursing Outcomes Classification) |

Suggested NOC Outcomes
Decision Making; Self-Esteem

Example NOC Outcome with Indicators

Self-Esteem as evidenced by the following indicators: Verbalizations of acceptance of self and limitations/ Open communication (Rate each indicator of **Self-Esteem:** 1 = never positive, 2 = rarely positive, 3 = sometimes positive, 4 = often positive, 5 = consistently positive [see Section I].)

Client Outcomes

Client Will (Specify Time Frame):
- State effect of life events on feelings about self
- State personal strengths
- Acknowledge presence of guilt and not blame self if an action was related to another person's appraisal
- Seek help when necessary
- Demonstrate self-perceptions that are accurate given physical capabilities
- Demonstrate separation of self-perceptions from societal stigmas

| NIC | Interventions (Nursing Interventions Classification) |

Suggested NIC Intervention
Self-Esteem Enhancement

Example NIC Activities—Self-Esteem Enhancement

Encourage the client to identify strengths; Assist the client in setting realistic goals to achieve higher self-esteem

---

Nursing Interventions and Rationales

- ▲ Assess the client for symptoms of depression and potential for suicide or violence. If present, immediately notify appropriate personnel of symptoms. See care plans for **Risk for other-directed Violence** and/or **Risk for Suicide.** *Safety measures and psychiatric interventions are essential when there is a risk of violence. Coping attempts may be ineffective during time of crisis.*
- Actively listen to, demonstrate respect for, and accept the client. *Clarification of thoughts and feelings promotes self-acceptance (LeMone, 1991).*
- Assist in the identification of problems and situational factors that contribute to problems, offering options for resolution. *Clients often expect professionals to recommend remedies to problems and need encouragement to participate in selecting treatment options (Pierce and Hicks, 2001).*
- Use statements such as, "No one can make you feel guilty without your consent," to help the client recognize that no one else can control the client's feelings.
- Mutually identify strengths, resources, and previously effective coping strategies. *Acknowledgment of competence enhances self-esteem (Miller, 1983) and reinforces previously intact self-esteem (Anderson, 1995). Knowledgeable clients make better decisions regarding their health care (Pierce and Hicks, 2001).*

- • = Independent; ▲ = Collaborative

- Have the client list strengths. **Nursing Research:** *Patients were found to use a variety of self-care strategies, medication management techniques and emotional supports to alleviate symptoms of CHF (Bennett et al, 2000).*
- Accept the client's own pace in working through grief or crisis situations. *Pressuring the client to prematurely resolve feelings increases the client's sense of inadequacy (Kus, 1985). Maladjustment to loss or change can have detrimental effects on the entire concept of self (Drench, 1994).*
- Accept the client's own defenses in dealing with the crisis. *Denial protects the self-concept by distorting reality in a self-enhancing way (Russell, 1993). Decision-making behaviors adapt and change with time and experience (Pierce and Hicks, 2001).*
- Assess for unhealthy coping mechanisms such as substance abuse. *Low self-esteem and anger in adolescents has been linked to health risk behaviors and negative life events (McGee and Williams, 2000; Modrcin-Talbott et al, 1998).*
- ▲ Assess the client for symptoms of depression and potential for suicide or violence. If present, immediately notify appropriate personnel of symptoms. See care plans for **Risk for other-directed Violence** and/or **Risk for self-directed Violence.** *Safety measures and psychiatric interventions are essential when there is a risk of violence. Coping attempts may be ineffective during time of crisis.*
- ▲ Provide information about support groups of people who have common experiences or interests. **Nursing Research:** *Social support was a strong predictor of resourcefulness, self-esteem, and well-being of postmastectomy patients (Dirsken, 2000).*
- Support problem-solving strategies but discourage decision-making when in crisis. *Crisis is a time of increased tension and disorganization.* **Nursing Research:** *Uncertainty is a significant negative predictor of resourcefulness (Dirsken, 2000).*
- Explore constructive outlets for frustration. *Exploration expands strategies for coping.*
- Encourage objective appraisal of self and life events and challenge negative or perfectionist expectations of self. *A positive adjustment to illness may be the result of the ability to lower ideal self-expectations (Heidrich and Ward, 1992).*
- ▲ Provide psychoeducation to the client and family. *Psychoeducation decreases symptomatology of the client and increases support by care providers (Biegel et al, 2000). Knowledge provides empowerment, which will increase self-esteem (Merrell, 2001).*
- Validate confusion when feeling ill but looking well. *Validation will decrease shame and guilt, and invites further verbalization (Gordon et al, 1998).*
- Acknowledge the presence of societal stigma. Teach management tools. *Health promotion requires modification of stigmas (O'Brien, 1998).*
- Validate the impact of past experiences on self-esteem and work on corrective measures. *Family dysfunction, child abuse, and other childhood stressors may lead to low self-esteem (Harter, 2000).*
- See care plan for **Chronic low Self-esteem.**

Geriatric

- Support the client in identifying and adapting to functional changes. *Accurate evaluation allows the client to establish realistic expectations of self.*
- Use reminiscence therapy to identify patterns of strength and accomplishment. *Identifying strengths and accomplishments counteracts pervasive negativity.*
- Encourage participation in peer group activities. *Withdrawal and social isolation are detrimental to feelings of self-worth.*

• = **Independent;** ▲ = **Collaborative**

- Encourage activities in which the client can support/help others. *Helping others increases self-esteem in older adults (Krause and Shaw, 2000).*

Multicultural

- Assess for the influence of cultural beliefs, norms, and values on the client's sense of self-esteem. **Nursing Research:** *How the client values self may be based on cultural perceptions (Cochran, 1998; Doswell and Erlen, 1998; Leininger and McFarland, 2002).*
- Validate the client's feelings regarding ethnic or racial identity. **Nursing Research:** *Validation lets the client know that the nurse has heard and understands what was said, and it promotes the nurse-client relationship (Heineken, 1998). Individuals with strong ethnic affiliation have higher levels of self-esteem than others (Phinney, 1995).*

Home care

- Above interventions may be adapted for home care use.
- Assist the client to initiate effective problem-solving toward current situation. *Ability to respond effectively to the situation will assist the client to regain previous level of self-esteem.*
- Establish an emergency plan and contract with the client for its use. *Having an emergency plan is reassuring to the client. Establishing a contract validates the worth of the client and provides a caring link between the client and society.*
- Access supplies that support the client's success at independent living.
- See care plan for **Chronic low Self-esteem.**

Client/Family Teaching

- Assess person's support system (family, friends, community) and involve if desired. Educate the client and family regarding the grief process. *Understanding this process normalizes responses of sadness, anger, guilt, and helplessness.*
- Teach the client and family that the crisis is temporary. *Knowing that the crisis is temporary provides a sense of hope for the future.*
- ▲ Refer to appropriate community resources or crisis intervention centers.
- ▲ Refer to resources for handicap and/or disability services.
- ▲ Refer to illness-specific consumer support groups.
- ▲ Refer to self-help support groups specific to needs.

evolve WEBSITES FOR EDUCATION

See the EVOLVE website for World Wide Web resources for client education.

REFERENCES

Anderson K: The effect of chronic obstructive pulmonary disease on quality of life, *Res Nurs Health* 18:547, 1995.
Biegel DE, Robinson EM, Kennedy M: A review of empirical studies of interventions of families of persons with mental illness. In Morrisey J, editor: *Research in community mental health: social facets in mental health and illness,* Vol 2, Greenwich, Conn, 2000, JAI Press.
Cochran M: Tears have no color, *Am J Nurs* 98(6):53, 1998.
Dirsken SR: Predicting well-being among breast cancer survivors, *J Adv Nurs* 32:4, 2000.

• = **Independent;** ▲ = **Collaborative**

Doswell W, Erlen J: Multicultural issues and ethical concerns in the delivery of revising care interventions, *Nurs Clin North Am* 33(2):353, 1998.

Drench ME: Changes in body image secondary to disease and injury, *Rehabil Nurs* 19:31, 1994.

Gordon P et al: The meaning of disability: how women with chronic illness view their experiences, *J Rehabil* 64:3, 1998.

Harter SL: Psychosocial adjustment of adult children of alcoholics, *Clin Psychol Rev* 20:3, 2000.

Heidrich SM, Ward SE: The role of the self in adjustment to cancer in elderly women, *Oncol Nurs Forum* 19: 1491, 1992.

Heineken J: Patient silence is not necessarily client satisfaction: Communication in home care nursing, *Home Healthc Nurse* 16(2):115, 1998.

Krause N, Shaw BA: Giving social support to others: socioeconomic status and self-esteem in late life, *J Gerontol B Psychol Sci Soc Sci* 55:11, 2000.

Kus RJ: Crisis intervention. In Bulechek GM, McCloskey JC, editors: *Nursing interventions: treatments for nursing diagnoses,* Philadelphia, 1985, WB Saunders.

Leininger MM, McFarland MR: *Transcultural nursing: concepts, theories, research and practices,* ed 3, New York, 2002, McGraw-Hill.

LeMone P: Analysis of a human phenomenon: self-concept, *Nurs Diagn* 2:126, 1991.

McGee R, Williams S: Does low self-esteem predict health compromising behaviors among adolescents, *J Adolesc* 23:569, 2000.

Merrell J: Social support for victims of domestic violence, *J Psychosoc Nurs* 39:11, 2001.

Miller JF: *Coping with chronic illness: overcoming powerlessness,* Philadelphia, 1983, FA Davis.

Modrcin-Talbott MA et al: A study of self-esteem among well adolescents: seeking a new direction, *Issues Compr Pediatr Nurs* 21:4, 1998.

O'Brien SM: Health promotion and schizophrenia: the year 2000 and beyond, *Holist Nurs Pract* 12:2, 1998.

Phinney JS: Ethnic identity and self-esteem. In Padilla A, editor: *Hispanic psychology: critical issues in theory and research,* Thousand Oaks, Calif, 1995, Sage.

Pierce P, Hicks F: Patient decision-making behavior: an emerging paradigm for nursing science, *Nurs Res* 50:5, 2001.

Puskar K et al: Optimism and its relationship to depression, coping, anger and life events in rural adolescents, *Issues Ment Health Nurs* 20:15, 1999.

Russell GC: The role of denial in clinical practice, *J Adv Nurs* 18:938, 1993.

Risk for situational low Self-esteem

Judith R. Gentz

NANDA Definition

At risk for developing negative perception of self-worth in response to a current situation (specify)

Risk Factors

Developmental changes (specify); disturbed body image; functional impairment (specify); loss (specify); social role changes (specify); history of learned helplessness; history of abuse, neglect, or abandonment; unrealistic self-expectations; behavior inconsistent with values; lack of recognition/rewards; failures/rejections; decreased power/control over environment; physical illness (specify)

NOC Outcomes (Nursing Outcomes Classification)

Suggested NOC Outcomes
Decision Making; Self-Esteem

• = Independent; ▲ = Collaborative

> ### Example NOC Outcome with Indicators
>
> **Self-Esteem** as evidenced by the following indicators: Verbalizations of acceptance of self and limitations/Open communication (Rate each indicator of **Self-Esteem:** 1 = never positive, 2 = rarely positive, 3 = sometimes positive, 4 = often positive, 5 = consistently positive [see Section I].)

Client Outcomes

Client Will (Specify Time Frame):
- State accurate self-appraisal
- Demonstrate the ability to self-validate
- Demonstrate the ability to make decisions independent of primary peer group
- Express effects of media on self-appraisal
- Express influence of substances on self-esteem
- Identify strengths and healthy coping skills
- State life events and change as influencing self-esteem

NIC   Interventions (Nursing Interventions Classification)

Suggested NIC Intervention
Self-Esteem Enhancement

> ### Example NIC Activities—Self-Esteem Enhancement
>
> Encourage the client to identify strengths; Help the client to set realistic goals to achieve higher self-esteem

Nursing Interventions and Rationales

- Help the client to identify environmental and/or developmental factors, which increase risk for low self-esteem. *Identification is early stage of problem-solving process. Preadolescence is a high-risk time for low self-esteem (McGee and Williams, 2000). Primary prevention includes community education in the schools (Merrell, 2001).*
- Help the client to identify current behaviors resulting from low self-esteem. *Low self-esteem increases risk for unhealthy behaviors (McGee and Williams, 2000).*
- Encourage creative problem solving through writing exercises. **Nursing Research:** *Creative writing increased self-efficacy and self-esteem among adolescents studied. Giving positive feedback can increase self-esteem (Chandler, 1999).*
- Encourage the client to maintain highest level of functioning, including work schedule. **Nursing Research:** *Social involvement and work were predictors of higher self-esteem among persons with mental illness (VanDongen, 1998).*
- Encourage the client to verbalize thoughts and feelings about the current situation, individually or in groups. *Allowing the client to clarify thoughts and feelings promotes self-acceptance (LeMone, 1991). Validation by others promotes acceptance of self (Linehan, 1993).*
- Help the client to identify what has helped maintain positive self-esteem thus far. *Identifying what works empowers the client and encourages positive outcomes.*
- Help the client to identify the resources and social support network available to him or her at this time. **Nursing Research:** *Greater resourcefulness positively impacted feeling of self-esteem in breast cancer patients (Dirksen, 2000).*

- = **Independent;** ▲ = **Collaborative**

▲ Encourage the client to find a self-help or therapy group that focuses on self-esteem enhancement. *Group therapy provides a safe place for feeling exploration, validation, positive role models, and to gain knowledge (Merrell, 2001).* **Nursing Research:** *Social support was a strong predictor of resourcefulness, self-esteem, and well-being in post mastectomy patients (Dirsken, 2000).*

• Encourage the client to create a sense of competence through short-term goal setting and goal achievement. *Sense of competence is related to global self-esteem (Willoughby et al, 2000).*

• Educate female clients about self-esteem differences between genders, and encourage exploration. *Females tend to have lower self-esteem than males no matter what domain is measured (Bolognini et al, 1996).*

▲ Assess the client for symptoms of depression and anxiety. Refer to specialist as needed. *Prompt and effective treatment can prevent exacerbation of symptoms or safety risks.*

• Teach the client a systematic problem-solving process. *Crisis provides an opportunity for effective change in coping skills.*

• See care plans for **Disturbed personal Identity** and **Situational low Self-esteem.**

Geriatric

• Help the client to identify age-related and/or developmental factors that may be affecting self-esteem. *Self-esteem levels vary with the normal aging process and tend to decrease with older age (Dietz, 1996).*

• Assist the client in life review and identifying positive accomplishments. *Life review is a developmental task that increases a person's sense of peace and serenity.*

• Help the client to establish a peer group and structured daily activities. *Social isolation and lack of structure increase a client's sense of feeling lost and worthless.*

Home care

• Above interventions may be adapted for home care use.

• Assess current environmental stresses and identify community resources. *Accessing resources to help decrease environmental stress will increase the client's ability to cope.*

• Assist the client to initiate effective problem solving toward current situation. *Ability to respond effectively to the situation will assist the client to regain previous level of self-esteem.*

• Encourage family members to acknowledge and validate the client's strengths. *Validation allows the client to increase self-reliance and to trust personal decisions.*

• Assess the need for establishing an emergency plan. *Openly assessing safety risks increases the client's sense of limits, boundaries, and safety.*

• See care plans for **Situational low Self-esteem** and **Chronic low Self-esteem.**

Client/Family Teaching

▲ Refer the client/family to community-based self-help and support groups.

▲ Refer to educational classes on stress management, relaxation training, etc.

▲ Refer to community agencies that offer support and environmental resources.

evolve WEBSITES FOR EDUCATION

See the EVOLVE website for World Wide Web resources for client education.

• = **Independent;** ▲ = **Collaborative**

REFERENCES

Bolognini M et al: Self-esteem and mental health in early adolescence: developmental and gender differences, *J Adolesc* 3:19, 1996.

Chandler GE: A creative writing program to enhance self-esteem and self-efficacy in adolescence, *J Child Adolesc Psychiatr Nurs* 2:12, 1999.

Dietz BE: The relationship of aging to self-esteem: the relative effects of maturation and role accumulation, *Int J Aging Hum Dev* 3:43, 1996.

Dirksen SR: Predicting well-being among breast cancer survivors, *J Adv Nurs* 4:32, 2000.

LeMone P: Analysis of a human phenomenon: self-concept, *Nurs Diagn* 2:126, 1991.

McGee R, Williams S: Does low self-esteem predict health compromising behaviours among adolescents? *J Adolesc* 5:23, 2000.

Merrell J: Social support for victims of domestic violence, *J Psychosoc Nurs* 39:11, 2001.

VanDongen CJ: Self-esteem among persons with severe mental illness, *Issues Ment Health Nurs* 1:19, 1998.

Willoughby C et al: Measuring the self-esteem of adolescents with mental health problems: theory meets practice, *Can J Occup Ther* 4:67, 2000.

Self-mutilation

Kathleen L. Patusky

NANDA Definition

Deliberate self-injurious behavior causing tissue damage with the intent of causing non-fatal injury to attain relief of tension

Defining Characteristics

Cuts/scratches on body; picking at wounds; self-inflicted burns (e.g., eraser, cigarette); ingestion/inhalation of harmful substances/objects; biting; abrading; severing; insertion of object(s) into body orifice(s); hitting; constricting a body part

Related Factors (r/t)

Psychotic state (command hallucinations); inability to express tension verbally; childhood sexual abuse; violence between parental figures; family divorce; family alcoholism; family history of self-destructive behaviors; adolescence; peers who self-mutilate; isolation from peers; perfectionism; substance abuse; eating disorders; sexual identity crisis; low or unstable self-esteem; low or unstable body image; labile behavior (mood swings); history of inability to plan solutions or see long-term consequences; use of manipulation to obtain nurturing relationship with others; chaotic/disturbed interpersonal relationships; emotionally disturbed, battered child; feels threatened with actual or potential loss of significant relationship (e.g., loss of parent/parental relationship); experiences dissociation or depersonalization; mounting tension that is intolerable; impulsivity; inadequate coping; irresistible urge to cut/damage self; needs quick reduction of stress; childhood illness or surgery; foster, group, or institutional care; incarceration; character disorder; borderline personality disorder; developmentally delayed or autistic individual; history of self-injurious behavior; feelings of depression, rejection, self-hatred, separation anxiety, guilt, depersonalization; poor parent-adolescent communication; lack of family confidant

• = Independent; ▲ = Collaborative

NOC   Outcomes (Nursing Outcomes Classification)

Suggested NOC Outcomes
Aggression Self-Control; Distorted Thought Self-Control; Impulse Self-Control; Mood Equilibrium; Risk Detection; Self-Mutilation Restraint

> **Example NOC Outcome with Indicators**
>
> **Self-Mutilation Restraint** as evidenced by the following indicators: Restrains from gathering means for self-mutilation/Seeks help when feeling urge to injure self/Requires no treatment for self-injury/Upholds contract not to harm self, maintains self-control without supervision, and does not injure self (Rate each indicator of **Self-Mutilation Restraint:** 1 = never demonstrated, 2 = rarely demonstrated, 3 = sometimes demonstrated, 4 = often demonstrated, 5 = consistently demonstrated [see Section I].)

Client Outcomes

Client Will (Specify Time Frame):
- Have injuries treated
- Refrain from further self-injury
- State appropriate ways to cope with increased psychological or physiological tension
- Express feelings
- Seek help when having urges to self-mutilate
- Maintain self-control without supervision
- Use appropriate community agencies when caregivers are unable to attend to emotional needs

NIC   Interventions (Nursing Interventions Classification)

Suggested NIC Interventions
Active Listening; Anger Control Assistance; Behavior Management: Self-Harm; Calming Technique; Environmental Management: Safety; Limit Setting; Mood Management; Mutual Goal Setting; Risk Identification; Self-Responsibility Facilitation

> **Example NIC Activities—Behavior Management: Self-Harm**
>
> Anticipate trigger situations that may prompt self-harm and intervene to prevent; Teach and reinforce effective coping behaviors and appropriate expression of feelings

Nursing Interventions and Rationales

NOTE: Prior to implementation of interventions in the face of self-mutilation, nurses should examine their own emotional responses to incidents of self-harm, to ensure that interventions will not be based on countertransference reactions. *Studies of staff working with individuals who self-mutilate have shown that staff members may experience feelings ranging from anger to inadequacy and guilt, with a subpopulation of staff holding punitive/negative beliefs toward the client (Fish, 2000; Gough and Hawkins, 2000; Horsfall, 1999).*
▲ Provide medical treatment for injuries. Use careful aseptic technique when caring for wounds. Care for the wounds in a matter-of-fact manner. *A significant impediment to wound healing is infection. Treatment of chronic wounds should be directed toward the main etiologic factors responsible for the wound. Moreover, factors that may impede healing*

• = Independent; ▲ = Collaborative

must be identified and, if possible, corrected for healing to occur (Stadelmann et al, 1998). A matter-of-fact approach does not promote inappropriate attention-getting behavior and may decrease repetition of behavior.

▲ Assess for risk of suicide. *While self-mutilation should not be viewed simply as failed suicide, it is a significant indicator of suicide risk (Cook, 1999).* **Clinical Research:** *A study of suicide attempters showed that individuals who mutilate themselves are at greater risk for suicide than those who do not (Stanley et al, 2001).* Refer to the care plan for **Risk for Suicide.**

▲ Assess for signs of depression, anxiety, and impulsivity. *These behaviors are identified in clients with a history of self-mutilation (Stanley et al, 2001).*

▲ Assess for presence of hallucinations. Ask specific questions such as, "Do you hear voices that other people do not hear? Are they telling you to hurt yourself?" *Command hallucinations occurring with schizophrenia or brief psychotic episodes may direct the client to hurt him or herself, or others. An accurate assessment of the client's contact with reality is important in planning care. Acknowledging that the client may hear something that others do not may open up communication and help establish trust. The presence of hallucinations may also indicate use of specific medications (i.e., antipsychotics) that can reduce the hallucinations more effectively than antianxiety medications.*

▲ Assure the client that he or she will not be alone and will be safe during hallucinations. Provide referrals for medication. *Hallucinations can be very frightening; therefore clients need reassurance that they will not be left alone. Significantly reduced rates of further self-harm were observed for depot flupentixol versus placebo in multiple repeaters (Hawton et al, 1998).*

• Monitor the client's behavior using 15-minute checks at irregular times so that the client does not notice a pattern. *When there is lack of control, client safety is an important issue and close observation is essential. Avoiding a pattern prevents clients from being self-abusive when they know a caregiver will not be present.*

• Establish trust. *Establishing trust appears to be the most critical component of assessing and treating the client who self-mutilates (Dallam, 1997). Discussing feelings of self-harm with a trusted person provides relief for the client.*

• Be extremely cautious about touching the client when he or she is experiencing an abreaction (reenactment of precipitating trauma). Sometimes physically holding a client is necessary to prevent self-injury. *Reexperiencing of a traumatic event may initiate self-mutilation behavior in individuals with this behavior pattern. Touch may be interpreted as coming from an abuser and could result in aggressive acting out. Even well-intentioned or consoling touching may further upset the client. A therapist who is attempting to be consoling should always ask abreacting clients whether they may be touched. Clients may initially refuse, but they generally appreciate the offer. An offer may be repeated several times and clients may eventually agree to be touched or held. If clients must be held to prevent self-injury, explain why it is necessary before touching them (Fike, 1990).*

▲ Assess the client's ability to enter into a no-suicide contract. Secure a written or verbal contract from the client to notify staff when experiencing the desire to self-mutilate. *A study indicated reduced repetition of self-harm when there is an emergency contact card in addition to standard care (Hawton et al, 1998). Discussing feelings of self-harm with a trusted person provides relief for the client. A contract gets the subject out in the open and places some of the responsibility for safety with the client. Some clients are not appropriate for a contract: those under the influence of drugs or alcohol, or unwilling to abstain from substance use; those who are isolated or alone without assistance to keep the environment safe*

• = **Independent;** ▲ = **Collaborative**

(Hauenstein, 2002). If the client will not contract, the risk of suicide should be considered. The lack of willingness for self-disclosure has been shown to discriminate the serious suicide attempter from clients with suicidal ideation or mild attempts (Apter et al, 2001). **Nursing Research:** *Contracting is a common practice in the psychiatric care setting. However, recent research has suggested that self-harm is not prevented by contracts (Drew, 2001). The researcher reported that 1) consistency of nursing assignment could be associated with lower probability of self-harm; and 2) a previous study showing positive effects, conducted with children, involved contracts that specified a positive contingency if clients refrained from self-harm. The researcher concluded that thorough, ongoing assessment of suicide risk is necessary, whether or not the client has a no self-harm contract.*

▲ Use a collaborative approach for care. *A collaborative approach to care is more helpful to the client (Clarke and Whittaker, 1998).*

▲ Refer for medication such as clozapine. **Clinical Research:** *In a study of seven subjects known to have a personality disorder and severe self-mutilation, there was a statistically significant reduction in incidents of self-mutilation with the use of medication (Chengappa et al, 1999).*

▲ Consider partial hospitalization with individual and group therapy. *Psychoanalytically oriented partial hospitalization is superior to standard psychiatric care for clients with borderline personality disorder. These clients had a decrease in self-mutilation (Bateman and Fonagy, 1999).*

• Refer to care plan for **Risk for Self-mutilation** for additional information.

Home care
• See care plan for **Risk for Self-mutilation.**

Client/Family Teaching
• See care plan for **Risk for Self-mutilation.**

evolve WEBSITES FOR EDUCATION

See the EVOLVE website for World Wide Web resources for client education.

REFERENCES

Apter A et al: Relationship between self-disclosure and serious suicidal behavior, *Comp Psychiatry* 42(1):70, 2001.

Bateman A, Fonagy P: Effectiveness of partial hospitalization in the treatment of borderline personality disorder: a randomized controlled trial, *Am J Psychiatry* 156(10):1563, 1999.

Chengappa KN et al: Clozapine reduces severe self-mutilation and aggression in psychotic patients with borderline personality disorder, *J Clin Psychiatry* 60(7):477, 1999.

Clarke L, Whittaker M: Self-mutilation: culture, contexts and nursing responses, *J Clin Nurs* 7(2):129, 1998.

Cook J: With serious intent: a review of the literature on non-fatal deliberate self-harm, *Ment Health Learn Disabil Care* 3(2):57, 1999.

Dallam SJ: The identification and management of self-mutilating patients in primary care, *Nurse Pract* 22(5): 151, 1997.

Drew BL: Self-harm behavior and no-suicide contracting in psychiatric inpatient settings, *Arch Psychiatr Nurs* 15:99, 2001.

Fike ML: Considerations and techniques in the treatment of persons with multiple personality disorder, *Am J Occup Ther* 44:999, 1990.

• = Independent; ▲ = Collaborative

Fish RM: Working with people who harm themselves in a forensic learning disability service: experiences of direct care staff, *J Learn Disabil* 4:193, 2000.

Gough K, Hawkins A: Staff attitudes to self-harm and its management in a forensic psychiatric service, *Br J Forens Pract* 2(4):22, 2000.

Hauenstein EJ: Case finding and care in suicide: children, adolescents, and adults. In Boyd MA, editor: *Psychiatric nursing. Contemporary practice*, ed 2, Philadelphia, 2002, Lippincott.

Hawton K et al: Deliberate self-harm: systematic review of efficacy of psychosocial and pharmacological treatments in preventing repetition, *BMJ* 317(7156):441, 1998.

Horsfall J: Towards understanding some complex borderline behaviors, *J Psychiatr Ment Health Nurs* 6:425, 1999.

Stadelmann WK, Digenis AG, Tobin GR: Impediments to wound healing, *Am J Surg* 176(2A suppl):39S, 1998.

Stanley B et al: Are suicide attempters who self-mutilate a unique population? *Am J Psychiatry* 158(3):427, 2001.

Risk for Self-mutilation

Kathleen L. Patusky

NANDA   Definition

At risk for deliberate self-injurious behavior causing tissue damage with the intent of causing nonfatal injury to attain relief of tension

Risk Factors

Psychotic state (command hallucinations); inability to express tension verbally; childhood sexual abuse; violence between parental figures; family divorce; family alcoholism; family history of self-destructive behaviors; adolescence; peers who self-mutilate; isolation from peers; perfectionism; substance abuse; eating disorders; sexual identity crisis; low or unstable self-esteem; low or unstable body image; history of inability to plan solutions or see long-term consequences; use of manipulation to obtain nurturing relationship with others; chaotic/disturbed interpersonal relationships; emotionally disturbed and/or battered child; feels threatened with actual or potential loss of significant relationship; loss of parent/parental relationships; experiences dissociation or depersonalization; experiences mounting tension that is intolerable; impulsivity; inadequate coping; experiences irresistible urge to cut/damage self; needs quick reduction of stress; childhood illness or surgery; foster, group, or institutional care; incarceration; character disorders; borderline personality disorders; loss of control of problem-solving situations; developmentally delayed or autistic individual; history of self-injurious behavior; feelings of depression, rejection, self-hatred, separation anxiety, guilt, and depersonalization

NOC   Outcomes (Nursing Outcomes Classification)

Suggested NOC Outcomes

Abuse Recovery: Emotional; Aggression Self-Control; Distorted Thought Self-Control; Impulse Self-Control; Mood Equilibrium; Risk Detection; Self-Mutilation Restraint

• = Independent; ▲ = Collaborative

Example NOC Outcome with Indicators

Self-Mutilation Restraint as evidenced by the following indicators: Restrains from gathering means for self-mutilation/Seeks help when feeling urge to injure self (Rate each indicator of **Self-Mutilation Restraint:** 1 = never demonstrated, 2 = rarely demonstrated, 3 = sometimes demonstrated, 4 = often demonstrated, 5 = consistently demonstrated [see Section I].)

Client Outcomes

Client Will (Specify Time Frame):
- Refrain from self-injury
- Identify triggers to self-mutilation
- State appropriate ways to cope with increased psychological or physiological tension
- Express feelings
- Seek help when having urges to self-mutilate
- Maintain self-control without supervision
- Use appropriate community agencies when caregivers are unable to attend to emotional needs

NIC   Interventions (Nursing Interventions Classification)

Suggested NIC Interventions

Active Listening; Anger Control Assistance; Behavior Management: Self-Harm; Calming Technique; Counseling; Environmental Management: Safety; Limit Setting; Mood Management; Mutual Goal Setting; Risk Identification; Self-Awareness Enhancement; Self-Esteem Enhancement; Self-Modification Assistance; Self-Responsibility Facilitation

---

Example NIC Activities—Behavior Management: Self-Harm

Anticipate trigger situations that may prompt self-harm and intervene to prevent; Teach and reinforce effective coping behaviors and appropriate expression of feelings

---

Nursing Interventions and Rationales

NOTE: Prior to implementation of interventions in the face of self-mutilation, nurses should examine their own emotional responses to incidents of self-harm, to ensure that interventions will not be based on countertransference reactions. *Studies of staff working with individuals who self-mutilate have shown that staff members may experience feelings ranging from anger to inadequacy and guilt, with a sub-population of staff holding punitive/negative beliefs toward the client (Fish, 2000; Gough and Hawkins, 2000; Horsfall, 1999).*

- Assessment data from the client and family members may have to be gathered at different times; allowing a family member or trusted friend with whom the client is comfortable to be present during the assessment may be helpful. *Self-mutilation sometimes occurs if clients have been victims of abuse. Clients or family members may be more willing to disclose the presence of abuse if greater privacy is afforded them. Presence of a trusted family member or friend may help clients to respond more comfortably to the interview situation.*

• = Independent; ▲ = Collaborative

- Assess for risk factors of self-mutilation, including the categories of psychiatric disorders (particularly borderline personality disorder, psychosis, eating disorders, autism); psychological precursors (e.g., low tolerance for stress, impulsivity, perfectionism); psychosocial dysfunction (e.g., presence of sexual abuse, divorce or alcoholism in the family; manipulative behavior to gain nurturing; chaotic interpersonal relationships), coping difficulties (e.g., inability to plan solutions or see long-term consequences of behavior), personal history (e.g., childhood illness or surgery, past self-injurious behavior), and peer influences (e.g., friends who mutilate, isolation from peers). *All of the risk factors listed above have been found to be associated with self-mutilation. A study of self-injurious behavior in women with eating disorders concluded that the occurrence of an eating disorder was sufficient to indicate the need for routine screening for self-injury (Paul et al, 2002).*
- ▲ Assess family dynamics and need for family therapy. *Impairment of adolescent-parental communication was associated with self-harm among a group of 14- to 19-year-olds (Tulloch et al, 1997).*
- ▲ Assess for presence of hallucinations. Ask specific questions such as, "Do you hear voices that other people do not hear? Are they telling you to hurt yourself?" *Command auditory hallucinations occurring with schizophrenia or with brief psychotic episodes may direct the client to hurt him or herself, or others. An accurate assessment of the client's contact with reality is important in planning care. Acknowledging that the client may hear something that others do not may open up communication and help establish trust. The presence of hallucinations may also indicate use of specific medications (i.e., antipsychotics) that can reduce the hallucinations more effectively than antianxiety medications.*
- ▲ Assure the client that he or she will not be alone and will be safe during hallucinations. Provide referrals for medication. *Hallucinations can be very frightening; therefore clients need reassurance that they will not be left alone. Significantly reduced rates of further self-harm were observed for depot flupentixol versus placebo in multiple repeaters (Hawton et al, 1998).*
- Be alert to other risk factors of self-mutilation in clients with psychosis, including acute intoxication, dramatic changes in body appearance, preoccupation with religion and sexuality, and anticipated or perceived object loss. **Clinical Research:** *A case study of a client with bipolar disorder who self-mutilated revealed the above list of risk factors, along with more usual risk factors of self-mutilation history and command auditory hallucinations. The client shaved his head, voiced literal interpretations of the Bible and profound feeling of guilt about his sexuality, and experienced rejection by his mother (Green et al, 2000).*
- Monitor clients with obsessive-compulsive disorder for possible self-mutilation. *Clients with high levels of obsessive-compulsive symptoms may self-mutilate (McKay et al, 2000).*
- Assess clients who have issues with gender identity for possible self-mutilation. *A study suggested that clients attending gender dysphoria clinics were at risk for self-mutilation (Wylie, 2000).*
- Maintain ongoing surveillance of the client and environment. Monitor the client's behavior using 15-minute checks at irregular times so that the client does not notice a pattern. *When there is lack of control, client safety is an important issue and close observation is essential. Not following a pattern prevents clients from being self-abusive when they know a caregiver will not be present.*
- ▲ When the client is experiencing extreme anxiety, use one-to-one staffing. Offer activi-

• = **Independent;** ▲ = **Collaborative**

ties that will serve as a distraction. **Nursing Research:** *The presence of a trusted individual may calm fears about personal safety. Distraction was reported by self-abusing women as one way of preventing a self-injury episode (Weber, 2002).*

- Implement active listening and early intervention. **Nursing Research:** *In one study, adolescent girls with a history of trauma found that cutting themselves communicated psychological distress when others would not listen to their verbal grievances, but lead to a pattern of self-harm when intervention was not forthcoming (Machoian, 2001).*

- When working with self-mutilative clients with borderline personality disorder, develop an effective therapeutic relationship by avoiding labeling, seeking to understand the meaning of the self-mutilation, and advocating for adequate opportunities for care. **Nursing Research:** *The lived experience of clients with borderline personality disorder identified despair, estrangement, and inadequacy as elements of that experience. Living with the diagnosis resulted in the following experiences: being labeled rather than diagnosed, leading to preconceived and unfavorable opinions by all health care providers and a sense of being marginalized and potentially mistreated; having self-mutilation viewed as deliberate attempts to manipulate others rather than a means of controlling emotional pain; and limited access to care when health care providers conclude nothing will help and clients should "help themselves" (Moffat, 1999; Nehls, 1999).*

- Maintain a consistent relational distance from the client with borderline personality disorder who self-mutilates: neither too close nor too distant, neither rewarding unacceptable behavior nor trying to control or avoid the client. **Nursing Research:** *Clients with borderline personality disorder recreate the chaos of their previous relationships in dealing with health care providers. Clients fear that they will be overwhelmed by or abandoned in relationships, and their reactions can change rapidly. The most effective posture is one that is consistent, allowing clients to react as they need to, while assuring clients that they will not be abandoned (Horsfall, 1999).*

- Inform the client of unit expectations for appropriate behavior and consequences. Emphasize that the client must comply with the rules of the unit. Contract with the client for no self-harm. Give positive reinforcement for compliance and minimize attention paid to disruptive behavior while setting limits. *Clients benefit from clear guidance regarding behavioral expectations and consequences, providing much-needed structure. The process emphasizes client responsibility for his or her own behavior. It is important to reinforce appropriate behavior to encourage repetition. The unit serves as a microcosm of client's outside world, so adherence to social norms while on the unit models adherence upon discharge, while providing the client with staff support to learn appropriate coping skills and alternate behaviors.*

- Assess the client's ability to enter into a no-suicide contract. Secure a written or verbal contract from the client to notify staff when experiencing the desire to self-mutilate. *A study indicated reduced repetition of self-harm when there is an emergency contact card in addition to standard care (Hawton et al, 1998). Discussing feelings of self-harm with a trusted person provides relief for the client. A contract gets the subject out in the open and places some of the responsibility for safety with the client. Some clients are not appropriate for a contract: those under the influence of drugs or alcohol, or unwilling to abstain from substance use; those who are isolated or alone without assistance to keep the environment safe (Hauenstein, 2002). If the client will not contract, the risk of suicide should be considered. The lack of willingness for self-disclosure has been shown to discriminate the serious suicide attempter from clients with suicidal ideation or mild attempts (Apter et al, 2001).* **Nursing Research:** *Contracting is a common practice in psychiatric care setting.*

- • = Independent; ▲ = Collaborative

However, recent research has suggested that self-harm is not prevented by contracts (Drew, 2001). The researcher reported that (1) consistency of nursing assignment could be associated with lower probability of self-harm; and (2) a previous study showing positive effects, conducted with children, involved contracts that specified a positive contingency if clients refrained from self-harm. The researcher concluded that thorough, ongoing assessment of suicide risk is necessary, whether or not the client has a no self-harm contract. Assist the client to identify and express the feelings that are being acted out in self-mutilation.

- Clients need to learn to recognize distress as it occurs and express it verbally rather than as a physical action against the self. **Nursing Research:** *Self-mutilation serves to act out feeling states that the client cannot express or process. Such acts may attempt to relieve pain or punish the self (Horsfall, 1999).*

- Assist the client to identify the motives/reasons for self-mutilation that have been perceived as positive. **Nursing and Clinical Research:** *Favazza (1989) identified the following gains of self-mutilation: tension release; returning to reality; regaining control of some aspect of self; expressing forbidden anger; escaping self-hatred associated with incest; aiming to decrease alienation from or influence others; relieve pressure from multiple personalities; sexual gratification; the sight of blood provides emotional release; the pain and the blood stop feelings of emptiness. The client must learn alternative ways of securing these gains if they are to give up self-mutilation as a means of obtaining the gains. The nurse should ask the client directly what is gained from continued self-mutilation, rather than assuming the motivation is already known (McAllister, 2001).*

- Help the client identify cues that precede impulsive behavior. *Early recognition of triggers permits the client to initiate self-calming procedures, such as relaxation techniques.* **Nursing Research:** *The Dialectical Behavior Therapy technique of behavioral chain analysis was found to reduce self-harm behaviors by 50% over a 4-week period, by processing events that precipitate self-mutilation (Alper and Peterson, 2001).*

- Give praise when the client identifies urges and delays self-destructive behavior. *Delaying destructive behavior and increasing awareness of urges to be self-destructive should both be acknowledged as progress (Gallop, 1992).*

- Assist clients to identify ways to sooth themselves and generate hopefulness when faced with painful emotions. **Nursing Research:** *Women with a history of childhood abuse may not have developed the internal ability to comfort themselves, or self-soothe, resulting in neurobiological disruptions that lead to self-harm as a means of relieving pain (Gallop, 2002). Generating hopefulness is an important self-comforting intervention (Weber, 2002).*

- Be extremely cautious about touching the client when he or she is experiencing an abreaction (reenactment of precipitating trauma). Sometimes physically holding a client is necessary to prevent self-injury. *Reexperiencing of a traumatic event, such as physical or sexual abuse, may initiate self-mutilative behavior in individuals with this behavior pattern. Touch may be interpreted as coming from an abuser and could result in aggressive acting out. Even well-intentioned or consoling touching may further upset the client. A therapist who is attempting to be consoling should always ask the reacting clients whether they may be touched. Clients may initially refuse, but they generally appreciate the offer. An offer may be repeated several times and clients may eventually agree to be touched or held. If clients must be held to prevent self-injury, explain why it is necessary before touching them (Fike, 1990; Weber, 2002).*

- Reinforce alternative ways of dealing with anxiety such as exercise, engaging in unit activities, or talking about feelings. **Clinical Research:** *In a study of exercise training in*

- = Independent; ▲ = Collaborative

adults 50 to 65 years of age, greater exercise participation was significantly related to less anxiety and fewer depressive symptoms (King et al, 1993).

- Keep environment safe; remove all harmful objects from the area. Use of unbreakable glass is recommended for the client at risk for self-injury. *Client safety is a nursing priority. Putting a hand through a window was the most frequent self-injuring behavior in one study. Unbreakable glass would eliminate this type of injury (Callias and Carpenter, 1994).*

- Encourage the client to seek out care providers to talk as urge to harm self occurs. Develop positive therapeutic relationship. *When the client seeks out staff, he or she is exercising self-responsibility and self-care management.* **Nursing Research:** *Even with a contract in place, clients are reassured that staff really do want to help. Self-abusing women have reported that caring relationships have kept them from hurting themselves, and that feeling comforted, supported, and believed would be helpful (Weber, 2002).*

- Anticipate trigger situations and intervene to assist the client in applying alternatives to self-mutilation. *When triggers occur, client stress level may obstruct ability to apply new learning. Assistance facilitates the ability to practice new skills in real situations.*

- If self-mutilation does occur, use a calm, nonpunitive approach. Whenever possible, assist the client to assume responsibility for consequences (e.g., dress self-inflicted wound) Refer to care plan for **Self-Mutilation.** *This approach does not promote inappropriate attention-getting behavior, may decrease repetition of behavior, and reinforces self-responsibility and self-care management.*

- If the client is unable to control behavior, provide interactive supervision, not isolation. *Isolation and deprivation take away individuals' coping abilities and place them at risk for self-harm. Implementing seclusion for clients who have injured themselves in the past may actually facilitate self-injury. Clients are extraordinarily resourceful at identifying environmental objects with which to self-mutilate.*

- ▲ Refer for medication such as clozapine. **Clinical Research:** *In a study of seven subjects known to have a personality disorder and severe self-mutilation, there was a statistically significant reduction in incidents of self-mutilation with use of medication (Chengappa et al, 1999).*

- Involve the client in planning of care and problem-solving, and emphasize that the client makes choices. *Individuals who self-mutilate can become caught up in power struggles with staff. A self-care management approach can circumvent such problems while emphasizing client responsibility and promoting active participation in therapeutic regimen. Individuals who self-mutilate also tend toward emotional impulsivity. Problem solving is a way to gain better emotional control by assisting clients with seeing the connection between problems and emotions (Miller et al, 1994).*

- ▲ Involve the client in group therapy. *Group members learn to identify patterns of behavior that were acquired as a result of painful past events. The past is not trivialized but acknowledged as leading to patterns that now influence all interactions (Gallop, 1992).*

- ▲ Use group therapy to exchange information about methods of coping with loneliness, self-destructive impulses, and interpersonal relationships, as well as housing, employment, and health care system issues directly and noninterpretively. *Individuals with multiple personality disorder/dissociative disorder (MPD/DD) often are estranged from abusive families and have difficulty with social connection. Group therapy can be a useful and successful adjunct to individual psychotherapy for relatively stable clients with MPD/DD. The group's focus should be here and now, supportive and psychoeducative (Dallam and Manderino, 1997).* **Nursing Research:** *Data suggest that an important*

• = Independent; ▲ = Collaborative

component of effective group treatment for a seriously ill person with borderline personality disorder is the meaningful exchange of information. The degree of structure may be a necessary condition for positive outcomes (Nehls, 1992).

▲ Refer to protective services if there is evidence of abuse. *It is the nurse's legal responsibility to report abuse.*

▲ Discharge planning: Provide follow-up to ensure clients attend mental health appointments. *Only a small fraction of people who present in general health care settings with self-mutilation actually follow through with mental health specialist appointments (Tobin et al, 2001).*

▲ Monitor the client for self-harm impulses that may progress to suicidal ideation. *Self-mutilation is a significant indicator of suicide risk (Cook, 1999).*

Geriatric

• Provide hand or back rubs, calming music when elderly client experiences symptoms of anxiety. **Nursing Research:** *In a study of older adults in nursing homes, calming music and hand massage were found to soothe agitation for up to one hour. No additional benefit was found from combining the two interventions (Remington, 2002).*

• Provide soft objects for elderly clients to hold and manipulate when self-mutilation occurs as a function of delirium or dementia. Apply mitts, splints, helmets, or restraints as appropriate. *Delirious or demented clients may unconsciously scratch or pick at themselves. Soft objects may provide a substitute object to pick at; mitts or restraints may be necessary if the client is unable to exercise self-restraint.*

• Older adults who show self-destructive behaviors should be evaluated for dementia. **Clinical Research:** *In a study of nursing home residents, self-destructive behaviors were common and more likely related to dementia than to depression (Draper et al, 2002).*

Home care

• Communicate degree of risk to family/caregivers; assess the family and caregiving situation for ability to protect the client, and to understand the client's self-mutilative behavior. Provide family and caregivers with guidelines on how to manage self-harm behaviors in the home environment. *Client safety between home visits is a nursing priority. Family/caregivers may become frightened by the client's self-mutilation, or may be angry with the client's perceived lack of self-control. Appropriate family/caregiver support is important to the client. Appropriate support will only be forthcoming if all parties understand the basis of the behavior and how to respond to it.*

• Establish an emergency plan, including when to use hotlines and 911. Develop a contract with the client and family for use of the emergency plan. Role-play access to the emergency resources with the client and caregivers. *Having an emergency plan reassures the client and caregivers and promotes client safety. Contracting gives guided control to the client and enhances self-esteem.*

• Assess the home environment for harmful objects. Have family remove or lock objects as able. *Client safety is a nursing priority.*

▲ If client behaviors intensify, institute emergency plan for mental health intervention. *The degree of disturbance and the ability to manage care safely at home determines the level of services needed to protect the client.*

▲ Refer for homemaker or psychiatric home health care services for respite, client reassurance, and implementation of therapeutic regimen. *Responsibility for a person at high risk for self-mutilation provides high caregiver stress. Respite decreases caregiver stress.*

• = **Independent;** ▲ = **Collaborative**

The presence of caring individuals is reassuring to both the client and caregivers, especially during periods of client anxiety. Self-mutilative behavior, especially if accompanied by depression, can make use of the interventions described above, modified for the home setting.

▲ If the client is on psychotropic medications, assess client and family knowledge of medication administration and side effects. Teach as necessary. *Knowledge of the medical regimen promotes compliance and promotes safe use of medications.*

▲ Evaluate the effectiveness and side effects of medications. *Accurate clinical feedback improves physician ability to prescribe an effective medical regimen specific to client needs.*

Client/Family Teaching

- Explain all relevant symptoms, procedures, treatments, and expected outcomes for self-mutilation that is illness-based (e.g., borderline personality disorder, autism). *By increasing knowledge and adapting new behaviors, clients learn that they have some control over their health (Hennessy-Harstad, 1999). Clients are more amenable to therapy and better able to initiate appropriate self-care if they know what to expect.*

- Provide written instructions for treatments and procedures for which the client will be responsible. *A written record provides a concrete reference so that the client and family can clarify any verbal information that was given.*

- Instruct the client in coping strategies (assertiveness training, impulse control training, deep breathing, progressive muscle relaxation). *Clients who self-mutilate have difficulty dealing with stress and painful emotions, which serve as triggers to self-harm. Once clients are able to identify these triggers, they need to learn how to respond to them more effectively through assertiveness, impulse control, or relaxation, as appropriate.*

- Role play (e.g., say, "Tell me how you will respond if someone ignores you"). *Role playing is the most commonly used technique in assertiveness training. It deconditions the anxiety that arises from interpersonal encounters by allowing the client to practice how they might respond in a given situation. Anxiety levels tend to be higher in situations that are unfamiliar.*

- Teach cognitive-behavioral activities, such as active problem solving, reframing (reappraising the situation from a different perspective), or thought-stopping (in response to a negative thought, picture a large stop sign and replace the image with a prearranged positive alternative). Teach the client to confront his or her own negative thought patterns (or cognitive distortions), such as catastophizing (expecting the very worst), dichotomous thinking (perceiving events in only one of two opposite categories), or magnification (placing distorted emphasis on a single event). *Clients who self-mutilate have a low tolerance for stress. Individuals with borderline personality disorder commonly engage in self-talk that is invalid and self-deprecating (Miller et al, 1994). Cognitive-behavioral activities address clients' assumptions, beliefs, and attitudes about their situations, fostering modification of these elements to be as realistic and optimistic as possible. Persons with negative cognitive styles tend to perceive situations as overwhelming, resistant to improvement, and all-encompassing. Through cognitive-behavioral interventions, clients become more aware of their cognitive choices in adopting and maintaining their belief systems, thereby exercising greater control over their own reactions (Hagerty and Patusky, 2003; Sinclair et al, 1998).*

▲ Provide the client and family with phone numbers of appropriate community agencies for therapy and counseling. *Continuous follow-up care should be implemented; therefore the method to access this care must be given to the client.*

▲ Give the client positive things on which to focus by referring to appropriate agencies

- • = **Independent;** ▲ = **Collaborative**

for job-training skills or education. *Alternative coping skills and the means to access them are essential for continued good mental health.*

evolve **WEBSITES FOR EDUCATION**

See the EVOLVE website for World Wide Web resources for client education.

REFERENCES

Alper G, Peterson SJ: Dialectical behavior therapy for patients with borderline personality disorder, *J Psychosoc Nurs Ment Health Serv* 39(10):38, 52, 2001.

Apter A et al: Relationship between self-disclosure and serious suicidal behavior, *Comp Psychiatry* 42(1):70, 2001.

Callias M, Carpenter M: Self-injurious behavior in a state psychiatric hospital, *Hosp Community Psychiatry* 45: 170, 1994.

Chengappa KN et al: Clozapine reduces severe self-mutilation and aggression in psychotic patients with borderline personality disorder, *J Clin Psychiatry* 60(7):477, 1999.

Cook J: With serious intent: a review of the literature on non-fatal deliberate self-harm, *Ment Health Learn Disabil Care* 3(2):57, 1999.

Dallam S, Manderino MA: "Free to be" peer group supports patients with MPD/DD, *J Psychosoc Nurs Ment Health Serv* 35(5):22, 1997.

Draper B et al: Self-destructive behaviors in nursing home residents, *J Am Geriatr Soc* 50:354, 2002.

Drew BL: Self-harm behavior and no-suicide contracting in psychiatric inpatient settings, *Arch Psychiatr Nurs* 15:99, 2001.

Favazza A: Why patients mutilate themselves, *Hosp Commun Psychiatry* 40:137, 1989.

Fike ML: Considerations and techniques in the treatment of persons with multiple personality disorder, *Am J Occup Ther* 44:999, 1990.

Fish RM: Working with people who harm themselves in a forensic learning disability service: experiences of direct care staff, *J Learn Disabil* 4:193, 2000.

Gallop R: Self-destructive and impulsive behavior in client with a borderline personality disorder: rethinking hospital treatment and management, *Arch Psychiatr Nurs* 6:178, 1992.

Gallop R: Failure of the capacity for self-soothing in women who have a history of abuse and self-harm, *J Am Psychiatr Nurses Assoc* 8:20, 2002.

Gough K, Hawkins A: Staff attitudes to self-harm and its management in a forensic psychiatric service, *Br J Forens Pract* 2(4):22, 2000.

Green CS, Knysz W, Tsuang MT: A homeless person with bipolar disorder and a history of serious self-mutilation, *Am J Psychiatry* 157:1392, 2000.

Hagerty B, Patusky K: Mood disorders: depression and mania, In Fortinash KM, Holoday-Worret PA, editors: *Psychiatric mental health nursing,* ed 3, St Louis, 2003, Mosby.

Hauenstein EJ: Case finding and care in suicide: children, adolescents, and adults. In Boyd MA, editor: *Psychiatric nursing. Contemporary practice,* ed 2, Philadelphia, 2002, Lippincott.

Hawton K et al: Deliberate self-harm: systematic review of efficacy of psychosocial and pharmacological treatments in preventing repetition, *BMJ* 317(7156):441, 1998.

Hennessy-Harstad EB: Empowering adolescents with asthma to take control through adaptation, *J Pediatr Health Care* 13:273, 1999.

Horsfall J: Towards understanding some complex borderline behaviors, *J Psychiatr Ment Health Nurs* 6:425, 1999.

King A, Taylor C, Haskell W: Effects of differing intensities and formats of 12 months of exercise training on psychological outcomes in older adults, *Health Psychol* 12(4):292, 1993.

Machoian L: Cutting voices: self-injury in three adolescent girls, *J Psychosoc Nurs Ment Health Serv* 39(11):22, 2001.

McAllister MM: In harm's way: a postmodern narrative inquiry, *J Psychiatr Ment Health Nurs* 8:391, 2001.

McKay D, Kulchycky S, Danyko S: Borderline personality and obsessive-compulsive symptoms, *J Personal Disord* 14(1):57, 2000.

Miller C, Eisner W, Allport C: Creative coping: a cognitive-behavioral group for borderline personality disorder, *Arch Psychiatr Nurs* 8:280, 1994.

● = **Independent; ▲** = **Collaborative**

Moffat C: Wound care. Self-inflicted wounding 1: psychosomatic concepts and physical conditions, *Br J Community Nurs* 4:502, 1999.

Nehls N: Group therapy for people with borderline personality disorder: interventions associated with positive outcomes, *Issues Ment Health Nurs* 13:255, 1992.

Nehls N: Borderline personality disorder: the voice of patients, *Res Nurs Health* 22:285, 1999.

Paul T et al: Self-injurious behavior in women with eating disorders, *Am J Psychiatry* 159:408, 2002.

Remington R: Calming music and hand massage with agitated elderly, *Nurs Res* 51:317, 2002.

Sinclair VG et al: Effects of a cognitive-behavioral intervention for women with rheumatoid arthritis, *Res Nurs Health* 21:315, 1998.

Tobin et al: From efficacy to effectiveness: managing organizational change to improve health services for young people with deliberate self harm behaviour, *Aust Health Rev* 24:143, 2001.

Tulloch AL, Blizzard L, Pinkus Z: Adolescent-parent communication in self-harm, *J Adolesc Health* 21:267, 1997.

Weber MT: Triggers for self-abuse: a qualitative study, *Arch Psychiatr Nurs* 16:118, 2002.

Wylie KR: Suction to the breasts of a transsexual male, *J Sex Marital Ther* 26(4):353, 2000.

Disturbed Sensory perception (specify: visual, auditory, kinesthetic, gustatory, tactile, olfactory)

Betty J. Ackley

NANDA Definition

Change in the amount or patterning of incoming stimuli accompanied by a diminished, exaggerated, distorted, or impaired response to such stimuli

Defining Characteristics

Poor concentration; auditory distortions; change in usual response to stimuli; restlessness; reported or measured change in sensory acuity; irritability; disoriented in time, in place, or with people; change in problem-solving abilities; change in behavior pattern; altered communication patterns; hallucinations; visual distortions

Related Factors (r/t)

Altered sensory perception; excessive environmental stimuli; psychological stress; altered sensory reception, transmission, and/or integration/insufficient environmental stimuli; biochemical imbalances for sensory distortion (e.g., illusions, hallucinations); electrolyte imbalance; biochemical imbalance

NOC Outcomes (Nursing Outcomes Classification) for Disturbed Sensory Perception: Visual

Suggested NOC Outcomes

Body Image; Cognitive Orientation; Sensory Function: Vision; Vision Compensation Behavior

• = Independent; ▲ = Collaborative

> ## Example NOC Outcome with Indicators
>
> **Vision Compensation Behavior** as evidenced by the following indicators: Uses adequate light for activity being performed/Wears eyeglasses correctly/Uses low-vision assistive devices/Uses computer assistive devices/Uses support services for low-vision (Rate each indicator of **Vision Compensation Behavior:** 1 = never demonstrated, 2 = rarely demonstrated, 3 = sometimes demonstrated, 4 = often demonstrated, 5 = consistently demonstrated [see Section I].)

NOC   Outcomes (Nursing Outcomes Classification) for Disturbed Sensory Perception: Auditory

Suggested NOC Outcomes

Cognitive Orientation; Communication: Receptive; Distorted Thought Self-Control; Hearing Compensation Behavior

> ## Example NOC Outcome with Indicators
>
> **Hearing Compensation Behavior** as evidenced by the following indicators: Reminds others to use techniques that advantage hearing/Eliminates background noise/Uses sign language/Uses lip reading/Uses hearing assistive devices/Uses hearing aid(s) correctly/Uses support services for hearing impaired (Rate each indicator of **Hearing Compensation Behavior:** 1 = never demonstrated, 2 = rarely demonstrated, 3 = sometimes demonstrated, 4 = often demonstrated, 5 = consistently demonstrated [see Section I].)

Client Outcomes

Client Will (Specify Time Frame):

- Demonstrate understanding by a verbal, written, or signed response
- Demonstrate relaxed body movements and facial expressions
- Explain plan to modify lifestyle to accommodate visual or hearing impairment
- Remain free of physical harm resulting from decreased balance or a loss of vision, hearing, or tactile sensation
- Maintain contact with appropriate community resources

NIC   Interventions (Nursing Interventions Classification)

Suggested NIC Interventions

Cognitive Stimulation; Communication Enhancement: Hearing Deficit, Visual Deficit; Environmental Management

> ## Example NIC Activities—Communication Enhancement: Visual Deficit
>
> Identify yourself when you enter the patient's space; Build on patient's remaining vision, as appropriate

Nursing Interventions and Rationales

Visual—loss of vision

- Identify name and purpose when entering the client's room. *Identification when entering the room helps the client feel secure and decreases social isolation.*

- = Independent; ▲ = Collaborative

- Orient to time, place, person, and surroundings. Provide a radio or talking books. *These actions help the client remain oriented and provide sensory stimulation.*
- Keep doors completely open or closed. Keep furniture out of path to bathroom, and do not rearrange furniture. *Consistency in placement of furniture and doors aids in location and decreases chances of injury (Beaver and Mann, 1995; Houde and Huff, 2003).*
- Feed the client at mealtimes if blindness is temporary.
- Keep side rails up using half or three-quarter rails, and maintain bed in a low position. Explain this precaution to the client.
- Converse with and touch the client frequently during care if frequent touch is within the client's cultural norm. *Appropriate touch can decrease social isolation.*
- Walk the client by having the client grasp nurse's elbow and walk partly behind nurse. Walk a frightened or confused client by having the client put both hands on nurse's shoulders; nurse backs up in desired direction while holding the client around the waist. *These methods help the client feel secure and ensure safety.*
- Keep call light button within client's reach, and check location of call light button before leaving the room.
- For blind client, consider referring to a clinic for use of a blind mobility aid device that utilizes ultrasound. *These devices can be helpful to the blind client to increase acuity to the environment and movement of objects in the environment (Bitjoka and Pourcelot, 1999).*
- Ensure access to eyeglasses or magnifying devices as needed.
- Pay attention to the client's emotional needs. Encourage expression of feelings and expect grieving behavior. *Blind people grieve the loss of vision and experience a loss of identity and control over their lives (Vader, 1992).*
- ▲ Refer to optometrist, ophthalmologist, or specialist in vision loss for vision care if needed. **Clinical Research:** *Photodynamic therapy for neovascular age-related changes is effective in preventing vision loss (Wormald et al, 2002).*

Auditory—hearing loss

- Keep background noise to a minimum. Turn off television and radio when communicating with the client. If noisy environment, take the client to a private room and shut the door. *Background noise significantly interferes with hearing in the hearing-impaired client (Jupiter and Spiver, 1997; Sommer and Sommer, 2002).*
- Stand or sit directly in front of the client when communicating. Make sure adequate light is on nurse's face, avoid chewing gum or covering mouth or face with hands while speaking, establish eye contact, and use nonverbal gestures. *These measures make it easier to read lips and see nonverbal communication, which is a large component of all communication (Jupiter and Spiver, 1997; Sommer and Sommer, 2002).*
- Speak distinctly in lower voice tones if possible. Do not over-enunciate or shout at the client. *In many kinds of hearing loss, clients lose the ability to hear higher-pitched tones but can still hear lower-pitched tones. Overenunciating makes it difficult to read lips. Shouting makes the words less clear and may be painful (Jupiter and Spiver, 1997).*
- State the topic of conversation before begin the conversation, make it clear when you change conversation topics. *This helps give the client a clear context for interpreting what you are speaking about (Sommer and Sommer, 2002).*
- Verify the client understands critical information by asking the client to repeat the information back. *Hearing impaired clients will often smile or nod when asked if they understand to avoid embarrassment, asking them to repeat the information back is the only way to verify they understand what is being said (Sommer and Sommer, 2002).*

- **= Independent; ▲ = Collaborative**

- If necessary, provide a communication board or personnel who know sign language. *Health care institutions are required to provide and pay for qualified interpreters under the Americans with Disabilities Act; an interpreter can be found through the Registry of Interpreters for the Deaf (703) (Sommer and Sommer, 2002).*
▲ Refer to appropriate resources such as a speech and hearing clinic; audiologist; or ear, nose, and throat physician. Refer children early for help. *Hearing loss can be treated with medical or surgical interventions or use of a hearing aid. Research demonstrates the positive effects of early diagnosis and intervention on the social and cognitive development of hearing impaired children (Meadow-Orland et al, 1997).*
- Encourage the client to wear hearing aid if available. **Clinical Research:** *A large study demonstrated that hearing impaired persons who wore hearing instruments, compared with those who did not, were more socially active, experienced more interpersonal warmth and less interpersonal negativity, communicated more effectively, had less self-criticism, frustration, anger and depression, and better health (Kochkin and Rogin, 2000).*
- Teach client to avoid excessive noise at work or at home, wearing hearing protection when necessary. Any noise that hurts the ears or is above 90 decibels is excessive. *Hearing loss from excessive noise is common and preventable (Lusk, 2002). The goal is to protect existing level of hearing.*
- Observe emotional needs and encourage expression of feelings. *Hearing impairments may cause frustration, anger, fear, and self-imposed isolation (Taylor, 1993).*
- For **Disturbed Sensory perception: kinesthetic and tactile,** see care plan for **Risk for Injury.** For **Disturbed Sensory perception: olfactory and gustatory,** see care plan for **Imbalanced Nutrition: less than body requirements.**

Geriatric
- Keep environment quiet, soothing, and familiar. Use consistent caregivers. *These measures are comforting to the elderly and help decrease confusion.*
- Avoid providing extremely hot or cold foods or using hot bath water if the client has decreased sensation in mouth, hands, or feet.
- If the client has a sensory deprivation, encourage family to provide sensory stimulation with music, voices, photographs, touch, and familiar smells.
- For a hearing impairment in the elderly, use the Hearing Handicap Inventory for the Elderly (HHIE-S) to determine how individuals perceive the emotional and social problems associated with a hearing loss. *The HHIE-S is a valid and reliable questionnaire to predict social and emotional effects of hearing loss (Demers, 2001).*
- If the client has a hearing or vision loss, work with the client to ensure contact with others and to strengthen the social network. **Nursing and Clinical Research:** *Severe loneliness can accompany vision loss in the elderly as a result of self-imposed isolation (Foxall et al, 1992). Loss of hearing has a negative impact on psychosocial function with loneliness and increased rate of depression (Carabellese et al, 1993; Wallhagen, 2001, 2002).*

Home care
- The listed interventions are applicable in the home care setting.

Client/Family Teaching
Low vision
- Teach the client how to use a lighted magnification device to increase the ability to read text or see details.

- = **Independent;** ▲ = **Collaborative**

- Teach the client to put a sheet of yellow acetate over text to make the text more visible. An alternative method is to highlight the text with a green or yellow highlighter (Beaver and Mann, 1995).
- Put red or yellow identifiers on important items that need to be seen, such as a red strip at the edge of steps, red behind a light switch, or a red dot on a stove or washing machine to indicate how far to turn knob. **Clinical Research:** *Color cues can improve the legibility of the environment and increase the ability to target objects quickly (Cooper, 1999).*
- Use a watch or clock that verbally tells time and a phone with large numbers and emergency numbers programmed in.
- Teach blind client how to feed self; associate food on plate with hours on a clock so that the client can identify location of food.
- Use low-vision aids including magnifying devices for near vision and telescopes for seeing objects at a distance, a closed-circuit television that magnifies print, guides for writing checks and envelopes. *Low vision aids can improve vision in clients with limited sight (Derrington, 2002).*
- Increase lighting in the home to help vision in the following ways:
  - Ensure adequate illumination of entire home, adding light fixtures and increase wattage of existing bulbs as needed
  - Decrease glare where light reflects on shiny surfaces, move or cover object
  - Use nonglare wax on the floor.
  - Use motion lights that come on automatically when a person enters the room for nighttime use
  - Add indoor strip or "runway" type of lighting to baseboards
  Visual acuity can be improved by taking steps to overcome age-related changes to vision (Beaver and Mann, 1995; Slay, 2002; Smith, 1998). **Clinical Research:** *Illumination can increase mobility in clients with age-related macular degeneration (Kuyk and Elliott, 1999).*
- ▲ Refer to low-vision clinics, or the Independent Living Program, which is designed for older individuals who are blind to help maintain independence (Moore et al, 2001). *Clients with vision loss should be referred to clinics early, before vision is gone, for help dealing with the loss (Brown, 1998).*

Hearing loss

- Suggest installation of devices such as ring signalers for the telephone and doorbell, sensors that detect an infant's cry, alarm clocks that vibrate the bed, and closed caption decoders for television sets. Other helpful devices include telephone amplifiers, speaker phones, pocket talker personal listening system, and FM and infrared amplification systems that connect directly to a TV or audio output jack. Also available is a telecommunication device—a typewriter keyboard with an alphanumeric display that allows the hearing impaired person to send typed messages over the telephone line, and software and modems are available that allow a home computer to be used in this fashion. Use of a hearing ear dogs—dogs specially trained to alert their owners to specific sound—may also be helpful. *These devices and the dogs can be helpful to increase communication and safety for the hearing impaired client (Committee on Disabilities, 1997; Jupiter and Spiver, 1997).*
- Teach family how to provide appropriate stimuli in the home environment to prevent disturbed sensory perception.
- ▲ Refer to hearing clinics.

- **• = Independent; ▲ = Collaborative**

evolve WEBSITES FOR EDUCATION

See the EVOLVE website for World Wide Web resources for client education.

REFERENCES

Beaver KA, Mann WC: Overview of technology for low vision, *Am J Occup Ther* 49:913, 1995.

Bitjoka L, Pourcelot L: New blind mobility aid devices based on the ultrasonic Doppler effect, *Int J Rehabil Res* 22(3):227, 1999.

Brown B: Five easy steps to helping your low vision patient, *J Ophthalmol Nurs Technol* 17(1):7, 1998.

Carabellese AH et al, Sensory impairment and quality of life in a community elderly population, *J Am Geriatr Soc* 41:401, 1993.

Committee on Disabilities: Issues to consider in deaf and hard-of-hearing patients, *Am Fam Physician* 56(8): 2057, 1997.

Cooper BA: The utility of functional colour cues: seniors' views, *Scand J Caring Sci* 13(3):186, 1999.

Demers K: Best practices in nursing care to older adults: hearing screening, *J Gerontol Nurs* 27(11):8, 2001.

Derrington D: Aids to low vision. *Nursing Residential Care* 4:5, 2002.

Foxall MJ et al: Predictors of loneliness in low vision adults, *West J Nurs Res* 14:86, 1992.

Houde SC, Huff MA: Age-related vision loss in older adults: a challenge for gerontological nurses, *J Gerontol Nurs* 29(4):25, 2003.

Jupiter T, Spiver V: Perception of hearing loss and hearing handicap on hearing aid use by nursing home residents: geriatric nursing, *Am J Care Aging* 18(5):201, 1997.

Kochkin W, Rogin CM: Quantifying the obvious: the impact of hearing instruments on quality of life, *Hearing Rev* 7:1, 2000.

Kuyk T, Elliott JL: Visual factors and mobility in persons with age-related macular degeneration, *J Rehabil Res Dev* 36(4):303, 1999.

Lusk SL: Preventing noise-induced hearing loss, *Nurs Clin North Am* 37(2):257, 2002.

Meadow-Orland KP et al: Support services for parents and their children who are deaf or hard of hearing, *Am Ann Deaf* 142(4):278, 1997.

Moore JE, Giesen JM, Weber JM: *J Visual Impairment Blindness* 95:7, 2001.

Slay DH: Home-based environmental lighting assessments for people who are visually impaired: developing techniques and tools, *J Visual Impairment Blindness* 96:2, 2002.

Smith SD: Aging, physiology, and vision, *Nurse Pract Forum* 9(1):19, 1998.

Sommer SK, Sommer NW: When your patient is hearing impaired, *RN* 65(12):28, 2002.

Taylor KS: Geriatric hearing loss: management strategies for nurses, *Geriatr Nurs* 14:74, 1993.

Vader LA: Vision and vision loss, *Nurs Clin North Am* 27:705, 1992.

Wallhagen MI, Strawbridge WJ, Kaplan GA: Five-year impact of hearing impairment on physical functioning, mental health and social relationships, *Br Soc Audiol News* 32:9, 2001.

Wallhagen MI: Hearing impairment, *Annu Rev Nurs Res* 20:341, 2002.

Wormald R et al: Photo dynamic therapy for neovascular age-related macular degeneration. *Cochrane Library* (CD002030, 2002).

Sexual dysfunction

Gail B. Ladwig

NANDA Definition

Change in sexual function that is viewed as unsatisfying, unrewarding, inadequate

Defining Characteristics

Change of interest in self and others; conflicts involving values; inability to achieve desired satisfaction; verbalization of problem; alteration in relationship with significant other; alteration in achieving sexual satisfaction; actual or perceived limitation imposed by

• = Independent; ▲ = Collaborative

disease or therapy; seeking confirmation of desirability; alteration in achieving perceived sex role

Related Factors (r/t)

Misinformation or lack of knowledge; vulnerability; value conflict; psychosocial abuse (e.g., harmful relationships); physical abuse; lack of privacy; ineffectual or absent role models; altered body structure of function (e.g., pregnancy, recent childbirth, drugs, surgery, anomalies, disease process, trauma, radiation); lack of significant other; biopsychosocial alterations of sexuality

NOC   Outcomes (Nursing Outcomes Classification)

Suggested NOC Outcomes

Abuse Recovery: Sexual; Child Development: Adolescence; Physical Aging Status; Risk Control: Sexually Transmitted Diseases (STD); Sexual Functioning

> #### Example NOC Outcome with Indicators
>
> **Sexual Functioning** as evidenced by the following indicators: Expresses comfort with sexual expression/ Expresses comfort with body/Expresses sexual interest (Rate each indicator of **Sexual Functioning**: 1 = never demonstrated, 2 = rarely demonstrated, 3 = sometimes demonstrated, 4 = often demonstrated, 5 = consistently demonstrated [see Section I].)

Client Outcomes

Client Will (Specify Time Frame):
- Identify individual cause of sexual dysfunction
- Identify stressors that contribute to dysfunction
- Discuss alternative, satisfying, and acceptable sexual practices for self and partner
- Discuss with partner concerns about body image and sex role

NIC   Interventions (Nursing Interventions Classification)

Suggested NIC Intervention

Sexual Counseling

> #### Example NIC Activities—Sexual Counseling
>
> Provide privacy and ensure confidentiality; Discuss modifications in sexual activity, as appropriate

Nursing Interventions and Rationales

- Gather the client's sexual history, noting normal patterns of functioning and the client's vocabulary. **Clinical Research:** *Health care professionals in urologic, gynecologic, and family practice offices and clinics are in key roles to identify females experiencing sexual dysfunction. Sexual identity is shaped throughout our life. It depends on religious and cultural beliefs and is strongly related to early sexual experiences (Brassil and Keller, 2002). Documentation of sexual function following all local treatments, including prostate brachytherapy, may help to clarify the etiology of treatment-induced erectile dysfunction (Stipetich et al, 2002).*

• = Independent; ▲ = Collaborative

- Determine the client's and partner's current knowledge and understanding. **Nursing Research:** *For patients, self-identity and communication were the predominant themes that emerged from the data. A lack of information related to issues of sexual functioning was the most prominent subcategory (Steinke and Patterson-Midgley, 1998). If unsure of a client's sexuality, use the term partner, which helps avoid making any assumptions or judgments about a relationship. A sexual relationship may be heterosexual or homosexual, and nurses must not lose sight of this (Taylor, 1994).*
- Observe for stress, anxiety, and depression as possible causes of dysfunction. **Clinical Research:** *Sexual dysfunction can be attributed to many psychological factors. Sexual problems are common in chronic-pain patients. Patients who reported symptoms of depression and distress had more sexual problems than others (Monga et al, 1998). Recognition of sexual dysfunction associated with depression and its treatment is critical for client satisfaction and medication compliance (Clayton, 2001).*
- Observe for grief related to loss (e.g., amputation, mastectomy, ostomy). *A change in body image often precedes sexual dysfunction (see care plan for* **Disturbed Body image***).* The trauma of being diagnosed and treated for breast cancer can impact greatly on women's psychosexual functioning and intimate relationships. Survivors of breast cancer report that issues of body image, sexuality, and partner communication are rarely addressed by traditional health care providers (Anllo, 2000). Sexuality concerns should be addressed with all clients undergoing ostomy placement (Sprunk and Alteneder, 2000).
- Explore physical causes such as diabetes, arteriosclerotic heart disease, arthritis, drug or medication side effects, or smoking (males). **Nursing Research:** *Sexual difficulties often occur as a result of cardiovascular disease (Papadopoulos, 1995). In this research study, women with arthritis and a high degree of morning stiffness worried more about their bodies and reported significantly more problems with sexuality than others (Gutweniger et al, 1999).* **Nursing Research:** *The literature review of 18 studies revealed the detrimental effect of smoking on erectile function. Smokers were 1.5 times more likely to suffer erectile dysfunction than were nonsmokers (Dorey, 2001).*
- Provide privacy and be verbally and nonverbally nonjudgmental. *Privacy is important to ensure confidentiality. To facilitate communication, it is also vital that the nurse clarify personal values and remain nonjudgmental.*
- Provide privacy to allow sexual expression between the client and partner (e.g., private room, "Do Not Disturb" sign for a specified length of time). *The hospital setting has little opportunity for privacy, so the nurse must ensure that it is available.*
- Explain the need for the client to share concerns with partner. **Nursing Research:** *This literature review demonstrated increasing recognition that the partner should be involved in the assessment, diagnosis, patient education, counseling and choice of treatment for long-term treatment to be successful, unless the informed patient is unwilling (Dorey, 2001).*
- Validate the client's feelings, let the client know that he or she is normal, and correct misinformation. *A sensitive nurse who has an understanding of sexual health and functioning and the conditions that interfere with them can direct those who need help toward treatment (Lewis, 1992).*
- ▲ Refer to appropriate medical providers for consideration of medication with premature ejaculation. **Clinical Research:** *This study examined the efficacy of citalopram, an SSRI, to 26 married patients diagnosed with premature ejaculation according to* Diagnostic and Statistical Manual of Mental Disorders Third Revised Version (DSM-III-R). *The patients were randomly assigned to two groups. The patients treated with citalopram showed*

- = **Independent;** ▲ = **Collaborative**

significantly greater improvement compared to the patients receiving placebo (Atmaca et al, 2002).

Geriatric

- Teach about normal changes that occur with aging: Female—reduction in vaginal lubrication, decrease in the degree and speed of vaginal expansion, reduction in duration and resolution of orgasm. Male—increase in time required for erection, increase in erection time without ejaculation, less firm erection, decrease in volume of seminal fluid, increase in time before another erection can occur (12 to 24 hours). **Nursing Research:** *The older adult experiences a number of physiological changes; however, these changes are gradual and vary from person to person (Shell and Smith, 1994). Erectile dysfunction may affect one in 10 men as they age (Sounes, 2001)*
- Suggest the following to enhance sexual functioning: Female—use water-based vaginal lubricant, increase foreplay time, avoid direct stimulation of the clitoris if painful (clitoris may be exposed because of atrophy of the labia), practice Kegel exercises (alternately contracting and relaxing the muscles in the pelvic area), urinate immediately after coitus to prevent irritation of the urethra and bladder, and consult with a physician about use of systemic estrogen therapy or topical estrogen cream. Male—have female partner try a new coital position by bending her knees and placing a pillow under her hips to elevate pelvis (will more easily accommodate a partially erect penis); massage penis down using pressure at base, which puts pressure on major blood vessel and keeps blood in the penis; ask the female partner to push the penis into the vagina herself and flex her vaginal muscles that have been strengthened by Kegel exercises. If one of the partners has a protruding abdomen, experiment to find a position that allows the penis to reach the vagina (e.g., have woman lie on her back with legs apart and knees sharply bent while the man places himself over her with his hips under the angle formed by the raised knees). **Nursing Research:** *These gender-specific sexual interventions for the elderly may help maintain sexual functioning (Shell and Smith, 1994).*
- Assess the possibility of erectile dysfunction. *Erectile dysfunction affects the lives of up to 30 million American men and their partners (Mayo Foundation for Medical Education and Research, 2003).*
- Explore with the client and partner various sexual gratification alternatives (e.g., caressing, sharing feelings). *There are many satisfying alternatives for expressing sexual feelings. The many losses associated with aging leave the elderly with special needs for love and affection.*
- Discuss the difference between sexual function and sexuality. *All individuals possess sexuality from birth to death, regardless of the changes that occur over the lifespan.*
- ▲ If prescribed, teach how to use nitroglycerin before sexual activity. *Pain inhibits satisfying sexual activity.*
- See care plan for **Ineffective Sexuality pattern.**

Multicultural

- Assess for the influence of cultural beliefs, norms, and values on the client's perceptions of normal sexual functioning. **Nursing Research:** *What the client considers normal sexual functioning may be based on cultural perceptions (Leininger and McFarland, 2002; Cochran, 1998; Doswell and Erlen, 1998).*
- Discuss with the client those aspects of sexual health/lifestyle that remain unchanged

• = **Independent;** ▲ = **Collaborative**

by his or her health status. **Nursing Research:** *Aspects of the client's life that are valuable to him or her should be understood and preserved without change (Leininger and McFarland, 2002).*

- Validate the client's feelings and emotions regarding the changes in sexual behavior. **Nursing Research:** *Validation lets the client know the nurse has heard and understands what was said, and it promotes the nurse-client relationship (Heineken, 1998).*

Home care

- Above interventions may be adapted for home care use.
- Identify specific sources of concern over sexual activity. Provide reassurance and instruction on appropriate expectations as indicated. **Nursing Research:** *In a study of heart transplantation clients' spouses (Bohachick et al, 2001), both clients and spouses reported large improvements in sexual function following transplant. A psychological influence prior to transplant was identified as concern over finding a donor.*
- Help the client and significant other to identify a place and time in the home and daily living for privacy to share sexual or relationship activity. If necessary, help the client to communicate the need for privacy to other family members. Consider periodic escapes to desirable surroundings. *The home setting can be one that affords little, if any, privacy without conscious effort on the part of members of the home.*
- ▲ Confirm that physical reasons for dysfunction have been addressed. Encourage participation in support groups or therapy if appropriate. **Nursing Research:** *Alterations in physical appearance can significantly influence people's perceptions of their sexual identities, attractiveness, and worthiness. Patients with lung cancer receiving chemotherapy may need sexual counseling. Therefore, patients and healthcare providers should create an environment that allows adequate time to discreetly discuss the impact that chemotherapy treatment may have on appearance, self-esteem, and sexuality (Schwartz and Plawecki, 2002)*
- Reinforce or teach the client about sexual functioning, alternative sexual practices, and necessary sexual precautions. Update teaching as the client status changes. **Nursing Research:** *In this Descriptive, qualitative study of the experiences of couples living with prostate cancer participants demonstrated a need for information and support. Both men and spouse-caregivers felt unprepared to manage treatment effects (Harden et al, 2002).*

Client/Family Teaching

- Teach the importance of resting before sexual activity. For some clients, mornings are the best time for sexual activity. *Clients may have a more satisfying experience if they are not tired.*
- Teach the client to resume intimate physical contact by using mutual touching 3 to 6 weeks after a MI. **Nursing Research:** *Sexual activity after a MI should not be demanding; therefore mutual touching is recommended (Papadopoulos, 1995).*
- Teach the client to begin vigorous sexual activity after a MI when the client can walk rapidly for 10 minutes and then climb two flights of stairs in 10 seconds. **Nursing Research:** *If this can be done without shortness of breath or other symptoms, then the client is ready to begin preestablished levels of sexual activity (Papadopoulos, 1995). The causes of erection problems after an MI can be physical, psychological, a result of medication or a combination of these factors (Jones and Nugent, 2001).* **Nursing Research:** *This study of 110 patients found all 110 had insufficient information about their future sexual functioning after an MI (myocardial infarction). Unnecessary limitations in sexual activities and mis-*

• = **Independent;** ▲ = **Collaborative**

takes in the reorganization of activities, such as resumption of sexual activity and frequency and positions of sexual intercourse were identified (Akdolun and Terakye, 2001).

▲ Teach the client to take prescribed pain medications before sexual activity. *Pain inhibits satisfying sexual activity.*

• Teach possible need for modifying positions (e.g., side-to-side, limited resting on arms, heavier person on bottom). *Changes in position can enhance satisfaction and comfort.*

▲ Refer to appropriate community resources, such as a clinical specialist, family counselor, or sexual counselor. If appropriate, include both partners in the discussion. *A high percentage of women report a need for more information after a cancer surgery that affected their sexual response. They also express a need for partners to be included in the discussions (Corney et al, 1992). Changes in the sexual relationship were described in the context of the effects of having interstitial cystitis and the centrality of maintaining relationships. Participation in support groups has a healing potential related to the woman's desire to maintain independence and to help others with the disease (Webster, 1997).*

• Teach vaginal dilation to prevent stenosis. Inform the client to expect a bit of spotting after first session of intercourse. *Clients with gynecological cancer and surgery, particularly cervical cancer, can reduce the number of physical problems if this information is taught (Laurent, 1994).*

▲ Teach how drug therapy affects sexual response (e.g., the possible side effects and the need to report them). **Nursing Research:** *SSRI-induced sexual dysfunction affects 30% to 50% or more of individuals who take these drugs for depression (Keltner et al, 2002).*

• Teach the importance of diabetic control and its effect on sexuality to clients with insulin-dependent diabetes. *Sexual functioning may be changed by alterations in glucose levels, infections that affect comfort during sexual intercourse, changes in vaginal lubrication and penile erection, and changes in sexual desire and arousal (Lemone, 1993).*

▲ Refer for medical advice for erectile dysfunction that lasts longer than 2 months or is recurring. *Erectile dysfunction can be treated, and underlying causes need to be investigated (Mayo Foundation for Medical Education and Research, 2003).*

• Teach the following interventions to decrease the likelihood of erectile dysfunction: limit or avoid the use of alcohol, stop smoking, exercise regularly, reduce stress, get enough sleep, deal with anxiety or depression, and see doctor for regular checkups and medical screening tests. *These interventions may prevent erectile dysfunction (Mayo Foundation for Medical Education and Research, 2003).*

▲ Refer for medication to treat erectile dysfunction if necessary. **Clinical Research:** *The oral agent sildenafil is now widely used, but not without concern about specific health risks (Mulhall, 2000). This study of 10 patients suggests that sildenafil use is effective and well-tolerated in patients with olanzapine-induced ED (Atmaca et al, 2002). In this prospective, parallel-group, randomized, double-blind, placebo-controlled trial, sildenafil effectively improved erectile function and other aspects of sexual function in men with sexual dysfunction associated with the use of SRI antidepressants (Nurnberg et al, 2003).*

• Teach specifics if the client has a stoma: do not substitute the stoma for an anus. *If a stoma is abused in this way, it can become traumatized and need further surgery (Taylor, 1994).*

• See geriatric interventions if there is a problem with erection associated with stoma surgery.

• = **Independent;** ▲ = **Collaborative**

ⓔⓥⓞⓛⓥⓔ WEBSITES FOR EDUCATION

See the EVOLVE website for World Wide Web resources for client education.

REFERENCES

Akdolun N, Terakye G: Sexual problems before and after myocardial infarction: patients' needs for information, *Rehabil Nurs* 26(4):152, 2001.

Anllo LM: Sexual life after breast cancer, *J Sex Marital Ther* 26(3):241, 2000.

Atmaca M, Kuloglu M, Tezcan E: Sildenafil use in patients with olanzapine-induced erectile dysfunction, *Int J Impot Res* 14(6):547, 2002.

Atmaca M et al: The efficacy of citalopram in the treatment of premature ejaculation: a placebo-controlled study, *Int J Impot Res* 14(6):502, 2002.

Brassil DF, Keller M: Female sexual dysfunction: definitions, causes, and treatment, *Urol Nurs* 22(4):237, 284; quiz 245, 248, 2002.

Bohachick P et al: Psychosocial impact of heart transplantation on spouses, *Clin Nurs Res* 10:6, 2001.

Clayton AH: Recognition and assessment of sexual dysfunction associated with depression, *J Clin Psychiatry* 62(suppl 3):5, 2001.

Cochran M: Tears have no color, *Am J Nurs* 98(6):53, 1998.

Corney R et al: The care of patients undergoing surgery for gynecological cancer: the need for information, emotional support and counseling, *J Adv Nurs* 17:667, 1992.

Dorey G: Is smoking a cause of erectile dysfunction? A literature review, *Br J Nurs* 12;10(7):455, 2001.

Dorey G: Partners' perspective of erectile dysfunction: literature review, *Br J Nurs* 8;10(3):187, 2001.

Doswell W, Erlen J: Multicultural issues and ethical concerns in the delivery of revising care interventions, *Nurs Clin North Am* 33(2):353, 1998.

Dupont S: Multiple sclerosis and sexual functioning: a review, *Clin Rehabil* 9:135, 1995.

Gutweniger S et al: Body image of women with rheumatoid arthritis, *Clin Exp Rheumatol* 17(4):413, 1999.

Harden J et al: Couples' experiences with prostate cancer: focus group research, *Oncol Nurs Forum* 29(4):701, 2002.

Heineken J: Patient silence is not necessarily client satisfaction: Communication in home care nursing, *Home Healthc Nurse* 16(2):115, 1998.

Jones C, Nugent P: The problem of erectile dysfunction following myocardial infarction, *Prof Nurse* 17(3):161, 2001.

Keltner NL, McAfee KM, Taylor CL: Mechanisms and treatments of SSRI-induced sexual dysfunction, *Perspect Psychiatr Care* 38(3):111, 2002.

Laurent C: Talking treatment: therapy for cervical cancer has left some women with severe sexual problems, *Nurs Times* 90:14, 1994.

Leininger MM, McFarland MR: *Transcultural nursing: concepts, theories, research and practices,* ed 3, New York, 2002, McGraw-Hill.

Lemone P: Human sexuality in adults with insulin-dependent diabetes mellitus, *Image* 25:101, 1993.

Lewis JH: Treatment options for men with sexual dysfunction, *J ET Nurs* 19:131, 1992.

Mayo Foundation for Medical Education and Research: Erectile dysfunction, retrieved from the World Wide Web February 27, 2003. Website: www.mayohealth.org/home?id=DS00162.

Monga TN et al: Sexuality and sexual adjustment of patients with chronic pain, *Disabil Rehabil* 20 (9), 1998.

Mulhall JP: Current concepts in erectile dysfunction, *Am J Manag Care* 6(12 suppl):S641-S643, 2000.

Nurnberg HG et al: Treatment of antidepressant-associated sexual dysfunction with sildenafil: a randomized controlled trial, *JAMA* 1;289(1):56, 2003.

Papadopoulos C: Sex and the cardiac patient, 1991, *Med Aspects Hum Sexuality* 24:55, 1991. In Quadagno D et al: Cardiovascular disease and sexual functioning, *Appl Nurs Res* 8:143, 1995.

Schwartz S, Plawecki HM: Consequences of chemotherapy on the sexuality of patients with lung cancer, *Clin J Oncol Nurs* 6(4):212, 2002.

Shell J, Smith C: Sexuality and the older person with cancer, *Oncol Nurs Forum* 21:553, 1994.

Steinke EE, Patterson-Midgley PE: Perspectives of nurses and patients on the need for sexual counseling of MI patients, *Rehabil Nurs* 23(2):64, 1998.

• = Independent; ▲ = Collaborative

Stipetich RL et al: Nursing assessment of sexual function following permanent prostate brachytherapy for patients with early-stage prostate cancer, *Clin J Oncol Nurs* 6(5):271, 2002.

Sounes P: Providing nursing care for erectile dysfunction, *Prof Nurse* 16(9):1374, 2001.

Sprunk E, Alteneder RR: The impact of an ostomy on sexuality, *Clin J Oncol Nurs* 4(2):85, 2000.

Taylor P: Beating the taboo, Stoma and sexual difficulty, *Nurs Times* 90:51, 1994.

Webster DC: Recontextualizing sexuality in chronic illness: women and interstitial cystitis, *Health Care Women Int* 18(6):575, 1997.

Ineffective Sexuality patterns

Gail B. Ladwig

NANDA Definition

Expressions of concern regarding own sexuality

Defining Characteristics

Reported difficulties, limitations, or changes in sexual behaviors or activities

Related Factors (r/t)

Lack of significant other; conflicts with sexual orientation or variant preferences; fear of pregnancy or of acquiring a sexually transmitted disease; impaired relationship with significant other; ineffective or absent role models; knowledge/skill deficit about alternative responses to health-related transitions, altered body function or structure, illness or medical treatment; lack of privacy

NOC Outcomes (Nursing Outcomes Classification)

Suggested NOC Outcomes

Abuse Recovery: Sexual; Child Development: Adolescence; Risk Control: Sexually Transmitted Diseases (STD); Role Performance; Self-Esteem; Sexual Functioning

> #### Example NOC Outcome with Indicators
>
> **Sexual Functioning** as evidenced by the following indicators: Expresses comfort with sexual expression/Expresses comfort with body/Expresses sexual interest (Rate each indicator of **Sexual Functioning:** 1 = never demonstrated, 2 = rarely demonstrated, 3 = sometimes demonstrated, 4 = often demonstrated, 5 = consistently demonstrated [see Section I].)

Client Outcomes

Client Will (Specify Time Frame):

- State knowledge of difficulties, limitations, or changes in sexual behaviors or activities
- State knowledge of sexual anatomy and functioning
- State acceptance of altered body structure or functioning
- Describe acceptable alternative sexual practices
- Identify importance of discussing sexual issues with significant other
- Describe practice of safe sex with regard to pregnancy and avoidance of STDs

• = Independent; ▲ = Collaborative

| **NIC** | **Interventions (Nursing Interventions Classification)** |

Suggested NIC Intervention

Sexual Counseling

> **Example NIC Activities—Sexual Counseling**
>
> Provide privacy and ensure confidentiality; Discuss modifications in sexual activity, as appropriate

Nursing Interventions and Rationales

- After establishing rapport or therapeutic relationship, give the client permission to discuss issues dealing with sexuality. Ask the client specifically, "Have you been or are you concerned about functioning sexually because of your health status?" **Nursing Research:** *For patients, self-identity and communication were the predominant themes that emerged from the data. A lack of information related to issues of sexual functioning was the most prominent subcategory (Steinke and Patterson-Midgley, 1998). Of 96 patients surveyed after a myocardial infarction, 71% believed that staff should address sexuality in the hospital setting (Steinke and Patterson-Midgley, 1996).*
- Determine the client's and partner's current knowledge and understanding. **Clinical Research:** *This survey indicated that in clinical practice and for those who have a partner, sexual disabilities and distress caused by them should be regarded from the partner relationship perspective (Sjvgren Fugl-Meyer and Fugl-Meyer, 2002).*
- Discuss alternative sexual expressions for altered body functioning or structure. Closeness and touching are other forms of expression. *Extensive touching, hugging, holding, huddling, and cuddling (3HC) in intimate (committed, close, and prolonged) relationships is important couple and family therapy (L'Abate, 2001).*
- Some clients choose masturbation for sexual release. **Clinical Research:** *Nearly 50% of staff who worked with clients with intellectual disability identified more training and clear policy guidelines as the two means of increasing their confidence in dealing with issues of client sexuality such as masturbation (McConkey and Ryan, 2001).*
- If mutual masturbation is a choice of expression, provide latex gloves. *Latex gloves prevent possible exposure to infection through cuts on hands (Tucker et al, 1996).*
- Discuss modifying positions to accommodate the altered physical state; instruct in the use of pillows for comfort. *Modified positions can enable and enhance sexual satisfaction otherwise impeded by physical disability.*
- Encourage the client to discuss concerns with his or her partner. *If unsure of a client's sexuality, use the term partner to avoid making any assumptions or judgments about the relationship. A sexual relationship may be heterosexual or homosexual, and nurses must not lose sight of this (Taylor, 1994). Communication between partners plays a direct key role in facilitating condom use and forms the basis for maintaining emotional intimacy (Parish et al, 2001).*
- Provide client privacy for sexual expression (e.g., closed door when significant other visits, "Do Not Disturb" sign on door). *The hospital environment needs to allow for sexual expression between partners.*
- Provide support for the client's chosen ways to cope with HIV or AIDS. **Nursing Research:** *This descriptive study was designed to assess coping strategies of female adolescents infected with Human Immunodeficiency Virus (HIV) or the Acquired Immunodeficiency Syndrome (AIDS) (N = 30). Results from the Adolescent Coping Orientation for Problem*

• = **Independent;** ▲ = **Collaborative**

Experiences Questionnaire (ACOPES) revealed that the most often utilized coping strategies identified by the adolescents were: listening to music, thinking about good things, making your own decisions, being close to someone you care about, sleeping, trying on your own to deal with problems, eating, watching television, daydreaming and praying (Lewis and Brown, 2002).

Geriatric

- Help the client redefine sexuality in broader terms such as sharing, communication, and intimacy. **Nursing Research:** *Sexuality is a primary part of being human and does not cease after age 65. Elderly persons need to continue to view themselves as masculine or feminine (Shell and Smith, 1994).*
- Explore possible changes in sexuality related to menopause. **Clinical Research:** *Evidence from existing research suggests a decline in sexual interest, frequency of sexual intercourse, and vaginal lubrication in association with menopause. Findings for variables such as capacity for orgasm, satisfaction with sex partner, and vaginal pain or discomfort are few and mixed (McCoy, 1998).*
- Allow the client to verbalize feelings regarding loss of sexual partner or significant other. Acknowledge problems such as disapproval of children, lack of available partner for women, and environmental variables that make forming new relationships difficult. **Nursing Research:** *Many individuals face loneliness when they lose a partner, and the loss of interpersonal intimacy is a sensitive problem. After a loss of this magnitude, elderly persons often find that forming new relationships is difficult. Privacy is also a problem (Shell and Smith, 1994).*
- Provide a milieu that allows for discussion of sexual issues and a higher level of sexual satisfaction. Allow couples to room together and bring in double beds from home. Place signs on the door to ensure privacy. **Nursing Research:** *Environmental variables have an impact on elderly people's ability to freely express sexuality (Shell and Smith, 1994).*
- Provide clients with the following information:
  - Exercise, such as walking, swimming, cycling, and riding a stationary bike, will help control flabby thighs and weak musculature and make people feel more sexually attractive.
  - Overindulgence in food or alcohol can affect sexual activity (see care plan for **Imbalanced Nutrition: less than body requirements**).
  - Resting and sleeping on a firm mattress may augment sexual desire.
  - Femininity and masculinity are still important.
  - Pay attention to cleanliness, skin care, and clothing.
  - Change environment.
  - Experiment with position changes.
  Because the majority of the elderly population maintains sexual interest, desire, and functioning, these interventions may be helpful during the rehabilitation process. Older adults may exercise aerobically 3 to 5 times a week for 15 to 30 minutes depending on physical status and treatment regimen (Steinke et al, 1986).
- See care plan for **Sexual dysfunction.**

Multicultural

- Assess for the influence of cultural beliefs, norms, and values on client's perceptions of normal sexual behavior. **Nursing Research:** *What the client considers normal sexual behavior may be based on cultural perceptions (Leininger and McFarland, 2002; Cochran,*

• = **Independent; ▲ = Collaborative**

1998; Doswell and Erlen, 1998). Religion may also influence one's perception of sexual be-havior (Lazoritz and McDermott, 2002).

- Discuss with the client those aspects of his or her sexual health/lifestyle that remain unchanged by their health status. **Nursing Research:** *Aspects of the client's life that are valuable to him or her should be understood and preserved without change (Leininger and McFarland, 2002).*
- Validate the client's feelings and emotions regarding the changes in sexuality patterns. **Nursing Research:** *Validation lets the client know the nurse has heard and understands what was said and promotes the nurse-client relationship (Heineken, 1998).*

Home care

- Above interventions may be adapted for home care use.
- Help the client and significant other to identify a place and time in the home and daily living for privacy in sharing sexual or relationship activity. If necessary, help the client to communicate the need for privacy to other family members. Consider periodic escapes to desirable surroundings. *The home setting can be one that affords little, if any, privacy without a conscious effort made by members of the home.*
- ▲ Confirm that physical reasons for dysfunction have been addressed. Encourage partici-pation in support groups or therapy if appropriate. **Clinical Research:** *Clients express embarrassment at continuing medical intervention or participation in groups once they are back in the community and know that peers may judge their activities. However, 22 fe-male psychiatric outpatients with experience of childhood sexual abuse took part in a 2-year group therapy, and at the end of the 2 years, group members evaluated their relationships as having improved (Lundquist and Ojehagen, 2001).*
- Reinforce or teach about sexual functioning, alternative sexual practices, and necessary sexual precautions. Update teaching as client status changes. *If the client or significant other has received information during an institutional stay, other stressors may have made the information a temporarily low priority or may have impaired learning. Depending on the cause for dysfunction, the client may experience changing status or feelings about the problem.*

Client/Family Teaching

- ▲ Refer to appropriate community agencies (e.g., certified sex counselor, Reach to Re-covery, Ostomy Association). *There may be needs that either are beyond the nurse's skill and ability to address or are related to a particular situation (e.g., presence of an ostomy that requires intervention from specialized sources) (Lewis, 1992).* **Nursing Research:** *Sexu-ality concerns should be addressed with all clients undergoing ostomy placement (Sprunk and Alteneder, 2000).*
- Provide information regarding self-care and sexuality for the woman who has cancer and her partner. **Nursing Research:** *Couples may hesitate to change their routines. Providing this kind of information in a sensitive way often gives permission to change (Shell and Smith, 1994).*
- ▲ Sexuality education is important to all populations, whether hearing or deaf, sighted or blind, disabled, or not disabled. Discuss contraceptive choices. Refer to appropriate health professional (e.g., gynecologist, nurse practitioner). *The need for accurate, com-prehensive, current sexuality education is present in all cultures and at all socioeconomic lev-els. The spread of myths, opinions, and stereotypes can be reduced by correctly educating*

- = **Independent;** ▲ = **Collaborative**

children. Sexuality education enables an individual to make the most appropriate decisions to advance his or her sexual and interpersonal health (Getch et al, 2001).

- Teach safe sex, which includes using latex condoms, washing with soap immediately after sexual contact, not ingesting semen, avoiding oral-genital contact, not exchanging saliva, avoiding multiple partners, abstaining from sexual activity when ill, and avoiding recreational drugs and alcohol when engaging in sexual activity. Contrary to previously published information, the use of a spermicide containing nonoxynol-9 (N-9) should not be recommended as a preventative strategy for HIV infection. *Accurate information regarding safe sex is essential for sexually active clients (Tucker et al, 1996).* **Clinical Research:** *In a study of 1000 women it was determined that N-9 has now been proven ineffective against HIV transmission. The possibility of risk, with no benefit, indicates that N-9, a product widely used in spermicides, should not be recommended as an effective means of HIV prevention (US Department of Health and Human Services, 2003).* **Nursing Research:** *Interventions that focus on self-efficacy are most likely to reduce anxiety related to condom use, increase positive perceptions about condoms, and increase the likelihood of adopting condom use behaviors (Dilorio et al, 2000).*

evolve WEBSITES FOR EDUCATION

See the EVOLVE website for World Wide Web resources for client education.

REFERENCES

Cochran M: Tears have no color, *Am J Nurs* 98(6):53, 1998.

Dilorio C et al: A social cognitive-based model for condom use among college students, *Nurs Res* 49(4):208, 2000.

Doswell W, Erlen J: Multicultural issues and ethical concerns in the delivery of revising care interventions, *Nurs Clin North Am* 33(2):353, 1998.

Getch YQ, Branca DL, Fitz-Gerald D: A rationale and recommendations for sexuality education in schools for students who are deaf, *Am Ann Deaf* 146(5):401, 2001.

Heineken J: Patient silence is not necessarily client satisfaction: Communication in home care nursing, *Home Healthc Nurse* 16(2):115, 1998.

L'Abate L: Hugging, holding, huddling and cuddling (3HC):a task prescription in couple and family therapy, *J Clin Activities Assignments Handouts Psychother Pract* 1(1):5, 2001.

Lazoritz S, McDermott RT: Adolescent sexuality, cultural sensitivity and the teachings of the Catholic Church, *J Reprod Med* 47(8):603, 2002.

Leininger MM, McFarland MR: *Transcultural nursing: concepts, theories, research and practices,* ed 3, New York, 2002, McGraw-Hill.

Lewis CL, Brown SC: Coping strategies of female adolescents with HIV/AI, *ABNF J* 13(4):72, 2002.

Lewis JH: Treatment options for men with sexual dysfunction, *J ET Nurs* 19:131, 1992.

Lundquist G, Ojehagen A: Childhood sexual abuse: an evaluation of a two-year group therapy in adult women, *Eur Psychiatry* 16(1):64, 2001.

McConkey R, Ryan D: Experiences of staff in dealing with client sexuality in services for teenagers and adults with intellectual disability, *J Intellectual Disabil Res* 45(1):83 2001.

McCoy N: Methodological problems in the study of sexuality and menopause, *Maturitas* 29(1):51, 1998.

Parish KL et al: Safer sex decision-making among men with haemophilia and HIV and their female partners, *Haemophilia* 7(1):72, 2001.

Shell J, Smith C: Sexuality and the older person with cancer, *Oncology* 21:553, 1994.

Sjvgren Fugl-Meyer K, Fugl-Meyer AR: Sexual disabilities are not singularities, *Int J Impot Res* 14(6):487, 2002.

Sprunk E, Alteneder RR: The impact of an ostomy on sexuality, *Clin J Oncol Nurs* 4(2):85, 2000.

• = **Independent;** ▲ = **Collaborative**

Steinke E, Patterson-Midgley P: Sexual counseling following acute myocardial infarction, *Clin Nurs Res* 5(4): 462, 1996.

Steinke EE, Patterson-Midgley PE: Perspectives of nurses and patients on the need for sexual counseling of MI patients, *Rehabil Nurs* 23(2):64, 1998.

Steinke EE et al: Sexuality and aging, *J Gerontol Nurs* 12(6):6, 1986.

Taylor P: Beating the taboo, *Nurs Times* 90:51, 1994.

Tucker M et al: *Patient care standards: collaborative practice planning,* ed 6, St Louis, 1996, Mosby.

US Department of Health and Human Services: *AIDS info:* available on-line at http://aidsinfo.nih.gov/ rwscripts/rwisapi.dll/@aidsinfo.env, accessed Feb 27, 2003.

Impaired Skin integrity

Diane L. Krasner

NANDA Definition

Altered epidermis and/or dermis

Defining Characteristics

Invasion of body structures; destruction of skin layers (dermis); disruption of skin surface (epidermis)

Related Factors (r/t)

External

Hyperthermia; hypothermia; chemical substance (e.g., incontinence); mechanical factors (e.g., friction, shearing forces, pressure, restraint); physical immobilization; humidity; extremes in age; moisture; radiation; medications

Internal

Altered metabolic state; altered nutritional state (e.g., obesity, emaciation); altered circulation; altered sensation; altered pigmentation; skeletal prominence; developmental factors; immunological deficit; alterations in skin turgor (change in elasticity); altered fluid status

NOC Outcomes (Nursing Outcomes Classification)

Suggested NOC Outcomes

Tissue Integrity: Skin and Mucous Membranes; Wound Healing: Primary Intention, Secondary Intention

> ### Example NOC Outcome with Indicators
>
> **Tissue Integrity: Skin and Mucous Membranes** will be intact as evidenced by the following indicators: Skin intactness/Tissue lesion-free/Tissue perfusion/Tissue temperature in expected range (Rate each indicator of **Tissue Integrity: Skin and Mucous Membranes:** 1 = extremely compromised, 2 = substantially compromised, 3 = moderately compromised, 4 = mildly compromised, 5 = not compromised [see Section I].)

• = Independent; ▲ = Collaborative

Client Outcomes

Client Will (Specify Time Frame):
- Regain integrity of skin surface
- Report any altered sensation or pain at site of skin impairment
- Demonstrate understanding of plan to heal skin and prevent reinjury
- Describe measures to protect and heal the skin and to care for any skin lesion

NIC　Interventions (Nursing Interventions Classification)

Suggested NIC Interventions

Incision Site Care; Pressure Ulcer Care; Skin Care: Topical Treatments; Skin Surveillance; Wound Care

---

Example NIC Activities—Pressure Ulcer Care

Monitor color, temperature, edema, moisture, and appearance of surrounding skin; Note characteristics of any drainage

---

Nursing Interventions and Rationales

- Assess site of skin impairment and determine etiology (e.g., acute or chronic wound, burn, dermatological lesion, pressure ulcer, skin tear) (Krasner and Sibbald, 1999a, 1999b). *Prior assessment of wound etiology is critical for proper identification of nursing interventions (van Rijswijk, 2001).*
- Determine that skin impairment involves skin damage only (e.g., partial-thickness wound, stage I or stage II pressure ulcer). Classify superficial pressure ulcers in the following manner:
  - Stage I: Observable pressure-related alteration of intact skin with indicators as compared with the adjacent or opposite area on the body that may include changes in one or more of the following: skin temperature (warmth or coolness), tissue consistency (firm or boggy feel), and/or sensation (pain, itching). The ulcer appears as a defined area of persistent redness in lightly pigmented skin, whereas in darker skin tones, the ulcer may appear with persistent red, blue, or purple hues (National Pressure Ulcer Advisory Panel, 1999).
  - Stage II: Partial-thickness skin loss involving epidermis or dermis superficial ulcer that appears as an abrasion, blister, or shallow crater (National Pressure Ulcer Advisory Panel, 1999).
  - NOTE: For wounds deeper into subcutaneous tissue, muscle, or bone (stage III or stage IV pressure ulcers), see the care plan for **Impaired Tissue integrity.**
- Monitor site of skin impairment at least once a day for color changes, redness, swelling, warmth, pain, or other signs of infection. Determine whether the client is experiencing changes in sensation or pain. Pay special attention to high-risk areas such as bony prominences, skinfolds, the sacrum, and heels. *Systematic inspection can identify impending problems early (Bryant, 1999).*
- Monitor the client's skin care practices, noting type of soap or other cleansing agents used, temperature of water, and frequency of skin cleansing.
- Individualize plan according to the client's skin condition, needs, and preferences. *Avoid harsh cleansing agents, hot water, extreme friction or force, or cleansing too frequently (Panel for the Prediction and Prevention of Pressure Ulcers in Adults, 1992).*

- = Independent; ▲ = Collaborative

- Monitor the client's continence status, and minimize exposure of skin impairment and other areas to moisture from incontinence, perspiration, or wound drainage.
- ▲ If the client is incontinent, implement an incontinence management plan to prevent exposure to chemicals in urine and stool that can strip or erode the skin. Refer to a urologist or gastroenterologist for incontinence assessment (Doughty, 2000; Wound, Ostomy, and Continence Nurses Society, 1992, 1994; Fantl et al, 1996). **Nursing and Clinical Research:** *Implementing an incontinence prevention plan with the use of a skin protectant or a cleanser protectant can significantly decrease skin breakdown and pressure ulcer formation (Clever et al, 2003; Warshaw et al, 2002).*
- For clients with limited mobility, use a risk-assessment tool to systematically assess immobility-related risk factors (van Rijswijk, 2001). *A validated risk-assessment tool such as the Norton or Braden scale should be used to identify clients at risk for immobility-related skin breakdown (Ayello and Braden, 2002; Panel for the Prediction and Prevention of Pressure Ulcers in Adults, 1992).* **Nursing Research:** *Targeting variables (such as age and Braden Scale Risk Category) can focus assessment on particular risk factors (e.g. pressure) and help guide the plan of prevention and care (Young et al, 2002).*
- Do not position the client on site of skin impairment. If consistent with overall client management goals, turn and position the client at least every 2 hours. Transfer the client with care to protect against the adverse effects of external mechanical forces such as pressure, friction, and shear.
- Evaluate for use of specialty mattresses, beds, or devices as appropriate (Fleck, 2001). *If the goal of care is to keep a client (e.g., a terminally ill client) comfortable, turning and repositioning may not be appropriate. Maintain the head of the bed at the lowest possible degree of elevation to reduce shear and friction, and use lift devices, pillows, foam wedges, and pressure-reducing devices in the bed. Evaluate for the use of specialty mattresses or beds as appropriate (Krasner et al, 2001; Panel for the Prediction and Prevention of Pressure Ulcers in Adults, 1992).*
- ▲ Implement a written treatment plan for topical treatment of the site of skin impairment. *A written plan ensures consistency in care and documentation (Maklebust and Sieggreen, 1996). Topical treatments must be matched to the client, wound, and setting (Krasner and Sibbald, 1999a, 1999b).*
- ▲ Select a topical treatment that will maintain a moist wound-healing environment and that is balanced with the need to absorb exudate. *Caution should always be taken not to dry out the wound (Bergstrom et al, 1994).*
- Avoid massaging around the site of skin impairment and over bony prominences. *Research suggests that massage may lead to deep-tissue trauma (Panel for the Prediction and Prevention of Pressure Ulcers in Adults, 1992).*
- ▲ Assess the client's nutritional status. Refer for a nutritional consult, and/or institute dietary supplements as necessary. *Inadequate nutritional intake places individuals at risk for skin breakdown and compromises healing (Demling and De Santi, 1998). Optimizing nutritional intake, including calories, fatty acids, protein, and vitamins, is needed to promote wound healing (Russell, 2001).*

Home care

- Identify the client's phase of wound healing (inflammation, proliferation, maturation) and stage of injury. *Accurate understanding of tissue status combined with knowledge of underlying diagnoses and product validity provide a basis for determining appropriate treat-*

• = **Independent;** ▲ = **Collaborative**

ment objectives (Ovington, 1998). There is no single wound dressing appropriate for all phases of wound healing (Ovington, 1998).

- Instruct and assist the client and caregivers to remove or control impediments to wound healing (e.g., management of underlying disease, improved approach to client positioning, improved nutrition). *Wound healing can be delayed or fail totally if impediments are not controlled (Krasner and Sibbald, 1999a, 1999b).*

▲ Initiate a consultation in a case assignment with a wound, ostomy, continence nurse (WOC nurse) to establish a comprehensive plan as soon as possible.

Client/Family Teaching

- Teach skin and wound assessment and ways to monitor for signs and symptoms of infection, complications, and healing. *Early assessment and intervention help prevent serious problems from developing.*

▲ Teach the client to use a topical treatment that is matched to client, wound, and setting. *The topical treatment must be adjusted as the status of the wound changes (van Rijswijk, 2001; Krasner and Sibbald, 1999a, 1999b; Ovington, 1998).*

- If consistent with overall client management goals, teach how to turn and reposition at least every 2 hours. *If the goal of care is to keep a client (e.g., terminally ill client) comfortable, turning and repositioning may not be appropriate (Krasner et al, 2001; Panel for the Prediction and Prevention of Pressure Ulcers in Adults, 1992).*

- Teach the client to use pillows, foam wedges, and pressure-reducing devices to prevent pressure injury. **Clinical Research:** *The use of effective pressure-reducing seat cushions for elderly wheelchair users significantly prevented sitting-acquired pressure ulcers (Geyer et al, 2001).*

evolve WEBSITES FOR EDUCATION

See the EVOLVE website for World Wide Web resources for client education.

REFERENCES

Ayello EA, Braden B: How and why to do pressure ulcer risk assessment, *Adv Skin Wound Care* 15(3):125, 2002

Bergstrom N et al: *Treatment of pressure ulcers, Clinical Practice Guideline No. 15,* Agency for Health Care Policy and Research, publication No. 95, Rockville, Md, 1994, Public Health Service, U.S. Department of Health and Human Services.

Bryant R: *Acute and chronic wounds,* ed 2, St Louis, 1999, Mosby.

Clever K et al: Evaluating the efficacy of a uniquely delivered skin protectant and its effect on the formation of sacral/buttock pressure ulcers, *Ostomy Wound Manag* 48(12):60, 2002.

Demling R, De Santi L: Closure of the non-healing wound corresponds with correction of weight loss using the anabolic agent oxandrolone, *Ostomy Wound Manag* 44(10):58, 1998.

Doughty D: *Urinary and fecal incontinence: nursing management,* ed 2, St Louis, 2000, Mosby.

Fantl JA et al: *Urinary incontinence in adults: acute and chronic management,* Clinical Practice Guideline, No. 2, 1996 Update, Agency for Health Care Policy and Research, publication No. 96, Rockville, Md, 1996, Public Health Service, U.S. Department of Health and Human Services.

Fleck C: Support surfaces: criteria and selection. In Krasner D, Rodeheaver G, Sibbald RG: *Chronic wound care: a clinical source book for healthcare professionals,* ed 2, Wayne, Penn, 2001, HMP Communications.

Geyer MJ et al: A randomized control trial to evaluate pressure-reducing seating cushions for elderly wheelchair users, *Adv Skin Wound Care* 14(3), 120, 2001.

Krasner D, Rodeheaver G, Sibbald RG: Advanced wound caring for a new millennium. In Krasner D, Rodeheaver G, Sibbald RG: *Chronic wound care: a clinical source book for healthcare professionals,* ed 2, Wayne, Penn, 2001, HMP Communications.

- = **Independent;** ▲ = **Collaborative**

Krasner D, Sibbald RG: Nursing management of chronic wounds: best practices across the continuum of care, *Nurs Clin North Am* 34(4):933, 1999a.

Krasner D, Sibbald RG, editors: Moving beyond the AHCPR guidelines: wound care evolution over the last five years, *Ostomy Wound Manag Spec Suppl* 45(1A):15, 1999b.

Maklebust J, Sieggreen M: *Pressure ulcers: guidelines for prevention and nursing management,* ed 2, Springhouse, Penn, 1996, Springhouse.

National Pressure Ulcer Advisory Panel, 1999. Website: www.npuap.org.

Ovington LG: The well-dressed wound: an overview of dressing types, *Wounds* 10(suppl)A: IA-IIA, 1998.

Panel for the Prediction and Prevention of Pressure Ulcers in Adults: *Pressure ulcers in adults: prediction and prevention,* Clinical Practice Guideline No. 3, Agency for Health Care Policy and Research, publication No. 92, Rockville, Md, 1992, Public Health Service, U.S. Department of Health and Human Services.

Russell L: The importance of patients' nutritional status in wound healing, *Br J Nurs* 10(6):S42, 2001.

van Rijswijk L: Wound assessment and documentation. In Krasner D, Rodeheaver G, Sibbald RG: *Chronic wound care: a clinical source book for healthcare professionals,* ed 2, Wayne, Penn, 2001, HMP Communications.

Warshaw E et al: Clinical and cost effectiveness of a cleanser protectant lotion for treatment of perineal skin breakdown in low-risk patients with incontinence. *Ostomy Wound Manag* 48(6):44, 2002.

Wound, Ostomy, and Continence Nurses Society: *Standards of care: patient with urinary incontinence,* Costa Mesa, Calif, 1992, The Society.

Wound, Ostomy, and Continence Nurses Society: *Standards of care: patient with fecal incontinence,* Costa Mesa, Calif, 1994, The Society.

Young J et al: Risk factors associated with pressure ulcer development at a major Western Australia teaching hospital from 1998 to 2000. *J WOCN* 29(5):234, 2002.

Risk for impaired Skin integrity

Diane L. Krasner

NANDA   Definition

At risk for skin being adversely altered

Risk Factors

External

Hypothermia; hyperthermia; chemical substance; excretions and/or secretions; mechanical factors (e.g., shearing forces, pressure, restraint); radiation; physical immobilization; humidity; moisture; extremes of age

Internal

Medication; altered nutritional state (e.g., obesity, emaciation); altered metabolic state; altered circulation; altered sensation; altered pigmentation; skeletal prominence; developmental factors; immunological deficit; alterations in skin turgor (change in elasticity); psychogenetic, immunological factors

NOTE: Risk should be determined by the use of a risk assessment tool (e.g., Norton scale, Braden scale).

Related Factors (r/t)

See Risk Factors.

NOC   Outcomes (Nursing Outcomes Classification)

Suggested NOC Outcomes

Immobility Consequences: Physiological; Tissue Integrity: Skin and Mucous Membranes

• = Independent; ▲ = Collaborative

Tissue Integrity: Skin and Mucous Membranes will be intact as evidenced by the following indicators: Skin intactness/Tissue lesion-free/Tissue perfusion/Tissue temperature in expected range (Rate each indicator of **Tissue Integrity: Skin and Mucous Membranes:** 1 = extremely compromised, 2 = substantially compromised, 3 = moderately compromised, 4 = mildly compromised, 5 = not compromised [see Section I].)

Client Outcomes

Client Will (Specify Time Frame):

- Report altered sensation or pain at risk areas
- Demonstrate understanding of personal risk factors for impaired skin integrity
- Verbalize a personal plan for preventing impaired skin integrity

NIC   Interventions (Nursing Interventions Classification)

Suggested NIC Interventions

Positioning; Pressure Management; Pressure Ulcer Care; Pressure Ulcer Prevention; Skin Surveillance

Monitor color, temperature, edema, moisture, and appearance of surrounding skin; Note characteristics of any drainage.

Nursing Interventions and Rationales

- Monitor skin condition at least once a day for color or texture changes, dermatological conditions, or lesions. Determine whether the client is experiencing loss of sensation or pain. *Systematic inspection can identify impending problems early (Krasner, Rodeheaver, Sibbald, 2001).*
- Identify clients at risk for impaired skin integrity as a result of compromised perfusion, immunocompromised status, or chronic medical condition such as diabetes mellitus or renal failure (Colburn, 2001). *These patient populations are known to be at high risk for impaired skin integrity (Bergstrom et al, 1987; Stotts and Wipke-Tevis, 2001).* **Nursing Research:** *Targeting variables (such as age and Braden Scale Risk Category) can focus assessment on particular risk factors (e.g. pressure) and help guide the plan of prevention and care (Young et al, 2002).*
- Monitor the client's skin care practices, noting type of soap or other cleansing agents used, temperature of water, and frequency of skin cleansing (Doughty, 2000). *Individualize plan according to the client's skin condition, needs, and preferences.*
- Avoid harsh cleansing agents, hot water, extreme friction or force, or too-frequent cleansing (Panel for the Prediction and Prevention of Pressure Ulcers in Adults, 1992).
- Monitor the client's continence status, and minimize exposure of the site of skin impairment and other areas to moisture from incontinence, perspiration, or wound drainage.

• = Independent; ▲ = Collaborative

▲ If the client is incontinent, implement an incontinence management plan to prevent exposure to chemicals in urine and stool that can strip or erode the skin; refer to a physician (e.g., urologist, gastroenterologist) for an incontinence assessment (Doughty, 2000; Wound, Ostomy and Continence Nurses Society, 1992, 1994; Fantl et al, 1996). **Nursing and Clinical Research:** *Implementing an incontinence prevention plan with the use of a skin protectant or a cleanser protectant can significantly decrease skin breakdown and pressure ulcer formation (Clever et al, 2003; Warshaw et al, 2002).*

• For clients with limited mobility, monitor condition of skin covering bony prominences. *Pressure ulcers usually occur over bony prominences, such as the sacrum, coccyx, trochanter, and heels, as a result of unrelieved pressure between the prominence and support surface (Maklebust and Sieggreen, 1996).*

• Use a risk-assessment tool to systematically assess immobility-related risk factors. *A validated risk-assessment tool such as the Norton or Braden scale should be used to identify clients at risk for immobility-related skin breakdown (Ayello and Braden, 2002; Bergstrom et al, 1987; Panel for the Prediction and Prevention of Pressure Ulcers in Adults, 1992; Sussman and Bates-Jensen, 1998).*

• Implement a written prevention plan. *A written plan ensures consistency in care and documentation (Maklebust and Sieggreen, 1996).* **Nursing Research:** *Implementing a prevention protocol can significantly reduce costs and incidence of skin breakdown and pressure ulcers in the long term care setting (Lyder et al, 2002).*

• If consistent with overall client management goals, turn and position the client at least every 2 hours. Transfer the client with care to protect against the adverse effects of external mechanical forces (e.g., pressure, friction, shear).

▲ Evaluate for use of specialty mattresses, beds, or devices as appropriate (Fleck, 2001). *If the goal of care is to keep the client (e.g., a terminally ill client) comfortable, turning and repositioning may not be appropriate. Maintain the head of the bed at the lowest possible degree of elevation to reduce shear and friction and use lift devices, pillows, foam wedges, and pressure-reducing devices in the bed (Krasner et al, 2001; Panel for the Prediction and Prevention of Pressure Ulcers in Adults, 1992).*

• Avoid massaging over bony prominences. *Research suggests that massage may lead to deep-tissue trauma (Panel for the Prediction and Prevention of Pressure Ulcers in Adults, 1992).*

▲ Assess the client's nutritional status; refer for a nutritional consult, and/or institute dietary supplements. *Inadequate nutritional intake places individuals at risk for skin breakdown and compromises healing (Demling and De Santi, 1998). Optimizing nutritional intake, including calories, fatty acids, protein, and vitamins, is needed to promote wound healing (Russell, 2001).*

Geriatric

• Limit number of complete baths to two or three per week, and alternate them with partial baths. Use a tepid water temperature (between 90° and 105° F) for bathing. *Excessive bathing, especially in hot water, depletes aging skin of moisture and increases dryness.*

• Use lotions and moisturizers to prevent skin from drying out, especially in the winter (Sibbald and Cameron, 2001). *Avoid skin care products that contain allergens such as lanolin, latex, and dyes (Sibbald and Cameron, 2001).*

• Increase fluid intake within cardiac and renal limits to a minimum of 1500 ml per day. *Dry skin is caused by loss of fluid; increasing fluid intake hydrates the skin.*

• = **Independent;** ▲ = **Collaborative**

- Increase humidity in the environment, especially during the winter, by using a humidifier or placing a container of water on a warm object. *Increasing the moisture in the air helps keep moisture in the skin (Sibbald and Cameron, 2001).*

Home care
- Assess caregiver vigilance and ability. **Nursing Research:** In a limited study of the Braden Scale, caregiver vigilance and ability were recognized as potentially significant variables for determining the risk of developing pressure sores (Ramundo, 1995).
- Initiate a consultation in a case assignment with a wound, ostomy, continence nurse (WOC nurse) to establish a comprehensive plan as soon as possible.
- See the care plan for **Impaired Skin integrity.**

Client/Family Teaching
- Teach the client skin assessment and ways to monitor for impending skin breakdown. *Early assessment and intervention help prevent the development of serious problems (Colburn, 2001).*
- If consistent with overall client management goals, teach how to turn and reposition the client at least every 2 hours. *If the goal of care is to keep the client (e.g., a terminally ill client) comfortable, turning and repositioning may not be appropriate (Panel for the Prediction and Prevention of Pressure Ulcers in Adults, 1992).*
- Teach the client to use pillows, foam wedges, and pressure-reducing devices to prevent pressure injury (Bryant, 1999; Krasner *and* Sibbald, 1999). **Clinical Research:** *The use of effective pressure-reducing seat cushions for elderly wheelchair users significantly prevented sitting-acquired pressure ulcers (Geyer et al, 2001).*

evolve WEBSITES FOR EDUCATION

See the EVOLVE website for World Wide Web resources for client education.

REFERENCES

Ayello EA, Braden B: How and why to do pressure ulcer risk assessment, *Adv Skin Wound Care* 15(3):125, 2002.
Bergstrom N et al: The Braden scale for prediction of pressure sore risk, *Nurs Res* 36:205, 1987.
Bryant R: *Acute and chronic wounds,* ed 2, St Louis, 1999, Mosby.
Clever K et al: Evaluating the efficacy of a uniquely delivered skin protectant and its effect on the formation of sacral/buttock pressure ulcers, *Ostomy Wound Manag* 48(12):60, 2002.
Colburn L: Prevention for chronic wounds. In Krasner D, Rodeheaver G, Sibbald RG: *Chronic wound care: a clinical source book for healthcare professionals,* ed 2, Wayne, Penn, 2001, HMP Communications.
Demling R, De Santi L: Closure of the non-healing wound corresponds with correction of weight loss using the anabolic agent oxandrolone, *Ostomy Wound Manag* 44(10):58, 1998.
Doughty D: *Urinary and fecal incontinence: nursing management,* ed 2, St Louis, 2000, Mosby.
Fantl JA et al: *Urinary incontinence in adults: acute and chronic management,* Clinical Practice Guideline No. 2, 1996 Update, Agency for Health Care Policy and Research, Publication No. 96, Rockville, Md, 1996, Public Health Service, U.S. Department of Health and Human Services.
Fleck C: Support surfaces: criteria and selection. In Krasner D, Rodeheaver G, Sibbald RG: *Chronic wound care: a clinical source book for healthcare professionals,* ed 2, Wayne, Penn, 2001, HMP Communications.
Geyer MJ et al: A randomized control trial to evaluate pressure-reducing seating cushions for elderly wheelchair users, *Adv Skin Wound Care* 14(3), 120, 2001.
Krasner D, Rodeheaver G, Sibbald RG: Advanced wound caring for a new millennium. In Krasner D, Rodeheaver G, Sibbald RG: *Chronic wound care: a clinical source book for healthcare professionals,* ed 2, Wayne, Penn, 2001, HMP Communications.

• = Independent; ▲ = Collaborative

Krasner D, Sibbald RG, editors: Moving beyond the AHCPR guidelines: wound care evolution over the last five years, *Ostomy Wound Manag Spec Suppl* 45(1A):1SS, 1999.

Lyder CH et al: A comprehensive program to prevent pressure ulcers in long-term care: exploring costs and outcomes, *Ostomy Wound Manage* 48(4):52, 2002.

Maklebust J, Sieggreen M: *Pressure ulcers: guidelines for prevention and nursing management,* ed 2, Springhouse, Penn, 1996, Springhouse.

Panel for the Prediction and Prevention of Pressure Ulcers in Adults: *Pressure ulcers in adults: prediction and prevention,* Clinical Practice Guideline No. 3, Agency for Health Care Policy and Research, publication No. 92, Rockville, Md, 1992, Public Health Service, U.S. Department of Health and Human Services.

Ramundo J: Reliability and validity of the Braden Scale in the home care setting, *J Wound Ostomy Cont Nurs* 22:3, 1995.

Russell L: The importance of patients' nutritional status in wound healing, *Br J Nurs* 10(6):S42, 2001.

Sibbald RG, Cameron J: Dermatological aspects of wound care. In Krasner D, Rodeheaver G, Sibbald RG: *Chronic wound care: a clinical source book for healthcare professionals,* ed 2, Wayne, Penn, 2001, HMP Communications.

Stotts NA, Wipke-Tevis: Co-factors in impaired wound healing. In Krasner D, Rodeheaver G, Sibbald RG: *Chronic wound care: a clinical source book for healthcare professionals,* ed 2, Wayne, Penn, 2001, HMP Communications.

Sussman C, Bates-Jensen BM: *Wound care: a collaborative practice manual for physical therapists and nurses,* Gaithersburg, Md, 1998, Aspen.

Warshaw E et al: Clinical and cost effectiveness of a cleanser protectant lotion for treatment of perineal skin breakdown in low-risk patients with incontinence. *Ostomy Wound Manag* 48(6):44, 2002.

Wound, Ostomy, and Continence Nurses Society: *Standards of care: patient with urinary incontinence,* Costa Mesa, Calif, 1992, The Society.

Wound, Ostomy, and Continence Nurses Society: *Standards of care: patient with fecal incontinence,* Costa Mesa, Calif, 1994, The Society.

Young J et al: Risk factors associated with pressure ulcer development at a major Western Australia teaching hospital from 1998 to 2000. *J WOCN* 29(5):234, 2002.

Sleep deprivation

Betty J. Ackley

NANDA Definition

Prolonged periods without sleep (sustained natural, periodic suspension of relative unconsciousness)

Defining Characteristics

Daytime drowsiness; decreased ability to function; malaise; tiredness; lethargy; restlessness; irritability; heightened sensitivity to pain; listlessness; apathy; slowed reaction; inability to concentrate; perceptual disorders (e.g., disturbed body sensation, delusions, feeling afloat); hallucinations; acute confusion; transient paranoia; agitated or combative; anxious; mild, fleeting nystagmus; hand tremors

Related Factors (r/t)

Prolonged physical discomfort; prolonged psychological discomfort; sustained inadequate sleep hygiene; prolonged use of pharmacological or dietary antisoporifics; aging-related sleep stage shifts; sustained circadian asynchrony; inadequate daytime activity; sustained environmental stimulation; sustained unfamiliar or uncomfortable sleep environment; nonsleep-inducing parenting practices; sleep apnea; periodic limb movement (e.g., restless leg syndrome, nocturnal myoclonus); sundowner's syndrome; narcolepsy; idiopathic central nervous system hypersomnolence; sleep walking; sleep terror; sleep-

• = Independent; ▲ = Collaborative

related enuresis; nightmares; familiar sleep paralysis; sleep-related painful erections; dementia

NOC Outcomes (Nursing Outcomes Classification)

Suggested NOC Outcomes
Rest; Sleep; Symptom Severity

> **Example NOC Outcome with Indicators**
>
> **Sleep** as evidenced by the following indicators: Hours of sleep/Sleep pattern/Sleep Quality/Sleep efficiency/ Feelings of rejuvenation after sleep/Napping appropriate for age (Rate each indicator of **Sleep:** 1 = extremely compromised, 2 = substantially compromised, 3 = moderately compromised, 4 = mildly compromised, 5 = not compromised [see Section I].)

Client Outcomes

Client Will (Specify Time Frame):
- Wake up less frequently during night
- Awaken refreshed and be less fatigued during day
- Fall asleep without difficulty
- Verbalize plan to implement bedtime routines
- Identify actions can take to improve quality of sleep

NIC Interventions (Nursing Interventions Classification)

Suggested NIC Intervention
Sleep Enhancement

> **Example NIC Activities—Sleep Enhancement**
>
> Monitor/record patient's sleep pattern and number of sleep hours; Encourage patient to establish a bedtime routine to facilitate transition from wakefulness to sleep

Nursing Interventions and Rationales

- Obtain a sleep history including bedtime routines, history of sleep problems, changes in sleep with present illness, and use of medications and stimulants. *Assessment of sleep behavior and patterns are an important part of any health status examination (Landis, 2002).*
- Ask the client to keep a sleep diary for several weeks, which includes bedtime, rise time, number of awakenings, naps, and more. *Often the client can find the cause of the sleep deprivation when the pattern of sleeping is examined (Pagel et al, 1997). A sleep diary is a necessary component of a behavioral assessment of sleep problems (Landis, 2002).* **Clinical Research:** *A study demonstrated that a daily sleep diary provided reliable and valid measurement of insomnia (Coates et al, 1982).*
- ▲ Observe for underlying physiological illnesses causing insomnia (e.g., cardiovascular, pulmonary, gastrointestinal, hyperthyroidism, nocturia occurring with benign hypertrophic prostatitis or pain). *Symptomatology of disease states can cause insomnia (Sateia et al, 2000).*

• = Independent; ▲ = Collaborative

▲ Determine level of anxiety. If the client is anxious, utilize relaxation techniques. See further Nursing Interventions and Rationales for **Anxiety. Nursing and Clinical Research:** *The use of relaxation techniques to promote sleep in people with chronic insomnia has been shown to be effective (Johnson, 1991a; Morin et al, 1994, Floyd et al, 2000).*

▲ Assess for signs of depression: depressed mood state, flat affect, statements of hopelessness, poor appetite. Refer for counseling/treatment as appropriate. *Many symptoms associated with sleep deprivation probably arise from central nervous system hyperarousal in the depressed client (Sateia et al, 2000).*

▲ Assess the client for other symptoms of bipolar disorder (mania, hypomania). Refer for mental health services as indicated. *Sleep disruption is part of the syndrome of bipolar disorder. Resumption of a normal sleep pattern is unlikely unless the underlying bipolar disorder is treated.*

▲ Monitor for presence of nocturnal symptoms of restless leg syndrome with uncomfortable restless sensations in legs that occur before sleep onset or during the night. Also monitor for nocturnal panic attacks, presence of headaches, or gastroesophageal reflux disease. Refer for treatment as appropriate. *Numerous nocturnal events and symptoms can contribute to problems with sleep (Sateia et al, 2000).*

• Observe the client's medication, diet, nicotine, and caffeine intake. Look for hidden sources of caffeine, such as over-the-counter medications. *Difficulty sleeping can be a side effect of medications such as bronchodilators. Caffeine can interfere with sleep (Epstein and Bootzin, 2002).*

• Provide measures to take before bedtime to assist with sleep (e.g., quiet time to allow the mind to slow down). *Simple measures can increase quality of sleep.*

• Provide a back massage before bedtime. **Nursing Research:** *Use of a back massage has been shown effective in promoting sleep (Richards, 1994).*

▲ Provide pain relief shortly before bedtime, and position the client comfortably for sleep. *Clients have reported that uncomfortable positions and pain are common factors in sleep disturbance (Sateia et al, 2000).*

▲ Monitor for presence of sleep disordered breathing as evidenced by loud snoring with periods of apnea, or other sleep disorders such as restless leg syndrome or periodic limb movement disorder. Refer to an accredited sleep disorder center. *Up to 15% of all chronic insomnia conditions are associated with breathing disturbances (Sateia et al, 2000). Polysomnography evaluation is recommended if there is a sleep disorder (Epstein and Bootzin, 2002).*

• Keep environment quiet (e.g., avoid use of intercoms, lower the volume on radio and television, keep beepers on nonaudio mode, anticipate alarms on IV pumps, talk quietly on unit). *Excessive noise causes sleep deprivation that can result in ICU psychosis (Barr, 1993).* **Nursing Research:** *Healthy volunteers exposed to recorded critical care noise levels experienced poor quality sleep (Topf et al, 1996).*

• Use soothing sound generators with sounds of the ocean, rainfall, or waterfall to induce sleep, or use "white noise" such as a fan to block out other sounds if desired by the client. **Nursing Research:** *Ocean sounds promoted sleep for a group of postoperative open-heart surgery clients (Williamson, 1992).*

Geriatric

▲ Determine if the client has a physiological problem that could result in insomnia such as pain, cardiovascular disease, pulmonary disease, neurological problems such as

• = **Independent;** ▲ = **Collaborative**

dementia, or urinary problems. *Sleep disturbances in the elderly may represent a complex interaction of age-related changes and pathological causes (Sateia et al, 2000).*

- Observe elimination patterns. Have the client decrease fluid intake in the evening, and ensure that diuretics are taken early in the morning. *Many elderly people void during the night. Increasing water intake at night or taking diuretics late in the day increases nocturia, which results in disrupted sleep.*
- ▲ If the client is waking frequently during the night with periods of apnea or increased leg movement, consider the presence of sleep apnea problems or periodic leg movements disorder and refer to a sleep clinic for evaluation. *Sleep apnea and periodic limb movement disorders interfering with sleep increase with aging (Floyd, 2002).*
- Encourage social activities. Help elderly get outside for increased light exposure and to enjoy nature. *Exposure to natural light and social interactions influence the circadian rhythms that control sleep (Labyak, 2002).*
- Suggest light reading or TV viewing that does not excite as an evening activity. *Soothing activities decrease stimulation of the reticular activating system and help sleep come naturally.*
- Increase daytime physical activity, and social activities to replace napping. Encourage walking as the client is able. **Nursing Research:** *Increasing activity during the day is effective in promoting sleep in residential care (Richards et al, 2001).*
- Reduce daytime napping in the late afternoon; limit naps to short intervals as early in the day as possible. *The majority of elderly nap during the day (Evans, Rogers, 1994). Avoiding naps in the late afternoon makes it easier to fall asleep at night.*
- Help the client take a warm bath in the evening. **Nursing Research:** *Passive heating by utilizing a warm bath has been shown to increase deep sleep in the elderly (Dorsey et al, 1999).*
- ▲ If the client continues to have insomnia despite developing good sleep hygiene habits, refer to a sleep clinic for further evaluation (Pagel et al, 1997).

Home care
- Above interventions may be adapted for home care use.
- Obtain a full current assessment and history of sleep activity, sleep disturbance, and sleep disturbance–related behaviors. *A complete assessment promotes accurate determination of the client's needs.*
- Instruct the client/family in expectations for normal sleep. Elicit expectations for sleep, previous sleep patterns; correct misconceptions that influence emotional responses to deviation from expectations. *Client/family may be unduly disturbed by normal changes in sleep patterns. Disturbances in sleep or frequent awakening may be misconstrued as lack of sleep.* **Nursing Research:** *As persons age, increased time is needed to fall asleep; frequency of waking after sleep onset increases; length of waking after sleep onset increases (which may be related to unrecognized sleep apnea); and nighttime sleep amount tends to decrease (Floyd et al, 2000).*
- Have the client maintain a sleep diary, describing daily activity levels, use of stimulants, activities or physical sensations around bedtime. Assess diary for potential areas of intervention. *Details about daily activities may yield clues to change sleep pattern (e.g., exercise timing or excessive coffee use, meals before bedtime, acid indigestion while lying flat).*
- Assess environment for possible hazards to the client during period of deprivation (e.g., appliances, stairs). *Client safety is a primary goal of care in the home setting.*

• = **Independent**; ▲ = **Collaborative**

- Obtain a listing of expected daily behaviors, before and since the onset of deprivation (e.g., mowing lawn, shaving, cooking). Identify tasks that may be delegated. Establish level of client participation in tasks. Use short task periods for the client. *Role changes may be necessary to protect client and family safety. Continued participation in family activities promotes sense of belonging.*
- Assess client support system for availability of psychological and task-related support. Refer to chore, homemaker, or home health aide services as necessary. *Home health aides can assist with ADLs; homemakers can do household tasks and shopping to support the family. Chore services can do major household cleaning and yard work.*
- ▲ Assess family/caregiver response to client status. Provide nursing support; refer to medical social services or mental health services/support groups as necessary. *Support of the family/caregiver structure can decrease caregiver burden.*
- If the client is taking medication, assess for effectiveness and safety in administration. Identify person administering medication if not the client. *Sleep-deprived persons may not be consistent in self-administration of medications.*
- Assist the family to arrange for supervision if the client presents confusion or perceptual dysfunction. *Client supervision provides for client safety and may provide additional caregiver respite if obtained from outside the usual support system.*
- ▲ Refer the client to medical social services or mental health/group support services such as I Can Cope. *Venting validates feelings of the client. Groups allow the client to recognize the love and caring of others and provide alternative ways of problem-solving.*
- ▲ In the presence of a psychiatric disorder, refer for psychiatric home health care services for client reassurance and implementation of therapeutic regimen. *Psychiatric home care nurses can address issues relating to the client's sleep deprivation and bipolar disorder. Behavioral interventions in the home can assist the client to participate more effectively in treatment plan (Patusky et al, 1996).*

Client/Family Teaching

- Encourage the client to avoid coffee and other caffeinated foods and liquids and to avoid eating large high-protein or high-fat meals close to bedtime. *Caffeine intake increases the time it takes to fall asleep and increases awake time during the night (Evans and Rogers, 1994). A full stomach interferes with sleep.*
- Advise the client to avoid use of alcohol or hypnotics to induce sleep. Avoid alcohol ingestion 4 to 6 hours before bedtime. *Sleep induced by alcohol is often disrupted later in the night (Epstein and Bootzin, 2002). Clients can easily become dependent on hypnotics for sleep, and develop rebound insomnia if they are discontinued. Nonpharmacological interventions to maintain sleep are more effective than pharmacological treatments in the long term (Epstein and Bootzin, 2002).*
- Teach somatic relaxation techniques to induce the relaxation response and facilitate sleep. **Nursing and Clinical Research:** *The use of relaxation techniques to promote sleep in people with chronic insomnia has been shown to be effective (Johnson, 1991; Morin et al, 1994, Floyd et al, 2000).*
- Teach the client need for increased exercise. Encourage to take a daily walk 5 to 6 hours before retiring. **Clinical Research:** *Moderate activity such as walking can increase the quality of sleep (King et al, 1997).*
- Encourage the client to develop a bedtime ritual that includes quiet activities such as reading, television, or crafts. **Nursing Research:** *The use of a bedtime routine has been*

• = **Independent;** ▲ = **Collaborative**

shown to be effective in inducing and maintaining sleep in a population of older women (Johnson, 1991).
- Teach the following sleep hygiene guidelines for improving sleep habits:
  - Go to bed only when sleepy.
  - When awake in the middle of the night, go to another room, do quiet activities, and go back to bed only when sleepy.
  - Use the bed only for sleeping—not for reading or snoozing in front of the television.
  - Avoid afternoon and evening naps.
  - Get up at the same time every morning.
  - Recognize that not everyone needs 8 hours of sleep.
  - Do not associate lulls in performance with sleeplessness; sleeplessness should not be blamed for everything that goes wrong during the day.

  Clinical Research: *These guidelines on sleep hygiene have been shown to effectively improve quality of sleep (Morin et al, 1994).*

evolve WEBSITES FOR EDUCATION

See the EVOLVE website for World Wide Web resources for client education.

REFERENCES

Barr WJ: Noise notes: working smart, *Am J Nurs* 93:16, 1993.

Coates TJ et al: Discriminating good sleepers from insomniacs using all-night polysomnograms conducted at home, *J Nerv Ment Dis* 170, 1982.

Dorsey CM et al: Effects of passive body heating on the sleep of older female insomniacs. *J Geriatr Psychiatry Neurol* 9, 83, 1996.

Epstein DR, Bootzin RR: Insomnia. *Nursing Clin North Am* 37:4, 2002.

Evans BD, Rogers AE: 24-hour sleep/wake patterns in healthy elderly persons, *Appl Nurs Res* 7:75, 1994.

Floyd JA: Sleep and aging. *Nurs Clin North Am* 37, 719, 2002.

Floyd JA, Falahee ML, Fhobir RH: Creation and analysis of a computerized database of interventions to facilitate adult sleep. *Nurs Res* 49:4, 2000.

Johnson JE: Progressive relaxation and the sleep of older noninstitutionalized women. *Appl Nurs Res* 4, 1991a.

Johnson JE: A comparative study of the bedtime routines and sleep of older adults. *J of Commun Nurs* 8 1991b.

King AC et al: Moderate-intensity exercise and self-rated quality of sleep in older adults, *JAMA* 277(1):32, 1997.

Labyak S: Sleep and circadian schedule disorders, *Nurs Clin North Am* 37, 599, 2002.

Landis CA: Sleep and methods of assessment, *Nurs Clin North Am* 37, 583, 2002.

Morin C et al: Behavioral and pharmacological therapies for late-life insomnia, *JAMA* 281(11):991, 1999.

Morin C, Culbert JP, Schwartz SM: Nonpharmacological interventions for insomnia: *Am J Psychiatry* 151, 1172, 1994.

Pagel JF, Zafralotfi S, Zammit G: How to prescribe a good night's sleep, *Patient Care* 31(4):87, 1997.

Patusky KL; Rodning C; Martinez-Kratz M: Clinical lessons in psychiatric home health care: a case study approach, *Home Healthc Manag Pract* 1996 9(1):18.

Richards KC: Sleep promotion in the critical care unit, *AACN Clin Issues* 5(2):152, 1994.

Richards KC et al: The effect of individualized activities on the sleep of nursing home residents who are cognitively impaired: a pilot study, *J Gerontol Nurs* 27(9):30 2001.

Sateia MJ et al: Evaluation of chronic insomnia, *Sleep* 23(2):243, 2000.

Topf M, Bookman M, Arand D: Effects of critical care unit noise on the subjective quality of sleep, *J Adv Nurs* 24:3, 1996.

Williamson J: The effect of ocean sounds on sleep after coronary artery bypass graft surgery, *Am J Crit Care* 1(1):91, 1992.

- = Independent; ▲ = Collaborative

Disturbed Sleep pattern

Betty J. Ackley

NANDA Definition

Time-limited disruption of sleep (natural periodic suspension of consciousness)

Defining Characteristics

Prolonged awakenings; sleep maintenance insomnia; self-induced impairment of normal pattern; sleep onset >30 minutes; early morning insomnia; awakening earlier or later than desired; verbal complaints of difficulty falling asleep; verbal complaints of not feeling well-rested; increased proportion of stage 1 sleep; dissatisfaction with sleep; less than age-normed total sleep time; three or more nighttime awakenings; decreased proportion of Stages 3 and 4 sleep (e.g., hyporesponsiveness, excess sleepiness, decreased motivation); decreased proportion of REM sleep (e.g., REM rebound, hyperactivity, emotional lability, agitation and impulsivity, atypical polysomnographic features); decreased ability to function

Related Factors (r/t)

Ruminative presleep thoughts; daytime activity pattern; thinking about home; body temperature; temperament; dietary; childhood onset; inadequate sleep hygiene; sustained use of antisleep agents; circadian asynchrony; frequently changing sleep-wake schedule; depression; loneliness; frequent travel across time zones; daylight/darkness exposure; grief; anticipation; shift work; delayed or advanced sleep phase syndrome; loss of sleep partner, life change; preoccupation with trying to sleep; periodic gender-related hormonal shifts; biochemical agents; fear; separation from significant others; social schedule inconsistent with chronotype; aging-related sleep shifts; anxiety; medications; fear of insomnia; maladaptive conditioned wakefulness; fatigue; boredom

Environmental

Noise; unfamiliar sleep furnishings; ambient temperature, humidity; lighting; other-generated awakening; excessive stimulation; physical restraint; lack of sleep privacy/control; interruptions for therapeutics, monitoring, lab tests; sleep partner; noxious odors

Parental

Mother's sleep-wake pattern; parent-infant interaction; mother's emotional support

Physiological

Urinary urgency, incontinence; fever; nausea; stasis of secretions; shortness of breath; position; gastroesophageal reflux

NOC Outcomes (Nursing Outcomes Classification)

Suggested NOC Outcomes

Comfort Level; Pain Level; Personal Well-Being; Psychosocial Adjustment: Life Change; Quality of Life; Rest; Sleep

• = Independent; ▲ = Collaborative

> ### Example NOC Outcome with Indicators
>
> **Sleep** as evidenced by the following indicators: Hours of sleep/Sleep pattern/Sleep quality/Sleep efficiency/ Feelings of rejuvenation after sleep/Napping appropriate for age (Rate each indicator of **Sleep:** 1 = extremely compromised, 2 = substantially compromised, 3 = moderately compromised, 4 = mildly compromised, 5 = not compromised [see Section I].)

Client Outcomes

Client Will (Specify Time Frame):
- Wake up less frequently during night
- Awaken refreshed and not be fatigued during day
- Fall asleep without difficulty
- Verbalize plan to implement bedtime routines

NIC   Interventions (Nursing Interventions Classification)

Suggested NIC Intervention
Sleep Enhancement

> ### Example NIC Activities—Sleep Enhancement
>
> Monitor/record patient's sleep pattern and number of sleep hours; Encourage patient to establish a bedtime routine to facilitate transition from wakefulness to sleep

Nursing Interventions and Rationales

- Obtain a sleep history including bedtime routines, history of sleep problems, changes in sleep with present illness, and use of medications and stimulants. *Assessment of sleep behavior and patterns are an important part of any health status examination (Landis, 2002).*
- Ask the client to keep a sleep diary for several weeks, which includes bedtime, rise time, number of awakenings, naps, and more. *Often the client can find the cause of the sleep deprivation when the pattern of sleeping is examined (Pagel et al, 1997). A sleep diary is a necessary component of a behavioral assessment of sleep problems (Landis, 2002).* **Clinical Research:** *A study demonstrated that a daily sleep diary provided reliable and valid measurement of insomnia (Coates et al, 1982).*
- ▲ Determine level of anxiety. If the client is anxious, utilize relaxation techniques. See further Nursing Interventions and Rationales for **Anxiety. Nursing and Clinical Research:** *The use of relaxation techniques to promote sleep in people with chronic insomnia has been shown to be effective (Johnson, 1991; Morin et al, 1994, Floyd et al, 2000).*
- ▲ Assess for signs of new onset of depression: depressed mood state, statements of hopelessness, poor appetite. Refer for counseling as appropriate. *Many symptoms associated with sleep deprivation probably arise from central nervous system hyperarousal in the depressed client (Sateia et al, 2000).*
- Observe the client's medication, diet, and caffeine intake. Look for hidden sources of caffeine, such as over-the-counter medications. *Difficulty sleeping can be a side effect of medications such as bronchodilators; caffeine can also interfere with sleep.*

- • = Independent; ▲ = Collaborative

- Provide measures to take before bedtime to assist with sleep (e.g., quiet time to allow the mind to slow down, carbohydrates such as crackers). *Simple measures can increase quality of sleep. Carbohydrates cause release of the neurotransmitter serotonin, which helps induce and maintain sleep (Somer, 1999).*
- Provide a back massage before bedtime. **Nursing Research:** *Use of a back massage has been shown effective in promoting sleep (Richards, 1998).*
- Provide pain relief shortly before bedtime and position the client comfortably for sleep. *Clients have reported that uncomfortable positions and pain are common factors of sleep disturbance (Sateia et al, 2000).*
- Keep environment quiet for sleeping (e.g., avoid use of intercoms, lower the volume on radio and television, keep beepers on nonaudio mode, anticipate alarms on IV pumps, talk quietly on unit). *Excessive noise causes sleep deprivation that can result in ICU psychosis (Barr, 1993)* **Nursing Research:** *Healthy volunteers exposed to recorded critical care noise levels experienced poor quality sleep (Topf et al, 1996).*
- Use soothing sound generators with sounds of the ocean, rainfall, or waterfall to induce sleep, or use "white noise" such as a fan to block out other sounds. **Nursing Research:** *Ocean sounds promoted sleep for a group of postoperative open-heart surgery clients (Williamson, 1992).*
- For hospitalized stable clients, consider instituting the following sleep protocol to foster sleep:
  - Night shift: Give the client the opportunity for uninterrupted sleep from 1 AM to 5 AM. Keep environmental noise to a minimum.
  - Evening shift: Limit napping between 4 PM and 9 PM. At 10 PM turn lights off, provide sleep medication according to individual assessment, and keep noise and conversation on the unit to a minimum.
  - Day shift: Encourage short naps before 11 AM. Enforce a physical activity regimen as appropriate. Schedule newly ordered medications to avoid waking the client between 1 AM and 5 AM. **Nursing Research:** *Critical care nurses can take effective actions to promote sleep (Edwards and Schuring, 1993b).*

Geriatric

▲ Determine if the client has new onset of a physiological problem that could result in insomnia such as pain, cardiovascular disease, pulmonary disease, neurological problems such as dementia, or urinary problems. *Sleep disturbances in the elderly may represent a complex interaction of age-related changes and pathological causes (Sateia et al, 2000).*

- Observe elimination patterns. Have the client decrease fluid intake in the evening, and ensure that diuretics are taken early in the morning. *Many elderly people void during the night. Increasing water intake at night or taking diuretics late in the day increases nocturia, which results in disrupted sleep.*
- Do a careful history of all medications including over-the-counter medications and alcohol intake. *Alcohol intake and medication effects are common causes of insomnia in the elderly. Rebound insomnia associated with the use of shorter-acting hypnotics may perpetuate a cycle of sleep disturbance and chronic hypnotic use (Sateia et al, 2000).*

▲ If the client is waking frequently during the night, consider the presence of sleep apnea problems and refer to a sleep clinic for evaluation. *Sleep apnea in the elderly may*

• = **Independent;** ▲ = **Collaborative**

be caused by changes in the respiratory drive of the central nervous system or may be obstructive and associated with obesity (Foyt, 1992).

▲ Evaluate the client for presence of depression or anxiety, which can result in insomnia. Refer for treatment as appropriate. *Anxiety and depression are common in the elderly and can result in insomnia (Sateia et al, 2000).*

• Encourage social activities. Help elderly get outside for increased light exposure and to enjoy nature. *Exposure to natural light and social interactions influence the circadian rhythms that control sleep (Labyak, 2002).*

• Suggest light reading or TV viewing that does not excite as an evening activity. *Soothing activities decrease stimulation of the reticular activating system and help sleep come naturally.*

• Increase daytime physical activity, and social activities to replace napping. Encourage walking as the client is able. **Nursing Research:** *Increasing activity during the day is effective in promoting sleep in residential care (Richards et al, 2001).*

▲ Avoid use of hypnotics and alcohol to sleep. *Long-term use of hypnotics can induce a drug-related insomnia. Alcohol also disrupts sleep and can exacerbate sleep apnea (Evans, Rogers, 1994).*

• Reduce daytime napping in the late afternoon; limit naps to short intervals as early in the day as possible. Avoid excessive napping. *The majority of elderly nap during the day (Evans, Rogers, 1994).* **Clinical Research:** *Excessive napping is associated with impaired sleep and health problems related to inactivity (Hays et al, 1996).*

• Help the client take a warm bath in the evening. **Nursing Research:** *Passive heating by utilizing a warm bath has been shown to increase deep sleep in the elderly (Dorsey et al, 1999; Liao, 2002).*

• Help the client recognize that there are changes in length of sleep with aging. Client may not be able to sleep for 8 hours as when younger, and more frequent awakening is part of the aging process (Floyd, 2002).

▲ If the client continues to have insomnia despite developing good sleep hygiene habits, refer to a sleep clinic for further evaluation (Pagel et al, 1997).

Home care

• Above interventions may be adapted for home care use.

• Provide support to the family of the client with chronic sleep pattern disturbance. *Ongoing sleep pattern disturbances can disrupt family patterns and cause sleep deprivation in client or family members, which creates increased stress on the family.*

• Instruct the client/family in expectations for normal sleep. Elicit expectations for sleep, previous sleep patterns; correct misconceptions that influence emotional responses to deviation from expectations. **Nursing Research:** *Client/family may be unduly disturbed by normal changes in sleep patterns. As persons age, increased time is needed to fall asleep; frequency of waking after sleep onset increases; length of waking after sleep onset increases (which may be related to unrecognized sleep apnea); and nighttime sleep amount tends to decrease (Floyd et al, 2000).*

▲ Assess the client for sleep apnea, particularly poststroke (e.g., interview partner regarding the client's sleep pattern and behaviors, have the client maintain sleep log). *Perceived sleep disturbance may be an indication of sleep apnea, which tends to increase with age. In one study poststroke, 59% of participants met criteria for sleep apnea. More clients with sleep apnea than without were delirious, depressed, or ADL-dependent; had a higher frequency of ischemic heart disease, and latency in reaction and in response to verbal stimuli.*

• = **Independent;** ▲ = **Collaborative**

Clients may benefit from continuous positive airway pressure (CPAP) treatment (Sandberg et al, 2001).

▲ Assess the client for depression or other psychiatric disorder. Refer for mental health services as indicated. *Sleep disturbance is part of the syndrome of depression and other psychiatric disorders. Improvement in sleep pattern is unlikely unless the underlying disorder is treated.*

• Have the client maintain a sleep diary, describing daily activity levels, use of stimulants, activities or physical sensations around bedtime. Assess diary for potential areas of intervention. *Details about daily activities may yield clues to change sleep pattern (e.g., exercise timing or excessive coffee use, meals before bedtime, acid indigestion while lying flat).*

• Initiate nonpharmacological interventions for insomnia: stimulus control, sleep restriction, relaxation techniques, increasing sunlight exposure, acupuncture; cognitive and educational interventions to address dysfunctional attitudes about sleep. **Nursing and Clinical Research:** *Nonpharmacological interventions can improve sleep efficiency and continuity, increase satisfaction with sleep pattern, while reducing hypnotic usage (Morin et al, 1999; Woodward, 1999). Nursing interventions are directed at making environments conducive to sleep, relaxing the client, or entraining the circadian sleep-wake cycle (Floyd, 1999).*

▲ In the presence of a psychiatric disorder, refer for psychiatric home health care services for client reassurance and implementation of therapeutic regimen. *Psychiatric home care nurses can address issues relating to client's sleep disturbance. Behavioral interventions in the home can assist client to participate more effectively in treatment plan (Patusky et al, 1996).*

• Provide support to the family of the client with chronic sleep pattern disturbance. *Ongoing sleep pattern disturbances can disrupt family patterns and cause sleep deprivation in the client or family members, which creates increased stress on the family.*

Client/Family Teaching

• Encourage the client to avoid coffee and other caffeinated foods and liquids and also to avoid eating large high-protein or high-fat meals close to bedtime. *Caffeine intake increases the time it takes to fall asleep and increases awake time during the night (Evans and Rogers, 1994). A full stomach interferes with sleep.*

• Advise the client to avoid use of alcohol or hypnotics to induce sleep. Avoid alcohol ingestion 4 to 6 hours before bedtime. *Sleep induced by alcohol is often disrupted later in the night (Epstein and Bootzin, 2002). Clients can easily become dependent on hypnotics for sleep, and develop rebound insomnia if they are discontinued. Nonpharmacological interventions to maintain sleep are more effective than pharmacological treatments in the long term (Epstein and Bootzin, 2002).*

• Ask the client to keep a sleep diary for several weeks. *Often the client can find the cause of the sleep deprivation when the pattern of sleeping is examined (Pagel et al, 1997).*

• Teach somatic and cognitive relaxation techniques to induce the relaxation response and facilitate sleep. **Nursing and Clinical Research:** *The use of relaxation techniques to promote sleep in people with chronic insomnia has been shown to be effective (Johnson, 1991; Morin et al, 1994, Floyd et al, 2000).*

• Teach the client need for increased exercise. Encourage to take a daily walk 5 to 6 hours before retiring. *Moderate activity such as walking can increase the quality of sleep (King et al, 1997).*

• Encourage the client to develop a bedtime ritual that includes quiet activities such as

• = **Independent;** ▲ = **Collaborative**

reading, television, or crafts. **Nursing Research:** *The use of a bedtime routine has been shown to be effective in inducing and maintaining sleep in a population of older women (Johnson, 1991).*

- Teach the following guidelines for good sleep hygiene to improve sleep habits:
  - Go to bed only when sleepy.
  - When awake in the middle of the night, go to another room, do quiet activities, and go back to bed only when sleepy.
  - Use the bed only for sleeping—not for reading or snoozing in front of the television.
  - Avoid afternoon and evening naps.
  - Get up at the same time every morning.
  - Recognize that not everyone needs 8 hours of sleep.
  - Move the alarm clock away from the bed so that it can not be seen.
  - Do not associate lulls in performance with sleeplessness; sleeplessness should not be blamed for everything that goes wrong during the day.

  Clinical Research: *These guidelines on sleep hygiene have been shown to effectively improve quality of sleep (Morin et al, 1994).*

evolve WEBSITES FOR EDUCATION

See the EVOLVE website for World Wide Web resources for client education.

REFERENCES

Barr WJ: Noise notes: working smart, *Am J Nurs* 93:16, 1993.

Coates TJ et al: Discriminating good sleepers from insomniacs using all-night polysomnograms conducted at home, *J Nerv Ment Dis* 170, 1982.

Dorsey CM et al: Effects of passive body heating on the sleep of older female insomniacs, *J Geriatr Psychiatry Neurol* 9, 83, 1996.

Edwards GB, Schuring LM: Pilot study: validating staff nurses' observations of sleep and wake states among critically ill patients using polysomnography, *Am J Crit Care* 2(2):125, 1993a.

Edwards GB, Schuring LM: Sleep protocol: a research-based practice change, *Crit Care Nurse* 13:84, 1993b.

Elmore SK, Betrus PA, Burr R: Light, social zeitgebers, and the sleep-wake cycle in the entrainment of human circadian rhythms, *Res Nurs Health* 17:471, 1994.

Epstein DR, Bootzin RR: Insomnia, *Nurs Clin North Am* 37:4, 2002.

Evans BD, Rogers AE: 24-hour sleep/wake patterns in healthy elderly persons, *Appl Nurs Res* 7:75, 1994.

Floyd JA: Sleep promotion in adults, *Annu Rev Nurs Res* 17:27, 1999.

Floyd JA: Sleep and aging. *Nurs Clin North Am* 37, 719, 2002.

Floyd JA, Falahee ML, Fhobir RH: Creation and analysis of a computerized database of interventions to facilitate adult sleep, *Nurs Res* 49:4, 2000.

Floyd JA et al: Age-related changes in initiation and maintenance of sleep: a meta-analysis, *Res Nurs Health* 23: 106, 2000.

Foyt MM: Impaired gas exchange in the elderly, *Geriatr Nurs* 13:262, 1992.

Hays JC; Blazer DG; Foley DJ: Risk of napping: excessive daytime sleepiness and mortality in an older community population, *J Am Geriatr Soc* 44(6):693, 1996.

Johnson JE: Progressive relaxation and the sleep of older noninstitutionalized women, *Appl Nurs Res* 4, 1991a.

Johnson JE: A comparative study of the bedtime routines and sleep of older adults, *J Commun Nurs* 8 1991b.

King AC et al: Moderate-intensity exercise and self-rated quality of sleep in older adults, *JAMA* 277(1):32, 1997.

Labyak S: Sleep and circadian schedule disorders, *Nurs Clin North Am* 37, 599, 2002.

Landis CA: Sleep and methods of assessment, *Nurs Clin North Am* 37, 583, 2002.

Liao WC: Effects of passive body heating on body temperature and sleep regulation in the elderly: a systematic review. *Int J Nurs Stud* 39(8), 803, 2002.

Morin C: Cognitive behavior therapy for late-life insomnia, *J Consult Clin Psychol* 61(1):137, 1993.

• = **Independent;** ▲ = **Collaborative**

Morin C, Culbert JP, Schwartz SM: Nonpharmacological interventions for insomnia, *Am J Psychiatry* 151, 1172, 1994.

Morin CM, Mimeault V, Gagne A: Nonpharmacological treatment of late-life insomnia, *J Psychosom Res* 46: 103, 1999.

Pagel JF, Zafralotfi S, Zammit G: How to prescribe a good night's sleep, *Patient Care* 31(4):87, 1997.

Patusky KL, Rodning C, Martinez-Kratz M: Clinical lessons in psychiatric home health care: a case study approach, *Home Healthc Manag Pract* 9(1):18, 1996.

Richards KC: Sleep promotion in the critical care unit, *AACN Clin Issues* 5(2):152, 1994.

Richards KC et al: The effect of individualized activities on the sleep of nursing home residents who are cognitively impaired: a pilot study, *J Gerontol Nurs* 27(9):30, 2001.

Sandberg O et al: Sleep apnea, delirium, depressed mood, cognition, and ADL ability after stroke, *J Am Geriatr Soc* 49:391, 2001.

Sateia MJ et al: Evaluation of chronic insomnia, *Sleep* 23(2):243, 2000.

Somer E: *Food and mood: the complete guide to eating well and feeling your best,* ed 2, New York, 1999, Henry Holt.

Topf M: Effects of personal control over hospital noise on sleep, *Res Nurs Health* 15:19, 1992.

Williamson J: The effect of ocean sounds on sleep after coronary artery bypass graft surgery, *Am J Crit Care* 1(1):91, 1992.

Woodward M: Insomnia in the elderly, *Aust Fam Phys* 28:653, 1999.

Readiness for enhanced Sleep

Betty Ackley

NANDA Definition

A pattern of natural, periodic suspension of consciousness that provides adequate rest, sustains a desired lifestyle, and can be strengthened

Defining Characteristics

Expresses willingness to enhance sleep; amount of sleep and REM sleep is congruent with developmental needs; expresses a feeling of being rested after sleep; follows sleep routines that promote sleep habits; occasional or infrequent use of medications to induce sleep

Related Factors (r/t)

Desire to improve sleep

NOC   Outcomes (Nursing Outcomes Classification)

Suggested NOC Outcomes
Personal Well-Being; Rest; Sleep

Example NOC Outcome with Indicators

Sleep as evidenced by the following indicators: Hours of sleep/Sleep pattern/Sleep quality/Sleep efficiency/Feelings of rejuvenation after sleep/Napping appropriate for age (Rate each indicator of **Sleep:** 1 = extremely compromised, 2 = substantially compromised, 3 = moderately compromised, 4 = mildly compromised, 5 = not compromised [see Section I].)

• = Independent; ▲ = Collaborative

Client Outcomes

Client Will (Specify Time Frame):
- Awaken refreshed and is not fatigued during day
- Fall asleep without difficulty
- Verbalize plan to implement improved bedtime routines

NIC | Interventions (Nursing Interventions Classification)

Suggested NIC Intervention
Sleep Enhancement

> **Example NIC Activities—Sleep Enhancement**
>
> Determine patient's sleep/activity pattern; Encourage patient to establish a bedtime routine to facilitate transition from wakefulness to sleep

Nursing Interventions and Rationales

- Obtain a sleep history including bedtime routines, sleep patterns, and use of medications and stimulants. *Assessment of sleep behavior and patterns is an important part of any health status examination (Landis, 2002).*
- Ask the client to keep a sleep diary for several weeks, which includes bedtime, rise time, number of awakenings, naps, and more. *A sleep diary is a necessary component of a behavioral assessment of sleep problems (Landis, 2002).* **Clinical Research:** *A study demonstrated that a daily sleep diary provided reliable and valid measurement of insomnia (Coates et al, 1982).*
- Determine level of anxiety. If the client is anxious, use relaxation techniques. See further Nursing Interventions and Rationales for **Anxiety. Nursing and Clinical Research:** *The use of relaxation techniques to promote sleep in people with chronic insomnia has been shown to be effective (Johnson, 1991a; Morin et al, 1994, Floyd et al, 2000).*
- Observe the client's medication, diet, and caffeine intake. Look for hidden sources of caffeine, such as over-the-counter medications. *Difficulty sleeping can be a side effect of medications such as bronchodilators; caffeine can also interfere with sleep.*
- Provide measures to take before bedtime to assist with sleep (e.g., quiet time to allow the mind to slow down, carbohydrates such as crackers). *Simple measures can increase quality of sleep. Carbohydrates cause release of the neurotransmitter serotonin, which helps induce and maintain sleep (Somer, 1999).*
- Provide a back massage before bedtime. **Nursing Research:** *Use of a back massage has been shown effective in promoting sleep (Richards, 1998).*
- Initiate nonpharmacological interventions for improved sleep: stimulus control, sleep restriction, increasing sunlight exposure, acupuncture; cognitive and educational interventions to address dysfunctional attitudes about sleep. **Nursing and Clinical Research:** *Nonpharmacological interventions can improve sleep efficiency and continuity, increase satisfaction with sleep pattern, while reducing hypnotic usage (Morin et al, 1999; Woodward, 1999). Nursing interventions are directed at making environments conducive to sleep, relaxing the client, or entraining the circadian sleep-wake cycle (Floyd, 1999).*

• = Independent; ▲ = Collaborative

Geriatric

- Encourage the client to develop a bedtime ritual that includes quiet activities such as reading, television, or crafts. **Nursing Research:** *The use of a bedtime routine has been shown to be effective in inducing and maintaining sleep in a population of older women (Johnson, 1991b).*
- Encourage the client take a warm bath in the evening. **Nursing Research:** *Passive heating by utilizing a warm bath has been shown to increase deep sleep in the elderly (Dorsey et al, 1999; Liao, 2002).*
- Observe elimination patterns. Have the client decrease fluid intake in the evening, and ensure that diuretics are taken early in the morning. *Many elderly people void during the night. Increasing water intake at night or taking diuretics late in the day increases nocturia, which results in disrupted sleep.*
- Encourage social activities. Help elderly get outside for increased light exposure and to enjoy nature. *Exposure to natural light and social interactions influence the circadian rhythms that control sleep (Labyak, 2002).*
- Increase daytime physical activity. Encourage walking as the client is able.
- ▲ Recommend avoid use of hypnotics and alcohol to sleep. *Long-term use of hypnotics can induce a drug-related insomnia. Alcohol also disrupts sleep and can exacerbate sleep apnea (Evans and Rogers, 1994).*
- Reduce daytime napping in the late afternoon; limit naps to short intervals as early in the day as possible. *The majority of elderly nap during the day (Evans and Rogers, 1994). Avoiding naps in the late afternoon makes it easier to fall asleep at night.*
- Help the client recognize that there are changes in length of sleep with aging. Client may not be able to sleep for 8 hours as when younger, and more frequent awakening is part of the aging process (Floyd et al, 2000).

Client/Family Teaching

- Teach somatic and cognitive relaxation techniques to induce the relaxation response and facilitate sleep. **Nursing and Clinical Research:** *The use of relaxation techniques to promote sleep in people with chronic insomnia has been shown to be effective (Johnson, 1991a; Morin et al, 1994, Floyd et al, 2000).*
- Advise the client to avoid use of alcohol or hypnotics to induce sleep. Avoid alcohol ingestion 4 to 6 hours before bedtime. *Sleep induced by alcohol is often disrupted later in the night (Epstein and Bootzin, 2002). Clients can easily become dependent on hypnotics for sleep, and develop rebound insomnia if they are discontinued. Nonpharmacological interventions to maintain sleep are more effective than pharmacological treatments in the long term (Epstein and Bootzin, 2002).*
- Teach the following guidelines for good sleep hygiene to improve sleep habits:
  - Go to bed only when sleepy.
  - When awake in the middle of the night, go to another room, do quiet activities, and go back to bed only when sleepy.
  - Use the bed only for sleeping—not for reading or snoozing in front of the television.
  - Avoid afternoon and evening naps.
  - Get up at the same time every morning.
  - Recognize that not everyone needs 8 hours of sleep.
  - Move the alarm clock away from the bed so that it can not be seen.
  - Do not associate lulls in performance with sleeplessness; sleeplessness should not be blamed for everything that goes wrong during the day.

- ● = **Independent;** ▲ = **Collaborative**

Clinical Research: *These guidelines on sleep hygiene have been shown to effectively improve quality of sleep (Morin et al, 1994).*

- Encourage the client to develop a bedtime ritual that includes quiet activities such as reading, television, or crafts. **Nursing Research:** *The use of a bedtime routine has been shown to be effective in inducing and maintaining sleep in a population of older women (Johnson, 1991b).*

evolve WEBSITES FOR EDUCATION

See the EVOLVE website for World Wide Web resources for client education.

REFERENCES

Coates TJ et al: Discriminating good sleepers from insomniacs using all-night polysomnograms conducted at home, *J Nerv Ment Dis* 170, 1982.

Dorsey CM et al: Effects of passive body heating on the sleep of older female insomniacs, *J Geriatr Psychiatry Neurol* 9:83, 1996.

Epstein DR, Bootzin RR: Insomnia, *Nurs Clin North Am* 37:4, 2002.

Evans BD, Rogers AE: 24-hour sleep/wake patterns in healthy elderly persons, *Appl Nurs Res* 7:75, 1994.

Floyd JA: Sleep promotion in adults, *Annu Rev Nurs Res* 17:27, 1999.

Floyd JA, Falahee ML, Fhobir RH: Creation and analysis of a computerized database of interventions to facilitate adult sleep, *Nurs Res* 49:4, 2000.

Floyd JA et al: Age-related changes in initiation and maintenance of sleep: a meta-analysis, *Res Nurs Health* 23:106, 2000.

Johnson JE: Progressive relaxation and the sleep of older noninstitutionalized women, *Appl Nurs Res* 4, 1991a.

Johnson JE: A comparative study of the bedtime routines and sleep of older adults, *J Commun Nurs* 8 1991b.

Labyak S: Sleep and circadian schedule disorders, *Nurs Clin North Am* 37, 599, 2002.

Landis CA: Sleep and methods of assessment, *Nurs Clin North Am* 37, 583, 2002.

Liao WC: Effects of passive body heating on body temperature and sleep regulation in the elderly: a systematic review. *Int J Nurs Stud* 39(8), 803, 2002.

Morin C, Culbert JP, Schwartz SM: Nonpharmacological interventions for insomnia, *Am J Psychiatry* 151, 1172, 1994.

Morin CM, Mimeault V, Gagne A: Nonpharmacological treatment of late-life insomnia, *J Psychosom Res* 46:103, 1999.

Richards KC: Sleep promotion in the critical care unit, *AACN Clin Issues* 5(2):152, 1994.

Somer E: *Food and mood: the complete guide to eating well and feeling your best,* ed 2, New York, 1999, Henry Holt.

Woodward M: Insomnia in the elderly, *Aust Fam Physician* 28:653, 1999.

Impaired Social interaction

Gail B. Ladwig

NANDA Definition

Insufficient or excessive quantity or ineffective quality of social exchange

Defining Characteristics

Verbalized or observed inability to receive or communicate a satisfying sense of belonging, caring, interest, or shared history; verbalized or observed discomfort in social situations; observed use of unsuccessful social interaction behaviors; dysfunctional inter-

- = Independent; ▲ = Collaborative

action with peers, family and/or others; family report of change of style or pattern of interaction

Related Factors (r/t)

Knowledge/skill deficit regarding ways to enhance mutuality; therapeutic isolation; sociocultural dissonance; limited physical mobility; environmental barriers; communication barriers; altered thought processes; absence of available significant others or peers; self-concept disturbance

NOC   Outcomes (Nursing Outcomes Classification)

Suggested NOC Outcomes

Child Development: 1 Month, 2 Months, 4 Months, 6 Months, 12 Months, 2 Years, 3 Years, 4 Years, Preschool, Middle Childhood, Adolescence; Play Participation; Role Performance; Social Interaction Skills; Social Involvement

> ### Example NOC Outcome with Indicators
>
> **Social Involvement** as evidenced by the following indicator: Interaction with close friends, neighbors, family members, and work groups (Rate each indicator of **Social Involvement:** 1 = Never demonstrated, 2 = Rarely demonstrated, 3 = Sometimes demonstrated 4 = Often demonstrated, 5 = Consistently demonstrated [see Section I].)

Client Outcomes

Client Will (Specify Time Frame):
- Identify barriers that cause impaired social interactions
- Discuss feelings that accompany impaired and successful social interactions
- Use available opportunities to practice interactions
- Use successful social interaction behaviors
- Report increased comfort in social situations
- Communicate, state feelings of belonging, demonstrate caring and interest in others
- Report effective interactions with others

NIC   Interventions (Nursing Interventions Classification)

Suggested NIC Intervention
Socialization Enhancement

> ### Example NIC Activities—Socialization Enhancement
>
> Encourage patience in developing relationships; Help the client increase awareness of strengths and limitations in communicating with others

Nursing Interventions and Rationales
- Observe for cause of discomfort in social situations; ask the client to explain when discomfort began and identify any losses (e.g., loss of health, job, or significant other; aging) and changes (e.g., marriage, birth or adoption of a child, change in body appearance). *Individualized assessment indicates specific interventions (Warren, 1993).*

• = Independent; ▲ = Collaborative

- Assess the client's social support system. **Nursing Research:** *Use a social support tool or validated assessment tool if possible (e.g., UCLA Loneliness Scale for adolescents [Mahon et al, 1995]).*
- Spend time with the client. **Nursing Research:** *In this study being truly present was listed as one behavior that demonstrated caring (Yonge and Molzahn, 2002).*
- Use active listening skills including assessment and clarification of the client's verbal and nonverbal responses and interactions. **Nursing Research:** *This article suggests that best practice with regard to communication in palliative care could be achieved by using a sensitive assessment of how each client chooses to cope with his or her situation rather than a uniform approach to care (Dean, 2002).*
- Encourage social support for patients with visual impairments. **Clinical Research:** *A large, nationwide study, conducted 1994 at the University of Amsterdam, on the meaning of personal networks and social support for Dutch adolescents with visual impairments indicate that social support, especially the support of peers, is important to adolescents with visual impairments (Kef, 2002).*
- Have the client list behaviors that are associated with being disconnected, and discuss alternative responses that may increase comfort. *Connections occur when a person is actively involved with another person, object, group, or environment; such involvement promotes a sense of comfort, well-being, and anxiety reduction (Hagerty et al, 1993).*
- Monitor the client's use of defense mechanisms, and support healthy defenses (e.g., the client focuses on present and avoids placing blame on others for personal behavior). *Solution-focused techniques have been demonstrated to be beneficial. Therapy focuses on client's present and future, capitalizing on the strengths and resources of the client and significant others around them (Bowles, 2002; University of Central Lancashire: Department of Nursing, 2003).*
- Have the client list behaviors that cause discomfort. Discuss alternative ways to alleviate discomfort (e.g., focusing on others and their interests, practicing making caring statements such as, "I understand you are feeling sad"). Encourage the client to express feelings to others (e.g., "I feel sad also"). *Self-expression invites involvement and increases connectedness (Hagerty et al, 1993).*
- Identify client strengths. Have the client make a list of strengths and refer to it when experiencing negative feelings. He or she may find it helpful to put the list on a note card to carry at all times. **Nursing Research:** *Extra stress in this study was reduced by positive thinking (Mkinen et al, 2000).*
- Have group members identify each other's strengths in a group setting. *This exercise encourages individuals to practice relating to each other on a more intimate level (Drew, 1991).*
- Role-play comfortable and uncomfortable social interactions with the client and appropriate responses (e.g., acknowledging a friendly greeting, responding to rude remarks with an "I" statement, such as, "I understand you may feel that way, but this is how I feel"). *Role-plays may help the client develop social interaction skills and identify feelings associated with isolation (Warren, 1993).*
- Model appropriate social interactions. Give positive verbal and nonverbal feedback for appropriate behavior (e.g., make statements such as, "I'm proud that you made it to work on time and did all the tasks assigned to you without saying that your supervisor was picking on you"; make eye contact). If not contraindicated, touch the client's arm or hand when speaking. One way to learn social skills is to observe the productive

• = **Independent;** ▲ = **Collaborative**

interactions of others (Drew, 1991). **Nursing Research:** *Shared feelings increased communication with stroke and aphasia clients without words (Sundin et al, 2000).*
- Use humor as appropriate. **Nursing Research:** *Humor is important for helping clients cope mentally (Mkinen et al, 2000).*
- Consider use of "animal" therapy; arrange for visitation. **Nursing Research:** *Equine-facilitated psychotherapy, while not a new idea, is a little-known experiential intervention that offers the opportunity to achieve healing (Vidrine et al, 2002).*

Geriatric
- Avoid assuming that social isolation is normal for elderly client. **Nursing Research:** *Caregiver bias and elderly client bias lead to a lack of recognition and treatment of the client's mental health needs (Dellasega, 1991).*
- ▲ Assess the client's potential or actual hearing loss or hearing impairment and make appropriate referrals if a problem is identified. *Because of the nature of the sensory deprivation, communication barriers are increased and human intimacy and self-esteem are negatively affected (Chen, 1994). In addition, it is important to note that hearing impairments often go unnoticed and may not be as obvious as more visibly recognized handicaps (Chen, 1994).* **Clinical Research:** *This study demonstrated declines in speech understanding in noise and central auditory processing are common, in the growing population of older women (Garstecki et al, 2001).*
- Monitor for depression, a particular risk in the elderly. *Age and its associated losses may cause formerly socially active people to be alone. Loneliness contributes to depression and social withdrawal (Warren, 1993).*
- Provide group situations for the client. *Group settings are necessary for the client to practice new skills.*
- Encourage physical activity such as aerobics or stretching and toning in a group. *These activities decreased loneliness in former sedentary adults (N = 174, median age = 65.5 years) (McAuley et al, 2000).* **Nursing Research:** *Extra stress was reduced for clients in this study (Mkinen et al, 2000).*
- Have clients reminisce. **Nursing Research:** *Through the process of reminiscence, older adults can actively evaluate life experiences and explore the meaning of memorable events (Harrand and Bollstetter, 2000).*
- Consider the use of the Internet to promote socialization. **Nursing Research:** *In this study there was a significant change toward improved self-esteem and depression when interactive computer use was accompanied with weekly nurse computer training. Weekly training with a significant other, as a substitute for the nurse trainer, significantly improved self-esteem scores but not depression scores (Heyn Billipp, 2001).*

Multicultural
- Acknowledge racial/ethnic differences at the onset of care. **Nursing Research:** *Acknowledgement of race/ethnicity issues will enhance communication, establish rapport, and promote positive treatment outcomes (D'Avanzo et al, 2001; Ludwick and Silva, 2000; Vontress and Epp, 1997).*
- Assess for the influence of cultural beliefs, norms, and values on the client's perception of social activity and relationships. **Nursing Research:** *What the client considers normal social interaction may be based on cultural perceptions (Leininger and McFarland, 2002; Cochran, 1998; Doswell and Erlen, 1998).*
- Approach individuals of color with respect, warmth, and professional courtesy. **Nurs-**

- **= Independent; ▲ = Collaborative**

ing Research: *Instances of disrespect and lack of caring have special significance for individuals of color and may impede efforts to increase social outlets (D'Avanzo et al, 2001; Vontress and Epp, 1997).*

- Assess the use of personal space needs, communication styles, acceptable body language, eye contact, perception of touch, and paraverbals when communicating with the client. **Nursing Research:** *Nurses need to consider these when interpreting verbal and nonverbal messages (Purnell, 2000). Native Americans may consider avoidance of direct eye contact as a sign of respect and asking questions to be rude and intrusive (Seiderman et al, 1996).*
- Validate the client's feelings regarding social interaction. **Nursing Research:** *Validation lets the client know that the nurse has heard and understands what was said, and it promotes the nurse-client relationship (Heineken, 1998).*

Home care

- Above interventions may be adapted for home care use.
- ▲ Assess family and living environment for social dynamics. Refer for medical social services to assist with family dynamics if appropriate. *The family is a socially significant cultural group that generates behavior, defines roles, and promotes values.*
- ▲ Assess the client for a psychiatric disorder. Refer for mental health services as indicated. *Impaired social interaction can occur with a number of psychiatric disorders (depression, bipolar disorder, schizophrenia). Improved social interaction is unlikely unless the underlying disorder is treated.*
- Assess the client social skills; provide feedback regarding maladaptive skills, and opportunities to role play alternative communication styles. *Social interaction is likely to be impaired if the client uses ineffective social skills. Experiencing how to interact with others differently is influential in creating new behaviors.*
- Suggest that the client avoid contact with negative persons. *Negative interactions reinforce undesired patterns.*
- Identify activities that the client does alone and assist the client with balancing solitary and social activities. *A healthy balance of social and private time supports positive coping.*
- Establish pattern of care and daily activities that involve the client socially (e.g., Meals on Wheels, home health aide visits). Give supportive feedback for positive and appropriate interactions. *The assumption of new patterns of interaction requires practice in safe situations. Feedback reinforces desired behaviors.*
- ▲ Refer to or support involvement with supportive groups and counseling. **Clinical Research:** *Cognitive behavioral group therapy was effective for social phobia in this group of 11 adolescent girls (Hayward et al, 2000). Group settings provide the opportunity to practice new skills. Counseling helps the client to define appropriate actions, and it is a source of support.*
- ▲ In the presence of a psychiatric disorder, refer for psychiatric home health care services for the client reassurance and implementation of therapeutic regimen. *Psychiatric home care nurses can address issues relating to the client's impaired social interaction. Behavioral interventions in the home can assist the client to participate more effectively in the treatment plan (Patusky et al, 1996).*

Client/Family Teaching

- Help the client accept responsibility for own behavior. Have the client keep a journal, and review it together at prescheduled intervals. Give the client positive feedback for

• = Independent; ▲ = Collaborative

appropriate behaviors, and suggest alternative approaches for behaviors that do not en-hance social interaction. Positive reinforcement perpetuates appropriate behaviors. Teach social interaction skills for use in actual situations the client is faced with daily. *Through productive connections with others, social skills are learned and a repertoire of roles for many social situations is developed, which leads to an increase in self-esteem and the capacity to interact with others (Drew, 1991).*

- Practice social skills one-to-one and, when the client is ready, in group sessions. *Practice improves performance and comfort level.*
▲ Refer to appropriate social agencies for assistance (e.g., family therapy, self-help groups, crisis intervention).

evolve WEBSITES FOR EDUCATION

See the EVOLVE website for World Wide Web resources for client education.

REFERENCES

Bowles N: A solution-focused approach to engagement in acute psychiatry, *Nurs Times,* 98(48):26, 2002.

Chen H: Hearing in the elderly, relation of healing loss, loneliness, and self-esteem, *J Gerontol Nurs* 20:22, 1994.

Cochran M: Tears have no color, *Am J Nurs* 98(6):53, 1998.

D'Avanzo CE et al: Developing culturally informed strategies for substance-related interventions. In Naegle MA, D'Avanzo CE, editors: *Addictions and substance abuse: strategies for advanced practice nursing,* St Louis, 2001, Mosby, pp 59.

Dean A: Talking to dying clients of their hopes and needs, *Nurs Times* 22;98(43):34, 2002.

Dellasega C: Meeting the mental health needs of elderly clients, *J Psychosoc Nurs Ment Health Serv* 29:10, 1991.

Doswell W, Erlen J: Multicultural issues and ethical concerns in the delivery of revising care interventions, *Nurs Clin North Am* 33(2):353, 1998.

Drew N: Combating the social isolation of chronic mental illness, *J Psychosoc Nurs Ment Health Serv* 29:14, 1991.

Garstecki D, Erler SF: Personal and social conditions potentially influencing women's hearing loss management, *Am J Audiol* 10(2):78, 2002.

Hagerty BM et al: An emerging theory of human relatedness, *Image* 25:291, 1993.

Harrand AG, Bollstetter JJ: Developing a community-based reminiscence group for the elderly, *Clin Nurse Spec* 14(1):17, 2000.

Hayward C et al: Cognitive-behavioral group therapy for social phobia in female adolescents: results of a pilot study, *J Am Acad Child Adolesc Psychiatry* 39(6):721, 2000.

Heineken J: Patient silence is not necessarily client satisfaction: Communication in home care nursing, *Home Healthc Nurse* 16(2):115, 1998.

Heyn Billipp S: The psychosocial impact of interactive computer use within a vulnerable elderly population: a report on a randomized prospective trial in a home health care setting, *Public Health Nurs* 18(2):138, 2001.

Kef S: Psychosocial adjustment and the meaning of social support for visually impaired adolescents, *J Visual Impairment Blindness* 96(1):22, 2002.

Leininger MM, McFarland MR: *Transcultural nursing: concepts, theories, research and practices,* ed 3, New York, 2002, McGraw-Hill.

Ludwick R, Silva M: Nursing around the world: Cultural values and ethical conflicts, *Online J Issues Nursing,* August 14, 2000, http://www.nursingworld.org/ojin/ethcol/ethics_4.htm accessed June 19, 2003.

Mahon NE, Yarcheski T, Yarcheski A: Validation of the revised UCLA loneliness scale for adolescents, *Res Nurs Health* 18:263, 1995.

Mkinen S, Suominen T, Lauri S: Self-care in adults with asthma: how they cope, *J Clin Nurs* 9(4):557, 2000.

McAuley E et al: Social relations, physical activity, and well-being in older adults, *Prev Med 31(5):608, 2000.*

Patusky KL, Rodning C, Martinez-Kratz M: Clinical lessons in psychiatric home care: a case study approach, *J Home Healthc Manag* 9:18, 1996.

- **= Independent; ▲ = Collaborative**

Purnell L: A description of the Purnell model for cultural competence, *J Transcult Nurs* 11(1):40, 2000.

Seiderman RY et al: Assessing American Indian families, *MCN Am J Matern Child Nurs* 21(6):274, 1996

Sundin K, Jansson L, Norberg A: Communicating with people with stroke and aphasia: understanding through sensation without words, *J Clin Nurs* 9(4):481, 2000.

University of Central Lancashire: Department of Nursing, Retrieved from www 1/18/03 http://www.uclan.ac.uk/courses/factsheets/health/nursing/3284.pdf

Vidrine M et al: Equine-facilitated group psychotherapy: applications for therapeutic vaulting, *Ment Health Nurs* 23(6):587, 2002.

Vontress CE, Epp LR: Historical hostility in the African American client: Implications for counseling, *J Multi-cult Counseling Dev* 25:170, 1997.

Warren BJ: Explaining social isolation through concept analysis, *Arch Psychiatr Nurs* 7:270, 1993.

Yonge O, Molzahn A: Exceptional nontraditional caring practices of nurses, *Scand J Caring Sci* 16(4):399, 2002.

Social isolation

Gail B. Ladwig

NANDA Definition

Aloneness experienced by the individual and perceived as imposed by others and as a negative or threatened state

Defining Characteristics

Objective

Absence of supportive significant others (e.g., family, friends, group); projection of hostility in voice and behavior; withdrawal; uncommunicativeness; demonstration of behavior unaccepted by dominant cultural group; desire to be alone or exist in a subculture; repetitive and meaningless actions; preoccupation with own thoughts; lack of eye contact; inappropriate or immature activities for developmental age/stage; evidence of physical/mental handicap or altered state of wellness; sad, dull affect

Subjective

Expression of feelings of aloneness imposed by others; expression of feelings of rejection; inappropriate or immature interests for developmental age/stage; inadequate or absent significant purpose in life; inability to meet expectations of others; expression of values acceptable to subculture but unacceptable to dominant cultural group; expression of interest inappropriate to developmental age/stage; feelings of differences from others; insecurity in public

Related Factors (r/t)

Alterations in mental status; inability to engage in satisfying personal relationships; unacceptable social values; unacceptable social behavior; inadequate personal resources; immature interests; factors contributing to absence of satisfying personal relationships (e.g., delay in accomplishing developmental tasks); alterations in physical appearance; altered state of wellness

NOC Outcomes (Nursing Outcomes Classification)

Suggested NOC Outcomes

Loneliness Severity; Mood Equilibrium; Personal Well-Being; Play Participation; Social Interaction Skills; Social Involvement; Social Support

• = Independent; ▲ = Collaborative

> ### Example NOC Outcome with Indicators
>
> **Social Involvement** as evidenced by the following indicator: Interaction with close friends, neighbors, family members, and work groups (Rate the indicator of **Social Involvement:** 1 = never demonstrated, 2 = rarely demonstrated, 3 = sometimes demonstrated, 4 = often demonstrated, 5 = consistently demonstrated [see Section I].)

Client Outcomes

Client Will (Specify Time Frame):
- Identify feelings of isolation
- Practice social and communication skills needed to interact with others
- Initiate interactions with others; set and meet goals
- Participate in activities and programs at level of ability and desire
- Describe feelings of self-worth

NIC   Interventions (Nursing Interventions Classification)

Suggested NIC Intervention
Socialization Enhancement

> ### Example NIC Activities—Socialization Enhancement
>
> Encourage patience in developing relationships; Help client increase awareness of strengths and limitations in communicating with others

Nursing Interventions and Rationales

- Establish a therapeutic relationship by being emotionally present and authentic. *Being emotionally present and authentic fosters growth in relationships and decreases isolation (Jordan, 2000).*
- Observe for barriers to social interaction (e.g., illness; incontinence; decreasing ability to form relationships; lack of transportation, money, support system, or knowledge). **Nursing Research:** *Causes of social isolation may be different for each individual; therefore adequate information must be gathered so that appropriate interventions can be planned (Badger, 1990).*
- Note risk factors (e.g., membership in ethnic/cultural minority, chronic physiological or psychological illness or deformities, advanced age). **Nursing Research:** *Clients with these risk factors may be at risk for social isolation (Warren, 1993).*
- Discuss causes of perceived or actual isolation. **Nursing Research:** *The individual's experience of illness; the circumstances of everyday living that influence quality of life; and emotions, fears, and concerns all have a bearing on the way illness is managed (Anderson, 1991).*
- Promote social interactions. Support grieving and verbalization of feelings. **Nursing Research:** *Women in one study needed health counseling for the management of illness, but some said they would have benefited from psychological counseling as well. They needed help with the emotional aspects of living with a chronic illness (Anderson, 1991).*
- Establish trust one on one and then gradually introduce the client to others. Allow the client opportunities to introduce issues and to describe his or her daily life. **Nursing**

- = **Independent;** ▲ = **Collaborative**

Research: *Individualization of care, or tailoring of care, involves taking into account the client's individuality and allowing that individuality to determine interpersonal approaches and health-illness management actions (Brown, 1994).*

- Use active listening skills. Establish a therapeutic relationship and spend time with the client. **Nursing Research:** *In one study, being truly present was listed as one behavior that demonstrated caring (Yonge and Molzahn, 2002).*
- Help the client experience success by working together with the client to establish easily attainable goals (e.g., spending 10 minutes conversing with peer). *Success encourages repetition of behaviors, and setting small, achievable goals can help the client be successful.*
- Provide positive reinforcement when the client seeks out others. **Nursing Research:** *Receiving instrumental social support such as practical help, advice, and feedback significantly contributes to positive well-being (White, 1992).*
- Help the client identify appropriate diversional activities to encourage socialization. *Active participation by the client is essential for behavioral changes.*
- Encourage physical closeness (e.g., use touch) if appropriate. **Nursing Research:** *Touch helps with integration and fosters social relatedness. Tactile stimulation benefits the older adult's psychological well-being (Jamison, 1997).*
- Identify available support systems and involve these individuals in the client's care. **Nursing Research:** *Clients cope more successfully with stressful life events if they have support (White, 1992).*
- Encourage liberal visitation for a client who is hospitalized or in an extended care facility. **Clinical Research:** *Visits from those in an emotionally close network were associated with perceived support, and this was associated with a decrease in depression (Oxman and Hull, 2001).*
- Help the client identify role models and others with similar interests. *Sometimes the client needs someone to model the appropriate behavior.*
- See the care plan for **Risk for Loneliness.**

Geriatric

- Observe for aggression or other interpersonal problems, poor self-image or signs of powerlessness, confusion of the past with the present, complaints about feeling confined or deserted, or difficulty setting goals and making decisions. **Nursing Research:** *Social isolation should be considered as a nursing diagnosis when these behaviors are observed (Meddaugh, 1991).*
- Assess for hearing deficit. Provide aids and use adaptive techniques such as facing the individual when speaking, speaking slowly, lowering the pitch of the voice, and enunciating clearly. **Clinical Research:** *There is a relationship between hearing acuity and loneliness. Hearing loss is one of the most prevalent chronic health problems of older adults, especially the very old. Adaptive techniques that facilitate communication must be used (Dugan and Kivett, 1994).*
- If the client is in a health care facility, visit him or her for at least 10 minutes every 2 to 3 hours. *The presence of a trusted individual provides emotional security for the client.*
- ▲ Involve nonprofessionals in activities, projects, and goal setting with the client. Practice interdisciplinary management for unit-based activities: engaging in arts and crafts projects, sewing, watching videos, reading large-print books, reading magazines, playing games, playing musical instruments, and using assistive listening devices. **Nursing Research:** *Nursing assistants are commonly concerned about the social support of*

• = Independent; ▲ = Collaborative

residents; therefore they can be a valuable resource for generating intervention ideas. (Alterations in job descriptions would be required.) Residents with visual, hearing, cognitive, and mobility impairments will participate more readily in events that involve a smaller number of people and in which the staff takes initiative and establishes rapport with each resident (Windriver, 1993). **Nursing Research:** *In a study of the use of calming music and hand massage, physically nonaggressive behaviors decreased during each of the interventions. At 1 hour following either intervention, agitated verbal behavior decreased (Remington, 2002).*

- Offer the client a choice of activities and persons with whom to sit and socialize. Introductions to strangers may need to be repeated several times. **Nursing Research:** *A recognized intervention for loneliness is to provide opportunities and assistance for making choices, setting goals, and making decisions. Cognitively impaired clients may require several repetitions (Windriver, 1993).*

- Put clients in groups according to activity preferences, abilities, age, life situations, personal and cultural characteristics, and social networks. **Nursing Research:** *Positive social interactions are enhanced by the aforementioned interventions (Windriver, 1993).*

- Develop and display a seating chart for the common areas of each personal care unit and develop a process for both identifying needed changes and executing them promptly. **Nursing Research:** *Personality factors that are difficult to predict affect the success of social groupings (Windriver, 1993).*

- Consider the use of simulated presence therapy (see the care plan for **Hopelessness**). **Nursing Research:** *Simulated presence therapy appears to be the most effective therapy for treating social isolation (Woods and Ashley, 1995).*

▲ Refer to programs such as Foster Grandparents and Senior Companions. **Clinical Research:** *Emotional isolation leads to social isolation. Social programs help increase contact with peers and decrease isolation. Programs to alleviate emotional isolation should focus on attachment loss (Dugan and Kivett, 1994).*

- Provide physical activity, either aerobic or stretching and toning. **Clinical Research:** *Physical activity increased social support in a group of older, formerly sedentary adults (McAuley et al, 2000).*

- Consider using computers and the Internet to alleviate or reduce loneliness and social isolation. **Nursing Research:** *A descriptive qualitative study used a web page questionnaire and chat room interviews with online participants aged 65 years and older living alone. Seven of the 10 participants used the computer to combat loneliness (Clark, 2002). In another study Internet use was found to decrease loneliness and depression significantly, while perceived social support and self-esteem increased significantly (Shaw and Gant, 2002).*

Multicultural

- Acknowledge racial/ethnic differences at the onset of care. **Nursing Research:** *Acknowledgment of race/ethnicity issues will enhance communication, establish rapport, and promote positive treatment outcomes (D'Avanzo et al, 2001; Ludwick and Silva, 2000, Vontress and Epp, 1997).* **Nursing Research:** Assess for the influence of cultural beliefs, norms, and values on the client's perception of social activity and relationships. *What the client considers normal social interaction may be based on cultural perceptions (Cochran, 1998; Doswell and Erlen, 1998; Leininger and McFarland, 2002).*

- Approach individuals of color with respect, warmth, and professional courtesy. **Nursing Research:** *Instances of disrespect and lack of caring have special significance for indi-*

• = **Independent;** ▲ = **Collaborative**

viduals of color and may impede efforts to increase social outlets (D'Avanzo et al, 2001; Vontress and Epp, 1997).

- Assess personal space needs, communication styles, acceptable body language, attitude toward eye contact, perception of touch, and paraverbal messages when communicating with the client. **Nursing Research:** *Nurses need to consider these aspects when interpreting verbal and nonverbal messages (Purnell, 2000). Native American clients may consider avoiding direct eye contact to be a sign of respect and asking questions to be rude and intrusive (Seiderman et al, 1996).*
- Use a family-centered approach when working with Latino, Asian, African American, and Native American clients. **Nursing Research:** *Latinos may perceive the family as source of support, solver of problems, and source of pride. Asian Americans may regard the family as the primary decision maker and influence on individual family members (D'Avanzo et al, 2001).*
- Promote a sense of ethnic attachment. **Nursing Research:** *Older Korean clients with strong ethnic attachments had higher levels of social involvement than others (Kim, 1999).*
- Validate the client's feelings regarding social isolation. **Nursing Research:** *Validation lets the client know that the nurse has heard and understood what was said, and it promotes the nurse-client relationship (Heineken, 1998).*

Home care

- The interventions described previously may be adapted for home care use.
- ▲ Assess the client for depression or other psychiatric disorder. Refer for mental health services as indicated. *Social isolation is part of the syndrome of depression or other psychiatric disorders. Increase in social activities is unlikely unless the underlying disorder is treated.*
- Confirm that the home setting has a telephone. Obtain one if necessary for medical safety. If the client lives alone, set up a Lifeline safety system that requires the client to answer the telephone. *The telephone can be used to achieve continuity of care and successful client/family interaction (Skinner, 2001). A Lifeline system can be a safety net for physical and psychological safety.*
- Consider the use of the computer and Internet to decrease isolation. **Nursing Research:** *In a qualitative exploratory, descriptive investigation of pregnant women on home bed rest for preterm labor, the women stated that their participation in a virtual online peer support group was valuable and beneficial in helping them to cope with the hardships of bed rest (Adler and Zarchin, 2002). A study of homebound older adults found that the Internet and e-mail were excellent sources of support and enjoyment, and their use resulted in an improved quality of life (Nahm and Resnick, 2001).*
- Encourage family involvement in daily life in small, nonthreatening activities such as short outings, assistance with shopping, and solicitation of input from the isolated person in decision making. *Reversing social isolation is a gradual process.*
- ▲ Establish a pattern of care and daily activities that involves the client socially (e.g., Meals-on-Wheels, home health aide visits). *Pattern changes encourage new behaviors.*
- Have the client keep a diary of social experiences. Discuss the diary during visits. *A review of social experiences helps the client identify those that are most comfortable.*
- Identify activities that the client does alone. Assist the client with balancing solitary and social activities, keeping alone time to a minimum. *A healthy balance of social and private time supports positive coping.*
- ▲ Refer for visiting volunteer services. *Spending time with the client enhances client self-esteem.*

- **• = Independent; ▲ = Collaborative**

- When the client is ready, encourage him or her to volunteer for short periods at community agencies in which contact is positive and nonthreatening (e.g., with hospitalized elders for 1 hr/wk). *Contributing to the welfare of others enhances self-esteem.*
▲ Assess options for living that allow the client privacy but not isolation (e.g., boarding home, congregate living, assertive community treatment programs). **Clinical Research:** *An exploratory qualitative study examined contexts and processes of social relationship development as experienced by adults with schizophrenia participating in assertive community treatment programs. Participants described their relationships with other mental health clients in primarily positive terms, yet several participants expressed dissatisfaction and desired greater integration into mainstream social networks (Angell, 2003).*
▲ In the presence of a psychiatric disorder, refer for psychiatric home health care services for client reassurance and implementation of a therapeutic regimen. **Nursing Research:** *Psychiatric home care nurses can address issues relating to the client's social isolation. Behavioral interventions in the home can help the client to participate more effectively in the treatment plan (Patusky, Rodning, and Martinez-Kratz, 1996).*

Client/Family Teaching

- Teach skills related to problem solving, communication, social interaction, activities of daily living, and positive self-esteem. *All of these skills are necessary to change isolating behavior.*
- Consider the use of telecommunication and group support via the Internet. **Clinical Research:** *One study delivered diabetes education and social support to rural women with diabetes. The women declared the computer-based social support to have positive effects of (Smith and Weinert, 2000).*
- Teach role playing (practicing communication skills in specific situations). **Nursing Research:** *Role playing may help clients develop social interaction skills and identify feelings associated with their isolation (Warren, 1993).*
▲ Encourage the client to initiate contacts with self-help groups, counselors, and therapists. **Nursing Research:** *If adjustment is to be successful and maintained, management of a chronic illness cannot occur in isolation; it requires a complex interaction of resources (White, 1992).*
- Provide information to the client about senior citizen services, house sharing, pets, day care centers, churches, and community resources. **Nursing Research:** *The well-documented negative effect of social isolation suggests that clients without confidants and supportive others must be referred to alternative sources, such as cardiac rehabilitation programs, support groups, and community agencies (McCauley, 1995).*
▲ Refer socially isolated caregivers to appropriate support groups as well. *Identification and recognition of the overwhelming task of caregiving are needed so that caregivers do not suffer in silence. Alzheimer's disease support groups offer participants an opportunity to share troubles and triumphs with others who truly understand the turmoil of caregiving (Bergman-Evans, 1994). (See the care plan for* **Caregiver role strain.***)*
- Teach caregivers methods to deal with troublesome behaviors related to memory disturbances, restlessness and agitation, catastrophic reactions, day/night disturbances, delusions, wandering, and physical violence. A general method for clinicians to manage these problems involves the identification of the behavior and its antecedent and consequent events. Stressors that may cause behavioral problems include fatigue, a change of routine, excessive demands, overwhelming stimuli, and acute illness or pain.

- = **Independent;** ▲ = **Collaborative**

Clinical Research: *Caregivers can be taught to identify these stressors to prevent or alleviate troublesome behaviors (Alessi, 1991).*

evolve WEBSITES FOR EDUCATION

See the EVOLVE website for World Wide Web resources for client education.

REFERENCES

Adler CL, Zarchin YR: The "virtual focus group": using the Internet to reach pregnant women on home bed rest, *J Obstet Gynecol Neonatal Nurs* 31(4):418, 2002.

Alessi C: Managing the behavioral problems of dementia in the home, *Clin Geriatr Med* 7(4):787, 1991.

Anderson JM: Immigrant women speak of chronic illness: the social construction of the devalued self, *J Adv Nurs* 16:710, 1991.

Angell B: Contexts of social relationship development among assertive community treatment clients, *Ment Health Serv Res* 5(1):13, 2003.

Badger VT: Men with cardiovascular diseases and their spouses, coping health and marital adjustment, *Arch Psychiatr Nurs* 4:319, 1990.

Bergman-Evans BF: Alzheimer's and related disorders: loneliness, depression, and social support of spousal caregivers, *J Gerontol Nurs* 20:6, 1994.

Brown S: Communication strategies used by an expert nurse, *Clin Nurs Res* 3(1):43, 1994.

Clark DJ: Older adults living through and with their computers, *Comput Inform Nurs* 20(3):117, 2002.

Cochran M: Tears have no color, *Am J Nurs* 98(6):53, 1998.

D'Avanzo CE et al: Developing culturally informed strategies for substance-related interventions. In Naegle MA, D'Avanzo CE, editors: *Addictions and substance abuse: strategies for advanced practice nursing,* St Louis, 2001, Mosby, pp 59-104.

Doswell W, Erlen J: Multicultural issues and ethical concerns in the delivery of nursing care interventions, *Nurs Clin North Am* 33(2):353, 1998.

Dugan E, Kivett V: The importance of emotional and social isolation to loneliness among very old rural adults, *Gerontologist* 34:340, 1994.

Heineken J: Patient silence is not necessarily client satisfaction: communication in home care nursing, *Home Healthc Nurse,* 16(2):115, 1998.

Jamison M: Failure to thrive in older adults, *J Gerontol Nurs* 23(2):13, 1997.

Jordan JV: The role of mutual empathy in relational/cultural therapy, *J Clin Psychol* 56(8):1005, 2000.

Kim O: Mediation effect of social support between ethnic attachment and loneliness in older Korean immigrants, *Res Nurs Health* 22(2):169, 1999.

Leininger MM, McFarland MR: *Transcultural nursing: concepts, theories, research and practices,* ed 3, New York, 2002, McGraw-Hill.

Ludwick R, Silva M: Nursing around the world: cultural values and ethical conflicts, *Online J Issues Nurs,* August 14, 2000, available online at http://www.nursingworld.org/ojin/ethcol/ethics_4.htm, accessed June 19, 2003.

McAuley E et al: Social relations, physical activity, and well-being in older adults, *Prev Med* 31(5):608, 2000.

McCauley K: Assessing social support in patients with cardiac disease, *J Cardiovasc Nurs* 10:73, 1995.

Meddaugh DJ: Before aggression erupts, *Geriatr Nurs* 12:114, 1991.

Nahm ES, Resnick B: Homebound older adults' experiences with the Internet and e-mail, *Comput Nurs* 19(6): 257, 2001.

Oxman TE, Hull JG: Social support and treatment response in older depressed primary care patients, *J Gerontol B Psychol Sci Soc Sci* 56(1):P35, 2001.

Patusky KL, Rodning C, Martinez-Kratz M: Clinical lessons in psychiatric home care: a case study approach, *J Home Health Case Manag* 9:18, 1996.

Purnell L: A description of the Purnell model for cultural competence, *J Transcult Nurs* 11(1):40, 2000.

Remington R: Calming music and hand massage with agitated elderly, *Nurs Res* 51(5):317, 2002.

Seiderman RY et al: Assessing American Indian families, *MCN Am J Matern Child Nurs* 21(6):274, 1996.

Shaw LH, Gant LM: In defense of the Internet: the relationship between Internet communication and depression, loneliness, self-esteem, and perceived social support, *Cyberpsychol Behav* 5(2):157, 2002.

Skinner D: Intimacy and the telephone, *Caring* 20(2):28, 2001.

• = **Independent;** ▲ = **Collaborative**

Smith L, Weinert C: Telecommunication support for rural women with diabetes, *Diabetes Educ* 26:645, 2000.

Vontress CE, Epp LR: Historical hostility in the African American client: implications for counseling, *J Multi-cult Counseling Dev* 25:170, 1997.

Warren B: Explaining social isolation through concept analysis, *Arch Psychiatr Nurs* 7:270, 1993.

White NE: Coping, social support and adaptation to chronic illness, *West J Nurs Res* 14:2, 1992.

Windriver W: Social isolation: unit-based activities for impaired elders, *J Gerontol Nurs* 19:15, 1993.

Woods P, Ashley J: Simulated presence therapy: using selected memories to manage problem behaviors in Alzheimer's disease patients, *Geriatr Nurs* 16:9, 1995.

Yonge O, Molzahn A: Exceptional nontraditional caring practices of nurses, *Scand J Caring Sci* 16(4):399, 2002.

Chronic Sorrow

Betty J. Ackley and Gail B. Ladwig

NANDA Definition

Cyclical, recurring, and potentially progressive pattern of pervasive sadness that is experienced (by client, parent or caregiver, or individual with chronic illness or disability) in response to continual loss throughout the trajectory of an illness or disability

Defining Characteristics

Feelings that vary in intensity, are periodic, may progress and intensify over time, and may interfere with client's ability to reach his or her highest level of personal and social well-being; expression of periodic, recurrent feelings of sadness; expression of one or more of the following feelings: anger, being misunderstood, confusion, depression, disappointment, emptiness, fear, frustration, guilt/self-blame, helplessness, hopelessness, loneliness, low self-esteem, recurring loss, being overwhelmed

Related Factors (r/t)

Death of a loved one; experience of chronic physical or mental illness or disability such as mental retardation, multiple sclerosis, prematurity, spina bifida or other birth defects, chronic mental illness, infertility, cancer, Parkinson's disease; experience of one or more trigger events (e.g., crises in management of illness, crises related to developmental stages and missed opportunities or milestones that bring comparisons with developmental, social, or personal norms); unending caregiving as constant reminder of loss

NOC   Outcomes (Nursing Outcomes Classification)

Suggested NOC Outcomes

Acceptance: Health Status; Depression Level; Depression Self-Control; Grief Resolution; Hope; Mood Equilibrium

> ### Example NOC Outcome with Indicators
>
> **Grief Resolution** with plans for a positive future as evidenced by the following indicators: Expresses feelings about loss/Verbalizes acceptance of loss/Describes meaning of loss or death/Reports decreased preoccupation with loss/Expresses positive expectations about the future (Rate each indicator of **Grief Resolution:** 1 = not at all, 2 = to a slight extent, 3 = to a moderate extent, 4 = to a great extent, 5 = to a very great extent [see Section I].)

• = Independent; ▲ = Collaborative

Client Outcomes

Client Will (Specify Time Frame):
- Express appropriate feelings of guilt, fear, anger, or sadness
- Identify problems associated with sorrow (e.g., changes in appetite, insomnia, nightmares, loss of libido, decreased energy, alteration in activity levels)
- Seek help in dealing with grief-associated problems
- Plan for future 1 day at a time
- Function at normal developmental level

NIC   Interventions (Nursing Interventions Classification)

Suggested NIC Interventions

Grief Work Facilitation; Grief Work Facilitation: Perinatal Death

Example NIC Activities—Grief Work Facilitation

Encourage client to verbalize memories of loss, both past and current; Assist client in identifying personal coping strategies

Nursing Interventions and Rationales

- Assess the client's degree of sorrow. Use the Burke/NCRS Chronic Sorrow Questionnaire (for the individual or caregiver as appropriate) if available. *This questionnaire is designed to determine the occurrence of chronic sorrow, cues that trigger sorrow, coping strategies, and factors that direct health care personnel to deal with the sorrowful client or caregiver (Hainsworth, Eakes, and Burke, 1994).*
- Identify problems of eating and sleeping; ensure that basic human needs are being met. *Losses often interrupt appetite and sleep (Bateman et al, 1992; Gifford and Cleary, 1990).* **Nursing Research:** *One study indicated that bereaved individuals, irrespective of whether they had counseling for grief resolution or not, had a moderate risk for poor nutrition). The implication is that food issues need to be included in grief resolution interventions (Johnson, 2002).*
- Spend time with the client and family. **Clinical Research:** *The main suggestion in a study of families who have a child with a chronic illness and are facing loss in their lives was the provision of an empathetic presence (Langridge, 2002).*
- Develop a trusting relationship with the client by using empathetic therapeutic communication techniques. *An empathetic person who takes the time to listen, offers support and reassurance, recognizes and focuses on feelings, and appreciates the uniqueness of each individual and family is helpful to clients experiencing chronic sorrow (Eakes, 1993; Eakes, Burke, and Hainsworth, 1998).*
- Help the client to understand that sorrow may be ongoing. Life may be characterized by good times and then bad times when sorrow is triggered by events. **Nursing Research:** *Studies have demonstrated that feelings of sadness, guilt, anger, frustration, and fear occur periodically throughout the lives of people experiencing chronic loss resulting in chronic sorrow (Eakes, Burke, and Hainsworth, 1998). In an analysis of 85 mourners' narratives, the most prominent theme was feeling the absence of the decedent (Gamino, Hogan, and Sewell, 2002).*
- Help the client recognize that, although sadness will occur at intervals for the rest of his or her life, it will become bearable. In time the client may develop a relation-

• = Independent; ▲ = Collaborative

ship with grief that is lifelong but livable, and as much filled with comfort as it is with sorrow (Moules, 1998). *The sadness associated with chronic sorrow is permanent, but as the grief resolves there can be times of satisfaction and even happiness (Grainger, 1990; Teel, 1991).*

- Encourage the use of positive coping techniques:
  - Taking action: Suggested strategies include keeping busy, keeping personal interests, going away, getting out of the house, doing something to gain a feeling of control over life.
  - Cognitive coping: Techniques include concentrating on the positive aspects of life, having a "can do" attitude, taking 1 day at a time, and taking responsibility for the quality of one's own life. Encourage the client to write about the experience.
  - Interpersonal coping: Techniques include talking to a close friend, a health care professional, or someone with the same condition or circumstance. Joining a support group can also help the sorrowful person to cope.
  - Emotional coping: Encourage the client to express feelings, cry as desired, give thanks, and pray if desired.

  Clients with chronic sorrow have found these coping techniques helpful. The techniques are arranged in order of effectiveness (Hainsworth, Eakes, and Burke, 1994). **Clinical Research:** *A group of 26 individuals with traumatic memories were instructed to write about the negative events they had experienced during five 45-minute sessions over a period of 2 weeks. The trauma-writing participants experienced fewer intrusions and showed less avoidance behavior from pretreatment to follow-up, whereas a waiting-list control group did not change significantly (Schoutrop et al, 2002).*

- Review past experiences, role changes, and coping skills. Use music if appropriate. **Nursing Research:** *One study revealed the theme of a need to remember and to hold onto the memory. Participants in this study found comfort in knowing that they were not alone (Hentz, 2002). One article presented four case studies that demonstrate the use of music therapy in assisting palliative care clients and families to cope with grief and loss (Hilliard, 2001b).* **Clinical Research:** *One investigator concluded that participation of grieving children in music therapy–based bereavement groups served to reduce grief symptoms among the participants as evaluated in the home (Hilliard, 2001a).*

- Expect the client to meet responsibilities; give positive reinforcement.

▲ Refer the client to spiritual counseling if desired. **Clinical Research:** *A prospective cohort study included people about to be bereaved, with follow-up continuing for 14 months after the death. Those who professed stronger spiritual beliefs seemed to resolve their grief more rapidly and completely after the death of a close person than people with no spiritual beliefs (Walsh et al, 2002).*

▲ Encourage the client to make time to talk to family members about the loss with the help of professional support as needed and without criticizing or belittling each other's feelings about the loss. Once these feelings are shared, family members can better begin to accept the chronic loss and develop coping strategies. **Nursing Research:** *In a study of adolescents dealing with the death of a loved one, the most important factors that helped adolescents cope with the grief were self-help and support from parents, relatives, and friends (Rask, Kaunonen, and Paunonen-Ilmonen, 2002). A study analyzing the grief and coping of mothers who had lost children under the age of 7 years found that the spouse, children, grandparents, next of kin, friends, and colleagues were the main sources of support (Laakso and Paunonen-Ilmonen, 2002).*

- Recognize that a stimulus for reactivation of sorrow in women is when a developmen-

• = **Independent**; ▲ = **Collaborative**

tally disabled child develops a health care crisis. In men, reactivation of sorrow is more associated with comparison with social norms (Mallow and Bechtel, 1999).

- Help the client determine the best way and place to find social support. *Social support is shown to help bereaved individuals as they reconstruct their lives and find new meaning in life (Hogan and Schmidt, 2002).*
- ▲ Identify available community resources, including grief counselors or support groups available for specific losses (e.g., Multiple Sclerosis Society). *Support groups can serve as a helpful means to improve interpersonal coping strategies to deal with the loss (Hainsworth, Eakes, and Burke, 1994).*
- ▲ Encourage the client to become active in interests such as volunteer work, service projects, or church activities. *When a grieving person can express caring for another, he or she gains a sense of being needed and an increased sense of purpose, which results in increased engagement in the world (Fischer and Hegge, 2000).*
- ▲ Identify whether the client is experiencing depression, suicidal tendencies, or other emotional disorders. Refer for counseling as appropriate. *Counseling, including the use of relaxation therapy, desensitization, and biofeedback, in addition to traditional psychotherapy, has been shown to be helpful (Arnette, 1996). Depression and the risk of suicide can accompany chronic grieving (Steen, 1998).*
- ▲ Consider the use of art for children in hospice care who are dying or dealing with the death of a parent, sibling, or other family member. **Nursing Research:** *The arts are being recognized as a powerful tool for psychological, emotional, and spiritual support. Through an "ART is the heART" approach, children learn to use the arts as a healthy and effective coping strategy (Rollins and Riccio, 2002).*

Geriatric

- Use reminiscence therapy in conjunction with the expression of emotions. *Reminiscence therapy can help the client look back at past experiences and use coping techniques that have been effective previously (Puentes, 1998).*
- Identify previous losses and assess the client for depression. *In older age losses and changes often occur in rapid succession without adequate recovery time. More than two concurrent losses increase the incidence of unresolved grief (Herth, 1990).*
- Evaluate the social support system of the elderly client. If the support system is minimal, help the client determine how to increase available support. *The elderly who have poor grieving outcomes often do not live with family members and have a minimal support system. The support of family (especially children) and friends is a common way for elderly widows to cope with a loss (Hegge and Fischer, 2000).*

Multicultural

- Assess for the influence of cultural beliefs, norms, and values on the client's expressions of sorrow. **Nursing Research:** *Expressions of sorrow may be based on cultural perceptions (Cochran, 1998; Doswell and Erlen, 1998; Leininger and McFarland, 2002). African Americans may be expected to act "strong" and go on with the business of life after a death; Native Americans may not talk about the death because of beliefs that such talk will detract from spirituality and bring bad luck; Latinos may wear black and act subdued during their* luto *(mourning) period; Southeast Asian families may wear white when mourning (McQuay, 1995).*
- Identify whether the client had been notified of the health status of the deceased and was able to be present during death and illness. **Nursing Research:** *Not being present*

• = **Independent;** ▲ = **Collaborative**

during terminal illness and death can disrupt the grieving process and contribute to chronic sorrow (McQuay, 1995).

- Validate the client's feelings regarding the loss. **Nursing Research:** *Validation is a therapeutic communication technique that lets the client know that the nurse has heard and understood what was said, and it promotes the nurse-client relationship (Heineken, 1998).*

Home care

- The interventions described previously may be adapted for home care use. Identify causes for chronic sorrow and observe the client's expression of this sorrow. *A clinician's ability to understand a client's perception of the impact of the illness is crucial to the clinician's ability to be therapeutic. Knowledge of a client's perceptions of chronic illness will help nurses intervene sensitively and effectively (Yuen-Juen, 1995).*
- ▲ Assess the client for depression. Refer for mental health services as indicated. *Sadness is part of the syndrome of depression. Increase in mood is unlikely unless the underlying depression is treated. Counseling services provide an opportunity for expression of feelings, increase coping skills, and provide respite for caregivers.*
- ▲ When sorrow is focused around loss of a pregnancy, encourage the client to follow through on a counseling referral. **Nursing and Clinical Research:** *Parents with a history of perinatal loss are at higher risk for depressive symptoms and pregnancy-specific anxiety during subsequent pregnancies, particularly before the third trimester. Mothers had a higher level of symptoms than fathers (Armstrong, 2002; Franche and Mikail, 1999).*
- Encourage the client to participate in activities that are diversionary and uplifting as tolerated (e.g., outdoor activities, hobby groups, church-related activities, pet care). *Diversionary activities decrease the time spent in sorrow, can give meaning to life, and provide a sense of well-being.*
- Encourage the client to participate in support groups appropriate to the area of loss or illness (e.g., Crohn's disease support group or Widow to Widow). *Support groups can increase an individual's sense of belonging. Group activity helps the client to identify alternative ways to problem solve and experience feelings.*
- Provide psychological support for family/caregivers. *Family/caregivers who feel supported are often able to provide greater and more consistent support to the affected person.*
- ▲ In the presence of a psychiatric disorder, refer for psychiatric home health care services for client reassurance and implementation of a therapeutic regimen. *Psychiatric home care nurses can address issues relating to the client's depression. Behavioral interventions in the home can help the client to participate more effectively in the treatment plan (Patusky, Rodning, and Martinez-Kratz, 1996).*
- ▲ See the care plans for **Impaired Adjustment, Chronic low Self-esteem, Risk for Loneliness,** and **Hopelessness.**

evolve WEBSITES FOR EDUCATION

See the EVOLVE website for World Wide Web resources for client education.

REFERENCES

Armstrong DS: Emotional distress and prenatal attachment in pregnancy after perinatal loss, *J Nurs Scholarsh* 34:339, 2002.

Arnette JD: Physiological effects of chronic grief: a biofeedback treatment approach, *Death Stud* 20:59, 1996.

• = **Independent;** ▲ = **Collaborative**

Bateman A et al: Dysfunctional grieving, *J Psychosoc Nurs Ment Health Serv* 30:5, 1992.

Cochran M: Tears have no color, *Am J Nurs* 98(6):53, 1998.

Doswell W, Erlen J: Multicultural issues and ethical concerns in the delivery of nursing care interventions, *Nurs Clin North Am* 33(2):353, 1998.

Eakes GG: Chronic sorrow: a response to living with cancer, *Oncol Nurs Forum* 20:1327, 1993.

Eakes GG, Burke ML, Hainsworth MA: Middle-range theory of chronic sorrow, *Image J Nurs Sch* 30:179, 1998.

Fischer C, Hegge M: The elderly woman at risk, *Am J Nurs* 100(6):54, 2000.

Franche R, Mikail S: The impact of perinatal loss on adjustment to subsequent pregnancy, *Soc Sci Med* 48:1613, 1999.

Gamino LA, Hogan NS, Sewell KW: Feeling the absence: a content analysis from the Scott and White grief study, *Death Stud* 26(10):793, 2002.

Gifford BJ, Cleary BB: Supporting the bereaved, *Am J Nurs* 90:49, 1990.

Grainger RD: Successful grieving, *Am J Nurs* 90:12, 1990.

Hainsworth MA, Eakes GG, Burke ML: Coping with chronic sorrow, *Issues Ment Health Nurs* 15:59, 1994.

Hegge M, Fischer C: Grief responses of senior and elderly widows: practice implications, *J Gerontol Nurs* 26(2):35, 2000.

Heineken J: Patient silence is not necessarily client satisfaction: communication in home care nursing, *Home Healthc Nurse* 16(2):115, 1998.

Hentz P: The body remembers: grieving and a circle of time, *Qual Health Res* 12(2):161, 2002.

Herth K: Relationship of hope, coping styles, concurrent losses, and setting to grief resolution in the elderly widow(er), *Res Nurs Health* 13:109, 1990.

Hilliard RE: The effects of music therapy–based bereavement groups on mood and behavior of grieving children: a pilot study, *J Music Ther* 38(4):291, 2001a.

Hilliard RE: The use of music therapy in meeting the multidimensional needs of hospice patients and families, *J Palliat Care* 17(3):161, 2001b.

Hogan NS, Schmidt LA: Testing the grief to personal growth model using structural equation modeling, *Death Stud* 26(8):615, 2002.

Johnson CS: Nutritional considerations for bereavement and coping with grief, *J Nutr Health Aging* 6(3):171, 2002.

Laakso H, Paunonen-Ilmonen M: Mothers' experience of social support following the death of a child, *J Clin Nurs* 11(2):176, 2002.

Langridge P: Reduction of chronic sorrow: a health promotion role for children's community nurses? *J Child Health Care* 6(3):157, 2002.

Leininger MM, McFarland MR: *Transcultural nursing: concepts, theories, research and practices,* ed 3, New York, 2002, McGraw-Hill.

Mallow GE, Bechtel GA: Chronic sorrow: the experience of parents with children who are developmentally disabled, *J Psychosoc Nurs* 37(7):31, 1999.

McQuay JE: Cross-cultural customs and beliefs related to health crises, death, and organ donation/transplantation: a guide to assist health care professionals understand different responses and provide cross-cultural assistance, *Crit Care Nurs Clin North Am* 7(3):581, 1995 (appendix).

Moules NJ: Legitimizing grief: challenging beliefs that constrain, *J Family Nurs* 4(2):142, 1998.

Patusky KL, Rodning C, Martinez-Kratz M: Clinical lessons in psychiatric home care: a case study approach, *J Home Health Case Manag* 9:18, 1996.

Puentes WJ: Incorporating simple reminiscence techniques into acute care nursing practice, *J Gerontol Nurs* 24(2):14, 1998.

Rask K, Kaunonen M, Paunonen-Ilmonen M: Adolescent coping with grief after the death of a loved one, *Int J Nurs Pract* 8(3):137, 2002.

Rollins JA, Riccio LL: ART is the heART: a palette of possibilities for hospice care, *Pediatr Nurs* 28(4):355, 2002.

Schoutrop MJ et al: Structured writing and processing major stressful events: a controlled trial, *Psychother Psychosom* 71(3):151, 2002.

Steen KF: A comprehensive approach to bereavement, *Nurse Pract* 23(3):54, 1998.

Teel CS: Chronic sorrow: analysis of the concept, *J Adv Nurs* 16:1311, 1991.

Walsh K et al: Spiritual beliefs may affect outcome of bereavement: prospective study, *BMJ* 324(7353):1551, 2002.

Yuen-Juen H: The impact of chronic illness on patients, *Rehabil Nurs* 20:221, 1995.

• = **Independent;** ▲ = **Collaborative**

Spiritual distress

Lisa Burkhart and Ann Solari-Twadell

NANDA **Definition**

Impaired ability to experience and integrate meaning and purpose in life through the individual's connectedness with self, others, art, music, literature, nature, or a power greater than oneself

Defining Characteristics

- Connections to self: Expresses lack of hope, meaning and purpose in life, peace/serenity, acceptance, love, forgiveness of self, courage; expresses anger, guilt, poor coping
- Connections with others: Refuses interactions with spiritual leaders; refuses interactions with friends and family; verbalizes being separated from their support system, expresses alienation
- Connections with art, music, literature, nature: Demonstrates inability to experience previous state of creativity (singing, listening to music, writing), disinterest in nature, and disinterest in reading spiritual literature
- Connections with power greater than oneself: Demonstrates inability to pray, inability to participate in religious activities, expressions of being abandoned by or having anger toward God; requests to see a religious leader; demonstrates sudden changes in spiritual practices, inability to be introspective/inward turning; expresses being hopeless and suffering

Related Factors (r/t)

Self-alienation; loneliness/social isolation; anxiety; sociocultural deprivation; death and dying of self or others; pain; life change; chronic illness of self or others

NOC **Outcomes (Nursing Outcomes Classification)**

Suggested NOC Outcomes

Acceptance: Health Status; Dignified Life Closure; Grief Resolution; Hope; Spiritual Health; Suffering Severity

> **Example NOC Outcome with Indicators**
>
> **Spiritual Health** as evidenced by the following indicators: Expression of faith, hope, meaning, and purpose in life/Connectedness with inner-self and with others to share thoughts, feelings, and beliefs (Rate each indicator of **Spiritual Health:** 1 = extremely compromised, 2 = substantially compromised, 3 = moderately compromised, 4 = mildly compromised, 5 = not compromised [see Section I].)

Client Outcomes

Client Will (Specify Time Frame):
- Express sense of connectedness with self, others, arts, music, literature, or power greater than oneself
- Express meaning and purpose in life

- = Independent; ▲ = Collaborative

- Express sense of optimism and hope in the future
- Express ability to forgive
- Express desire to discuss health state and integrate care in lifestyle
- Discuss personal response to dying
- Discuss personal response to grieving

NIC   Interventions (Nursing Interventions Classification)

Suggested NIC Interventions

Forgiveness Facilitation; Grief Work Facilitation; Hope Instillation; Humor; Music Therapy; Presence; Reminiscence Therapy; Simple Guided Imagery; Simple Massage; Simple Relaxation Therapy; Spiritual Support; Therapeutic Touch; Touch

---

Example NIC Activities—Spiritual Support

Encourage use of spiritual resources if desired; Be available to listen to client's expression of feelings

---

Nursing Interventions and Rationales

- Observe the client for loss of meaning, purpose, and hope in life. **Nursing Research:** *A qualitative study of mental health nursing professionals found that it is important for health care providers to identify and assess for spiritual needs (Greasley, Chiu, and Gartland, 2001). Spirituality is associated with meaning and purpose in life and hope (Burkhart and Solari-Twadell, 2001).*
- Respect the client's beliefs; avoid imposing your own spiritual beliefs on the client. Be aware of your own belief systems and accept the client's spirituality. Allow for self-disclosure. Promote a sense of love, caring, and compassion. **Nursing Research:** *In a literature study of AIDS clients in pain, Newshan (1998) found that disclosure of the self could be comforting and healing. In a study of mental health nursing professionals, Greasley, Chiu, and Gartland (2001) found that love, caring, and compassion are interpersonal values that promote spiritual care. Respecting the client's beliefs promotes trust and connectedness (Engebretson, 1996).*
- Monitor and promote supportive social contacts. **Nursing Research:** *Social supports are positively correlated with spiritual well-being (Coyle, 2002). Coward (1995) found in a study of self-transcendence in women with AIDS that successful nursing interventions include preventing emotional and environmental isolation. In a phenomenological study, clients found spiritual support from family and friends (Smucker, 1996). Also, by definition, spirituality, or the expression of the spirit, is enhanced through a sense of connectedness with other people (Burkhart and Solari-Twadell, 2001).*
- ▲ Refer the client to a support group. **Nursing Research:** *In a study of battered women, the women participated in spiritual discussion and other practices once a week (Humphreys, 2000). The findings indicated that, among these sheltered battered women, spirituality may be associated with greater internal resources that buffer distressing feelings and calm the mind. Cultivating relationships that promote transformation, empowerment, and healing promotes spiritual well-being (Lauver, 2000).*
- Be physically present and actively listen to the client. **Nursing Research:** *In a phenomenological study, Smucker (1996) found that listening is an important nursing intervention. A survey of parish nurses demonstrated that listening and presence support clients spiritually (Tuck, Wallace, and Pullen, 2001). Another study demonstrated that the client's*

- = Independent; ▲ = Collaborative

faith and trust in nurses produces a positive effect on the client and family. Listening attentively and being physically present can be spiritually nourishing (Berggren-Thomas and Griggs, 1995). Physical presence can decrease separation and aloneness, which clients often fear (Dossey et al, 1995). Being present and actively listening to the client promotes nurse-client connectedness and helps the client feel valued (Lauver, 2000).

- Support meditation, guided imagery, therapeutic touch, journaling, relaxation, and involvement in art, music, or poetry. Support outdoor activities. **Nursing Research:** *In a survey of parish nurses, the nurses were found to use guided imagery to support clients spiritually (Tuck, Wallace, and Pullen, 2001). All these techniques have been used to promote spiritual well-being (Newshan, 1998). By definition, spirituality includes connectedness with art, music, literature, and nature (Burkhart and Solari-Twadell, 2001).*

▲ Offer or suggest visits with spiritual and/or religious advisors. **Nursing Research:** *The number one need expressed by clients who had been hospitalized, which was declared by persons of all denominations and faiths, was for their pastor/rabbi/spiritual advisor to not abandon them. For those who did not belong to a religious/spiritual group, the number one need was at least to be asked about some type of religious/spiritual preference (Moller, 1999). Clients are experts on their own paths, and knowing their values helps in exploring their uniqueness (Dossey et al, 1995).*

- Help the client make a list of important and unimportant values. **Nursing Research:** *In a survey of parish nurses, the nurses were found to implement values clarification to support clients spiritually (Tuck, Wallace, and Pullen, 2001).*

- Assist the client in identifying and creating his or her own meaningful experiences. Help the client develop skills to deal with illness or lifestyle changes. Include the client in care planning. **Nursing Research:** *In a phenomenological study, Smucker (1996) found that nurses assist clients in finding clients' own strategies to meet their spiritual needs. Clients perceived the experience of healing as an active process and expressed a desire to take conscious control (Criddle, 1993). Meaningful experiences promote spiritual well-being (Lauver, 2000).*

- Ask how to be most helpful; encourage the client to look inward, look outward, reflect, and seek clarification. **Nursing Research:** *Tuck, Pullen, and Lynn (1997) suggested that spiritual interventions include doing things for clients and encouraging inward and outward reflection.*

- If the client is comfortable with touch, hold the client's hand or place a hand gently on the client's arm. **Nursing Research:** *A survey of parish nurses found that touch supports clients spiritually (Tuck, Wallace, and Pullen, 2001).*

- Help the client find a reason for living and be available for support. Promote hope. **Nursing Research:** In one study, *"the need for a positive attitude for optimum healing was by far the most commonly mentioned subtheme by these participants and the strongest area of literature" (Criddle, 1993). Instilling hope is a common strategy to promote spiritual well-being (Baldacchino and Draper, 2001).*

- Listen to the client's feelings about suffering and/or death. Be nonjudgmental and allow time for grieving. *Being with the person who is suffering gives meaning to his or her experience (O'Brien, 1999).*

- Provide appropriate religious materials, artifacts, or music as requested. **Nursing Research:** *In a survey of battered women, church attendance and reading the Bible were rated highly in promoting spiritual well-being (Humphreys, 2000). In a survey of parish nurses, religious rites and rituals (e.g., ministering, offering communion, laying on of hands, and anointing) supported clients spiritually (Tuck, Wallace, and Pullen, 2001). Helping a*

- = **Independent;** ▲ = **Collaborative**

client incorporate religious rites and rituals can enhance meaning in life and promote a sense of connectedness with a faith community and/or a higher power (Conrad, 1985; Lauver, 2000).

- Promote forgiveness. **Nursing Research:** *In a survey of battered women, forgiveness was rated as an important part of spirituality (Humphreys, 2000). In a survey of parish nurses, the nurses promoted forgiveness (Tuck, Wallace, and Pullen, 2001).*
- Provide privacy or a "sacred space." *Sacred spaces promote spiritual well-being by enhancing a sense of connectedness with self and/or others (Lauver, 2000).*
- Allow time and a place for prayer. **Nursing Research:** *In a survey of battered women, prayer was highly rated in promoting spiritual well-being (Humphreys, 2000). A survey of parish nurses found that prayer supports clients spiritually (Tuck, Wallace, and Pullen, 2001). In a double-blind experiment, Byrd (1988) found that intercessory prayer improved clinical outcomes in coronary bypass clients. Engebretson (1996) also supported prayer, or looking upward, to promote spiritual well-being.*

Geriatric

- Discuss personal definitions of spiritual wellness with the client. *Listening attentively and helping elderly clients identify past coping strategies is part of helping with life review and finding meaning in life (Berggren-Thomas and Griggs, 1995).*
- Identify the client's past sources of spirituality. Help the client explore his or her life and identify those experiences that are noteworthy. Clients may want to read the Bible or other religious text or have it read to them. *Older adults often identify spirituality as a source of hope (Gaskins and Forte, 1995). Religious belief has been associated with higher levels of well-being and lower levels of depression and suicide (Van Ness and Larson, 2002).*

Multicultural

- Assess for the influence of cultural beliefs, norms, and values on the client's ability to cope with spiritual distress. **Nursing Research:** *How the client copes with spiritual distress may be based on cultural perceptions (Cesario, 2001; Cochran, 1998; Doswell and Erlen, 1998; Leininger and McFarland, 2002; Zapata and Shippee-Rice, 1999).*
- Acknowledge the value conflicts from acculturation stresses that may contribute to spiritual distress. **Nursing Research:** *Challenges to traditional beliefs are anxiety provoking and can produce distress (Charron, 1998).*
- Encourage spirituality as a source of support. **Nursing Research:** *African Americans and Latinos may identify spirituality, religiousness, prayer, and church-based approaches as coping resources (Bourjolly, 1998; Mapp and Hudson, 1997; Samuel-Hodge et al, 2000).*
- Validate the client's spiritual concerns and convey respect for his or her beliefs. **Nursing Research:** *Validation is a therapeutic communications technique that lets the client know the nurse has heard and understood what was said (Heineken, 1998).*

Home care

- All of the nursing interventions described previously apply in the home setting.

evolve WEBSITES FOR EDUCATION

See the EVOLVE website for World Wide Web resources for client education.

- = Independent; ▲ = Collaborative

REFERENCES

Baldacchino D, Draper P: Spiritual coping strategies: a review, *J Adv Nurs* 34:83, 2001.

Berggren-Thomas P, Griggs M: Spirituality in aging: spiritual need or spiritual journey? *J Gerontol Nurs* 21:5, 1995.

Bourjolly JN: Differences in religiousness among black and white women with breast cancer, *Soc Work Health Care* 28(1):21, 1998.

Burkhart L, Solari-Twadell PA: Spirituality and religiousness: differentiating the diagnoses through a review of the nursing literature, *Nurs Diagn* 12:45, 2001.

Byrd RC: Positive therapeutic effects of intercessory prayer in a coronary care unit population, *South Med J* 81: 826, 1988.

Cesario S: Care of the Native American woman: strategies for practice, education, and research, *J Gynecol Neonat Nurs* 30(1):13, 2001.

Charron HS: Anxiety disorders. In Varcarolis EM, editor: *Foundations of psychiatric mental health nursing,* ed 3, Philadelphia, 1998, WB Saunders.

Cochran M: Tears have no color, *Am J Nurs* 98(6):53, 1998.

Conrad NJ: Spiritual support for the dying, *Nurs Clin North Am* 20:415, 1985.

Coward DD: The lived experience of self-transcendence in women with AIDS, *J Obstet Gynecol Neonat Nurs* 24: 314, 1995.

Coyle J: Spirituality and health: towards a framework for exploring the relationship between spirituality and health, *J Adv Nurs* 37:589, 2002.

Criddle L: Healing from surgery: a phenomenological study, *Image* 25:208, 1993.

Dossey BM et al: *Holistic nursing: a handbook for practice,* 1 ed, Rockville, Md, 1988, Aspen.

Dossey BM et al: *Holistic nursing: a handbook for practice,* 2 ed, Gaithersburg, Md, 1995, Aspen.

Doswell W, Erlen J: Multicultural issues and ethical concerns in the delivery of nursing care interventions, *Nurs Clin North Am* 33(2):353, 1998.

Engebretson J: Considerations in diagnosing in the spiritual domain, *Nurs Diagn* 7:100, 1996.

Gaskins S, Forte L: The meaning of hope: implications for nursing practice and research, *J Gerontol Nurs* 21:17, 1995.

Greasley P, Chiu LF, Gartland RM: The concept of spiritual care in mental health nursing, *J Adv Nurs* 33:629, 2001.

Heineken J: Patient silence is not necessarily client satisfaction: communication in home care nursing, *Home Healthc Nurse* 16(2):115, 1998.

Humphreys J: Spirituality and distress in sheltered battered women, *J Nurs Scholarsh* 32:273, 2000.

Lauver D: Commonalities in women's spirituality and women's health, *Adv Nurs Sci* 22:76, 2000.

Leininger MM, McFarland MR: *Transcultural nursing: concepts, theories, research and practices,* ed 3, New York, 2002, McGraw-Hill.

Mapp I, Hudson R: Stress and coping among African American and Hispanic parents of deaf children, *Am Ann Deaf* 142(1):48, 1997.

Moller MD: Meeting spiritual needs on an inpatient unit, *J Psychosoc Nurs Ment Health Serv* 37(11):5, 1999.

Newshan G: Transcending the physical: spiritual aspects of pain in patients with HIV and/or cancer, *J Adv Nurs* 28:1236, 1998.

O'Brien ME: *Spirituality in nursing: standing on holy ground,* Boston, 1999, Jones and Bartlett.

Samuel-Hodge CD et al: Influences on day-to-day self-management of type 2 diabetes among African-American women: spirituality, the multi-caregiver role, and other social context factors, *Diabetes Care* 23(7): 928, 2000.

Smucker C: A phenomenological description of the experience of spiritual distress, *Nurs Diagn* 7:81, 1996.

Tuck I, Pullen L, Lynn C: Spiritual interventions provided by mental health nurses, *West J Nurs Res* 19:351, 1997.

Tuck I, Wallace D, Pullen L: Spirituality and spiritual care provided by parish nurses, *West J Nurs Res* 23:144, 2001.

Van Ness PH, Larson DB: Religion, senescence, and mental health: the end of life is not the end of hope, *Am J Geriatr Psychiatry* 10:386, 2002.

Zapata J, Shippee-Rice R: The use of folk healing and healers by six Latinos living in New England, *J Transcult Nurs* 10(2):136, 1999.

• = **Independent;** ▲ = **Collaborative**

Risk for Spiritual distress

Lisa Burkhart and Ann Solari-Twadell

NANDA **Definition**

At risk for altered sense of harmonious connectedness with all of life and the universe in which dimensions that transcend and empower the self may be disrupted

Risk Factors

Energy-consuming anxiety; low self-esteem; mental illness; physical illness; blocks to self-love; poor relationships; physical or psychological stress; substance abuse; loss of loved one; natural disaster; situational loss; maturational loss; inability to forgive

NOC **Outcomes (Nursing Outcomes Classification)**

Suggested NOC Outcomes

Acceptance: Health Status; Dignified Life Closure; Health Beliefs; Hope; Grief Resolution; Quality of Life; Spiritual Health; Suffering Severity

---

Example NOC Outcome with Indicators

Spiritual Health as evidenced by the following indicators: Expression of faith, hope, meaning, and purpose in life/Connectedness with inner self and with others to share thoughts, feelings, and beliefs (Rate each indicator of **Spiritual Health:** 1 = extremely compromised, 2 = substantially compromised, 3 = moderately compromised, 4 = mildly compromised, 5 = not compromised [see Section I].)

Client Outcomes

Client Will (Specify Time Frame):

- Express sense of connectedness with self, others, arts, music, literature, or power greater than oneself
- Express meaning and purpose in life
- Express sense of optimism and hope in the future
- Express ability to forgive
- Express desire to discuss health state and integrate care in lifestyle
- Discuss personal response to dying
- Discuss personal response to grieving
- Express satisfaction with life circumstances

NIC **Interventions (Nursing Interventions Classification)**

Suggested NIC Interventions

Forgiveness Facilitation; Grief Work Facilitation; Hope Instillation; Humor; Music Therapy; Presence; Reminiscence Therapy; Simple Guided Imagery; Simple Massage; Simple Relaxation Therapy; Spiritual Support; Touch; Therapeutic Touch

• = Independent; ▲ = Collaborative

Example NIC Activities—Spiritual Support
Encourage use of spiritual resources if desired; Be available to listen to client's feelings

Nursing Interventions and Rationales

- Observe the client for loss of meaning, purpose, and hope in life. **Nursing Research:** *A qualitative study of mental health nursing professionals found that it is important for health care providers to identify and assess for spiritual needs (Greasley, Chiu, and Gartland, 2001). Spirituality is associated with meaning and purpose in life and with hope (Burkhart and Solari-Twadell, 2001).*

- Respect the client's beliefs; avoid imposing your own spiritual beliefs on the client. Be aware of your own belief systems and accept the client's spirituality. Allow for self-disclosure. Promote a sense of love, caring, and compassion. **Nursing Research:** *In a literature study of AIDS clients in pain, Newshan (1998) found that disclosure of self could be comforting and healing. In a study of mental health nursing professionals, Greasley, Chiu, and Gartland (2001) found that love, caring, and compassion are interpersonal values that promote spiritual care. Respecting the client's beliefs promotes trust and connectedness (Engebretson, 1996).*

- Monitor and promote supportive social contacts. **Nursing Research:** *Social supports are positively correlated with spiritual well-being (Coyle, 2002). Coward (1995) found in a study of self-transcendence in women with AIDS that successful nursing interventions include preventing emotional and environmental isolation. In a phenomenological study, clients found spiritual support from family and friends (Smucker, 1996). Also, by definition, spirituality, or the expression of the spirit, is enhanced through a sense of connectedness with other people (Burkhart and Solari-Twadell, 2001).*

- ▲ Inform the client about available support groups. **Nursing Research:** *In a study of battered women, the women participated in spiritual discussion and other practices once a week (Humphreys, 2000). Cultivating relationships that promote transformation, empowerment, and healing promotes spiritual well-being (Lauver, 2000).*

- Be physically present and actively listen to the client. **Nursing Research:** *In a phenomenological study, Smucker (1996) found that listening is an important nursing intervention. A survey of parish nurses found that listening and presence support clients spiritually (Tuck, Wallace, and Pullen, 2001). Listening attentively and being physically present can be spiritually nourishing (Berggren-Thomas, Griggs, 1995). Physical presence can decrease separation and aloneness, which clients often fear (Dossey et al, 1995). Being present and actively listening to the client promotes nurse-client connectedness and helps the client feel valued (Lauver, 2000).*

- Support meditation, guided imagery, therapeutic touch, journaling, relaxation, and involvement in art, music, or poetry. Support outdoor activities. **Nursing Research:** *In a survey of parish nurses, the nurses were found to use guided imagery to support clients spiritually (Tuck, Wallace, and Pullen, 2001). All these techniques have been used to promote spiritual well-being (Newshan, 1998). By definition, spirituality includes connectedness with art, music, literature, and nature (Burkhart and Solari-Twadell, 2001).*

- ▲ Offer or suggest visits with spiritual and/or religious advisors. **Nursing Research:** *The number one need expressed by clients who had been hospitalized, which was declared by persons of all denominations and faiths, was for their pastor/rabbi/spiritual advisor to not abandon them. For those who did not belong to a religious/spiritual group, their number one*

• = Independent; ▲ = Collaborative

need was at least to be asked for some type of religious/spiritual preference (Moller, 1999). Clients are experts on their own paths and knowing their values helps in exploring their uniqueness (Dossey et al, 1995).

- Help the client make a list of important and unimportant values. **Nursing Research:** *In a survey of parish nurses, the nurses implemented values clarification to support clients spiritually (Tuck, Wallace, and Pullen, 2001).*

- Assist the client in identifying and creating his or her own meaningful experiences. Help the client develop skills to deal with illness or lifestyle changes. Include the client in care planning. **Nursing Research:** *In a phenomenological study, Smucker (1996) found that nurses help clients to find their own strategies to meet their spiritual needs. Clients perceived the experience of healing as an active process and expressed a desire to take conscious control (Criddle, 1993). Meaningful experiences promote spiritual well-being (Lauver, 2000).*

- Ask how to be most helpful; encourage the client to look inward, look outward, reflect, and seek clarification. **Nursing Research:** *Tuck, Pullen, and Lynn (1997) suggested that spiritual interventions include doing things for clients and encouraging inward and outward reflection.*

- If the client is comfortable with touch, hold the client's hand or place a hand gently on the client's arm. **Nursing Research:** *A survey of parish nurses found that touch supports clients spiritually (Tuck, Wallace, and Pullen, 2001).*

- Help the client find a reason for living and be available for support. Promote hope. **Nursing Research:** In one study, *"the need for a positive attitude for optimum healing was by far the most commonly mentioned subtheme by these participants and the strongest area of literature" (Criddle, 1993). Instilling hope is a common strategy to promote spiritual well-being (Baldacchino and Draper, 2001).*

- Listen to the client's feelings about suffering and/or death. Be nonjudgmental and allow time for grieving. *Being with the person who is suffering gives meaning to his or her experience (O'Brien, 1999).*

- Provide appropriate religious materials, artifacts, or music as requested. **Nursing Research:** *In a survey of battered women, church attendance and reading the Bible were rated highly in promoting spiritual well-being (Humphreys, 2000). In a survey of parish nurses, religious rites and rituals (e.g., ministering, offering communion, laying on of hands, and anointing) supported clients spiritually (Tuck, Wallace, and Pullen, 2001). Helping a client incorporate religious rites and rituals can enhance meaning in life and promote a sense of connectedness with a faith community and/or a higher power (Conrad, 1985; Lauver, 2000).*

- Promote forgiveness. **Nursing Research:** *In a survey of battered women, forgiveness was rated as an important part of spirituality (Humphreys, 2000). In a survey of parish nurses, the nurses promoted forgiveness (Tuck, Wallace, and Pullen, 2001).*

- Provide privacy or a "sacred space." *Sacred spaces promote spiritual well-being by enhancing a sense of connectedness with self and/or others (Lauver, 2000).*

- Allow time and a place for prayer. **Nursing Research:** *In a survey of battered women, prayer was highly rated in promoting spiritual well-being (Humphreys, 2000). A survey of parish nurses found that prayer supports clients spiritually (Tuck, Wallace, and Pullen, 2001). In a double-blind experiment, Byrd (1988) found that intercessory prayer significantly improved clinical outcomes of coronary bypass clients. Engebretson (1996) also supported prayer, or looking upward, to promote spiritual well-being.*

• = Independent; ▲ = Collaborative

Multicultural

- Assess for the influence of cultural beliefs, norms, and values on the client's ability to cope with spiritual distress. **Nursing Research:** *How the client copes with spiritual distress may be based on cultural perceptions (Cesario, 2001; Cochran, 1998; Doswell and Erlen, 1998; Leininger and McFarland, 2002; Zapata and Shippee-Rice, 1999).*
- Acknowledge the value conflicts from acculturation stresses that may contribute to spiritual distress. **Nursing Research:** *Challenges to traditional beliefs are anxiety provoking and can produce distress (Charron, 1998).*
- Encourage spirituality as a source of support. **Nursing Research:** *African Americans and Latinos may identify spirituality, religiousness, prayer, and church-based approaches as coping resources (Bourjolly, 1998; Mapp and Hudson, 1997; Samuel-Hodge et al, 2000). Studies indicate that African American caregivers cite religion and spirituality as their greatest source of support (Poindexter and Linsk, 1998).*
- Validate the client's spiritual concerns and convey respect for his or her beliefs. **Nursing Research:** *Validation is a therapeutic communication technique that lets the client know the nurse has heard and understood what was said (Heineken, 1998).*

Home care

- Interventions mentioned under other subheadings in this nursing diagnosis also apply to home care.

evolve WEBSITES FOR EDUCATION

See the EVOLVE website for World Wide Web resources for client education.

REFERENCES

Baldacchino D, Draper P: Spiritual coping strategies: a review, *J Adv Nurs* 34:83, 2001.

Berggren-Thomas P, Griggs M: Spirituality in aging: spiritual need or spiritual journey? *J Gerontol Nurs* 21:5, 1995.

Bourjolly JN: Differences in religiousness among black and white women with breast cancer, *Soc Work Health Care* 28(1):21, 1998.

Burkhart L, Solari-Twadell PA: Spirituality and religiousness: differentiating the diagnoses through a review of the nursing literature, *Nurs Diagn* 12:45, 2001.

Byrd RC: Positive therapeutic effects of intercessory prayer in a coronary care unit population, *South Med J* 81:826, 1988.

Cesario S: Care of the Native American woman: strategies for practice, education, and research, *J Gynecol Neonat Nurs* 30(1):13, 2001.

Charron HS: Anxiety disorders. In Varcarolis EM, editor: *Foundations of psychiatric mental health nursing*, ed 3, Philadelphia, 1998, WB Saunders.

Cochran M: Tears have no color, *Am J Nurs* 98(6):53, 1998.

Conrad NJ: Spiritual support for the dying, *Nurs Clin North Am* 20:415, 1985.

Coward DD: The lived experience of self-transcendence in women with AIDS, *J Obstet Gynecol Neonat Nurs* 24:314, 1995.

Coyle J: Spirituality and health: towards a framework for exploring the relationship between spirituality and health, *J Adv Nurs* 37:589, 2002.

Criddle L: Healing from surgery: a phenomenological study, *Image* 25:208, 1993.

Dossey BM et al: *Holistic nursing: a handbook for practice*, Gaithersburg, Md, 1995, Aspen.

Doswell W, Erlen J: Multicultural issues and ethical concerns in the delivery of nursing care interventions, *Nurs Clin North Am* 33(2):353, 1998.

Engebretson J: Considerations in diagnosing in the spiritual domain, *Nurs Diagn* 7:100, 1996.

• = **Independent;** ▲ = **Collaborative**

Greasley P, Chiu LF, Gartland RM: The concept of spiritual care in mental health nursing, *J Adv Nurs* 33:629, 2001.

Heineken J: Patient silence is not necessarily client satisfaction: communication in home care nursing, *Home Healthc Nurse* 16(2):115, 1998.

Humphreys J: Spirituality and distress in sheltered battered women, *J Nurs Scholarsh* 32:273, 2000.

Lauver D: Commonalities in women's spirituality and women's health, *Adv Nurs Sci* 22:76, 2000.

Leininger MM, McFarland MR: *Transcultural nursing: concepts, theories, research and practices,* ed 3, New York, 2002, McGraw-Hill.

Mapp I, Hudson R: Stress and coping among African American and Hispanic parents of deaf children, *Am Ann Deaf* 142(1):48, 1997.

Moller MD: Meeting spiritual needs on an inpatient unit, *J Psychosoc Nurs Ment Health Serv* 37(11):5, 1999.

Newshan G: Transcending the physical: spiritual aspects of pain in patients with HIV and/or cancer, *J Adv Nurs* 28:1236, 1998.

O'Brien ME: *Spirituality in nursing: standing on holy ground,* Boston, 1999, Jones and Bartlett.

Poindexter CC, Linsk NL: Sources of support in a sample of HIV-affected older minority caregivers, *Fam Soc J Contemp Hum Serv* Sep/Oct:491, 1998.

Samuel-Hodge CD et al: Influences on day-to-day self-management of type 2 diabetes among African-American women: spirituality, the multi-caregiver role, and other social context factors, *Diabetes Care* 23(7): 928, 2000.

Smucker C: A phenomenological description of the experience of spiritual distress, *Nurs Diagn* 7:81, 1996.

Tuck I, Pullen L, Lynn C: Spiritual interventions provided by mental health nurses, *West J Nurs Res* 19:351, 1997.

Tuck I, Wallace D, Pullen L: Spirituality and spiritual care provided by parish nurses, *West J Nurs Res* 23:144, 2001.

Zapata J, Shippee-Rice R. The use of folk healing and healers by six Latinos living in New England, *J Transcult Nurs* 10(2):136, 1999.

Readiness for enhanced Spiritual well-being

Ann Solari-Twadell and Lisa Burkhart

NANDA Definition

Ability to experience and integrate meaning and purpose in life through connectedness with self, others, art, music, literature, nature, or a power greater than oneself

Defining Characteristics

- Connections to self: Desires enhanced connections; expresses hope, meaning and purpose in life, peace and serenity, acceptance, surrender, love, forgiveness of self, satisfying philosophy of life, joy, courage, heightened coping, and meditation
- Connections with others: Provides service to others, requests interaction with spiritual leaders, requests forgiveness of others, requests interaction with friends and family
- Connections with art, music, literature, nature: Displays creative energy (e.g., writing poetry), sings, listens to music, reads spiritual literature, spends time outdoors
- Connection with a power greater than self: Prays, reports mystical experiences, participates in religious activities, expresses reverence and awe

Related Factors (r/t)

Health-seeking behaviors; empathy; self-care; self-awareness; desire for harmonious interconnectedness; desire to find meaning and purpose in life

• = Independent; ▲ = Collaborative

| NOC | Outcomes (Nursing Outcomes Classification) |

Suggested NOC Outcomes

Acceptance: Health Status; Adherence Behavior; Caregiver Emotional Health; Caregiver Well-Being; Caregiver-Patient Relationship; Comfort Level; Coping; Dignified Life Closure; Endurance; Family Integrity; Grief Resolution; Health Beliefs; Health-Promoting Behavior; Hope; Knowledge: Health Behavior; Leisure Participation; Personal Well-Being; Psychosocial Adjustment: Life Change; Quality of Life; Self-Esteem; Social Involvement; Spiritual Health

---

Example NOC Outcome with Indicators

Hope as evidenced by the following indicators: Expression of positive future orientation/Faith/Optimism/Belief in self/Sense of meaning in life/Belief in others/Inner peace (Rate each indicator of **Hope:** 1 = never demonstrated, 2 = rarely demonstrated, 3 = sometimes demonstrated, 4 = often demonstrated, 5 = constantly demonstrated [see Section I].)

Client Outcomes

Client Will (Specify Time Frame):

- Express hope
- Express sense of meaning and purpose in life
- Express peace and serenity
- Express acceptance
- Express surrender
- Express forgiveness of self and others
- Express satisfaction with philosophy of life
- Express joy
- Express courage
- Describe being able to cope
- Describe practicing meditation
- Describe being in service to others
- Describe interaction with spiritual leaders, friends, and family
- Describe appreciation for art, music, literature, and nature

| NIC | Interventions (Nursing Interventions Classification) |

Suggested NIC Interventions

Active Listening; Animal-Assisted Therapy; Anticipatory Guidance; Anxiety Reduction; Art Therapy; Coping Enhancement; Counseling; Crisis Intervention; Decision-Making Support; Dying Care; Emotional Support; Forgiveness Facilitation; Grief Work Facilitation; Guilt Work Facilitation; Hope Instillation; Humor; Meditation Facilitation; Music Therapy; Mutual Goal Setting; Presence; Religious Ritual Enhancement; Reminiscence Therapy; Security Enhancement; Self-Awareness Enhancement; Self-Esteem Enhancement; Simple Guided Imagery; Simple Relaxation Therapy; Socialization Enhancement; Spiritual Growth Facilitation; Spiritual Support; Support Group; Support System Enhancement; Touch; Truth Telling; Values Clarification

• = Independent; ▲ = Collaborative

Example NIC Activities—Spiritual Support
Encourage use of spiritual resources if desired; Be available to listen to client's feelings

Nursing Interventions and Rationales

- Perform a spiritual assessment that includes the client's relationship with God, meaning and purpose in life, religious affiliation, and any other significant beliefs. *Autonomy, the right of client self-determination, encompasses a client's needs whether physical, psychosocial, or spiritual. Autonomy requires nurses to assess what clients desire regarding spiritual care, setting aside personal beliefs and values to meet clients' needs from clients' own perspective of meaning (Wright, 1998). Meaning and purpose in life are associated with spirituality (Burkhart and Solari-Twadell, 2001).* **Nursing Research:** *Many nurses feel they have assessed spiritual needs when in reality they have only determined religious affiliation. Spiritual assessment reveals clients' deeper feelings about the meaning of life, love, hope, and forgiveness (Newshan, 1998).*

- Be present for the client. **Nursing Research:** *For staff to acknowledge spiritual issues, a more holistic approach to care is necessary that would entail multidisciplinary education and training in spiritual care (Greasely, Chiu, and Gartland, 2001). Eliminating expectations is essential to true presence (Bunkers, 1999). A wisdom is required in practicing presence; the nurse strives to be a caregiver, not a caretaker (Montgomery, 1992). Presencing is effective not only for clients who are dying or in severe pain but also for those who are experiencing spiritual or emotional discomfort (Taylor, 2002).*

- Listen actively to the client. **Nursing Research:** *In a phenomenological study, Smucker (1996) found that listening is an important nursing intervention. A survey of parish nurses found that listening and presence were the most frequently used interventions (Tuck, Wallace, and Pullen, 2001). Listening attentively and being physically present can be spiritually nourishing (Berggren-Thomas and Griggs, 1995). Listening is an element of presencing (Taylor, 2002).*

- Encourage the client to pray, setting the example by praying with and for the client. **Nursing Research:** *Parish nurses reported prayer to be the intervention used most frequently with clients (Tuck, Wallace, and Pullen, 2001). Frequent prayer is associated with high mental scores regardless of age and gender (Meisenhelder and Chandler, 2000). Prayer is considered an adjunct therapy in some critical care settings (Holt-Ashley, 2000). Shared prayer can be one of the deepest forms of communication (Shelly, 2000).*

- ▲ Encourage involvement in group religious practices. **Nursing Research:** *Socialization and support found through participation in personal and/or group religious practices may decrease feelings of withdrawal and isolation (Baldacchino and Draper, 2001).*

- Encourage increased quality of life through social support. **Nursing Research:** *Quality of life was potentially related to social support; physical, social, and functional well-being; and appraisal-focused coping in persons living with HIV (Tuck, McCain, and Elswick, 2001). Connectedness, defined as "a relationship one forms with self, others, nature, higher power," was identified as an important element that enhanced spirituality (Cavendish et al, 2001).*

- Assist the client in identifying religious or spiritual beliefs that encourage integration of meaning and purpose in the client's life. **Nursing Research:** *Beliefs were identified as an important theme that enhanced spirituality (Cavendish et al, 2001). Religious and/or spiritual beliefs were presented as important in interviews conducted with focus groups of us-*

• = Independent; ▲ = Collaborative

ers, caregivers, and mental health nursing professionals (Greasely, Chiu, and Gartland, 2001).

- Encourage the client to use music as a means of reducing stress. **Nursing Research:** *Participants in one study used music listening as a means of stress reduction in the home. They were facilitated by a music therapist visit and a self-administered program using the same techniques with a phone call by the therapist. These subjects performed significantly better than controls on standardized tests of depression, distress, self-esteem, and mood (Hanser and Thompson, 1994). Music is known to relieve stress and promote an interest in the transcendent (O'Brien, 1999).*
- Encourage the client to engage regularly in bibliotherapy. *Reading spiritually uplifting materials, including sacred writings, enhances well-being (Taylor, 2002).*
- Encourage storytelling. *This is an intervention nurses can use to promote spiritual health. Stories are a medium for assessment and intervention in areas that essentially reflect an individual's spirituality (Taylor, 1997).*
- Offer to read to the client. *Some clients cannot read because they are illiterate, have a pathological problem that prevents reading, or are taking medications that cause visual problems or drowsiness. Reading to clients, regardless of whether the material is religious or not, is an act of care because time is being spent with them (Bolander, 1994).*
- Support involvement in expressive art. *Sculpture, painting, knitting, and dance are all forms of expressive art that can boost the spirit (Taylor, 2002).*
- Support the use of humor by the client. *Laughter and humor increase physiological production of endorphins and shorten the distance between people (Dossey et al, 1995).*
- Encourage the client to use journal writing as a means of reflection on his or her life. *Journaling guides the client in tapping into inner realities through use of reflection and writing (Dossey et al, 1995).*
- Encourage the client to practice forgiveness. **Nursing Research:** *In a survey of battered women, forgiveness was rated as an important part of spirituality (Humphreys, 2000). In a survey of parish nurses, the nurses promoted forgiveness (Tuck, Wallace and Pullen, 2001). Caregivers agreed that forgiveness is an important part of spirituality (Kaye and Robinson, 1994).*
- Support the client in contemplating, viewing, and/or experiencing nature. **Nursing Research:** *Postoperative hospital stay was shorter and use of analgesics was lower with natural surroundings than with an urban view (Travis and McCauley, 1998).*
- Encourage expressions of spirituality. **Nursing Research:** *African Americans and Latinos may identify spirituality, religiousness, prayer, and church-based approaches as coping resources (Bourjolly, 1998; Mapp and Hudson, 1997; Samuel-Hodge et al, 2000).*
- Validate the client's spiritual concerns and convey respect for his or her beliefs. *Validation lets the client know that the nurse has heard and understood what was said (Giger and Davidhizar, 1995; Stuart and Laraia, 2001).*
- ▲ Help the client participate in religious rites or obtain spiritual guidance. *Support in spiritual beliefs (belief in a divine being or God) was identified as a factor that contributed to initiation and maintenance of behavior changes after an illness (McSweeney, 1993). The nurse is rarely the client's primary spiritual caregiver. No single approach to spiritual care is satisfactory for all clients; many kinds of resources are needed (Bolander, 1994).*
- Assist the client in developing spirituality. List the most valuable qualities he or she can bring from within, the circumstances most helpful for unfolding these qualities, and the ways of incorporating these circumstances into the client's lifestyle. *Interventions assist clients in bringing forth courage, compassion, inner peace, and creative insight (spirituality) (Macrae, 1995).*

Multicultural

- Assess for the influence of cultural beliefs, norms, and values on the client's perceptions of spirituality. **Nursing Research:** *The client's expressions of spirituality may be based on cultural perceptions (Cesario, 2001; Cochran, 1998; Doswell and Erlen, 1998; Leininger and McFarland, 2002; Zapata and Shippee-Rice, 1999).*
- Encourage expressions of spirituality. **Nursing Research:** *African Americans and Latinos may identify spirituality, religiousness, prayer, and church-based approaches as coping resources (Bourjolly, 1998; Mapp and Hudson, 1997; Samuel-Hodge et al, 2000). Studies indicate that African American caregivers cite religion and spirituality as their greatest source of support (Poindexter and Linsk, 1998).*
- Validate the client's spiritual concerns and convey respect for his or her beliefs. **Nursing Research:** *Validation is a therapeutic communication technique that lets the client know the nurse has heard and understood what was said (Heineken, 1998).*

Home care

- All of the nursing interventions mentioned previously apply in the home setting.
- ▲ Refer the client to parish nurses. *Parish nurses are experienced registered nurses committed to helping people meet the health needs of the mind, body, and spirit (Stewart, 2000).*

evolve WEBSITES FOR EDUCATION

See the EVOLVE website for World Wide Web resources for client education.

REFERENCES

Baldacchino D, Draper P: Spiritual coping strategies: a review, *J Adv Nurs* 34:83, 2001.

Berggren-Thomas P, Griggs M: Spirituality in aging: spiritual need or spiritual journey? *J Gerontol Nurs* 21:5, 1995.

Bolander V: *Sorensen and Luckmann's basic nursing: a psychophysiologic approach,* Philadelphia, 1994, WB Saunders.

Bourjolly JN: Differences in religiousness among black and white women with breast cancer, *Soc Work Health Care* 28(1):21, 1998.

Bunkers S: Learning to be still, *Nurs Sci Q* 12(2):172, 1999.

Burkhart L, Solari-Twadell A: Spirituality and religiousness: differentiating the diagnosis through a review of the literature, *Nurs Diagn* 12(2):45, 2001.

Cavendish R et al: Recognizing opportunities for spiritual enhancement in young adults: *Nurs Diagn* 12(3):77, 2001.

Cesario S: Care of the Native American woman: strategies for practice, education, and research, *J Gynecol Neonat Nurs* 30(1):13, 2001.

Cochran M: Tears have no color, *Am J Nurs* 98(6):53, 1998.

Dossey BM et al: *Holistic nursing: a handbook for practice,* Gaithersburg, Maryland, 1995, Aspen.

Doswell W, Erlen J: Multicultural issues and ethical concerns in the delivery of nursing care interventions, *Nurs Clin North Am* 33(2):353, 1998.

Giger JN, Davidhizar RE: *Transcultural nursing,* ed 2, St Louis, 1995, Mosby.

Greasley P, Chiu LF, Gartland RM: The concept of spiritual care in mental health nursing, *J Adv Nurs* 33:629, 2001.

Hanser SB, Thompson L: Effects of a music therapy strategy on depressed older adults, *J Gerontol* 49(6):P265, 1994.

Heineken J: Patient silence is not necessarily client satisfaction: communication in home care nursing, *Home Healthc Nurse* 16(2):115, 1998.

Holt-Ashley M: Nurses pray: use of prayer and spirituality as complementary therapy in the intensive care setting, *AACN Clin Issues* 11(1):60, 2000.

- = Independent; ▲ = Collaborative

Humphreys J: Spirituality and distress in sheltered battered women, *Image: J Nurs Sch* 32:273, 2000.

Kaye J, Robinson KM: Spirituality among caregivers, *Image J Nurs Sch* 26(3):218, 1994.

Leininger MM, McFarland MR: *Transcultural nursing: concepts, theories, research and practices,* ed 3, New York, 2002, McGraw-Hill.

Macrae J: Nightingale's spiritual philosophy and its significance for modern nursing, *Image* 27:8, 1995.

Mapp I, Hudson R: Stress and coping among African American and Hispanic parents of deaf children, *Am Ann Deaf* 142(1):48, 1997.

McSweeney J: Making behavior changes after a myocardial infarction, *West J Nurs Res* 15:441, 1993.

Meisenhelder JB, Chandler EN: Prayer and health outcomes in church lay leaders, *West J Nurs Res* 22:706, 2000.

Montgomery CL: The spiritual connection: nurses perceptions of the experience of caring. In Gaur DA, editor: *The presence of caring in nursing,* New York, 1992, National League for Nursing, Pub No. 15-2465, pp 9-52.

Newshan G: Transcending the physical: spiritual aspects of pain in patients with HIV and/or cancer, *J Adv Nurs* 28(6):1236, 1998.

O'Brien ME: *Spirituality in nursing: standing on holy ground,* Boston, 1999, Jones and Bartlett.

Poindexter CC, Linsk NL: Sources of support in a sample of HIV-affected older minority caregivers, *Fam Soc J Contemp Hum Serv* Sep/Oct:491, 1998.

Samuel-Hodge CD et al: Influences on day-to-day self-management of type 2 diabetes among African-American women: spirituality, the multi-caregiver role, and other social context factors, *Diabetes Care* 23(7): 928, 2000.

Shelly J: *Spiritual care: a guide for caregivers,* Downers Grove, Ill, 2000, InterVarsity Press.

Stewart LE: Parish nursing: renewing a long tradition of caring, *Gastroenterol Nurs* 23(3):116, 2000.

Stuart GW, Laraia MT: Therapeutic nurse-patient relationship. In Stuart GW, Laraia MT, editors: *Principles and practice of psychiatric nursing,* St Louis, 2001, Mosby, p 30.

Smucker C: A phenomenological description of the experience of spiritual distress, *Nurs Diagn* 7:81, 1996.

Taylor E: *Spiritual care: nursing theory, research and practice,* Upper Saddle River, NJ, 2002, Prentice Hall.

Taylor E: The story behind the story: the use of storytelling in spiritual caregiving, *Semin Oncol Nurs* 13(4):252, 1997.

Travis S, McCauley W: Mentally restorative experience supporting rehabilitation of high functioning elders recovering from hip surgery, *J Adv Nurs,* 27:977, 1998.

Tuck I, McCain NL, Elswick RK: Spirituality and psychosocial factors in persons living with HIV, *J Adv Nurs* 33(6):776, 2001.

Tuck I, Wallace D, Pullen L: Spirituality and spiritual care provided by parish nurses, *West J Nurs Res* 23:144, 2001.

Wright KB: Professional, ethical and legal implications for spiritual care in nursing, *Image J Nurs Sch* 30(1):81, 1998.

Zapata J, Shippee-Rice R: The use of folk healing and healers by six Latinos living in New England, *J Transcult Nurs* 10(2):136, 1999.

Risk for Suffocation

T. Heather Herdman and Betty J. Ackley

NANDA **Definition**

Accentuated risk of accidental suffocation (inadequate air available for inhalation)

Risk Factors

External

Vehicle warming in closed garage; use of fuel-burning heaters not vented to outside; smoking in bed; children's playing with plastic bags or inserting small objects into their mouths or noses; placement of propped bottle in infant's crib; placement of pillow in infant's crib; consumption of large mouthfuls of food; failure to remove doors on discarded or unused refrigerators or freezers; leaving children unattended in bathtubs or pools; household gas leaks; low-strung clothesline; hanging of pacifier around infant's neck

• = **Independent;** ▲ = **Collaborative**

Internal

Reduced olfactory sensation; reduced motor abilities; cognitive or emotional difficulties; disease or injury process; lack of safety education; lack of safety precautions

Related Factors (r/t)

See Risk Factors.

NOC   Outcomes (Nursing Outcomes Classification)

Suggested NOC Outcomes

Knowledge: Child Physical Safety, Personal Safety; Parenting: Adolescent Physical Safety, Early/Middle Childhood Physical Safety, Infant/Toddler Physical Safety; Risk Control; Risk Detection; Safe Home Environment; Substance Addiction Consequences

---

Example NOC Outcome with Indicators

Knowledge: Child Physical Safety as evidenced by the following indicators: Description of methods to prevent choking on object/Description of appropriate activities for child's developmental level/Demonstration of first aid techniques (Rate each indicator of **Knowledge: Child Physical Safety:** 1 = none, 2 = limited, 3 = moderate, 4 = substantial, 5 = extensive [see Section I].)

Client Outcomes

Client Will (Specify Time Frame):

- Explain and undertake appropriate measures to prevent suffocation
- Demonstrate correct techniques for emergency rescue maneuvers (e.g., Heimlich maneuver, rescue breathing, cardiopulmonary resuscitation [CPR]) and describe situations that require them

NIC   Interventions (Nursing Interventions Classification)

Suggested NIC Interventions

Aspiration Precautions; Environmental Management: Safety; Infant Care; Positioning; Security Enhancement; Surveillance; Surveillance: Safety; Teaching: Infant Safety

---

Example NIC Activities—Environmental Management: Safety

Identify safety hazards in environment (e.g., physical, biological, and chemical); Remove hazards from environment when possible

---

Nursing Interventions and Rationales

NOTE: Management of a risk diagnosis necessitates approaches using primary and secondary prevention. Primary prevention interventions, which include activities such as safety instruction, focus on thwarting the development of a disease or condition. Secondary prevention is achieved through screening, monitoring, and surveillance (Shortridge and Valanis, 1992).

- Conduct risk factor identification, noting special circumstances in which preventive or

• = **Independent;** ▲ = **Collaborative**

protective measures are indicated. Note the presence of environmental hazards, including the following:

- Plastic bags (e.g., dry cleaner's bags, bags used for mattress protection)
- Cribs with slats wider than $2^3/_8$ inches
- Ill-fitting crib mattresses that can allow the infant to become wedged between the mattress and crib
- Pillows in cribs
- Abandoned large appliances such as refrigerators, dishwashers, or freezers
- Clothing with cords or hoods that can become entangled
- Bibs, pacifiers on a string, drapery cords, pull-toy strings
- Earth cave-ins
- Food items

  Suffocation by airway obstruction is a leading cause of death in children younger than 6 years of age. Cords longer than 12 inches can lead to strangulation. Clients and families identified as at risk need special teaching and referral (Green, 1993; Jones, 1993; McCloskey and Bulechek, 1992). **Clinical Research:** *Children between the ages of 4 and 36 months of age are at risk for suffocation by hollow, semirigid hemispherical/ellipsoidal objects through suction formation and complete airway obstruction (Nakamura, Pollack-Nelson, and Chidekel, 2003).*

- Identify hospitalized clients at particular risk for suffocation, including the following:
  - Clients with altered levels of consciousness
  - Infants or young children
  - Clients with developmental delays
- Institute safety measures such as proper positioning and feeding precautions. See the care plans for **Risk for Aspiration** and **Impaired Swallowing** for additional interventions. *Vigilance and special protective measures are necessary for clients at greater risk for suffocation (Green, 1993).*

Geriatric

- Assess the status of the swallow reflex and dentition; offer appropriate foods and beverages accordingly.
- Observe the client for pocketing of food in the side of the mouth; remove food as needed.
- Position the client in high Fowler's position when eating and for 1 hour afterward. *Elderly clients may be at risk for suffocation that results from dysphagia and poor dental health.*
- Use care in pillow placement when positioning frail elderly clients who are on bed rest. *Frail elderly clients are at risk for suffocation if pillows become lodged in the bed and the client cannot reposition them because of weakness.*

Home care

- Assess the home for potential safety hazards in systems that are not likely to be fixed (e.g., faulty pilot lights or gas leaks in gas stoves, carbon monoxide release from heating systems, kerosene fumes from portable heaters). Assist the family in having these areas assessed and making appropriate safety arrangements (e.g., installing detectors, making repairs). *Assessment and correction of system problems prevents accidental suffocation.*

• = **Independent;** ▲ = **Collaborative**

Client/Family Teaching

- Counsel families on the following:
  - Following general safety practices such as not smoking in bed, properly disposing of large appliances, using properly functioning heating systems and ventilation, having functional smoke detectors, and opening garage doors when warming up a car
  - Taking safety measures appropriate to the functional or developmental age of the client (with emphasis on crib safety in particular)
  - Not placing the infant in the prone position but instead positioning on the back and not placing any soft bedding near the infant's airway. *Population studies have demonstrated a striking trend in decreased incidence of sudden infant death syndrome (SIDS) since parents have been taught to not place infants in the prone position (Ponsonby, Dwyer, and Cochrane, 2002).* **Clinical Research:** *The introduction of the "Back to Sleep" program has not brought about an increase in the incidence of aspiration-related deaths. The rate of infant death related to SIDS has declined (Malloy, 2002).*
  - Not allowing the infant or small child to sleep in the same bed as adults and avoiding consuming alcohol or illicit drugs, or smoking if the infant is sleeping with an adult. **Clinical Research:** *In one study of SIDS deaths, over half of the infants were sleeping in the same bed as an adult, which suggests that some of the deaths were due to unintentional suffocation by the adult or by compressible bedding (Person, Lavezzi, and Wolf, 2002). Another study demonstrated that parents who were under the influence of alcohol or illicit drugs, or were smoking were more likely to have an infant experiencing SIDS (James, Klenka, and Manning, 2003).*
- Advise parents to avoid food that can be inhaled (e.g., peanuts, popcorn, hard candy, gum, whole or large pieces of hot dog, whole grapes). Nonfood items smaller than $1\frac{1}{4}$ inches in diameter (e.g., coins, latex balloons, small parts on toys) also present a hazard. *Mechanical suffocation and asphyxia caused by foreign objects in the respiratory tract are the leading cause of death in children under 1 year of age. Children under 2 years of age have a high level of hand-to-mouth behavior. This behavior, combined with a lack of fear, puts them at risk even in a child-safe environment (Gotsch, Annest and Holmgreen, 2002; Green, 1993; Holida, 1993).* **Clinical Research:** *Rigid items that are of a spherical or cylindrical shape can cause upper airway occlusion (Nakamura, Pollack-Nelson, and Chidekel, 2003).*
- ▲ Provide information to parents about obtaining the "no-choke test tube" if desired. *This tube teaches parents about safe sizes of toys and other small objects (Jones, 1993).*
- Stress water and pool safety precautions, including vigilant, uninterrupted parental supervision. *An intense drive for exploration combined with a lack of awareness of danger makes drowning a threat to small children. A child's high center of gravity and poor coordination make buckets and toilets a threat because a child looking inside either can fall over and become lodged (Green, 1993; Jones, 1993).*
- Underscore the necessity of not allowing children to play with or near electric garage doors and of keeping garage door openers out of the reach of young children. *Children close to the ground may not be large enough to trigger reversal mechanisms on the door and may become trapped.*
- ▲ Recommend that families who are seeking day care or in-home care for children, geriatric family members, or at-risk family members with developmental or functional disabilities inspect the environment for hazards and examine the first aid preparation and vigilance of providers. *Many working families must trust others to care for family members.*

- • = Independent; ▲ = Collaborative

▲ Involve family members in learning and practicing rescue techniques, including treatment of choking and lack of breathing, and CPR. Initiate referral to formal training classes. *Family members need adequate preparation to deal with emergency situations and should take part in the American Heart Association Basic Lifesaving Course or the American Red Cross Infant/Child CPR Course (Gotsch, Annest, and Holmgreen, 2002).*

evolve WEBSITES FOR EDUCATION

See the EVOLVE website for World Wide Web resources for client education.

REFERENCES

Gotsch K, Annest JL, Holmgreen P: Nonfatal choking-related episodes among children—United States, 2001, *MMWR* 51(42), 2002.

Green PM: High risk for suffocation. In McFarland GK, McFarlane EA, editors: *Nursing diagnosis and intervention*, St Louis, 1993, Mosby.

Holida DL: Latex balloons: they can take your breath away, *Pediatr Nurs* 19:39, 1993.

James C, Klenka H, Manning D: Sudden infant death syndrome: bed sharing with mothers who smoke, *Arch Dis Child* 88(2):112, 2003.

Jones NE: Childhood residential injuries, *MCN Am J Matern Child Nurs* 18:168, 1993.

Malloy MS: Trends in postneonatal aspiration deaths and reclassification of sudden infant death syndrome: impact of the "Back to Sleep" program, *Pediatrics* 109(4):661, 2002.

McCloskey JC, Bulechek GM, editors: *Nursing interventions classification*, St Louis, 1992, Mosby.

Nakamura S, Pollack-Nelson C, Chidekel A: Suction-type suffocation incidents in infants and toddlers, *Pediatrics* 111(1):e12-6, 2003.

Person TL, Lavezzi WA, Wolf BC: Cosleeping and sudden unexpected death in infancy, *Arch Pathol Lab Med* 126(3):343, 2002.

Ponsonby A, Dwyer T, Cochrane J. Population trends in sudden infant death syndrome, *Semin Perinatol* 26(4): 296, 2002.

Shortridge L, Valanis B: The epidemiological model applied in community health nursing. In Stanhope M, Lancaster J, editors: *Community health nursing: process and practice for promoting health*, ed 3, St Louis, 1992, Mosby.

Risk for Suicide

Kathleen L. Patusky

NANDA Definition

At risk for self-inflicted, life-threatening injury

Related Factors (r/t)

Behavioral

History of previous suicide attempt; impulsiveness; purchase of gun; stockpiling of medicines; making or changing of a will; giving away of possessions; sudden euphoric recovery from major depression; marked changes in behavior, attitude, or school performance

Verbal

Threats of killing oneself; statement of desire to die/end it all

• = Independent; ▲ = Collaborative

Situational

Living alone; retirement; relocation, institutionalization; economic instability; loss of autonomy/independence; presence of gun in home; residence of adolescent in nontraditional setting (e.g., juvenile detention center, prison, half-way house, group home)

Psychological

Family history of suicide; alcohol and substance use/abuse; psychiatric illness/disorder (e.g., depression, schizophrenia, bipolar disorder); abuse in childhood; guilt; gay or lesbian orientation in youth

Demographic

Age: elderly, young adult male, adolescent; race: white, Native American; gender: male; marital status: divorced, widowed

Physical

Physical illness; terminal illness; chronic pain

Social

Loss of important relationship; disrupted family life; grief, bereavement; poor support systems; loneliness; hopelessness; helplessness; social isolation; legal or disciplinary problems; cluster suicides

NOC Outcomes (Nursing Outcomes Classification)

Suggested NOC Outcomes

Depression Level; Distorted Thought Self-Control; Impulse Self-Control; Loneliness Severity; Mood Equilibrium; Risk Detection; Self-Mutilation Restraint; Suicide Self-Restraint

---

Example NOC Outcome with Indicators

Suicide Self-Restraint as evidenced by the following indicators: Expresses feelings/Seeks help when feeling self-destructive/Verbalizes and controls suicidal ideas and impulses (Rate each indicator of **Suicide Self-Restraint:** 1 = never demonstrated, 2 = rarely demonstrated, 3 = sometimes demonstrated, 4 = often demonstrated, 5 = consistently demonstrated [see Section I].)

Client Outcomes

Client Will (Specify Time Frame):

- Not harm self
- Maintain connectedness in relationships
- Disclose and discuss suicidal ideas if present; seek help
- Express decreased anxiety and control of impulses
- Talk about feelings; express anger appropriately
- Refrain from using mood-altering substances
- Obtain no access to harmful objects
- Yield access to harmful objects
- Maintain self-control without supervision

• = **Independent;** ▲ = **Collaborative**

NIC   Interventions (Nursing Interventions Classification)

Suggested NIC Interventions

Anger Control Assistance; Anxiety Reduction; Calming Technique; Coping Enhancement; Crisis Intervention; Delusion Management; Medication Administration; Mood Management; Substance Use Prevention; Suicide Prevention; Support System Enhancement; Surveillance

> **Example NIC Activities—Suicide Prevention**
>
> Determine presence and degree of suicide risk; Encourage client to seek out care providers to talk when urge to harm self occurs

Nursing Interventions and Rationales

NOTE: Prior to implementation of interventions in the face of suicidal behavior, nurses should examine their own emotional responses to incidents of suicide to ensure that interventions will not be based on countertransference reactions. **Nursing and Clinical Research:** *Suicidal behavior can lead to stigmatization and discrediting of the client, as it may tap into the nurse's fears about mental illness, concerns about being able to respond effectively, and expectations that persons with mental illness tend toward violence (Joachim and Acorn, 2000; Steadman et al, 1998; Wilson et al, 1999). In one study, medical nurses reported that they could not understand why people harm themselves, and they felt they did not have the skills to deal with suicidal clients (Hopkins, 2002).*

- Establish a therapeutic relationship with the client. Use a direct, nonjudgmental approach in discussing suicide. **Clinical Research:** *A study has demonstrated the importance of the therapeutic relationship in identifying risk for and preventing suicide (Rudd et al, 2000). Clients who perceive that nurses are responding negatively to suicidal behavior are less likely to self-disclose.*
- Monitor, document, and report the client's potential for suicide. *All members of the health care team need to be aware of a client's potential risk for suicide and to be prepared to respond in the event of suicidal behavior.*
- Be alert for warning signs of suicide:
  - Making statements such as, "I can't go on," "Nothing matters anymore," "I wish I were dead"
  - Becoming depressed or withdrawn
  - Behaving recklessly
  - Getting affairs in order and giving away valued possessions
  - Showing a marked change in behavior, attitudes, or appearance
  - Abusing drugs or alcohol
  - Suffering a major loss or life change
  - Manifesting a psychiatric disorder associated with suicidal behavior, including depression, substance abuse, bipolar disorder, schizophrenia, panic disorder, dissociative disorder, antisocial personality disorder, or borderline personality disorder

  Suicide is rarely a spur-of-the-moment decision. In the days and hours before people kill themselves, there are usually clues and warning signs (Befrienders International, 2003). Ideation precedes planning, which may result in an attempt leading to death. If nonfatal, the attempt may increase the likelihood of subsequent ideation, planning, and attempts (Vilhjalmsson, Kristjansdottir, and Sveinbjarnardottir, 1998). The current

• = **Independent; ▲ = Collaborative**

presence of psychiatric disorders has been associated with suicidal behavior (Henriksson et al, 1996).

- Question family members regarding the preparatory actions mentioned. *Clinicians should be alert for suicide when these factors are present in asymptomatic persons (National Guideline Clearing House, 2001). Family members may have noted preparatory actions.*
- Assess for suicidal ideation when the history reveals the following:
  - Depression, substance abuse, or other psychiatric disorders
  - Attempted suicide, current or past
  - Recent stressful life events (divorce and/or separation, relocation, problems with children)
  - Recent unemployment
  - Recent bereavement
  - Chronic pain or physical illness
  - Childhood physical or sexual abuse
  - Gay, lesbian, or bisexual gender orientation
  - Family history of suicide

  Clinicians should be alert for suicide when the aforementioned factors are present in asymptomatic persons (National Guideline Clearing House, 2001). **Clinical Research:** *A study revealed that clients with chronic pain and depression expressed suicidal ideation (Fisher et al, 2001; Gilman et al, 2001). Sexual orientation has been implicated as a factor in some suicide attempts (Fergusson, Horwood, and Beautrais, 1999). The process leading to suicide in young people often involves untreated depression (Houston, Hawton, and Shepperd, 2001). Suicide assessment may be aided by having the client complete screening instruments such as the Center for Epidemiological Studies Depression Scale (CES-D), which indicates degree of depressed mood, or the Beck Suicide Intent Scale, which identifies a strong intent to die. The Risk of Suicide Questionnaire (RSQ) is available for children and adolescents (Horowitz et al, 2001).*

- Determine the presence and degree of suicidal risk. A number of questions will elicit the necessary information:
  - Have you been thinking about hurting or killing yourself?
  - How often do you have these thoughts and how long do they last?
  - Do you have a plan? What is it?
  - Do you have access to the means to carry out that plan?
  - How likely is it that you could carry out the plan?
  - Are there people or things that could prevent you from hurting yourself?
  - What do you see in your future a year from now? Five years from now?
  - What do you expect would happen if you died?
  - What has kept you alive up to now?

  Using the acronym SAL, the nurse can evaluate the client's suicide plan for its Specificity (how detailed and clear is the plan?), Availability (does the client have immediate access to the planned means?), and Lethality (could the plan be fatal or does the client believe it would be fatal?). Assessment of reasons for living is another important part of evaluating suicidal clients (Malone et al, 2000).

- ▲ Refer to mental health counseling and refer for possible hospitalization if there is evidence of suicidal intent, which may include evidence of preparatory actions (e.g., obtaining a weapon, making a plan, putting affairs in order, giving away prized possession, preparing a suicide note).
- ▲ Assign a hospitalized client to a room located near the nursing station. *Close assign-*

• = Independent; ▲ = Collaborative

ment increases ease of observation and availability for a rapid response in the event of a suicide attempt.

▲ Search the newly hospitalized client and the client's personal belongings for weapons or potential weapons and hoarded medications during the inpatient admission procedure, as appropriate. *Clients intent on suicide may bring the means with them.*

▲ Initiate suicide precautions (e.g., ongoing observation and monitoring of the client, provision of a protective environment) for a client who is at serious risk of suicide. Place the client in the least restrictive environment that allows for the necessary level of observation. Assess suicidal risk at least daily. *Close observation of the client is necessary for safety as long as intent remains high. Suicide risk should be assessed periodically to adjust suicide precautions and limitations on the client's freedom of movement and to ensure that restrictions continue to be appropriate.*

▲ Assess the client's ability to enter into a no-suicide contract. Contract (verbally or in writing) with the client for no self-harm; recontract at appropriate intervals. *Discussing feelings of self-harm with a trusted person provides relief for the client. A contract gets the subject out in the open and places some of the responsibility for safety with the client. A contract is not appropriate for some clients: those who are under the influence of drugs or alcohol, or are unwilling to abstain from substance use; those who are isolated or alone without assistance to keep the environment safe; those who are unwilling to dismantle a suicide plan or disclose alternative plans (Hauenstein, 2002). If the client will not contract, the risk of suicide should be considered higher. The lack of willingness to self-disclose has been shown to discriminate the serious suicide attempter from the client with suicidal ideation or the mild attempter (Apter et al, 2001).* **Nursing Research:** NOTE: *Contracting is a common practice in psychiatric care settings. However, recent research has suggested that self-harm is not prevented by contracts (Drew, 2001). The researcher reported that (1) consistency of nursing assignment could be associated with lower probability of self-harm, and (2) a previous study involving children that showed beneficial effects of contracts used contracts that specified a positive contingency if clients refrained from self-harm. The researcher concluded that thorough, ongoing assessment of suicide risk is necessary, whether or not the client has entered into a no-self-harm contract.*

▲ Increase surveillance of a hospitalized client at times when staffing is predictably low (e.g., staff meetings, change of shift report, periods of unit disruption). *Clients who remain intent on suicide will be watchful of periods when staff surveillance lessens to permit completion of a suicide plan.*

▲ Consider strategies to decrease isolation and opportunity to act on harmful thoughts (e.g., use of a sitter). **Nursing Research:** *Continuous staff-client contact may be necessary to prevent suicidal behavior and to provide the availability that will help the client experience a sense of support (Cleary et al, 1999). Clients have reported feeling safe and having their hope restored in response to close observation (Bowers and Park, 2001).*

▲ Observe, record, and report any changes in mood or behavior that may signify increasing suicide risk and document results of regular surveillance checks. *Suicidal ideation often is not continuous; it may decrease then increase in response to negative thinking or exposure to stressors (e.g., family visits). Documentation of surveillance will alert all members of the health care team to changes in the client's potential risk for suicide so they may be prepared to respond in the event of suicidal behavior.*

▲ Explain suicide precautions and relevant safety issues to the client and family (e.g., purpose, duration, behavioral expectations, and behavioral consequences). **Nursing Research:** *Suicide precautions may be viewed as restrictive. Clients have reported the loss of*

• = **Independent;** ▲ = **Collaborative**

privacy as distressing (Bowers and Park, 2001). Explanations will highlight the importance of taking suicidal behavior seriously as well as emphasize that the client makes choices and is an integral part of his or her own care.

▲ Refer for treatment and participate in the management of any psychiatric illness or symptoms that may be contributing to the client's suicidal ideation or behavior. *Psychiatric disorders have been associated with suicidal behavior (Henriksson et al, 1996). Symptoms of the disorder may require treatment with antidepressant, antipsychotic, or antianxiety medications.*

▲ Verify that the client has taken medications as ordered (e.g., conduct mouth checks following medication administration). *The client may attempt to hoard medications for a later suicide attempt.*

▲ Maintain increased surveillance of the client whenever use of an antidepressant has been initiated or the dosage increased. *Antidepressant medications take anywhere from 2 to 6 weeks to achieve full efficacy. During that period, the client's energy level may increase although the depression has not yet lifted, which increases the potential for suicide.*

• Search the environment routinely and remove dangerous items. *Action is necessary to maintain a hazard-free environment and client safety. Controlling the environment may be a viable strategy for preventing suicide (Leenaars et al, 2000).*

• Limit access to windows and exits unless locked and shatterproof, as appropriate. *Suicidal behavior may include attempts to jump out of windows or to escape the unit to find other means of suicide (e.g., gaining roof access for a jump). Hospitals should ensure that exits are secure.*

• Monitor the client during the use of potential weapons (e.g., razor, scissors). *Clients with suicidal intent may take advantage of any opportunity to harm themselves.*

• Involve the client in treatment planning and self-care management of psychiatric disorders. *Self-care management promotes feelings of self-efficacy (Lorig et al, 2001), particularly for clients with depression (Allen and Hagerty, 2003). Suicidal ideation may occur in response to a sense of hopelessness, a sense that the client has no control over life circumstances. The more clients participate in their own care, the less powerless and hopeless they feel. Refer to the care plan for* **Powerlessness.**

• Develop a positive therapeutic relationship with the client; *do not* make promises that may not be kept. *Clients will speak of their suicidal ideation more readily if they feel a connection with the nurse. Be aware that some clients may offer to self-disclose if the nurse will promise not to tell anyone what they have said. Clarify with the client that anything they share will be communicated only to other staff, but that secrets cannot be kept.*

• Interact with the client at regular intervals to convey caring and openness, and to provide opportunities for the client to talk about feelings. *Emotional safety is promoted when the nurse helps the client to become aware of feelings, name them, and develop strategies to express distress more constructively (Marcus, 1998).*

• Explore with the client all circumstances and motivations related to the suicidality. *Interpersonal conflict is a frequent precipitating factor in suicidal ideation and should be addressed, even if the primary focus of treatment is to be an underlying psychiatric disorder (Isacsson and Rich, 2001).*

• Explore with the client all perceived consequences that could act as a barrier to suicide (e.g., impact on family, religious beliefs). Be aware that resources should not be assumed to be barriers to suicide without exploring the client's feelings toward them. **Nursing Research:** *A study of older white men revealed that the most common barrier to suicide was consequences to family members (Bell, 2000). When familial relations are*

• = **Independent;** ▲ = **Collaborative**

strained, however, consequences to family members may not be a barrier if the client perceives suicide as a way to punish others.

- Encourage the client to seek out care providers to talk whenever the urge to harm himself or herself occurs. *Listening, being supportive, exploring antecedents to suicidal ideation, and helping the client verbalize pain and fear provide an alternative to suicide (Horsfall, 1999). Much of suicidality results from the client's frustrated efforts at affiliation (Schneidman, 2001); thus the nurse-client relationship provides needed empathetic contact.*

- Avoid repeated discussion of the client's suicide history by keeping discussion oriented to the present and future. *Clients under stress have difficulty focusing their thoughts, which leads to a sense of being overwhelmed by problems. Focusing on the present and future helps the client to address problem solving with regard to current stressors, while avoiding secondary gain from idealizing past behavior.*

▲ Discuss plans for dealing with suicidal ideation in the future (e.g., how to identify precipitating factors, whom to contact, where to go for help, how to respond to desire for self-harm) and for dealing with questions from friends and others about the client's hospitalization/suicide attempt. *Clients are supported in self-care management when they are helped to identify actions they can take if suicidal ideation recurs. However, the social stigma attached to the client's behavior can create stress and discomfort, potentially leading to additional feelings of alienation and suicidal ideation.*

▲ Assist the client in identifying a network of supportive persons and resources (e.g., clergy, family, care providers). *Clients who are suicidal often feel alienated from others and benefit from actions that facilitate support of the client by family and friends.*

▲ Refer family members and friends to local mental health agencies and crisis intervention centers if the client has suicidal ideation or there is a suspicion of suicidal thoughts. *Clients at risk should receive evaluation and help (National Guideline Clearing House, 2001).*

▲ Consider outpatient commitment or an overnight psychiatric observation program for an actively suicidal client. *Involuntary outpatient commitment can improve treatment, reduce the likelihood of hospital readmission, and reduce episodes of violent behavior in persons with severe psychiatric illnesses (Torrey and Zdanowicz, 2001). Overnight psychiatric observation followed by outpatient referral also can be an effective alternative to traditional hospitalization without leading to an increase in suicide gestures or attempts (Francis et al, 2000).*

▲ If imminent suicide is suspected or an attempt has occurred, call for assistance and do not leave the client alone. *Client and staff safety will be served by assistance in the response. The client may attempt additional self-harm if left alone.*

▲ With the client's consent, facilitate family-oriented crisis intervention. *Family-oriented crisis intervention can clarify stresses and allow assessment of family dynamics. A study of depressed adult inpatients revealed that the families of suicidal clients were considered more dysfunctional than the families of clients with no history of attempted suicide (McDermut et al, 2001).*

▲ Involve the family in discharge planning (e.g., illness/medication teaching, recognition of increasing suicidal risk, client's plan for dealing with recurring suicidal thoughts, community resources). *Suicidal clients often are ambivalent about hurting themselves; they may not want to die so much as to escape an intolerable situation. Consequently they often leave clues about their state of mind. Family members can learn to respond to clues early, support the treatment regimen, and encourage the client to initiate the emergency plan.*

- = Independent; ▲ = Collaborative

▲ Prior to discharge from the hospital, ensure that the client has a supply of ordered medications, has a plan for outpatient follow-up, understands the plan or has a caregiver able and willing to follow the plan, and has the ability to access outpatient treatment. *With shortened hospital stays, clients may be discharged before they have recovered substantial functional ability and may have difficulty concentrating on the plan for follow-up. They may need the assistance of others to ensure that prescriptions are filled, that they attend appointments, or that they have transportation to the outpatient care setting. Lack of adequate follow-up has been associated with repeated suicide attempts among adolescents (Hulten et al, 2001).*

▲ In the event of successful suicide, refer the family to a therapy group for survivors of suicide. **Nursing Research:** *Survivors of suicide may be reluctant to contact health care professionals, out of fear that they will be blamed or stigmatized. Group counseling addresses the blame, anger, guilt, shame, and search for a reason for the suicide that occurs in suicide survivors (Barlow, 2002).*

• See the care plans for **Risk for self-directed Violence, Hopelessness,** and **Risk for Self-Mutilation.** *Clients with suicidal ideation often are reacting to a feeling of hopelessness (D'Zurilla et al, 1998).*

Multicultural

• Assess for the influence of cultural beliefs, norms, and values on the individual's perceptions of suicide. **Nursing Research:** *What the individual believes about suicide may be based on cultural perceptions (Cochran, 1998; Doswell and Erlen, 1998; Leininger and McFarland, 2002).*

• Facilitate modeling and role playing for the client and family regarding healthy ways to start a discussion about the client's suicide attempt. *It is helpful for families and the client to practice communication skills in a safe environment before trying them in a real-life situation (Rivera-Andino and Lopez, 2000).*

• Identify and acknowledge the stresses unique to culturally diverse individuals. *Financial difficulties and maintaining cultural values are two of the most common family stressors cited by women of color (Majumdar and Ladak, 1998). Suicide rates among African American male teenagers increased 105% from 1980 to 1986 (Surgeon General, 1999), with "suicide by cop" speculated to increase these rates (Daugherty, 1999). A high rate of suicidal ideation has been reported as a result of the social discrimination experienced by gay and bisexual Latino men in the United States (Diaz et al, 2001).*

• Identify and acknowledge unique cultural responses to stressors in determining sensitive interventions to prevent suicide. **Nursing Research:** *In a study of African American, Hispanic/Latina, and white adolescent girls, the Hispanic/Latina girls had a significantly higher percentage of suicide attempts. Relationships were found between recent suicide attempts and family history of suicide attempts, friend's history of suicide attempt, history of physical or sexual abuse, and environmental stress. For all three groups, rate of recent suicide attempts was also associated with stress level, social connectedness, and religious influence (Rew et al, 2001).*

• Encourage family members to demonstrate and offer caring and support to each other. *The familial characteristics of care and support may be associated with fostering resilience in African American families. Resilience is the ability to experience adverse conditions and successfully overcome them (Calvert, 1997).*

• Foster the client's use of available family and religious supports. *Christian religious roots and family closeness, while eroding among many young African Americans, traditionally*

• = **Independent;** ▲ = **Collaborative**

have worked against suicidal behavior among African Americans (Neeleman, Wessely, and Lewis, 1998).

- Validate the individual's feelings regarding concerns about the current crisis and family functioning. *Validation lets the client know that the nurse has heard and understood what was said, and it promotes the nurse-client relationship (Giger and Davidhizar, 1995; Stuart and Laraia, 2001).*

Geriatric

- Perform careful assessment and ongoing evaluation of the potential for suicidal ideation in the older adult, particularly the older man. *The highest incidence of completed suicide occurs in older white men, and a gun is often involved (Quan and Arboleda-Florez, 1999).*
- Evaluate the older client's mental and physical health status and financial stressors. *Mental disorders have been associated with suicide in older women (Agbayewa, Marion, and Wiggins, 1998). Physical illness, particularly that accompanied by chronic or unremitting pain, and financial difficulties can precipitate suicide in older men (Uncapher et al, 1998a).*
- Monitor the older adult for subtle signs of suicidal risk. *The elderly, who experience multiple losses and have fragile support systems, are at greatest risk for suicide. Assess death wishes and suicidal thoughts. Consider noncompliance with medical treatment to be a possible means of suicide. Also assess stress, social support, and vulnerability to guide interventions (Valente, 1994).*
- Explore triggers of and barriers to suicidal behavior, with particular attention to real and perceived losses (e.g., professional role, health). **Nursing Research:** *A study of older white men revealed that losing connections initiated a process of loss and depression, and triggered a decision point that could include suicidal ideation. The decision point was characterized by a balance of triggers and barriers, modulated by ambivalence. Triggers included death of a spouse, emotional pain, health problems, and feelings of uselessness or hopelessness. A strong barrier was consequences to family members. Religion and social isolation were not relevant (Bell, 2000).*
- An older adult who shows self-destructive behaviors should be evaluated for dementia. **Clinical Research:** *In one study of older men in nursing homes, depression rather than medical illness or functional disability predicted suicidal ideation (Uncapher et al, 1998b). In another study of nursing home residents, however, self-destructive behaviors were common; these behaviors were more likely related to dementia than to depression, and were only weakly associated with suicidal intent (Draper et al, 2002).*
- ▲ Advocate for the older client with other professionals in securing treatment for suicidal states. *Primary care physicians have been noted to underrecognize and undertreat older adult clients with depression.* **Clinical Research:** *A study of primary care providers reported that, although physicians recognized depression and suicidal risk in both adults and geriatric clients, they were less willing to treat or refer the older suicidal client, viewing the suicidal ideation as rational and normal (Uncapher and Arean, 2000).*

Home care

- Communicate the degree of risk to family/caregivers; assess the family and caregiving situation for ability to protect the client and to understand the client's suicidal behavior. Provide the family and caregivers with guidelines on how to manage self-harm behaviors in the home environment. *Client safety between home visits is a nursing priority. Family/caregivers may become frightened by the client's suicidal ideation, may be angry*

- = **Independent;** ▲ = **Collaborative**

at the client's perceived lack of self-control, or may feel as if they are walking on eggshells awaiting another suicide attempt. Appropriate family/caregiver support is important to the client. Appropriate support will be forthcoming only if all parties understand the basis of the behavior and how to respond to it.

▲ Establish an emergency plan, including when to use hotlines and 911. Develop a contract with the client and family for use of the emergency plan. Role play access to the emergency resources with the client and caregivers. *Having an emergency plan reassures the client and caregivers and promotes client safety. Contracting gives guided control to the client and enhances self-esteem.*

• Assess the home environment for harmful objects. Have the family remove or lock up objects as possible. *Client safety is a nursing priority.*

• Counsel parents and homeowners to restrict unauthorized access to potentially lethal prescription drugs and firearms within the home. *Identifying teens at high risk of firearm suicide and limiting access to firearms is a type of public health intervention likely to be successful in preventing firearm suicides (Shah, 2000).*

• Identify the client's concerns and implement interventions to address the consequences of disability in a client with medical illness. **Clinical Research:** *In a study of cancer clients being cared for at home, primary factors influencing vulnerability to suicide were identified as real or feared loss of autonomy and independence, concerns about being a burden on others, hopelessness about the health condition, and fear of suffering (Filiberti et al, 2001). Hopelessness and demoralization in conjunction with dependence have been noted as precursors to suicidal ideation in palliative care clients (Kissane, Clarke, and Street, 2001). Refer to the care plans for* **Hopelessness** *and* **Powerlessness.**

▲ If the client's suicidal ideation intensifies, or if a suicide plan with access to means becomes evident, institute an emergency plan for mental health intervention. *The degree of disturbance and the ability to manage care safely at home determines the level of services needed to protect the client. Approximately 25% of clients who are hospitalized after a suicide attempt kill themselves within 3 months following hospitalization (Appleby et al, 1999).*

▲ Refer for homemaker or psychiatric home health care services for respite, client reassurance, and implementation of a therapeutic regimen. *Having responsibility for a person at risk for suicide creates high caregiver stress. Respite decreases caregiver stress. The presence of caring individuals is reassuring to both the client and caregivers, especially during periods of client anxiety. A client with suicidal ideation, especially if it is accompanied by depression or other psychiatric disorders, can benefit from use of the interventions described earlier, modified for the home setting.*

▲ If the client is on psychotropic medications, assess the client's and family's knowledge of medication administration and side effects. Teach as necessary. *Knowledge of the medical regimen promotes compliance and promotes safe use of medications.*

▲ Evaluate the effectiveness and side effects of medications, and adherence to the medication regimen. Review with the client and family all medications kept in the home; encourage discarding of old prescriptions. Monitor the amount of medications ordered/provided by the physician; limiting the amount of medications to which the client has access may be necessary. *Accurate clinical feedback improves the physician's ability to prescribe an effective medical regimen specific to the client's needs. At home, clients may have greater access to medications, including old prescriptions, that may be used to overdose.*

• = Independent; ▲ = Collaborative

Client/Family Teaching

- Establish a supportive relationship with family members. **Nursing Research:** *When families with a suicidal member experienced mental health care personnel as reaching out to them, they reported an ability to trust the personnel, treatment, and care; a feeling of being trusted; and a sense of hope (Talseth, Gilje, and Norberg, 2001).*

- Explain all relevant symptoms, procedures, treatments, and expected outcomes for suicidal ideation that is illness based (e.g., depression, bipolar disorder). *Self-care management has been posited to empower clients with depression and suicidal ideation (Allen and Hagerty, 2003). By increasing knowledge and adapting new behaviors, clients learn that they have some control over their health (Hennessy-Harstad, 1999). Clients are more amenable to therapy and better able to initiate appropriate self-care if they know what to expect.*

- Teach the family how to recognize that the client is at increased risk for suicide (changes in behavior and verbal and nonverbal communication, withdrawal, depression, or sudden lifting of depression). *A client may be at peace because a suicide plan has been made and the client has the energy to carry it out. Therefore, when depression lifts, increased vigilance is necessary.*

- Provide written instructions for treatments and procedures for which the client will be responsible. *A written record provides a concrete reference so that the client and family can clarify any verbal information that was given.*

- Instruct the client in coping strategies (assertiveness training, impulse control training, deep breathing, progressive muscle relaxation). *Suicidal ideation may be triggered by stress and painful emotions. Once clients are able to identify these triggers, they need to learn how to respond to them more effectively through assertiveness, impulse control, or relaxation techniques, as appropriate.*

- Role play (e.g., say, "Tell me how you will respond if a friend asks why you were in the hospital"). *Role playing is the most commonly used technique in assertiveness training. It deconditions the anxiety that arises from interpersonal encounters by allowing the client to practice how he or she might respond in a given situation. Anxiety levels tend to be higher in situations that are unfamiliar.*

- Teach cognitive behavioral activities, such as active problem solving, reframing (reappraising the situation from a different perspective), or thought stopping (in response to a negative thought, picturing a large stop sign and replacing the image with a prearranged positive alternative). Teach the client to confront his or her own negative thought patterns (or cognitive distortions), such as catastophizing (expecting the very worst), dichotomous thinking (perceiving events in only one of two opposite categories), or magnification (placing distorted emphasis on a single event). *Depressed and suicidal clients often have negative perceptions of themselves, their circumstances, and their future. Cognitive behavioral activities address clients' assumptions, beliefs, and attitudes about their situations, and foster modification of these elements to be as realistic and optimistic as possible. Persons with negative cognitive styles tend to perceive situations as overwhelming, resistant to improvement, and all encompassing. Through cognitive behavioral interventions, clients become more aware of their cognitive choices in adopting and maintaining their belief systems, and thereby exercise greater control over their own reactions (Hagerty and Patusky, 2003; Sinclair et al, 1998).*

- ▲ Provide the client and family with phone numbers of appropriate community agencies for therapy and counseling. *Continuous follow-up care should be implemented; therefore, the method to access this care must be given to the client.*

- **= Independent; ▲ = Collaborative**

WEBSITES FOR EDUCATION

evolve

See the EVOLVE website for World Wide Web resources for client education.

REFERENCES

Agbayewa MO, Marion SA, Wiggins S: Socioeconomic factors associated with suicide in elderly populations in British Columbia: an 11-year review, *Can J Psychiatry* 43:829, 1998.

Allen KS, Hagerty BM: Depression in primary care: empowering depressed patients to monitor their recurrent depression, in preparation, 2003.

Appleby L et al: Suicide within 12 months of contact with mental health services: national clinical survey, *Br Med J* 318:1235, 1999.

Apter A et al: Relationship between self-disclosure and serious suicidal behavior, *Compr Psychiatry* 42(1):70, 2001.

Barlow CA: Survivors of suicide: emerging counseling strategies, *J Psychosoc Nurs Ment Health Serv* 40:28, 2002.

Befrienders International: *The warning signs of suicide,* available online at http://www.befrienders.org/ suicide.htm, accessed June 22, 2003.

Bell MA: Losing connections: a process of decision-making in late-life suicidality, doctoral dissertation, Tucson, Ariz, 2000, University of Arizona.

Bowers L, Park A: Special observation in the care of psychiatric inpatients: a literature review, *Issues Ment Health Nurs* 22:769, 2001.

Calvert WJ: Protective factors within the family, and their role in fostering resiliency in African American adolescents, *J Cult Divers* 4(4):110, 1997.

Cleary M et al: Suicidal patients and special observation, *J Psychiatr Ment Health Nurs* 6:461, 1999.

Cochran M: Tears have no color, *Am J Nurs* 98(6):53, 1998.

Daugherty M: Suicide by cop, *J Calif Alliance Ment Ill* 10(2):79, 1999.

Diaz RM et al: The impact of homophobia, poverty, and racism on the mental health of gay and bisexual Latino men: findings from 3 US cities, *Am J Public Health* 91:927, 2001.

Doswell W, Erlen J: Multicultural issues and ethical concerns in the delivery of nursing care interventions, *Nurs Clin North Am* 33(2):353, 1998.

Draper B et al: Self-destructive behaviors in nursing home residents, *J Am Geriatr Soc* 50:354, 2002.

Drew BL: Self-harm behavior and no-suicide contracting in psychiatric inpatient settings, *Arch Psychiatr Nurs* 15:99, 2001.

D'Zurilla TJ et al: Social problem-solving deficits and hopelessness, depression, and suicidal risk in college students and psychiatric inpatients, *J Clin Psychol* 54:1091, 1998.

Fergusson DM, Horwood LJ, Beautrais AL: Is sexual orientation related to mental health problems and suicidality in young people? *Arch Gen Psychiatry* 56:883, 1999.

Filiberti A et al: Characteristics of terminal cancer patients who committed suicide during a home palliative care program, *J Pain Symptom Manage* 22:544, 2001.

Fisher BJ et al: Suicidal intent in patients with chronic pain, *Pain* 89(2-3):199, 2001.

Francis E et al: Utilization and outcome in an overnight psychiatric observation program at a Veterans Affairs medical center, *Psychiatr Serv* 51:92, 2000.

Giger JN, Davidhizar RE: *Transcultural nursing,* ed 2, St Louis, 1995, Mosby.

Gilman SE et al: Risk of psychiatric disorders among individuals reporting same-sex sexual partners in the National Comorbidity Survey, *Am J Public Health* 91:933, 2001.

Hagerty B, Patusky K: Mood disorders: depression and mania. In Fortinash KM, Holoday-Worret PA, editors: *Psychiatric mental health nursing,* ed 3, St Louis, 2003, Mosby.

Hauenstein EJ: Case finding and care in suicide: children, adolescents, and adults. In Boyd MA, editor: *Psychiatric nursing: contemporary practice,* ed 2, Philadelphia, 2002, Lippincott, p 1019.

Hennessy-Harstad EB: Empowering adolescents with asthma to take control through adaptation, *J Pediatr Health Care* 13:273, 1999.

Henriksson MM et al: Panic disorder in completed suicide, *J Clin Psychol* 57(7):275, 1996.

Hopkins C: "But what about the really ill, poorly people?" *J Psychiatr Ment Health Nurs* 9:147, 2002.

Horowitz LM et al: Detecting suicide risk in a pediatric emergency department: development of a brief screening tool, *Pediatrics* 107:1133, 2001.

• = **Independent;** ▲ = **Collaborative**

Horsfall J: Towards understanding some complex borderline behaviors, *J Psychiatr Ment Health Nurs* 6:425, 1999.

Houston K, Hawton K, Shepperd R: Suicide in young people aged 15-24: a psychological autopsy study, *J Affect Disord* 63(1-3):159, 2001.

Hulten A et al: Repetition of attempted suicide among teenagers in Europe: frequency, timing and risk factors, *Eur Child Adolesc Psychiatry* 10:161, 2001.

Isacsson G, Rich CL: Management of patients who deliberately harm themselves, *Br Med J* 322:213, 2001.

Joachim G, Acorn S: Stigma of visible and invisible chronic conditions, *J Adv Nurs* 32(1):243, 2000.

Kissane DW, Clarke DM, Street AF: Demoralization syndrome— relevant psychiatric diagnosis for palliative care, *J Palliat Care* 17(1):12, 2001.

Leenaars A et al: Controlling the environment to prevent suicide: international perspectives, *Can J Psychiatry* 45(7):639, 2000.

Leininger MM, McFarland MR: *Transcultural nursing: concepts, theories, research and practices,* ed 3, New York, 2002, McGraw-Hill.

Lorig K et al: Chronic disease self-management program: 2-year health status and health care utilization outcomes, *Med Care* 39:1217, 2001.

Majumdar B, Ladak S: Management of family and workplace stress experienced by women of color from various cultural backgrounds, *Can J Public Health* 89(1):48, 1998.

Malone KM et al: Protective factors against suicidal acts in major depression: reasons for living, *Am J Psychiatry* 157:1084, 2000.

Marcus P: Personality disorders. In Burgess A, editor: *Advanced practice psychiatric nursing,* Stamford, Conn, 1998, Appleton and Lange, pp 347-370.

McDermut W et al: Family functioning and suicidality in depressed adults, *Compr Psychiatry* 42:96, 2001.

National Guideline Clearing House: *Practice parameter for the assessment and treatment of children and adolescents with suicidal behavior,* available on-line at http://www.ngc.gov/FRAMESETS/guideline_fs.asp?guideline= 002245&sSearch_string=screening+for+suicide+risk, accessed June 22, 2003.

Neeleman J, Wessely S, Lewis G: Suicide acceptability in African and white Americans: the role of religion, *J Nerv Ment Dis* 186:12, 1998.

Quan H, Arboleda-Florez J: Elderly suicide in Alberta: difference by gender, *Can J Psychiatry* 44:762, 1999.

Rew L et al: Correlates of recent suicide attempts in a triethnic group of adolescents, *J Nurs Scholarsh* 33:361, 2001.

Rivera-Andino J, Lopez L: When culture complicates care, *RN* 63(7):47, 2000.

Rudd MD et al: Personality types and suicidal behavior: an exploratory study, *Suicide Life Threat Behav* 30(3): 199, 2000.

Schneidman E: *Contemporary suicide,* Washington, DC, 2001, American Psychological Association.

Shah S et al: Adolescent suicide and household access to firearms in Colorado: results of a case-control study, *J Adolesc Health* 26(3):157, 2000.

Sinclair VG et al: Effects of a cognitive-behavioral intervention for women with rheumatoid arthritis, *Res Nurs Health* 21:315, 1998.

Steadman HJ et al: Violence by people discharged from acute psychiatric inpatient facilities and by others in the same neighborhoods, *Arch Gen Psychiatry* 55:393, 1998.

Stuart GW, Laraia MT: Therapeutic nurse-patient relationship. In Stuart GW, Laraia MT, editors: *Principles and practice of psychiatric nursing,* St Louis, 2001, Mosby, p 30.

Surgeon General: *The Surgeon General's call to action to prevent suicide,* 1999, available at http://www.surgeongeneral.gov/library/calltoaction/fact3.htm, accessed Dec 1, 2002.

Talseth A, Gilje F, Norberg A: Being met—a passageway to hope for relatives of patients at risk of committing suicide: a phenomenological hermeneutic study, *Arch Psychiatr Nurs* 15:249, 2001.

Torrey EF, Zdanowicz M: Outpatient commitment: what, why, and for whom, *Psychiatr Serv* 52(3):337, 2001.

Uncapher H, Arean PA: Physicians are less willing to treat suicidal ideation in older patients, *J Am Geriatr Soc* 48:188, 2000.

Uncapher H et al: Hopelessness and suicidal ideation in older adults, *Gerontologist* 38:62, 1998a.

Uncapher H et al: Suicidal thoughts in male nursing home residents, *Ann Long Term Care* 6:301, 1998b.

Valente S: Suicide and elderly people: assessment and intervention, *J Death Dying* 28:317, 1994.

Vilhjalmsson R, Kristjansdottir G, Sveinbjarnardottir E: Factors associated with suicide ideation in adults, *Soc Psychiatry Psychiatr Epidemiol* 33(3):97, 1998.

Wilson C et al: Constructing mental illness as dangerous: a pilot study, *Austr N Z J Psychiatry* 33:240, 1999.

• = **Independent;** ▲ = **Collaborative**

Delayed Surgical recovery

Gail B. Ladwig

NANDA Definition

Extension in number of postoperative days required for individuals to initiate and perform on their own behalf activities that maintain life, health, and well-being

Defining Characteristics

Evidence of interrupted healing of surgical area (e.g., redness, induration, draining, immobility); loss of appetite with or without nausea; difficulty in moving about; need for help to complete self-care; fatigue; report of pain or discomfort; postponement in resumption of employment activities; perception that more time is needed to recover

Related Factors (r/t)

To be developed

NOC Outcomes (Nursing Outcomes Classification)

Suggested NOC Outcomes

Endurance; Infection Severity; Mobility; Pain Control; Self-Care: Activities of Daily Living (ADL); Wound Healing: Primary Intention, Secondary Intention

Example NOC Outcome with Indicators

Wound Healing: Primary Intention as evidenced by the following indicators: Skin approximation/Resolution of signs of infection of wound (Rate each indicator of **Wound Healing: Primary Intention:** 1 = none, 2 = limited, 3 = moderate, 4 = substantial, 5 = extensive [see Section I].)

Client Outcomes

Client Will (Specify Time Frame):

- Have surgical area that shows evidence of healing: no redness, induration, draining, or immobility
- State that appetite is regained
- State that no nausea is present
- Demonstrate ability to move about
- Demonstrate ability to complete self-care activities
- State that no fatigue is present
- State that pain is controlled or relieved after nursing interventions
- Resume employment activities/ADLs

NIC Interventions (Nursing Interventions Classification)

Suggested NIC Interventions

Incision Site Care; Nutrition Management; Pain Management; Self-Care Assistance

• = Independent; ▲ = Collaborative

> ## Example NIC Activities—Incision Site Care and Nutrition Management
>
> Teach client and/or family how to care for the incision, including how to recognize signs and symptoms of infection; Provide client with high-protein, high-calorie, nutritious finger foods and drinks that can be readily consumed, as appropriate

Nursing Interventions and Rationales

- Perform a thorough assessment of the client, including risk factors. **Nursing Research:** *Nursing interventions can either enhance or delay the healing process (King, 2001).* **Clinical Research:** *A hospital-based preoperative assessment clinic run by a highly qualified nurse on an outpatient basis can more efficiently use hospital resources and decrease preoperative inpatient time. The assessment of discharge requirements, which starts at the clinic, further reduces length of stay (Golubtsov et al, 1998).*

▲ Assess for the presence of medical conditions and treat appropriately before surgery. If the client is diabetic, maintain normal blood glucose levels before surgery. **Clinical Research:** *Good blood glucose control promotes faster healing (Cavanaugh et al, 1999). Some of the most commonly encountered and clinically significant impediments to healing include conditions such as diabetes mellitus (Stadelmann, Digenis, and Tobin, 1998).*

- Provide preoperative teaching by a nurse to decrease postoperative problems of anxiety, pain, nausea, and lack of independence. **Nursing Research:** *One study showed a significant decrease in anxiety 24 to 72 hours postoperatively for the group who had preoperative teaching by a nurse. The author recommends that all surgical clients receive a visit from theater nurses before their operations (Martin, 1996).* **Nursing Research:** *Those who displayed high fear wanted informational support from nurses more often than clients who showed lower fear. It was concluded that the fear and anxiety of clients awaiting coronary artery bypass grafting (CABG) are connected with their social support resources (Koivula et al, 2002).*

- Provide preoperative information in verbal and written form. **Nursing Research:** *Receipt of preparatory information of various types and in different forms appears to have positive effects on clients' ability to cope with and recover physically from a total hip replacement. Clients who received such information required significantly less postoperative intramuscular analgesia and were mobilized sooner with a Zimmer frame and walking sticks. In addition, their length of stay was, on average, 2 days shorter than that of the control group (Gammon and Mulholland, 1996).*

- Play music of the client's choice before surgery. **Nursing Research:** *Music listening by hospital clients reduces their anxiety, produces a small reduction in the respiratory rate, improves mood, and reduces the need for sedation and analgesia (Joanna Briggs Institute, 2001).*

▲ Consider using healing touch in the perianesthesia setting. **Nursing Research:** *Energy-medicine therapy such as healing touch is a powerful way to promote relaxation and enhance the healing process in the perianesthesia setting (King, 2000).*

- For female premenopausal clients, assess the date when the menstrual cycle is most likely to occur and schedule surgery on alternate dates if possible. **Clinical Research:** *Menstruation at the time of surgery increases the likelihood of vomiting to four times higher than normal (Haynes and Bailey, 1996).*

- Consider the use of an adjustable recliner if not contraindicated for recovery. **Nursing Research:** *Postsurgical laparoscopy clients who recovered in adjustable recliner-chairs*

- **= Independent; ▲ = Collaborative**

reached home readiness sooner and experienced greater comfort levels than clients who recovered in traditional hospital beds. Furthermore, clients in the recliner-chair group had fewer adverse symptoms such as nausea, severe pain, and delayed voiding (Agodoa, Holder, and Fowler, 2002).

- Do not offer fluids in the immediate postoperative period. **Clinical Research:** *Early ingestion of fluids in the postoperative period contributes to emesis. Oral intake before discharge from an ambulatory surgery unit increased the incidence of vomiting to four times that of the control group and prolonged the hospital stay (Haynes and Bailey, 1996).*

▲ In a client with postoperative nausea and vomiting, consider the use of multiple antiemetic medications (double or triple combinations of antiemetic agents acting at different neuroreceptor sites), less emetogenic anesthesia techniques, and adequate intravenous hydration. **Clinical Research:** *The combination of antiemetic therapy and the other measures mentioned improved efficacy of prevention and treatment of postoperative nausea and vomiting (Kovac, 2000).*

- The client should be provided with a complete, balanced therapeutic diet after the immediately postoperative period (24 to 48 hours). **Clinical Research:** *Suggestive evidence exists that improvement in nutritional status can improve outcomes of wound healing (Thomas, 1996).* **Nursing Research:** *Good nutrition is important for effective wound healing (Casey, 1998).*

- The client should have a nutritious diet with adequate protein intake that restores normal weight for the client. **Clinical Research:** *In a study that examined restoration of weight loss and healing of a "nonhealing wound," the rate of wound healing was most prominent after 50% of the weight loss had been restored. This finding reflects the key relationship between restoration of body weight, body protein stores, and wound healing (Demling and De Santi, 1998).*

- Use careful aseptic technique when caring for wounds. **Clinical Research:** *A significant impediment to wound healing is infection. Treatment of chronic wounds should be directed at the main causal factors responsible for the wound. Moreover, factors that may impede healing must be identified and corrected, if possible, for healing to occur (Stadelmann, Digenis, and Tobin, 1998).*

▲ Suggest the use of a semipermeable dressing and suction drainage for selected orthopedic clients. **Clinical Research:** *A combination of a semipermeable dressing and suction drainage was used successfully in 20 orthopedic clients without any wound complication and with satisfactory comfort to the client. This form of postoperative wound management appears to retain the nursing and hygiene advantages of suction drainage while avoiding the client discomfort and possibilities of wound infection associated with deep internal drainage (Strover and Thorpe, 1997).*

▲ Carefully consider the use of alternative therapy with a physician's order, such as application of aloe vera or aqueous cream to promote wound healing. **Nursing Research:** *Aloe vera gel or aqueous cream was used in a randomized study involving 225 clients with breast cancer who required a course of radiation therapy after lumpectomy or partial mastectomy. Aloe vera gel did not significantly reduce radiation-induced skin side effects. Aqueous cream was useful in reducing dry desquamation and pain related to radiation therapy (Heggie et al, 2002).*

- Clients should be allowed to shower after surgery to maintain cleanliness if not contraindicated because of the presence of pacemaker wires, etc. **Clinical Research:** *Clients undergoing open hernia repair who were allowed to shower showed no manifest infection*

● = Independent; ▲ = Collaborative

and no difference in wound healing compared to those who were not allowed to shower (Riederer and Inderbitzi, 1997).

- Provide supportive telephone calls from nurse to client as a means of decreasing anxiety and providing the psychosocial support necessary for recovery from surgery. **Clinical Research:** *Telephone calls are an effective method of providing supportive psychosocial care for individuals who may not be able to access this care because of geographic isolation, physical limitations, or discomfort with face-to-face interventions (Gotay and Bottomley, 1998).*

▲ Assess and treat for depression and anxiety in a client complaining of continuing fatigue after surgery. **Clinical Research:** *Level of fatigue at 30 days after coronary bypass surgery correlated with concurrent levels of depression and anxiety (Pick et al, 1994).*

▲ Consider the use of alternative therapies: hypnosis, aromatherapy, music, guided imagery, and massage. **Nursing Research:** *Alternative therapies offer high-touch balance when integrated with high-tech surgical treatments and may decrease anxiety (Norred, 2000).*

- Encourage the client to use prayer as a form of spiritual coping if this is comfortable for the client. **Clinical Research:** *Results of one study show that most clients pray about their postoperative problems and that private prayer appears to significantly decrease depression and general distress 1 year after CABG (Ai et al, 1998).*

- See the care plans for **Anxiety, Acute Pain, Fatigue,** and **Impaired physical Mobility.**

Geriatric

▲ Carefully assess the fluid and electrolyte status and glomerular filtration rate (GFR) of elderly clients before surgery. Provide fluid and electrolyte replacement per the physician's order. **Clinical Research:** *In many cases acute renal failure (ARF) can be prevented in older clients (e.g., by correcting any sodium deficit and hypovolemia before a surgical procedure and by considering the true GFR of a given client before prescribing a potentially nephrotoxic drug). Recovery is delayed in older clients and in those whose oliguric period is prolonged. The high cost of therapy for ARF justifies the use of all current preventive measures in clients at risk. The incidence of ARF is five times higher in elderly clients than in younger clients (Kleinknecht and Pallot, 1998).*

- Carefully evaluate the client's temperature. Know what is normal and abnormal for each client. Check baseline temperature and monitor trends. *Even a normal temperature (37° C [98.6° F]) can indicate an infection because many older adults have subnormal body temperatures (averaging 36° C [96.8° F]) (Faherty, 1994).*

▲ To maximize the recovery of walking ability in elderly clients with hip fracture, a multidisciplinary approach using skilled medical, nursing, and paramedical care appears to be optimal. **Clinical Research:** *In today's cost-cutting environment, caution must be used to prevent short-term cost-saving measures from compromising long-term outcome (Lyons, 1997).*

- Offer spiritual support. **Clinical Research:** *In a qualitative study, religion and spirituality were found to help older adults maintain and recover both physical and mental health (Mackenzie et al, 2000).*

Client/Family Teaching

▲ To decrease postoperative nausea and vomiting, the client should be instructed to fast before surgery, with the time frame to be determined by the physician. **Nursing Research:** *Fasting times for fluids should not normally be longer than 4 hours or less than*

- = **Independent;** ▲ = **Collaborative**

2 hours. Fasting times for solid food should not normally be longer than 6 hours or less than 4 hours. Inappropriately prolonged preoperative fasting might result in dehydration, electrolyte imbalance, hypoglycemia, discomfort, and confusion (Dean and Fawcett, 2002).
Nursing Research: *Fasting overnight or up to 8 hours before surgery can cause dehydration, electrolyte imbalance, malnutrition, and general malaise. Evidence shows that clients can benefit from receiving clear liquids up to 3 hours before surgery (Watson and Rinomhota, 2002).*

evolve WEBSITES FOR EDUCATION

See the EVOLVE website for World Wide Web resources for client education.

REFERENCES

Agodoa SE, Holder MA, Fowler SM: Effects of recliner-chair versus traditional hospital bed on postsurgical diagnostic laparoscopic recovery time, *J Perianesth Nurs* 17(5):318, 2002.

Ai AL et al: The role of private prayer in psychological recovery among midlife and aged patients following cardiac surgery, *Gerontologist* 38(5):591, 1998.

Casey G: The importance of nutrition in wound healing, *Nurs Stand* 13(3):51, 1998.

Cavanaugh P et al: Consensus development conference on diabetic wound foot care, American Diabetes Association, Boston Mass, April 7-8, 1999, available on-line at http://care.diabetesjournals.org/cgi/reprint/22/8/1354.pdf?ijkey=ae4410ea6195e10bbe290d5ada6908966f5739d7, accessed June 22, 2003.

Dean A, Fawcett T: Nurses' use of evidence in pre-operative fasting, *Nurs Stand* 17(12):33, 2002.

Demling R, De Santi L: Closure of the "non-healing wound" corresponds with correction of weight loss using the anabolic agent oxandrolone, *Ostomy Wound Manage* 44(10):58, 1998.

Faherty B: Myths and facts about older adults, *Nursing* 24(4):75, 1994.

Gammon J, Mulholland CW: Effect of preparatory information prior to elective total hip replacement on postoperative physical coping outcomes, *Int J Nurs Stud* 33(6):589, 1996.

Golubtsov BV et al: Pre-operative orthopaedic assessment clinic for major joint replacement operations: an assessment of value, *Health Bull* 56(3):648, 1998.

Gotay CC, Bottomley A: Providing psycho-social support by telephone: what is its potential in cancer patients? *Eur J Cancer Care* 7(4):225, 1998.

Haynes G, Bailey M: Charleston, South Carolina: postoperative nausea and vomiting—review and clinical approaches, *South Med J* Oct 1996, available online at http://www.sma.org/smj/96oct2.htm, accessed Feb 25, 2003.

Heggie S et al: A phase III study on the efficacy of topical aloe vera gel on irradiated breast tissue, *Cancer Nurs* 25(6):442, 2002.

Joanna Briggs Institute: Music as an intervention in hospitals, *Evidence Based Practice Information Sheets for Health Professionals* 5(4), 2001.

King CE: Healing pathways through energy work in the perianesthesia care setting, *CRNA* 11(4):180, 2000.

King L: Impaired wound healing in patients with diabetes, *Nurs Stand* 15(38):39, 2001.

Kleinknecht D, Pallot JL: Epidemiology and prognosis of acute renal insufficiency in 1997, *Nephrologie* 19(2):49, 1998.

Koivula M et al: Social support and its relation to fear and anxiety in patients awaiting coronary artery bypass grafting, *J Clin Nurs* 11(5):622, 2002.

Kovac AL: Prevention and treatment of postoperative nausea and vomiting, *Drugs* 59(2):213, 2000.

Lyons AR: Clinical outcomes and treatment of hip fractures, *Am J Med* 103(2A):51S (discussion 63S), 1997.

Mackenzie ER et al: Spiritual support and psychological well-being: older adults' perceptions of the religion and health connection, *Altern Ther Health Med* 6(6):37, 2000.

Martin D: Pre-operative visits to reduce patient anxiety: a study, *Nurs Stand* 10(23):33, 1996.

Norred CL: Minimizing preoperative anxiety with alternative caring-healing therapies, *AORN J* 72(5):838, 2000.

Pick B et al: Post-operative fatigue following coronary artery bypass surgery: relationship to emotional state and to the catecholamine response to surgery, *J Psychosom Res* 38(6):599, 1994.

• = Independent; ▲ = Collaborative

Riederer SR, Inderbitzi R: [Does a shower put postoperative wound healing at risk]? *Chirurg* 68(7):715 (discussion 717), 1997.

Stadelmann WK, Digenis AG, Tobin GR: Impediments to wound healing, *Am J Surg* 176(2A suppl):39S, 1998.

Strover AE, Thorpe R: Suction dressings: a new surgical dressing technique, *J R Coll Surg Edinb* 42(2):119, 1997.

Thomas DR: Nutritional factors affecting wound healing, *Ostomy Wound Manage* 42(5):40, 1996.

Watson K, Rinomhota S: Preoperative fasting: we need a new consensus, *Nurs Times* 98(15):36, 2002.

Impaired Swallowing

Roslyn Fine and Betty J. Ackley

NANDA Definition

Abnormal functioning of the swallowing mechanism associated with deficits in oral, pharyngeal, or esophageal structure or function

Defining Characteristics

- Oral phase impairment: Lack of tongue action to form bolus; weak suck resulting in inefficient nippling; incomplete lip closure; pushing of food out of mouth; slow bolus formation; falling of food from mouth; premature entry of bolus; nasal reflux; inability to clear oral cavity; long meals with little consumption; coughing, choking, or gagging before a swallow; abnormality in oral phase of swallow study; piecemeal deglutition; lack of chewing; pooling in lateral sulci; sialorrhea or drooling
- Pharyngeal phase impairment: Altered head position; inadequate laryngeal elevation; food refusal; unexplained fever; delayed swallow; recurrent pulmonary infections; gurgly voice quality; nasal reflux; choking, coughing, or gagging; multiple swallows; abnormality in pharyngeal phase by swallowing study
- Esophageal phase impairment: Heartburn or epigastric pain; acidic-smelling breath; unexplained irritability surrounding mealtime; vomitus on pillow; repetitive swallowing or ruminating; regurgitation of gastric contents or wet belches; bruxism; nighttime coughing or awakening; observed evidence of difficulty in swallowing (e.g., stasis of food in oral cavity, coughing, or choking); hyperextension of head, arching during or after meals; abnormality in esophageal phase by swallow study; odynophagia; food refusal or volume limiting; complaints of "something stuck"; hematemesis; vomiting

Related Factors (r/t)

Congenital deficits; upper airway anomalies; failure to thrive; protein energy malnutrition; conditions with significant hypotonia; respiratory disorders; history of tube feeding; behavioral feeding problems; self-injurious behavior; neuromuscular impairment (e.g., decreased or absent gag reflex, decreased strength or excursion of muscles involved in mastication, perceptual impairment, or facial paralysis); mechanical obstruction (e.g., edema, tracheotomy tube, or tumor); congenital heart disease; cranial nerve involvement; neurological problems; upper airway anomalies; laryngeal abnormalities; achalasia; gastroesophageal reflux disease; acquired anatomic defects; cerebral palsy; internal or external traumas; tracheal, laryngeal, or esophageal defects; traumatic head injury; developmental delay; nasal or nasopharyngeal cavity defects; oral cavity or oropharynx abnormalities; prematurity

• = Independent; ▲ = Collaborative

| NOC | Outcomes (Nursing Outcomes Classification) |

Suggested NOC Outcomes

Swallowing Status; Swallowing Status: Esophageal Phase, Oral Phase, Pharyngeal Phase

---

Example NOC Outcome with Indicators

Swallowing Status as evidenced by the following indicators: Delivery of bolus to hypopharynx commensurate with swallow reflex/Ability to clear oral cavity/Number of swallows appropriate for bolus size and texture/Normal voice quality/Absence of choking, coughing, gagging/Normal swallow effort (Rate each indicator of **Swallowing Status:** 1 = extremely compromised, 2 = substantially compromised, 3 = moderately compromised, 4 = mildly compromised, 5 = not compromised [see Section I].)

Client Outcomes

Client Will (Specify Time Frame):
- Demonstrate effective swallowing without choking or coughing
- Remain free from aspiration (e.g., lungs clear, temperature within normal range)

| NIC | Interventions (Nursing Interventions Classification) |

Suggested NIC Interventions

Aspiration Precautions; Swallowing Therapy

Example NIC Activities—Swallowing Therapy

Assist client to sit in erect position (as close to 90 degrees as possible) for feeding/exercise; Instruct client not to talk during eating, if appropriate

---

Nursing Interventions and Rationales

- Determine the client's readiness to eat. The client needs to be alert, able to follow instructions, able to hold the head erect, and able to move the tongue in the mouth. *If one of these elements is missing, it may be advisable to withhold oral feeding and use enteral feeding for nourishment (McHale et al, 1998). Cognitive deficits can result in aspiration even if the client is able to swallow adequately (Poertner and Coleman, 1998).*
- ▲ If the swallowing impairment is of new onset, ensure that the client receives a diagnostic workup. *There are multiple causes of swallowing impairment, some of which are treatable (Schechter, 1998).*
- Assess ability to swallow by positioning the thumb and index finger on the client's laryngeal protuberance. Ask the client to swallow; feel the larynx elevate. Ask the client to cough; test for a gag reflex on both sides of the posterior pharyngeal wall (lingual surface) with a tongue blade. Do not rely on the presence of a gag reflex to determine when to feed. *Normally the time required for the bolus to move from the point at which the reflex is triggered to the esophageal entry (pharyngeal transit time) is <1 second (Logemann, 1983). Clients can aspirate even if they have an intact gag reflex (Baker, 1993; Lugger, 1994).* **Clinical Research:** *Cerebrovascular accident (CVA) clients with prolonged pharyngeal transit times (prolonged swallowing) have a greatly increased chance of developing aspiration pneumonia (Johnson, McKenzie, and Sievers, 1993).*
- Consider the use of the Massey Bedside Swallowing Screen to screen for swallowing

• = Independent; ▲ = Collaborative

dysfunction. **Nursing Research:** *The Massey Bedside Swallowing Screen demonstrated high sensitivity and specificity in predicting dysphagia, compared to assessment by experts in the field (Massey and Jedlicka, 2002).*

- Observe for signs associated with swallowing problems (e.g., coughing, choking, spitting of food, drooling, difficulty handling oral secretions, double swallowing or major delay in swallowing, watering eyes, nasal discharge, wet or gurgly voice, decreased ability to move the tongue and lips, decreased mastication of food, decreased ability to move food to the back of the pharynx, slow or scanning speech). *These are all signs of swallowing impairment (Lugger, 1994; Terrado, Russell, and Bowman, 2001).*

▲ If the client has impaired swallowing, refer to a speech pathologist for bedside evaluation as soon as possible. Ensure that the client is seen by a speech pathologist within 72 hours after admission if the client has had a CVA. *Speech pathologists specialize in impaired swallowing. Early referral of CVA clients to a speech pathologist, along with early initiation of nutritional support, results in decreased length of hospital stay, shortened recovery time, and reduced overall health costs (Scott, 1998).* **Clinical Research:** *Research demonstrates that a program of diagnosis and treatment of dysphagia in acute stroke management decreases the incidence of pneumonia (AHCPR, 1999).*

▲ To manage impaired swallowing, use a dysphagia team composed of a rehabilitation nurse, speech pathologist, dietitian, physician, and radiologist who work together. *The dysphagia team can help the client learn to swallow safely and maintain a good nutritional status (Davies, 2002; Poertner and Coleman, 1998).*

▲ If the client has impaired swallowing, do not feed until an appropriate diagnostic workup is completed. Ensure proper nutrition by consulting with a physician regarding enteral feedings, preferably using a percutaneous endoscopic gastrostomy (PEG) tube in most cases. *Feeding a client who cannot adequately swallow results in aspiration and possibly death.* **Clinical Research:** *Enteral feedings via PEG tube are generally preferable to nasogastric tube feedings because studies have demonstrated that nutritional status is better and survival rates are possibly improved (Bath, Bath, and Smithard, 2000).*

- If the client has an intact swallowing reflex, attempt to feed. Observe the following feeding guidelines:
  - Position the client upright at a 90-degree angle with the head flexed forward at a 45-degree angle (Galvan, 2001). This position forces the trachea to close and the esophagus to open, which makes swallowing easier and reduces the risk of aspiration.
  - Ensure that the client is awake, alert, and able to follow sequenced directions before attempting to feed. As the client becomes less alert, the swallowing response decreases, which increases the risk of aspiration.
  - Begin by feeding the client one third of a teaspoon of applesauce. Provide sufficient time to masticate and swallow.
  - Place the food on the unaffected side of the tongue.
  - During feeding, give the client specific directions (e.g., "Open your mouth, chew the food completely, and when you are ready, tuck your chin to your chest and swallow").
  ▲ Watch for uncoordinated chewing or swallowing; coughing immediately after eating or delayed coughing, which may indicate silent aspiration; pocketing of food; wet-sounding voice; sneezing when eating; delay of more than 1 second in swallowing; or a change in respiratory patterns. If any of these signs is present, put on gloves, remove all food from the oral cavity, stop feedings, and consult with a speech

• = **Independent;** ▲ = **Collaborative**

and language pathologist and a dysphagia team. *These are signs of impaired swallowing and possible aspiration (Baker, 1993; Galvan, 2001).*

- If the client tolerates single-textured foods such as pudding, hot cereal, or strained baby food, advance to a soft diet with guidance from the dysphagia team. Avoid foods such as hamburgers, corn, and pastas that are difficult to chew. Also avoid sticky foods such as peanut butter and white bread. *The dysphagia team should determine the appropriate diet for the client based on progression in swallowing and need to ensure that the client is nourished and hydrated.*
- Avoid providing liquids until the client is able to swallow effectively. Add a thickening agent to liquids to obtain a soft consistency that is similar to nectar, honey, or pudding, depending on the degree of swallowing problems. *Liquids can be easily aspirated; thickened liquids form a cohesive bolus that the client can swallow with increased efficiency (Langmore and Miller, 1994; Poertner and Coleman, 1998).*
- Preferably use prepackaged thickened liquids, or use a viscosimeter to ensure appropriate thickness. *Often staff members overthicken liquids, which results in decreased palatability with decreased intake.* **Clinical Research:** *Using prepackaged thickened liquids or a viscosimeter to determine appropriate thickness can increase intake, which increases hydration and nutrition (Boczko, 2000; Goulding and Bakheit, 2000).*
- ▲ Work with the client on swallowing exercises prescribed by the dysphagia team (e.g., touching the palate with the tongue, stimulating the tonsillar arch and soft palate with a cold metal examination mirror [thermal stimulation], labial/lingual range-of-motion exercises). *Swallowing exercises can improve the client's ability to swallow (Langmore and Miller, 1994). Exercises need to be done at intervals, which necessitates nursing involvement (Poertner and Coleman, 1998).*
- ▲ For many adult clients, avoid the use of straws if recommended by the speech pathologist. *Use of straws can increase the risk of aspiration because straws can result in spilling of a bolus of fluid in the oral cavity as well as decrease control of the posterior transit of fluid to the pharynx (Travers, 1999).*
- Provide meals in a quiet environment away from excessive stimuli such as a community dining room. *A noisy environment can be an aversive stimulus and can decrease effective mastication and swallowing. Talking and laughing while eating increase the risk of aspiration (Galvan, 2001).*
- Ensure that there is adequate time for the client to eat. *Clients with swallowing impairments often take two to four times longer than others to eat, if they are being fed. Often, food is offered rapidly to speed up the task, and this can increase the chance of aspiration (Poertner and Coleman, 1998).*
- ▲ Have suction equipment available during feeding. If choking occurs and suctioning is necessary, discontinue oral feeding until the client is safely assessed with a videofluoroscopic swallow study and fiberoptic endoscopic evaluation of swallowing, whichever the client can safely tolerate. *Suctioning may be necessary if the client is choking on food and could aspirate.*
- Check the oral cavity for proper emptying after the client swallows and after the client finishes the meal. Provide oral care at the end of the meal. It may be necessary to manually remove food from the client's mouth. If this is the case, use gloves and keep the client's teeth apart with a padded tongue blade. *Food may become pocketed on the affected side and cause stomatitis, tooth decay, and possible later aspiration.*
- Praise the client for successfully following directions and swallowing appropriately. *Praise reinforces behavior and sets up a positive atmosphere in which learning takes place.*

- = Independent; ▲ = Collaborative

- Keep the client in an upright position for 45 minutes to an hour after a meal. *Maintaining an upright position ensures that food stays in the stomach until it has emptied and decreases the chance of aspiration following meals (Galvan, 2001).* **Clinical Research:** *A study demonstrated that the number of elderly clients developing a fever was significantly reduced when clients were kept sitting upright after eating (Matsui et al, 2002).*
- ▲ Watch for signs of aspiration and pneumonia. Auscultate lung sounds after feeding. Note new crackles or wheezing, and note elevated temperature. Notify the physician as needed. *The presence of new crackles or wheezing, an elevated temperature or white blood cell count, and a change in sputum could indicate aspiration of food (Murray and Brzozowski, 1998). It could also indicate the presence of pneumonia (Galvan, 2001). Clients with dysphagia are at serious risk for aspiration pneumonia (Kedlaya and Brandstater, 2002; Langmore, 1999).*
- Watch for signs of malnutrition and dehydration. Keep a record of food intake. *A food intake record will allow the nurse, speech and language pathologist, and dietitian to determine the adequacy of nutritional intake (Beadle, Townsend, and Palmer, 1995). Malnutrition is common in dysphagic clients (Galvan, 2001). Clients with dysphagia are at serious risk for malnutrition and dehydration, which can lead to aspiration pneumonia resulting from depressed immune function and weakness, lethargy, and decreased cough (Langmore, 1999).*
- Weigh the client weekly to help evaluate nutritional status. Evaluate nutritional status daily. If the client is not adequately nourished, work with the dysphagia team to determine whether the client needs to avoid oral intake with therapeutic feeding only or needs enteral feedings until the client can swallow adequately. **Clinical Research:** *One study demonstrated that dysphagic stroke clients who received thickened-fluid dysphagia diets failed to meet their needs for fluids, whereas a group receiving enteral feeding and intravenous fluid did meet fluid requirements (Finestone et al, 2001).* **Nursing Research:** *Four independent risk factors for dysphagia—hypoglossal nerve dysfunction, National Institutes of Health Stroke Scale score, incomplete oral labial closure, and wet voice after swallowing water—predicted the need for tube feedings in stroke clients with dysphagia (Wojner and Alexandrov, 2000).*
- ▲ If the client has a tracheotomy, ask for a diagnostic workup before attempting to feed and ensure that all staff members know the appropriate feeding technique. *Aspiration is common in clients with tracheotomies, and care must be used in feeding (Murray and Brzozowski, 1998). See the care plan for* **Risk for Aspiration.**

Pediatric
- ▲ Refer to a physician a child who has difficulty swallowing and symptoms such as difficulty manipulating food, delayed swallow response, and pocketing of a bolus of food. *Research has indicated that surgery should be used to correct structural deficits (e.g., those related to pyloric stenosis, neurological disorders that involve cranial nerve pathways, and disorders resulting in swallowing changes, such as brain injury and cerebral palsy [Rosenthal, Sheppard, and Lotze, 1995]). Respiratory and gastrointestinal system disorders (gastroesophageal reflux disease) and esophagitis can affect swallowing and nutrition. These systemic disorders are diagnosed by a physician and treated with medications.*
- When feeding an infant or child, place the infant/child in a 90-degree position with the head slightly flexed. Change the consistency of the diet as needed, and use a curly

• = **Independent;** ▲ = **Collaborative**

straw for young children to facilitate tucking the chin, which helps improve swallowing ability (Arvedson and Brodsky, 1993).

- Give oral motor stimulation that increases oral-sensory awareness by waking the mouth using exercises that focus on temperature, taste, and texture. *Many of these infants require supplemental tube feedings as well as special nipples or bottles to boost oral intake.*
- For infants with poor sucking and swallowing, do the following:
  - Support the cheeks and jaw to increase sucking skills. Pace or rhythmically move the bottle, which encourages better suck-swallow-breath synchrony.
- ▲ Work with the dietitian. Some infants may need a high-calorie formula so that food volume can be decreased (which requires the infant to expend less energy) while still meeting nutritional requirements (Klein and Tracey, 1994). Some infants may also need to have the tongue brushed, which provides tongue stimulation (tongue tip and tongue lateralization) and promotes lip seal and lip pursing.
- Watch for indicators of aspiration: coughing, a change in web vocal quality while feeding, perspiration and color changes during feeding, sneezing, and increased heart rate and breathing.
- Watch for warning signs of reflux: sour-smelling breath after eating, sneezing, lack of interest in feeding, crying and fussing extraordinarily when feeding, pained expressions when feeding, and excessive chewing and swallowing after eating.

  Many premature and medically fragile children experience growth deficits and respiratory problems from an underlying dysphagia. Some infants may need to work harder to breathe than others and as a result develop a decreased tolerance for food intake. They also demonstrate inconsistent arousal and poor/uncoordinated suck-swallow-breath synchrony. Many of these infants require supplemental tube feedings, as well as the use of special nipples or bottles to boost oral intake.

Geriatric

- ▲ Evaluate medications the client is presently taking, especially if elderly. Consult with the pharmacist for assistance in monitoring for incorrect dosages and drug interactions that could result in dysphagia. *Dysphagia is more prevalent in the elderly than in younger persons because of the coexistence of a variety of neurological, neuromuscular, or oncological conditions (Kosta and Mitchell, 1998). Most elderly clients take numerous medications, which when taken individually can slow motor function, cause anxiety and depression, and reduce salivary flow. When taken together, these medications can interact, resulting in impaired swallowing function. Drugs that reduce muscle tone for swallowing and can cause reflux include calcium channel blockers and nitrates. Drugs that can reduce salivary flow include antidepressants, antiparkinsonism drugs, antihistamines, antispasmodics, antipsychotic agents or major tranquilizers, antiemetics, antihypertensives, and drugs for treating diarrhea and anxiety (Schechter, 1998; Sliwa and Lis, 1993; Sonies, 1992).*
- Recognize that the elderly client with dementia needs a longer time to eat. *The dementia client has decreased cognition, distractibility, and decreased efficiency in chewing and is likely to have problems with swallowing (Granville, 2002).*
- Recognize that the loss of teeth can cause problems with chewing and swallowing. *Without teeth, three to four times more effort may be required to chew food so that it is able to be swallowed (Granville, 2002).*

• = Independent; ▲ = Collaborative

Client/Family Teaching

▲ Teach the client and family exercises prescribed by the dysphagia team.

• Teach the client a step-by-step method of swallowing effectively.

• Educate the client, family, and all caregivers about rationales for food consistency and choices. *It is common for family members to disregard necessary dietary restrictions and give the client inappropriate foods that predispose to aspiration (Poertner and Coleman, 1998).*

• Teach the family how to monitor the client to prevent aspiration during eating.

evolve WEBSITES FOR EDUCATION

See the EVOLVE website for World Wide Web resources for client education.

REFERENCES

AHCPR: *Diagnosis and treatment of swallowing disorders (dysphagia) in acute-care stroke patients,* Evidence Report/Technology Assessment No. 8, AHCPR Pub No. 99-E024, 1999.

Arvedson JC, Brodsky L: *Pediatric swallowing and feeding assessment and management,* San Diego, 1993, Singular.

Baker DM: Assessment and management of impairments in swallowing, *Nurs Clin North Am* 28:793, 1993.

Bath PM, Bath FJ, Smithard EG: Interventions for dysphagia in acute stroke, *Cochrane Database Syst Rev* 2(CD000323), DJ9, 2000.

Beadle L, Townsend S, Palmer D: The management of dysphagia in stroke, *Nurs Stand* 9:37, 1995.

Boczko T: Increasing liquid consumption in patients with dysphagia, *Adv Speech Language Pathol Audiol* 10(45), 2000.

Davies S: An interdisciplinary approach to the management of dysphagia, *Prof Nurse* 18(1):22, 2002.

Finestone HM et al: Quantifying fluid intake in dysphagic stroke patients: a preliminary comparison of oral and nonoral strategies, *Arch Phys Med Rehabil* 82(12):1744, 2001.

Galvan TJ: Dysphagia: going down and staying down, *Am J Nurs* 101(1):37, 2001.

Goulding R, Bakheit A: Evaluation of the benefits of monitoring fluid thickness in the dietary management of dysphagic stroke patients, *Clin Rehabil* 14:119, 2000.

Granville L: *Introduction to comprehensive geriatric assessment,* Presented at the Florida Speech-Language-Hearing Association Convention, Orlando, Fla, Sept 21-22, 2002.

Johnson ER, McKenzie SW, Sievers A: Aspiration pneumonia in stroke, *Arch Phys Med Rehabil* 74:973, 1993.

Kedlaya D, Brandstater ME: Swallowing, nutrition and hydration during acute stroke care, *Top Stroke Rehabil* 9(2):23, 2002.

Klein MD, Tracey A: *Feeding and nutrition for the child with special needs,* Tucson, Ariz, 1994, Therapy Skill Builders.

Kosta JC, Mitchell CA: Current procedures for diagnosing dysphagia in elderly clients, *Geriatr Nurs* 19(4):195, 1998.

Langmore SE: Risk factors for aspiration pneumonia, *Nutr Clin Pract* 14(5):S41, 1999.

Langmore SE, Miller RM: Behavioral treatment for adults with oropharyngeal dysphagia, *Arch Phys Med Rehabil* 75:1154, 1994.

Logemann JA: *Evaluation and treatment of swallowing disorders,* San Diego, 1983, College Hill.

Lugger KE: Dysphagia in the elderly stroke patient, *J Neurosci Nurs* 26:78, 1994.

Massey R, Jedlicka D: The Massey Bedside Swallowing Screen, *J Neurosci Nurs* 34(5):252, 2002.

Matsui T et al: Sitting position to prevent aspiration in bed-bound patients, *Gerontology* 48:194, 2002.

McHale JM et al: Expert nursing knowledge in the care of the patients at risk of impaired swallowing, *Image J Nurs Sch* 30(2):237, 1998.

Murray KA, Brzozowski LA: Swallowing in patients with tracheotomies, *AACN Clin Issues* 9(3):416, 1998.

Poertner LC, Coleman RF: Swallowing therapy in adults, *Otolaryngol Clin North Am* 31(3):561, 1998.

Rosenthal WR, Sheppard JJ, Lotze M: *Dysphagia and the child with developmental disabilities,* San Diego, 1995, Singular.

• = **Independent**; ▲ = **Collaborative**

Schechter GL: Systemic causes of dysphagia in adults, *Otolaryngol Clin North Am* 31(3):525, 1998.

Scott A: Swallowing in strokes, *Adv Speech Pathol Audiol* Oct 26:15, 1998.

Sliwa JA, Lis S: Drug-induced dysphagia, *Arch Phys Med Rehabil* 74:445, 1993.

Sonies BC: Oropharyngeal dysphagia in the elderly. In Baum BJ, editor: *Clinics in geriatric medicine,* Philadelphia, 1992, WB Saunders.

Terrado M, Russell C, Bowman JF: Dysphagia: an overview, *Medsurg Nurs* 10(5):233, 2001.

Travers P: Poststroke dysphagia: implications for nurses, *Rehabil Nurs* 24(2):69, 1999.

Wojner AW, Alexandrov AV: Predictors of tube feeding in acute stroke patients with dysphagia, *AACN Clin Issues* 11(4):531, 2000.

Effective Therapeutic regimen management

Margaret Lunney

NANDA Definition

Pattern of regulating and integrating into daily living a program for treatment of illness and its sequelae that is satisfactory for meeting specific health goals

Defining Characteristics

Appropriate choices of daily activities for meeting goals of a treatment or prevention program; illness symptoms within normal range of expectation; verbalization of desire to manage treatment of illness and prevention of sequelae; verbalization of intent to reduce risk factors for progression of illness and sequelae

Related Factors (r/t)

None. Related factors are not relevant with strength diagnoses.

NOC Outcomes (Nursing Outcomes Classification)

Suggested NOC Outcomes

Knowledge: Treatment Regimen; Participation in Health Care Decisions; Risk Control; Symptom Control

---

Example NOC Outcome with Indicators

Knowledge: Treatment Regimen (select the level of achievement on the following scale: 1 = none, 2 = limited, 3 = moderate, 4 = substantial, 5 = extensive [see Section I]) as evidenced by the following indicator: Description of prescribed medication, activity, exercise, and disease process (Rate the indicator of **Knowledge: Treatment Regimen** on the same five-point scale.)

Client Outcomes

Client Will (Specify Time Frame):

- Acknowledge appropriateness of choices for meeting goals of treatment or prevention programs
- Agree to continue making appropriate choices
- Verbalize intent to contact health provider(s) for additional information, support, or resources as needed

• = Independent; ▲ = Collaborative

| **NIC** | **Interventions (Nursing Interventions Classification)** |

Suggested NIC Interventions

Anticipatory Guidance; Health Education; Health Screening; Health System Guidance; Learning Facilitation; Learning Readiness Enhancement; Risk Identification; Self-Modification Assistance

| **Example NIC Activities—Learning Facilitation** |

Relate information in a stimulating manner; Encourage client's active participation

Nursing Interventions and Rationales

NOTE: Little or no research is being done to investigate interventions to maintain strengths. Theoretical rationales are provided as evidence rather than as research findings.

- Acknowledge the congruence of activities of daily living (ADLs) with health-related goals. **Theoretical Rationale:** *Support from health provider(s) in efforts made to manage therapeutic regimens motivates individuals to continue these efforts despite difficulties (Miller, 2000).*
- Support decisions regarding methods of integrating therapeutic regimens into ADLs. **Theoretical Rationale:** *Support from health providers for previous decisions provides evidence of continued ability to successfully manage therapeutic regimens (Miller, 2000).*
- Provide information on possible illness trajectories to allow planning for future management. **Theoretical Rationale:** *Knowledge and awareness of illness trajectories enables the individual to plan for future management of therapeutic regimens (Lubkin and Larsen, 2002).*
- Assist the client in resolving ambivalent feelings about illness and management of the therapeutic regimen. **Theoretical Rationale:** *Wide variations may exist in attitudes and ambivalence toward illness and management of illness regimens. Ambivalence interferes with effective decision making regarding illness care (Chinn et al, 2000).*
- Review methods of contacting health provider(s) for changes in therapeutic regimen and/or methods of incorporating therapeutic regimens into ADLs. **Theoretical Rationale:** *The partnership process includes continued contact as changes occur; people with chronic illnesses need to know how to obtain interventions that are needed in the future (Gallant, Beaulieu, and Carnevale, 2002; Lubkin and Larsen, 2002).*
- Record the effectiveness of managing the therapeutic regimens. **Theoretical Rationale:** *For clients who are at risk of ineffective management of therapeutic regimens, health providers may continue to assess and diagnose this phenomenon unnecessarily. It saves the health care system time, effort, and money if the assessment and diagnosis of effective management is communicated to other health providers.*

Multicultural

- Assess for the influence of cultural beliefs, norms, and values on the individual's perceptions of the therapeutic regimen. **Nursing Research:** *What the individual considers therapeutic may be based on cultural perceptions (Leininger and McFarland, 2002).*
- Use a family-centered approach when working with Latino, Asian, African American, and Native American clients. **Nursing Research:** *Latinos may perceive the family as a source of support, solver of problems, and source of pride (Leininger and McFarland, 2002). Asian Americans may regard the family as the primary decision maker and influence on indi-*

• = **Independent;** ▲ = **Collaborative**

vidual family members (D'Avanzo et al, 2001). Native American families may have extended structures and exert powerful influences over functioning (Leininger and McFarland, 2002).

- Discuss with the client those aspects of health and lifestyle that will remain unchanged by his or her health status. **Theoretical Rationale:** *Aspects of the client's life that are meaningful and valuable to him or her should be understood and preserved without change (Leininger and McFarland, 2002).*
- Validate the client's feelings regarding the ability to manage his or her own care and the impact on current lifestyle. **Theoretical Rationale:** *Validation of feelings lets the client know that the nurse has heard and understood what was said, and it promotes the nurse-client relationship (Stuart and Laraia, 2001).*

Client/Family Teaching

- Teach about the disease trajectory and ways to manage disease symptoms as the trajectory changes.

evolve WEBSITES FOR EDUCATION

See the EVOLVE website for World Wide Web resources for client education.

REFERENCES

Chinn MH et al: Developing a conceptual framework for understanding illness and attitudes in older, urban African Americans with diabetes, *Diabetes Educ* 26(3):439, 2000.

D'Avanzo CE et al: Developing culturally informed strategies for substance-related interventions. In Naegle MA, D'Avanzo CE, editors: *Addictions and substance abuse: strategies for advanced practice nursing,* St Louis, 2001, Mosby.

Gallant MH, Beaulieu MC, Carnevale FA: Partnership: an analysis of the concept within the nurse-client relationship, *J Adv Nurs* 40(2):149, 2002.

Leininger MM, McFarland MR: *Transcultural nursing: concepts, theories, research and practices,* ed 3, New York, 2002, McGraw-Hill.

Lubkin IM, Larsen PD: *Chronic illness: impact and interventions,* ed 5, Boston, 2002, Jones and Bartlett.

Miller JF: *Coping with chronic illness: overcoming powerlessness,* ed 3, Philadelphia, 2000, FA Davis.

Stuart GW, Laraia MT: Therapeutic nurse-patient relationship. In Stuart GW, Laraia MT, editors: *Principles and practice of psychiatric nursing,* St Louis, 2001, Mosby.

Ineffective Therapeutic regimen management

Margaret Lunney

NANDA Definition

Pattern of regulating and integrating into daily living a program for treatment of illness and its sequelae that is unsatisfactory for meeting specific health goals

Defining Characteristics

Choices of daily living ineffective for meeting goals of a treatment or prevention program; verbalization that client did not take action to reduce risk factors for progression of illness and sequelae; verbalization of desire to manage treatment of illness and prevention of sequelae; verbalization of difficulty with regulation of one or more prescribed regimens

- = Independent; ▲ = Collaborative

for prevention of complications and treatment of illness or its effects; verbalization that client did not take action to include treatment regimens in daily routines

Related Factors (r/t)

Perceived barriers; social support deficits; powerlessness; perceived susceptibility; perceived benefits; mistrust of regimen and/or health care personnel; knowledge deficit; family patterns of health care; family conflict; excessive demands made on individual or family; economic difficulties; decisional conflicts; complexity of therapeutic regimen; complexity of health care system; faulty perception of illness seriousness; inadequate number and types of cues to action

NOC Outcomes (Nursing Outcomes Classification)

Suggested NOC Outcomes
Decision Making; Knowledge: Disease Process, Treatment Regimen; Participation in Health Care Decisions; Symptom Severity; Treatment Behavior: Illness or Injury

---

Example NOC Outcome with Indicators

Knowledge: Treatment Regimen (select the level of achievement on the following scale: 1 = none, 2 = limited, 3 = moderate, 4 = substantial, 5 = extensive [see Section I]) as evidenced by the following indicator: Description of prescribed medication, activity, exercise, and disease process (Rate the indicator of **Knowledge: Treatment Regimen** on the same five-point scale.)

Client Outcomes

Client Will (Specify Time Frame):
- Describe daily food and fluid intake that meets therapeutic goals
- Describe activity/exercise patterns that meet therapeutic goals
- Describe scheduling of medications that meets therapeutic goals
- Verbalize ability to manage therapeutic regimens
- Collaborate with health providers to decide on therapeutic regimen that is congruent with health goals and lifestyle

NIC Interventions (Nursing Interventions Classification)

Suggested NIC Interventions
Anticipatory Guidance; Health Education; Health Screening; Health System Guidance; Learning Facilitation; Learning Readiness Enhancement; Risk Identification; Self-Modification Assistance

---

Example NIC Activities—Learning Facilitation

Relate information in a stimulating manner; Encourage client's active participation

---

Nursing Interventions and Rationales

NOTE: This diagnosis does not have the same meaning as the diagnosis **Noncompliance.** This diagnosis is made with the client. If the client does not agree with the diagnosis, it should not be made (Bakker, Kastermans, and Dassen, 1995). The emphasis is on

• = Independent; ▲ = Collaborative

helping the client to direct his or her own life and health, not on the client's compliance with the provider's instructions (Kastermans and Bakker, 1999).

- See the care plans for **Effective Therapeutic regimen management** and **Ineffective family Therapeutic regimen management.**
- Establish a collaborative partnership with the client for purposes of meeting health-related goals. **Nursing Research:** *The U.S. Healthy People 2010 goals and objectives (http://www.healthypeople.gov) suggest that collaborative partnerships should be established to promote health. This approach differs from a traditional health care model in which the provider assumes authoritative and paternalistic roles. A nurse-consumer partnership "embodies power sharing and negotiation" (Gallant, Beaulieu, and Carnevale, 2002). In a grounded theory study, a caring partnership was used to control hypertension; the authors suggest that this model should also be used with other chronic illnesses (Mohammadi et al, 2002). In clinical trials, it was shown that self-efficacy is enhanced when people solve problems that they themselves identify (Bodenheimer et al, 2002).*
- Discuss all strategies with the client in the context of the client's culture. **Nursing Research:** *Research studies involving culture and health behavior show that culture significantly affects decision making for meeting therapeutic goals (Degazon, 2000).*
- Assist the client in resolving ambivalent feelings. **Nursing Research:** *In a grounded theory study of 19 African Americans over 65 years of age, wide variation existed in attitudes and ambivalence toward the illness and self-management (Chinn et al, 2000).*
- Review factors of the Health Belief Model with the client (i.e., individual perceptions of seriousness and susceptibility, demographic and other modifying factors, and perceived benefits and barriers). **Nursing Research:** *Studies using the Health Belief Model support the view that individual perceptions and a variety of modifying factors affect the likelihood of changing health behaviors (Pender, Murdaugh, and Parsons, 2002).*
- Identify the reasons for actions that are not therapeutic and discuss alternatives. **Nursing Research:** *There are many possible reasons for actions that do not meet therapeutic goals. Older women, for example, may not increase their activity levels because they have inaccurate perceptions of the related risks (Cousins, 2000). Fatigue and pain can have profound effects on the ability to perform therapeutic actions (Thorne and Paterson, 2000). Perceptions may differ according to diseases (e.g., people with pulmonary diseases are more likely than others to blame themselves for their condition) (Thorne and Paterson, 2000). Substantial numbers of older adults are fatalistic about their diseases (Goodwin, Black, and Satish, 1999).*
- Provide in-depth explanations of the therapeutic regimen to meet health-related goals, including pathophysiology and scientific rationales. **Nursing Research:** *In a prospective, randomized, controlled trial involving 77 clients with asthma, participants with moderate and severe asthma in the group that received additional client education experienced significant improvements in quality of life and symptoms (Marabini et al, 2002).*
- Use various formats to provide information about the therapeutic regimen (e.g., brochures, videotapes, written instructions, computer-based programs). **Nursing Research:** *Adequate resources are needed to enhance learning (Lubkin and Larsen, 2002). In a study with older adults using a three-group design, users of computer-based software for education about self-medication had significantly greater knowledge and self-efficacy scores as well as fewer adverse self-medication behaviors over time than conventional education and control groups (Neafsey et al, 2002).*
- Help the client to develop a positive attitude toward the disease and therapeutic regimen management. **Nursing Research:** *In a study of 29 adults with asthma, more posi-*

• = Independent; ▲ = Collaborative

tive attitudes were associated with higher knowledge and self-efficacy scores, and greater compliance with the use of peak flow meters (Scherer and Bruce, 2001). In a quasi-experimental study of the regimen adherence patterns of 249 people with osteoarthritis, self-efficacy and beliefs were contributing factors to adherence (Belza et al, 2002).

- Deliberate with the client on changes that are possible to meet therapeutic goals. **Nursing Research:** *Although decisions about actions to meet therapeutic goals are made by the client, the collaborative nature of the nurse-client interaction strengthens the relationship and contributes to the effectiveness of primary care (Wilkinson and Williams, 2002).*

- Help the client to self-manage his or her own health through teaching about strategies for changing habits such as overeating, sedentary lifestyle, and smoking. **Nursing Research:** *Teaching about the disease process includes teaching strategies for changing unhealthful habits (McCloskey and Bulechek, 2000). Evidence from controlled clinical trials indicates that teaching self-management skills is more effective for improving health outcomes than just providing information (Bodenheimer et al, 2002). In a quasi-experimental study involving 83 diabetic clients on a dialysis unit, the group that received self-management education showed a higher rate of significantly improved or maintained health outcomes than did those in the control group (McMurray et al, 2002). Aspects such as glycemic control and foot risk were significantly different for the two groups.*

- Develop a contract with the client to maintain motivation for changes in behavior. **Nursing Research:** *Developing a contract between nurse and client, or helping the client to develop a contract with himself or herself, provides a concrete means of keeping track of actions to meet health-related goals (McCloskey and Bulechek, 2000).*

- Help the client to maintain consistency in therapeutic regimen management for optimum results. **Nursing Research:** *In a randomized quasi-experimental study of 249 adults with osteoarthritis, the group that consistently participated in the aquatic exercise program (attended 16 of 20 weeks) had improved quality of well-being, physical functioning, and changes in arthritis quality of life compared to those who were inconsistent in participation (Belza et al, 2002).*

- ▲ Review methods of contacting health provider(s) as needed for changes in therapeutic regimen. **Theoretical Rationale:** *The partnership process includes continued contact as changes occur; people with chronic illnesses need to know how to obtain interventions that are needed in the future (Gallant, Beaulieu, and Carnevale, 2002; Lubkin and Larsen, 2002).*

Multicultural

- Conduct a self-assessment of the relation of culture to ethically based care. **Clinical Research:** *A tool was developed by the Midwest Bioethics Center Cultural Diversity Task Force (2001) to help providers conduct self-reflection and examination for ethically based care.*

- Assess the influence of cultural beliefs, norms, values, and attitudes on the client's ability to modify health behavior. **Theoretical Rationale:** *What the client considers normal and abnormal health behavior may be based on cultural perceptions (Leininger, 2001, Leininger and McFarland, 2002). Studies have shown wide variations in attitudes, including ambivalence and uncertainty (Chinn et al, 2000).*

- Discuss with the client those aspects of his or her health behavior/lifestyle that will remain unchanged by the therapeutic regimen. **Theoretical Rationale:** *Aspects of the client's life that are meaningful and valuable to him or her should be understood and preserved without change (Leininger, 2001; Leininger and McFarland, 2002).*

- Assess temporal orientation and its relationship to the management of the therapeutic

- = **Independent;** ▲ = **Collaborative**

regimen. **Nursing Research:** *Temporal orientation differs among cultures. The client's orientation to the present or the future was shown to affect management of hypertension and may also affect other therapeutic regimens (Brown and Segal, 1996).*

- Assess the effect of fatalism on the client's ability to adopt the therapeutic regimen. **Nursing Research:** *Fatalistic perspectives, which involve the belief that one cannot control one's own fate, may influence health behaviors in some African American and Latino populations (Harmon, Castro, and Coe, 1996; Phillips, Cohen, and Moses, 1999).*
- Validate the client's feelings regarding the impact of the therapeutic regimen on current lifestyle. **Theoretical Rationale:** *Validation lets the client know that the nurse has heard and understood what was said, and it promotes the nurse-client relationship (Leininger, 2001; Stuart and Laraia, 2001).*

Client/Family Teaching

- Identify what the client and/or family knows and adjust teaching accordingly. *Teach the client and family about all aspects of the therapeutic regimen, providing as much knowledge as the client and family will accept, in a culturally congruent manner.*
- Teach ways to adjust daily activities for inclusion of therapeutic regimens.
- Teach safety in taking medications.
- Teach the client to act as a self-advocate with health providers who prescribe therapeutic regimens.

evolve WEBSITES FOR EDUCATION

See the EVOLVE website for World Wide Web resources for client education.

REFERENCES

Bakker RH, Kastermans MC, Dassen TWN: An analysis of the nursing diagnosis ineffective management of therapeutic regimen compared to noncompliance and Orem's self-care deficit theory of nursing, *Nurs Diagn* 6:161, 1995.

Belza B et al: Does adherence make a difference: results from a community-based aquatic exercise program, *Nurs Res* 51(5):285, 2002.

Bodenheimer T et al: Patient self-management of chronic disease in primary care, *JAMA* 288(19):2469, 2002.

Brown CM, Segal R: Ethnic differences in temporal orientation and its implications for hypertension management, *J Health Soc Behav* 37:350, 1996.

Chinn MH et al: Developing a conceptual framework for understanding illness and attitudes in older, urban African Americans with diabetes, *Diabetes Educ* 26(3):439, 2000.

Cousins SO: "My heart can't take it": older women's beliefs about exercise benefits and risks, *J Gerontol B Psychol Sci Soc Sci* 55B(5):283, 2000.

Degazon C: Cultural diversity and community-oriented nursing practice. In Stanhope M, Lancaster J: *Community and public health nursing*, ed 5, St Louis, 2000, Mosby.

Gallant MH, Beaulieu MC, Carnevale FA: Partnership: an analysis of the concept within the nurse-client relationship, *J Adv Nurs* 40(2):149, 2002.

Goodwin JS, Black SA, Satish S: Aging versus disease: the opinions of older black, Hispanic, and non-Hispanic white Americans about the causes and treatment of common medical conditions, *J Am Geriatr Soc* 47(8): 973, 1999.

Harmon MP, Castro FG, Coe K: Acculturation and cervical cancer: knowledge, beliefs, and behaviors of Hispanic women, *Women Health* 24(3):37, 1996.

Kastermans MC, Bakker RH: Managing the impact of health problems on daily living. In Ranz MJ, Lemone P, editors: *Classification of nursing diagnoses: proceedings of the thirteenth conference*, Glendale, Calif, 1999, CINAHL Information Systems.

Leininger MM: *Culture care diversity and universality: a theory of nursing*, Boston, 2001, Jones and Bartlett.

• = Independent; ▲ = Collaborative

Leininger MM, McFarland MR: *Transcultural nursing: concepts, theories, research and practices,* ed 3, New York, 2002, McGraw-Hill.

Lubkin IM, Larsen PD: *Chronic illness: impact and interventions,* ed 5, Boston, 2002, Jones and Bartlett.

Marabini A et al: Short term effectiveness of an asthma educational program: results of a randomized controlled trial, *Respir Med* 96(12):933, 2002.

McCloskey JC, Bulechek GM, editors: Patient contracting; teaching: disease process. In *Nursing Interventions Classification (NIC),* ed 3, St Louis, 2000, Mosby.

McMurray SD et al: Diabetes education and care management significantly improve patient outcomes in a dialysis unit, *Am J Kidney Dis* 40(3):566, 2002.

Midwest Bioethics Center: Healthcare narratives from diverse communities—a self-assessment tool for healthcare providers, *Bioethics Forum* 17(3-4):SS1, 2001.

Mohammadi E et al: Partnership caring: a theory of high blood pressure control in Iranian hypertensives, *Int J Nurs Pract* 8(6):324, 2002.

Neafsey PJ et al: An interactive technology approach to educate older adults about drug interactions arising from over-the-counter self medication practices, *Public Health Nurs* 19(4):255, 2002.

Pender NJ, Murdaugh CL, Parsons MA: *Health promotion in nursing practice,* ed 4, Upper Saddle River, NJ, 2002, Prentice Hall.

Phillips JM, Cohen MZ, Moses G: Breast cancer screening and African American women: fear, fatalism, and silence, *Oncol Nurs Forum* 26(3):561, 1999.

Scherer YK, Bruce S: Knowledge, attitudes, and self-efficacy and compliance with medical regimen, number of emergency visits, and hospitalizations in adults with asthma, *Heart Lung* 30(4):250, 2001.

Stuart GW, Laraia MT: Therapeutic nurse-patient relationship. In Stuart GW, Laraia MT, editors: *Principles and practice of psychiatric nursing,* St Louis, 2001, Mosby, p 30.

Thorne SE, Paterson BL: Two decades of insider research: what we know and don't know about chronic illness experience, *Annu Rev Nurs Res* 18:3, 2000.

Wilkinson CR, Williams M: Strengthening patient-provider relationships, *Lippincotts Case Manag* 7(3):86, 2002.

Readiness for enhanced Therapeutic regimen management

Margaret Lunney

NANDA Definition

Pattern of regulating and integrating into daily living a program(s) for treatment of illness and its sequelae that is sufficient for meeting health-related goals and can be strengthened

Defining Characteristics

Expression of desire to manage treatment of illness and prevention of sequelae; choices of daily living that are appropriate for meeting goals of treatment or prevention; expression of little to no difficulty with regulation/integration of one or more prescribed regimens for treatment of illness or prevention of complications; reduction of risk factors for progression of illness and sequelae; lack of unexpected acceleration of illness symptoms

NOC Outcomes (Nursing Outcomes Classification)

Suggested NOC Outcomes

Health-Promoting Behavior; Health-Seeking Behavior; Knowledge: Health Behavior, Health Promotion, Health Resources, Illness Care, Medication, Prescribed Activity, Treatment Regimen

• = Independent; ▲ = Collaborative

Example NOC Outcome with Indicators

Health-Promoting Behavior (select the level of achievement on the following scale: 1 = never demonstrated, 2 = rarely demonstrated, 3 = sometimes demonstrated, 4 = often demonstrated, 5 = consistently demonstrated [see Section I]) as evidenced by the following indicators: Monitors personal behavior for risks/Seeks balance among exercise, work, leisure, rest, and nutrition/Performs health activities correctly/Uses financial and physical resources to promote health (Rate each indicator of **Health-Promoting Behavior** on the same five-point scale.)

Client Outcomes

Client Will (Specify Time Frame):
- Describe integration of therapeutic regimen into daily living
- Demonstrate continued commitment to integration of therapeutic regimen into daily living routines

NIC   Interventions (Nursing Interventions Classification)

Suggested NIC Interventions
Anticipatory Guidance; Mutual Goal Setting; Patient Contracting; Self-Modification Assistance; Self-Responsibility Facilitation; Support System Enhancement; Teaching: Disease Process

---

Example NIC Activities—Mutual Goal Setting

Assist client in prioritizing identified goals; Clarify roles of client and health care provider, respectively

---

Nursing Interventions and Rationales

- Explore attitudes toward the illness/disease and the need for management of a therapeutic regimen. **Clinical Research:** *In a qualitative study of 19 African American clients 65 years of age and older, ambivalence toward illness care was an identified theme (Chinn et al, 2000).*
- Review the factors contributing to the likelihood of taking action for health promotion and health protection. Use Pender's Health Promotion Model and Becker's Health Belief Model to identify contributing factors (Pender, Murdaugh, and Parsons, 2002). **Nursing Research:** *Studies using both the Health Promotion Model and the Health Belief Model support the view that individual perceptions and a variety of modifying factors affect the likelihood of improving health behaviors (Pender, Murdaugh, and Parsons, 2002). For example, in a study of 179 African American women 20 to 49 years old, the frequency of breast self-examination was related to the perceived seriousness of breast cancer, perceived benefits of breast self-examination, and health motivation, and was inversely related to perceived barriers.*
- Further develop and reinforce contributing factors that might change with ongoing management of the therapeutic regimen, e.g., knowledge, self-efficacy, self-esteem, and perceived benefits. **Nursing Research:** *Illness care is associated with ongoing changes and, over time, management of therapeutic regimens can become increasingly tedious and difficult (Lubkin and Larsen, 2002). For example, in a study of the education of hypertensive clients and their compliance with the medication regimen (N = 40), a negative correla-*

• = Independent; ▲ = Collaborative

tion was seen between duration of treatment and compliance. Ongoing support and assistance from health care providers is needed to identify and enhance factors that contribute to the likelihood of taking action for health promotion and health protection (Pender, Murdaugh, and Parsons, 2002). In a study examining whether adherence to regular aquatic exercise made a difference for 249 adults with osteoarthritis, it was found that exercise benefited the participants and that increased attention by health providers to improving clients' self-efficacy and belief systems would likely facilitate adherence (Belza et al, 2002).

- Review the client's strengths in the management of the therapeutic regimen. **Theoretical Rationale:** *People who are doing the work of managing a therapeutic regimen may not even realize that they are doing it well (Lubkin and Larsen, 2002).*
- Collaborate with the client to identify strategies to maintain strengths and develop additional strengths as indicated. **Theoretical Rationale:** *The client and provider working in partnership can facilitate, support, and reinforce the client's strengths (Gallant, Beaulieu, and Carnevale, 2002).*
- Identify contributing factors that may need to be improved now or in the future. **Theoretical Rationale:** *Health promotion and protection are complex behaviors that are difficult to implement on a daily basis. Based on the complexity of achieving these behaviors and the perceived barriers to implementation (e.g., time, energy, money), usually one or more contributing factors would benefit from increased focus and attention (Pender, Murdaugh, and Parsons, 2002).*
- Provide knowledge as needed related to the pathophysiology of the disease/illness, prescribed activities, prescribed medications, and nutrition. **Nursing Research:** *Knowledge is a factor that contributes significantly to the client's taking action for health promotion and protection (Pender, Murdaugh, and Parsons, 2002). It is important to remember, however, that knowledge is necessary but not sufficient to explain why people perform or do not perform actions for health promotion and protection (Pender, Murdaugh, and Parsons, 2002).*
- Use coaching strategies such as educational reinforcement, psychosocial support, and motivational guidance. **Nursing Research:** *In a study involving individuals newly diagnosed with type 2 diabetes, nurse coaching yielded a modest increase in health-promoting behaviors and a decrease in fasting blood glucose level (Whittemore et al, 2001).*
- Support positive health-promotion and health-protection behaviors. **Theoretical Rationale:** *Ongoing support may be needed to maintain these behaviors (Pender, Murdaugh, and Parsons, 2002).*
- Help the client to maintain existing support and seek additional supports as needed. **Nursing Research:** *In numerous research studies, social support was shown to be a factor contributing to ongoing maintenance of positive health behaviors (Lubkin and Larsen, 2002; Pender, Murdaugh, and Parsons, 2002). For example, in a study of long-term survivors of cancer, social support and self-esteem were two of the three variables that explained 53% of the variance in health-related quality of life (Pedro, 2001).*

Multicultural

- Acknowledge the cultural dimensions of health promotion and protection behaviors. **Nursing Research:** *For success in health promotion and health protection, nurses must demonstrate full acceptance of and respect for the cultural aspects of the client's therapeutic regimen management (Leininger, 2001; Leininger and McFarland, 2002).*
- Assist the client in integrating cultural patterns with prescribed activities, prescribed

• = **Independent; ▲** = **Collaborative**

medications, and prescribed diet. **Nursing Research:** *Clients who are trying to achieve optimum behaviors for health need assistance from nurses to integrate cultural patterns with knowledge of pathophysiology, the prescribed activity, medications, and diet (Leininger, 2001; Leininger and McFarland, 2002).*

- Manipulate community factors that may affect the management of the therapeutic regimen, e.g., barriers, supports, insurance, education about the illness, and provider-client relationships. **Clinical Research:** *A study involving African American diabetic clients concluded that complex environmental factors can indirectly affect glycemic control and management of the therapeutic regimen (Brody et al, 2001).*

Community Teaching

- Review therapeutic regimens and their optimum integration with daily living routines.
- Teach disease processes and therapeutic regimens for management of these disease processes.

evolve WEBSITES FOR EDUCATION

See the EVOLVE website for World Wide Web resources for client education.

REFERENCES

Belza B et al: Does adherence make a difference? Results from a community-based aquatic exercise program, *Nurs Res* 51(5):285, 2002.

Brody GH et al: Heuristic model linking contextual processes to self-management in African American adults with types 2 diabetes, *Diabetes Educ* 27(5):685, 2001.

Chinn MH et al: Developing a conceptual framework for understanding illness and attitudes in older, urban African Americans with diabetes, *Diabetes Educ* 26(3):439, 2000.

Gallant MH, Beaulieu MC, Carnevale FA: Partnership: an analysis of the concept within the nurse-client relationship, *J Adv Nurs* 40(2):149, 2002.

Leininger MM: *Culture care diversity and universality: a theory of nursing,* Boston, 2001, Jones and Bartlett.

Leininger MM, McFarland MR: *Transcultural nursing: concepts, theories, research and practices,* ed 3, New York, 2002, McGraw-Hill.

Lubkin IM, Larsen PD: *Chronic illness: impact and interventions,* ed 5, Boston, 2002, Jones and Bartlett.

Pedro LW: Quality of life for long-term survivors of cancer: influencing variables, *Cancer Nurs* 24(1):1, 2001.

Pender NJ, Murdaugh CL, Parsons MA: *Health promotion in nursing practice,* ed 4, Upper Saddle River, NJ, 2002, Prentice Hall.

Whittemore R et al: The content, integrity and efficacy of a nurse coaching intervention in type 2 diabetes, *Diabetes Educ* 27(6):887, 2001.

Ineffective community Therapeutic regimen management

Margaret Lunney

NANDA Definition

Pattern of regulating and integrating into community processes programs for the treatment of illness and its sequelae that is unsatisfactory for meeting health-related goals

Defining Characteristics

Illness symptoms above norm expected for number and type of population; unexpected acceleration of illness(es); number of health care resources insufficient for incidence or

- **= Independent; ▲ = Collaborative**

prevalence of illness(es); deficits in aggregates for specific groups; deficits in people and programs to be accountable for illness care of specific groups; deficits in community activities for secondary and tertiary prevention; unavailability of health care resources for illness care

Related Factors (r/t)

To be developed.

NOC Outcomes (Nursing Outcomes Classification)

Suggested NOC Outcomes

Decision Making; Knowledge: Disease Process, Treatment Regimen; Participation in Health Care Decisions; Symptom Severity; Treatment Behavior: Illness or Injury

> **Example NOC Outcome with Indicators**
>
> **Knowledge: Treatment Regimen** (select the level of achievement using the following scale: 1 = none, 2 = limited, 3 = moderate, 4 = substantial, 5 = extensive [see Section I]) as evidenced by the following indicator: Description of prescribed medication, activity, exercise, and disease process (Rate the indicator of **Knowledge: Treatment Regimen** using the same five-point scale.)

Community Outcomes

Community Will (Specify Time Frame):

- Secure community members and/or health providers who will be accountable for illness care of specific groups
- Remain involved in advocacy for illness care and prevention programs
- Develop health care plans for effective prevention and treatment of illnesses
- Make resources available for illness care and prevention
- Initiate or improve strategies for prevention of the sequelae of illness

NIC Interventions (Nursing Interventions Classification)

Suggested NIC Interventions

Community Health Development; Environmental Management: Community; Health Policy Monitoring; Teaching: Disease Process

NOTE: NIC interventions that were developed for use with individuals can be adapted for use with communities

> **Example NIC Activities—Community Health Development**
>
> Identify health concerns, strengths, and priorities with community partners; Facilitate implementation and revision of community plans

Nursing Interventions and Rationales

NOTE: Nursing interventions are conducted in collaboration with key members of the community, community/public health nurses, and members of other disciplines (Anderson and McFarlane, 2000; Bolton et al, 1998; Chinn, 2001; Reuter, Neufeld, and Harrison, 1995).

- ● = Independent; ▲ = Collaborative

- Seek community leaders (e.g., community board members) who are willing to learn about community assessment data and diagnoses and have the potential to work in partnership with nurses and other providers in planning for positive change. **Clinical Research:** *Through randomized telephone interviews with 286 households in poor neighborhoods, it was determined that the health priorities of district health council members were consistent with those of community residents (Conway, Hu, and Harrington, 1997). Only services that are valued and perceived as needed by community members are used effectively. Community health interventions are complex and often require multidisciplinary strategies (Bolton et al, 1998).*
- Examine the perceptions of community members regarding service needs. **Clinical Research:** *In a study to determine the congruence of the perceptions of consumers (N = 385) and case managers, the correlations were low between the perceptions of these two groups; consumers perceived that service needs were unmet, whereas case managers perceived that service needs were overly met (Crane-Ross, Roth, and Lauber, 2000).*
- Apply the concept of caring to the community as client. **Nursing Research:** *A systematic case study approach illustrated a community model of caring and showed that the concept of caring applies to communities as well as individuals (Smith-Campbell, 1999).*
- Advocate for and with the community in multiple arenas (e.g., newspapers, television, legislative bodies, community boards). **Theoretical Rationale:** *The community benefits from the advocacy of nurses and other health providers whose opinions are respected (Anderson and McFarlane, 2000).*
- Provide information to public and private sources about community assessment, diagnosis, and plans of care. **Theoretical Rationale:** *The commitment that is needed for improvements in health services can be obtained only when others have adequate information (Anderson and McFarland, 2000).*
- Mobilize support for the community to obtain the resources necessary for illness care and prevention. **Clinical Research:** *In a study of the Cardiovascular Health Network Project using focus groups with women participants, a lack of community support was identified as a barrier for women from some communities to practice health-promoting activities such as physical exercise (Eyler et al, 2002).*
- Provide informal helping roles as health educator and/or change agent. **Theoretical Rationale:** *Nurses are often sought out by friends and neighbors as informal helpers and, as such, can play important roles in helping communities to make behavioral and social changes for health (Tessaro, 1997).*
- ▲ Recruit additional health providers as needed. **Theoretical Rationale:** *If health providers are aware of inadequate community services, they may be able to contribute the necessary services (Anderson and McFarland, 2000). In applying the caring model to a community, Smith-Campbell (1999) was able to enlist additional health providers to participate in supplying community services.*
- Determine the cultural appropriateness of all programs. **Nursing Research:** *The cultural appropriateness of a program is an indicator of the potential success of the program (Leininger and McFarland, 2002).*
- Write grant proposals for the funding of new programs or the expansion of existing programs. (See Coley and Scheinberg [2000] for grant-writing methods.) **Theoretical Rationale:** *Public and private sources of funds can often supply the financial bases of health care programs (Anderson and McFarland, 2000).*
- Conduct research studies to convince others of the need to improve services or change policy. **Nursing Research:** *Research findings may be needed to obtain broad support for*

• = Independent; ▲ = Collaborative

needed changes (Anderson and McFarland, 2000). For example, in the last few decades, nurses have conducted research studies on the topic of battered women that were successful in influencing legislators to change laws and public policies in ways that positively affected the prevention and treatment of violence against women. A recent example of this type of research showed that there is a definite link between abuse during pregnancy and attempted and completed femicide (homicide of females) (McFarlane et al, 2002).

- With other persons and groups, obtain changes in health policy as indicated. **Theoretical Rationale:** *Health policies set the stage for effective health programs (Chaffee, Mason, and Leavitt, 2002; Milio, 1996). Policy evaluation and development is a core public health function (Turnock, Handler, and Miller, 1998; US Public Health Service, 1993).*
- Avoid victim-blaming stances in efforts to promote community responsibility for health. **Theoretical Rationale:** *A literature review of health promotion work with communities showed that health promotion strategies may lead to blaming the community for not taking responsibility for problems (Lowenberg, 1995).*

Multicultural

- Identify the health services and information resources that are currently available in the community. **Theoretical Rationale:** *This will assist in focusing efforts and promote the wise use of valuable resources. Many communities of color lack access to culturally competent health care providers, pharmacies, and grocery stores (National Institutes of Health, 1998).*
- Identify cultural barriers such as acculturation issues, lack of community support, and lack of past experience with a health behavior. **Clinical Research:** *Cultural barriers to exercise regimens were identified in a series of focus groups with women in the Cardiovascular Health Network Project (Eyler et al, 2002).*
- Work with members of the community to prioritize and target health goals specific to the community. **Theoretical Rationale:** *This will increase feelings of control and sense of ownership of programs and interventions (National Institutes of Health, 1998).*
- Approach community leaders and members of color with respect, warmth, and professional courtesy. **Theoretical Rationale:** *Instances of disrespect and lack of caring have special significance for individuals of color (D'Avanzo et al, 2001).*
- Establish and sustain partnerships with key individuals within the community in developing and implementing programs. **Theoretical Rationale:** *Local leaders are excellent sources of information, and their participation will enhance the credibility of the programs (National Institutes of Health, 1998).*
- Use community church settings as a forum for advocacy, teaching, and program implementation. **Nursing Research:** *A review of church-based health promotion programs shows that they are successful in helping people to adopt health-promoting behaviors (Peterson, Atwood, and Yates, 2002). Church-based interventions have been very successful in communities of color (Kotecki, 2002).*

evolve **WEBSITES FOR EDUCATION**

See the EVOLVE website for World Wide Web resources for client education.

• = **Independent; ▲ = Collaborative**

REFERENCES

Anderson ET, McFarlane J: *Community as partner: theory and practice in nursing,* ed 3, Philadelphia, 2000, Lippincott.

Bolton LB et al: Community health collaboration models for the 21st century, *Nurs Admin Q* 22(3):6, 1998.

Chaffee MW, Mason DJ, Leavitt JK: *Policy and politics in nursing and health care,* ed 4, Philadelphia, 2002, WB Saunders.

Chinn PL: Making a difference in health care, *ANS Adv Nurs Sci* 24(1), 2001.

Coley SM, Scheinberg CA: *Proposal writing,* ed 2, Thousand Oaks, Calif, 2000, Sage.

Conway T, Hu TC, Harrington T: Setting health priorities: community boards accurately reflect the preferences of the community residents, *J Community Health* 22(1):57, 1997.

Crane-Ross D, Roth D, Lauber BG: Consumers' and case managers' perceptions of mental health and community support service needs, *Community Ment Health J* 36(2):161, 2000.

D'Avanzo CE et al: Developing culturally informed strategies for substance related interventions. In Naegle MA, D'Avanzo CE, editors: *Addictions and substance abuse: strategies for advanced practice nursing,* St Louis, 2001, Mosby, pp 59-104.

Eyler AA et al: Environmental, policy, and cultural factors related to physical activity in a diverse sample of women: the Women's Cardiovascular Health Network Project—summary and discussion, *Women Health* 36(2):123, 2002.

Kotecki CN: Developing a health promotion program for faith-based communities, *Holist Nurs Pract* 16(3):61, 2002.

Leininger MM, McFarland MR: *Transcultural nursing: concepts, theories, research and practices,* ed 3, New York, 2002, McGraw-Hill.

Lowenberg JS: Health promotion and the "ideology of choice," *Public Health Nurs* 12(5):319, 1995.

McFarlane J et al: Abuse during pregnancy and femicide: urgent implications for women's health, *Obstet Gynecol* 100(1):27, 2002.

Milio N: *Engines of empowerment: using information technology to create healthy communities and challenge public policy,* Ann Arbor, Mich, 1996, Health Administration Press.

National Institutes of Health: *Salud para su corazón: bringing heart health to Latinos—a guide for building community programs,* DHHS Pub No. 98-3796, Washington, DC, 1998, US Government Printing Office.

Peterson J, Atwood JR, Yates B: Key elements for church-based health promotion programs: outcome-based literature review, *Public Health Nurs* 19(6):401, 2002.

Reuter L, Neufeld A, Harrison MJ: Using critical feminist principles to analyze programs for low-income urban women, *Public Health Nurs* 12:424, 1995.

Smith-Campbell B: A case study on expanding the concept of caring from individuals to communities, *Public Health Nurs* 16(6):405, 1999.

Tessaro I: The natural helping role of nurses in promoting healthy behaviors in communities, *Adv Pract Nurs Q* 2(4):73, 1997.

Turnock BJ, Handler AS, Miller CA: Core function-related public health practice effectiveness, *J Public Health Manag Pract* 4(5):26, 1998.

US Public Health Service: *The core functions project,* Washington, DC, 1993, Office of Disease Prevention and Health Promotion.

Ineffective family Therapeutic regimen management

Margaret Lunney

NANDA Definition

Pattern of regulating and integrating into family processes a program for treatment of illness and its sequelae that is unsatisfactory for meeting specific health goals

Defining Characteristics

Inappropriate family activities for meeting goals of treatment or prevention program; acceleration of illness symptoms of family member; lack of attention to illness and its sequelae; verbalization of difficulty with regulation/integration of one or more activities or prevention of complications; verbalization of desire to manage treatment of illness and prevention of its sequelae; verbalization that family did not take action to reduce risk factors for progression of illness and sequelae

Related Factors (r/t)

Complexity of health care system; complexity of therapeutic regimen; decisional conflicts; economic difficulties; excessive demands on individual or family; family conflict

| NOC | Outcomes (Nursing Outcomes Classification) |

Suggested NOC Outcomes

Health Orientation; Health-Promoting Behavior; Health-Seeking Behavior; Knowledge: Treatment Regimen; Participation in Health Care Decisions; Treatment Behavior: Illness or Injury

---

Example NOC Outcome with Indicators

Knowledge: Treatment Regimen (select the level of achievement on the following scale: 1 = none, 2 = limited, 3 = moderate, 4 = substantial, 5 = extensive [see Section I]) as evidenced by the following indicator: Description of prescribed medication, activity, exercise, and disease process (Rate the indicator of **Knowledge: Treatment Regimen** on the same five-point scale.)

Family Outcomes

Family Will (Specify Time Frame):
- Make adjustments in usual activities (e.g., diet, activity, stress management) to incorporate therapeutic regimens of its members
- Reduce illness symptoms of family members
- Desire to manage therapeutic regimens of its members
- Describe a decrease in the difficulties of managing therapeutic regimens
- Describe actions to reduce risk factors

| NIC | Interventions (Nursing Interventions Classification) |

Suggested NIC Interventions

Family Involvement Promotion; Family Mobilization; Family Process Maintenance; Teaching: Disease Process

---

Example NIC Activities—Family Involvement Promotion

Identify and respect family's coping mechanisms; Provide information to family members about client in accordance with client's preference

---

Nursing Interventions and Rationales

- Base family interventions on your knowledge of the family, family context, and family function. **Nursing Research:** *Family research has established that families differ widely from one another, even within cultures (Denham, 2002; Friedman, Bowden, and Jones, 2002). Family context "includes all aspects of the larger societal systems. The context is the stage for interactive relationships and discourse, the place where functional relationships occur, and the settings for enacting family health routines" (Denham, 2002, p 52).*

- • = Independent; ▲ = Collaborative

- Use a family approach when helping an individual with a health problem that requires therapeutic management. **Nursing Research:** *In a family health model developed from three qualitative studies involving Appalachian families from Ohio, it was shown that health habits are largely taught and defined within the family, so therapeutic regimens need to be addressed with the family (Denham, 2002).*
- Ensure that all strategies for working with the family are congruent with the culture of the family. **Nursing Research:** *Many nursing studies among people of a variety of cultures show that cultural variations exist in the management of therapeutic regimens, and these differences should be taken into account when working with families (Degazon, 2000; Leininger, 2001; Leininger and McFarland, 2002).*
- Support religious beliefs and the comfort role of religion. **Nursing Research:** *Studies have shown that there is a strong relationship between religion and subjective health and that subjective health is predictive of health outcomes. There seems to be a stronger relationship between religion and subjective health for African Americans than for whites (Kotecki, 2002; Musick, 1996).*
- Identify family interactions and their embedded contexts relative to specific health objectives. **Nursing Research:** *Family-focused practice requires viewing each interaction to accomplish health objectives as an opportunity to address the household production of health or work toward health objectives (Denham, 2002).*
- Review with family members the congruence and incongruence of family behaviors and health-related goals. **Nursing Research:** *To attain the motivation that is needed for changes in health habits, family members should understand the relationship of daily habits to health-related goals (Miller, 1999). Family goals are stable and take precedence over health-related goals (Stetz, Lewis, and Houck, 1994).*
- Help family members make decisions regarding ways to integrate therapeutic regimens into daily living. Provide advice or suggestions as solicited and accepted by the family. **Nursing Research:** *Decisions made by the family rather than by health providers or others guide everyday actions (Denham, 2002; Friedman, Bowden, and Jones, 2002). The advice of others, including nurses, will not be followed unless it is valued and respected by the family.*
- Demonstrate respect for and trust in family decisions. **Theoretical Rationale:** *People make decisions that they believe are appropriate for them. Family members who are respected and trusted by health providers are more likely to collaborate effectively with them.*
- Acknowledge the challenge of integrating therapeutic regimens with family behaviors. **Nursing Research:** *Therapeutic regimens require modifications of daily activities that have already been established based on family values and beliefs. Acknowledging the difficulty of changing family habits supports families through the process (Friedman, Bowden, and Jones, 2002).*
- Review the symptoms of specific illness(es) and work with the family toward development of greater self-efficacy in relation to these symptoms. **Nursing Research:** *Knowledge of symptoms improves the ability of family members to adjust behaviors to prevent and manage symptoms (Lubkin and Larsen, 2002). In a study of 197 family caregivers of people with Alzheimer's disease, higher symptom management self-efficacy scores were associated with fewer depressive symptoms and fewer physical health symptoms (Fortinsky, Kercher, and Burant, 2002).*
- Provide sufficient knowledge to support family decisions regarding therapeutic regimens. **Nursing Research:** *Knowledge deficits are obstacles to effective management of therapeutic regimens (Fujita and Duncan, 1994).*

- = **Independent;** ▲ = **Collaborative**

- Selectively support family decisions to adjust therapeutic regimens as indicated. **Nursing Research:** *Sometimes families do not have access to health providers and should make independent decisions because of side effects or adverse effects of therapeutic regimens. Family members need to make informed decisions that are in their best interests (Lubkin and Larsen, 2002). Providing support for appropriate decisions made by the family and caregivers improves the ability of the family to make such decisions.*
- Advocate for the family in negotiating therapeutic regimens with health providers. **Theoretical Rationale:** *Illness regimens generally are neither arbitrary nor absolute; therefore modifications can be discussed as needed to fit with the family lifestyle (Lubkin and Larsen, 2002).*
- Help the family to mobilize social supports. **Nursing Research:** *Increased social support helps families to meet health-related goals (Pender, Murdaugh, and Parsons, 2002).*
- Help family members to modify perceptions as indicated. **Nursing Research:** *Individual perceptions of the seriousness of, susceptibility to, and threat of illness may be distorted or inaccurate and perhaps can be modified with new information (Pender, Murdaugh, and Parsons, 2002).*
- Use one or more theories of the family to describe, explain, or predict family dynamics (e.g., theories of Bowen, Satir, Minuchin). **Theoretical Rationale:** *Family systems are complex and may not be understood by the nurse without adequate knowledge of family theory (Denham, 2002; Friedman, Bowden, and Jones, 2002).*
- Collaborate with nurses or other consultants regarding strategies for working with families. **Nursing Research:** *For some families, the knowledge and skills of nurses with advanced degrees or other specialists may be needed to design effective interventions (Kang, Barnard, and Oshio, 1994).*

Multicultural

- Acknowledge racial/ethnic differences at the onset of care. **Nursing Research:** *Acknowledgment of race/ethnicity issues will enhance communication, establish rapport, and promote treatment outcomes (D'Avanzo et al, 2001).*
- Approach families of color with respect, warmth, and professional courtesy. **Nursing Research:** *Instances of disrespect and lack of caring have special significance for families of color (D'Avanzo et al, 2001).*
- Assess for the influence of cultural beliefs, norms, and values on the family's perceptions of the therapeutic regimen. **Nursing Research:** *How the family views the therapeutic regimen may be based on cultural perceptions (Leininger, 2001).*
- Give a rationale when assessing African American families about sensitive issues. **Nursing Research:** *Many African Americans expect white caregivers to hold negative and preconceived ideas about African Americans. Giving a rationale for questions asked will help reduce this perception (D'Avanzo et al, 2001).*
- Use a family-centered approach when working with Latino, Asian, African American, and Native American clients. **Nursing Research:** *Latinos may perceive the family as a source of support, solver of problems and source of pride. Asian Americans may regard the family as the primary decision maker and influence on individual family members (D'Avanzo et al, 2001). Native American families may have extended structures and exert powerful influences over functioning (Seiderman et al, 1996).*
- Facilitate modeling and role-playing for the family regarding healthy ways to communicate and interact. **Nursing Research:** *It is helpful for families and the client to practice*

• = **Independent;** ▲ = **Collaborative**

communication skills in a safe environment before trying them in a real-life situation (Rivera-Andino, Lopez, 2000).

- Validate family members' feelings regarding the impact of the therapeutic regimen on the family lifestyle. **Nursing Research:** *Validation lets the client know that the nurse has heard and understood what was said, and it promotes the nurse-client relationship (Leininger and McFarland, 2002; Stuart and Laraia, 2001).*

Client/Family Teaching

- Teach about all aspects of therapeutic regimens. Provide as much knowledge as family members will accept, adjust instruction to account for what the family already knows, and provide information in a culturally congruent manner.
- Teach ways to adjust family behaviors to include therapeutic regimens.
- ▲ Teach safety in taking medications.
- ▲ Teach family members to act as self-advocates with health providers who prescribe therapeutic regimens.

evolve WEBSITES FOR EDUCATION

See the EVOLVE website for World Wide Web resources for client education.

REFERENCES

D'Avanzo CE et al: Developing culturally informed strategies for substance related interventions. In Naegle MA, D'Avanzo CE, editors: *Addictions and substance abuse: strategies for advanced practice nursing,* St Louis, 2001, Mosby, pp 59-104.

Degazon C: Cultural diversity and community-oriented nursing practice. In Stanhope M, Lancaster J: *Community and public health nursing,* ed 5, St Louis, 2000, Mosby, pp 138-156.

Denham SA: Family routines: a structural perspective for viewing family health, *ANS Adv Nurs Sci* 24(4):60, 2002.

Fortinsky RH, Kercher K, Burant CJ: Measurement and correlates of family caregiver self-efficacy for managing dementia, *Aging Ment Health* 6(2):153, 2002.

Friedman M, Bowden V, Jones E: *Family nursing: research, theory and practice,* ed 5, New York, 2002, Prentice Hall.

Fujita LJ, Duncan J: High risk for ineffective management of therapeutic regimen: a protocol study, *Rehabil Nurs* 19(2):75, 1994.

Kang R, Barnard K, Oshio S: Description of the clinical practice of advanced practice nurses in family-centered early intervention in two rural settings, *Public Health Nurs* 11:376, 1994.

Kotecki CN: Developing a health promotion program for faith-based communities, *Holist Nurs Pract* 16(3):61, 2002.

Leininger MM: *Culture care diversity and universality: a theory of nursing,* Boston, 2001, Jones and Bartlett.

Leininger MM, McFarland MR: *Transcultural nursing: concepts, theories, research and practices,* ed 3, New York, 2002, McGraw-Hill.

Lubkin IM, Larsen PD: *Chronic illness: impact and interventions,* ed 5, Boston, 2002, Jones and Bartlett.

Miller JF: *Coping with chronic illness: overcoming powerlessness,* ed 3, Philadelphia, 1999, FA Davis.

Musick MA: Religion and subjective health among black and white elders, *J Health Soc Behav* 37:221, 1996.

Pender NJ, Murdaugh CL, Parsons MA: *Health promotion in nursing practice,* ed 4, Upper Saddle River, NJ, 2002, Prentice Hall.

Rivera-Andino J, Lopez L: When culture complicates care, *RN* 63(7):47, 2000.

Seiderman RY et al: Assessing American Indian families, *MCN Am J Matern Child Nurs* 21(6):274, 1996.

Stetz KM, Lewis FM, Houck GM: Family goals as indicants of adaptation during chronic illness, *Public Health Nurs* 11:385, 1994.

Stuart GW, Laraia MT: Therapeutic nurse-patient relationship. In Stuart GW, Laraia MT, editors: *Principles and practice of psychiatric nursing,* St Louis, 2001, Mosby, p 30.

- **• = Independent; ▲ = Collaborative**

Ineffective Thermoregulation

Betty J. Ackley

NANDA Definition

Temperature fluctuation between hypothermia and hyperthermia

Defining Characteristics

Fluctuations in body temperature above or below normal range; cool skin; cyanotic nail-beds; flushed skin; hypertension; increased respiratory rate; pallor (moderate); pilo-erection; reduction in body temperature below normal range; seizures/convulsions; shivering (mild); slow capillary refill; tachycardia; warmth to touch

Related Factors (r/t)

Trauma; illness; immaturity; aging; fluctuating environmental temperature

NOC Outcomes (Nursing Outcomes Classification)

Suggested NOC Outcomes

Thermoregulation; Thermoregulation: Newborn

Example NOC Outcome with Indicators

Thermoregulation as evidenced by the following indicators: Body temperature WNL/Skin temperature IER/Skin color changes not present/Hydration adequate/Reported thermal comfort (Rate each indicator of **Thermoregulation:** 1 = extremely compromised, 2 = substantially compromised, 3 = moderately compromised, 4 = mildly compromised, 5 = not compromised [see Section I].)

IER, In expected range; *WNL,* within normal limits.

Client Outcomes

Client Will (Specify Time Frame):
- Maintain temperature within normal range
- Explain measures needed to maintain normal temperature
- Explain symptoms of hypothermia or hyperthermia

NIC Interventions (Nursing Interventions Classification)

Suggested NIC Interventions

Temperature Regulation; Temperature Regulation: Inoperative

Example NIC Activities—Temperature Regulation

Institute use of a continuous core temperature–monitoring device, as appropriate; Promote adequate fluid and nutritional intake

---

• = Independent; ▲ = Collaborative

Nursing Interventions and Rationales

- Monitor temperature every 1 to 4 hours or use continuous temperature monitoring as appropriate. *Normal adult temperature is usually identified as 37° C (98.6° F), but in actuality the normal temperature fluctuates throughout the day. In the early morning it may be as low as 35.8° C (96.4° F) and in the late afternoon or evening as high as 37.3° C (99.1° F) (Bates, Bickley, and Hoekelman, 1998). Disease, injury, or pharmacological agents may impair regulation of body temperature (Dennison, 1995; Holtzclaw, 1993).*
- If the client is awake, measure the oral temperature, instead of the tympanic or axillary temperature. **Nursing Research:** *Oral temperature measurement provides a more accurate temperature reading than tympanic measurement (Fisk and Arcona, 2001; Giuliano et al, 2000; Lee, McKenzie, and Cathcart, 1999). Axillary temperatures are often inaccurate (Fulbrook, 1997). The oral temperature is usually accurate even in the intubated client (Fallis, 2002).*
- Take vital signs every 1 to 4 hours, noting changes associated with hypothermia: first, increased blood pressure, pulse, and respirations; then, decreased values as hypothermia progresses (Edwards, 1999).
- Note changes in vital signs associated with hyperthermia: rapid, bounding pulse; increased respiratory rate; and decreased blood pressure accompanied by orthostatic hypotension (Worfolk, 2000). *Consistent monitoring promotes prevention and early intervention in clients with altered cardiopulmonary status associated with hypothermia or hyperthermia.*
- Monitor the client for signs of hyperthermia (e.g., headache, nausea and vomiting, weakness, absence of sweating, delirium, and coma) (Worfolk, 2000). *Monitoring for the defining characteristics of hypothermia and hyperthermia allows for prevention and/or early intervention.*
- Note vital sign changes associated with hypothermia: first increased and then decreased blood pressure, pulse rate, and respiratory rate. *Mild hypothermia activates the sympathetic nervous system, which can increase the levels of vital signs; as hypothermia progresses, the heart becomes suppressed, with decreased cardiac output and lowering of vital sign readings (Ruffolo, 2002).*
- Monitor the client for signs of hypothermia (e.g., shivering, cool skin, piloerection, pallor, slow capillary refill, cyanotic nailbeds, decreased mentation, dysrhythmias) (Edwards, 1999).
- Maintain a consistent room temperature (22.2° C [72° F]). *A consistent temperature limits environmental effects on thermoregulation.*
- Promote adequate nutrition and hydration. *These measures help maintain a normal body temperature.*
- Adjust clothing to facilitate passive warming or cooling as appropriate. *This will help maintain a normal body temperature.*
- See the Nursing Interventions and Rationales for **Hypothermia** or **Hyperthermia** as appropriate.

Geriatric

- Do not allow an elderly client to become chilled. Keep the client covered when giving a bath and offer socks to wear in bed. Be aware of factors such as room temperature (heating/air conditioning), clothing (layered/loose), and fluid intake. *Older adults have a decreased ability to adapt to temperature extremes and need protection from extreme environmental temperatures. They also have a higher threshold of central temperature for*

• = **Independent;** ▲ = **Collaborative**

sweating, diminished or absent sweating, impaired warmth or cold perception, an impaired shiver response, diminished thermogenesis, an abnormal peripheral blood flow response to warmth or cold, and a compromised cardiovascular reserve (Ballester and Harchelroad, 1999; Florez-Duquet and McDonald, 1998).

▲ Assess the medication profile for the potential risk of drug-related altered body temperature. *Anesthetics, barbiturates, salicylates, nonsteroidal anti-inflammatory drugs, diuretics, antihistamines, anticholinergics, beta-blockers, and thyroid hormones have been linked to altered body temperature (Haskell et al, 1997).*

Pediatric

• Recognize that pediatric clients have a decreased ability to adapt to temperature extremes. Take the following actions to maintain body temperature in the infant/child:
  ■ Keep the head covered.
  ■ Use blankets to keep the client warm.
  ■ Keep the client covered during procedures, transport, and diagnostic testing.
  ■ Keep the room temperature at 22.2°C (72° F).
  These measures can help prevent hypothermia in the child, which is a very possible occurrence, especially in the pediatric trauma client (Bernardo and Henker, 1999). The combination of a relatively larger body surface area, smaller body fluid volume, less well developed temperature control mechanisms, and smaller amount of protective body fat limits the pediatric client's ability to maintain normal temperatures (Noerr, 1997; Roncoli and Medoff-Cooper, 1992).

Home care
Prevention of Hypothermia in Cold Weather

• Instruct the client to avoid prolonged exposure outdoors. When outdoors, the client should wear gloves and a cap on the head. Wool or fleece clothing can help to maintain body heat.
• Keep the room temperature at 20° to 22.2 °C (68° to 72° F).
▲ Ensure an adequate source of heat. Refer to social services if the client/family has a low income and the heat could be turned off.
• Help the elderly client locate a warm environment to which the client can go for safety in cold weather if the home environment is no longer warm.

Prevention of Hyperthermia in Hot Weather

• Encourage the client to wear lightweight cotton clothing. Help the elderly client remove the usual sweater.
• Ensure that the client drinks adequate amounts of fluids—2000 ml/day—and avoids caffeine and alcohol. *Adequate fluids are needed during hot weather to replace fluids lost from sweating. Fluids containing caffeine and alcohol can serve as a diuretic and decrease fluid volume in the body.*
• Help the client obtain a fan or an air conditioner to increase evaporation, as needed.
• Take the temperature of the elderly client in hot weather. *Elderly clients may not be able to tell that they are hot because of decreased sensation (Worfolk, 2000).*
• Help the elderly client locate a cool environment to which the client can go for safety in hot weather.

• = Independent; ▲ = Collaborative

Client/Family Teaching

- Teach the client and family the signs of hypothermia and hyperthermia and appropriate actions to take if either condition develops. *Adequate teaching improves compliance and reduces anxiety.*
- Teach the client and family an age-appropriate method for taking the temperature. *Optimal placement of the appropriate device is essential for accurate monitoring.*
- Teach the client to avoid alcohol and medications that depress cerebral function. *When the client is sedated or under the influence of alcohol, mentation is depressed, which results in decreased activities to maintain an adequate body temperature.*

evolve WEBSITES FOR EDUCATION

See the EVOLVE website for World Wide Web resources for client education.

REFERENCES

Ballester JM, Harchelroad FP: Hypothermia: an easy-to-miss, dangerous disorder in winter weather, *Geriatrics* 54(2):51, 1999.

Bates B, Bickley LS, Hoekelman RA: *A guide to physical examination and history taking*, ed 7, Philadelphia, 1998, Lippincott.

Bernardo LM, Henker R: Thermoregulation in pediatric trauma: an overview, *Int J Trauma Nurs* 5(3):101, 1999.

Dennison D: Thermal regulation of patients during the perioperative period, *AORN J* 61:827, 1995.

Edwards SL: Hypothermia, *Prof Nurse* 14(4):253, 1999.

Fallis WM, Oral measurement of temperature in orally intubated critical care patients: state-of-the-science review, *Am J Crit Care* 9(5):2000.

Fisk J, Arcona S: Comparing tympanic membrane and pulmonary artery catheter temperatures, *Dimens Crit Care Nurs* 20(2):44, 2001.

Florez-Duquet M, McDonald RB: Cold-induced thermoregulation and biological aging, *Physiol Rev* 78(2):339, 1998.

Fulbrook P: Core body temperature measurement: a comparison of axilla, tympanic membrane and pulmonary artery blood temperature, *Intensive Crit Care Nurs* 13(5):1997.

Giuliano KK et al: Temperature measurement in critically ill adults: a comparison of tympanic and oral methods, *Am J Crit Care* 9(4):254, 2000.

Haskell RM et al: Hypothermia, *AACN Clin Issues* 8(3):368, 1997.

Holtzclaw BJ: Monitoring body temperature, *AACN Clin Issues* 4:44, 1993.

Lee VK, McKenzie NE, Cathcart M: Ear and oral temperatures under usual practice conditions, *Res Nurs Pract* 1(1):8, 1999.

Noerr B: Keeping the newborn warm: understanding thermoregulation, *Mother Baby J* 2(5):6, 1997.

Roncoli M, Medoff-Cooper B: Thermoregulation in low-birth-weight infants, *NAACOGS Clin Issu Perinat Womens Health Nurs* 3:25, 1992.

Ruffolo D: Hypothermia in trauma: the cold hard facts, *RN* 65(2):2002.

Worfolk JB: Heat waves: their impact on the health of elders, *Geriatr Nurs* 21(2):70, 2000.

Disturbed Thought processes

Judith R. Gentz and Gail B. Ladwig

NANDA Definition

Disruption in cognitive operations and activities

- • = Independent; ▲ = Collaborative

Defining Characteristics

Cognitive dissonance; memory deficit/problems; inaccurate interpretation of environment; hypovigilance; hypervigilance; distractibility; egocentricity; inappropriate non–reality-based thinking

Related Factors (r/t)

Organic brain changes (specify); changes in physical health (specify); mental illness (specify)

NOC Outcomes (Nursing Outcomes Classification)

Suggested NOC Outcomes

Cognition; Cognitive Orientation; Concentration; Decision Making; Distorted Thought Self-Control; Identity; Information Processing; Memory; Neurological Status: Consciousness

> **Example NOC Outcome with Indicators**
>
> **Distorted Thought Self-Control** as evidenced by the following indicators: Recognizes that hallucinations or delusions are occurring/Refrains from attending to or responding to hallucinations or delusions/Exhibits reality-based thinking (Rate each indicator of **Distorted Thought Self-Control:** 1 = never demonstrated, 2 = rarely demonstrated, 3 = sometimes demonstrated, 4 = often demonstrated, 5 = consistently demonstrated [see Section I].)

Client Outcomes

Client Will (Specify Time Frame):

- Demonstrate orientation to time, place, and person; demonstrate improved cognitive function.
- Be free from physical harm
- Perform activities of daily living (ADLs) appropriately and independently
- Identify community resources for help

NIC Interventions (Nursing Interventions Classification)

Suggested NIC Interventions

Delusion Management; Dementia Management

> **Example NIC Activities—Delusion Management**
>
> Provide opportunity for client to discuss delusions with caregivers; Focus discussion on underlying feelings, rather than content of the delusion ("It appears as if you may be feeling frightened")

Nursing Interventions and Rationales

- Observe for causes of altered thought processes (see Related Factors). *Differential diagnosis is important because physical and mental health problems, substance abuse, neoplasms, and medication side effects may effect cognitive status (Ungvarski and Trzcianowska, 2000).*
- Monitor, record, and report changes in the client's neurological status (level of con-

• = **Independent;** ▲ = **Collaborative**

sciousness, increased intracranial pressure), mental status (memory, cognition, judgment, concentration), vital signs, laboratory results, and ability to follow commands. *Assessing cognitive, physical, and behavioral symptoms helps to determine the relationship between brain anatomy, neurochemical systems, and symptoms (Garand, Buckwalter, and Hall, 2000).*

- Obtain a medical history to rule out physical illness causes for mental status changes. *Changes in behavior, cognitive functioning, and functional level occur with organic brain disease and other physiological changes in the body (Garand, Buckwalter, and Hall 2000).*
- Complete a mental status examination of the client. **Clinical Research:** *A mental status examination is a recommended procedure in assessing any cognitive difficulties (Boise et al, 1999).*
- Report any new onset or sudden increase in confusion. **Nursing Research:** *Postoperative acute confusional state is a significant problem among older surgical clients; its incidence is higher in orthopedic surgery than in general surgery (Wong, Wong, and Brooks, 2002).* **Nursing Research:** *In one study acute confusion was determined on the basis of observation of clients' behavior, functioning, and orientation as well as nurses' knowledge of factors that predispose clients to the development of acute confusion (Rogers and Gibson, 2002).*
- Adjust communication style to the client. Speak slowly and calmly; use short phrases and concrete, nontechnical words; use writing if appropriate; allow time for thinking; use face-to-face communication; listen carefully; and seek clarification. *Basic interactions provide the nurse with the opportunity to assess the client's agitation and response level (Kozub and Skidmore, 2001).*
- Assess pain and promptly provide comfort measures. **Nursing Research:** *Confused clients cannot accurately report pain (Buffman et al, 2001). Pain control reduces suffering and adverse health effects related to pain (Huffman and Kunik, 2000).*
- Identify and remove potentially dangerous items in the environment. **Clinical Research:** *Alteration of thoughts can lead to misinterpretation of the environment and decreased judgment and impulse control. Cognitive impairment can result in a number of problems, such as communication difficulties, compromised safety, self-care deficits, and behavioral problems (Day, Carreon, and Stump, 2000).*
- ▲ Limit the use of sedatives and drugs affecting the nervous system. *Sedation, imbalance, slowed reaction time, hypotension and parkinsonism side effects all increase the risk of falls and confusion (Lieu et al, 1997).*
- ▲ Use soft restraints with discretion and with a physician's order. *Seclusion, restraint, and/or other behavioral management interventions must be used in accordance with the client's plan of care and regulatory guidelines (Health Care Financing Administration, 2000; Joint Commission on Accreditation of Healthcare Organizations, 2000).*
- Orient the client and call the client by name; introduce yourself on each contact; frequently mention time, date, and place; prominently display in the room a clock and calendar that are easy to read and refer to them; and request the family to bring in familiar pictures and articles from home. **Clinical Research:** *These steps help reinforce reality and provide cues that maintain orientation. External, written reminders are more effective than verbal reinforcement as memory aids (Davis and Burgio, 1999; Day, Carreon, and Stump, 2000).*
- Provide validation of the client's thoughts and feelings. *Validation seeks to help the caregiver understand the care receiver and encourages empathy (Linehan, 1993).*
- Stay with the client if the client is agitated and likely to be injured. *One-on-one contact*

• = **Independent;** ▲ = **Collaborative**

between staff and client is the first step in successful de-escalation (Kozub and Skidmore, 2001).

- Assess the client's assault potential and maintain staff safety. *Client resistance to staff direction requires immediate consideration of staff safety (Kozub and Skidmore, 2001).*
- Establish predictable care routines and maintain continuity of the client's nursing staff. *Routines promote feelings of security.*
- Frequently check on the client and have brief interactions to prevent sensory deprivation. *Avoid an overstimulating or a sensory-deprived environment. Provide adequate lighting that is not too bright. Alternate short, frequent visits with defined rest periods. Monitor noise levels.* **Clinical Research:** *Excessive environmental stimuli can adversely affect the client's level of orientation and increase disorganization (Day, Carreon, and Stump, 2000).*
- Assist the client with daily hygiene as needed; encourage self-care. *Good hygiene and self-care increase self-esteem and autonomy.*
- Provide support and education to the family during the client's period of cognitive change. Involve the family in current care and in planning of postdischarge care, recognizing the family members' strengths and needs. **Nursing Research:** *Family members may also have cognitive symptoms related to age or mental illness (Wuerker, 2000). Family involvement promotes continuity of care.*
- ▲ Initiate a social service referral to find help for the client following discharge. **Clinical Research:** *An adequate level of client supervision following discharge may reduce risk of readmission (Mercer et al, 1999).*
- Observe for hallucinations as evidenced by behavioral response to internal stimuli, inappropriate laughter, slow verbal responses, lip movements without sound, smiling at inappropriate times, or grimacing. **Clinical Research:** *Provide support and reality orientation to increase the client's sense of personal power (Williams and Collins, 1999).*
- Ask direct questions such as, "Are you seeing or hearing something now?" or "Do you sometimes hear or see things that other people don't hear or see?" **Nursing Research:** *Validation of symptoms increases empathy and the client's perception of safety (Forchuk et al, 2000).*
- Do not attempt to argue or change the client's beliefs, but do not imply agreement. Without implying agreement, attend to the client's reaction or response to his or her beliefs. **Nursing Research:** *Attending to reactions or responses promotes a trusting relationship with the client (Forchuk et al, 2000).*
- Accept that the client is seeing or hearing things that are not there, but tactfully tell the client that only he or she is hearing or seeing these things. Focus on the feelings that accompany hallucinations and delusions rather than on the content of delusions (e.g., "You look frightened"). **Nursing Research:** *Acceptance promotes trust and understanding (Forchuk et al, 2000).*
- Set limits on delusional conversations (e.g., "We discussed that; let's talk about what is happening now on the unit"). **Nursing Research:** *Balancing control and caring behaviors fosters rapport between the nurse and client (Forchuk et al, 2000).*
- Ask for clarification when necessary.
- Help the client state needs and ask for assistance.
- Involve the client in short activities. *Distraction is a positive coping skill (Linehan, 1993).*
- See the care plans for **Risk for self-directed Violence** and **Risk for other-directed Violence** for further nursing interventions and rationales.

• = **Independent;** ▲ = **Collaborative**

Geriatric

- Monitor for dementia, as evidenced by a gradual onset and a progressive deterioration, or for delirium, as evidenced by an acute onset and generally reversible course. **Nursing Research:** *States of confusion require careful assessment (Milisen et al, 1998; Vermeersch, 1990).*
- Focus on the feelings associated with hallucinations and delusions rather than their content. *Nurses should not engage with clients regarding the meaning of auditory hallucinations (Coffey and Higgon, 2001).*

Multicultural

- Assess for the influence of cultural beliefs, norms, and values on the family's or caregiver's understanding of disturbed thought processes. **Nursing Research:** *What the family considers normal and abnormal behavior may be based on cultural perceptions (Cochran, 1998; Doswell and Erlen, 1998; Guarnaccia, 1998; Leininger and McFarland, 2002).*
- Inform the client's family or caregiver of the meaning of and reasons for common behaviors observed in client with disturbed thought processes. *An understanding of behavior will enable the client's family or caregiver to provide the client with a safe environment.*
- Validate the family members' feelings regarding the impact of the client's behavior on family lifestyle. **Nursing Research:** *Validation is a therapeutic communication technique that lets the individual know that the nurse has heard and understood what was said, and it promotes the relationship between the nurse and the individual (Heineken, 1998).*

Home care

- The interventions described previously may be adapted for home care use.
- ▲ Assess the client for the presence of a psychiatric disorder. Refer for mental health services as indicated. *Disturbed thought processes are part of several psychiatric disorders. Improvement in thought processes is unlikely unless the underlying disorder is treated.*
- Assess the family's knowledge of the disease process and plan of care; teach as necessary. Encourage participation. *Illnesses associated with thought process disorders generally affect the family and family life as much as they do the client. Misinterpretation of the client's behavior is common, and instruction regarding the disease process is necessary to secure understanding of and cooperation with the treatment plan.*
- Identify the strengths of the caregiver and the caregiver's efforts to gain control of unpredictable situations. Help the caregiver to stay connected with a client who may be behaving differently than usual, to make life as routine as possible, to help the client set goals and sustain hope, and to allow the client space to experience progress. **Nursing Research:** *Identifying and acknowledging positive caregiver responses to the client's illness will assist the caregiver in maintaining a positive relationship with the client. Family members of persons with severe mental illness have found it helpful to work at staying connected to the person with mental illness, finding a role that they can feel comfortable with, and helping the relative move forward (Rose, 1998).*
- ▲ Assess the client's functional status as it relates to the ability for self-care; refer to a physician for evaluation of medication levels as indicated. *Negative symptoms, abnormal movements, and use of antiparkinsonism agents may increase the likelihood of functional impairment in older adults with schizophrenia. These elements may be treatable with new antipsychotic medications and psychological approaches (e.g., social skills training) (Cohen and Talavera, 2000).*

- • = Independent; ▲ = Collaborative

- Assess the home environment for the availability of distractions from hallucinations, such as playing music over headphones. **Clinical Research:** *One study showed that having schizophrenics listen to music produced beneficial effects (Glicksohn and Cohen, 2000).*
▲ If the client's condition deteriorates, seek acute medical or mental health intervention immediately, as appropriate. *Acute behavioral change could place the client or caregivers at risk; behavioral change often responds to sedation or increase in medications.*
▲ Identify an emergency plan and discuss criteria for its use with the family or caregivers. *An appropriate level of clinical intervention supports client and family well-being.*
▲ Assess the client's ability to manage his or her own medications. If the client is unable, identify a responsible caregiver for medication administration. Teach the purpose, administration, and side effects of medications based on level of knowledge. Identify a plan for response to side effects if they occur. **Nursing Research:** *Assistance, such as the use of a medication box or reminder telephone calls, may be sufficient to allow the client to perform care activities independently (Beebe, 2001).*
- Assess and modify environmental stimuli that could be misinterpreted (e.g., use a night light, evaluate placement of mirrors). *Clients may tend toward illusory experiences, misinterpreting actual stimuli. Night lights help clients reorient themselves and decrease fear if clients awaken during the night.*
- Allow the client control over aspects of his or her environment, as he or she is able. *Control enhances self-esteem, although sometimes only for a short time. Refer to the care plan for* **Powerlessness.**
- Identify the client's interests and skills. Provide an opportunity for the client to pursue interests and use skills without taxing the client's judgment and cognitive ability. *Diversionary activities decrease anxiety and give meaning to life.*
▲ Refer the client and family to community support groups (e.g., psychosocial rehabilitation programs for the client, National Alliance for the Mentally Ill for the client and family). Groups that include older adults with mental illness would be particularly useful. *Coping strategies described by older adults with mental illness were similar to those of younger clients but were used more effectively in conjunction with greater acceptance of the mental illness. Older adults may serve as a helpful resource to younger clients struggling with adjustment to their illness (Solano and Whitbourne, 2001).*
▲ In the presence of chronic thought process disorder, institute case management of frail elderly to support continued independent living. *Difficulties with thought disorder can lead to increasing needs for assistance in using the health care system effectively. Case management combines the nursing activities of client and family assessment, planning and coordination of care among all health care providers, delivery of direct nursing care, and monitoring of care and outcomes. These activities can address continuity of care, mutual goal setting, behavior management, and prevention of worsening health problems (Guttman, 1999).*
▲ When the client has a psychiatric disorder, pay special attention to the presence of comorbid medical conditions and the need for medical care. *Clients with schizophrenia have higher mortality rates and generally have received less than optimal health care. They are in particular need of assessment, health instruction, and involvement in their own care (Folsom and Jeste, 2001).*
▲ When the client has a psychiatric disorder, refer for psychiatric home health care services for client reassurance and implementation of a therapeutic regimen. *Psychiatric home care nurses can address issues relating to the client's thought process disorder. Behavioral interventions in the home can help the client to participate more effectively in the treatment plan (Patusky, Rodning, and Martinez-Kratz, 1996).*

- = **Independent;** ▲ = **Collaborative**

Client/Family Teaching

- Teach family members reorientation techniques and the need to repeat instructions frequently.
- Teach the client distraction techniques to manage hallucinations.
- Teach family members ways to support the client without supporting delusional beliefs.
- Help the family identify coping skills, environmental supports, and community services for dealing with the chronically mentally ill client.
- Discuss the caregiver's need for respite. Offer support, encouragement, and information for meeting that need.

evolve WEBSITES FOR EDUCATION

See the EVOLVE website for World Wide Web resources for client education.

REFERENCES

Beebe LH: Community nursing support for clients with schizophrenia, *Arch Psychiatr Nurs* 15:214, 2001.

Boise L et al: Diagnosing dementia: perspectives of primary care physicians, *Gerontologist* 39(4):457, 1999.

Buffman MD et al: A pilot study of the relationship between discomfort and agitation in patients with dementia, *Geriatr Nurs* 22(2):2001.

Cochran M: Tears have no color, *Am J Nurs* 98(6):53, 1998.

Coffey M, Higgon J: Auditory hallucinations, *Ment Health Nurs* 21(2):2001.

Cohen CI, Talavera N: Functional impairment in older schizophrenic persons, *Am J Geriatr Psychiatry* 8:237, 2000.

Davis L, Burgio L: Planning cognitive behavioral management for long-term care, *Issues Ment Health Nurs* 20:587, 1999.

Day K, Carreon D, Stump C: The therapeutic design of environments for people with dementia: a review of the empirical research, *Gerontologist* 40:4, 2000.

Doswell W, Erlen J: Multicultural issues and ethical concerns in the delivery of nursing care interventions, *Nurs Clin North Am* 33(2):353, 1998.

Folsom DP, Jeste DV: Medical comorbidity in patients with schizophrenia, *Home Health Care Consult* 8(9):17, 2001.

Forchuk C et al: The developing nurse-client relationship: nurses' perspective, *J Am Psychiatr Nurses Assoc* 6:1, 2000.

Garand L, Buckwater K, Hall G: The biological basis of behavioral symptoms in dementia, *Issues Ment Health Nurs* 21:21, 2000.

Glicksohn J, Cohen Y: Can music alleviate cognitive dysfunction in schizophrenia? *Psychopathology* 33(1):43, 2000.

Guarnaccia P: Multicultural experiences of family caregiving: a study of African American, European American, and Hispanic American families, *New Dir Ment Health Serv* 77:45, 1998.

Guttman R: Case management of the frail elderly in the community, *Clin Nurs Spec* 13(4):174, 1999.

Heineken J: Patient silence is not necessarily client satisfaction: communication in home care nursing, *Home Healthc Nurse* 16(2):115, 1998.

Huffman J, Kunik M: Assessment and understanding of pain in patients with dementia, *Gerontologist* 40:5, 2000.

Kozub M, Skidmore R: Least to most restrictive interventions, *J Psychosoc Nurs Ment Health Serv* 39: 3, 2001.

Leininger MM, McFarland MR: *Transcultural nursing: concepts, theories, research and practices,* ed 3, New York, 2002, McGraw-Hill.

Lieu PK et al: Prevention of falls in a geriatric ward, *Ann Acad Med Singapore* 26(3):266, 1997.

Linehan M: *Cognitive-behavioral treatment of borderline personality disorder,* New York, 1993, Guilford Press.

Mercer G et al: Rehospitalization of older psychiatric inpatients: an investigation of predictors, *Gerontologist* 39:5, 1999.

Milisen K et al: Delirium in the hospitalized elderly, *Nurs Clin North Am* 33:3, 1998.

• = Independent; ▲ = Collaborative

Patusky KL, Rodning C, Martinez-Kratz M: Clinical lessons in psychiatric home care: a case study approach, *J Home Health Case Manag* 9:18, 1996.

Rogers AC, Gibson CH: Experiences of orthopaedic nurses caring for elderly patients with acute confusion, *J Orthopaed Nurs* 6(1):9, 2002.

Rose LE: Gaining control: family members relate to persons with severe mental illness, *Res Nurs Health* 21:363, 1998.

Solano NH, Whitbourne SK: Coping with schizophrenia: patterns in later adulthood, *Int J Aging Hum Dev* 53:1, 2001.

Ungvarski P, Trzcianowska H: Neurocognitive disorders seen in HIV disease, *Issues Ment Health Nurs* 21:51, 2000.

Vermeersch PE: The clinical assessment of confusion, *Appl Nurs Res* 3(3):128, 1990.

Williams CC, Collins AA: Defining new frameworks for psychosocial intervention, *Psychiatry* 62:61, 1999.

Wong J, Wong S, Brooks E: A study of hospital recovery pattern of acutely confused older patients following hip surgery, *J Orthopaed Nurs* 6(2):2002.

Wuerker A: The family and schizophrenia, *Issues Ment Health Nurs* 21:1, 2000.

Impaired Tissue integrity

Diane L. Krasner

NANDA Definition

Damage to mucous membrane, corneal, integumentary, or subcutaneous tissues

Defining Characteristics

Damaged or destroyed tissue (e.g., cornea, mucous membrane, integumentary or subcutaneous tissue)

Related Factors (r/t)

Mechanical factors (e.g., pressure, shear, friction); radiation (including therapeutic radiation); nutritional deficit or excess; thermal factors (temperature extremes); knowledge deficit; chemical irritants (including body excretions, secretions, medications); impaired physical mobility; altered circulation; fluid deficit or excess

NOC Outcomes (Nursing Outcomes Classification)

Suggested NOC Outcomes

Tissue Integrity: Skin and Mucous Membranes; Wound Healing: Primary Intention, Secondary Intention

> ### Example NOC Outcome with Indicators
>
> Intact Tissue Integrity: Skin and Mucous Membranes as evidenced by the following indicators: Skin intactness/ Absence of tissue lesions/Tissue perfusion/Tissue temperature in expected range (Rate each indicator of **Tissue Integrity: Skin and Mucous Membranes: 1** = extremely compromised, 2 = substantially compromised, 3 = moderately compromised, 4 = mildly compromised, 5 = not compromised [see Section I].)

Client Outcomes

Client Will (Specify Time Frame):

- Report any altered sensation or pain at site of tissue impairment

• = **Independent;** ▲ = **Collaborative**

- Demonstrate understanding of plan to heal tissue and prevent injury
- Describe measures to protect and heal the tissue, including wound care
- Experience a wound that decreases in size and has increased granulation tissue

NIC   Interventions (Nursing Interventions Classification)

Suggested NIC Interventions
Incision Site Care; Pressure Ulcer Care; Skin Care: Topical Treatments; Skin Surveillance; Wound Care

Example NIC Activities—Pressure Ulcer Care

Monitor color, temperature, edema, moisture, and appearance of surrounding skin; Note characteristics of any drainage

Nursing Interventions and Rationales

- Assess the site of impaired tissue integrity and determine the cause (e.g., acute or chronic wound, burn, dermatological lesion, pressure ulcer, leg ulcer). *Prior assessment of wound cause is critical for proper identification of nursing interventions (van Rijswijk, 2001).*
- Determine the size and depth of the wound (e.g., full-thickness wound, stage III or stage IV pressure ulcer). *Serial wound assessments are more reliable when performed by the same caregiver, with the client in the same position, and using the same techniques (Krasner and Sibbald, 1999; Sussman and Bates-Jensen, 1998).*
- Classify pressure ulcers in the following manner (National Pressure Ulcer Advisory Panel, 1989):
  - Stage III: Full-thickness skin loss involving damage to or necrosis of subcutaneous tissue that may extend down to but not through underlying fascia; ulcer appears as a deep crater with or without undermining of adjacent tissue
  - Stage IV: Full-thickness skin loss with extensive destruction; tissue necrosis; or damage to muscle, bone, or supporting structures (e.g., tendons, joint capsules)
- Monitor the site of impaired tissue integrity at least once daily for color changes, redness, swelling, warmth, pain, or other signs of infection. Determine whether the client is experiencing changes in sensation or pain. Pay special attention to all high-risk areas such as bony prominences, skin folds, sacrum, and heels. *Systematic inspection can identify impending problems early (Bryant, 1999).* **Nursing and Clinical Research:** *Pain secondary to dressing changes can be managed by interventions aimed at reducing trauma and other sources of wound pain (European Wound Management Association, 2001; Krasner 2001).*
- Monitor the status of the skin around the wound. Monitor the client's skin care practices, noting type of soap or other cleansing agents used, temperature of water, and frequency of skin cleansing. *Individualize the plan according to the client's skin condition, needs, and preferences. Avoid harsh cleansing agents, hot water, extreme friction or force, or too frequent cleansing (Bergstrom et al, 1994; Panel for the Prediction and Prevention of Pressure Ulcers in Adults, 1992).*
- Monitor the client's continence status and minimize exposure of the skin impairment site and other areas to moisture from urine or stool, perspiration, or wound drainage. *If the client is incontinent, implement an incontinence management plan to prevent ex-*

• = Independent; ▲ = Collaborative

posure to chemicals in urine and stool that can strip or erode the skin. Refer to a physician (e.g., urologist, gastroenterologist) for an incontinence assessment (Doughty, 2000; Wound, Ostomy, and Continence Nurses Society, 1992, 1994). **Nursing and Clinical Research:** *Implementing an incontinence prevention plan with the use of a skin protectant or a cleanser-protectant can significantly decrease skin breakdown and pressure ulcer formation (Clever et al, 2002; Warshaw et al, 2002).*

- Monitor for correct placement of tubes, catheters, and other devices. Assess the skin and tissue affected by the tape that secures these devices (Faller and Beitz, 2001). *Mechanical damage to skin and tissues as a result of pressure, friction, or shear is often associated with external devices.*

- In an orthopedic client, check every 2 hours for correct placement of foot boards, restraints, traction, casts, or other devices, and assess skin and tissue integrity. Be alert for symptoms of compartment syndrome (see the care plan for **Risk for Peripheral neurovascular dysfunction**). *Mechanical damage to skin and tissues (pressure, friction, or shear) is often associated with external devices.*

- For a client with limited mobility, use a risk assessment tool to systematically assess immobility-related risk factors. *A validated risk assessment tool such as the Norton or Braden scale should be used to identify clients at risk for immobility-related skin breakdown (Ayello and Braden, 2002; Bergstrom et al, 1987; Krasner and Sibbald, 1999; Panel for the Prediction and Prevention of Pressure Ulcers in Adults, 1992).* **Nursing Research:** *Targeting variables (such as age and Braden Scale risk category) can focus assessment on particular risk factors (e.g., pressure) and help guide the plan of prevention and care (Young et al, 2002).*

- Implement a written treatment plan for the topical treatment of the skin impairment site. *A written treatment plan ensures consistency in care and documentation (Maklebust and Sieggreen, 1996). Topical treatments must be matched to the client, wound, and setting (Krasner and Sibbald, 1999; Ovington, 1998).*

- ▲ Identify a plan for débridement if necrotic tissue (eschar or slough) is present and if consistent with overall client management goals. *Healing does not occur in the presence of necrotic tissue (Bergstrom et al, 1994; Krasner and Sibbald, 1999; Panel for the Prediction and Prevention of Pressure Ulcers in Adults, 1992).*

- Select a topical treatment that maintains a moist wound-healing environment but that also allows absorption of exudate and filling of dead space. *Caution should always be taken to not dry out the wound (Bergstrom et al, 1994; Ovington, 1998; Panel for the Prediction and Prevention of Pressure Ulcers in Adults, 1992).*

- Do not position the client on the site of impaired tissue integrity. If it is consistent with overall client management goals, turn and position the client at least every 2 hours and transfer the client carefully to avoid adverse effects of external mechanical forces (i.e., pressure, friction, and shear).

- Evaluate for the use of specialty mattresses, beds, or devices as appropriate (Fleck, 2001).

- If the goal of care is to keep the client comfortable (e.g., for a terminally ill client), turning and repositioning may not be appropriate. Maintain the head of the bed at the lowest degree of elevation possible to reduce shear and friction, and use lift devices, pillows, foam wedges, and pressure-reducing devices in the bed (Krasner, Rodeheaver, and Sibbald, 2001; Panel for the Prediction and Prevention of Pressure Ulcers in Adults, 1992).

- Avoid massaging around the site of impaired tissue integrity and over bony promi-

• **= Independent; ▲ = Collaborative**

nences. *Research suggests that massage may lead to deep tissue trauma (Panel for the Prediction and Prevention of Pressure Ulcers in Adults, 1992).*

▲ Assess the client's nutritional status; refer for a nutritional consultation and/or institute use of dietary supplements. *Inadequate nutritional intake places the client at risk for skin breakdown and compromises healing (Demling and De Santi, 1998). Optimizing nutritional intake, including calories, fatty acids, protein, and vitamins, is needed to promote wound healing (Russell, 2001).*

Home care

- Some of the interventions described previously may be adapted for home care use.
- Assess the client's current phase of wound healing (inflammation, proliferation, maturation) and stage of injury; initiate appropriate wound management. *Accurate understanding of tissue status combined with knowledge of underlying diagnoses and product validity provide a basis for determining appropriate treatment objectives (Ovington, 1998). A variety of advanced dressings (e.g., films, foams, hydrocolloids, hydrogels) have replaced standard wet-to-dry dressings (Ovington, 2001a) in a cost-effective manner (Ovington and Schaum, 2001). Wound cleansing and débridement advances offer additional support (Ovington, 2001b).*
- Instruct and assist the client and caregivers with removing or controlling impediments to wound healing (e.g., management of underlying disease, improvement in approach to client positioning, improved nutrition). *Wound healing can be delayed or can fail totally if impediments are not controlled (Krasner and Sibbald, 1999).*
- ▲ Initiate a consultation in a case assignment with a wound, ostomy, and continence nurse to establish a comprehensive plan as soon as possible. Plan case conferencing to promote optimal wound care. *Case conferencing ensures that cases are reviewed regularly to discuss and implement the most effective wound care management to meet client needs (Biala, 2002).*
- ▲ Refer for consideration of treatment options for leg ulcers: *A wide variety of modalities can be tailored to the client's needs (Longobardi, Huthison, and Caputo, 2001). Physical therapists, occupational therapists, enterostomal therapists, and dietitians can be helpful resources (Spoelhof, 2001).*

Client/Family Teaching

- Teach skin and wound assessment and ways to monitor for signs and symptoms of infection, complications, and healing. *Early assessment and intervention help prevent the development of serious problems (van Rijswijk, 2001).*
- Teach the use of a topical treatment that is matched to the client, wound, and setting. *The topical treatment needs to be adjusted as the status of the wound changes (Krasner and Sibbald, 1999).*
- If it is consistent with overall client management goals, teach how to turn and reposition the client at least every 2 hours. *If the goal of care is to keep the client comfortable (e.g., for a terminally ill client), turning and repositioning may not be appropriate (Krasner, Rodeheaver, and Sibbald, 2001; Panel for the Prediction and Prevention of Pressure Ulcers in Adults, 1992).*
- Teach the use of pillows, foam wedges, and pressure-reducing devices to prevent pressure injury. **Clinical Research:** *The use of effective pressure-reducing seat cushions for elderly wheelchair users significantly prevented sitting-acquired pressure ulcers (Geyer et al, 2001).*

- = Independent; ▲ = Collaborative

evolve WEBSITES FOR EDUCATION

See the EVOLVE website for World Wide Web resources for client education.

REFERENCES

Ayello EA, Braden B: How and why to do pressure ulcer risk assessment, *Adv Skin Wound Care* 15(3):125, 2002.

Bergstrom N et al: The Braden scale for prediction of pressure sore risk, *Nurs Res* 36:205, 1987.

Bergstrom N et al: *Treatment of pressure ulcers,* Clinical Practice Guideline No. 15, Agency for Health Care Policy and Research Pub. No. 95-0652, Rockville, Md, 1994, Public Health Service, US Department of Health and Human Services.

Biala KY: Case conferencing for wound care patients, *Home Healthc Nurs* 20(2):120, 2002.

Bryant R: *Acute and chronic wounds,* ed 2, St Louis, 1999, Mosby.

Clever K et al: Evaluating the efficacy of a uniquely delivered skin protectant and its effect on the formation of sacral/buttock pressure ulcers, *Ostomy Wound Manage* 48(12):60, 2002.

Demling R, De Santi L: Closure of the "non-healing wound" corresponds with correction of weight loss using the anabolic agent oxandrolone, *Ostomy Wound Manage* 444(10):58, 1998.

Doughty D: *Urinary and fecal incontinence: nursing management,* St Louis, 2000, Mosby.

European Wound Management Association: *Pain at wound dressing changes,* position document, London, 2001, Medical Education Partnership, available online at http://www.tendra.com/index.asp?id=1321&lang=2, accessed Feb 10, 2003.

Faller N, Beitz J: When a wound isn't a wound: tubes, drains, fistulas and draining wounds. In Krasner D, Rodeheaver G, Sibbald RG: *Chronic wound care: a clinical source book for healthcare professionals,* ed 2, Wayne, Penn, 2001, HMP Communications.

Fleck D: Support surfaces: criteria and selection. In Krasner D, Rodeheaver G, Sibbald RG: *Chronic wound care: a clinical source book for healthcare professionals,* ed 2, Wayne, Penn, 2001, HMP Communications.

Geyer MJ et al: A randomized control trial to evaluate pressure-reducing seating cushions for elderly wheelchair users, *Adv Skin Wound Care* 14(3):120, 2001.

Krasner D: Caring for the person experiencing chronic wound pain. In Krasner D, Rodeheaver G, Sibbald RG: *Chronic wound care: a clinical source book for healthcare professionals,* ed 2, Wayne, Penn, 2001, HMP Communications.

Krasner D, Rodeheaver G, Sibbald RG: Advanced wound caring for a new millennium. In Krasner D, Rodeheaver G, Sibbald RG: *Chronic wound care: a clinical source book for healthcare professionals,* ed 2, Wayne, Penn, 2001, HMP Communications.

Krasner D, Sibbald RG: Moving beyond the AHCPR guidelines: wound care evolution over the last five years, *Ostomy Wound Manage* 45(suppl 1A):1S, 1999.

Longobardi S, Huthison R, Caputo WJ: Considerations in the local treatment of diabetic lower extremity ulcers, *Home Health Care Consult* 8(7):23, 2001.

Maklebust J, Sieggreen M: *Pressure ulcers: guidelines for prevention and nursing management,* ed 2, Springhouse, Penn, 1996, Springhouse.

National Pressure Ulcer Advisory Panel: *Consensus development conference statement,* Buffalo, NY, 1989, The Panel.

Ovington LG: The well-dressed wound: an overview of dressing types, *Wounds* 10(suppl A):1A, 1998.

Ovington LG: Hanging wet-to-dry dressings out to dry, *Home Healthc Nurse* 19(8):477, 2001a.

Ovington LG: Battling bacteria in wound care, *Home Healthc Nurse* 19(10):622, 2001b.

Ovington LG; Schaum KD: Wound care products: how to choose, *Home Healthc Nurse* 19(4):224, 2001.

Panel for the Prediction and Prevention of Pressure Ulcers in Adults: *Pressure ulcers in adults: prediction and prevention,* Clinical Practice Guideline No. 3, Agency for Health Care Policy and Research Pub No. 92-0047, Rockville, Md, 1992, US Department of Health and Human Services, Public Health Service.

Russell L: The importance of patients' nutritional status in wound healing, *Br J Nurs* 10(6):S42, 2001.

Spoelhof GD: Treatment of pressure ulcers, *Home Health Care Consult* 8(3):10, 2001.

Sussman C, Bates-Jensen BM: *Wound care: a collaborative practice manual for physical therapists and nurses,* Gaithersburg, Md, 1998, Aspen.

van Rijswijk L: Wound assessment and documentation. In Krasner D, Rodeheaver G, Sibbald RG: *Chronic wound care: a clinical source book for healthcare professionals,* ed 2, Wayne, Penn, 2001, HMP Communications.

• = **Independent;** ▲ = **Collaborative**

Warshaw E et al: Clinical and cost effectiveness of a cleanser protectant lotion for treatment of perineal skin breakdown in low-risk patients with incontinence, *Ostomy Wound Manage* 48(6):44, 2002.

Wound, Ostomy, and Continence Nurses Society: *Standards of care: dermal wounds: pressure ulcers,* Costa Mesa, Calif, 1992, The Society.

Wound, Ostomy, and Continence Nurses Society: *Standards of care: patient with fecal incontinence,* Costa Mesa, Calif, 1994, The Society.

Young J et al: Risk factors associated with pressure ulcer development at a major Western Australia teaching hospital from 1998 to 2000, *J Wound Ostomy Continence Nurs* 29(5):234, 2002.

Ineffective Tissue perfusion (specify type: renal, cerebral, cardiopulmonary, gastrointestinal, peripheral)

Betty J. Ackley

NANDA Definition

Decrease in oxygen resulting in failure to nourish tissues at capillary level

Defining Characteristics

Renal

Altered blood pressure outside of acceptable parameters; hematuria; oliguria or anuria; elevation in blood urea nitrogen/creatinine ratio

Cerebral

Speech abnormalities; changes in pupillary reactions; extremity weakness or paralysis; altered mental status; difficult in swallowing; changes in motor response; behavioral changes

Cardiopulmonary

Altered respiratory rate outside of acceptable parameters; use of accessory muscles; capillary refill longer than 3 seconds; abnormal arterial blood gas levels; chest pain; sense of impending doom; bronchospasms; dyspnea; dysrhythmias; nasal flaring; chest retraction

Gastrointestinal

Hypoactive or absent bowel sounds; nausea; abdominal distention; abdominal pain or tenderness

Peripheral

Edema; positive Homans' sign; altered skin characteristics (hair, moisture) or nails; weak or absent pulses; skin discolorations; skin temperature changes; altered sensations; diminished arterial pulsations; pale skin color upon elevation of leg with color not returning upon lowering of leg; slow healing of lesions; cold extremities; dependent, blue, or purple skin color

Related Factors (r/t)

Hypovolemia; interruption of arterial flow; hypervolemia; exchange problems; interruption of venous flow; mechanical reduction of venous and/or arterial blood flow; hypoventilation; impaired transport of oxygen across alveolar and/or capillary membrane; mismatch of ventilation with blood flow; decreased hemoglobin concentration in blood; enzyme poisoning; altered affinity of hemoglobin for oxygen

• = Independent; ▲ = Collaborative

| **NOC** | Outcomes (Nursing Outcomes Classification) |

Suggested NOC Outcomes

Cardiac Pump Effectiveness; Circulation Status; Fluid Balance; Hydration; Tissue Perfusion: Cardiac, Cerebral, Peripheral; Urinary Elimination

> **Example NOC Outcome with Indicators**
>
> Demonstrates adequate **Circulation Status** as evidenced by the following indicators: Peripheral pulses strong/Peripheral pulses symmetrical/Peripheral edema not present (Rate each indicator of **Circulation Status:** 1 = extremely compromised, 2 = substantially compromised, 3 = moderately compromised, 4 = mildly compromised, 5 = not compromised [see Section I].)

Client Outcomes

Client Will (Specify Time Frame):

- Demonstrate adequate tissue perfusion as evidenced by palpable peripheral pulses, warm and dry skin, adequate urinary output, and absence of respiratory distress
- Verbalize knowledge of treatment regimen, including appropriate exercise and medications and their actions and possible side effects
- Identify changes in lifestyle that are needed to increase tissue perfusion

| **NIC** | Intervention (Nursing Interventions Classification) |

Suggested NIC Intervention

Circulatory Care: Arterial Insufficiency

> **Example NIC Activities—Circulatory Care: Arterial Insufficiency**
>
> Evaluate peripheral edema and pulses; Inspect skin for arterial ulcers and tissue breakdown

Nursing Interventions and Rationales

Cerebral perfusion

- If the client experiences dizziness because of postural hypotension when getting up, teach methods to decrease dizziness, such as remaining seated for several minutes before standing, flexing feet upward several times while seated, rising slowly, sitting down immediately if feeling dizzy, and trying to have someone present when standing. *Postural hypotension can be detected in up to 30% of elderly clients. These methods can help prevent falls (Tinetti, 2003).*
- ▲ Monitor neurological status; perform a neurological examination; if symptoms of a cerebrovascular accident occur (e.g., hemiparesis, hemiplegia, or dysphasia), call 911 and send the client to the emergency department. **Clinical Research:** *New onset of these neurological symptoms can signify a stroke. If the stroke is caused by a thrombus and the client receives thrombolytic treatment within 3 hours, effects can often be reversed and function improved, although there is an increased risk of intracranial hemorrhage (Wardlaw, 2001; Wardlaw, Zoppo, and Yamaguchi, 2000).*
- ▲ If an ischemic stroke is present, consider keeping the head of the bed lower or flat as long as the airway is maintained, after consulting with the physician. **Nursing Research:** *A pilot study examining the velocity of blood flow in the middle cerebral artery dem-*

- • = Independent; ▲ = Collaborative

onstrated increased flow when the head was lower than 30 degrees or flat (Wojner, El-Mitwalli, and Alexandrov, 2002). This study must be replicated before the change in position can be advocated for general practice.

- See the care plans for **Decreased Intracranial adaptive capacity, Risk for Injury,** and **Acute Confusion.**

Peripheral perfusion

▲ Check the dorsalis pedis, posterior tibial, and popliteal pulses bilaterally. If unable to find them, use a Doppler stethoscope and notify the physician immediately if new onset of pulses is not present. *Diminished or absent peripheral pulses indicate arterial insufficiency with resultant ischemia (Harris, Brown-Etris, and Troyer-Caudle, 1996; Karthikeshwar and Ouriel, 2002).*

- Note skin color and feel the temperature of the skin. *Skin pallor or mottling, cool or cold skin temperature, or an absent pulse can signal arterial obstruction, which is an emergency that requires immediate intervention (Dillon, 2003). Rubor (reddish-blue color accompanied by dependency) indicates dilated or damaged vessels. Brownish discoloration of the skin indicates chronic venous insufficiency (Bright and Georgi, 1992; Feldman, 1998).*

- Check capillary refill. *Nailbeds usually return to a pinkish color within 2 to 3 seconds after nailbed compression (Dillon, 2003).*

- Note skin texture and the presence of hair, ulcers, or gangrenous areas on the legs or feet. *Thin, shiny, dry skin with hair loss; brittle nails; and gangrene or ulcerations on toes and anterior surfaces of the feet are seen in clients with arterial insufficiency. If ulcerations are on the side of the leg, they are usually associated with venous insufficiency (Bickley, Szilagyi, and Stackhouse, 2003).*

- Note the presence of edema in the extremities and rate it on a four-point scale. Measure the circumference of the ankle and calf at the same time each day in the early morning (Cahall and Spence, 1995).

- Assess for pain in the extremities, noting severity, quality, timing, and exacerbating and alleviating factors. Differentiate venous from arterial disease. *In clients with venous insufficiency the pain lessens with elevation of the legs and exercise. In clients with arterial insufficiency the pain increases with elevation of the legs and exercise (Black, 1995). Some clients have both arterial and venous insufficiency. Arterial insufficiency is associated with pain when walking (claudication) that is relieved by rest. Clients with severe arterial disease have foot pain while at rest, which keeps them awake at night. Venous insufficiency is associated with aching, cramping, and discomfort (Bright and Georgi, 1992).*

Arterial insufficiency

▲ Monitor peripheral pulses. If there is new onset of loss of pulses with bluish, purple, or black areas and extreme pain, notify a physician immediately. *These are symptoms of arterial obstruction that can result in loss of a limb if not immediately reversed.*

- Do not elevate the legs above the level of the heart. *With arterial insufficiency, leg elevation decreases arterial blood supply to the legs.*

▲ For early arterial insufficiency, encourage exercise such as walking or riding an exercise bicycle from 30 to 60 min/day as ordered by the physician. *Exercise therapy should be the initial intervention in nondisabling claudication (Zafar, Farkouh, and Chesebro, 2000).* **Clinical Research:** *Participation in an exercise program was shown to increase walking times more effectively than angioplasty and antiplatelet therapy (Leng, Fowler, and Ernst,*

• = **Independent;** ▲ = **Collaborative**

2000). Aerobic exercise training can reverse age-related peripheral circulatory problems in otherwise healthy older men (Beere et al, 1999).

- Keep the client warm and have the client wear socks and shoes or sheepskin-lined slippers when mobile. Do not apply heat. *Clients with arterial insufficiency complain of being constantly cold; therefore, keep extremities warm to maintain vasodilation and blood supply. Heat application can easily damage ischemic tissues.*

▲ Pay meticulous attention to foot care. Refer to a podiatrist if the client has a foot or nail abnormality. *Ischemic feet are very vulnerable to injury; meticulous foot care can prevent further injury.*

- If the client has ischemic arterial ulcers, see the care plan for **Impaired Tissue integrity** but avoid use of occlusive dressings. *Occlusive dressings should be used with caution in clients with arterial ulceration because of the increased risk for cellulitis (Cahall and Spence, 1995).*

Venous insufficiency

- Elevate edematous legs as ordered and ensure that there is no pressure under the knee. *Elevation increases venous return and helps decrease edema. Pressure under the knee decreases venous circulation.*
- Apply graduated compression stockings as ordered. Ensure proper fit by measuring and remove the stocking at least twice a day, in the morning with the bath and in the evening, to assess the condition of the extremity, then reapply. **Nursing and Clinical Research:** *A meta-analysis of 11 studies encompassing 1752 subjects demonstrated that the use of graduated compression stockings reduced the incidence of deep vein thrombosis in a high-risk orthopedic surgical population and that implementation of additional antithrombotic measures along with stocking use decreased the incidence even further (Joanna Briggs Institute, 2001). Graduated compression stockings, alone or used in conjunction with other prevention modalities, help prevent deep vein thrombosis in hospitalized patients (Amarigiri and Lees, 2000).*
- Encourage the client to walk with support hose on and perform toe-up and point-flex exercises. *Exercise helps to increase venous return, build up collateral circulation, and strengthen the calf muscle pumps (Cahall and Spence, 1995).*
- If the client is overweight, encourage weight loss to decrease venous disease. *Obesity is a risk factor for development of chronic venous disease (Kunimoto et al, 2001).*
- If the client has venous leg ulcers, encourage the client to avoid prolonged sitting, standing, and elevation of the involved leg. **Nursing Research:** *A study demonstrated that wound perfusion was lower when the client with venous leg ulcers was sitting, standing, or elevating the involved leg than when the client was lying supine (Wipke-Tevis et al, 2001).*
- Discuss lifestyle with the client to determine if the client's occupation requires prolonged standing or sitting, which can result in chronic venous disease (Kunimoto et al, 2001). *If the client is mostly immobile, consult with the physician regarding use of a calf-high pneumatic compression device for prevention of deep vein thrombosis. Pneumatic compression devices can be effective in preventing deep vein thrombosis in the immobile client (Hyers, 1999).*
- Observe for signs of deep vein thrombosis, including pain, tenderness, swelling in the calf and thigh, and redness in the involved extremity. Take serial leg measurements of the thigh and calf circumferences. In some clients a tender venous cord can be felt in the popliteal fossa. Do not rely on Homans' sign. *Thrombosis with clot formation is*

• = **Independent;** ▲ = **Collaborative**

usually first detected as swelling of the involved leg and then as pain. Leg measurement discrepancies of more than 2 cm warrant further investigation (Herzog, 1992; Launius and Graham, 1998). Homans' sign is not reliable (Dillon, 2003). Unfortunately, symptoms of existing deep vein thrombosis will not be found in 25% to 50% of client examinations even when a thrombus is present (Eftychiou, 1996; Launius and Graham, 1998).

- Note the results of a d-dimer test. *High levels of d-dimer, a fibrin degradation fragment, are found in deep vein thrombosis, pulmonary embolism, and disseminated intravascular coagulation (Pagana and Pagana, 2001; Sullano and Ortiz, 2001).*
- If deep vein thrombosis is present, observe for symptoms of a pulmonary embolism, especially if there is history of trauma. **Clinical Research:** *Based on data from 16 studies, fatal pulmonary embolisms are reported in one third of trauma clients (Agency for Healthcare Research and Quality, 2000).*

Geriatric

- Change the client's position slowly when getting the client out of bed. *Postural hypotension can be detected in up to 30% of elderly clients (Tinetti, 2003).*
- Recognize that the elderly have an increased risk of developing pulmonary embolism and that, if it is present, the symptoms are nonspecific and often mimic those of heart failure or pneumonia (Berman, 2001; Hyers, 1999).

Home care

- The interventions described previously may be adapted for home care use.
- Differentiate between arterial and venous insufficiency. *Accurate diagnostic information clarifies clinical assessment and allows for more effective care.*
- If arterial disease is present and the client smokes, aggressively encourage smoking cessation. See the care plan for **Health-seeking behaviors.**
- Examine the feet carefully at frequent intervals for changes and new ulcerations. *Lower Extremity Amputation Prevention Program (LEAP) documentation forms are available at http://www.bphc.hrsa.gov/leap/ (Feldman, 1998).*
- ▲ Assess the client's nutritional status, paying special attention to obesity, hyperlipidemia, and malnutrition. Refer to a dietitian if appropriate. *Malnutrition contributes to anemia, which further compounds the lack of oxygenation to tissues. Obese clients encounter poor circulation in adipose tissue, which can create increased hypoxia in tissue (Rolstad, 1990).*
- Monitor for development of gangrene, venous ulceration, and symptoms of cellulitis (redness, pain, and increased swelling in an extremity). *Cellulitis often accompanies peripheral vascular disease and is related to poor tissue perfusion (Marrelli, 1994).*

Client/Family Teaching

- Explain the importance of good foot care. Teach the client and family to wash and inspect the feet daily. Recommend that the diabetic client wear padded socks, special insoles, and jogging shoes. *Use of cushioned footwear can decrease pressure on the feet, decrease callus formation, and help save the feet (Feldman, 1998; George, 1993).*
- ▲ Teach the diabetic client that he or she should have a comprehensive foot examination at least annually, including assessment of sensation using the Semmes-Weinstein monofilaments. If good sensation is not present, refer to a footwear professional for fitting of therapeutic shoes and inserts, the cost of which is covered by Medicare. **Clinical Research:** */Testing with Semmes-Weinstein monofilaments is effectively diagnos-*

• = **Independent;** ▲ = **Collaborative**

tic of impaired sensation, especially when combined with clinical examination (Pham et al, 2000).

- For arterial disease, stress the importance of not smoking, following a weight loss program (if the client is obese), carefully controlling a diabetic condition, controlling hyperlipidemia and hypertension, and reducing stress. *All of these risk factors for atherosclerosis can be modified (Bright and Georgi, 1992).*
- Teach the client to avoid exposure to cold, to limit exposure to brief periods if going out in cold weather, and to wear warm clothing. *For venous disease, teach the importance of wearing support hose as ordered, elevating the legs at intervals, and watching for skin breakdown on the legs.*
- Teach the client to recognize the signs and symptoms that should be reported to a physician (e.g., change in skin temperature, color, or sensation, or the presence of a new lesion on the foot).

NOTE: If the client is receiving anticoagulant therapy, see the care plan for **Ineffective Protection.**

evolve WEBSITES FOR EDUCATION

See the EVOLVE website for World Wide Web resources for client education.

REFERENCES

Agency for Healthcare Research and Quality: *Prevention of venous thromboembolism after injury: summary,* Evidence Report/Technology Assessment Number 22, Rockville, Md, August 2000, The Agency, available online at http://www.ahrq.gov/clinic/epcsums/vtsumm.htm, accessed Jan 12, 2003.

Amarigiri SV, Lees TA: Elastic compression stockings for prevention of deep vein thrombosis. *Cochrane Database Syst Rev* 3(CD001484), 2000.

Bickley LS, Szilagyi PG, Stackhouse JG: *Bates guide to physical examination and history taking,* ed 8, Philadelphia, 2003, Lippincott.

Beere PA et al: Aerobic exercise training can reverse age-related peripheral circulatory changes in healthy older men, *Circulation* 100(10):1085, 1999.

Berman AR: Pulmonary embolism in the elderly, *Clin Geriatr Med* 17:1, 2001.

Black SB: Venous stasis ulcers: a review, *Ostomy Wound Manage* 41:20, 1995.

Bright LD, Georgi S: Peripheral vascular disease, is it arterial or venous? *Am J Nurs* 92:34, 1992.

Cahall E, Spence RK: Practical nursing measures for vascular compromise in the lower leg, *Ostomy Wound Manage* 41:16, 1995.

Dillon PM: *Nursing health assessment,* Philadelphia, 2003, FA Davis.

Eftychiou V: Clinical diagnosis and management of the patient with deep venous thromboembolism and acute pulmonary embolism, *Nurse Pract* 21:50, 1996.

Feldman CB: Caring for feet: patients and nurse practitioners working together, *Nurse Pract Forum* 9(2):87, 1998.

George NE: Give 'em the old soft shoe: working smart, *Am J Nurs* 93:16, 1993.

Harris AH, Brown-Etris M, Troyer-Caudle J: Managing vascular leg ulcers, *Am J Nurs* 1:38, 1996.

Herzog JA: Deep vein thrombosis in the rehabilitation client, *Rehabil Nurs* 17:196, 1992.

Hyers TM: Venous thromboembolism, *Am J Respir Crit Care Med* 159:1, 1999.

Joanna Briggs Institute: Best practice: graduated compression stockings for the prevention of post-operative venous thromboembolism, *Evidenced Based Practice Information Sheets for Health Professions* 5:2, 2001.

Karthikeshwar K, Ouriel K: Current options in the diagnosis and management of acute limb ischemia, *Prog Cardiovasc Nurs* 17:1, 2002.

Kunimoto B et al: Best practices for the prevention and treatment of venous leg ulcers, *Ostomy Wound Manage* 47(2):34, 2001.

Launius BK, Graham BD: Understanding and preventing deep vein thrombosis and pulmonary embolism, *AACN Clin Issues* 9(1):91, 1998.

- = **Independent;** ▲ = **Collaborative**

Leng GC, Fowler B, Ernst E: Exercise for intermittent claudication, *Cochrane Library*, 2(CD000990), 2000.

Marrelli TM: *Handbook of home health standards and documentation guidelines for reimbursement*, ed 2, St Louis, 1994, Mosby.

Pagana KD, Pagana TJ: *Mosby's diagnostic and laboratory test reference*, ed 5, St Louis, 2001, Mosby.

Pham H et al: Screening techniques to identify people at high risk for diabetic foot ulceration: a prospective multicenter trial, *Diabetes Care* 23(5):606, 2000.

Rolstad BS: Treatment objectives in chronic wound care, *Home Healthc Nurse* 9:6, 1990.

Sullano ME, Ortiz EJ: Deep vein thrombosis and anticoagulant therapy, *Nurs Clin North Am* 36(4):645, 2001.

Tinetti ME: Preventing falls in elderly persons, *N Engl J Med* 348(1):421, 2003.

Wardlaw JM: Overview of Cochrane thrombolysis meta-analysis, *Neurology* 57:5, 2001.

Wardlaw JM, Zoppo G, Yamaguchi T: Thrombolysis for acute ischaemic stroke, *Cochrane Database Syst Rev* CD000213, 2000.

Wipke-Tevis DD et al: Tissue oxygenation, perfusion, and position in patients with venous leg ulcers, *Nurs Res* 50(1):24, 2001.

Wojner AW, El-Mitwalli A, Alexandrov AV: Effect of head positioning on intracranial blood flow velocities in acute ischemic stroke: a pilot study, *Crit Care Nurs Q* 24(4):57, 2002.

Zafar MU, Farkouh ME, Chesebro JH: A practical approach to lower-extremity arterial disease, *Patient Care* 30:96, 2000.

Impaired Transfer ability

Brenda Emick-Herring

NANDA Definition

Limitation of independent movement between two nearby surfaces

Defining Characteristics

Impaired ability to transfer: from bed to chair and chair to bed/on or off toilet or commode/between uneven levels/from chair to car or car to chair/from chair to floor or floor to chair/from standing to floor or floor to standing

Related Factors (r/t)

See Defining Characteristics

NOC Outcomes (Nursing Outcomes Classification)

Suggested NOC Outcomes

Balance; Body Positioning: Self-Initiated

Example NOC Outcome with Indicators

Body Positioning: Self-Initiated as evidenced by the following indicators: Transfers from chair to bed and back/Transfers from chair to commode and back/Transfers from chair to car and back (Rate each indicator of **Body Positioning: Self-Initiated:** 1 = dependent—does not participate, 2 = requires assistive person and device, 3 = requires assistive person, 4 = independent with assistive device, 5 = completely independent [see Section I].)

Outcome adapted from NOC.

• = Independent; ▲ = Collaborative

Client Outcomes

Client Will (Specify Time Frame):

- Transfer from bed to chair and back successfully
- Transfer from chair to chair successfully
- Transfer from chair to toilet and back successfully
- Transfer from chair to car and back successfully

NIC Interventions (Nursing Interventions Classification)

Suggested NIC Interventions

Exercise Promotion: Strength Training; Exercise Therapy: Muscle Control

> **Example NIC Activities—Exercise Promotion: Strength Training**
>
> Obtain medical clearance for initiating a strength-training program, as appropriate; Assist client in setting realistic short- and long-term goals and taking ownership of the exercise plan

Nursing Interventions and Rationales

▲ Request a consult for a physical therapist (PT) and/or occupational therapist (OT) for an upper and lower extremity exercise and strengthening program early in the client's progressive mobilization and recovery. *Lower extremity and trunk strengthening will be key for persons doing partial or full weight-bearing transfers; upper extremity and trunk strength will be important for sliding-board transfers.*

▲ Obtain a consult for a PT, OT, or orthotist to evaluate, prescribe, measure, and fit the client with the proper orthoses, braces, splints, walking aids, raised toilet seats, etc. *Assistive devices and walking aids must be individualized to help clients move and function safely, comfortably, effectively, and as independently as possible (Hoeman, 2002).*

▲ Inquire about and learn the specific techniques and instructions the OT and PT have taught the client to reinforce and assist the client as he or she transfers to various surfaces. *Clear communication and a consistent team approach are needed to promote client/ family learning and to monitor the client's progress so that the approach can be updated as needed (Rehabilitation Nursing Standards Task Force, 2000).*

▲ Ergonomically assess the client's dependence level, size, weight, strength, movement abilities in bed, balance, tolerance to position change, sensation, behavior, and cognition, as well as equipment availability and staff ratios and experience to decide whether to perform a manual or device-assisted lift, transfer, or weighing of the client. (If a PT has already evaluated and identified a specific transfer method and it is compatible with the nursing assessment, use that method.) **Nursing Research:** *Redesigning a task with the use of equipment reduced the physical stress on staff and provided comfort and security to clients. Use of a wheelchair ramp or hoist scale to weigh clients reduced perceived stress on employees' shoulders, backs, and whole bodies, and objectively reduced compressive and shear forces to L5 to S1 discs (Owen and Garg, 1994). Staff subjectively reported that work fatigue, demands, and back and shoulder pain decreased and safety increased with a "safe lifting" approach (staff education and use of assistive devices such as transfer belts and slide devices) and "no strenuous lifting" approach (staff training and consistent availability and use of mechanical lift and transfer devices) to lift and transfer hospitalized clients. Actual musculoskeletal injuries of staff did not change with either approach (Yassi et al, 2001). A pilot study using a nursing staff trained lift team to transfer clients*

- = Independent; ▲ = Collaborative

needing maximal assistance reported a high volume of requests and successful completion of transfers, lack of nurse injury, and positive staff evaluation of the team. Potential long-range implications were raised, such as injury over time, monotony, cost effectiveness, and need for rotation of team members (Caska, Patnode, and Clickner, 1998).

- Do not use the under-axilla method to transfer, lift, and weigh a physically dependent client. Rather, use mechanical devices such as hydraulic or battery-operated mechanical lifts, stand-assist lifts, and bed or wheelchair ramp scales. **Nursing Research:** *Under-axilla lifts can cause overexertion back injuries to staff because of the lateral bending, trunk rotation, and full vertical weight lift that it induces. Mechanical devices may be more comfortable physically and psychologically for the clients, yet nursing educators continue to teach the under-axilla method and see it used clinically by staff nurses (Owen, Welden, and Kane, 1999).*

- Apply a gait belt or walking belt with handles before manually transferring the client to counteract unsteadiness and weakness and to help prevent client falls. Keep the belt and client close to the staff member, not at arm's length. *Using a belt at arm's length moves the client's base of support away from the staff member, prevents proper support of the client, and places the staff member at risk for back and arm injury (Minor and Minor, 1999).* **Nursing Research:** *Use of a belt decreases staff exertion, back stress, and compressive force to L5 to S1 (Owen and Garg, 1993).*

- Enforce and verbally cue the client on how to comply with any weight-bearing restrictions ordered.

- Assist the client in donning the appropriate orthoses, braces, collars, prostheses, immobilizers, splints, gait belts, and binders while in bed (always loosen or remove the abdominal binder after the client returns to bed). *These devices stabilize and align necessary body parts during motion. Abdominal binders help prevent postural hypotension.*

- Adjust surfaces so that they are as similar in height as possible. For example, lower a hospital bed or use a tub seat, commode, or shower/bowel care chair that is nearly the same height as the wheelchair. **Clinical Research:** *Arranging equal heights between seat surfaces requires much less upper extremity muscular effort during transfers to and from wheelchairs (Wang et al, 1994).*

- Help the client put on shoes or socks with nonskid soles before transfers. *To prevent falls during transfers, have the client avoid wearing footwear with a smooth or fabric sole, such as antiembolic stockings. Negotiate with diabetic clients always to wear shoes or slippers because their feet heal poorly if injured (Yetzer, 2002).*

- Remove or swivel a chair's leg rests, arm rests, and foot plates to the side before transferring the client. *This gives the client's and nurse's feet more space in which to maneuver and provides fewer obstacles to trip over (Minor and Minor 1999; Ossman and Campbell, 1990).*

- Place the wheelchair, commode, or shower chair at a 20- to 45-degree angle next to the surface onto which the client will transfer (e.g., bed, chair, toilet). *Such an angle gets the two transfer surfaces close to one another yet allows room for client and staff or family to adjust the client's movements during the transfer (Hoeman, 2002; Kumagai, 1998; Ossman and Campbell, 1990).*

- Teach the client to consistently lock the brakes on wheelchairs, commodes, shower chairs, and beds before transfer. *These devices are often portable and have wheels. If wheels are not locked, the devices can roll as the client transfers into or out of them, which thus creates a risk for falls. Pneumatic wheelchair tires must be adequately inflated for the brakes to lock effectively (Minor and Minor, 1999).*

- • = Independent; ▲ = Collaborative

- Position walking aids logistically so that the client can grasp and use them once he or she is standing. Walking aids provide support, balance, and stability to help the client stand and step safely and functionally (Bohannon, 1997). **Clinical Research:** *Elderly persons with diagnosed peripheral neuropathy had less risk of losing their balance standing on an unstable (suddenly tilting) surface in normal-light and low-light conditions when using a cane in the nondominant hand (Ashton-Miller et al, 1996).*
- Strongly encourage the client to practice transfer techniques in a consistent manner, whether during therapy or during functional activities such as toileting. *Transfers will be individualized depending on the client's diagnoses, joint range of motion, strength, tone, pain, medical restrictions, etc.*
- Give clear, simple instructions; allow time to process the information; and let the client do as much of the transfer as possible.
- ▲ Implement and document the interdisciplinary plan of care, including the type of transfer (sitting, squatting, pivoting, etc.), weight-bearing status (none, partial, full), equipment (lift, sliding board, crutches, etc.), level of assistance (standby, moderate, etc.), and type of assistance to provide (manual guidance, balance control, physical levering, verbal cueing, etc.). *Team collaboration, communication, consistency, and repetitive practice are critical for learning, motor recovery, and safety (Gee and Passarella, 1985; Minor and Minor 1999; Kumagai, 1998; Rehabilitation Nursing Standards Task Force, 2000).*
- Incorporate set positions before transferring the client (e.g., sitting on the edge of the surface/seat with bilateral weight bearing, hips and knees flexed, the front [balls] of the feet aligned under the knees, and the head in midline). *These are the normal movements/postures that prepare humans for weight bearing. These postures permit shifting of weight from the pelvis to the feet as the center of gravity changes during standing (Gee and Passarella, 1985; Kumagai, 1998).*
- Recognize the normal sequence of movements for standing (i.e., hips and knees flex; back extends; trunk, head, and finally knees lean forward over feet; weight shifts to the feet, thus lifting up hips and buttocks; standing occurs as the knees, hips, and trunk extend). *Knowing the normal movements of standing may help nurses identify key points to emphasize and at which to give assistance to the client during transfers (Gee and Passarella, 1985; Kumagai, 1998).*
- Support or stabilize the client's knee(s) with one or both of your knees next to or encircling the client's knee(s) rather than "blocking" the client's knee(s). *This allows the client to flex the knee(s) and to lean forward during transfers.*
- Four methods of transferring the client are described below.
  - Squat transfer: Stand in front of the client and guide him or her in the following manner: (1) guide the client into the set position for standing. (2) The nurse stands with one foot forward as his or her arms lie over the client's shoulders with the hands on the gait belt around the client's lower back or on the pelvic girdle. (3) The nurse shifts weight from his or her front foot to the back foot while reminding the client to lean well forward. (4) The client pivots as his or her flexed hips raise from the surface. (5) The nurse rocks forward while lowering the client onto the intended surface. *This technique can be used for clients who have sensorimotor disturbances but some muscle control (Kumagai, 1998; Ossman and Campbell, 1990).*
  - Seated to standing transfer: Stand in front of the client to help unless he or she is using a walker, then stand on the weakest side of the client. Help the client to do the following: (1) attain the set position and lean well forward; (2) slowly stand

• = **Independent**; ▲ = **Collaborative**

when instructed to, with the nurse placing pressure with his or her hands on the client's buttocks to help extend the hips or on the chest to move the shoulders gently back once erect, or assisting with knee extension and stability as the client "unfolds" to stand up (a second nurse may be needed if the client needs help in all three areas). *Clients may have difficulty with balance, weight shifting, extension, achievement of neutral trunk alignment, or knee buckling or hyperextension. This method is appropriate for clients whose legs and feet are starting to bear weight (Kumagai, 1998).*

■ Standing pivot transfer: Stand in front or to the side of the client and assist the client with the following actions: (1) get in the set position; (2) place the palms of the hands on the surface from which the client is transferring (the chair arm rests or mattress), or else on the closest part of the surface to which the client is transferring; (3) lean forward and flex the hips so that weight shifts to the feet; (4) push with the hands; (5) bear weight on both feet while arising to an erect position; (6) pivot by shifting and centering weight on the foot next to the chair or surface to which the client is transferring, which unweights the opposite foot so that it can be slid or pivoted; (7) reposition the foot back on the floor, centering the weight on it; (8) unweight the opposite foot; (9) repeat the weight shift and pivot maneuver until the backside of the client touches the desired surface; (10) grasp or place the hands on the arm rest or the surface to which the client is transferring for steadiness; and (11) flex the hips, lean forward, and sit down. (Using a gait belt, a nurse may need to help the client arise, maintain standing balance, and sit back down; a second nurse can help move/control the pelvis from behind the client.) *This method is appropriate for clients with some weight-bearing capability. Unless weight bearing is restricted, it is important for bilateral weight bearing to take place during the sequence of movements, especially in hemiplegics. Pivoting should be done with both feet if possible; if not, with one foot at a time (Kumagai, 1998).*

■ Sliding board transfer: (1) Ensure that the client has pants on or put a pillowcase over the board. (2) Remove the arm and leg rests from the chair and securely lock all brakes. (3) Place the chair angled up to 45 degrees alongside the surface on which the client is sitting. (4) Help the client to shift weight onto the hip opposite the angled chair and place the sliding board under the raised buttock. (5) Have the client shift weight back to a normal sitting posture. (6) Ensure that the board lies angled across both transferring surfaces and that the client will miss hitting the wheel of the chair. (7) Have the client place one hand on the sliding board and other hand on the surface on which he or she is sitting. (8) Instruct the client to perform a series of pushups with the arms, leaning forward slightly to help lift the buttocks onto the board. (9) Move by lifting, not sliding, the body a bit at a time with each pushup. (10) The nurse(s) may need to stand in front and/or in back of the client and use a gait belt to help lift the client's buttocks with each pushup. Clothing prevents the skin from sticking to the board. *This type of transfer is beneficial for those who cannot move the lower extremities and those who are extremely weak (Hoeman, 2002; Minor and Minor, 1999).*

▲ Procure extra staff and special equipment to help a debilitated bariatric client (extremely obese person) establish balance and lean forward as he or she transfers. Help the client get set by placing both knees level with the thighs so they do not drift downward. The feet may need to be placed on a stool to help get them level. Place the bed against the wall and lock the brakes. *Specialized equipment may include bed, lift, commode, wheelchair, and shower/bowel care chair. A large room with a wide doorway may be*

• = Independent; ▲ = Collaborative

necessary. The bariatric client will likely need bilevel or continuous airway pressure therapy at night. Fear of falling is a grave concern of the bariatric client. Past falls may have evoked embarrassment when help arrived to get the client up. Center-of-gravity and balance skills must be learned so the client will lean forward and staff can use this momentum to help transfer the client. Obesity is a causative factor in obstructive sleep apnea, which can contribute to poor endurance and activity tolerance (Daus, 2001).

▲ Investigate and offer current devices to safely transfer the bariatric client based on individual needs. Such devices may include an air mattress overlay, Gore-Tex or silicone transfer sheet, 60-inch-long gait belt, supine sliding or roller board, high-low chair, bedside sling-lift device, bedside weight-bearing or standing-lift device, overhead ceiling-mounted lift, or overhead A-frame lift (Dionne, 2000, 2002).

Home care

▲ Obtain a referral for an OT and/or PT to develop home exercise and transfer regimes and evaluate the need for home modifications such as wider doorways, safe floor surface, grab bars, clutter elimination, adequate lighting, adequate seating (proper chair height, stability, support, and firmness), optimum furniture placement (for maneuverability and stability in using to assist in getting up if a fall occurs), fitted bedspreads and blankets so that the client does not trip, etc. *Home evaluation and treatment help meet the unique mobility needs of clients within their personal environments. Therapists can help families understand, choose, access, and evaluate needed adaptive equipment to promote independence (Aiello et al, 2001).* **Clinical Research:** *Nonuse of prescribed equipment may be prevented by ensuring that home visits are made by the therapists prior to discharge; tub transfers were frightening and difficult at home even with teaching prior to hospital discharge (Finlayson and Havixbeck, 1992).*

▲ Involve a social worker to educate the client and family about equipment costs and financial benefits and regulations associated with Medicare, Medicaid, and third-party payers, as well as local community options for securing durable medical equipment and home care services. *Such information can help families understand the financial implications of desired services and equipment.*

▲ Coordinate with therapy services to reinforce client and family education regarding safe and effective transfer methods; equipment; application, removal, and care of assistive devices; skin checks and care associated with the use of braces, splints, immobilizers, etc.; and proper fit and use of transfer aids such as canes, walkers, and crutches. *Repetition and a consistent approach reinforce learning and follow-through. Overassisting the client may decrease learning, self-esteem, and independence.*

• Use an ergonomic approach and implement ongoing research findings to safely handle and transfer clients in their homes. *Risk of back, shoulder, and neck injury is high because home health care staff work alone and often without mechanical lifts or aids, work in crowded spaces, use nonadjustable beds and chairs, and use awkward postures to move or care for clients (Galinsky, Waters, and Malit, 2001).*

• For further information see the care plans for **Impaired physical Mobility** and **Impaired Walking.**

Client/Family Teaching

▲ Begin discharge planning as soon as possible with the case manager or social worker to assess the need for home support systems, assistive devices, and community or home health services.

• = **Independent;** ▲ = **Collaborative**

▲ Obtain referral for an OT and/or PT to develop home exercise and transfer regimes, and evaluate home modification and equipment needs such as wheelchairs, tub seats, hand rails, and raised toilet seats. *Home evaluation and treatment helps meet the unique mobility needs of clients within their personal environments. Therapists can help families understand, choose, and access needed adaptive equipment to promote independence (Aiello et al, 2001).* **Nursing Research:** *The ability to perform bed transfer was shown to be the most important factor in enabling frail elderly clients to live independently (Seidenfeld, Eberle, and Potter, 2000).*

▲ Involve a social worker to educate the client and family about equipment costs and financial benefits and regulations associated with Medicare, Medicaid, and third-party payers, as well as local community options for securing durable medical equipment and home care services. *Such information can help families understand the financial implications of desired services and equipment.*

▲ Coordinate with therapy services to reinforce client and family education regarding safe and effective transfer methods; application, removal, and care of assistive devices; skin checks and care associated with the use of braces, splints, immobilizers, etc.; and proper fit and use of transfer aids such as canes, walkers, and crutches. *Repetition and a consistent approach reinforce learning and follow-through. Overassisting the client may decrease learning, self-esteem, and independence.*

• Demonstrate and encourage supervised practice using hydraulic lifts or battery-operated mechanical or stand-assist lifts to transfer dependent clients into and out of bed and chairs. *This may help prevent back stress and injuries in family caregivers.*

• Teach, model, and monitor the client's and family's consistent performance of safety precautions for transfers, including wearing proper shoes, placing equipment and chairs correctly, locking brakes, applying gait belts, swiveling leg rests out of the way, etc. *Such actions will help prevent falls and injury to clients and caregivers.*

▲ Reinforce teaching given to the family about how to transfer the client left and right, and to and from various surfaces; collaborate with the PT and OT if home visits will not be made. Encourage supervised practice before facility discharge and the client's return home. *The basic principles for transfers are constant from surface to surface; however, individuals often need special instruction from a therapist to individualize the approaches for the home. Repetitive practice may help use of these techniques become habitual (Gee and Passarella, 1985; Ossman and Campbell, 1990).*

• Teach the client and family how to check brakes on chairs to make sure they engage and how to check that tires have adequate air pressure. Recommend routine inspection and an annual tune-up of the wheelchair. *Long-term use may loosen brakes or cause them to slip. The brakes work only if they make sound contact with the tire or wheel; therefore it is important that pneumatic tires be adequately inflated (Minor and Minor, 1999).*

• Offer information to promote the use of a safe shower/bowel care chair to prevent serious complications such as discomfort, pressure ulcers, falls during transfer or transport, and inaccessibility for bowel care and hygiene (bowel care may take 30 minutes to 3 hours in persons with neurogenic bowel). **Nursing Research:** *Three shower/ bowel care chairs were evaluated by clients and caregivers for comfort and safety (cushion padding, seam placement, seat opening, support and mobility of foot and arm rests), transportability, accessibility for bowel care/showering, and repeated use in the shower. Many inadequacies and unsafe features were identified, especially regarding development of pressure ulcer and falls (Malassigné et al, 1993). Based on these data the research team designed,*

• = **Independent;** ▲ = **Collaborative**

tested, and marketed a new shower/bowel chair to minimize such risks and client error in using the chair (Nelson et al, 2000).

• For further information, see the care plans for **Impaired physical Mobility** and **Impaired Walking.**

evolve WEBSITES FOR EDUCATION

See the EVOLVE website for World Wide Web resources for client education.

REFERENCES

Aiello DD et al: Safety in the home, *Rehab Manag* 14(5):54, 2001.

Ashton-Miller JA et al: A cane reduces loss of balance in patients with peripheral neuropathy: results from a challenging unipedal balance test, *Arch Phys Med Rehabil* 77:446, 1996.

Bohannon RW: Gait performance with wheeled and standard walkers, *Percept Mot Skills* 85:1185, 1997.

Caska BA, Patnode RE, Clickner D: Feasibility of a nurse staffed lift team, *AAOHN J* 46(6):283, 1998.

Daus C: Rehab and the bariatric patient, *Rehab Manag* 14(9):42, 2001.

Dionne M: Maximizing efficiency with minimum effort: transferring the bariatric patient, *Rehab Manag* 13(6):64, 2000.

Dionne M: Ten tips for safe mobility in the bariatric population, *Rehab Manag* 15(8):28, 2002.

Finlayson M, Havixbeck K: A post-discharge study on the use of assistive devices, *Can J Occup Ther* 59(4):201, 1992.

Galinsky T, Waters T, Malit B: Overexertion injuries in home health care workers and the need for ergonomics, *Home Health Care Serv Q* 20(3):57, 2001.

Gee AL, Passarella PM: *Nursing care of the stroke patient: a therapeutic approach,* Pittsburgh, 1985, Harmarville Rehabilitation Center.

Hoeman SP: Movement, functional mobility, and activities of daily living. In Hoeman SP, editor: *Rehabilitation nursing: process, application, and outcomes,* ed 3, St Louis, 2002, Mosby, pp 211-258.

Kumagai KAS: Physical management of the neurologically involved client: techniques for bed mobility and transfers. In Chin PA, Finocchiaro D, Rosebrough A, editors: *Rehabilitation nursing practice,* New York, 1998, McGraw-Hill, pp 524-601.

Malassigné P et al: Toward the design of a new bowel care chair for the spinal cord injured: a pilot study, *SCI Nurs* 10(3):84, 1993.

Minor MAD, Minor SD: *Patient care skills,* ed 4, Stamford, Conn, 1999, Appleton and Lange.

Nelson A et al: Promoting safe use of equipment for neurogenic bowel management, *SCI Nurs* 17(3):119, 2000.

Ossman NJH, Campbell M: *Adult positions, transitions, and transfers: reproducible instruction cards for caregivers,* Therapist Guide No. 4166, Tucson, Ariz, 1990, Therapy Skill Builders.

Owen BD, Garg A: Back stress isn't part of the job, *Am J Nurs* 93(2):48, 1993.

Owen BD, Garg A: Reducing back stress through an ergonomic approach: weighing a patient, *Int J Nurs Stud* 31(6):511, 1994.

Owen BD, Welden N, Kane J: What are we teaching about lifting and transferring patients? *Res Nurs Health* 22(1):3, 1999.

Rehabilitation Nursing Standards Task Force: *Standards and scope of rehabilitation nursing practice,* ed 2, Glenview, Ill, 2000, Association of Rehabilitation Nurses.

Seidenfeld SE, Eberle CM, Potter JF: Functional abilities of frail elderly that enable return to the community, *Home Health Care Consult* 7(8):29, 2000.

Wang YT et al: Reaction force and EMG analyses of wheelchair transfers, *Percep Mot Skills* 79:763, 1994.

Yassi A et al: A randomized controlled trial to prevent patient lift and transfer injuries of health care workers, *Spine* 26(16):1739, 2001.

Yetzer EA: Causes and prevention of diabetic foot skin breakdown, *Rehabil Nurs* 27(2):52, 2002.

• = **Independent**; ▲ = **Collaborative**

Risk for Trauma

Gail B. Ladwig and Michele Walters

NANDA Definition

Accentuated risk of accidental tissue injury (e.g., wound, burn, fracture)

Risk Factors

External

High-crime neighborhood and client vulnerability; pot handles facing toward front of stove; knives stored uncovered; inappropriate call-for-aid mechanisms for bed-resting client; inadequately stored combustibles or corrosives (e.g., matches, oily rags, lye); highly flammable children's toys or clothing; obstructed passageways; high beds; large icicles hanging from roof; nonuse or misuse of seat restraints; overexposure to sun, sunlamps, or radiotherapy; overloaded electrical outlets; overloaded fuse boxes; play or work near vehicle pathways (e.g., driveways, lane ways, railroad tracks); playing with fireworks or gunpowder; unlocked storage of guns or ammunition; contact with rapidly moving machinery, industrial belts, or pulleys; litter or liquid spills on floors or stairways; defective appliances; bathing in very hot water (e.g., unsupervised bathing of young children); bathtub without hand grip or antislip equipment; children's playing with matches, candles, cigarettes, or sharp-edged toys; children's playing at top of stairs without gates; children's riding in front seat of car; delayed lighting of gas burner or oven; contact with intense cold; collection of grease waste on stove; operation of mechanically unsafe vehicle; driving after use of alcoholic beverages or drugs; driving at excessive speeds; entry into unlighted rooms; experimentation with chemicals or gasoline; exposure to dangerous machinery; faulty electrical plugs; frayed wires; contact with acids or alkalis; unsturdy or absent stair rails; use of unsteady ladders or chairs; use of cracked dishware or glasses; wearing of plastic apron or flowing clothes around open flame; lack of screening on fires or heaters; unsafe window protection in homes with young children; sliding on coarse bed linen or struggling within bed restraints; use of thin or worn potholders; unanchored electric wires; misuse of necessary headgear for motor cyclists or young children carried on adult bicycles; gas leaks; unsafe road or road-crossing conditions; slippery floors (e.g., wet or highly waxed); smoking in bed or near oxygen-delivery system; snow or ice on stairs or walkways; unanchored rugs; driving without necessary visual aids

Internal

Lack of safety education; insufficient finances to purchase safety equipment or effect repairs; history of trauma; lack of safety precautions; poor vision; reduced temperature and/or tactile sensation; balancing difficulties; cognitive or emotional difficulties; reduced large or small muscle coordination; weakness; reduced hand-eye coordination

Related Factors (r/t)

See Risk Factors.

NOC Outcomes (Nursing Outcomes Classification)

Suggested NOC Outcomes

Risk Control; Fall Prevention Behavior

• = Independent; ▲ = Collaborative

> ### Example NOC Outcome with Indicators
>
> Accomplishes **Risk Control** as evidenced by the following indicators: Monitors environmental risk factors/Develops effective risk control strategies/Modifies lifestyle to reduce risk (Rate each indicator of **Risk Control:** 1 = never demonstrated, 2 = rarely demonstrated, 3 = sometimes demonstrated, 4 = often demonstrated, 5 = consistently demonstrated [see Section I].)

Client Outcomes

Client Will (Specify Time Frame):
- Remain free from trauma
- Explain actions that can be taken to prevent trauma

NIC   Interventions (Nursing Interventions Classification)

Suggested NIC Interventions
Environmental Management: Safety; Skin Surveillance

> ### Example NIC Activities—Environmental Management
>
> Provide family/significant other with information about making home environment safe for client; Remove harmful objects from environment

Nursing Interventions and Rationales
- Provide vision aids for visually impaired clients. *Vision aids, including good lighting, eyeglasses if necessary, and reduction of physical barriers, can make it safer for the client to participate in the activities of daily living (ADLs) (St. Pierre, 1998). A client with a sensory loss must be protected from injury; therefore the visually impaired client must use vision aids (Potter and Perry, 2003).*
- Assist the client with ambulation. *Allow the client to use assistive devices in ADLs as needed. Assistive devices can augment the client's ability to perform ADLs (Mion and Mercurio, 1992).*
- Have a family member evaluate water temperature for the client. *A client with a tactile sensory impairment resulting from age or psychological or physiological factors must be protected from burns (Potter and Perry, 2003).*
- Assess the client for causes of impaired cognition. *Early identification of delirium assists in early intervention, including education and collaboration with other disciplines such as occupational and physical therapy (St. Pierre, 1998).*
- Use reality orientation to improve the client's cognition. *Clients who are confused lack the insight and judgment to consider physical disabilities and may attempt to walk without assistance (Capezuti et al, 1998).*
- Teach safety measures to prevent trauma. Ensure that the client can read if using written materials. *The home care nurse can act as advocate, teacher, and caregiver to help clients reach the goals of maintaining function and improving quality of life (Wright, 1998). Health care professionals have a legal and ethical obligation to provide clients with self-care instructions they can understand (Wong, 1992).*
- Keep walkways clear of snow, debris, and household items. *These are personal safety measures to prevent falls (Wright, 1998).*

- **• = Independent; ▲ = Collaborative**

- Provide assistive devices in bathrooms (e.g., hand rails, nonslip decals on the floor of the shower and bathtub). *Assistive devices are personal safety measures to prevent falls (Wright, 1998). These interventions promote mobility, assist in the maintenance of function, and prevent falls (St. Pierre, 1998).* **Clinical Research:** *Two or more hazards were found in the majority of bathrooms in the homes of the elderly (Gill et al, 1999).*
- Ensure that call-light systems are functioning and that the client is able to use them. *Hospital injuries often result from a client's attempt to get out of bed and use the bathroom when a caregiver cannot be contacted.*
- Use a night light after dark. *A night light provides some light in the room to assist in orientation (Hammond and Levine, 1999).*
- Never leave young children unsupervised around water or cooking areas. *Young children are at risk for drowning even in small amounts of water. Heat and fire from cooking are a hazard to young children (Potter and Perry, 2003).*
- Keep flammable and potentially flammable articles out of the reach of young children.
- Lock up harmful objects such as guns. *Increased access to guns and limited parental supervision significantly increase the risk of youths' exposure to gun violence (Slovak, 2002).*
- Teach the client to observe safety precautions in high-crime neighborhoods (e.g., lock doors, do not leave home at night without a companion, keep entryways well lighted). *Adequate lighting helps protect the home and its inhabitants from crime (Potter and Perry, 2003).* **Clinical Research:** *Dim lighting was found to be one of the most frequent hazards in the homes of the elderly (Gill et al, 1999).*
- Instruct the client not to drive under the influence of alcohol or drugs. Assess for a substance abuse problem and refer to appropriate resources for drug and alcohol education. *Approximately 1 out of every 16 hospitalized clients is admitted because of an injury in which alcohol played a role; therefore a brief intervention for all trauma clients can significantly affect this group of clients (Gentilello et al, 1999). A well-supported relationship exists between alcohol consumption and traumatic deaths from falls, fires, burns, and motor vehicle accidents.*
- Assess all clients for the use of alcohol and observe for alcohol withdrawal as appropriate. *Approximately 1 out of every 16 hospitalized clients is admitted because of an injury in which alcohol played a role; therefore a brief intervention for all trauma clients can significantly affect this group of clients (Gentilello et al, 1999). Alcohol withdrawal can be fatal (Mudd et al, 1994).*
- Review drug profile for potential side effects that may inhibit performance of ADLs. *Drug side effects can alter cognition and gait (St. Pierre, 1998).*
- Keep frequently used items within the client's reach. *This makes manipulating the environment easier for the client (St. Pierre, 1998).*
- See Nursing Interventions and Rationales in the care plans for **Risk for Aspiration, Impaired Home maintenance, Risk for Injury, Risk for Poisoning,** and **Risk for Suffocation.**

Geriatric

- Assess the geriatric client's level of functioning both at admission and periodically. *Deconditioning or the physiological changes related to prolonged inactivity are a common problem among the hospitalized elderly (Spencer et al, 1999). Admission assessment of the elderly client's optimal functional status is critical and serves as the goal for functional maintenance and rehabilitation. The key lies in frequent reassessment to detect deviation from the client's baseline (St. Pierre, 1998).*

- = Independent; ▲ = Collaborative

- Perform a home safety assessment and recommend the following preventive measures: keep electrical cords out of the flow of traffic; remove small rugs or make sure they are slip resistant; increase lighting in hallways and other dark areas; place a light in the bathroom; keep towels, curtains, and other items that might catch fire away from the stove; store harmful products away from food products; provide at least one grab bar in tubs and showers; check prescribed medications for appropriate labels; store medications in original containers or in a dispenser of some type (e.g., egg carton, seven-day plastic dispenser); if the client cannot administer medications according to directions, secure someone to administer medications. **Clinical Research:** *Home hazard assessment and modification are personal safety measures to prevent falls (Gillespie et al, 2002). Identifying risks and implementing changes decreases risk of injury (National Center for Injury Prevention and Control, 2000; Wright, 1998).*
- Mark stove knobs with bright colors (yellow or red), and outline the borders of steps. *Easily visible markings are helpful for clients with decreased depth perception (Potter and Perry, 2003).*
- Discourage driving at night. *A decline in depth perception, slower recovery from glare, and night blindness are common in the elderly and make night driving a difficult and unsafe task (Ringsven and Bond, 1991).*
- Encourage family members to reminisce with an agitated client. *Reminiscence can be used to increase self-esteem, assist in coping, decrease anxiety, and change an altered self-concept (Nugent, 1995). Agitation was the second most common behavior among 1000 residents sampled in 42 skilled nursing homes. Agitated individuals are prone to injury. Engaging in reminiscence with a special family member was the only intervention that effectively calmed severely agitated clients observed over a 24-hour period (Woods and Ashley, 1995).*
- Encourage the client to participate in resistance and impact exercise programs as tolerated. **Clinical Research:** *Muscle strengthening and balance retraining are beneficial in preventing falls (Gillespie et al, 2002). These types of exercise have been found to delay bone loss in the hip (Snow et al, 2000).*
- Implement fall and injury prevention strategies in residential care facilities. **Clinical Research:** *An interdisciplinary and multifactorial prevention program targeting residents, staff, and the environment may reduce falls and femoral fractures (Jensen et al, 2002).*

Client/Family Teaching

- Educate the family regarding age-appropriate child safety precautions, environmental safety precautions, and intervention in an emergency. *Education in these areas helps to prevent falls and injuries from occurring and enables caregivers to help in an emergency situation (Wright, 1998).*
- Educate the client and family regarding helmet use during recreation and sports activities. *Each year 1.5 million people sustain traumatic brain injuries, which account for one third of all injury deaths (National Center for Injury Prevention and Control, 2002).*
- Teach the family to assess a day care center's or babysitter's knowledge regarding child safety, environmental safety precautions, and assistance of a child in an emergency.
- Encourage the use of proper car seats and safety belts. *The risk of fatal injury in motor vehicle accidents is decreased by 45% when a shoulder and lap safety belt is worn (Segui-Gomez, 2000). Every state requires that children ride buckled up, and using a car safety seat or belt correctly can prevent injuries to children (American Academy of Pediatrics, 2002).*

• = **Independent;** ▲ = **Collaborative**

- Teach how to plan safe prom and graduation parties. *Guests can have fun and live to tell about it (Mothers Against Drunk Driving, 2002).*
- Teach parents the importance of monitoring youths after school. *Firearm injuries increase after school and violent crimes by youths peak between 3:00 PM and 4:00 PM (Slovak, 2002).*
- Teach firearm safety. Encourage the family to keep firearms and ammunition in locked storage. *Trauma is a major cause of death in young people. Every day, hundreds of young people die from firearm injuries in inner cities across the country.*
- Educate that the use of psychotropic medications may increase the risk of falls and that withdrawal of psychotropic medications should be considered. **Clinical Research:** *Withdrawal of psychotropic medication decreased risk of falls in the elderly (Gillespie et al, 2002).*
- For further information, see the care plans for **Risk for Aspiration, Impaired Home maintenance, Risk for Injury, Risk for Poisoning,** and **Risk for Suffocation.**

evolve WEBSITES FOR EDUCATION

See the EVOLVE website for World Wide Web resources for client education.

REFERENCES

American Academy of Pediatrics: *Car safety seats: a guide for families,* 2002, available online at http://www.aap.org/advocacy/releases/car.html, accessed June 23, 2003.

Capezuti E et al: The relationship between physical restraint removal and falls and injuries among nursing home residents, *J Gerontol* 53(1):M47, 1998.

Gentilello LM et al: Alcohol interventions in a trauma center as a means of reducing the risk of injury recurrence, *Ann Surg* 230(4):473, 1999.

Gill T et al: A population-based study of environmental hazards in the homes of older persons, *Am J Public Health* 89(4):553, 1999.

Gillespie LD et al: Interventions for preventing falls in elderly people (Cochrane Review), *Cochrane Library* 2, 2003.

Hammond M, Levine JM: Bedrails: choosing the best alternative, *Geriatr Nurs* 20(6):297, 1999.

Jensen J et al: Fall and injury prevention in older people living in residential care facilities, *Ann Intern Med* 136: 733, 2002.

Mion LC, Mercurio AT: Methods to reduce restraints: process, outcomes, and future directions, *J Gerontol Nurs* 18(11):5, 1992.

Mothers Against Drunk Driving: *Prom/graduation party guide,* 2002, available online at http://www.madd.org/madd_programs/0,1056,1494,00.html, accessed Jan 11, 2003.

Mudd SA et al: Alcohol withdrawal and related nursing care in older adults, *J Gerontol Nurs* 20(10):17, 1994.

National Center for Injury Prevention and Control: *Traumatic brain injury,* 2002, available online at http://www.cdc.gov/ncipc/factsheets/tbi.htm, accessed Jan 11, 2003.

National Center for Injury Prevention and Control: *Falls and hip fractures among older adults,* available on-line at http://www.cdc.gov/ncipc/factsheets/falls.htm, accessed June 23, 2003.

Nugent E: Reminiscence as a nursing intervention, *J Psychosoc Nurs* 33(11):7, 1995.

Potter P, Perry A: *Basic nursing: essentials for practice,* St Louis, 2003, Mosby.

Ringsven M, Bond D: *Gerontology and leadership skills for nurses,* Albany, NY, 1991, Delmar.

Segui-Gomez M: Evaluating worksite-based interventions that promote safety belt use, *Am J Prev Med* 18(4S): 11, 2000.

Slovak K: Gun violence and children: factors related to exposure and trauma, *Health Soc Work* 27(2):104, 2002.

• = Independent; ▲ = Collaborative

Snow CM et al: Long-term exercise using weighted vests prevents hipbone loss in postmenopausal women, *J Gerontol* 55(9):M489, 2000.

Spencer J et al: Outcomes of protocol-based and adaptation-based occupational therapy interventions for low-income elderly persons on a transitional unit, *Am J Occup Ther* 53(2):159, 1999.

St. Pierre J: Functional decline in hospitalized elders: preventive nursing measures, *AACN Clin Issues* 9(1):109, 1998.

Wong M: Self-care instructions: do patients understand educational materials? *Focus Crit Care* 19:47, 1992.

Woods P, Ashley J: Simulated presence therapy: using selected memories to manage problem behaviors in Alzheimer's disease patients, *Geriatr Nurs* 16:9, 1995.

Wright A: Nursing interventions with advanced osteoporosis, *Home Healthc Nurse* 16(3):145, 1998.

Readiness for enhanced Urinary elimination

Mikel Gray

NANDA Definition

A pattern of urinary functions that is sufficient for meeting eliminatory needs and can be strengthened

Defining Characteristics

Expresses willingness to enhance urinary elimination; urine is straw colored with no odor; specific gravity is within normal limits; amount of output is within normal limits for age and other factors; positions self for emptying of bladder; fluid intake is adequate for daily needs

NOC Outcomes (Nursing Outcomes Classification)

Suggested NOC Outcomes

Urinary Continence, Urinary Elimination

> **Example NOC Outcome with Indicators**
>
> **Urinary Continence** as evidenced by the following indicators: Voids >150 ml each time/Empties bladder completely/Absence of postvoid residual >100 to 200 ml (Rate each indicator of **Urinary Continence**: 1 = never demonstrated, 2 = rarely demonstrated, 3 = sometimes demonstrated, 4 = often demonstrated, 5 = consistently demonstrated [see Section I].)

Client Outcomes

Client Will (Specify Time Frame):
- Eliminate or reduce incontinent episodes
- Recognize sensory stimulus indicating readiness for urine elimination
- Respond to prompts for toileting

NIC Interventions (Nursing Interventions Classification)

Suggested NIC Intervention

Urinary Elimination Management

• = Independent; ▲ = Collaborative

> **Example NIC Activities—Urinary Elimination Management**
>
> Monitor urinary elimination—including frequency, consistency, odor, volume, and color—as appropriate; Teach client signs and symptoms of urinary tract infection

Nursing Interventions and Rationales

- Assess the client for readiness for improving urine elimination patterns, focusing on need for physical assistance to access toilet, cognitive awareness of sensations indicating readiness for urine elimination and current continence status (bladder management strategy, frequency of incontinent episodes). *Definitions of urinary continence and incontinence applied to ambulatory adults must be modified for the frail, elder client who is homebound or who resides in a long-term care setting (Palmer et al, 1997).*
- Complete a bladder diary of diurnal and nocturnal urine elimination patterns and patterns of urinary leakage. *A bladder diary provides a more objective verification of urine elimination patterns than a history (Resnick et al, 1994).* Nursing Research: *A bladder diary is an integral portion of the evaluation of urinary incontinence in the client who is homebound or residing in a long-term setting, and it provides a baseline against which outcomes of treatment can be evaluated (Pfister, 1999).*
- Begin a scheduled toileting program (usually every 2 to 3 hours) for the client who is normally continent (recognizes cues to toilet and expresses readiness to toilet) but requires physical assistance to access the toilet.
- Remove environmental barriers to toilet access.
- Provide a urinal or bedside toilet as indicated.
- Assist client to remove clothing, transfer to the toilet, cleanse the perineal skin, and redress as indicated.
- Ensure that toileting opportunities are offered both during daytime hours and during hours of sleep. *Certain clients who are homebound or reside in a long-term care facility have the potential for continence but experience urine loss because they lack adequate physical assistance needed to access the toilet, remove clothing, and redress after toileting is finished. The level of assistance varies significantly and depends on the client's mobility and dexterity and the availability of bedside toileting aids (Palmer et al, 1997).*
- For the client experiencing urinary incontinence who has mild cognitive deficits, begin a prompted voiding program or patterned urge response toileting program. Begin a prompted toileting program based on the results of bladder log over a period of 2 to 3 days, using a check and change system as indicated (Palmer et al, 1997; Kilpatrick, 2001):
    - Approach the client and briefly explain that it is time to toilet.
    - Assist the client to the toilet, provide assistance removing clothing and urine-containment devices (pads or adult urine-containment briefs), and check for urinary leakage since the last scheduled toileting.
    - Praise the client when toileting occurs with prompting.
    - If the client does not toilet or has evidence of an incontinence episode, refrain from praise, gently inform the client of the urine loss, remove and replace the soiled containment device, and assist the client to redress and rejoin activities or return to bed.

  Nursing Research: *Prompted voiding or patterned urge response toileting has been shown*

• = **Independent;** ▲ = **Collaborative**

> *to markedly reduce or eliminate functional incontinence in selected clients in the long-term care facility and in the community setting.*

- Institute regular use of incontinence-containment devices combined with routine perineal skin care for the client with severe cognitive impairment, significant functional impairment, or no reduction in urinary incontinence frequency or severity with a scheduled or prompted toileting program. (Refer to **Total urinary Incontinence.**) *Urine-containment products include a variety of absorptive pads, incontinent briefs, underpads for bedding, absorptive inserts that fit into specially designed undergarments, and condom catheters. Careful selection of an absorptive device and education concerning its use maximizes its effectiveness in controlling urine loss in a particular individual (Dunn et al, 2002).*

evolve WEBSITES FOR EDUCATION

See the EVOLVE website for World Wide Web resources for client education.

REFERENCES

Dunn S et al: Systematic review of the effectiveness of urinary continence products, *J Wound Ostomy Continence Nurs* 29(3):129, 2002.

Kilpatrick JA: Urinary elimination, health promotion. In Potter PA, Perry AG, editors: *Fundamentals of nursing*, ed 5, St Louis, 2001, Mosby.

Palmer MH et al: Urinary outcomes in older adults: research and clinical perspective, *Urol Nurs* 17(1):2, 1997.

Pfister SM: Bladder diaries and voiding patterns in older adults, *J Gerontol Nurs* 25(3):36, 1999.

Resnick NM et al: Short term variability of self-report of incontinence in older persons, *J Am Geriatr Soc* 42:202, 1994.

Impaired Urinary elimination

Mikel Gray

NANDA Definition

Disturbance in urine elimination

NOTE: This broad diagnosis may be used to describe many dysfunctional voiding conditions. Refer to **Functional urinary Incontinence, Reflex urinary Incontinence, Stress urinary Incontinence, Total urinary Incontinence, Urge urinary Incontinence** and **Urinary retention** for information on these more specific diagnoses.

Defining Characteristics

The term *lower urinary tract symptoms* (LUTS) is now used to describe the variety of complaints associated with disorders of bladder filling/storage or altered patterns of urine elimination (Jackson, 1999). Bothersome bladder filling/storage symptoms include diurnal frequency (voiding more than every 2 hours), infrequent urination (voiding less then every 6 hours), nocturia (arising from sleep more than once or twice to urinate), as well as sensations of excessive urgency or pain associated with bladder filling. Bothersome voiding symptoms include reduced force of the urinary stream, intermittency of the stream, hesitancy and the need to strain to evacuate the bladder. Other voiding symptoms

• = Independent; ▲ = Collaborative

are postvoid dribbling, feelings of incomplete bladder emptying, or the total inability to urinate (acute urinary retention).

Urinary incontinence is the uncontrolled loss of urine of sufficient magnitude to constitute a problem for the client, family, or caregivers (Hunskaar et al, 1999). Stress urinary incontinence is the loss of urine with physical exertion. Urge urinary incontinence is the loss of urine associated with unstable (hyperactive) detrusor contractions and a precipitous desire to urinate. Reflex urinary incontinence is urine loss associated with hyperreflexic detrusor contractions, diminished or absent sensations of bladder filling, and dyssynergia between the detrusor and striated sphincter. Functional urinary incontinence is urine loss associated with deficits of mobility, dexterity, cognition, or environmental barriers to timely toileting. Urine loss from an extraurethral source can be defined as total incontinence, and urinary retention is the condition where the client is unable to completely evacuate urine from the bladder despite micturition. Chronic urinary retention is defined as the inability to completely evacuate urine from the bladder after voiding, and acute urinary retention is the inability to urinate (Gray, 2000).

The term *overactive bladder* is used to define a cluster of LUTS often associated with urge incontinence (Anonymous, 2000). These LUTS include diurnal frequency, excessive episodes of nocturia, and excessive urgency to urinate, with or without the symptom of urge incontinence.

Related Factors (r/t)

Bothersome lower urinary tract symptoms (urological disorders, neurological lesions, gynecological conditions, dysfunction of bowel elimination); incontinence (refer to specific diagnosis); urinary retention (refer to specific diagnosis); acute urinary retention (refer to **Urinary retention**)

NOC   Outcomes (Nursing Outcomes Classification)

Suggested NOC Outcomes

Urinary Continence; Urinary Elimination; Knowledge: Medication

---

Example NOC Outcome with Indicators

Urinary Continence as evidenced by the following indicators: Has no urine loss with physical activity or exertion, coughing, sneezing, or other maneuvers that precipitously raise abdominal pressure/Voids in appropriate receptacle/Is able to move to toilet after strong desire to urinate perceived/Keeps underclothing dry during day/Keeps underclothing or bedding dry during night (Rate each indicator of **Urinary Continence:** 1 = never demonstrated, 2 = rarely demonstrated, 3 = sometimes demonstrated, 4 = often demonstrated, 5 = consistently demonstrated [see Section I].)

Client Outcomes

Client Will (Specify Time Frame):

- Demonstrate diurnal frequency no more than every 2 hours
- Demonstrate nocturia zero to one time per night for adults younger than 70 years and no more than two times per night for persons 70 years or older
- Be able to postpone voiding until toileting facility is accessed and clothing is removed

• = **Independent;** ▲ = **Collaborative**

- Be able to perceive and recognize cues for toileting, move to toilet or use urinal or portable toileting apparatus, and remove clothing as necessary for toileting
- Demonstrate postvoiding residual volumes less than 200 ml or 25% of total bladder capacity
- State absence of pain or excessive urgency with bladder filling and with urination

NIC   Interventions (Nursing Interventions Classification)

Suggested NIC Intervention
Urinary Elimination Management

> **Example NIC Activities—Urinary Elimination Management**
>
> Monitor urinary elimination—including frequency, consistency, odor, volume, and color—as appropriate; Teach client signs and symptoms of urinary tract infection

Nursing Interventions and Rationales

- Routinely screen all adult women and aging men for urinary incontinence or lower urinary tract symptoms including bothersome urgency. *Urinary incontinence and overactive bladder dysfunction are prevalent problems, particularly among women and aging males in the sixth decade of life or older (Gray, 2003). Routine screening is justified because urinary incontinence is prevalent, negatively impacts physical health and psychosocial function, and is amenable to treatment (Gray, 2003).*
- Assess bladder function using the following techniques:
  - Take a focused history including duration of bothersome LUTS, characteristics of symptoms, patterns of diurnal and nocturnal urination, frequency and volume of urine loss, alleviating and aggravating factors, and exploration of possible causative factors
  - Perform a focused physical assessment of perineal skin integrity, evaluation of the vaginal vault, evaluation of urethral hypermobility, and neurological evaluation including bulbocavernosus reflex and perineal sensations
  - Review results of urinalysis for the presence of urinary infection, polyuria, hematuria, proteinuria, and other abnormalities, or obtain urine for analysis
  A history, focused physical assessment, and urinalysis are the essential components of evaluation for any client with dysfunctional voiding complaints (Urinary Incontinence Guideline Panel, 1996; Shull et al, 2002).
- Complete a more detailed assessment on selected clients including a bladder log and functional/cognitive assessment. (Refer to **Functional urinary Incontinence, Reflex urinary Incontinence, Stress urinary Incontinence, Total urinary Incontinence,** and **Urge urinary Incontinence.**)
- Assess the client for urinary retention. (Refer to **Urinary retention.**)
- Teach the client general guidelines for bladder health:
  - Clients should avoid dehydration and its irritative effects on the bladder; fluid consumption for the ambulatory, normally active adult should be approximately 30 ml/kg of body weight.
  - Clients with irritative lower urinary tract symptoms, overactive bladder dysfunction,

• = Independent; ▲ = Collaborative

or urinary incontinence should reduce or eliminate bladder irritants (including caffeine) from the diet (Gray, 2002) and alcohol (Parazzinni et al, 2000).

- Clients with lower urinary tract pain or interstitial cystitis should eliminate bladder irritants including caffeine, alcohol, aspartame, carbonated beverages, alcohol, citrus juices, chocolate, vinegar, and highly spiced foods such as those flavored with curries or peppers to determine their effects of bothersome LUTS (Bade, Peeters, and Mensink, 1997; Interstitial Cystitis Association, 1999). These foods should be introduced singly to the diet to determine their effect (if any) on bothersome symptoms.

- All clients should be counseled about measures to alleviate or prevent constipation including adequate consumption of dietary fluids, dietary fiber, exercise, and regular bowel elimination patterns.

- All clients should be strongly advised to stop smoking.

Dehydration increases irritating voiding symptoms and may enhance the risk of urinary infection. Constipation predisposes the individual to urinary retention, and it increases the risk of urinary infection. Smoking may increase the severity and risk of stress incontinence, and it is clearly linked with an increased risk for bladder cancer (Tampakoudis et al, 1995). **Nursing Research:** *Multiple randomized clinical trials and noncontrolled clinical trials demonstrate that client education, alteration of fluid volume intake, reduction of caffeine consumption, and bladder training and pelvic floor muscle training administered by generic and advanced practice nurses reduce the frequency of urinary incontinence, pad use, and perceived severity of bothersome lower urinary tract symptoms (Dougherty et al, 2002; Borrie et al, 2002; Sampselle et al, 2000; Dowd, Kolcaba, and Steiner, 2000).*

▲ Consult the physician for culture and sensitivity testing and antibiotic treatment in the individual with evidence of a urinary infection. *Urinary tract infection is a transient, reversible condition that is associated with urge urinary incontinence and overactive bladder syndrome (Brown et al, 2001). Although the precise nature of this relationship remains unclear, it is known that eradication of urinary tract infection will alleviate or reverse lower urinary tract symptoms including suprapubic pressure and discomfort, bothersome urgency, daytime voiding frequency, and dysuria (Malterud and Baerheim, 1999).*

▲ Refer the individual with irritative symptoms; chronic, burning bladder; and urethral pain to a urologist or specialist in the management of pelvic pain. *Bladder pain and irritative voiding symptoms, in the absence of an acute urinary infection, may indicate the presence of interstitial cystitis, a chronic condition requiring ongoing treatment (Gray Hufstuttler, and Albo, 2002).*

- Teach the client to recognize symptoms of urinary tract infection (dysuria that crescendos as the bladder nears complete evacuation; urgency to urinate followed by micturition of only a few drops; suprapubic aching discomfort; malaise; voiding frequency; sudden exacerbation of urinary incontinence with or without fever, chills, and flank pain). *Qualitative research focusing on women with a history of recurring urinary tract infections reveals a variety of typical and unexpected symptoms (Malterud and Baerheim, 1999).*

- Teach the client to recognize and to seek help promptly if hematuria occurs. *Hematuria in the presence of irritative voiding symptoms typically indicates urinary infection; however, gross painless hematuria (and bleeding with irritative symptoms) may indicate a bladder cancer (Mazhari and Kimmel, 2002).*

• = **Independent;** ▲ = **Collaborative**

- Assist the individual with urinary leakage to select a product that adequately contains urine, avoids soiling clothing, is not apparent when worn under clothing, and protects the underlying skin. (Refer to **Total urinary Incontinence.**)
- Teach perineal care including judicious use of soaps and use of vaginal douches only under special circumstances. (Refer to **Total urinary Incontinence.**)

Geriatric

- Provide an environment that encourages toileting for the elderly client cared for in the home or in acute care, long-term care, or critical care units. *Insufficient toileting opportunities, medications, acute or chronic illnesses, and environmental factors may contribute to functional incontinence or exacerbate other forms of urinary leakage in the elderly client (Morris, Browne, and Saltmarche, 1992; Jirovec and Wells, 1990; Gray and Burns, 1996).*
- ▲ Perform urinalysis in all elderly persons who experience a sudden change in urine elimination patterns, lower abdominal discomfort, acute confusion, or a fever of unclear origin. *Elderly persons, particularly adults aged 80 years and older, often experience atypical symptoms with a urinary tract infection or pyelonephritis (Bostwick, 2000; Suchinski et al, 1999).*
- Encourage elderly women to drink at least 10 ounces of cranberry juice daily, regularly consume one to two servings of fresh blueberries, or supplement the diet with cranberry concentrate capsules (usually taken in 500 mg doses with each meal). *Cranberry juice has been reported to exert a bacteriostatic effect on* Escherichia coli, *the most common pathogen associated with urinary infection among community-dwelling adult women (Gray, 2002; Avorn et al, 1994).*

Client/ Family Teaching

- Provide all clients with the basic principles for optimal bladder function.
- Teach the community and health care providers that urinary incontinence is not a normal part of aging and that incontinence can be corrected or managed with proper evaluation and care.
- Provide information to health care providers and the community about the signs, symptoms, and management of urinary tract infections and interstitial cystitis.
- Teach all persons the signs and symptoms of urinary tract infection and its management.
- Teach all persons to recognize hematuria and to promptly seek care if this symptom occurs.

evolve WEBSITES FOR EDUCATION

See the EVOLVE website for World Wide Web resources for client education.

REFERENCES

Anonymous: Overactive bladder and its treatment consensus conference, *Urology* 55(suppl 5A):1, 2000.

Avorn J et al: Reduction of bacteriuria and pyuria after ingestion of cranberry juice, *JAMA* 271:751, 1994.

Bade JJ, Peeters JM, Mensink HJ: Is the diet of patients with interstitial cystitis related to their disease? *Eur Urol* 32:179, 1997.

Borrie MJ et al: Interventions led by nurse continence advisers in the management of urinary incontinence: a randomized controlled trial, *Can Med Assoc J* 166(10):1267, 2002.

• = **Independent;** ▲ = **Collaborative**

Bostwick JM: The many faces of confusion. Timing and collateral history often hold the key to diagnosis, *Postgrad Med* 108(6):60, 2000.

Brown JS et al: Heart and Estrogen/Progestin Replacement Study Research Group. Urinary tract infections in postmenopausal women: effect of hormone therapy and risk factors, *Obstet Gynecol* 98(6):1045, 2001.

Dougherty MC et al: A randomized trial of behavioral management for continence with older rural women, *Res Nurs Health* 25:3, 2002.

Dowd T, Kolcaba K, Steiner R: Using cognitive strategies to enhance bladder control and comfort, *Holist Nurs Pract* 14(2):91, 2000.

Gray M: Urinary retention: management in the acute care setting, Part 1, *Am J Nurs* 100:40, 2000.

Gray M: Are cranberry juice or cranberry products effective in the prevention or management of urinary tract infection? *J Wound Ostomy Continence Nurs* 29:122, 2002.

Gray M: The importance of screening, assessing and managing urinary incontinence in primary care, *J Am Acad Nurse Practit* 15(3):102, 2003.

Gray M, Hufstuttler S, Albo M: Interstitial cystitis: a guide to recognition, evaluation and management for the nurse practitioner, *J Wound Ostomy Continence Nurs* 29:93, 2002.

Gray ML, Burns SB: Continence management, *Crit Care Clin North Am* 8:29, 1996.

Hunskaar S et al: Epidemiology and natural history of urinary incontinence. In Abrams P, Khoury S, Wein A, editors: *Incontinence,* Plymouth, UK, 1999, Plymbridge, Health Publications.

Interstitial Cystitis Association: *Interstitial cystitis and diet,* Rockville, Md, 1999, The Association.

Jackson S: Lower urinary tract symptoms and nocturia in men and women: prevalence, etiology and diagnosis, *Br J Urol Int* 84(suppl 1):5, 1999.

Jirovec MM, Wells TJ: Urinary incontinence in nursing home residents with dementia: the mobility-cognition paradigm, *Appl Nurs Res* 3:11, 1990.

Malterud K, Baerheim A: Peeing barbed wire. Symptom experiences in women with lower urinary tract infection, *Scand J Prim Health Care* 17(1):49, 1999.

Mazhari R, Kimmel PL: Hematuria: an algorithmic approach to finding the cause, *Cleve Clin J Med* 69(11): 870, 2002.

Morris A, Browne G, Saltmarche A: Urinary incontinence among cognitively impaired elderly veterans, *J Gerontol Nurs* 18:33, 1992.

Parazzinni F et al: Risk factors for urinary incontinence in women, *Eur Urol* 37:637, 2000.

Sampselle CM et al: Continence for women: evaluation of AWHONN's third research utilization project, *J Obstet Gynecol Neonat Nurs* 29:9, 2000.

Shull BL et al: Physical examination. In Abrams P, Khoury S, Wein AJ, editors: *Incontinence: 2nd International Consultation on Incontinence,* ed 2, Plymouth, UK, 2002, Plymbridge, Health Publications.

Suchinski GA et al: Treating urinary tract infections in the elderly, *Dimens Crit Care Nurs* 18(1):21, 1999.

Tampakoudis P et al: Cigarette smoking and urinary incontinence in women—a new calculative method of estimating the exposure to smoke, *Eur J Obstet Gynecol Reprod Biol* 63(1):27, 1995.

Urinary Incontinence Guideline Panel: Urinary incontinence in adults: clinical practice guideline, ed 2, Rockville, Md, 1996, Agency for Health Care Policy and Research.

Urinary retention

Mikel Gray

NANDA Definition

Incomplete emptying of the bladder

Defining Characteristics

Measured urinary residual greater than 150 to 200 ml or 25% of total bladder capacity; obstructive lower urinary tract symptoms (poor force of stream, intermittency of stream, hesitancy of urination, postvoiding dribbling, feelings of incomplete bladder emptying); irritative lower urinary tract symptoms (urgency to urinate, diurnal frequency of uri-

• = Independent; ▲ = Collaborative

nation, nocturia); overflow incontinence (dribbling urine loss caused when intravesical pressure overwhelms the sphincter mechanism)

Related Factors (r/t)

Bladder outlet obstruction (benign prostatic hyperplasia, prostate cancer, prostatitis, urethral stricture, bladder neck dyssynergia, bladder neck contracture, detrusor striated sphincter dyssynergia, obstructing cystocele or urethral distortion, urethral tumor, urethral polyp, posterior urethral valves, postoperative complication)

Deficient detrusor contraction strength (sacral level spinal lesions, cauda equina syndrome, peripheral polyneuropathies, herpes zoster or simplex affecting sacral nerve roots, injury or extensive surgery causing denervation of pelvic plexus, medication side effect, complication of illicit drug use, impaction of stool)

NOC   Outcomes (Nursing Outcomes Classification)

Suggested NOC Outcomes

Urinary Continence; Urinary Elimination

Example NOC Outcome with Indicators

Urinary Continence as evidenced by the following indicators: Absence of urinary leakage between catheterizations or containment of micturition by condom catheter and drainage bag/Absence of UTI (negative leukocytes and bacterial growth negative or <100,000 CFU/ml)/Underclothing dry during day/Underclothing or bedding dry during night (Rate each indicator of **Urinary Continence:** 1 = never demonstrated, 2 = rarely demonstrated, 3 = sometimes demonstrated, 4= often demonstrated, 5 = consistently demonstrated [see Section I].)

CFU, Colony-forming units; *UTI,* urinary tract infection.

Client Outcomes

Client Will (Specify Time Frame):

- Completely and regularly eliminate urine from the bladder; measured urinary residual volume is less than 150 to 200 ml or 25% of total bladder capacity (voided volume plus urinary residual volume)
- Experience correction or relief from obstructive symptoms
- Experience correction or alleviation of irritative symptoms
- Be free of upper urinary tract damage (renal function remains sufficient; febrile urinary infections are absent)

NIC   Interventions (Nursing Interventions Classification)

Suggested NIC Interventions

Urinary Catheterization; Urinary Retention Care

Example NIC Activities—Urinary Retention Care

Perform a comprehensive urinary assessment focusing on incontinence (e.g., urinary output, urinary voiding pattern, cognitive function, and preexistent urinary problems); Use the power of suggestion by running water or flushing the toilet

---

• = Independent; ▲ = Collaborative

Nursing Interventions and Rationales

- Obtain a focused urinary history emphasizing the character and duration of lower urinary symptoms. Query the client about episodes of acute urinary retention (complete inability to void) or chronic retention (documented elevated postvoid residual volumes). *Although the presence of obstructive or irritative voiding symptoms is not diagnostic of urinary retention (Roehrborn et al, 2002), a focused nursing history can provide clues to the likely etiology of retention and its management (Gray, 2000a).*
- Question the client concerning specific risk factors for urinary retention including:
  - Disorders affecting the sacral spinal cord such as spinal cord injuries of vertebral levels T12 to L2, disk problems, cauda equina syndrome, tabes dorsalis
  - Acute neurological injury causing sudden loss of mobility such as spinal shock
  - Metabolic disorders such as diabetes mellitus, chronic alcoholism, and related conditions associated with polyuria and peripheral polyneuropathies
  - Heavy-metal poisoning (lead, mercury) causing peripheral polyneuropathies
  - Advanced stage HIV
  - Medications including antispasmodics/parasympatholytics, alpha-adrenergics, antidepressants, sedatives, narcotics, psychotropic medications, illicit drugs
  - Recent surgery requiring general or spinal anesthesia
  - Bowel elimination patterns, history of fecal impaction, encopresis
  - Current or recent surgical procedures

  Urinary retention is related to multiple factors affecting either detrusor contraction strength or urethral obstruction (Gray, 2000a; Kruse, Bray, and deGroat, 1995; Pertek and Haberer, 1995; Anders and Goebel, 1998; Ginsberg et al, 1998). **Nursing Research:** *Multiple factors in the surgical patient are associated with an increased risk of postoperative urinary retention including preoperative voiding difficulty, advanced age, total amount of fluid replacement during a 24-hour postoperative period, type of anesthesia, pain management medications, and route and length of medication administration (Wynd et al, 1996).*
- ▲ Perform a focused physical assessment or review results of a recent physical including perineal skin integrity; inspection, percussion, and palpation of the lower abdomen for obvious bladder distension; a neurological examination including perineal skin sensation and the bulbocavernosus reflex; and vaginal vault examination in women and digital rectal examination in men. *The physical assessment provides clues to the likely etiology of urinary retention and its management.*
- ▲ Determine the urinary residual volume by catheterizing the client immediately after urination or by obtaining a bladder ultrasound after micturition. *Although catheterization provides the most accurate method to determine urinary residual volume, it is invasive, produces discomfort, and carries a risk of infection (Gray, 2000b).* **Nursing Research:** *A study of 30 clients treated in an acute care unit found a high correlation between catheterized volumes and volumes estimated by bladder ultrasound. In addition, results of the ultrasonic measurement changed nursing practice in 51% of instances, reducing unneeded catheterizations by 32% (O'Farrell et al, 2001).*
- Complete a bladder log including patterns of urine elimination, urine loss (if present), nocturia, and volume and type of fluids consumed for a period of 3 to 7 days. *The bladder log provides an objective verification of urine elimination patterns and allows comparison of fluids consumed versus urinary output during a 24-hour period (Nygaard and Holcomb, 2000).*

- = Independent; ▲ = Collaborative

▲ Consult with the physician concerning eliminating or altering medications suspected of producing or exacerbating urinary retention. *Medication side effects may cause or greatly exacerbate urinary retention in susceptible individuals (Gray, 2000a,b).*

• Teach the client with mild to moderate obstructive symptoms to double void by urinating, resting in the bathroom for 3 to 5 minutes, and then trying again to urinate. *Double voiding promotes more efficient bladder evacuation by allowing the detrusor to contract initially and then rest and contract again (Gray, 2000b).*

• Teach the client with urinary retention and infrequent voiding to urinate by the clock. *Timed or scheduled voiding may reduce urinary retention by preventing bladder overdistention (Gray, 2000b).*

• Advise the male client with urinary retention related to benign prostatic hyperplasia (BPH) to avoid risk factors associated with acute urinary retention as follows:
  ▪ Avoid over-the-counter cold remedies containing a decongestant (alpha-adrenergic agonist)
  ▪ Avoid taking over-the-counter dietary medications (frequently contain alpha-adrenergic agonists)
  ▪ Discuss voiding problems with a health care provider before beginning new prescription medications
  ▪ After prolonged exposure to cool weather, warm the body before attempting to urinate
  ▪ Avoid overfilling the bladder by regular urination patterns and refrain from excessive intake of alcohol

  These modifiable factors predispose the client to acute urinary retention by overdistending the bladder and compromising detrusor contraction strength or by increasing outlet resistance (Gray, 2000b).

▲ Teach the elderly male client with BPH to self-administer finasteride or an alpha-adrenergic–blocking agent such as doxazosin, terazosin, or tamsulosin as directed. Provide careful instruction concerning the dosage, administration schedule, and side effects of these drugs including possible adverse side effects when multiple doses are inadvertently missed. *Finasteride is a 5-alpha-reductase inhibitor that reduces the risk of acute urinary retention when taken by men with BPH over a prolonged period (McConnell et al, 1998). The magnitude of obstruction associated with BPH is also reduced by routine administration of alpha-adrenergic–blocking agents including tamsulosin, terazosin, or doxazosin. However, these agents must be taken regularly to reduce the risk of side effects including postural hypotension (Narayan and Tewari, 1998; Lepor et al, 1997, 1998).*

▲ Teach the client who is unable to void specific strategies to manage this potential medical emergency as follows:
  ▪ Attempt urination in complete privacy
  ▪ Place the feet solidly on the floor
  ▪ If unable to void using these strategies, take a warm sitz bath or shower and void (if possible) while still in the tub or shower
  ▪ Drink a warm cup of coffee or tea to stimulate the bladder, which may promote voiding
  ▪ If unable to void within 6 hours or if bladder distention is producing significant pain, seek urgent or emergency care

  Attempting urination in complete privacy and placing the feet solidly on the floor help relax the pelvic muscles and may encourage voiding. Warm water also stimulates the bladder

• = Independent;   ▲ = Collaborative

and may produce voiding; the cooling experienced by leaving the tub or shower may again inhibit the bladder (Gray, 2000b).

▲ Remove the indwelling urethral catheter at midnight in the hospitalized client to reduce the risk of acute urinary retention. *Removal of indwelling catheters offers several advantages to "morning removal" including a larger initial voided volume (Crowe et al, 1994) and earlier hospital discharge with no increased risk for readmission compared with those undergoing morning removal (McDonald and Thompson, 1999).*

▲ Consult the physician about bladder stimulation in the client with urinary retention caused by deficient detrusor contraction strength. **Nursing Research:** *Electrical stimulation of the bladder neck has been reported to provide beneficial results in persons with urinary retention that is caused by deficient detrusor contraction strength (Moore and Rayome, 1995).*

▲ Teach the client with significant urinary retention to perform self-intermittent catheterization as directed. **Nursing Research:** *Intermittent catheterization allows regular, complete bladder evacuation without serious complications (Horsley, Crane, and Reynolds, 1982).*

• Advise clients who undergo intermittent catheterization that bacteria are likely to colonize the urine but that this condition does not indicate a clinically significant urinary tract infection. *Bacteriuria frequently occurs in the client undergoing intermittent catheterization; only symptoms producing infections warrant treatment (Wyndaele, 2002).*

▲ Insert an indwelling catheter for the individual with urinary retention who is not a suitable candidate for intermittent catheterization. *An indwelling catheter provides continuous drainage of urine; however, the risks of serious urinary complications with prolonged use are significant (Anson and Gray, 1993; Weld et al, 2000).*

• Advise clients with indwelling catheters that bacteria in the urine is an almost universal finding after the catheter has remained in place for a period of 30 days or longer and that only symptomatic infections warrant treatment. *The long-term indwelling catheter is inevitably associated with bacterial colonization. Most bacteriuria does not produce significant infection, and attempts to eradicate bacteriuria often produce subsequent morbidity because resistant bacteria are encouraged to reproduce while more easily managed strains are eradicated (Moore and Rayome, 1995).*

▲ Consult the physician about the catheter change schedule, and institute routine catheter care for the client with urinary retention managed by a long-term indwelling catheter. **Nursing Research:** *The risk of symptomatic urinary tract infection is significant when long-term catheterization is used to manage chronic urinary retention. The risk of symptomatic catheterization is reduced by a program of regular cleansing of the urethral meatus and exposed catheter, combined with routine catheter changes (typically every 4 weeks). Excessively frequent changes are only indicated if encrustation occurs (White and Ragland, 1995).*

Geriatric

• Aggressively assess elderly clients, particularly those with dribbling urinary incontinence, urinary tract infections, and related condition for urinary retention. *Elderly women (and men) may experience urinary retention of 1500 ml or more with few or no apparent symptoms; a urinary residual volume and related assessments are necessary to determine the presence of retention in this population (Williams, Wallhagen, and Dowling, 1993).*

• Assess elderly clients for impaction when urinary retention is documented or sus-

• = Independent; ▲ = Collaborative

pected. *Fecal impaction and urinary retention frequently coexist in elderly clients and, unless reversed, may lead to acute delirium, urinary tract infection, or renal insufficiency (Waale, Bruijns, and Dautzenberg, 2001).*

- Assess elderly male clients for retention related to BPH or prostate cancer. *Prostate enlargement in elderly men increases the risk of acute and chronic urinary retention (McNeill and Hargreave, 2000; Loh and Chin, 2002).*

Home care

- The interventions listed previously may be adapted for home care use.
- Encourage the client to report any inability to void. *Pathophysiological factors of urinary retention require follow-up.*
- ▲ Maintain an up-to-date medication list; evaluate side-effect profiles for risk of urinary retention. *New medications or changes in dosage may cause urinary retention.*
- ▲ Refer the client for physician evaluation if there is a new occurrence of urinary retention. *Identification of cause is important. Left untreated, urinary retention may lead to urinary tract infection or kidney failure.*

Client/ Family Teaching

- Teach techniques for intermittent catheterization including use of clean rather than sterile technique, washing using soap and water or a microwave technique, and reuse of the catheter.
- Teach the client with an indwelling catheter to assess the tube for patency, maintain the drainage system below the level of the symphysis pubis, and routinely cleanse the bedside bag.
- Teach the client with an indwelling catheter or undergoing intermittent catheterization the symptoms of a significant urinary infection including hematuria, acute-onset incontinence, dysuria, flank pain, or fever.

evolve WEBSITES FOR EDUCATION

See the EVOLVE website for World Wide Web resources for client education.

REFERENCES

Anders HJ, Goebel FD: Cytomegalovirus polyradiculopathy in patients with AIDS, *Clin Infect Dis* 27:345, 1998.

Anson C, Gray ML: Secondary complications after spinal cord injury, *Urol Nurs* 13:107, 1993.

Crowe H et al: Randomized study of the effect of midnight removal of urinary catheter, *Urol Nurs* 14:18, 1994.

Ginsberg PC et al: Rare presentation of acute urinary retention secondary to herpes zoster, *J Am Osteopath Assoc* 95:508, 1998.

Gray M: Urinary retention: management in the acute care setting, Part 1, *Am J Nurs* 100(7):40, 2000a.

Gray M: Urinary retention: management in the acute care setting, Part 2, *Am J Nurs* 100(8):36, 2000b.

Horsley JA, Crane J, Reynolds MA: *Clean intermittent catheterization: conduct and utilization of research in nursing project,* New York, 1982, Grune & Stratton.

Kruse MN, Bray LA, deGroat WC: Influence of spinal cord injury in the morphology of bladder afferent and efferent neurons, *J Autonom Nerv Sys* 54:215, 1995.

Lepor H et al: Doxazosin for benign prostatic hyperplasia: long-term efficacy and safety in hypertensive and normotensive patients, *J Urol* 157:525, 1997.

Lepor H et al: The impact of medical therapy due to symptoms, quality of life and global outcome, and factors predicting response, *J Urol* 160: 1358, 1998.

● = **Independent;** ▲ = **Collaborative**

Loh SY, Chin CM: A demographic profile of patients undergoing transurethral resection of the prostate for benign prostate hyperplasia and presenting in acute urinary retention, *Br J Urol Int* 89(6):531, 2002.

McConnell JD et al: The effect of finasteride on the risk of acute urinary retention and the need for surgical treatment among men with benign prostatic hyperplasia. Finasteride Long-Term Efficacy Safety Study Group, *N Engl J Med* 338:557, 1998.

McDonald C, Thompson J: A comparison of midnight versus early morning removal of urinary catheters following transurethral resection of the prostate, *J Wound Ostomy Continence Nurs* 26:94, 1999.

McNeill SA, Hargreave TB: Efficacy of PSA in the detection of carcinoma of the prostate in patients presenting with acute urinary retention, *J R Coll Surg Edinb* 45(4):227, 2000.

Moore KN, Rayome RG: Problem solving and trouble shooting: the indwelling catheter, *J Wound Ostomy Continence Nurs* 22:242, 1995.

Narayan P, Tewari A: A second phase III multicenter placebo study of 2 dosages of modified release tamsulosin in patients with symptoms of benign prostatic hyperplasia. United States 93-01 study group, *J Urol* 160:1701, 1998.

Nygaard I, Holcomb R: Reproducibility of the seven day voiding diary in women with stress urinary incontinence, *Int Urogynecol J Pelvic Floor Dysfunct* 11:15, 2000.

O'Farrell B et al: Evaluation of portable bladder ultrasound: accuracy and effect on nursing practice in an acute neuroscience unit, *J Neurosci Nurs* 33(6):301, 2001.

Pertek JP, Haberer JP: Effects of anesthesia on postoperative micturition and urinary retention, *An Franc Anesthesis Reanimation* 14:340, 1995.

Roehrborn CG et al: Proscar Long-term Efficacy and Safety Study. Storage (irritative) and voiding (obstructive) symptoms as predictors of benign prostatic hyperplasia progression and related outcomes, *Eur Urol* 42(1):1, 2002.

Waale WH, Bruijns E, Dautzenberg PJ: Delirium due to urinary retention: confusing for both the patient and the doctor, *Tijdschr Gerontol Geriatr* 32(3):100, 2001.

Weld KJ et al: Influences on renal function in chronic spinal cord injured patients, *J Urol* 164(5):1490, 2000.

White MC, Ragland KE: Urinary catheter—related infections among home care patients, *J Wound Ostomy Continence Nurs* 22:286, 1995.

Williams MP, Wallhagen M, Dowling G: Urinary retention in elderly hospitalized women, *J Gerontol Nurs* 19:7, 1993.

Wynd CA et al: Factors influencing postoperative urinary retention following orthopaedic surgical procedures, *Orthop Nurs* 15(1):43, 2002.

Wyndaele JJ: Complications of intermittent catheterization: their prevention and treatment, *Spinal Cord* 40(10):536, 2002.

Impaired spontaneous Ventilation

Betty Ackley

NANDA Definition

Decreased energy reserves result in an individual's inability to maintain breathing adequate for supporting life

Defining Characteristics

Dyspnea; increased metabolic rate; increased heart rate, decreased Po_2, increased Pco_2, decreased Sao_2; increased restlessness; apprehension; increased use of accessory muscles; decreased tidal volume; decreased cooperation

Related Factors (r/t)

Metabolic factors; respiratory muscle fatigue

• = Independent; ▲ = Collaborative

| NOC | Outcomes (Nursing Outcomes Classification) |

Suggested NOC Outcomes

Neurological Status: Central Motor Control; Respiratory Status: Gas Exchange, Ventilation

Example NOC Outcome with Indicators

Achieves appropriate **Respiratory Status: Ventilation** as evidenced by the following indicators: Respiratory rate IER/Respiratory rhythm IER/Depth of inspiration/Chest expansion symmetrical/Ease of breathing/ Sputum moves out of airways/Accessory muscle use not present/Adventitious breath sounds not present/Chest retraction not present/Auscultated breath sounds IER/Tidal volume IER/Vital capacity IER (Rate each indicator of **Respiratory Status: Ventilation:** 1 = extremely compromised, 2 = substantially compromised, 3 = moderately compromised, 4 = mildly compromised, 5 = not compromised [see Section I].)

IER, In expected range.

Client Outcomes

Client Will (Specify Time Frame):

- Maintain arterial blood gases within safe parameters
- Remain free of dyspnea or restlessness
- Effectively maintain airway
- Effectively mobilize secretions

| NIC | Interventions (Nursing Interventions Classification) |

Suggested NIC Interventions

Artificial Airway Management; Mechanical Ventilation; Respiratory Monitoring; Resuscitation: Neonate; Ventilation Assistance

Example NIC Activities—Mechanical Ventilation

Monitor for respiratory muscle fatigue; Consult with other health care personnel in selection of a ventilator mode

Nursing Interventions and Rationales

▲ Collaborate with the client, family, and physician regarding possible intubation and ventilation. Ask whether the client has advanced directives and, if so, integrate them into the plan of care in conjunction with clinical data regarding overall health and reversibility of the medical condition. *Many clients and their families make decisions about the level of therapy aggressiveness that they desire. Health care providers have a responsibility to allow the client to participate in care decisions (Campbell and Thill-Baharozian, 1994).*

- Assess and respond to changes in the client's respiratory status. Monitor the client for dyspnea including respiratory rate, use of accessory muscles, intercostal retractions, flaring of nostrils, and subjective complaints. *It is essential to monitor for these signs of impending respiratory failure (McCord and Cronin-Stubbs, 1992).*

- Have the client use a numerical scale (0 to 10) to describe dyspnea. **Nursing Research:**

• = **Independent;** ▲ = **Collaborative**

The numerical rating scale is a valid measure of dyspnea. This allows measurement of the intensity, progression, and resolution of dyspnea (Gift and Narsavage, 1998).

- Assess for chronic respiratory disorders when administering oxygen. With chronic obstructive pulmonary disease (COPD) the respiratory drive is primarily in response to hypoxia, not hypercarbia; oxygenating too aggressively can result in respiratory depression. *When managing acute respiratory failure in clients with COPD, use caution in administering oxygen because hyperoxygenating can lead to respiratory depression.*

▲ Collaborate with the physician and respiratory therapists in determining the appropriateness of noninvasive positive pressure ventilation (NPPV) for the decompensated client with COPD.

▲ Assist with implementation, client support, and monitoring if NPPV is used. *In a client with exacerbation of COPD, NPPV should be used and can be as effective as intubation with use of a ventilator or else the client has other complications such as hypotension or severely impaired mental status (Perkins and Shortall, 2000; Pierson, 2002).*

▲ If the client has apnea, pH <7.25, $Paco_2$ >50 mm Hg, Pao_2 <50 mm Hg, respiratory muscle fatigue, or somnolence, prepare the client for intubation and placement on a ventilator. *These indicators are predictive of the need for invasive mechanical ventilation (Burns, 2001; Pierson, 2002).*

Ventilator support

- Explain the intubation intervention to the client and family as appropriate and, during the procedure, administer sedation for client comfort according to the physician's orders. *Explanation of the procedure decreases anxiety and increases understanding; premedication allows for a more controlled intubation with decreased incidence of insertion problems (Burns, 2001).*

- Secure the endotracheal tube in place using either tape or a device, auscultate bilateral breath sounds, use a CO_2 detector, and obtain a chest x-ray to confirm endotracheal tube placement. *Secure taping is needed to prevent inadvertent extubation; correct placement of the endotracheal tube in the trachea must be confirmed by a number of means (Burns, 2001).* **Nursing Research:** *Nursing studies have shown conflicting results regarding the preferable way to secure the endotracheal tube, including finding advantage to using the Haid Holder (Chinea Rodriguez et al, 1999), no advantage to using either adhesive or twill tape (Barnason et al, 1998), preference for the bow method versus tying of the endotracheal tube (Clarke et al, 1998), and increased nurse satisfaction with use of the SecureEasy device (Kaplow and Bookbinder, 1994).*

- Suction as needed, and hyperoxygenate and hyperventilate according to policy. Refer to **Ineffective Airway clearance** for further information on suctioning.

- Ensure activation of all monitor alarms each shift. *This action helps ensure client safety (Burns, 2001).*

- Respond to ventilator alarms promptly. If unable to rapidly locate the source of alarm, use a manual self-inflating resuscitation bag to ventilate the client while waiting for assistance. *Common causes of a high-pressure alarm include secretions, condensation, biting of the endotracheal tube, decreased compliance of the lungs, and tubing compression. Common causes of a low-pressure alarm are ventilator disconnection, leaks in the circuit, and changing compliance and resistance. Using a manual self-inflating resuscitation bag with supplemental oxygen, the nurse can provide immediate ventilation and oxygenation as needed (Burns, 2001).*

• = Independent; ▲ = Collaborative

▲ Prevent unplanned extubation by maintaining stability of endotracheal tube and using soft wrist restraints on the client if needed and ordered. *The client's hands are often immobilized to prevent inadvertent dislodgment of the tube (Burns, 2001).*

• Drain collected fluid from condensation out of ventilator tubing as needed. *This action reduces the risk of infection by decreasing potential inhalation of contaminated fluid (Burns, 2001).*

• Note ventilator settings of flow of inspired oxygen, peak inspiratory pressure, tidal volume, and alarm activation at intervals and when removing the client from the ventilator for any reason. *Checking the settings ensures that safety measures are taken and that the client is not left on 100% oxygen after suctioning (Burns, 2001).*

▲ Administer analgesics and sedatives as needed with a defined protocol to facilitate client comfort and rest. **Clinical Research:** *A study demonstrated that a nurse-implemented sedation protocol decreased the number of days of intubation, the need for a tracheotomy, and the length of hospital stay (Brook et al, 1999). Oral intubation and inadequate sedation have been noted to be indicators for unplanned extubation (Chevron et al, 1998).*

• To decrease anxiety, use music therapy with selections of client's choice played on headphones at intervals. **Nursing Research:** *A study demonstrated that playing music that was chosen by the client decreased anxiety and increased relaxation as shown by reduced heart and respiratory rate in intubated adults (Chlan, 1998).*

• Analyze and respond to arterial blood gas results. *Ventilatory support must be closely monitored to ensure adequate oxygenation and acid-base balance.*

• Use an effective means of communication with the client. Use nonverbal communication, an electronic voice output communication aid, an alphabet board, a picture board, a computer, or a writing slate. Ask the client for input into care as able. Ensure client's human rights are met. *Inability to communicate can lead to client frustration, insecurity, and sometimes panic (Happ, 2001).* **Clinical Research:** *Use of a voice-output communication device was shown to be effective in a group of intubated surgery clients (Costello, 2000).* **Nursing Research:** *Use of a picture board increased nurse-client communication in intubated cardiothoracic surgical clients (Stovsky, Rudy, and Dragonette, 1988). A study of young ventilator-dependent clients demonstrated that social and educational exclusion was experienced during their hospital stays (Noyes, 2000).*

• Move the endotracheal tube from side to side every 24 hours, and tape it or secure it with a device. Assess and document client's skin condition, and ensure correct tube placement at lip line. *These steps help prevent skin breakdown at the lip line resulting from endotracheal tube pressure (Chang, 1995).*

• Provide oral care every 4 hours and prn.

• Position the client in a semirecumbent position with the head of the bed at a 45-degree angle. **Clinical Research:** *Studies have shown that mechanically ventilated clients have a decreased incidence of pneumonia if the client is positioned at a 45-degree semirecumbent position as opposed to a supine position (Torres et al, 1992; Drakulovic et al, 1999; Collard, Saint, and Matthay, 2003).*

• Turn the client from side to side every 2 hours or more often if possible. *Changing position frequently decreases the incidence of atelectasis, pooling of secretions, and resultant pneumonia (Burns, 2001).*

• Assess bilateral anterior and posterior breath sounds every 2 to 4 hours and prn; respond to any relevant changes.

• = **Independent;** ▲ = **Collaborative**

- Assess responsiveness to ventilator support; monitor for subjective complaints and sensation of dyspnea (Ferrin and Tino, 1997).
▲ Collaborate with the interdisciplinary team in treating and responding to the cause of underlying acute respiratory failure. *The mechanical ventilator is usually a temporary support until the underlying pathology can be effectively resolved.*

Geriatric
- Recognize that elderly have a high rate of morbidity when mechanically ventilated. *Implement interventions to prevent decline such as positioning, nutrition maintenance early to prevent decline (Phelen, Cooper, and Sangkachand, 2002).*

Client/Family Teaching
- Explain to the client the potential sensations that will be experienced including relief of dyspnea, the feeling of lung inflations, the noise of the ventilator, and the reality of alarms. **Nursing Research:** *Knowledge of potential sensations and experiences before they are encountered can help to decrease anxiety (Johnson, 1972).*
- Explain to the client and family about being unable to speak, and work out an alternative system of communication. See previous intervention.
- Demonstrate to the family how to perform simple procedures such as suctioning the mouth with a Yankeur catheter, providing range-of-motion exercises, and reconnecting the ventilator immediately if it becomes disconnected. *Families often need to be part of the client's care (Burns, 2001) and may be present at the bedside for prolonged periods of time.*
- Offer both the client and family explanations of how the ventilator works and answer any questions asked. *Having questions answered is often cited as an important need of clients and families when a client is on a ventilator (Burns, 2001).*

Home care
- Some of the interventions listed previously may be adapted for home care use.
▲ Begin discharge planning as soon as possible with the case manager or social worker to assess the need for home support systems, assistive devices, and community or home health services.
▲ With help from a medical social worker, assist the client and family to determine the fiscal impact of home care vs. an extended care facility.
- Assess the home setting during the discharge process to ensure the home can safely accommodate ventilator support (e.g., adequate space and electricity).
- Have the family contact the electric company and place the client residence on a high-risk list in case of a power outage (Humphrey, 1994). *Some home-based care requires special conditions for safe home administration.*
- Assess the caregivers for commitment to support a ventilator-dependent client in the home. *Commitment to care and valuing home as a healing place provide meaning for participating in caregiving and decrease caregiver role strain (Boland and Sims, 1996).*
- Be sure that the client and family or caregivers are familiar with operation of all ventilation devices, know how to suction if needed, are competent in doing tracheostomy care, and know schedules for cleaning equipment. Have the designated caregiver or caregivers demonstrate care before discharge. *Some home-based care involves specialized technology and requires specific skills for safe and appropriate care.*

- = Independent; ▲ = Collaborative

- Assess client and caregiver knowledge of the disease, client needs, and medications to be administered via ventilation-assistive devices. Avoid analgesics. Assess knowledge of how to use equipment. Teach as necessary. *A client receiving ventilation support may not be able to articulate needs. Respiratory medications can have side effects that change the client's respiration or level of consciousness.*
- Establish an emergency plan and criteria for use. Identify emergency procedures to be used until medical assistance arrives. Teach and role-play emergency care. *A prepared emergency plan reassures the client and family and ensures client safety.*
- Institute case management of frail elderly clients to support continued independent living. *Respiratory difficulties represent and can lead to increasing needs for assistance in using the health care system effectively. Case management combines nursing activities of the client and family assessment, planning and coordination of care among all health care providers, delivery of direct nursing care, and monitoring of care and outcomes. These activities are able to address continuity of care, mutual goal setting, behavior management, and prevention of worsening health problems (Guttman, 1999).*

evolve WEBSITES FOR EDUCATION

See the EVOLVE website for World Wide Web resources for client education.

REFERENCES

Barnason S et al: Comparison of two endotracheal tube securement techniques on unplanned extubation, oral mucosa, and facial skin integrity, *Heart Lung* 27(6):409, 1998.

Boland D, Sims S: Family caregiving at home as a solitary journey, *Image* 28:1, 1996.

Brook AD et al: Effect of a nursing-implemented sedation protocol on the duration of mechanical ventilation, *Crit Care Med* 27(12):2609, 1999.

Burns SM: Ventilatory management—volume and pressure modes. In Lynn-McHale DJ, Carolson KK, editors: *AACN procedure manual for critical care*, ed 4, Philadelphia, 2001, WB Saunders.

Campbell M, Thill-Baharozian M: Impact of the DNR therapeutic plan on patient care requirements, *Am J Crit Care* 3:202, 1994.

Chang V: Protocol for prevention of complications of endotracheal intubation, *Crit Care Nurs* 15:19, 1995.

Chevron V et al: Unplanned extubation risk factors of development and predictive criteria for reintubation, *Crit Care Med* 26(6):1049, 1998.

Chinea Rodriguez CD et al: Comparative evaluation of four methods of endotracheal tube holder, *Enferm Intensiva* 10(3):110, 1999.

Chlan L: Effectiveness of a music therapy intervention on relaxation and anxiety for patients receiving ventilatory assistance, *Heart Lung* 27(3):169, 1998.

Clarke T et al: A comparison of two methods of securing an endotracheal tube, *Aust Crit Care* 11(2):45, 1998.

Collard HR, Saint S, Matthay MA: Prevention of ventilator-associated pneumonia: an evidence-based systemic review, *Ann Intern Med* 138(6):494, 2003.

Costello JM: AAC intervention in the intensive care unit: the Children's Hospital Boston model, *Augment Alternative Comm* 16, 2000.

Drakulovic MB et al: Supine body position as a risk factor for nosocomial pneumonia in mechanically ventilated patients: a randomised trial, *Lancet* 354(9193):1851, 1999.

Ferrin MS, Tino G: Acute dyspnea, *AACN Clin Issues* 8(3):398, 1997.

Gift A, Narsavage G: Validity of the numeric rating scale as a measure of dyspnea, *Am J Crit Care* 7(3):200, 1998.

Guttman R: Case management of the frail elderly in the community, *Clin Nurs Spec* 13(4):174, 1999.

Happ MB: Communicating with mechanically ventilated patients: state of the science, *AACN Clin Issues* 12(2):247, 2001.

Humphrey C: *Home care nursing handbook*, ed 2, Gaithersburg, Md, 1994, Aspen.

• = Independent; ▲ = Collaborative

Johnson J: Effects of structuring patient's expectations on their reactions to threatening events, *Nurs Res* 21(6): 499, 1972.

Kaplow R, Bookbinder M: A comparison of four endotracheal tube holders, *Heart Lung* 23:59, 1994.

McCord M, Cronin-Stubbs D: Operationalizing dyspnea, *Heart Lung* 21:167, 1992.

Noyes J: Enabling young ventilator-dependent people to express their views and experiences of their care in hospital, *J Adv Nurs* 31:1206, 2000.

Perkins LA, Shortall SP: Ventilation without intubation, *RN* 63(1):34, 2000.

Phelan BA, Cooper DA, Sangkachand P: Prolonged mechanical ventilation and tracheostomy in the elderly, *AACN Clin Issues* 13:1, 2002.

Pierson DJ: Indications for mechanical ventilation in adults with acute respiratory failure, *Respir Care* 47:3, 2002.

Stovsky B, Rudy E, Dragonette P: Comparison of two types of communication methods used after cardiac surgery with patients with endotracheal tubes, *Heart Lung* 17(3):281, 1988.

Torres A et al: Pulmonary aspiration of gastric contents in patients receiving mechanical ventilation: the effect of body position, *Ann Intern Med* 116:540, 1992.

Dysfunctional Ventilatory weaning response

Betty Ackley

NANDA Definition

Inability to adjust to lowered levels of mechanical ventilator support that interrupts and prolongs the weaning process

Defining Characteristics

Severe

Deterioration in arterial blood gases from current baseline; respiratory rate increases significantly from baseline; increase from baseline blood pressure (20 mm Hg); agitation; increase from baseline heart rate (20 beats/min); paradoxical abdominal breathing; adventitious breath sounds, audible airway secretions; cyanosis; decreased level of consciousness; full respiratory accessory muscle use; shallow, gasping breaths; profuse diaphoresis; breathing uncoordinated with the ventilator

Moderate

Slight increase from baseline blood pressure (<20 mm Hg); baseline increase in respiratory rate (<5 breaths/min); slight increase from baseline heart rate (<20 beats/min); pale, slight cyanosis; slight respiratory accessory muscle use; inability to respond to coaching; inability to cooperate; apprehension; color changes; decreased air entry on auscultation; diaphoresis; eye widening, wide-eyed look; hypervigilance to activities

Mild

Warmth; restlessness; slight increase of respiratory rate from baseline; queries about possible machine malfunction; expressed feelings of increased need for oxygen; fatigue; increased concentration on breathing

Related Factors (r/t)

Physiological

Ineffective airway clearance; sleep pattern disturbance; inadequate nutrition; uncontrolled pain or discomfort

• = Independent; ▲ = Collaborative

Psychological

Knowledge deficit of the weaning process and client role; perceived inefficacy about the ability to wean; decreased motivation; decreased self-esteem; moderate or severe anxiety or fear; hopelessness; powerlessness; insufficient trust in nurse

Situational

Uncontrolled episodic energy demands or problems; inappropriate pacing of diminished ventilator support; inadequate social support; adverse environment (e.g., noise, activity, negative events in the room); low nurse-client ratio; extended nurse absence from bedside; unfamiliar nursing staff; history of ventilator dependence for >4 days to 1 week; history of multiple unsuccessful weaning attempts

NOC Outcomes (Nursing Outcomes Classification)

Suggested NOC Outcomes

Respiratory Status: Gas Exchange, Ventilation

Example NOC Outcome with Indicators

Respiratory Status: Ventilation as evidenced by the following indicators: Respiratory rate IER/Respiratory rhythm IER/Depth of inspiration/Chest expansion symmetrical/Ease of breathing/Moves sputum out of airways/Accessory muscle use not present/Adventitious breath sounds not present/Chest retraction not present/Auscultated breath sounds IER/Tidal volume IER/Vital capacity IER (Rate each indicator of **Respiratory Status: Ventilation:** 1 = extremely compromised, 2 = substantially compromised, 3 = moderately compromised, 4 = mildly compromised, 5 = not compromised [see Section I].)

IER, In expected range.

Client Outcomes

Client Will (Specify Time Frame):

- Wean from ventilator with adequate arterial blood gases
- Remain free of unresolved dyspnea or restlessness
- Effectively clear secretions

NIC Interventions (Nursing Interventions Classification)

Suggested NIC Interventions

Mechanical Ventilation; Mechanical Ventilatory Weaning

Example NIC Activities—Mechanical Ventilatory Weaning

Monitor for optimal fluid and electrolyte status; Monitor to ensure client is free of significant infection before weaning

---

Nursing Interventions and Rationales

- Assess client's readiness for weaning as evidenced by the following:
  - Hemodynamic stability with adequate heart function
  - Resolution of initial medical problem that led to ventilator dependence
  - Adequate nutritional status with serum albumin levels >2.5 g/dl

- = Independent; ▲ = Collaborative

- Adequate sleep
- Psychological readiness, alertness, and stable vital signs

Adequate respiratory parameters include the following: a negative inspiratory pressure <-20 cm, positive expiratory pressure >+30 cm H_2O, spontaneous tidal volume >5 ml/kg, vital capacity >10 to 15 ml/kg, fraction of inspired oxygen <50%/min, and ventilation <10 L/min (Burns, 2001).

Fluid and electrolyte balance

- For best results ensure that the client is in an optimal physiological and psychological state before introducing the stress of weaning (Burns, 2001; Martensson and Fridlund, 2002; MacIntyre et al, 2002). *For more information on weaning assessment, please refer to the Burns Weaning Assessment Program (Burns, 2001).*
- Initiate conditioning for the client including strength training where the client uses a T piece or low intermittent mandatory ventilation for short durations or endurance training where the client uses pressure support ventilation on inspiration to prepare for weaning. *Strength training helps increase muscle function; endurance training helps the client maintain a level of work of breathing for a progressively longer period of time (Burns, 2001).*
- Identify reasons for previous unsuccessful weaning attempts, and include that information in development of the weaning plan. *Analyzing client responses after each weaning attempt prevents repeated unsuccessful weanings (Clochesy et al, 1997). A search for all causes of ventilator dependence should be done, and reversing the cause if possible is key to weaning (MacIntyre et al, 2002).*
- ▲ Collaborate with an interdisciplinary team (physician, nurse, respiratory therapist, nutritionist) to develop a weaning plan with a timeline and goals; revise this plan throughout the weaning period. Use a communication device such as a weaning board or flow sheet. **Nursing Research:** *A nurse-led weaning program following a defined protocol has been shown to be effective in weaning (Crocker, 2002; Henneman, 2001; Kollef et al, 1997). Effective interdisciplinary collaboration can positively affect client outcomes (Baggs et al, 1992).*
- Assist client to identify personal strategies that result in relaxation and comfort (e.g., music, visualization, relaxation techniques, reading, television, family visits). Support implementation of these strategies. **Nursing Research:** *Personal strategies for relaxation are effective (Gift, Moore, and Soeken, 1992). A study demonstrated that playing music that was relaxing decreased anxiety and increased relaxation as shown by reduced heart and respiratory rate in intubated adults (Chlan, 1998).*
- Provide a safe and comfortable environment. Stay with the client during weaning if at all possible. If unable to stay, make the call light button readily available, and assure the client that needs will be met responsively. *A client who feels safe and trusts the health care providers can focus on the immediate work of weaning; support from the nurse helps decrease anxiety (Burns, 2001).*
- ▲ Do not administer narcotics immediately before weaning; coordinate any pain management routine to effectively offer analgesia with minimal sedative effects (Kollef et al, 1998).
- Schedule weaning periods for the time of day when the client is most rested. Cluster care activities to promote successful weaning. Avoid other procedures during weaning: keep the environment quiet and promote restful activities between weaning periods.

• = Independent; ▲ = Collaborative

It is important that the client receive adequate rest between weaning periods. Control of external noises and stimuli can promote restful periods (Cropp et al, 1994).

- Promote a normal sleep-wake cycle, allowing uninterrupted periods of nighttime sleep (Higgins, 1998). *Limit visitors during weaning to close and supportive persons; ask visitors to leave if they are negatively affecting the weaning process.*

- During weaning, monitor the client's physiological and psychological responses; acknowledge and respond to fears and subjective complaints. Validate that the client is doing the work of weaning. **Nursing Research:** *Weaning is a stressful experience that requires active participation by the client. The client's work needs to be understood and supported by clinicians to facilitate recovery from mechanical ventilation and weaning (Logan, 1997).*

- Monitor subjective and objective data (breath sounds, respiratory pattern, respiratory effort, heart rate, blood pressure, oxygen saturation per oximetry, amount and type of secretions, anxiety, energy level) throughout weaning to determine client tolerance and responses. *Continued assessment and maintenance of airway clearance throughout weaning supports client comfort, safety, and trust (Carroll and Milikowski, 1996).*

- Coach the client through episodes of increased anxiety. Remain with client or place a supportive and calm significant other in this role. Give positive reinforcement, and with permission use touch to communicate support and concern. *It is not unusual for a client with lung disease to experience self-limiting episodes of increased shortness of breath. Supporting and coaching a client through such episodes allows weaning to continue.*

- Terminate weaning when the client demonstrates predetermined criteria or when the following signs of weaning intolerance occur:
  - Tachypnea, dyspnea, or chest and abdominal asynchrony
  - Agitation or mental status changes
  - Decreased oxygen saturation: Sao_2 <90%
  - Increased or decreased pulse rate or blood pressure or presence of new onset of dysrhythmias
  Continuing the weaning trial when the client has intolerance leads to fatigue and possible cardiovascular failure (Burns, 2001).

▲ If the dysfunctional weaning response is severe, consider slowing weaning to brief increments of time (e.g., 5 minutes). Continue to collaborate with the team to determine whether an untreated physiological cause for the dysfunctional weaning pattern remains. Consider an alternative care setting (subacute, rehabilitation facility, home) for clients with prolonged ventilator dependence as a strategy that can positively affect outcomes. **Clinical Research:** *One study indicated that half of the clients admitted to a rehabilitation facility were weaned from the ventilator (Modawal et al, 2002).*

Geriatric

- Recognize that older clients may require longer periods of time to wean. **Nursing Research:** *A study demonstrated that older clients required a longer period of time to wean, especially if they were older than 80 years (Epstein, Modadem, and Peerless, 2002).*

Home care

NOTE: Weaning from a ventilator at home should be based on client stability and comfort of the client and caregivers under an intermittent care plan. The client and/or family may be more comfortable having the client rehospitalized for the process.

• = **Independent;** ▲ = **Collaborative**

- Assess comfort and coping ability of the client and/or family to wean at home, as well as fiscal implications and home care coverage. *Compromises in respiratory function are frightening for clients and family who perceive the availability of a high-technology, structured environment as a more appropriate environment for weaning (Sevick et al, 1997).*

- Establish an emergency plan and methods of implementation. Include emergency aeration and reestablishment of the ventilation assistive device. *Having a prepared emergency plan reassures the client and family and provides for client safety.*

▲ Obtain orders for alternative routes of medication administration when medications have been administered via a ventilation device. Instruct the client and family in changes.

evolve WEBSITES FOR EDUCATION

See the EVOLVE website for World Wide Web resources for client education.

REFERENCES

Baggs J et al: The association between interdisciplinary collaboration and patient outcomes in a medical intensive care unit, *Heart Lung* 21(1):18, 1992.

Burns SM: Standard weaning criteria. In Lynn-McHale DJ, Carolson KK, editors: *AACN procedure manual for critical care,* ed 4, Philadelphia, 2001, WB Saunders.

Carroll P, Milikowski K: Getting your patient off a ventilator, *RN* 96(6):42, 1996.

Chlan L: Effectiveness of a music therapy intervention on relaxation and anxiety for patients receiving ventilatory assistance, *Heart Lung* 27(3):169, 1998.

Clochesy J et al: Volunteers in participatory sampling of weaning practices: the Third National Study Group on Weaning from Mechanical Ventilation, *Crit Care Nurs* 17(2):72, 1997.

Crocker C: Nurse-led weaning from ventilatory and respiratory support, *Intens Crit Care Nurs* 18:272, 2002.

Cropp A et al: Name that tone: the proliferation of noise in the intensive care unit, *Chest* 105:1217, 1994.

Epstein CD, El-Modadem N, Peerless JR: Weaning older patients from long-term mechanical ventilation: a pilot study, *Am J Crit Care* 11:4, 2002.

Gift A, Moore T, Soeken K: Relaxation to reduce dyspnea and anxiety in COPD patients, *Nurs Res* 41:242, 1992.

Henneman EA: Liberating patients from mechanical ventilation, a team approach, *Crit Care Nurs* 21(3):25, 2001.

Higgins P: Patient perception of fatigue while undergoing long term mechanical ventilation: incidence and associated factors, *Heart Lung* 27(3):177, 1998.

Kollef M et al: The use of continuous IV sedation is associated with prolongation of mechanical ventilation, *Chest* 114(2):541, 1998.

Kollef MH et al: A randomized controlled trial of protocol-directed versus physician-directed weaning from mechanical ventilation, *Crit Care Med* 25(4):567, 1997.

Logan J: Qualitative analysis of patient's work during mechanical ventilation and weaning, *Heart Lung* 26(2):140, 1997.

MacIntyre NR et al: Evidence-based guidelines for weaning and discontinuing ventilatory support, *Respir Care* 47(1):69, 2002.

Martensson IE, Fridlund B: Factors influencing the patient during weaning from mechanical ventilation: a national survey, *Intensive Crit Care Nurs* 18:223, 2002.

Modawal A et al Weaning success among ventilator-dependent patients in a rehabilitation facility, *Arch Phys Med Rehabil* 83(2):154, 2002.

Sevick M et al: Economic value of caregiver effort in maintaining long term ventilatory assisted individuals, *Heart Lung* 26(2):148, 1997.

• = **Independent;** ▲ = **Collaborative**

Risk for other-directed Violence

Kathleen L. Patusky

NANDA   Definition

At risk for behaviors in which an individual demonstrates that he or she can be physically, emotionally, and/or sexually harmful to others

Risk Factors

Body language: rigid posture, clenching of fists and jaw, hyperactivity, pacing, breathlessness, threatening stances; history of violence against others (e.g., hitting someone, kicking someone, spitting at someone, scratching someone, throwing objects at someone, biting someone, attempted rape, rape, sexual molestation, urinating/defecating on someone); history of threats of violence (e.g., verbal threats against property, verbal threats against person, social threats, cursing, threatening notes/letters, threatening gestures, sexual threats); history of violent antisocial behavior (e.g., stealing, insistent borrowing, insistent demanding of privileges, insistent interrupting of meetings, refusing to eat, refusing to take medication, ignoring instructions); history of violence, indirect (e.g., tearing off clothes, ripping objects off walls, writing on walls, urinating on floor, defecating on floor, stamping feet, displaying temper tantrum, running in corridors, yelling, throwing objects, breaking a window, slamming doors, making sexual advances); neurological impairment (e.g., positive EEG, CAT, or MRI; head trauma; positive neurological findings; seizure disorders); cognitive impairment (e.g., learning disabilities, attention deficit disorder, decreased intellectual functioning); history of childhood abuse; history of witnessing family violence; cruelty to animals; fire setting; prenatal/perinatal complications or abnormalities; history of drug or alcohol abuse; pathological intoxication; psychotic symptomatology (e.g., auditory, visual, command hallucinations; paranoid delusions; loose, rambling, or illogical thought processes); motor vehicle offenses (e.g., frequent traffic violations, use of a motor vehicle to release anger); suicidal behavior; impulsivity; availability/possession of weapon(s)

NOC   Outcomes (Nursing Outcomes Classification)

Suggested NOC Outcomes

Abuse Cessation; Abusive Behavior Self-Restraint; Aggression Self-Control; Distorted Thought Self-Control; Impulse Self-Control; Parenting: Psychosocial Safety; Risk Detection

> **Example NOC Outcome with Indicators**
>
> **Aggression Self-Control** as evidenced by the following indicators: Restrains from harming others/ Communicates needs and feelings appropriately/Identifies when angry (Rate each indicator of **Aggression Self-Control:** 1 = never demonstrated, 2 = rarely demonstrated, 3 = sometimes demonstrated, 4 = often demonstrated, 5 = consistently demonstrated [see Section I].)

• = Independent; ▲ = Collaborative

Client Outcomes

Client Will (Specify Time Frame):

- Stop all forms of abuse (physical, emotional, sexual; neglect; financial exploitation)
- Have cessation of abuse reported by victim
- Display no aggressive activity
- Refrain from verbal outbursts
- Refrain from violating others' personal space
- Refrain from antisocial behaviors
- Maintain relaxed body language and decreased motor activity
- Identify factors contributing to abusive/aggressive behavior
- Demonstrate impulse control or state feelings of control
- Identify impulsive behaviors
- Identify feelings/behaviors that lead to impulsive actions
- Identify consequences of impulsive actions to self or others
- Avoid high-risk environments and situations
- Identify and talk about feelings; express anger appropriately
- Express decreased anxiety and control of hallucinations as applicable
- Displace anger to meaningful activities
- Communicate needs appropriately
- Identify responsibility to maintain control
- Express empathy for victim
- Obtain no access or yield access to harmful objects
- Use alternative coping mechanisms for stress
- Obtain and follow through with counseling
- Demonstrate knowledge of correct role behaviors

Victim (and Children If Applicable) Will (Specify Time Frame):

- Have safe plan for leaving situation or avoiding abuse
- Resolve depression or traumatic response

Parent Will (Specify Time Frame):

- Monitor social/play contacts
- Provide supervision and nurturing environment
- Intervene to prevent high-risk social behaviors

NIC Interventions (Nursing Interventions Classification)

Suggested NIC Interventions

Abuse Protection Support; Anger Control Assistance; Behavior Management; Calming Technique; Coping Enhancement; Crisis Intervention; Delusion Management; Dementia Management; Distraction; Environmental Management: Violence Prevention; Mood Management; Physical Restraint; Seclusion; Substance Use Prevention

> **Example NIC Intervention—Environmental Management: Violence Prevention**
>
> Remove other individuals from the vicinity of a violent or potentially violent client; Provide ongoing surveillance of all client access areas to maintain client safety; Therapeutically intervene as needed

• = Independent; ▲ = Collaborative

Nursing Interventions and Rationales

▲ Monitor the environment, evaluate situations that could become violent, and intervene early to de-escalate the situation. Enlist support from other staff rather than attempting to handle the situation alone. *Violent situations can arise any time that anger or frustration occurs and need not limit participation to clients. Family members or other staff can initiate violence, especially around disagreements over a client's treatment plan or if kept waiting for prolonged periods (Duncan, Estabrookes, Reimer, 2000). Most psychiatric facilities identify specific policies and offer training in crisis intervention or conflict resolution. Participation in such training for all staff is highly recommended.*

▲ Know and follow institution's policies and procedures concerning violence. *Being familiar with and following policies and procedures of the department prevents violence. Policies should be developed, and training programs should be provided in proper use and application of restraints (Daum, 1994). All nursing units should develop a proactive plan for dealing with violent situations.*

▲ Assess the client for risk factors of violence including those in the following categories: psychiatric disorders (particularly paranoid or bipolar disorders, substance abuse), neurological disorders (e.g., head injury, temporal lobe epilepsy), psychological precursors (e.g., low tolerance for stress, impulsivity), coping difficulties (e.g., inability to plan solutions or see long-term consequences of behavior), and personal history (e.g., past violent behavior). *All of these risk factors have been implicated in aggressive, agitated, or violent behavior. Additional potential triggers include confusion, anxiety/frustration, boredom, heat, excessive or constant noise, lack of information, having no right or appeal, lack of choice, lack of space, or group/peer pressure (Graham, 2001). Medical history and physical findings should be considered carefully for elements that may decrease the client's anger threshold or influence the client's thought processes (e.g., chronic medical condition, neoplasm) (Citrome and Volavka, 1999; Corrigan, Yudofsky, and Silver, 1993).*

▲ Assess for potential indicators of impending violence against others: frequent medication change, high use of sedative drugs, past violent behavior, a *Diagnostic and Statistical Manual of Mental Health IV* diagnosis of antisocial personality or borderline personality disorder, and long hospitalization. Other indicators include hypervigilance, hostility, substance use, and lack of adherence to medication regimen. *A study indicated that behaviors and situations in the first list are the most powerful predictors of violence (Soliman and Reza, 2001). Knowing, recognizing, and promptly intervening in early precipitating factors prevents violence.*

• Assess the client with history of previous assaults. Listen to and acknowledge feelings of anger, observe for increased motor activity, and prepare to intervene if the client becomes aggressive. **Nursing Research:** *In one study, physically assaultive clients had significantly more previous assaults and more difficulty appropriately verbalizing angry feelings on their units than did control group members. Before the assault, assaultive clients were more verbally hostile and showed more increased motor activity than control subjects (Lanza et al, 1996).*

• Assess for the client's experience of physiological signs and for external signs of anger. *Internal signs of anger include increased pulse, respirations, and blood pressure; chills; prickly sensations; numbness; choking sensation; nausea; and vertigo. External signs include increased muscle tone, changes in body posture (clenched fists, set jaw), eye changes (eyebrows lower and drawn together, eyelids tense, eyes assuming a "hard" appearance), lips pressed together, flushing or pallor, goose bumps, twitching, and sweating (Harper-Jacques and Reimer, 2002).*

• = Independent; ▲ = Collaborative

- Assess for the presence of hallucinations. *Command hallucinations may direct the client to behave violently, and assessment of their presence is important when evaluating the risk for violence in clients with major mental disorders (McNeil, Eisner, and Binder, 2000).*
- Determine the presence and degree of homicidal risk. A number of questions will elicit the necessary information:
  - Have you been thinking about harming someone? If yes, who?
  - How often do you have these thoughts, and how long do they last?
  - Do you have a plan? What is it?
  - Do you have access to the means to carry out that plan?
  - What has kept you from hurting the person until now?

  Psychotherapists are required to report harm or threats of harm to another person; this is referred to as the duty to warn. State laws and mental health codes should be checked to determine local mandates for threat reporting by specific types of health care professionals.

▲ Screen for possible abuse in women or children with a pattern of injury, particularly if there is any suspicion that the physical findings are inconsistent with the explanation of how the injuries were incurred. Report suspected child abuse to Child Protective Services. Refer women suspected of being in a spouse abuse situation to an area crisis center. Rapid screening tools are needed to identify intimate partner violence. *Screening for battering was demonstrated as an effective tool in this study (Coker et al, 2001). All nurses are required by law to report suspected child abuse.*

- Take action to minimize personal risk:
  - Use nonthreatening body language
  - Respect personal space and boundaries
  - Do not allow the client to block access to an exit
  - If speaking with the client alone, keep the door to the room open
  - Be aware of where other staff are at all times
  - Notify other staff of where you are at all times
  - Take verbal threats seriously, and notify other staff
  - Wear clothing and accessories that are not restricting and that will not be dangerous (e.g., sandals or shoes with heels can lead to twisted ankles; necklaces or dangling earrings could be grabbed).

  Actions must be taken by nurses to minimize personal risk if they are to be available to respond to violence (Harper-Jacques and Reimer, 2002). Other staff must be notified so they can also take proper precautions and be alert to the potential for violence.

- Maintain at least an arm's length distance from the client; do not touch the client without permission (unless physical restraint is the goal). *Encroaching on the client's personal space is likely to increase fear, anger, or paranoia and thus increase the magnitude of the reaction. Touching may be perceived as initiation of an attack; the client may strike out in self-defense.*
- Remove potential weapons from the environment. Be prepared to remove obstructions to staff response from the environment. *Clients prone to violence may use available weapons opportunistically. If client restraint becomes necessary, environmental hazards (e.g., chairs, wastebaskets) should be moved out of the way to prevent injuries.*
- Search the client and his or her belongings for weapons or potential weapons on admission to the hospital as appropriate. *Clients prone to violence may carry a weapon routinely (e.g., knife). Weapons should be removed for safety of clients and staff.*
- Inform the client of unit expectations for appropriate behavior and the consequences of not meeting these expectations. Emphasize that the client must comply with the

- = **Independent;** ▲ = **Collaborative**

rules of the unit. Give positive reinforcement for compliance. *Clients benefit from clear guidance regarding behavioral expectations and consequences, providing much-needed structure. The process emphasizes client responsibility for his or her own behavior. It is important to reinforce appropriate behavior to encourage repetition. The unit serves as a microcosm of the client's outside world, so adherence to social norms while on the unit models adherence upon discharge, while providing the client with staff support to learn appropriate coping skills and alternative behaviors.*

- Increase surveillance of the hospitalized client at smoking, meal, and medication times. **Nursing Research:** *A study of temporal patterns of physical control use (mechanical restraint and locked seclusion) at a state psychiatric hospital revealed that the use of control increased at clients' smoking, meal, and medication times. Increased demands on clients, difficulty adjusting to shifts in activity, close proximity to other clients, or denial of privileges (e.g., smoking) may have accounted for the increases (Vittengl, 2002).*

- Assign a single room to the client with a potential for violence toward others. *The client will be able to take time away from unit stimulation to calm self as needed. Another client will not be placed at risk as a roommate.*

- Maintain a secluded area for the client to be placed when violent. *The violent client is removed from a potentially overstimulating environment. Violence on a unit can frighten other persons present.*

- Maintain a calm attitude in response to the client. *Anxiety is contagious.*

- Provide a low level of stimulation in the client's environment; place the client in a safe, quiet place, and speak slowly and quietly. *A safe, quiet environment that provides structure decreases the outside stimuli that may be precipitating violent behavior (Citrome and Volavka, 1999).*

- Redirect possible violent behaviors into physical activities (e.g., walking, jogging) if the client is physically able. *Using a punching bag or hitting a pillow may not be indicated because they are not calming activities and they continue patterning violent behavior. However, activities that distract while draining excess energy are appropriate. They help to build a repertoire of alternative behaviors for stress reduction.*

- Provide sufficient staff if a show of force is necessary to demonstrate control to the client. *When staff respond to an escalating or violent situation, it can reassure clients that they will not be allowed to lose control. On the other hand, leave immediately if the client becomes violent and you are not trained to handle it.*

- Protect other clients in the environment from harm. Remove other individuals from the vicinity of a violent or potentially violent client. Follow safety protocols of the department. *Proper preparation, training, and implementation of strict protocols can save nurses' and others' lives when violence occurs.* Others can be injured during a violent outburst; therefore their safety must be considered. *The risk of a violent client to others in the area (other clients, visitors) should be anticipated, even as efforts proceed to de-escalate the situation with the client.*

▲ Use chemical restraints as ordered. Obtain an order for medication, and administer it immediately. *Medications should be offered before physical restraints or seclusion is considered; the medications used most often are haloperidol (Haldol) and lorazepam (Ativan).*

▲ Use mechanical restraints if ordered and as necessary. **Nursing Research:** *Physical restraint of children can be therapeutic for the child (Morales and Duphorne, 1995). Clients externalize why restraining occurred ("I was out of control"). Most can verbalize the reason they were restrained (Outlaw and Lowery, 1994).*

▲ Follow institution's protocol for releasing restraints. Observe client closely, remain

• = Independent; ▲ = Collaborative

calm, and provide positive feedback as client's behavior becomes controlled. *The period during which restraints are removed can be dangerous for staff if they do not recognize that the client may choose to reinitiate violence. Protocols will specify safe procedures for removing restraints.*

▲ If restraints are necessary, provide the client with musical tapes and a headset. *Music can provide a distraction from negative thoughts or auditory hallucinations.* **Nursing Research:** *Use of taped music via a headset can decrease negative behaviors (Janelli et al, 1995). Listening to music of their own choosing may help produce positive behaviors in previously restrained clients (Janelli and Kanski, 1997).*

• Encourage clients to eat a balanced diet instead of junk food. *In clients with a poor dietary history, particularly indigent clients or clients with alcoholism, deficiencies of thiamine and niacin may lead to irritability, disorientation, and paranoia (Harper-Jacques and Reimer, 2002).*

• Form a therapeutic alliance with the client, identifying the source of anger as external to both nurse and client. *The development of a therapeutic relationship before aggressive behavior occurs provides an alternative for working through anger and frustration. Assisting the client to identify a source of anger or frustration that is external to both the nurse and client prevents the need for defensiveness by both and directs energy at solving an external problem.*

• Allow and encourage the client to verbalize feelings either one on one or in a group setting. *When clients' feelings are not addressed, intense emotions can obstruct the ability to consider alternatives to violence (Wright and Leahey, 2000). Violence is a physical manifestation of feelings (e.g., anger, frustration, fear). When clients verbalize their feelings, they are not only exercising a more appropriate means of expressing feelings; they are entering into an opportunity to examine the source of those feelings. Clients can then problem-solve to determine a more effective way to address the situation.*

• Recognize that anger is generally purposeful and situation dependent. Actively listen to the client; explore the source of the client's anger, and negotiate resolution when possible. *Anger can be a normal response when an individual feels threatened or experiences delay or denial of gratification. Concern arises when anger escalates to the extent that it becomes intimidating or behavioral control may be lost. Conflict resolution before anger is expressed behaviorally is the goal of listening to the individual. For example, the visitor who becomes angry when told visiting hours are over has the potential to become violent. Listening to the visitor may reveal that he just arrived from out of town and is very concerned about the well-being of a client. Negotiating a brief visit and providing visiting hours for the next day can avert escalation of anger. A paranoid client who is becoming agitated because he believes another client is watching him generally calms when he is encouraged to discuss his fears and is reassured that staff will keep him safe.*

• Teach healthy ways to express feelings/anger, appropriate gender roles, and how to communicate needs appropriately. *Instruction that expands young men's conceptions of manhood and appropriate gender roles can reduce the likelihood of their engaging in sexually or physically violent behavior (Hong, 2000). Clients may become violent if their perceived needs are thwarted. Instruction that prepares them to express their needs appropriately, while recognizing that others are under no obligation to meet their needs, prepares them to defuse this anger trigger.*

• Help the client identify when anger develops. Have the client keep an anger diary and discuss alternative responses together. Teach cognitive-behavioral techniques. *Clients with anger management difficulties may not be alert to physiological changes or cues that*

• = Independent; ▲ = Collaborative

they are becoming angry. They may not be aware of any time delay between the stimulus and their angry response. Instruction in cognitive-behavioral techniques and review of the diary with staff assists clients in identifying thought processes leading to anger and the space between stimulus and response.

- Identify stimuli that initiate violence and means of dealing with the stimuli. *Assisting the client to identify situations and people that upset him or her provides information needed for problem solving. The client may then identify alternative responses; e.g., leaving the stimulus, using relaxation techniques (e.g., deep breathing), initiating thought stopping; initiating a distracting activity, responding assertively rather than aggressively.*

- Emphasize that the client is responsible for his or her choices and behavior. Introduce descriptions of possible effects of client's aggressive/violent behavior on others. *In most cases clients are capable of learning to control angry impulses. In many cases clients operate from a world view that perceives others as instruments of the clients' gratification. A difficult but important insight that clients must gain is that they are dealing with other human beings who experience pain. Clients' behaviors influence how others respond to them.*

▲ In cases where spouse or child abuse accompanies substance abuse, refer the abusive client to a substance abuse treatment program and refer the spouse receiving abuse to Al Anon. *Use of drugs or alcohol decreases impulse control and aggravates abusive behavior.*

▲ In dealing with abused wives, maintain a nonjudgmental response when clients refuse to leave husbands or return to them. *An estimated 90% to 95% of abused partners are women battered by men (Sisley et al, 1999). Reasons for remaining in or returning to the relationship include economic concerns (especially with children), socialization about the women's role, political or legal obstacles, traumatic bonding that leaves the woman feeling powerless, and realistic fear of retaliation or death (Boyd and Mackey, 2000; Dutton, 1995; Wallace, 1999). Refer to care plan for* **Powerlessness.**

▲ In cases of potential child abuse, refer the client to parenting classes or a parental counseling support group. *Early intervention may prevent abuse from occurring. Young parents in particular may have difficulty dealing with the stresses of parenthood combined with other life stresses; sharing their concerns with others can help normalize the stress. Support from others can help prevent the need to displace anger and frustration onto the child.*

▲ Always follow up a violent episode with a debriefing of clients and staff. *Allowing discussion of a violent episode, either individually or in a group, among other clients present reveals clients' responses to the event and provides the opportunity for staff to offer reassurance and support. Clients may have concerns that staff will attempt to restrain them without reason or may feel uncertain whether staff can keep them safe. Staff debriefing offers a calming influence while providing the opportunity to evaluate the effectiveness of the reaction to violence and to brainstorm any necessary changes in procedure. Recent evidence has suggested that more extensive psychological debriefing, of the type used for individuals who experience extreme trauma, may not be warranted for all individuals. Providing comfort, support, and information and meeting immediate practical needs is useful; assumptions that global psychological debriefing would prevent subsequent psychopathology (e.g., posttraumatic stress disorder) have not been supported. Intervention beyond the initial screening and psychological first aid should be individualized (Litz et al, 2002).*

Geriatric

- Assess for changes in physiological functions (e.g., constipation, dehydration) or impairment of the ability to meet basic needs (e.g., inadequate toileting, decreased

• = Independent; ▲ = Collaborative

mobility). *In older adults subtle physiological changes can lead to observable changes in behavior, including agitation. Interruptions of or changes in routine can unsettle the older adult and be expressed as frustration or anger. Fears about medical disorders or potential loss of independence can be transformed into anger, irritability, or agitation.*

- Observe for dementia and delirium. *Clients with dementia or delirium may strike out if they are frustrated or if they have the sense that their personal space is being violated. However, this may not occur within a cognitive capacity that permits discussion of the behavior.*
- Assess sensory impairments and the influence they may have on the client's behavior. *Agitation and striking out may be precipitated in older adults who are experiencing either sensory impairment or difficulty communicating (Allen, 1999).*
- Observe for signs of fear, anxiety, anger, and agitation, and intervene immediately. *Gerontological nurses can prevent the incidence of assault by recognizing the potential risks, preventing clients' fear and anxiety, reducing the outburst of anger, and decreasing clients' agitation (Chou, Kaas, and Richie, 1996).*
- ▲ Monitor for paradoxical drug reactions, and report any to the physician. *Violent behavior can be stimulated by a medication intended to calm the client.*
- ▲ Assess for brain insults such as recent falls or injuries, strokes, or transient ischemic attacks. *Clients with brain injuries need specific interventions such as stimulus control, problem solving, social skills training, relaxation training, and anger management to reduce aggressive behaviors (Teichner, Golden, and Giannaris, 1999). Maintenance of a structured environment limits confusing external stimuli. Brain injuries, which are related to ambivalence, lowered impulse control, and reduced coping, can cause violent reactions to self or others. Brain injury symptoms may be mistaken for mental illness.*
- Decrease environmental stimuli if violence is directed at others. *Removal of the client to a quiet area can reduce violent impulses. Use a calm voice to "talk down" the client.*
- Provide hand or back rubs and calming music when elderly client experiences agitation. **Nursing Research:** *In a study of older adults in nursing homes, calming music and hand massage were found to soothe agitation for up to 1 hour. No additional benefit was found from combining the two interventions (Remington, 2002).*
- ▲ If abuse or neglect of an elderly client is suspected, report the suspicion to a local Adult Protective Services agency. *The telephone number for the Adult Protective Services office can be found by checking the blue governmental section of the phone book or by calling directory assistance and asking for the department of social services or aging services. It is essential to call the office with jurisdiction over the geographical area where the client lives.*

Home care

- Assess family members or caregivers for their ability to protect the client and themselves. *The safety of the client between home visits is a nursing priority. Caregivers often need assistance with recognizing or admitting fear of or danger from a loved one.*
- Include an initial and ongoing assessment and evaluation of potential abuse and neglect. Photograph evidence of abuse or neglect when possible. *Victims of abuse perceive themselves to be powerless to change the situation. Indeed, the abuser fosters this perception and may threaten violence or death if the victim attempts to leave. Chronic abuse and neglect by a spouse or other family among the elderly is often hidden until home care is actively involved. Refer to the care plan for* **Powerlessness.**
- ▲ If neglect or abuse is suspected, identify an emergency plan that addresses the problem immediately, ensures client safety, and includes a report to the appropriate authori-

• = Independent; ▲ = Collaborative

ties. Discuss when to use hotlines and 911. Role-play access to emergency resources with the client and caregivers. *Client safety is a nursing priority. An emergency plan should address either immediate removal to a safe environment or identification of appropriate steps to take in the event of abuse and the securing of resources for the anticipated action (e.g., available phone, packed bag, alternative living arrangements). Reporting is a legal requirement of health care workers.*

- Encourage appropriate safety behaviors in abused women; call the client at intervals during a 6-month period to determine whether safety behaviors are being carried out. **Nursing Research:** *A study of telephone contacts to women who sought help through the district attorney's office demonstrated that safety behaviors increased dramatically. Calls were initiated within 48 to 72 hours of initial contact. Safety behaviors included hiding money; hiding an extra set of house and car keys; establishing a code for abuse occurrence with family or friends; asking neighbors to call police if violence occurred; removing weapons; keeping available family social security numbers, rent and utility receipts, family birth certificates, identification or drivers licenses, bank account numbers, insurance policies and numbers, marriage license, valuable jewelry, important phone numbers, and a hidden bag with extra clothing (McFarlane et al, 2002).*
- Assess the home environment for harmful objects. Have the family remove or lock objects as able. *The safety of the client and caregivers is a nursing priority.*
- ▲ Refer for homemaker or psychiatric home health care services for respite, client reassurance, and implementation of a therapeutic regimen. *Responsibility for a person who may become violent provides high caregiver stress. Respite decreases caregiver stress. The presence of caring individuals is reassuring to both the client and caregivers, especially during periods of client anxiety. Violent behaviors can respond to the interventions described above, modified for the home setting.*
- ▲ If the client is taking psychotropic medications, assess client and family knowledge of medication and its administration and side effects. Teach as necessary. *Knowledge of the medical regimen supports compliance.*
- ▲ Evaluate effectiveness and side effects of medications. *Accurate clinical feedback improves physician ability to prescribe an effective medical regimen specific to client needs.*
- If client displays mildly intensifying aggressive behavior, attempt to diffuse anger or violence (e.g., ask for a glass of water to distract client). Later in the visit explain that aggressive behavior is not acceptable and present consequences of continued aggressive behavior (i.e., right of agency to discontinue services). *Mild aggression can be diffused safely. Confronting the client before severe aggression is evident places responsibility on the client and family for respectful partnership in care.*
- Document all acts or verbalizations of aggression. *Safety of the staff is a primary responsibility of home health agencies. Law enforcement intervention may be necessary.*
- ▲ If client verbalizes or displays threatening behavior, notify supervisor and plan to make joint visits with another staff person or a security escort. *Having a second person at the visit is a show of power and control used to subdue aggressive behavior.*
- ▲ If the client behaves in such a manner as to make the nurse uncomfortable without overt threat, a meeting may be held outside the home in sight of others (e.g., front porch). *The nurse should trust a "gut" reaction that prompts concern regarding the client's potential for aggressive or violent behavior. Such intuitive reactions are often the result of subliminal cues that are not readily voiced.*
- ▲ Never enter a home or remain in a home if aggression threatens your well-being. Never challenge a show of force such as a gun threat. Leave and notify your supervisor

• = Independent; ▲ = Collaborative

and the appropriate authorities. Document the incident. *Safety of the staff is a primary responsibility of home health agencies. Law enforcement intervention may be necessary.*

▲ If client behaviors intensify, refer for immediate mental health intervention. *The degree of disturbance and ability to manage care safely at home determines the level of services needed to protect the client.*

Client/Family Teaching

• Teach relaxation and exercise as ways to release anger.

• Teach cognitive-behavioral activities such as active problem solving, reframing (reappraising the situation from a different perspective), or thought stopping (in response to a negative thought, picture a large stop sign and replace the image with a prearranged positive alternative). Teach the client to confront his or her own negative thought patterns (or cognitive distortions) such as catastophizing (expecting the very worst), dichotomous thinking (perceiving events in only one of two opposite categories), magnification (placing distorted emphasis on a single event), or unrealistic expectations (e.g., "I should get what I want when I want it."). *Aggressive clients often have negative, even paranoid, perceptions of others and unrealistic expectations of how they should be treated, leading to their anger. The client may or may not be capable of empathy for others. Cognitive-behavioral activities address clients' assumptions, beliefs, and attitudes about their situations, fostering modification of these elements to be as realistic as possible. Through cognitive-behavioral interventions, clients become more aware of their cognitive choices in adopting and maintaining their belief systems, thereby exercising greater control over their own reactions (Hagerty and Patusky, 2003; Sinclair et al, 1998).*

• For religious couples, encourage the use of prayer. *Prayer may invoke a couple-God system, which significantly influences couple interaction during conflict. Prayer appears to be a significant "softening" event for religious couples, facilitating reconciliation and problem solving. It de-escalates hostile emotions and reduces emotional reactivity (Butler, Gardner, and Bird, 1998).*

▲ Refer to individual or group therapy.

• Teach the adolescent client violence prevention and encourage him or her to become involved in community service activities. *School programs that couple community service with classroom health instruction can have a measurable impact on violent behaviors of young adolescents at high risk for being both the perpetrators and victims of peer violence. Community service programs may be an effective supplement to curricular interventions and a valuable component of multicomponent violence-prevention programs (O'Donnell et al, 1999).*

• Teach caregivers and family members of clients with dementia to use expressive physical touch and verbalization (EPT/V) when caring for these clients. **Nursing Research:** *One study found that (1) anxiety is lower immediately after EPT/V, and (2) EPT/V causes decreasing episodes of dysfunctional behavior. It is cost-effective and simple to learn and practice, and it is most effective in improving and maintaining a client's high quality of life (Kim and Buschmann, 1999).*

▲ Teach the use of appropriate community resources in emergency situations (e.g., hotline, community mental health agency, emergency department, 911 in most places in the United States, the toll-free National Domestic Violence Hotline [1-800-799-SAFE]). *It is necessary to get immediate help when violence occurs.*

▲ Encourage the use of self-help groups in nonemergency situations.

▲ Inform the client and family about medication actions, side effects, target symptoms, and toxic reactions.

• = Independent; ▲ = Collaborative

evolve WEBSITES FOR EDUCATION

See the EVOLVE website for World Wide Web resources for client education.

REFERENCES

Allen LA: Treating agitation without drugs, *Am J Nurs* 99(4):36, 1999.

Boyd MR, Mackey M: Alienation from self and others: the psychosocial problem of rural alcoholic women, *Arch Psychiatr Nurs* 14:134, 2000.

Butler MH, Gardner BC, Bird MH: Not just a time-out: change dynamics of prayer for religious couples in conflict situations, *Fam Process* 37(4):451, 1998.

Chou K, Kaas M, Richie M: Assaultive behavior in geriatric patients, *J Gerontol Nurs* 22(11):30, 1996.

Citrome L, Volavka J: Violent patients in the emergency setting, *Psychiatr Clin North Am* 22(4):789, 1999.

Coker AL et al: Assessment of clinical partner violence screening tools, *J Am Med Womens Assoc* 56(1):19, 2001.

Corrigan PW, Yudofsky SC, Silver JM: Pharmacological and behavioral treatment for aggressive psychiatric inpatients, *Hosp Commun Psychiatr* 44(3):125, 1993.

Daum A: Disruptive antisocial patient: management strategies, *Nurs Manage* 8:46, 1994.

Duncan S, Estabrookes CA, Reimer M: Violence against nurses, *Alberta RN* 56(2):13, 2000.

Dutton DG: *The domestic assault of women*, Vancouver, Canada, 1995, UBC Press.

Graham P: Understanding and dealing with anger, aggression and violence, *Nurs Stand* 16:37, 2001.

Hagerty B, Patusky K: Mood disorders: depression and mania. In Fortinash KM, Holoday-Worret PA, editors: *Psychiatric mental health nursing*, ed 3, St Louis, 2003, Mosby.

Harper-Jacques S, Reimer M: Management of aggression. In Boyd MA, editor: *Psychiatric nursing. Contemporary practice*, ed 2, Philadelphia, 2002, Lippincott.

Hong L: Toward a transformed approach to prevention: breaking the link between masculinity and violence, *J Am Coll Health* 48(6):269, 2000.

Janelli LM, Kanski GW: Music intervention with physically restrained patients, *Rehabil Nurs* 22(1):14, 1997.

Janelli LM et al: Exploring music intervention with restrained patients, *Nurs Forum* 30(4):12, 1995.

Kim EJ, Buschmann MT: The effect of expressive physical touch on patients with dementia, *Int J Nurs Stud* 36(3):235, 1999.

Lanza M et al: The relationship of behavioral cues to assaultive behavior, *Clin Nurs Res* 5(1):6, 1996.

Litz BT et al: Early intervention for trauma: current status and future directions, *Clin Psychol Sci Pract* 9(2):112, 2002.

McFarlane J et al: An intervention to increase safety behaviors of abused women, *Nurs Res* 51:347, 2002.

McNeil DE, Eisner JP, Binder RL: The relationship between command hallucinations and violence, *Psychiatr Serv* 51(10):1288, 2000.

Morales E, Duphorne P: Least restrictive measures: alternatives to four-pt. restraints and seclusion, *J Psychosoc Nurs Ment Health Serv* 33:13, 1995.

O'Donnell L et al: Violence prevention and young adolescents' participation in community youth service, *J Adolesc Health* 24(1):28, 1999.

Outlaw F, Lowery B: An attributional study of seclusion and restraint of psychiatric patients, *Arch Psychiatr Nurs* 8:69, 1994.

Remington R: Calming music and hand massage with agitated elderly, *Nurs Res* 51:317, 2002.

Sinclair VG et al: Effects of a cognitive-behavioral intervention for women with rheumatoid arthritis, *Res Nurs Health* 21:315, 1998.

Sisley A et al: Violence in America: a public health crisis—domestic violence, *J Trauma* 46:1105, 1999.

Soliman AE, Reza H: Risk factors and correlates of violence among acutely ill adult psychiatric inpatients, *Psychiatr Serv* 52(1):75, 2001.

Teichner G, Golden CJ, Giannaris WJ: A multimodal approach to treatment of aggression in a severely brain-injured adolescent, *Rehabil Nurs* 24(5):207, 1999.

Vittengl JR: Temporal regularities in physical control at a state psychiatric hospital, *Arch Psychiatr Nurs* 16:80, 2002.

Wallace H: *Family violence: legal, medical, and social perspectives*, ed 2, Boston, 1999, Allyn & Bacon.

Wright LM, Leahey M: *Nurses and families: a guide to family assessment and intervention*, ed 3, Philadelphia, 2000, FA Davis.

• = **Independent;** ▲ = **Collaborative**

Risk for self-directed Violence

Kathleen L. Patusky

NANDA Definition

At risk for behaviors in which an individual demonstrates that he or she can be physically, emotionally, and/or sexually harmful to self

Risk Factors

Body language: rigid posture, clenching of fists and jaw, hyperactivity, pacing, breathlessness, threatening stances; history of violence against others (e.g., hitting someone, kicking someone, spitting at someone, scratching someone, throwing objects at someone, biting someone, attempted rape, rape, sexual molestation, urinating/defecating on someone); history of threats of violence (e.g., verbal threats against property, verbal threats against person, social threats, cursing, threatening notes/letters, threatening gestures, sexual threats); history of violent antisocial behavior (e.g., stealing, insistent borrowing, insistent demanding of privileges, insistent interrupting of meetings, refusing to eat, refusing to take medication, ignoring instructions); history of violence, indirect (e.g., tearing off clothes, ripping objects off walls, writing on walls, urinating on floor, defecating on floor, stamping feet, displaying temper tantrum, running in corridors, yelling, throwing objects, breaking a window, slamming doors, making sexual advances); neurological impairment (e.g., positive EEG, CAT, or MRI; head trauma; positive neurological findings; seizure disorders); cognitive impairment (e.g., learning disabilities, attention deficit disorder, decreased intellectual functioning); history of childhood abuse; history of witnessing family violence; cruelty to animals; fire setting; prenatal/perinatal complications or abnormalities; history of drug or alcohol abuse; pathological intoxication; psychotic symptomatology (e.g., auditory, visual, command hallucinations; paranoid delusions; loose, rambling, or illogical thought processes); motor vehicle offenses (e.g., frequent traffic violations, use of a motor vehicle to release anger); suicidal behavior; impulsivity; availability/possession of weapon(s)

NOC Outcomes (Nursing Outcomes Classification)

Suggested NOC Outcomes

Depression Self-Control; Distorted Thought Self-Control; Impulse Self-Control; Loneliness Severity; Mood Equilibrium; Risk Detection; Self-Mutilation Restraint; Suicide Self-Restraint

> **Example NOC Outcome with Indicators**
>
> **Suicide Self-Restraint** as evidenced by the following indicators: Expresses feelings and seeks help when feeling self-destructive/Verbalizes and controls suicidal ideas and impulses (Rate each indicator of **Suicide Self-Restraint:** 1 = never demonstrated, 2 = rarely demonstrated, 3 = sometimes demonstrated, 4 = often demonstrated, 5 = consistently demonstrated [see Section I].)

• = Independent; ▲ = Collaborative

Client Outcomes

Client Will (Specify Time Frame):

- Refrain from self-injury
- State appropriate ways to cope with increased psychological or physiological tension
- Talk about feelings; express anger appropriately
- Seek help when feeling self-destructive or having urges to self-mutilate
- Maintain self-control without supervision
- Use appropriate community agencies when caregivers are unable to attend to emotional needs
- Maintain connectedness in relationships
- Express decreased anxiety and control of impulses
- Refrain from using mood-altering substances
- Obtain no access to harmful objects
- Yield access to harmful objects
- Maintain self-control without supervision

NIC Interventions (Nursing Interventions Classification)

Suggested NIC Interventions

Anger Control Assistance; Anxiety Reduction; Behavior Management: Self-Harm; Calming Technique; Coping Enhancement; Crisis Intervention; Mood Management; Substance Use Prevention; Suicide Prevention; Surveillance

---

Example NIC Activities—Suicide Prevention

Determine presence and degree of suicide risk; Encourage client to seek out care providers to talk as urge to harm self occurs

---

Nursing Interventions and Rationales

- Refer to care plan for **Risk for Suicide.**
- Refer to care plans for **Self-mutilation** and **Risk for Self-mutilation.**

Impaired Walking

Brenda Emick-Herring

NANDA Definition

Limitation of independent movement within the environment on foot (or artificial limb)

Defining Characteristics

Impaired ability to climb stairs; walk on uneven surface; walk required distances; walk on even surfaces; walk on an incline or decline; navigate curbs

Related Factors (r/t)

Intolerance to activity; decreased strength and endurance; pain or discomfort; perceptual or cognitive impairment; neuromuscular impairment; musculoskeletal impairment; depression; severe anxiety; lower extremity amputation

- **= Independent; ▲ = Collaborative**

NOTE: These are the same as the etiologies for **Impaired physical Mobility** with the addition of lower extremity amputation.

Suggested functional level classifications follow:

0—Completely independent

1—Requires use of equipment or device

2—Requires help from another person for assistance, supervision, or teaching

3—Requires help from another person and equipment device

4—Dependent (does not participate in activity)

NOC   Outcomes (Nursing Outcomes Classification)

Suggested NOC Outcomes

Ambulation; Mobility

> ### Example NOC Outcome with Indicators
>
> **Ambulation** as evidenced by the following indicators: Walks with effective gait/Walks at moderate pace/Walks up and down steps/Walks moderate distance (Rate each indicator of **Ambulation:** 1 = dependent [does not participate], 2 = requires assistive person and device, 3 = requires assistive person, 4 = independent with assistive device, 5 = completely independent [see Section I].)

Client Outcomes/Goals

Client Will (Specify Time Frame):

- Demonstrate optimal independence and safety in walking
- Demonstrate the ability to direct others on how to assist with walking
- Demonstrate the ability to properly and safely use and care for assistive walking devices

NIC   Interventions (Nursing Interventions Classification)

Suggested NIC Intervention

Exercise Therapy: Ambulation

> ### Example NIC Activities—Exercise Therapy: Ambulation
>
> Assist client to use footwear that facilitates walking and prevents injury; Encourage client to sit in bed, on side of bed ("dangle"), or in chair, as tolerated

Nursing Interventions and Rationales

▲ Reinforce or request physical therapy consult to teach "bridging"; have client use the technique to move side to side in bed and to raise buttocks off bed. *This bed activity prepares a person for walking because it involves hip extension with simultaneous weight bearing through the lower extremity. It is particularly helpful for hemiplegics (Bobath, 1978; Gee and Passarella, 1985).*

▲ Apply antiembolic stockings, leg bandage wraps, and abdominal binders; elevate the head of the bed in small increments to as high a degree as tolerated; and change positions slowly and provide adequate hydration to persons who are at risk for or who initially display postural hypotension when standing, sitting, and walking. Assess by

• = Independent; ▲ = Collaborative

comparing lying, sitting, and standing blood pressure changes. If there is a blood pressure discrepancy (lower in upright positions) or symptoms occur, consult the physician for medication review. *These measures promote circulatory redistribution to prevent blood volume from pooling in the lower extremities. Adjustment of medications including antihypertensives, vasodilators, diuretics, and neuroleptics may improve postural hypotension (Halm, 2001).*

▲ Remind clients of physician orders regarding weight-bearing limitations during walking (e.g., "non–weight bearing on left foot" or "partial weight bearing on right wrist"). *Weight bearing may retard bone healing in fractured extremities.*

• Explain meaning and goals of progressive mobilization (gradual elevation of head of bed, tilt table, reclined chair sitting, etc.) to the client who has been on prolonged bedrest and who has poor cardiovascular functioning. *These measures help the client adapt to upright position changes. The tilt table incrementally allows passive standing in physical therapy. It provides relief of pressure, stimulates postural reflexes, and promotes chest expansion and cardiovascular, bowel, and bladder functioning. Cardiopulmonary assessment is critical while the client is on the tilt table (Hoeman, 2002).*

• Implement the following interventions as the client resumes weight-bearing activities after prolonged bedrest: adequate protein intake, analgesics other than nonsteroidal anti-inflammatory drugs (NSAIDs) for about 1 week, avoidance of infections, and client education that depression may result from fatigue and short-term muscle soreness. *Protein is needed for muscle repair and growth. Use of NSAIDs may disturb macrophage activity (removal of injured myofibers) and therefore delay muscle recovery. Soreness results from the inflammatory response (release of prostaglandins and kinins) that occurs with muscle damage (St. Pierre and Flaskerud, 1995).* **Nursing Research:** *Animal studies indicated that muscle fiber damage occurred with non–weight bearing. On the second day of recovery, two types of macrophages increased, around day 4 myofiber formation began, and by day 7 myofibers had returned to normal size (St. Pierre and Tidball, 1994).*

• Encourage frequent weight bearing and walking in persons who have no physician restrictions. *Weight bearing and skeletal muscle contraction stimulate bone growth and calcium resorption, thus helping to maintain bone density; prevent disuse osteoporosis; increase oxygen-carrying capacity; and regulate many physiological processes in the body (Sims and Olson, 2002; International Food Information Council Foundation, 2002).* **Clinical Research:** *The risk of hip fracture was reduced by 20% to 40% in older persons who were physically active versus those who were sedentary (Gregg, Pereira, and Casperson, 2000).*

• Assist clients to properly apply orthoses, immobilizers, splints, and braces before walking. *These devices maintain joint stability, immobilization, and alignment during movement, especially when the wearer is upright (e.g., an ankle foot orthosis maintains the ankle in neutral alignment to prevent ankle twisting, foot drop, and potential falls (Hoeman, 2002).*

• Assist clients with lower extremity amputations to correctly don a lower extremity sheath, stump socks, liner, and prosthesis before walking. *Prostheses increase a client's functional ability to walk, and they cosmetically look similar to lost lower limbs. A thin nylon sheath is often applied over the residual limb to prevent it from turning in the socket of the prosthesis. Stump socks of varying thickness are used to establish a proper fit between the residual limb and the socket of the prosthesis. A liner is put on last before putting the stump into the socket of the prosthesis. The stump should not touch the bottom of the socket because a pressure ulcer may form (Kipnis 1993; Yeltzer, 1998).*

• = **Independent;** ▲ = **Collaborative**

- Collect a baseline pulse rate and rhythm before walking the client, and then check the pulse 5 minutes after walking. *Pulse monitoring indicates cardiac tolerance to walking. If an abnormal pulse occurs, stop walking and let the client sit and rest about 5 minutes before taking the pulse again. If the pulse is still abnormal, walking may need to be done more slowly, with more help, or for a shorter period. If the pulse rises too high after a few walking trials, it is probably too difficult a task, and the physician should be notified (Radwanski and Hoeman, 1996).*
- ▲ Monitor the client's tolerance for walking by assessing his or her physical status. Initiate a 5-minute rest period if any of the following are noted: shortness of breath, use of accessory muscles to breathe, chest pain, nausea, cold sweat, pale or flushed skin, dizziness, syncope, diaphoresis, or mental confusion. If signs persist, notify the physician. *For more information on assessing vital sign changes with activity, refer to the care plan for* **Activity intolerance.**
- Use appropriate assistive devices when walking the client, including gait (walking) belts, walkers, crutches, wheelchairs, and canes. *Snug gait belts may help prevent staff back injuries and provide a surface for nurses to grasp to steady a client who begins to fall or lose balance (therapists call this "guarding"). The gait belt and client should remain close to the staff member. Walking devices help compensate for poor balance, coordination, and strength and provide stability and support (Minor and Minor, 1999).* **Nursing Research:** *Use of a belt decreased staff exertion, back stress, and compressive force from L5 to S1 of the spine (Owen and Garg, 1993).*
- Obtain the appropriate number of assistants to help walk the client. One team member should give simple instructions to the client and assistants (e.g., verbally cue the client to raise the head, straighten the trunk, or lift a foot higher, for example; or cue the assistant to help the client lean a certain direction or stabilize a knee while stepping). *Having one spokesperson give directions prevents confusion and mixed messages. Walking takes concentration and thinking, especially if the client is learning to use an assistive device for the first time (Minor and Minor, 1999). Ingvor and Philipson (1977) and Yonekura (1981) found that blood flow increased about 20% when a participant was thinking. Adequate helpers are needed to prevent client falls and injury and to relieve client fear and anxiety. Fear, anxiety, and fatigue can cause hypertonicity (Gee and Passarella, 1985).*
- ▲ Ask the physical therapist where to stand in relation to client as the client walks. Assistants commonly stand slightly behind and to the side of the client, holding on to his or her gait belt with one supinated hand. The assistant's other hand then can rest lightly on the client's closest shoulder. *The assistant needs to be nearby and ready to assist in case the client begins to fall but should not stand so close that the assistant interferes with the client's movements. The forearms have more strength when supinated (Minor and Minor, 1999).*
- Limit distractions and environmental clutter while the client walks. Staff should monitor the environment for safety because the client needs to concentrate on walking and often looks at where his or her feet are and where the assistive device is while stepping. *Active attending, thinking, and visualization give the client necessary input about where the feet and assistive device are in relation to the body (Minor and Minor, 1999).*
- Allow distractions and obstacles as the client's balance, gait, coordination, endurance, and concentration improve. *This prepares clients for walking in real-life situations.*
- Indicate on the care plan how many assistants it takes to walk the client, the level of assistance needed (e.g., maximum, moderate, or minimal assistance or standby as-

- = Independent; ▲ = Collaborative

sistance), the type of assistance needed (e.g., physical support, instructional cues [verbal and/or tactile], balance control, actual lifting), and the specific assistive devices needed to walk. *Clear communication establishes a consistent approach to client care and motor relearning. Consistent practice (repetition and rehearsal) of the motor task promotes learning.*

• Perform initial screening and subsequent assessments to detect hospitalized clients at high risk for falls. If high risk is present, develop focused interventions to prevent falls and overuse of restraints. **Nursing Research:** *Many falls occurred in client rooms while the client was trying to get to the bathroom; use of bed side rails and restraints did not prevent falls; and a recent history of falls, depression, altered elimination patterns (frequency, nocturia, or incontinence), dizziness/vertigo, a primary diagnosis of cancer, confusion, and altered mobility (lower extremity weakness or decreased mobility) were factors that placed clients at high risk for falls either at admission or as their health status changed (Hendrich et al, 1995).*

Geriatric

• Monitor pulse, respirations, and blood pressure before and 5 minutes after beginning a new activity. Stop activity if any of the following are detected: resting heart rate >100 beats/min, exercise heart rate that is 35% greater than the resting rate, exercise systolic blood pressure >25 to 35 mm Hg above resting pressure, or a decrease in systolic blood pressure that is >20 mm Hg (Radwanski and Hoeman, 1996). *Realize and teach the benefits of walking to clients, and be patient when walking them, because they have a slow gait pattern. Muscle strength in the hip extensors, abductors, and plantar flexors decreases as a normal part of aging. Knee flexion contractures are not uncommon. Declining visual acuity and balance, foot pain, and fear of falling may also slow walking speed (Jones, 2001; Sims and Olson, 2002).*

• Recognize that the use of a walking aid increases energy and therefore may raise pulse and blood pressure; however, they are often prescribed to give stability and support to clients with lower extremity weakness, poor balance, or weight-bearing restrictions (Jones, 2001). **Clinical Research:** *Elderly subjects with peripheral neuropathy had less risk of losing their balance standing on an unstable (suddenly tilting) surface in normal light and low-light conditions when using a cane in the nondominant hand than control subjects with no aid (Ashton-Miller et al, 1996). A literature review found that wheeled walkers were preferred over standard walkers by clients and "...were associated with faster speeds and cadences, lower energy demands and a more normal appearing gait" (Bohannon, 1997, p 1185).*

• For elderly clients use safety and fall precautions such as the following: visual identification (arm bands, etc.), especially in clients at high risk of falling; a call system within reach; client education to call for help before standing and walking; a bed/chair alarm or one-to-one observation, especially for clients with cognitive or memory impairment; obstacle clearance; and assistive devices that are properly chosen and measured specifically for client. *Assessment and preventative implementation of safety measures are appropriate for elderly clients because many experience impaired balance and unsteadiness when changing positions or walking. Postural control disturbances occur with aging, chronic disease, visual function changes, and medications, all of which place clients at risk for falls (Alexander, 1994; Ulfarsson and Robinson, 1997).* **Clinical Research:** *Elderly residents who went to the emergency department after a fall were placed in an intervention group in which education about fall prevention, safety at home, and ideas for modification and*

• = Independent; ▲ = Collaborative

equipment were compared with a control group. The intervention group had significantly fewer falls and recurrent falls the next year than did the control group (Close et al, 1999). Two factors, lower limb weakness and poor tandem walk ability, were predictive for elderly hospitalized clients who fell; these two tests could potentially be used to screen those at risk for falls (Chu et al, 1999).

- If the client experiences dizziness resulting from orthostatic hypotension when arising, teach methods to decrease dizziness such as rising slowly, remaining seated several minutes before standing, flexing feet upward several times while sitting, sitting immediately if feeling dizzy, and trying to have someone present when standing. *The elderly develop arterial stiffness and reduced autonomic nervous system functioning; therefore their baroreceptors respond more slowly and have less ability to maintain blood pressure when standing. This results in postural hypotension (Fluckiger et al, 1999).*

- Emphasize the importance of wearing firm, low-heeled shoes with nonskid and non-friction soles and seeking medical care for foot pain and problems. **Clinical Research:** *Elderly women had more foot problems than men. Persons with foot pain did worse with leaning, stair climbing/descent, alternate step up, and timed 6-meter walk testing. Medical treatment and preventative foot care could potentially improve pain and function (Menz and Lord, 2001).*

Home care

- Assess the client and obtain a complete history with reference to reasons for impairment. *Complete understanding of the client problem promotes accurate determination of client needs and individualized care.*

- Explain the importance of having adequate lighting both day and night; tacking carpet edges down, removing throw rugs from traffic flow areas, and having nonskid backings on those that are used; applying nonskid wax on floors; and removing clutter, especially small objects, from the floor. *Removal of potential environmental hazards is a means of preventing falls in the elderly (Ulfarsson and Robinson, 1997).*

- Assess the home environment for all barriers to walking.

- If the client lives alone, assess his or her support system for emergency and contingency care (e.g., Lifeline). *Impaired walking mobility may pose a life threat during a crisis (e.g., falls, fire).* **Clinical Research:** *There was a positive association of two variables—living alone and high mastery (belief in self)—with walking, even if clients had physical difficulty. Negative factors for walking included old age, black race, fatigue, obesity, and use of a cane (Simonsick, Guralnik, and Fried, 1999).*

- Use safety devices such as a gait belt when assisting the client in ambulation. *Client safety is a primary goal in home care.*

- ▲ Refer to physical and occupational therapists for skills building, strength building, options for restructuring the environment, and present alternative mobility options. *Referral to specialty services may be a key component of the nursing care plan. A multidisciplinary approach supports total needs assessment and planning (Sloan, Haslam, and Foret, 2001).*

- ▲ Refer to home health aide services as appropriate for assistance with activities of daily living. *Mobility impairments may serve as a barrier to self-care.*

- ▲ Provide support to the client and caregivers during long-term impairment. Refer to case manager/medical social services or mental health/support group services as necessary. *Long-term impairment may necessitate role changes and create anger and frustra-*

• = **Independent;** ▲ = **Collaborative**

tion. Counseling and support groups provide validation of feelings and alternative methods of problem solving.

▲ Ensure that the client has information on advocacy, options for disability access, and related issues (e.g., education, personnel, equipment availability) under the Americans with Disabilities Act. *The more informed a person is, the more potential he or she has for being independent (Minor and Minor, 1999).*

● Introduce and reinforce positive perceptions of old age. *A study of older adults exposed to a protocol of positive and negative stereotypes of aging found that significant improvements in walking gait were associated with positive images; no change was seen with the negative stereotypes (Hausdorff, Levy, and Wei, 1999).*

▲ Provide support to the client and caregivers during long-term impairment. Refer to case manager/medical social services or mental health/support group services as necessary. *Long-term impairment may necessitate role changes and create anger and frustration. Counseling and support groups provide validation of feelings and alternative methods of problem solving.*

Client/Family Teaching

● Recommend that the client and family check assistive devices to keep them in safe working order. *Replace rubber tips if worn and remove dirt in grooves of walkers, crutches, and canes, otherwise they will not grip the floor. Check push button locks on walkers with telescoping legs (Minor and Minor, 1999). Inspect and repair prostheses for cracks, rough spots inside the socket, and odd noises or movement at the joints or foot (Yeltzer, 1998).*

● Recommend daily weight-bearing activity and walking, calcium and vitamin D supplementation if dietary intake is low, and avoidance of smoking to prevent osteoporosis and related fractures. Assess for and strongly encourage client *not* to substitute beverages with caffeine (including cola) and alcohol for milk at meal time. Estrogen-replacement therapy may be helpful; therefore the client may need to consult with a physician (Franzen-Korzendorfer, 2002). **Clinical Research:** *Fifty of 52 studies concluded that high calcium intake increased accumulation of bone, promoted bone mass during growth, prevented bone loss in elderly persons, and lessened risk of fractures (Heaney, 2000).*

evolve WEBSITES FOR EDUCATION

See the EVOLVE website for World Wide Web resources for client education.

REFERENCES

Alexander NB: Postural control in older adults, *J Am Geriatr Soc* 42(1):93, 1994.

Ashton-Miller JA et al: A cane reduces loss of balance in patients with peripheral neuropathy: results from a challenging unipedal balance test, *Arch Phys Med Rehabil* 77:446, 1996.

Bobath B: *Adult hemiplegia: evaluation and treatment,* London, 1978, William Heinemann.

Bohannon RW: Gait performance with wheeled and standard walkers, *Percept Mot Skills* 85:1185, 1997.

Chu L-W et al: Risk factors for falls in hospitalized older medical patients, *J Gerontol* 54(1):M38, 1999.

Close J et al: Prevention of falls in the elderly trial (PROFET): a randomised controlled trial, *Lancet* 353:93, 1999.

Fluckiger L et al: Differential effects of aging on heart rate variability and blood pressure variability, *J Gerontol* 54A(5):B219, 1999.

Franzen-Korzendorfer H: The silent disease, *Rehabil Manage* 15(8):30, 2002.

● = **Independent;** ▲ = **Collaborative**

Gee ZL, Passarella PM: *Nursing care of the stroke patient: a therapeutic approach*, Pittsburgh, 1985, AREN.

Gregg EW, Pereira MA, Casperson CJ: Physical activity, falls, and fractures among older adults: a review of the epidemiologic evidence, *J Am Geriatr Soc* 48:883, 2000.

Halm M: Altered tissue perfusion. In Maas ML et al, editors: *Nursing care of older adults: diagnosis, outcomes, & interventions*, St Louis, 2001, Mosby.

Hausdorff JM, Levy BR, Wei JY: The power of ageism on physical function of older persons: reversibility of age-related gait changes, *J Am Geriatr Soc* 47:1346, 1999.

Heaney RP: Calcium, dairy products and osteoporosis, *J Am Coll Nutr* 19:835, 2000.

Hendrich A et al: Hospital falls: development of a predictive model for clinical practice, *Appl Nurs Res* 8(3):129, 1995.

Hoeman SP: Movement, functional mobility, and activities of daily living. In Hoeman SP editor: *Rehabilitation nursing: process, application, & outcomes*, ed 3, St Louis, 2002.

Ingvor DH, Philipson L: Distribution of cerebral blood flow in the dominant hemisphere during motor ideation and motor performance, *Ann Neurol* 2:230, 1977.

International Food Information Council Foundation (IFIC): *IFIC review: physical activity, nutrition and bone health*, available on-line at *http://ific.org/healthybones*, April 2002.

Jones DA: Successful aging: maintaining mobility in a geriatric patient population, *Rehabil Manage* 14(9):46, 2001.

Kipnis ND: Musculoskeletal/orthopedic disorders. In McCourt A, editor: *The specialty practice of rehabilitation nursing: a core curriculum*, ed 3, Skokie, Ill, 1993, Rehabilitation Foundation.

Menz HB, Lord SR: Foot pain impairs balance and functional ability in community-dwelling older people, *J Am Podiatr Med Assoc* 91(5):222, 2001.

Minor MAD, Minor SD: *Patient care skills*, ed 4, Stamford, Conn, 1999, Appleton & Lange.

Owen BD, Garg A: Back stress isn't part of the job, *Am J Nurs* 93(2):48, 1993.

Radwanski MB, Hoeman SP: Geriatric rehabilitation nursing. In Hoeman SP, editor: *Rehabilitation nursing: process and application*, ed 2, St Louis, 1996, Mosby.

Simonsick EM, Guralnik JM, Fried LP: Who walks? Factors associated with walking behavior in disabled older women with and without self-reported walking difficulty, *J Am Geriatr Soc* 47(6):672, 1999.

Sims GL, Olson RS: Muscle and skeletal function. In Hoeman SP, editor, *Rehabilitation nursing: process, application, & outcomes*, ed 3, St Louis, 2002, Mosby.

Sloan HL, Haslam K, Foret CM: Teaching the use of walkers and canes, *Home Healthc Nurs* 19:241, 2001.

St. Pierre BA, Flaskerud JH: Clinical nursing implications for the recovery of atrophied skeletal muscle following bed rest, *Rehabil Nurs* 20(6):314, 1995.

St. Pierre BA, Tidball JG: Differential response of macrophage subpopulations to soleus muscle reloading after rat hindlimb suspension, *J Appl Physiol* 77:290, 1994.

Ulfarsson J, Robinson BE: Falls and falling. In Ham RJ, Sloane PD, editors: *Primary care geriatrics: a case-based approach*, ed 3, St Louis, 1997, Mosby.

Yeltzer EA: Care of the client with an amputation. In Chin PA, Finocchiaro D, Rosebrough A, editors: *Rehabilitation nursing practice*, New York, 1998, McGraw-Hill.

Yonekura M: Evaluation of cerebral blood flow in patients with transient attacks and minor strokes, *J Neurosurg* 15:58, 1981.

Wandering

Donna Algase

NANDA Definition

Meandering; aimless or repetitive locomotion that exposes the individual to harm; frequently incongruent with boundaries, limits, or obstacles

Defining Characteristics

Frequent or continuous movement from place to place, often revisiting the same destinations; persistent locomotion in search of "missing" or unattainable people or places;

• = Independent; ▲ = Collaborative

haphazard locomotion; locomotion in unauthorized or private spaces; locomotion resulting in unintended leaving of a premise; long periods of locomotion without an apparent destination; fretful locomotion or pacing; inability to locate significant landmarks in a familiar setting; locomotion that cannot be easily dissuaded or redirected; following behind or shadowing a caregiver's locomotion; trespassing; hyperactivity; scanning, seeking, or searching behaviors; periods of locomotion interspersed with periods of nonlocomotion (e.g., sitting, standing, sleeping); getting lost

Related Factors (r/t)

Cognitive impairment, specifically memory and recall deficits, disorientation, poor visuoconstructive (or visuospatial) ability, and language (primarily expressive) defects; cortical atrophy; premorbid behavior (e.g., outgoing, sociable personality); premorbid dementia; separation from familiar people and places; sedation; emotional state, especially frustration, anxiety, boredom, or depression (agitation); overstimulating/understimulating social or physical environment; physiological state or need (e.g., hunger/thirst, pain, urination, constipation); time of day

NOC Outcomes (Nursing Outcomes Classification)

Suggested NOC Outcomes

Caregiver Home Care Readiness; Fall Prevention Behavior; Falls Occurrence

---

Example NOC Outcome with Indicators

Caregiver Home Care Readiness as evidenced by the following indicators: Knowledge of recommended treatment regimen/Knowledge of prescribed activity/Knowledge of emergency care/Confidence in ability to manage care at home (Rate each indicator of **Caregiver Home Care Readiness:** 1 = none, 2 = limited, 3 = moderate, 4 = substantial, 5 = extensive [see Section I].)

Client Outcomes

Client Will (Specify Time Frame):
- Decrease incidence of falls (preferably free of falls)
- Decrease incidence of elopements
- Maintain appropriate body weight

Caregiver Will (Specify Time Frame):
- Be able to explain interventions he or she can use to provide a safe environment for a care receiver who displays wandering behavior

NIC Interventions (Nursing Interventions Classification)

Suggested NIC Intervention

Dementia Management

Example NIC Activities—Dementia Management

Place identification bracelet on the client; Provide space for safe pacing and wandering

---

• = Independent; ▲ = Collaborative

Nursing Interventions and Rationales

- Assess and document the amount (frequency and duration), pattern (random, lapping, or pacing), and 24-hour distribution of wandering behavior over a 3-day interval. **Nursing Research:** *Assessment over time provides a baseline against which behavior change can be evaluated (Algase et al, 1997). Such assessment can also reveal the time of day when wandering is greatest and when surveillance or other precautionary measures are most necessary.*

- Document particular aspects of wandering that are troubling. **Nursing Research:** *Instruments such as the Algase Wandering Scale (Algase et al, 2001) can indicate whether the behavior is persistent, spatially disordered, or prone to elopement. Such information can direct caregivers toward more appropriate intervention strategies.*

- Obtain a history of personality characteristics and behavioral responses to stress. **Nursing and Clinical Research:** *Information about long-standing behavioral tendencies may reveal circumstances under which wandering will occur and can aid in interpreting both positive and negative meanings of wandering behavior of the client (Kolanowski, Strand, and Whall, 1997; Monsour and Robb, 1982; Thomas, 1997).*

- Evaluate for neurocognitive strengths and limitations, particularly language, attention, visuospatial skills, and perseveration. **Nursing Research:** *Wanderers may have expressive language deficits that hamper their ability to communicate needs (Algase, 1992; Dawson and Reid, 1987).* **Nursing and Clinical Research:** *Knowledge of attentional and visuospatial deficits, which may account for certain patterns of wandering or way-finding deficits and can lead to identification of appropriate environmental modifications that could enhance functional ambulation such as elimination of distractions and enhancement of cues marking desired destinations (Chiu, 2002; Fischer, Marterer, and Danielczyk, 1990; Henderson, Mack, and Williams, 1989; Passini et al, 1995; Passini et al, 2000).* **Clinical Research:** *The presence of perseveration may indicate that the wanderer is unable to voluntarily stop his or her behavior (Passini et al, 1995; Ryan et al, 1995), thus calling for nursing judgment as to when wandering should be interrupted to enhance the wanderer's safety, comfort, or well-being.*

- Assess for physical distress or needs such as hunger, thirst, pain, discomfort, or elimination. **Nursing Research:** *Although physical needs have not been documented in relation to wandering, the Need-Driven Dementia-Compromised Model hypothesizes this relationship (Algase et al, 1996).*

- Assess for emotional or psychological distress such as anxiety, fear, or feeling lost. **Clinical Research:** *Anxiety and depression frequently accompany wandering (Teri et al, 1999).*

- Observe wandering episodes for antecedents and consequences. **Nursing and Clinical Research:** *People, events, or circumstances surrounding the onset or conclusion of wandering may provide cues about triggers or rewards that are stimulating or reinforcing wandering behavior (Heard and Watson, 1999; Hirst and Metcalf, 1989; Hussain, 1981, 1982).*

- Apply observed consequences of wandering such as personal attention, food, and so forth at times when the person is *not* wandering, and withhold them while the person is wandering. **Clinical Research:** *Differential reinforcement of other behavior (non-wandering) can reduce wandering episodes by 50% to 80% (Heard and Watson, 1999).*

- Assess regularly for the presence of or potential for negative outcomes of wandering such as weight change, declining social skills, falls, and elopement. **Clinical Research:** *Wanderers are at greater risk for falls than other cognitively impaired persons (Kippenbrock*

- **= Independent; ▲ = Collaborative**

and Soja, 1993; Morse, Tylko, and Dixon, 1987). Wanderers have also shown greater loss in social skills over time than nonwandering counterparts (Cornbleth, 1977).

- Provide for safe ambulation with comfortable and well-fitting clothes, shoes with non-skid soles and foot support, and any necessary walking aids (such as a cane, walker, or Merry-Walker). **Clinical Research:** *Falls in persons with advanced dementia are often related to a decline in vigor in persons who had been previously active (Brody et al, 1984).*

- Provide safe and secure surroundings that deter accidental elopements using perimeter control devices, camouflage, or electronic tracking systems. **Nursing Research:** *Eloping can have hazardous outcomes, including death (Rowe and Glover, 2001).* **Clinical Research:** *Perimeter control devices can effectively reduce or prevent exiting behavior (Negley, Molla, and Obenchain, 1990).* **Nursing and Clinical Research:** *However, under some circumstances, these devices are viewed as unnecessarily restrictive, and more passive means such as camouflage have been substituted. Camouflage techniques such as masking the doorknob or creating striped floor patterns in front of exits have been used with success (Hussain and Brown, 1987; Namazi, Rosner, and Calkins, 1989), particularly in subjects with Alzheimer's disease (Hewewasam, 1996), but the effectiveness may be mitigated by other architectural features of the setting (Chafetz, 1990; Hamilton, 1993). Newer electronic monitoring and tracking systems are highly effective and reduce caregiver burden (Altus et al, 2000).*

- During periods of inactivity, position the wanderer so that desirable destinations (such as the bathroom) are within the client's line of vision and undesirable destinations (such as exits or stairwells) are out of sight. **Nursing and Clinical Research:** *Functional, nonwandering ambulation is possible even into late-stage dementia and may be facilitated by keeping appropriate visual cues accessible (Algase, 1999; Martino-Saltzman et al, 1991; Passini et al, 2000).*

- If wandering takes a random or haphazard route, reduce environmental distractions and increase relevant environmental cues. Note and eliminate stimuli that distract the wanderer while in route. Provide afternoon rest periods if assessment reveals that random-pattern wandering worsens as the day progresses. **Nursing Research:** *Random-pattern wandering may be affected by environmental stimuli (Algase, 1999). The proportion of wandering that is random increases as the day progresses (Algase et al, 1997; Algase, 1999) and may indicate fatigue.*

- Enhance institutional settings with areas that provide interesting views and opportunities to sit. **Clinical Research:** *Enhanced environments can improve mood, and they encourage wanderers to linger or sit more than purely institutional surroundings do (Cohen-Mansfield and Werner, 1998).*

- Engage wanderers in social interaction and structured activity, especially when wanderers appear distressed or otherwise uncomfortable or their wandering presents a challenge to others in the setting. **Nursing and Clinical Research:** *Wandering and social interaction are inversely related. Wanderers often have an outgoing or sociable personality and also have deficits in expressive language skills. Thus while they may prefer social interaction, their ability to initiate it may be compromised (Algase, 1992; Thomas, 1997).*

- If wandering has a pacing quality, attempt to identify and address any underlying problems or concerns. Offer stress-reducing approaches such as music, massage, or rocking. Attempts to distract or redirect the pacing wanderer may worsen wandering. **Nursing Research:** *Pacing, as a wandering pattern, is not associated with level of cognitive impairment and may reflect anxiety, agitation, pain, or another internal process (Algase, Beattie, and Therrien, 2001; Gerdner, 2000; Snyder and Olson, 1996).*

- = **Independent;** ▲ = **Collaborative**

- If wandering is a new or recently acquired behavior or if it increases in intensity over previous levels, evaluate for constipation, pneumonia, or acute physical problems. **Nursing and Clinical Research:** *Persons who first exhibit wandering within 3 months after admission to a nursing home are more likely than others to have developed physical problems that stimulate wandering (Keily, Morris, and Algase, 2000).*
- If wandering has a lapping or circuitous pattern, signs or labels may be effective. Substitute another repetitive activity such as folding or rocking if lapping becomes problematic or excessive. **Nursing Research:** *Not all wanderers display lapping-pattern wandering, and when it does occur, it tends to occur early in the day or to follow rest periods. Thus it may be a more functional pattern than random wandering and may indicate a slightly better level of cognitive function for the individual, even if transient. Thus wanderers who lap may be better able to make use of information in the environment (Algase, Beattie, and Therrien, 2001).* **Clinical Research:** *However, this pattern of wandering may also be a form of perseveration, and therefore the person may be unable to disengage voluntarily (Passini et al, 1995; Ryan et al, 1995).*
- Provide a regularly scheduled and supervised exercise or walking program, particularly if wandering occurs excessively during the night or at times that are inconvenient in the setting. **Nursing and Clinical Research:** *Although exercise or walking programs do not reduce daytime wandering, they have been shown to reduce or eliminate nighttime wandering (Robb, 1987; Carillon Nursing and Rehabilitation Center, 2000) and to decrease general agitation levels (Holmberg, 1997).*
- Use slow-stroke, hand, or foot massage before the times of day or events that induce wandering. **Nursing and Clinical Research:** *Various massage techniques have been shown to reduce wandering and diffuse agitation in persons with dementia (Kilstoff and Chenoweth, 1998; Malaquin-Pavan, 1997; Rowe and Alfred, 1999; Snyder, Egan, and Burns, 1995; Sutherland Reakes, and Bridges, 1999).*

Multicultural

- Assess for the influence of cultural beliefs, norms, and values on the family's understanding of wandering behavior. **Nursing Research:** *What the family considers normal and abnormal health behavior may be based on cultural perceptions (Leininger and McFarland, 2002; Cochran, 1998; Doswell and Erlen, 1998; Guaranccia, 1998).*
- ▲ Refer the family to social services or other supportive services to assist with the impact of caregiving for the wandering client. **Nursing Research:** *African-American caregivers of dementia clients may evidence less desire than other caregivers to institutionalize their family members and are more likely to report unmet service needs (Hinrichsen and Ramirez, 1992). African-American and white families of dementia clients may report restricted social activity (Haley et al, 1995).*
- ▲ Encourage the family to use support groups or other service programs. **Nursing Research:** *Studies indicate that minority families of clients with dementia use few support programs even though these programs could have a positive impact on caregiver well-being (Cox, 1999).*
- Validate the family's feelings regarding the impact of client wandering on family lifestyle. **Nursing Research:** *Validation is a therapeutic communication technique that lets the client know that the nurse has heard and understands what was said (Heineken, 1998).*

• = Independent; ▲ = Collaborative

Home care

- Help the caregiver set up a plan to deal with wandering behavior using the interventions mentioned in Nursing Interventions and Rationales.
- Assess the home environment for modifications that will protect the client and prevent elopement. *Security devices are available to notify the caregiver of the client's movements (e.g., alarms at doors, bed alarms).*
- ▲ Enroll wanderers in the Safe Return Program of the Alzheimer's Association, and help the caregiver develop a plan of action to use if the client elopes. **Nursing Research:** *The Safe Return Program has assisted in locating numerous persons who have eloped from their homes or other residential care settings. Mortality rates are high if there is failure to locate elopers within the first 24 hours (Rowe and Glover, 2001).*
- Help the caregiver develop a plan of action to use if the client elopes.
- ▲ Institute case management of frail elderly clients to support continued independent living. *Wandering behavior represents and can lead to increasing needs for assistance in using the health care system effectively. Case management combines nursing activities of client and family assessment, planning and coordination of care among all health care providers, delivery of direct nursing care, and monitoring of care and outcomes. These activities are able to address continuity of care, mutual goal setting, behavior management, and prevention of worsening health problems (Guttman, 1999).*
- ▲ Refer for homemaker or psychiatric home health care services for respite, client reassurance, and implementation of a therapeutic regimen. Refer to the care plan for **Caregiver role strain.** *Responsibility for a person at high risk for wandering provides high caregiver stress. Respite decreases caregiver stress. The presence of caring individuals is reassuring to both the client and caregivers, especially during periods of client anxiety. Wandering behavior can make use of the interventions described above, modified for the home setting.*

Client/Family Teaching

- Inform the client and family of the meaning of and reasons for wandering behavior. An understanding of wandering behavior will enable the client and family to provide the client with a safe environment.
- Teach the caregiver/family methods to deal with wandering behavior using the interventions mentioned in Nursing Interventions and Rationales.

evolve WEBSITES FOR EDUCATION

See the EVOLVE website for World Wide Web resources for client education.

REFERENCES

Algase DL: Cognitive discriminants of wandering among nursing home residents, *Nurs Res* 41(2):78, 1992.

Algase DL: Wandering: a dementia-compromised behavior, *J Gerontol Nurs* 25(9):10, 1999.

Algase DL, Beattie ERA, Therrien B: Impact of cognitive impairment on wandering behavior, *West J Nurs Res* 23:283, 2001.

Algase DL et al: Need-driven dementia-compromised behavior: an alternative view of disruptive behavior, *Am J Alzheimers Dis* 11(6):10, 1996.

Algase DL et al: Estimates of stability of daily wandering behavior among cognitively impaired long-term care residents, *Nurs Res* 46(3):172, 1997.

• = **Independent;** ▲ = **Collaborative**

Algase DL et al: The Algase wandering scale: initial psychometrics of a new caregiver reporting tool, *Am J Alzheimers Dis Other Demen* 16(3):141, 2001.

Altus DE et al: Evaluating an electronic monitoring system for people who wander, *Am J Alzheimers Dis* 15(2): 121, 2000.

Brody E et al: Predictors of falls among institutionalized females with Alzheimer's disease, *J Am Geriatr Soc* 32: 877, 1984.

Carillon Nursing and Rehabilitation Center: Nature walk: from aimless wandering to purposeful walking, *Nurs Homes Long Term Care Manage* 49(11):50, 2000.

Chafetz PK: Two dimensional grid is ineffective against demented patients' exiting through glass doors, *Psychol Aging* 5:146, 1990.

Chiu Y: *Getting lost behavior & directed attention impairments in Taiwanese patients with early Alzheimer's disease*, Ann Arbor, 2002, University of Michigan (doctoral dissertation).

Cochran M: Tears have no color, *Am J Nurs* 98(6):53, 1998.

Cohen-Mansfield J, Werner P: The effects of an enhanced environment on nursing home residents who pace, *Geronotologist* 38(2):199, 1998.

Cornbleth T: Effects of a protected hospital ward area on wandering and non-wandering geriatric patients, *J Gerontol* 32:573, 1977.

Cox C: Race and caregiving: patterns of service use by African American and white caregivers of persons with Alzheimer's, *J Gerontol Soc Work* 32(2):5, 1999.

Dawson P, Reid DW: Behavioral dimensions of patients at risk for wandering, *Gerontologist* 27:104, 1987.

Doswell W, Erlen J: Multicultural issues and ethical concerns in the delivery of revising care interventions, *Nurs Clin North Am* 33(2):353, 1998.

Fischer P, Marterer A, Danielczyk W: Right-left disorientation in dementia of the Alzheimer's type, *Neurology* 40:1619, 1990.

Gerdner LA: Effects of individualized versus classical "relaxation" music on the frequency of agitation in elderly persons with Alzheimer's disease and related disorders, *Int Psychogeriatr* 12(1):49, 2000.

Guarnaccia P: Multicultural experiences of family caregiving: a study of African American, European American, and Hispanic American families, *New Direct Ment Health Serv* 77:45, 1998.

Guttman R: Case management of the frail elderly in the community, *Clin Nurs Spec* 13(4):174, 1999.

Haley WE et al: Psychological, social, and health impact of caregiving: a comparison of black and white dementia family caregivers and noncaregivers, *Psychol Aging* 10(4):540, 1995.

Hamilton C: *The use of tape patterns as an alternative method for controlling wanderers' exiting behavior in a dementia care unit*, Blacksburg, Va, 1993, Virginia Polytechnic Institute and State University (unpublished master's thesis).

Heard K, Watson TS: Reducing wandering by persons with dementia using differential reinforcement, *J Appl Behav Anal* 32(9):381, 1999.

Heineken J: Patient silence is not necessarily client satisfaction: communication in home care nursing, *Home Healthc Nurse* 16(2):115, 1998.

Henderson V, Mack W, Williams BW: Spatial disorientation in Alzheimer's disease, *Arch Neurol* 46:391, 1989.

Hewewasam L: Floor patterns limit wandering of people with Alzheimer's, *Nurs Times* 92:41, 1996.

Hinrichsen GA, Ramirez M: Black and white dementia caregivers: a comparison of their adaptation, *Gerontologist* 32(3):375, 1992.

Hirst ST, Metcalf BJ: Whys and whats of wandering, *Geriatr Nurs Am J Care Aging* 10(5):237, 1989.

Holmberg SK: Evaluation of a clinical intervention for wanderers on a geriatric nursing unit, *Arch Psychiatr Nurs* 11:21, 1997.

Hussain RA: Psychotherapeutic intervention: organic mental disorders. In *Geriatric psychology: a behavioral perspective*, New York, 1981, Van Nostrand Reinhold.

Hussain RA: Stimulus control in the modification of problematic behavior in elderly institutionalized patients, *Int J Behav Geriatr* 1:33, 1982.

Hussain RA, Brown DC: Use of two dimensional grid patterns to limit hazardous ambulation in demented patients, *J Gerontol* 42:558, 1987.

Keily DK, Morris JN, Algase DL: Resident characteristics associated with wandering in nursing homes, *Int J Geriatr Psychiatry* 15:1013, 2000.

Kilstoff K, Chenoweth L: New approaches to health and well-being for dementia day-care clients, family carers and day care staff, *Int J Nurs Pract* 4(2):72, 1998.

Kippenbrock T, Soja M: Preventing falls in the elderly: interviewing patients who have fallen, *Geriatr Nurs* 14: 205, 1993.

• = **Independent;** ▲ = **Collaborative**

Kolanowski AM, Strand G, Whall A: A pilot study of the relation in premorbid characteristics to behavior in dementia, *J Gerontol Nurs* 23:21, 1997.

Leininger MM, McFarland MR: *Transcultural nursing: concepts, theories, research and practices,* ed 3, New York, 2002, McGraw-Hill.

Malaquin-Pavan E: Therapeutic benefit of touch-massage in the overall management of demented elderly, *Recherche en Soins Infirmiers* 49:11, 1997 (in French).

Martino-Saltzman D et al: Travel behavior of nursing home residents perceived as wanderers and nonwanderers, *Gerontologist* 31:666, 1991.

Monsour N, Robb S: Wandering behavior in old age: a psychosocial study, *Soc Work* 27:411, 1982.

Morse J, Tylko S, Dixon H: Characteristics of the fall-prone patient, *Gerontologist* 27:516, 1987.

Namazi KH, Rosner TT, Calkins MP: Visual barriers to prevent ambulatory Alzheimer's patients from exiting through an emergency door, *Gerontologist* 29:699, 1989.

Negley E, Molla PM, Obenchain J: No exit: the effects of an electronic security system on confused patients, *J Gerontol Nurs* 16:21, 1990.

Passini R et al: Wayfinding in dementia of the Alzheimer's type: planning abilities, *J Clin Exp Neuropsychol* 17: 820, 1995.

Passini R et al: Wayfinding in a nursing home for advanced dementia of the Alzheimer's type, *Environ Behav* 32(5):684, 2000.

Robb SS: Exercise treatment for wandering. In Altman HJ, editor: *Alzheimer's disease: problems, prospects, and perspectives,* New York, 1987, Plenum.

Rowe M, Alfred D: The effectiveness of slow stroke massage in diffusing agitated behaviors in individuals with Alzheimer's disease, *J Gerontol Nurs* 25(6):22, 1999.

Rowe MA, Glover JC: Antecedents, descriptions and consequences of wandering in cognitively-impaired adults and the Safe Return (SR) program, *Am J Alzheimers Dis* 16(6):344, 2001.

Ryan JP et al: Graphomotor perseveration and wandering in Alzheimer's disease, *J Geriatr Psychiatry Neurol* 8:209, 1995.

Snyder M, Egan E, Burns K: Interventions for decreasing agitation behaviors in persons with dementia, *J Gerontol Nurs* 21(7):34, 1995.

Snyder M, Olson J: Music and hand massage interventions to produce relaxation and reduce aggressive behaviors in cognitively impaired elders: a pilot study, *Clin Gerontol* 17(1):64, 1996.

Sutherland JA, Reakes J, Bridges C: Foot acupressure and massage for patients with Alzheimer's disease and related dementias, *J Nurs Sch* 31(4):34, 1999.

Teri L et al: Anxiety of Alzheimer's disease: prevalence and comorbidity, *J Gerontol A Biol Sci Med Sci* 54(7): M348, 1999.

Thomas DW: Understanding the wandering patient: a continuity of personality perspective, *J Gerontol Nurs* 23(1):16, 1997.

• = **Independent;** ▲ = **Collaborative**

Appendix A

Nursing Diagnoses Arranged by Maslow's Hierarchy of Needs

Because human beings adapt in many ways to establish and maintain the self, health problems are much more than simple physical matters. Maslow's Hierarchy of Needs (see diagram below) is a system of classifying human needs. Maslow's hierarchy is based on the idea that lower level physiological needs must be met before higher level, abstract needs can be met.

For nurses, Maslow's hierarchy has special significance in decision making and planning for care. By considering need categories as you identify client problems, you will be able to provide more holistic care. For example, a client who demands frequent attention for a seemingly trivial matter may require help with self-esteem needs. Need levels vary from client to client. If a client is short of breath, the client is probably not interested in or capable of discussing spirituality. In addition, a client's need level may change throughout planning and intervention, so you will need to be vigilant in your assessment.

Read the descriptions of each category in the diagram, and see how you would relate them to nursing diagnoses. Compare your evaluation with how the authors categorized the nursing diagnoses according to this hierarchy. Be sure to assess clients for potential problems at all levels of the pyramid, regardless of their initial complaint.

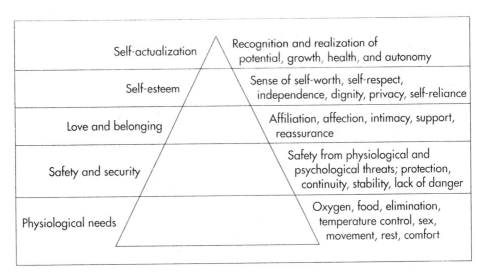

Self-actualization	Recognition and realization of potential, growth, health, and autonomy
Self-esteem	Sense of self-worth, self-respect, independence, dignity, privacy, self-reliance
Love and belonging	Affiliation, affection, intimacy, support, reassurance
Safety and security	Safety from physiological and psychological threats; protection, continuity, stability, lack of danger
Physiological needs	Oxygen, food, elimination, temperature control, sex, movement, rest, comfort

Physiological Needs

Activity intolerance
Activity intolerance, risk for
Airway clearance, ineffective
Aspiration, risk for
Body temperature, risk for imbalanced
Bowel incontinence
Breastfeeding, effective
Breastfeeding, ineffective
Breastfeeding, interrupted
Breathing pattern, ineffective
Cardiac output, decreased
Comfort, impaired
Confusion, acute
Confusion, chronic
Constipation
Constipation, perceived
Constipation, risk for
Dentition, impaired
Diarrhea
Environmental interpretation syndrome,
   impaired
Fatigue
Fluid balance, readiness for enhanced
Fluid volume, deficient
Fluid volume, excess
Fluid volume, risk for deficient
Fluid volume, risk for imbalanced
Gas exchange, impaired
Hyperthermia
Hypothermia
Incontinence, functional urinary
Incontinence, reflex urinary
Incontinence, stress urinary
Incontinence, total urinary
Incontinence, urge urinary
Incontinence, risk for urge urinary
Infant behavior, disorganized
Infant behavior, risk for disorganized
Infant behavior, readiness for enhanced
   organized
Infant feeding pattern, ineffective
Intracranial adaptive capacity, decreased
Memory, impaired
Mobility, impaired bed
Mobility, impaired physical
Mobility, impaired wheelchair
Nausea
Nutrition, readiness for enhanced
Nutrition, imbalanced: less than body
   requirements

Nutrition, imbalanced: more than body
   requirements
Nutrition, imbalanced: risk for more than
   body requirements
Oral mucous membrane, impaired
Pain, acute
Pain, chronic
Protection, ineffective
Self-care deficit, bathing/hygiene
Self-care deficit, dressing/grooming
Self-care deficit, feeding
Self-care deficit, toileting
Sensory perception, disturbed (specify):
   visual, auditory, kinesthetic, gustatory,
   tactile, olfactory
Sexual dysfunction
Sexuality patterns, ineffective
Skin integrity, impaired
Skin integrity, risk for impaired
Sleep deprivation
Sleep pattern, disturbed
Sleep, readiness for enhanced
Surgical recovery, delayed
Swallowing, impaired
Thermoregulation, ineffective
Thought processes, disturbed
Tissue integrity, impaired
Tissue perfusion, ineffective (specify type):
   cerebral, renal, cardiopulmonary, gas-
   trointestinal, peripheral
Transfer ability, impaired
Urinary elimination, readiness for
   enhanced
Urinary elimination, impaired
Urinary retention
Ventilation, impaired spontaneous
Ventilatory weaning response,
   dysfunctional
Walking, impaired

Safety and Security Needs

Allergy response, latex
Allergy response, risk for latex
Anxiety, death
Autonomic dysreflexia
Autonomic dysreflexia, risk for
Communication, readiness for enhanced
Communication, impaired verbal
Death syndrome, risk for sudden infant
Disuse syndrome, risk for

Falls, risk for
Fear
Grieving, anticipatory
Grieving, dysfunctional
Growth, risk for disproportionate
Health maintenance, ineffective
Home maintenance, impaired
Infection, risk for
Injury, risk for
Injury, risk for perioperative-positioning
Knowledge, deficient
Knowledge of (specify), readiness for
  enhanced
Neglect, unilateral
Peripheral neurovascular dysfunction,
  risk for
Poisoning, risk for
Sorrow, chronic
Suffocation, risk for
Therapeutic regimen management,
  ineffective
Therapeutic regimen management,
  readiness for enhanced
Therapeutic regimen management,
  ineffective community
Therapeutic regimen management,
  ineffective family
Trauma, risk for
Wandering

Love and Belonging Needs

Anxiety
Attachment, risk for impaired
  parent/infant/child
Caregiver role strain
Caregiver role strain, risk for
Conflict, parental role
Coping, compromised family
Coping, disabled family
Coping, readiness for enhanced
Coping, readiness for enhanced family
Failure to thrive, adult
Family processes, readiness for enhanced
Family processes, interrupted
Grieving
Loneliness, risk for
Parenting, readiness for enhanced
Parenting, impaired
Parenting, risk for impaired
Relocation stress syndrome

Relocation stress syndrome, risk for
Social interaction, impaired
Social isolation

Self-Esteem Needs

Adjustment, impaired
Body image, disturbed
Conflict, decisional
Coping, ineffective
Coping, defensive
Coping, ineffective community
Coping, readiness for enhanced
  community
Denial, ineffective
Diversional activity, deficient
Family processes, dysfunctional:
  alcoholism
Hopelessness
Identity, disturbed personal
Noncompliance
Post-trauma syndrome
Post-trauma syndrome, risk for
Powerlessness
Powerlessness, risk for
Rape-trauma syndrome
Rape-trauma syndrome: compound
  reaction
Rape-trauma syndrome: silent reaction
Role performance, ineffective
Self-esteem, chronic low
Self-esteem, situational low
Self-esteem, risk for situational low
Self-mutilation
Self-mutilation, risk for
Suicide, risk for
Violence, risk for other-directed
Violence, risk for self-directed

Self-Actualization Needs

Development, risk for delayed
Energy field, disturbed
Growth and development, delayed
Health-seeking behaviors
Self-concept, readiness for enhanced
Spiritual distress
Spiritual distress, risk for
Spiritual well-being, readiness for
  enhanced
Therapeutic regimen management,
  effective

Appendix B

Taxonomy II: NANDA's Domains, Classes, and Diagnoses

Domain	Class	Approved Diagnoses
1. Health promotion The awareness of well-being or normality of function and the strategies used to maintain control of and enhance that well-being or normality of function	*1. Health awareness* Recognition of normal function and well-being	
	2. Health management Identifying, controlling, performing, and integrating activities to maintain health and well-being	Effective Therapeutic regimen management Ineffective Therapeutic regimen management Ineffective family Therapeutic regimen management Ineffective community Therapeutic management Health-seeking behaviors (specify) Ineffective Health maintenance Impaired Home maintenance Readiness for enhanced Therapeutic regimen management Readiness for enhanced Nutrition
2. Nutrition The activities of taking in, assimilating, and using nutrients for the purpose of tissue maintenance, tissue repair, and production of energy	*1. Ingestion* Taking food or nutrients into the body	Ineffective Infant feeding pattern

From North American Nursing Diagnosis Association: *Nursing diagnoses: definitions and classification 2003-2004,* Philadelphia, 2003, The Association.

Domain	Class	Approved Diagnoses
		Impaired Swallowing Imbalanced Nutrition: less than body requirements Imbalanced Nutrition: more than body requirements Risk for imbalanced Nutrition: more than body requirements
	2. Digestion The physical and chemical activities that convert foodstuffs into substances suitable for absorption and assimilation	
	3. Absorption The act of taking up nutrients through body tissues	
	4. Metabolism The chemical and physical processes occurring in living organisms and cells for the development and use of protoplasm and production of waste and energy, with the release of energy for all vital processes	
	5. Hydration The taking in and absorption of fluids and electrolytes	Deficient Fluid volume Risk for deficient Fluid volume Excess Fluid volume Risk for Fluid imbalanced fluid volume Readiness for enhanced Fluid balance
3. Elimination Secretion and excretion of waste products from the body	*1. Urinary system* The process of secretion and excretion of urine	Impaired Urinary elimination Urinary retention Total urinary Incontinence Functional urinary Incontinence Stress urinary Incontinence Urge urinary Incontinence Reflex urinary Incontinence Risk for urge urinary Incontinence Readiness for enhanced Urinary elimination

Continued

Taxonomy II: NANDA's Domains, Classes, and Diagnoses—cont'd

Domain	Class	Approved Diagnoses
	2. Gastrointestinal system Excretion and expulsion of waste products from the bowel	Bowel incontinence
		Diarrhea Constipation Risk for Constipation Perceived Constipation
	3. Integumentary system Process of secretion and excretion through the skin	
	4. Pulmonary system Removal of byproducts of metabolic processes, secretions, and foreign material from the lungs or bronchi	Impaired Gas exchange
4. Activity/rest The production, conservation, expenditure, or balance of energy resources	**1. Sleep/rest** Slumber, repose, ease, or inactivity	Disturbed Sleep pattern
		Sleep deprivation Readiness for enhanced Sleep Risk for Disuse syndrome
	2. Activity/exercise Moving parts of the body (mobility), doing work, or performing actions often (but not always) against resistance	
		Impaired physical Mobility Impaired bed Mobility Impaired wheelchair Mobility Impaired Transfer ability Impaired Walking Deficient Diversional activity Dressing/grooming Self-care deficit Bathing/hygiene Self-care deficit Feeding Self-care deficit

Domain	Class	Approved Diagnoses
		Toileting Self-care deficit
		Delayed Surgical recovery
	3. Energy balance	Disturbed Energy field
	A dynamic state of harmony be-tween intake and expenditure of resources	
		Fatigue
	4. Cardiovascular/pulmonary responses	Decreased Cardiac output
	Cardiopulmonary mechanisms that support activity/rest	
		Impaired spontaneous Ventilation
		Ineffective Breathing pattern
		Activity intolerance
		Risk for Activity intolerance
		Dysfunctional Ventilatory weaning response
		Ineffective Tissue perfusion (specify type: cerebral, renal, cardiopulmonary, gastrointestinal, peripheral)
5. Perception/ cognition The human information-processing system including attention, orientation, sensation, perception, cognition, and communication	*1. Attention* Mental readiness to notice or observe	Unilateral Neglect
	2. Orientation Awareness of time, place, and person	Impaired Environmental interpretation syndrome
	3. Sensation/perception Receiving information through the senses of touch, taste, smell, vision, hearing, and kinesthesia and the comprehension of sense data resulting in naming, associating, and/or pattern recognition	Wandering Disturbed Sensory perception (specify: visual, auditory, kinesthetic, gustatory, tactile, olfactory)

Continued

Taxonomy II: NANDA's Domains, Classes, and Diagnoses—cont'd

Domain	Class	Approved Diagnoses
	4. Cognition Use of memory, learning, thinking, problem solving, abstraction, judgment, insight, intellectual capacity, calculation, and language	Deficient Knowledge (specify)
		Readiness for enhanced Knowledge of (specify) Acute Confusion Chronic Confusion Impaired Memory Disturbed Thought processes
	5. Communication Sending and receiving verbal and nonverbal information	Impaired verbal Communication
6. Self-perception Awareness about the self	**1. Self-concept** The perception(s) about the total self	Readiness for enhanced Communication Disturbed personal Identity
		Powerlessness Risk for Powerlessness Hopelessness Risk for Loneliness Readiness for enhanced Self-concept
	2. Self-esteem Assessment of one's own worth, capability, significance, and success	Chronic low Self-esteem
	3. Body image A mental image of one's own body	Situational low Self-esteem Risk for situational low Self-esteem Disturbed Body image

Domain	Class	Approved Diagnoses
7. Role relationships The positive and negative connections or associations between persons or groups of persons and the means by which those connections are demonstrated	*1. Caregiving roles* Socially expected behavior patterns by persons providing care who are not health care professionals	Caregiver role strain
		Risk for Caregiver role strain Impaired Parenting Risk for impaired Parenting Readiness for enhanced Parenting Interrupted Family processes
	2. Family relationships Associations of people who are biologically related or related by choice	
		Readiness for enhanced Family processes Dysfunctional Family processes: alcoholism Risk for impaired parent/infant/child Attachment Effective Breastfeeding
	3. Role performance Quality of functioning in socially expected behavior patterns	
		Ineffective Breastfeeding Interrupted Breastfeeding Ineffective Role performance Parental role Conflict Impaired Social interaction
8. Sexuality Sexual identity, sexual function, and reproduction	*1. Sexual identity* The state of being a specific person in regard to sexuality or gender	
	2. Sexual function The capacity or ability to participate in sexual activities	Sexual dysfunction
		Ineffective Sexuality patterns
	3. Reproduction Any process by which new individuals (people) are produced	

Continued

Taxonomy II: NANDA's Domains, Classes, and Diagnoses—cont'd

Domain	Class	Approved Diagnoses
9. Coping/stress tolerance Contending with life events/life processes	*1. Post-trauma responses* Reactions occurring after physical or psychological trauma	Relocation stress syndrome
		Risk for Relocation stress syndrome Rape-trauma syndrome Rape-trauma syndrome: silent reaction Rape-trauma syndrome: compound reaction Post-trauma syndrome Risk for Post-trauma syndrome
	2. Coping responses The process of managing environmental stress	Fear
		Anxiety Death Anxiety Chronic Sorrow Ineffective Denial Anticipatory Grieving Dysfunctional Grieving Impaired Adjustment Ineffective coping Disabled family Coping Compromised family Coping Defensive Coping Ineffective community Coping Readiness for enhanced Coping Readiness for enhanced family Coping Readiness for enhanced community Coping
	3. Neurobehavioral stress Behavioral responses reflecting nerve and brain function	
		Autonomic dysreflexia Risk for Autonomic dysreflexia Disorganized Infant behavior Risk for disorganized Infant behavior Readiness for enhanced organized Infant behavior Decreased Intracranial adaptive capacity

Domain	Class	Approved Diagnoses
10. Life principles Principles underlying conduct, thought, and behavior about acts, customs, or institutions viewed as being true or having intrinsic worth	*1. Values* The identification and ranking of preferred modes of conduct or end states	
	2. Beliefs Opinions, expectations, or judgments about acts, customs, or institutions viewed as being true or having intrinsic worth	Readiness for enhanced Spiritual well-being
	3. Value/belief/action congruence The correspondence or balance achieved between values, beliefs, and actions	Spiritual distress
		Risk for Spiritual distress Decisional Conflict (specify) Noncompliance
11. Safety/ protection Freedom from danger, physical injury, or immune system damage; preservation from loss; and protection and safety and security	*1. Infection* Host responses following pathogenic invasion	Risk for Infection
	2. Physical injury Bodily harm or hurt	Impaired Oral mucous membrane
		Risk for Injury Risk for perioperative positioning Injury Risk for Falls Risk for Trauma Impaired Skin integrity Risk for impaired Skin integrity Impaired Tissue integrity Impaired Dentition Risk for Suffocation

Continued

Taxonomy II: NANDA's Domains, Classes, and Diagnoses—cont'd

Domain	Class	Approved Diagnoses
		Risk for Aspiration
		Ineffective Airway clearance
		Risk for Peripheral neurovascular dysfunction
		Ineffective Protection
		Risk for sudden infant Death syndrome
	3. Violence The exertion of excessive force or power so as to cause injury or abuse	Risk for Self-mutilation
		Self-mutilation
		Risk for other-directed Violence
		Risk for self-directed Violence
		Risk for Suicide
	4. Environmental hazards Sources of danger in the surroundings	Risk for Poisoning
	5. Defensive process The processes by which the self protects itself from the nonself	Latex Allergy response
		Risk for latex Allergy response
	6. Thermoregulation The physiological process of regulating heat and energy within the body for purposes or protecting the organism	Risk for imbalanced Body temperature
		Ineffective Thermoregulation
		Hypothermia
		Hyperthermia

Domain	Class	Approved Diagnoses
12. Comfort Sense of mental, physical, or social well-being or ease	*1. Physical comfort* Sense of well-being or ease	Acute Pain
		Chronic Pain Nausea
	2. Environmental comfort Sense of well-being or ease in/ with one's environment	
	3. Social comfort Sense of well-being or ease with one's social situations	Social isolation
13. Growth/ development Age-appropriate increases in physical dimensions, organ systems, and/or attainment of developmental milestones	*1. Growth* Increases in physical dimensions or maturity of organ systems	Risk for disproportionate Growth
		Adult Failure to thrive Delayed Growth and development
	2. Development Attainment, lack of attainment, or loss of developmental milestone	
		Risk for delayed Development

Appendix C

Nursing Outcomes Classification (NOC) Labels

2500	Abuse Cessation	2200	Caregiver Adaptation to Patient
2501	Abuse Protection		Institutionalization
2502	Abuse Recovery: Emotional	2506	Caregiver Emotional Health
2503	Abuse Recovery: Financial	2202	Caregiver Home Care Readiness
2504	Abuse Recovery: Physical	2203	Caregiver Lifestyle Disruption
2505	Abuse Recovery: Sexual	2204	Caregiver-Patient Relationship
2514	Abuse Recovery Status	2205	Caregiver Performance:
1400	Abusive Behavior Self-Restraint		Direct Care
1300	Acceptance: Health Status	2206	Caregiver Performance:
0005	Activity Tolerance		Indirect Care
1308	Adaptation to Physical Disability	2507	Caregiver Physical Health
1600	Adherence Behavior	2208	Caregiver Stressors
1401	Aggression Self-Control	2508	Caregiver Well-Being
0705	Allergic Response: Localized	2210	Caregiving Endurance Potential
0706	Allergic Response: Systemic	1301	Child Adaptation to
0200	Ambulation		Hospitalization
0201	Ambulation: Wheelchair	0120	Child Development: 1 Month
1211	Anxiety Level	0100	Child Development: 2 Months
1402	Anxiety Self-Control	0101	Child Development: 4 Months
1014	Appetite	0102	Child Development: 6 Months
1918	Aspiration Prevention	0103	Child Development: 12 Months
0704	Asthma Self-Management	0104	Child Development: 2 Years
0202	Balance	0105	Child Development: 3 Years
0409	Blood Coagulation	0106	Child Development: 4 Years
2300	Blood Glucose Level	0107	Child Development: Preschool
0413	Blood Loss Severity	0108	Child Development: Middle
0700	Blood Transfusion Reaction		Childhood
1200	Body Image	0109	Child Development: Adolescence
1616	Body Mechanics Performance	0401	Circulation Status
0203	Body Positioning: Self-Initiated	3000	Client Satisfaction: Access to Care
1104	Bone Healing		Resources
0500	Bowel Continence	3001	Client Satisfaction: Caring
0501	Bowel Elimination	3002	Client Satisfaction:
1000	Breastfeeding Establishment:		Communication
	Infant	3003	Client Satisfaction: Continuity
1001	Breastfeeding Establishment:		of Care
	Maternal	3004	Client Satisfaction: Cultural Needs
1002	Breastfeeding Maintenance		Fulfillment
1003	Breastfeeding Weaning	3005	Client Satisfaction: Functional
1617	Cardiac Disease Self-Management		Assistance
0400	Cardiac Pump Effectiveness	3006	Client Satisfaction: Physical Care

3007	Client Satisfaction: Physical Environment	0001	Endurance
3008	Client Satisfaction: Protection of Rights	0002	Energy Conservation
		1909	Fall Prevention Behavior
3009	Client Satisfaction: Psychological Care	1912	Falls Occurrence
		2600	Family Coping
3010	Client Satisfaction: Safety	2602	Family Functioning
3011	Client Satisfaction: Symptom Control	2606	Family Health Status
		2603	Family Integrity
3012	Client Satisfaction: Teaching	2604	Family Normalization
3013	Client Satisfaction: Technical Aspects of Care	2605	Family Participation in Professional Care
0900	Cognition	2607	Family Physical Environment
0901	Cognitive Orientation	2608	Family Resiliency
2100	Comfort Level	2601	Family Social Climate
2007	Comfortable Death	2609	Family Support During Treatment
0902	Communication	1210	Fear Level
0903	Communication: Expressive	1213	Fear Level: Child
0904	Communication: Receptive	1404	Fear Self-Control
2700	Community Competence	0111	Fetal Status: Antepartum
2804	Community Disaster Readiness	0112	Fetal Status: Intrapartum
2701	Community Health Status	0601	Fluid Balance
2800	Community Health Status: Immunity	0603	Fluid Overload Severity
		1304	Grief Resolution
2801	Community Risk Control: Chronic Disease	0110	Growth
		1700	Health Beliefs
2802	Community Risk Control: Communicable Disease	1701	Health Beliefs: Perceived Ability to Perform
2803	Community Risk Control: Lead Exposure	1702	Health Beliefs: Perceived Control
		1703	Health Beliefs: Perceived Resources
2805	Community Risk Control: Violence	1704	Health Beliefs: Perceived Threat
2702	Community Violence Level	1705	Health Orientation
1601	Compliance Behavior	1602	Health-Promoting Behavior
0905	Concentration	1603	Health-Seeking Behavior
0212	Coordinated Movement	1610	Hearing Compensation Behavior
1302	Coping	1105	Hemodialysis Access
0906	Decision Making	1201	Hope
1208	Depression Level	0602	Hydration
1409	Depression Self-Control	0915	Hyperactivity Level
1619	Diabetes Self-Management	1202	Identity
1307	Dignified Life Closure	0204	Immobility Consequences: Physiological
0311	Discharge Readiness: Independent Living	0205	Immobility Consequences: Psychocognitive
0312	Discharge Readiness: Supported Living	0707	Immune Hypersensitivity Response
1403	Distorted Thought Self-Control	0702	Immune Status
0600	Electrolyte and Acid-Base Balance	1900	Immunization Behavior

1405	Impulse Self-Control
0703	Infection Severity
0708	Infection Severity: Newborn
0907	Information Processing
0213	Joint Movement: Ankle
0214	Joint Movement: Elbow
0215	Joint Movement: Fingers
0216	Joint Movement: Hip
0217	Joint Movement: Knee
0218	Joint Movement: Neck
0207	Joint Movement: Passive
0219	Joint Movement: Shoulder
0220	Joint Movement: Spine
0221	Joint Movement: Wrist
0504	Kidney Function
1827	Knowledge: Body Mechanics
1800	Knowledge: Breastfeeding
1830	Knowledge: Cardiac Disease Management
1801	Knowledge: Child Physical Safety
1821	Knowledge: Conception Prevention
1820	Knowledge: Diabetes Management
1802	Knowledge: Diet
1803	Knowledge: Disease Process
1804	Knowledge: Energy Conservation
1828	Knowledge: Fall Prevention
1816	Knowledge: Fertility Promotion
1805	Knowledge: Health Behavior
1823	Knowledge: Health Promotion
1806	Knowledge: Health Resources
1824	Knowledge: Illness Care
1819	Knowledge: Infant Care
1807	Knowledge: Infection Control
1817	Knowledge: Labor and Delivery
1808	Knowledge: Medication
1829	Knowledge: Ostomy Care
1826	Knowledge: Parenting
1809	Knowledge: Personal Safety
1818	Knowledge: Postpartum Maternal Health
1822	Knowledge: Preconception Maternal Health
1810	Knowledge: Pregnancy
1811	Knowledge: Prescribed Activity
1815	Knowledge: Sexual Functioning
1812	Knowledge: Substance Use Control

1814	Knowledge: Treatment Procedure(s)
1813	Knowledge: Treatment Regimen
1604	Leisure Participation
1203	Loneliness Severity
2509	Maternal Status: Antepartum
2510	Maternal Status: Intrapartum
2511	Maternal Status: Postpartum
0411	Mechanical Ventilation Response: Adult
0412	Mechanical Ventilation Weaning Response: Adult
2301	Medication Response
0908	Memory
0208	Mobility
1204	Mood Equilibrium
1209	Motivation
1618	Nausea and Vomiting Control
2106	Nausea and Vomiting: Disruptive Effects
2107	Nausea and Vomiting Severity
2513	Neglect Cessation
2512	Neglect Recovery
0909	Neurological Status
0910	Neurological Status: Autonomic
0911	Neurological Status: Central Motor Control
0912	Neurological Status: Consciousness
0913	Neurological Status: Cranial Sensory/Motor Function
0914	Neurological Status: Spinal Sensory/Motor Function
0118	Newborn Adaptation
1004	Nutritional Status
1005	Nutritional Status: Biochemical Measures
1007	Nutritional Status: Energy
1008	Nutritional Status: Food and Fluid Intake
1009	Nutritional Status: Nutrient Intake
1100	Oral Hygiene
1615	Ostomy Self-Care
1306	Pain: Adverse Psychological Response
1605	Pain Control
2101	Pain: Disruptive Effects
2102	Pain Level

2105	Symptom Severity: Premenstrual Syndrome (PMS)	1609	Treatment Behavior: Illness or Injury
2302	Systemic Toxin Clearance: Dialysis	0502	Urinary Continence
0800	Thermoregulation	0503	Urinary Elimination
0801	Thermoregulation: Newborn	1611	Vision Compensation Behavior
1101	Tissue Integrity: Skin and Mucous Membranes	0802	Vital Signs
		1006	Weight: Body Mass
0404	Tissue Perfusion: Abdominal Organs	1612	Weight Control
		1206	Will to Live
0405	Tissue Perfusion: Cardiac	1102	Wound Healing: Primary Intention
0406	Tissue Perfusion: Cerebral		
0407	Tissue Perfusion: Peripheral	1103	Wound Healing: Secondary Intention
0408	Tissue Perfusion: Pulmonary		
0210	Transfer Performance		

From Moorehead S, Johnson M, Maas ML, editors: *Nursing outcomes classification (NOC),* ed 3, St Louis, 2004, Mosby (in press).

Appendix D

Nursing Interventions Classification (NIC) Labels

Abuse Protection Support
Abuse Protection Support: Child
Abuse Protection Support: Domestic
  Partner
Abuse Protection Support: Elder
Abuse Protection Support: Religious
Acid-Base Management
Acid-Base Management: Metabolic
  Acidosis
Acid-Base Management: Metabolic
  Alkalosis
Acid-Base Management: Respiratory
  Acidosis
Acid-Base Management: Respiratory
  Alkalosis
Acid-Base Monitoring
Active Listening
Activity Therapy
Acupressure
Admission Care
Airway Insertion and Stabilization
Airway Management
Airway Suctioning
Allergy Management
Amnioinfusion
Amputation Care
Analgesic Administration
Analgesic Administration: Intraspinal
Anaphylaxis Management
Anesthesia Administration
Anger Control Assistance
Animal-Assisted Therapy
Anticipatory Guidance
Anxiety Reduction
Area Restriction
Aromatherapy
Art Therapy
Artificial Airway Management
Aspiration Precautions

Assertiveness Training
Asthma Management
Attachment Promotion
Autogenic Training
Autotransfusion
Bathing
Bed Rest Care
Bedside Laboratory Testing
Behavior Management
Behavior Management: Overactivity/
  Inattention
Behavior Management: Self-Harm
Behavior Management: Sexual
Behavior Modification
Behavior Modification: Social Skills
Bibliotherapy
Biofeedback
Bioterrorism Preparedness
Birthing
Bladder Irrigation
Bleeding Precautions
Bleeding Reduction
Bleeding Reduction: Antepartum Uterus
Bleeding Reduction: Gastrointestinal
Bleeding Reduction: Nasal
Bleeding Reduction: Postpartum Uterus
Bleeding Reduction: Wound
Blood Products Administration
Body Image Enhancement
Body Mechanics Promotion
Bottle Feeding
Bowel Incontinence Care
Bowel Incontinence Care: Encopresis
Bowel Irrigation
Bowel Management
Bowel Training
Breast Examination
Breastfeeding Assistance
Calming Technique

Capillary Blood Sample
Cardiac Care
Cardiac Care: Acute
Cardiac Care: Rehabilitative
Cardiac Precautions
Caregiver Support
Case Management
Cast Care: Maintenance
Cast Care: Wet
Cerebral Edema Management
Cerebral Perfusion Promotion
Cesarean Section Care
Chemical Restraint
Chemotherapy Management
Chest Physiotherapy
Childbirth Preparation
Circulatory Care: Arterial Insufficiency
Circulatory Care: Mechanical Assist
   Device
Circulatory Care: Venous Insufficiency
Circulatory Precautions
Circumcision Care
Code Management
Cognitive Restructuring
Cognitive Stimulation
Communicable Disease Management
Communication Enhancement:
   Hearing Deficit
Communication Enhancement:
   Speech Deficit
Communication Enhancement:
   Visual Deficit
Community Disaster Preparedness
Community Health Development
Complex Relationship Building
Conflict Mediation
Constipation/Impaction Management
Consultation
Contact Lens Care
Controlled Substance Checking
Coping Enhancement
Cost Containment
Cough Enhancement
Counseling
Crisis Intervention
Critical Path Development
Culture Brokerage
Cutaneous Stimulation

Decision-Making Support
Delegation
Delirium Management
Delusion Management
Dementia Management
Dementia Management: Bathing
Deposition Testimony
Developmental Care
Developmental Enhancement: Adolescent
Developmental Enhancement: Child
Dialysis Access Maintenance
Diarrhea Management
Diet Staging
Discharge Planning
Distraction
Documentation
Dressing
Dying Care
Dysreflexia Management
Dysrhythmia Management
Ear Care
Eating Disorders Management
Electroconvulsive Therapy Management
Electrolyte Management
Electrolyte Management: Hypercalcemia
Electrolyte Management: Hyperkalemia
Electrolyte Management:
   Hypermagnesemia
Electrolyte Management: Hypernatremia
Electrolyte Management:
   Hyperphosphatemia
Electrolyte Management: Hypocalcemia
Electrolyte Management: Hypokalemia
Electrolyte Management:
   Hypomagnesemia
Electrolyte Management: Hyponatremia
Electrolyte Management:
   Hypophosphatemia
Electrolyte Monitoring
Electronic Fetal Monitoring: Antepartum
Electronic Fetal Monitoring: Intrapartum
Elopement Precautions
Embolus Care: Peripheral
Embolus Care: Pulmonary
Embolus Precautions
Emergency Care
Emergency Cart Checking
Emotional Support

Endotracheal Extubation
Energy Management
Enteral Tube Feeding
Environmental Management
Environmental Management: Attachment
  Process
Environmental Management: Comfort
Environmental Management: Community
Environmental Management: Home
  Preparation
Environmental Management: Safety
Environmental Management: Violence
  Prevention
Environmental Management: Worker
  Safety
Environmental Risk Protection
Examination Assistance
Exercise Promotion
Exercise Promotion: Strength Training
Exercise Promotion: Stretching
Exercise Therapy: Ambulation
Exercise Therapy: Balance
Exercise Therapy: Joint Mobility
Exercise Therapy: Muscle Control
Eye Care
Fall Prevention
Family Integrity Promotion
Family Integrity Promotion: Childbearing
  Family
Family Involvement Promotion
Family Mobilization
Family Planning: Contraception
Family Planning: Infertility
Family Planning: Unplanned Pregnancy
Family Presence Facilitation
Family Process Maintenance
Family Support
Family Therapy
Feeding
Fertility Preservation
Fever Treatment
Financial Resource Assistance
Fire-Setting Precautions
First Aid
Fiscal Resource Management
Flatulence Reduction
Fluid Management
Fluid Monitoring

Fluid Resuscitation
Fluid/Electrolyte Management
Foot Care
Forgiveness Facilitation
Gastrointestinal Intubation
Genetic Counseling
Grief Work Facilitation
Grief Work Facilitation: Perinatal Death
Guilt Work Facilitation
Hair Care
Hallucination Management
Health Care Information Exchange
Health Education
Health Policy Monitoring
Health Screening
Health System Guidance
Heat Exposure Treatment
Heat/Cold Application
Hemodialysis Therapy
Hemodynamic Regulation
Hemofiltration Therapy
Hemorrhage Control
High-Risk Pregnancy Care
Home Maintenance Assistance
Hope Instillation
Hormone Replacement Therapy
Humor
Hyperglycemia Management
Hypervolemia Management
Hypnosis
Hypoglycemia Management
Hypothermia Treatment
Hypovolemia Management
Immunization/Vaccination Management
Impulse Control Training
Incident Reporting
Incision Site Care
Infant Care
Infection Control
Infection Control: Intraoperative
Infection Protection
Insurance Authorization
Intracranial Pressure (ICP) Monitoring
Intrapartal Care
Intrapartal Care: High-Risk Delivery
Intravenous (IV) Insertion
Intravenous (IV) Therapy
Invasive Hemodynamic Monitoring

Kangaroo Care
Labor Induction
Labor Suppression
Laboratory Data Interpretation
Lactation Counseling
Lactation Suppression
Laser Precautions
Latex Precautions
Learning Facilitation
Learning Readiness Enhancement
Leech Therapy
Limit Setting
Lower Extremity Monitoring
Malignant Hyperthermia Precautions
Mechanical Ventilation
Mechanical Ventilatory Weaning
Medication Administration
Medication Administration: Intraspinal
Medication Administration: Nasal
Medication Administration: Ear
Medication Administration: Enteral
Medication Administration: Eye
Medication Administration: Inhalation
Medication Administration: Interpleural
Medication Administration: Intradermal
Medication Administration: Intramuscular (IM)
Medication Administration: Intraosseous
Medication Administration: Intravenous (IV)
Medication Administration: Oral
Medication Administration: Rectal
Medication Administration: Skin
Medication Administration: Subcutaneous
Medication Administration: Vaginal
Medication Administration: Ventricular Reservoir
Medication Management
Medication Prescribing
Meditation Facilitation
Memory Training
Milieu Therapy
Mood Management
Multidisciplinary Care Conference
Music Therapy
Mutual Goal Setting
Nail Care
Nausea Management

Neurological Monitoring
Newborn Care
Newborn Monitoring
Nonnutritive Sucking
Normalization Promotion
Nutrition Management
Nutrition Therapy
Nutritional Counseling
Nutritional Monitoring
Oral Health Maintenance
Oral Health Promotion
Oral Health Restoration
Order Transcription
Organ Procurement
Ostomy Care
Oxygen Therapy
Pain Management
Parent Education: Adolescent
Parent Education: Childrearing Family
Parent Education: Infant
Parenting Promotion
Pass Facilitation
Patient Contracting
Patient Rights Protection
Patient-Controlled Analgesia (PCA) Assistance
Peer Review
Pelvic Muscle Exercise
Perineal Care
Peripheral Sensation Management
Peripherally Inserted Central (PIC) Catheter Care
Peritoneal Dialysis Therapy
Pessary Management
Phlebotomy Cannulated Vessel
Phlebotomy: Arterial Blood Sample
Phlebotomy: Blood Unit Acquisition
Phlebotomy: Venous Blood Sample
Phototherapy: Mood/Sleep Regulation
Phototherapy: Neonate
Physical Restraint
Physician Support
Pneumatic Tourniquet Precautions
Positioning
Positioning: Intraoperative
Positioning: Neurological
Positioning: Wheelchair
Postanesthesia Care

Postmortem Care
Postpartal Care
Preceptor: Employee
Preceptor: Student
Preconception Counseling
Pregnancy Termination Care
Premenstrual Syndrome Management
Prenatal Care
Preoperative Coordination
Preparatory Sensory Information
Presence
Pressure Management
Pressure Ulcer Care
Pressure Ulcer Prevention
Product Evaluation
Program Development
Progressive Muscle Relaxation
Prompted Voiding
Prosthesis Care
Pruritus Management
Quality Monitoring
Radiation Therapy Management
Rape-Trauma Treatment
Reality Orientation
Recreation Therapy
Rectal Prolapse Management
Referral
Religious Addiction Prevention
Religious Ritual Enhancement
Relocation Stress Reduction
Reminiscence Therapy
Reproductive Technology Management
Research Data Collection
Resiliency Promotion
Respiratory Monitoring
Respite Care
Resuscitation
Resuscitation: Fetus
Resuscitation: Neonate
Risk Identification
Risk Identification: Childbearing Family
Risk Identification: Genetic
Role Enhancement
Seclusion
Security Enhancement
Sedation Management
Seizure Management
Seizure Precautions

Self-Awareness Enhancement
Self-Care Assistance
Self-Care Assistance: IADL
Self-Care Assistance: Transfer
Self-Care Assistance: Bathing/Hygiene
Self-Care Assistance: Dressing/Grooming
Self-Care Assistance: Feeding
Self-Care Assistance: Toileting
Self-Esteem Enhancement
Self-Hypnosis Facilitation
Self-Modification Assistance
Self-Responsibility Facilitation
Sexual Counseling
Shift Report
Shock Management
Shock Management: Cardiac
Shock Management: Vasogenic
Shock Management: Volume
Shock Prevention
Sibling Support
Simple Guided Imagery
Simple Massage
Simple Relaxation Therapy
Skin Care: Donor Site
Skin Care: Graft Site
Skin Care: Topical Treatments
Skin Surveillance
Sleep Enhancement
Smoking Cessation Assistance
Socialization Enhancement
Specimen Management
Spiritual Growth Facilitation
Spiritual Support
Splinting
Sports-Injury Prevention: Youth
Staff Development
Staff Supervision
Subarachnoid Hemorrhage Precautions
Substance Use Prevention
Substance Use Treatment
Substance Use Treatment: Alcohol
   Withdrawal
Substance Use Treatment: Drug
   Withdrawal
Substance Use Treatment: Overdose
Suicide Prevention
Supply Management
Support Group

Support System Enhancement
Surgical Assistance
Surgical Precautions
Surgical Preparation
Surveillance
Surveillance: Community
Surveillance: Late Pregnancy
Surveillance: Remote Electronic
Surveillance: Safety
Sustenance Support
Suturing
Swallowing Therapy
Teaching: Foot Care
Teaching: Infant Stimulation
Teaching: Toilet Training
Teaching: Disease Process
Teaching: Group
Teaching: Individual
Teaching: Infant Nutrition
Teaching: Infant Safety
Teaching: Preoperative
Teaching: Prescribed Activity/Exercise
Teaching: Prescribed Diet
Teaching: Prescribed Medication
Teaching: Procedure/Treatment
Teaching: Psychomotor Skill
Teaching: Safe Sex
Teaching: Sexuality
Teaching: Toddler Nutrition
Teaching: Toddler Safety
Technology Management
Telephone Consultation
Telephone Follow-up
Temperature Regulation
Temperature Regulation: Intraoperative
Temporary Pacemaker Management
Therapeutic Play
Therapeutic Touch
Therapy Group
Total Parenteral Nutrition (TPN)
  Administration

Touch
Traction/Immobilization Care
Transcutaneous Electrical Nerve Stimula-
  tion (TENS)
Transport
Trauma Therapy: Child
Triage: Disaster
Triage: Emergency Center
Triage: Telephone
Truth Telling
Tube Care
Tube Care: Chest
Tube Care: Gastrointestinal
Tube Care: Umbilical Line
Tube Care: Urinary
Tube Care: Ventriculostomy/Lumbar
  Drain
Ultrasonography: Limited Obstetric
Unilateral Neglect Management
Urinary Bladder Training
Urinary Catheterization
Urinary Catheterization: Intermittent
Urinary Elimination Management
Urinary Habit Training
Urinary Incontinence Care
Urinary Incontinence Care: Enuresis
Urinary Retention Care
Values Clarification
Vehicle Safety Promotion
Venous Access Devices (VAD)
  Maintenance
Ventilation Assistance
Visitation Facilitation
Vital Signs Monitoring
Vomiting Management
Weight Gain Assistance
Weight Management
Weight Reduction Assistance
Wound Care
Wound Care: Closed Drainage
Wound Irrigation

From McCloskey JC, Bulechek GM, editors: *Nursing interventions classification (NIC)*, ed 4, St Louis, 2004, Mosby (in press).

Index

Boldfaced entries indicate care plan titles; page numbers in *italics* indicate care plan locations.

J

Jaundice, 73
Jaw surgery, 73
Jittery, 73
Jock itch, 73
Joint replacement, 74
JRA (juvenile rheumatoid arthritis), 107
Juvenile diabetes mellitus, 49
Juvenile rheumatoid arthritis (JRA), 107

K

Kaposi's sarcoma, 74
Kawasaki syndrome, 74
Kegel exercise, 74
Ketoacidosis, 74
    diabetic, 49
Kidney(s)
    failure of, 74, 105
    transplantation of, 105
Kidney stone, 74
Knee replacement, 74
Knowledge
    deficient, 74, *607–612*
    enhanced, readiness for, 74, *612–617*
Kock pouch, 42, 74
Korsakoff's syndrome, 74

L

Labor
    induction of, 70
    normal, 75
    preterm, 100–101
    suppression of, 116
    uterine atony in, 124
Laminectomy, 75
Laparoscopic laser cholecystectomy, 75
Laparotomy, 75
Laryngectomy, 75
Laser surgery, 75
Latex allergy, 75
Latex allergy response, *148–154*
    risk for, 75, *154–157*
Laxative abuse, 75
Legionnaires' disease, 76
Lens implant, 76
Lethargy, 76
Leukemia, 76
Leukopenia, 76
Lice, 41, 76
Lifestyle, sedentary, 109
Limb reattachment procedures, 76
Lip, cleft, 39
Listlessness, 76
Liver
    biopsy of, 76

Liver *(Continued)*
    disease of, 76
Living will, 76
Lobectomy, 76
Loneliness, risk for, 76, *617–623*
Low back pain, 76
Lumbar fusion, 58–59
Lumbar puncture, 76
Lung(s)
    cancer of, 77
    crackles in, 44
    edema of, 1–2
    left, hypoplastic, 68
Lupus erythematosus, 77
Lyme disease, 77
Lymphedema, 77
Lymphoma, 77

M

Mad cow disease, 77
Magnetic resonance imaging (MRI), 82
Malabsorption syndrome, 77
Maladaptive behavior, 77
Malaria, 77
Malnutrition, 77
Manic disorder, bipolar, 77–78
Manipulation of organs, 78
Manipulative behavior, 78
Marasmus, 78
Marshall-Marchetti-Krantz operation, 78
Mastectomy, 78
    modified radical, 81
Mastitis, 78
Maternal infection, 78
Maturational issues, adolescent, 78–79
Maze III procedure, 79
MD (muscular dystrophy), 83
Measles, 41, 79
Meconium aspiration, 79, 105–106
Melanoma, 79
Melena, 79
Membranes, premature rupture of, 99–100
Memory, impaired, 79, *624–630*
Meningitis, 79
Meningocele, 79, 86
Menopause, 79–80
Menorrhagia, 80
Mental disorders, organic, 89
Mental illness, 80
Mental retardation, 80
Mental status, altered. *See* Confusion; Memory
Metabolic acidosis, 80
MI (myocardial infarction), 80–81
Miscarriage, 81
Mitral stenosis, 81

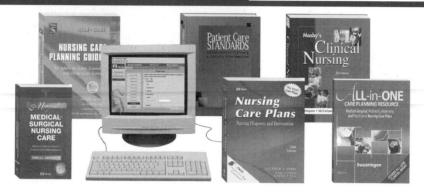